The American Urological Association Educational Review Manual in Urology

Second Edition • 2010

Editors-in-Chief

Daniel A. Shoskes, MD
Professor of Surgery, Cleveland Clinic Lerner College of Medicine
Director, The Novick Center for Clinical & Translational Research
Glickman Urological and Kidney Institute
The Cleveland Clinic
Cleveland, OH

Allen F. Morey, MD
Professor, Department of Urology
University of Texas Southwestern Medical Center
Dallas, TX

Watson®

CCGMP

Castle Connolly Graduate Medical Publishing

Castle Connolly Graduate Medical Publishing, Ltd.

17 Battery Place, Suite 643 • New York, NY 10004 • Tel: 212.644.9696 • Fax: 646.827.6443 • www.ccgmp.com • e-mail: info@ccgmp.com

Castle Connolly Graduate Medical Publishing, Ltd. publishes review manuals to assist residents and fellows in preparing for board certification exams, and practicing physicians in preparing for board recertification.

NOTICE

ISBN: 978-0-9840551-4-2

Our thanks to Copy Editor Sarah Herndon

Cover Illustration: InViVo Communications

Contents

List of Contributors

Second Edition

Kenneth W. Angermeier, MD
Associate Professor
Section of Prosthetic Surgery
The Cleveland Clinic
Genitourethral Reconstruction
9500 Euclid Ave., Q-10-1
Cleveland, OH 44195-0001

Kathleen Beekman, MD
University of Michigan Comprehensive Cancer Center
1500 East Medical Center Drive
CCC 6-303
Ann Arbor, MI 48109-0330

Jay T. Bishoff, MD
Director Endourology
Urology San Antonio
18729 Brookwood Forest
San Antonio, TX 78258

Jeffrey A. Cadeddu, MD
Professor of Urology & Radiology
UT Southwestern Medical Center
Dept. of Urology UT Southwestern Medical Center
5323 Harry Hines Blvd.
Dallas, TX 75390-9110

Fergus V. Coakley, MD
Professor of Radiology
University of California, San Francisco
505 Parnassus Ave., Rm. M372
San Francisco, CA 94143

Jose J. Correa
Fellow
Moffitt Cancer Ctr.
12902 Magnolia Dr.
4th Fl., Office 4035
Tampa, FL 33612

Alain Duclos, MD
The Cleveland Clinic
9500 Euclid Avenue
Cleveland, OH 44195

Deborah R. Erickson, MD
Professor of Surgery
University of Kentucky
Division of Urology
3038 Windermere Rd.
Lexington, KY 40502

Gary J. Faerber, MD
Professor
University of Michigan
1500 E. Medical Center Drive
Dept. of Urology
Ann Arbor, MI 48109-0330

Howard B. Goldman, MD
Co-Head, Section of Female Urology
Glickman Urological Institute
The Cleveland Clinic
9500 Euclid Ave., A100
Cleveland, OH 44195-0001

Brent K. Hollenbeck, MD
Department of Urology
University of Michigan Health System
3875 Taubman Center
1500 E. Medical Center Drive
Ann Arbor, MI 48109-0330

Maha Hussain, MD
University of Michigan Comprehensive Cancer Center
1500 East Medical Center Drive
CCC 6-303
Ann Arbor, MI 48109-0330

Martin A. Koyle, MD
Professor
Chief, Division of Pediatric Urology
Seattle Children's Hospital/
University of Washington
4800 Sandy Point Way NW
MS W-7729
Seattle, WA 98105

Jo Ellen Cottey-Krueger, MD
Medical City Dallas Hospital
3307 Beverly Drive
Dallas, TX 75205-2906

Joseph Lattanzi, MD
Department of Radiation Oncology
Community Medical Center
99 Hwy 37W
Toms River, NJ 08755-6423

Una J. Lee, MD
Urology Resident
The Cleveland Clinic
9500 Euclid Ave., A100
Cleveland, OH 44195-0001

Seth P. Lerner, MD
Professor
Baylor College of Medicine
Scott Department of Urology
6620 Main, Ste. 1325
Houston, TX 77030

Allen F. Morey, MD
Professor, Department of Urology
University of Texas Southwestern Medical Center
5323 Harry Hines Blvd.
Dallas, TX 75390-9110

Judd W. Moul, MD
Professor of Surgery
Duke University
Division of Urologic Surgery
Duke Univ Med Ctr. Box 3707
Durham, NC 27710-0001

Hiep Thieu Nguyen, MD
Assistant Professor
Children's Hospital and Harvard Medical School
Department of Urology
300 Longwood Ave., HU353
Boston, MA 02115

Victor W. Nitti, MD
Professor and Vice-Chairman,
Department of Urology
New York University School of Medicine
150 East 32nd St.
New York, NY 10016

Michael A. O'Donnell, MD
Professor of Urology, Director of Urologic
Oncology Research
University of Iowa
200 Hawkins Drive, 3 RCP Urology
Iowa City, IA 52242-1089

Dana A. Ohl, MD
Professor of Urology, Head of Division of Andrology &
Microsurgery
University of Michigan
TC3875 Urology
1500 E. Medical Center Drive
Ann Arbor, MI 48109-0330

Sean Anthony Pierre, MD
Clinical Associate/Fellow, Urology
Duke University Medical Center
DUMC 3167 Room 1576, Duke South
Durham, NC 27710

Glenn M. Preminger, MD
Professor, Urologic Surgery/Director, Comprehensive
Kidney Stone Center
Duke University Medical Center
Room 1572D White Zone, Duke South
DUMC Box 3167
Durham, NC 27710-0001

Susanne A. Quallich, MD

Raymond R. Rackley, MD
Professor of Surgery
The Cleveland Clinic Lerner College of Medicine at
CWRU and the Glickman Urological Institute
Cleveland Clinic Foundation
Glickman Urological Institute, A100
9500 Euclid Ave.
Cleveland, OH 44195-0001

Richard A. Santucci, MD
Clinical Professor
Wayne State University School of Medicine
Harper Professional Building, Suite 1017
4160 John R St.
Detroit, MI 48201-2017

Wade J. Sexton, MD
Assistant Professor of Surgery & Urology
H. Lee Moffitt Cancer Center and Research Institute
Department of Interdisciplinary Oncology Genitourinary
Oncology Program
12902 Magnolia Drive
Tampa, FL 33612

Daniel A. Shoskes, MD
Professor of Surgery
Glickman Urological and Kidney Institute
The Cleveland Clinic
9500 Euclid Ave., A100
Cleveland, OH 44195-0001

Warren T. Snodgrass, MD
Professor of Urology, Chief of Pediatric Urology
UT Southwestern Medical Center
2350 Stemmons Freeway
Ste. F4300, MS F4.04
Dallas, TX 75207

Jens Sønksen, MD

Alexis E. Te, MD
Associate Professor of Urology, Director, Brady Prostate Center, Dept of Urology
Weill Medical College of Cornell University
1300 York Avenue
Suite F-9 West, Box 261
New York, NY 10021

Paul J. Turek, MD
Director
The Turek Clinic
55 Francisco St.
Ste. 300
San Francisco, CA 94133

James C. Ulchaker, MD, FACS
Co-Director, Prostate Center
Cleveland Clinic Foundation
9500 Euclid Ave, Q-10-1
Cleveland, OH 44195

Robert G. Uzzo, MD
Chairman of Surgery
Fox Chase Cancer Center
333 Cottman Avenue, Rm C-302
Philadelphia, PA 19111

J. Christian Winters, MD
Professor & Department Head
Louisiana State University Health Science Ctr.
1542 Tulane Ave #547
New Orleans, LA 70112

Hadley M. Wood, MD
Renovascular Disease
Cleveland Clinic Foundation
9500 Euclid Ave., A100
Cleveland, OH 44195-0001

Faculty Disclosure

According to the American Urological Association's (AUA) Disclosure policy, speakers and authors involved in continuing medical education activities are required to complete an online AUA Disclosure. This information is presented to meeting participants so that they may make their own judgments about a speaker's presentation or an author's chapter.

The AUA does not view the existence of these interests or relationships as necessarily implying bias or decreasing the value of the presentation or chapter. Prior to planning the program, directors review all speaker conflicts and implement a variety of mechanisms to resolve.

Each faculty member presenting a chapter has submitted a copy of his/her online disclosure to the AUA. These copies are on file in the AUA Office of Education.

This review manual has been planned to be well balanced, objective, and scientifically rigorous. Information and opinions offered by the authors represented their viewpoints. Conclusion drawn by the readers should be derived from careful consideration of all available scientific information.

The following faculty members declare a relationship with the commercial concerns listed below, related directly or indirectly to this program. Readers may form their own judgments about the chapters in light of full disclosure of the facts.

Kenneth W. Angermeier	American Medical Systems- Consultant or Advisor
Jay T. Bishoff	Pfizer-Meeting Participant or Lecturer; Perc Systems-Consultant or Advisor
Jeffrey A. Cadeddu	Ethicon Endosurgery, Inc.-Scientific Study or Trial, Other: intellectual property licensing; MedTrials, Inc.-Consultant or Advisor
Fergus Coakley	Nothing to disclose
Jose J. Correa	Nothing to disclose
Jo Ellen Cottey-Krueger	Nothing to disclose
Deborah R. Erickson	NeurAxon- Consultant or Advisor; Trillium Therapeutics Inc. Consultant or Advisor
Gary J. Faerber	Olympus North America-Consultant or Advisor
Howard B. Goldman	Johnson and Johnson – Meeting Participant or Lecturer, Consultant or Advisor; American Medical Systems – Consultant or Advisor; Allergan – Scientific Study or Trial; Pfizer – Meeting Participant or Lecturer, Consultant or Advisor; Novartis – Meeting Participant or Lecturer; Astellas – Meeting Participant or Lecturer; Endogun Medical Systems – Consultant or Advisor, Investment Interest
Martin A. Koyle	Nothing to disclose

Seth P. Lerner	GE Healthcare – Meeting Participant or Lecturer, Scientific Study or Trial; Pfizer – Scientific Study or Trial, Consultant or Advisor; Eli Lilly – Scientific Study or Trial; Bristol-Meyers Squibb – Scientific Study or Trial; Tengion – Consultant or Advisor; Imalux-Scientific Study or Trial, Consultant or Advisor; Photocure-Scientific Study or Trial; Spectrum-Investigator
Allen F. Morey	AMS-Meeting Participant or Lecturer; Glaxo Smith Klein-Meeting Participant or Lecturer; Pfizer-Meeting Participant or Lecturer
Judd W. Moul	Astra Zeneca- Meeting Participant or Lecturer; Sanofi-Aventis-Scientific Study or Trial; Theralogix-Consultant or Advisor; Glaxo Smith Kline-Other: Safety Monitoring Committee for Clinical Trial; Ferring Pharmaceuticals Inc-Consultant or Advisor
Hiep Thieu Nguyen	Nothing to disclose
Victor W. Nitti	Ethicon-Consultant or Advisor; Allergan-Consultant or Advisor, Scientific Study or Trial; Pfizer-Consultant or Advisor; Astellas- Consultant or Advisor, Investigator; Coloplast-Scientific Study or Trial, Consultant or Advisor; American Medical Systems-Other: Preceptor; Serenity Pharmaceuticals-Consultant or Advisor; Uroplasty-Consultant or Advisor; Alita Pharmaceuticals – Consultant or Advisor; Uromedia - Consultant or Advisor.
Michael A. O'Donnell	Abbott-Investigator; Endo Pharmaceuticals-Consultant or Advisor; Viventia-Consultant or Advisor; Spectrum Pharmaceuticals-Consultant or Advisor; Medical Enterprises-Consultant or Advisor; Amplimmune-Other: Grant Research
Dana Alan Ohl	Solvay-Meeting Participant or Lecturer; Auxilium-Meeting Participant or Lecturer; GSK/Schering-Consultant Advisor; Pfizer-Consultant or Advisor; Lilly-ICOS-Consultant or Advisor, Meeting Participant or Lecturer; Colopast-Investigator, Meeting Participant or Lecturer; Endo-Consultant or Advisor
Margaret Sue Pearle	Cook Urological-Consultant or Advisor; Percutaneous Systems, Inc-Consultant or Advisor; Karl Storz-Other: Course Faculty
Glenn M. Preminger	Nothing to disclose
Raymond R. Rackley	Novartis Pharmaceuticals Corp-Meeting Participant or Lecturer, Consultant or Advisor; Pfizer-Consultant or Advisor, Meeting Participant or Lecturer
Richard A. Santucci	Nothing to disclose
Wade J. Sexton	Endocare-Other: proctor
Daniel A. Shoskes	Triurol-Investment Interest; Pfizer-Scientific Study or Trial

Warren T. Snodgrass	Nothing to disclose
Paul J. Turek	Gilead Sciences-Consultant or Advisor; MandalMed-Board Member, Officer, Trustee; Medical Board of California-Consultant or Advisor
James C. Ulchaker	Astellas-Meeting Participant or Lecturer; Olympus-Scientific Study or Trial; AMS-Scientific Study or Trial; Fortec Medical-Board Member, Officer, Trustee; Pfizer-Meeting Participant or Lecturer; GSK-Meeting Participant or Lecturer
Robert G. Uzzo	Pfizer-Meeting Participant or Lecturer
J. Christian Winters	Solace Thera – Scientific Study or Trial; Astellas, inc. – Consultant or Advisor; Contura – Scientific Study or Trial; Pfizer – Consultant or Advisor

Preface

Second Edition

Dear Colleague,

We are delighted to present to you the second edition of the Board Review Manual for Urology to be included as part of the AUA Annual Review Course. This manual is intended to be a unique reference, both comprehensive and focused on the salient, practical material geared to test preparation but also of value to clinical practice. Our goal is that you will find this information valuable whether you are preparing for the ABU Qualifying Examination, recertifying, or just interested in a refresher course.

We applaud the heroic efforts of our authors, all of whom are nationally recognized experts in their topic areas, who prepared their chapters on very short notice. Some of the included material duplicates information in the lectures but much is additional and supplementary.

Many thanks to Michael D. Wolf, Ph.D. and his staff at Castle Connolly Graduate Medical Publishing for their tireless efforts in bringing this project to completion. Thanks also to our sponsor, Watson Pharmaceuticals, whose generous support of this manual represents a major contribution to the specialty of urology.

We continue to look forward to your feedback. Authors were free to use textbook style or point form outline, and we are eager to learn which you found easier to study from. Best of luck in your exams and in all your future endeavors.

Sincerely,

Daniel A. Shoskes, MD
Glickman Urological and Kidney Institute
The Cleveland Clinic

Allen F. Morey, MD
University of Texas Southwestern Medical Center
Department of Urology

American
Urological
Association
Education and Research, Inc.

The American Urological Association Annual Review Course was established with one simple mission: To provide the most up-to-date information regarding the practice of Urology on an annual basis. The Course was originally designed to provide a thorough review of pertinent urologic information for Chief Residents who were about to take their written American Board of Urology Examination. Since that time, the Course has grown to include a comprehensive review for those Urologists who are participating in the Maintenance of Certification process and also for those practicing Urologists who want a general review in the field.

Now accommodating over 800 participants per year, this Annual Review Course has become one of the most popular and perhaps, most important offerings from the AUA Office of Education. By assembling the best and the brightest to present this message, Co-Directors Dan Shoskes and Al Morey have made this the premier Review Course in Urology. Moreover, they have also added urologic pathology and radiology modules, as well as an expansion of the course syllabus to this already comprehensive offering.

This volume was envisioned as an additional study aid to those preparing for the American Board of Urology examinations, but can also be used as a general Review of the entire field of Urology. I believe that this mission has been accomplished with the production of the AUA EDUCATIONAL REVIEW MANUAL IN UROLOGY. This is the third edition of the Review Manual, now with updated basic science and clinical information for all Urologists.

The support of Watson Pharmaceuticals has been instrumental to the development of this valuable educational compendium and the AUA Office of Education is grateful for their continued assistance.

Finally, thanks to Michael D. Wolf, Ph.D. and his excellent staff at Castle Connolly Graduate Medical Publishing, Ltd., who were able to efficiently and effectively design, implement and publish this compendium.

The AUA Office of Education is proud to support this valuable endeavor.

Elspeth M. McDougall, MD, FRCSC, MHPE
Chair, AUA Officer of Education

Watson®

To our colleagues in Urology:

Watson Pharmaceutical, Inc. is proud to sponsor The American Urological Association Educational Review Manual in Urology and Companion CD-Rom, a thorough and up to the minute review of the field.

This manual and CD-Rom are tools that will assist you through your preparation for board certification or recertification. It was prepared under the expert guidance of Allen F. Morey, MD and Daniel A. Shoskes, MD. Written by a superb faculty of specialists and educators from medical centers around the United States, the manual and CD will be an invaluable tool for you in the months and years ahead.

As a leader in Urology, Watson Pharmaceutical, Inc. is dedicated to providing patients with safe and effective treatments, unsurpassed quality, and support for the specialty of Urology. Watson is committed to improving the quality of life for patients around the world through the development and distribution of advanced branded and trusted generic pharmaceuticals.

Watson Pharmaceutical, Inc. recognizes the value of continuing education in the field of Urology, and commends the authors and the editors for an outstanding effort in developing this review. We hope that the wealth of information presented herein will enrich your understanding of Urology and help you confidently complete your training.

Regards,

Gary D. Kozloski, PharmD
Vice President, Medical Affairs
Watson Pharmaceuticals, Inc.

American Urological Association (AUA) Educational Programs and Services

Medical Journal
The most widely read publication in the field, *The Journal of Urology*® brings solid coverage — all the clinically relevant information needed to stay at the forefront of this dynamic field. This top-ranking journal in the urology field presents investigative studies on critical areas of research and practice; survey articles providing short condensations of the best and most important urology literature worldwide; and practice-oriented reports on interesting clinical observations. This is the Official Journal of the American Urological Association.
Visit www.jurology.com for more details.

News and Information

AUANews®
AUANews®, the Official Newsmagazine of the American Urological Association, is written for urologists by urologists and is provided to AUA members as a benefit. It features current, highly relevant, cutting-edge news of practical value to urologists, while also serving as a vehicle for prompt and current communication between the AUA and its members. Visit www.AUAnet.org/AUANews to view current issues or visit www.AUAnet.org/catalog to order.

Health Policy Brief
The *Health Policy Brief* is a monthly newsletter covering the latest issues in coding and reimbursement, regulatory changes to Medicare, national legislation, tips for guarding against fraud and abuse and practice management issues. This publication keeps urologists abreast of important issues and engages them in the legislative arena affecting urology practice. To subscribe, call 1-866-RING-AUA (1-866-746-4282).

AUAnet.org
AUAnet.org is the AUA's Web site – designed for members and residents searching for information on our educational programs and services. The site also features clinical guidelines, code of ethics, policy statements and membership information. For information about the 2010 Annual Meeting, including Webcasts of plenary sessions and other valuable educational information, visit www.AUA2010.org.

Coding Tips for the Urologist's Office
Everything urologists, practice managers and coders need to know about urology coding is featured on line – from coding basics to the Medicare fee schedule. Coding tips are featured on our Web site at www.AUAnet.org/CodingTips.

AUA Coding Hotline
Consider us an extension of your coding staff. An AUA coding specialist is on hand to answer your toughest coding questions. Just dial 1-866-RING-AUA (1-866-746-4282), select option 2 and receive answers to your toughest coding questions from the certified professional coders on our staff. Each call is $25, but unlimited calls are free to members of the AUA Practice Managers' Network (PMN).

Educational Offerings

AUA Annual Meeting

The American Urological Association's Annual Meeting is the world's largest meeting of urologic professionals. With more than 10,000 urologists and health care professionals and more than 5,000 representatives from more than 350 companies in attendance, there is no better place to learn about the advances in urology.

Join us next year in Washington, DC from May 14 - 19, 2011. Visit www.AUA2011.org for more details when the website launches in August, 2010.

Year-round Subject-oriented and Surgical Learning Courses

The AUA offers many Subject-oriented and Surgical Learning Center courses on a variety of topics essential to the urologist. Visit www.AUAnet.org/calendar to view a complete list of upcoming courses.

Coding and Practice Management Seminars

By possessing the most up-to-date information on coding and practice management, urologists and their staff members will manage their practices more effectively, spend less time on paperwork and more time devoted to patient care. The AUA offers seminars on coding and practice management at various times and locations during the year. Visit the urology calendar at www.AUAnet.org/calendar for details.

The AUA Update Series

The 2010 Update Series is the most professional self-study product in urology. Now in its 29th installment, this invaluable tool continues the tradition of providing up-to-date information that's relevant to you. Improve your practice and patient care by staying abreast of the latest in treatments and surgical techniques. The *AUA Update Series* includes 40 new lessons with content-related, five-question posttests. For CME credit, subscribers must receive a minimum score of 80 percent for the posttests. The *AUA Update Series* is available in print format and online (with four new lessons posted as they are published for 10 months). This innovative CME program helps urologists meet the core curriculum standards and CME required by states and the American Board of Urology (ABU). Visit www.AUAnet.org/UpdateSeries for more information.

Self-Assessment Study Program

The *Self-Assessment Study Program (SASP)* has been a leading educational resource for practicing urologists and urology residents since 1977. Each year, a new 150 multiple choice item examination is developed and includes discussions and references from current literature in clinical areas of interest to urologists. Sharpen your clinical skills, prepare for an examination or fulfill ABU MOC requirements with this annually developed study program. The SASP is an excellent way to prepare for the American Board of Urology (ABU) Re-certification Examination because 20 percent of the content for the exam comes from this product. **The 2010 SASP is now available on your iPhone and iPod touch via the new, innovative Spaced Education format**—a new online platform that provides an easy, effective and enjoyable method to learn and retain urology content.

Product can also help fulfill the CME requirements mandated by the ABU Maintenance of Certification (MOC)® process. You can earn *20 AMA PRA Category 1 Credits™* by successfully completing this annually developed examination. Visit http://www.auanet.org/content/products/self-assessment-study-program.cfm for more details.

Clinical Guidelines
All AUA guidelines are accessible to the public online – visit www.AUAnet.org/Guidelines to view.

***The Journal of Urology*® Home Study Course**
Earn credits while you read *The Journal of Urology*® with the *JU Home Study Course*. Designed by a team of educators, academicians and clinicians, this program is the AUA's most convenient and affordable self-study program and allows physicians to immediately test their knowledge and apply this knowledge to improve the quality of patient care. Course is available only to subscribers of *The Journal of Urology*®. Journal subscribers will receive 12 individual five-question answer sheets or they can go on line to receive instant credit. A maximum of 24 CME credits per year can be earned. This course is available to JU subscribers for just $60 per year. Visit www.auanet.org to order.

Membership
AUA membership offers unique benefits and experiences that enhance not only your career, but also your personal growth. AUA is the largest and most prestigious organization of urology professionals in the world. We work to represent you in government on the vital issues that impact your practice and your ability to offer the best possible urologic care. The AUA also provides unparalleled information resources, such as standards of quality, clinical guidelines and research advances in urology. Join today at www.AUAnet.org/join.

Join the American Urological Association (AUA) – the AUA offers the following categories of membership:

Active/Associate – practicing urologists within the AUA Section boundaries

- Affiliate – scientists and researchers
- International – practicing urologists outside the AUA Section boundaries
- Candidate – residents-in-training within the U.S., Canada and Mexico
- International Residents-in-training – residents-in-training outside the U.S., Canada and Mexico
- Allied – other health care professionals
- Honorary – AUA members who have achieved outstanding prominence in a field of medicine related to Urology, Officers of the Association, and/ or distinguished urologists

For more information or to complete an application, visit www.AUAnet.org/join.

Practice Managers' Network (PMN)

Whether you are a solo practitioner running your own business or you employ a professional administrator, the challenges of running a urology practice today requires access to expert advice and updates on the ever-changing healthcare environment. This network of urologists and practice managers is a fee-based program that every urology practice should belong to. Visit www.AUAnet.org for more details.

AUA CME Credit Registry

The AUA's free, online, self-reporting AUA CME Credit Registry is a benefit for all AUA members, allowing you to self-report and track your AMA PRA Category 1 Credits™ online and print a CME transcript anytime. The AUA CME Credit Registry offers an economical, fast and convenient way to keep track of their Maintenance of Certification credits.

Career Development

AUA Jobfinder, the online source for careers in urology, is our most popular program for members on the move. Visit www.AUAnet.org/JobFinder for more details.

Chapter 1: Applied Anatomy of the Genitourinary Tract

Howard B. Goldman, MD, FACS

Contents

Introduction

A thorough knowledge of genitourinary anatomy is the foundation upon which we base our understanding of the pathophysiology of urologic disease. Furthermore, it is the surgeon's roadmap, illuminating the arena in which they practice every day. At some point during medical school or residency, we all memorized general anatomy—at least for a short time. As our interest in urology deepened many of these anatomic principles were reviewed.

Oftentimes, however, the integration of anatomic knowledge regarding the genitourinary organs, the supporting and surrounding structures, and their physiologic function does not completely occur. This review will focus on that integration by providing a generous overview of the genitourinary supporting structures—specifically the bones, muscles, vessels and nerves—and the urologic organs themselves. This review should be beneficial for those studying for exams as well as those interested in refreshing their understanding of genitourinary anatomy.

Anatomy requires illustration and for that reason this review is accompanied by references only to the *Atlas of Human Anatomy* (4th ed) by Frank Netter and the *Atlas of Urosurgical Anatomy* by Frank Hinman Jr. This chapter will thus be most beneficial if it is reviewed alongside a copy of Netter's atlas. There are fewer references to Hinman's so if this book is not readily available that should not impact the review significantly. Ideally, it would be best to have all the Figures reproduced alongside the text; however, because of copyright issues and space, that is not possible.

1. Skeletal Structures

A number of structures of the bony skeleton are involved in urologic anatomy and help support the various genitourinary structures.

Ribs

A number of ribs—specifically ribs 6 through 10 which are connected to the sternum by a cartilaginous costal arch—are important to urologists. When making a thoracoabdominal incision the costal arch may be cut. Ribs eleven and twelve are not joined anteriorly and are sometimes referred to as the "floating" ribs. It is these ribs that are intimately associated with the various flank incisions that are made to access the retroperitoneum. Each rib has a costal groove on the inner inferior surface within which the intercostal vessels and nerve travel. When making a flank incision and especially when removing a portion of the rib it is important to try to keep these structures intact to prevent abdominal wall or flank muscle weakness (Netter 186, 248).

Vertebral Bodies

A number of the vertebral bodies are significant as well. The thoracic eleventh and twelfth, the lumbar first through fifth and the sacrococcygeal bones are particularly relevant to urologic anatomy. Most of the nerves that innervate the pelvis and urologic organs travel through these vertebral bones. It is important to recognize that the spinal nerves are named for the vertebral body just above its foramen of exit and that while the spinal cord terminates at the lumbar first and second level in the adult the nerves continue on as a structure called the cauda equina. Thus, for example, the S2 nerve leaves the sacral spinal cord just below the S2 vertebral body and then travels as part of the cauda equina. Therefore, the area which is called the sacral cord, which is the portion of the spinal cord from which the spinal nerves emanate, is not near the sacral vertebral bodies, but is more rostral, at the termination of the cord at the L1-L2 level. Again the important factor when naming the cord level is the site of exit of the nerves emanating from that portion of the cord. Similarly the lumbar cord runs through the T11 to L1 bodies after which the nerves that emanate from it continue on and exit near the L1-L5 vertebral bodies. This becomes important when classifying spinal cord injuries. Though the actual fracture may be at the L1 level, the spinal cord injury itself may be to the sacral cord since the sacral cord is at the L1 level. Similarly, an injury to the T11 or T12 vertebral body can produce a lumbar cord injury (Netter 161).

Pelvis

The bones that make up the pelvis help support and protect many of the urologic organs. The innominates of the pelvis are three sets of paired bones—a right and left ilium, right and left ischium, as well as right and left pubic bones. Posteriorly the sacrum and the coccyx lay between the paired iliac bones and below the L5 vertebral body (Netter 248).

In the past much of this anatomy was not clinically relevant, however, neuromodulation techniques which have recently entered the urologist's armamentarium utilize some of the foramina of the sacrum and the knowledge of the sacral anatomy has become important.

Within the pelvis there are a number of openings (foramina), one of which is completely within and bordered by pelvic skeletal structures and others which are formed by portions of the bony structure as well as various ligaments (Table 1). The obturator foramen is bounded anteriorly and anteromedially by portions of the pubis while posteriorly a portion of the ischium surrounds it. The obturator vessels and nerves travel through the superiolateral portion of the obturator foramen through the obturator canal. The obturator foramen is clinically relevant to urologists as it is a thoroughfare for the passage of trocars used in incontinence and prolapse surgery. The other pelvic foramina or openings within the pelvis are formed by ligaments and bone. The sacrotuberous ligament bridges the ischial tuberosity to the sacrum and coccyx while the sacrospinous ligament travels from the ischial spine to the sacrum. Knowledge of the anatomy of the sacrospinous ligament is especially important for those utilizing it as an anchor during vaginal vault suspension procedures. The greater sciatic foramen is bounded by bone and the sacrospinous ligament inferiorly while the lesser sciatic foramen is bounded by the sacrospinous ligament superiorly, the sacrotuberous ligament inferiorly and the ischium laterally (Netter 353).

Table 1

Pelvic Foramina

Within bone

1. Obturator foramen

Formed by ligaments
-sacrotuberous (ischial tuberosity to sacrum/coccyx)
-sacrospinous (ischial spine to lower sacrum)

2. Greater sciatic foramen

3. Lesser sciatic foramen

2. Muscles

Subcutaneous Tissues

The abdominal wall is composed of muscle groups covered by layers of subcutaneous tissue and skin (Table 2). Immediately beneath the skin is Camper's fascia which is a layer of loose fatty tissue. Just deep to Camper's is Scarpa's fascia which is not real fascia but a thickening of tissue which superiorly and laterally blends with Camper's fascia, inferiorly fuses with the fascia of the thigh and medially is continuous with Colle's fascia. Colle's fascia is continuous with Scarpa's superiorly and with the Dartos fascia overlying the penis and scrotum and runs to the posterior edge of the urogenital diaphragm (Netter 380).

Musculature

The abdominal wall musculature can be divided into four groups: anterior, anterolateral, posterior and pelvic floor (Table 3).

Table 2

Skin and Subcutaneous Fascia

Camper's fascia	- loose layer of fatty tissue beneath skin
Scarpa's fascia	- deep to Camper's - superior/lateral—blends with Camper's - inferior—fuses with fascia of thigh - medially—continuous with Colle's
Colle's fascia	- continuous with Scarpa's and Dartos - until posterior edge of UG diaphragm
Dartos fascia	- superficial layer of penis and scrotum - continuous with Colle's and Scarpa's

Table 3

Abdominal Wall Musculature

Anterior
- Rectus
- Aponeurosis of oblique and transversus muscules

Anteriolateral
- External oblique
- Internal oblique
- Transversus abdominus
- Intercostals

Posterior
- Outer layer
  - Latissimus dorsi
  - External oblique
- Middle layer
  - Internal oblique
  - Serratus posterior inferior
  - Sacrospinalis
- Inner layer
  - Quadratus lumborum
  - Iliacus
- Innermost layer
  - Psoas
  - Diaphragm

Anterior Abdominal Wall

The most medial muscle which makes up part of the anterior abdominal wall is the rectus muscle which runs from ribs 5, 6, and 7 down to the pubic crest. The other primary component of the anterior abdominal wall is the fascial aponeurosis of the external and internal oblique and transversus abdominus muscles. There are anterior and posterior fascial sheaths around the rectus from its origin in the upper abdominal wall to a point one-third of the way from the umbilicus to the pubis. Further than one-third of the way down the fascia is only anterior to the rectus muscles. This area of transition about one-third of the distance from the umbilicus to the pubis is called the arcuate line. Cephalad to the arcuate line the external and internal oblique fascia covers the rectus anteriorly while a portion of the internal oblique and transverses abdominus fascia cover it posteriorly. Caudad to the arcuate line all of the various fascial layers are anterior to the rectus muscle (Netter 251).

Anteriolateral Abdominal Wall

The anterolateral group of abdominal wall muscles is made up of the external oblique, internal oblique, transverses abdominus and intercostal muscles. The external oblique fibers run caudad and medially. The free inferior border of the muscle is the inguinal ligament and a portion of it continues as the external spermatic fascia (Netter 249). The internal oblique upper fibers run cranially while the lower fibers run medially. Some of the lower fibers form part of the conjoined tendon and a portion continues as the cremaster muscle (Netter 250). The transverses abdominus fibers run medially and some of its lowest fibers form the conjoined tendon as well. The intercostal muscles connect the ribs and are made up of both external and internal muscle layers (Netter 251).

Posterior Abdominal Wall

The posterior abdominal wall muscles can be subdivided into four layers: the outer, middle, inner and innermost layers. The outer layer is made up of the latissimus dorsi—a large triangular shaped muscle that covers most of the lower back—and the external oblique. Petit's triangle is an area bounded medially by the latissimus dorsi, laterally by the external oblique, and inferiorly by the iliac crest, and is an area with a relative dearth of musculature, and which has been used as an easy access route to the retroperitoneum (Netter 254). The middle layer of the posterior abdominal wall muscle group is made of the internal oblique, the serratus posterior inferior, and the sacrospinalis muscle. The inner layer of the posterior abdominal wall is made up of the quadratus lumborum muscle and the iliacus. The innermost layer is made up of the psoas and the diaphragm (Netter 254, 263).

Layers Encountered During Surgical Incisions

When making a flank incision, many of these muscle groups are encountered and incised (Table 4). Posteriorly, the latissimus dorsi may be incised and sometimes portions of the serratus posterior inferior as well. Anterolaterally the layers from out to in consist of the external oblique, internal oblique, transverses abdominus layer—which is where one would find the rib—the transversalis fascia, thoracolumbar fascia, the pararenal connective tissue, Gerota's fascia, the perirenal fat and finally the kidney itself. The neurovascular bundle coming out of the intercostal groove lies between the internal oblique and the transversus abdominus (Netter 237, Hinman 8.5b).

When making an anterior subcostal or chevron incision, the various layers encountered include the skin, Camper's fascia, external oblique, internal oblique, rectus muscles, the transversus abdominus muscle, transversalis fascia and finally the parietal peritoneum (Netter 252).

Table 4

Layers of a Flank Incision

Posteriorly	-Latissimus dorsi
	-Serratus posterior inferior
Anterolaterally	-External oblique
	-Internal oblique
	neurovascular bundle
	-Transversus abdominus (+/-rib)
	-Transversalis fascia
	-Thoracolumber fascia
	-Pararenal connective tissue fat
	-Gerota's fascia
	-Perirenal fat
	-Kidney

Layers of Anterior Subcostal or Chevron Incision

External oblique
Internal oblique and rectus
Transversus abdominus
Transversalis fascia
Parietal peritoneum

Strata of Retroperitoneal Tissue

The layers of retroperitoneal tissue are sometimes separated into different "strata" based on embryologic origin. The tissues that are divided in this way are the so-called "fascial" layers of the retroperitoneum. In truth, none of these are true fascia but instead are thin layers of tissue similar to Scarpa's fascia. The strata are divided into the outer, intermediate, and inner layers. The important points are as follows. The outer layer is made up of those "fascial" layers which invest the body wall muscles. Therefore, the endopelvic fascia and the transversalis fascia are part of the outer stratum of the retroperitoneal tissue. The components of the inner layer are those tissues that invest the intestinal tract. For example, Denonvillier's fascia is part of the inner stratum.

Finally, those layers that invest the urologic organs are part of the intermediate layer and thus Gerota's fascia is part of the intermediate stratum.

Pelvic Musculature

The pelvic musculature is made up of the psoas muscle which originates outside of the pelvis but then passes through the pelvis, as well as the iliacus which originates within the pelvis but likewise passes through the pelvis and inserts on the proximal portion of the femur. Muscles that are entirely contained within the pelvis include the obturator internus, the piriformis, the coccygeus, and the levator ani group, which is made up primarily of the puborectalis, pubococcygeus and the iliococcygeus muscles (Netter 263). The levator ani group provides support to the pelvic organs. The puborectalis muscle originates from the pubis, is horseshoe shaped, wraps around the rectum, and comes back to the pubic bone. The pubococcygeus originates lateral to the puborectalis on the pubic bone and then travels to the coccyx where it ends. The iliococcygeus originates from the side wall of the pelvis from the arcus tendineus and then runs to the coccyx (Table 5). The arcus tendineus is a condensation of tissue which runs from the pubis to the ischial spine and is readily palpable. For those more interested in the pelvic anatomy there is actually the arcus tendineus fascia pelvis (ATFP) to which the various "fascial" layers that are of most importance in female pelvic anatomy attach, as well as the arcus tendineus levator ani (ATLA) to which the levator muscles attach. The coccygeus muscle and the piriformis muscle make up more of the posterior pelvic floor. On the inner surface of the obturator foramen is the obturator internus muscle, and more superficially, external to the obturator foreman is the obturator externus muscle. On the superiolateral portion of the obturator foramen is the obturator canal through which the obturator nerve and vessels travel (Netter 356, 358). Recently, the obturator foramen has become more important for urologists as a number of midurethral sling and pelvic floor reconstructive procedures make use of the obturator foramen to pass various needles, trocars and mesh.

Perineum and Urogenital Diaphragm

At first glance there are obvious striking differences between the structures of the male and female perineum. However, on closer inspection they are really almost the same—the major difference being that the proportions have changed. Most of the area of interest for urologists is within the urogenital triangle, which is a triangle contained by the symphysis pubis and the right and left ischial tuberosities.

When evaluating the female perineum superficially one can identify the superficial transverse perineal muscles running from the ischial tuberosities to the

Table 5

Pelvic Musculature

Iliacus		
Psoas		
Obturator internus		
Piriformis		
Coccygeus		
Levator ani -	puborectalis pubococcygeus iliococcygeus	} Arise from arcus tendineus and pubis

perineal body in the midline. The ischiocavernosus muscles run from the area of the ischial tuberosities towards the pubis while the bulbospongiosus muscles run from the perineum towards the pubis passing lateral to the vaginal wall. The perineal membrane is the central point in the midline where many of these muscles connect, and inferior to that is the external anal sphincter. It is at this superficial level that the Bartholin's glands lay at the inferior aspect of the vagina (Netter 379). In the male perineum we find the same structures, differently proportioned. The superficial transverse perineal muscles and the external anal sphincter are relatively unchanged. However, the ischiocavernosus muscles now wrap around the corporal bodies while the bulbospongiosus muscles cover the corpus spongiosum, and these muscles are part of the penis (Netter 382).

Deeper in the perineum is where the deep transverse perineal muscles lay, as do the levator ani, and it is at this level that the membranous urethra in the male and what is sometimes referred to as the external urethral sphincter in the female exist. In addition, Cowper's glands in the male are at this deep perineal level (Netter 383) (Table 6).

Table 6

Perineum

Superficial	- superficial transverse perineal muscles - ischiocavernosus muscles - bulbospongiosus muscles - perineal body - external anal sphincter [Bartholin's glands [F])
Deep	- deep transverse perineal muscles - levator ani - perineal body - membranous urethra (M)/ext. urethral sphincter (F) (Cowper's glands (M])

3. Vasculature

The vascular anatomy will be divided into three sections: the arterial, venous and lymphatic.

Arterial Anatomy

The abdominal branches of the aorta as well as the pelvic arteries are of primary importance to the urologist.

The inferior phrenic arteries which originate above the celiac trunk give off the superior suprarenal (adrenal) arterial branches. This is one of the arterial supplies to the adrenal gland. The next branch of the aorta is the celiac trunk which gives off the common hepatic artery. The common hepatic artery supplies the liver and gives off the gastroduodenal branch, which gives off the right gastroepiploic artery that supplies much of the stomach and omentum. For practical purposes, if one needs to utilize an omental flap during surgery it is best to base the omentum on a pedicle originating from the right gastroepiploic artery as that artery is of larger caliber than the left gastroepiploic artery. Furthermore, it originates more caudad and thus one is able to pull the omental flap further into the pelvis when the flap is based on the right gastroepiploic artery. The splenic artery branches off of the celiac trunk and gives off the left gastroepiploic artery which supplies a portion of the stomach and omentum. Finally, the left gastric artery comes from the celiac trunk as well. Moving further along the aorta, the middle suprarenal (adrenal) arteries come off the aorta to supply the adrenal glands. In addition, along the aorta at this point are four pairs of lumbar arteries which have the potential to cause troublesome bleeding particularly during a retroperitoneal lymph node dissection (Netter 264, 300).

The superior mesenteric artery arises from the anterior portion of the aorta and supplies much of the small and large bowel. The various details regarding the arterial supply to the bowel are particularly important when utilizing bowel segments for urinary diversion. The superior mesenteric artery gives rise to various intestinal arteries that supply the jejunum and the ileum, as well as the ileocolic artery that supplies the distal ileum, appendix and cecum, the right colic artery that supplies the ascending colon, and the middle colic artery that supplies the transverse colon. Just beneath the take off of the superior mesenteric artery the renal arteries leave the aorta bilaterally to supply the kidneys, while the gonadal arteries leave the aorta, just caudal to that. Further down the aorta the inferior mesenteric artery comes off the anterior portion of the aorta and gives off a number of branches: the left colic artery supplies the descending colon, the sigmoid arteries supply the sigmoid and various rectal arteries supply the rectum (Netter 306, 307).

The aorta then divides into the common iliacs which themselves divide at the junction of L5 and the sacrum into the external iliac and the internal iliac (hypogastric) arteries (Netter 401).

The external iliac artery gives off the inferior epigastric medially and the deep circumflex artery laterally. It then passes beneath the inguinal ligament and becomes the femoral artery (Table 7).

The internal iliac (hypogastric) artery is responsible for most of the pelvic blood supply. It gives off a posterior and an anterior branch. The posterior branch gives off an iliolumbar artery, a lateral sacral artery, and then continues as the superior gluteal artery supplying the gluteal muscles. Loss of the superior gluteal blood supply can lead to cramping and pain in the gluteal muscles and buttocks. Therefore, if one were to attempt to tie off the hypogastric arteries in an effort to stop or diminish pelvic bleeding it is preferable to do that distal to the origin of the posterior branch, therefore sparing the blood supply to the gluteal muscles. Currently, it is much more common to utilize the skills of our interventional radiology colleagues to selectively embolize a particular artery in an effort to stop pelvic bleeding. The anterior division of the internal iliac artery gives off the obturator artery, followed by the umbilical artery, which itself becomes the obliterated umbilical and the superior vesical artery. The superior vesical artery is one of the primary blood supplies to the pedicle of the bladder. During surgery, one way to easily find it is to follow the obliterated umbilical to its origin which is where the superior vesical artery originates as well. In women, the vaginal and uterine arteries come off soon after the umbilical artery. Distal to that is the origin of the inferior vesical artery which supplies much of the bladder as well as the prostate. The internal pudendal artery then comes off and leaves the pelvis through Alcock's canal and gives off penile and perineal branches (Netter 402, 403).

Venous Anatomy

In most cases the venous structures parallel the arteries. Some of the exceptions include the left gonadal and adrenal veins that empty into the left renal vein. In many cases multiple veins or plexii accompany single arteries (Netter 265).

Lymphatic Anatomy

The retroperitoneal lymph nodes are important landing sites, primarily for metastatic testis tumors. Because of the embryologic origin of the testicles in the retroperitoneum, that is where their vascular and lymphatic structures are based and to where their tumors metastasize. It is important to recall that while left-sided tumors stay on either the left side of the retroperitoneum or in the interaortocaval area, right-sided tumors can cross over and occasionally involve even the left side of the retroperitoneum. That is why the templates for lymph node dissections are different, based on whether the tumor is from the right or left testicle. The retroperitoneum can also be a landing site for renal tumors. The prostatic lymphatics drain through the internal and external iliac chains and many of the prostatic metastases may be found within the obturator node group (Netter 408). The bladder drains through a similar pathway. There are inguinal lymph nodes which serve as landing sites for scrotal and penile carcinoma. Superficial lymph nodes are external to the fascia lata, while the deep chain lies along the femoral vessels, deep to the fascia lata (Hinman 3.4, Netter 266).

Table 7

Branches of Iliac Artery

External iliac
- Inferior epigastric
- Deep circumflex (lateral)

Internal iliac (Hypogastric)
- Posterior Division
  - Iliolumbar
  - Lateral sacral
  - Superior gluteal
- Anterior Division
  - Obturator
  - Umbilical
    - obliterated umbilical
    - superior vesical
  - Vaginal/uterine
  - Inferior vesical
  - Internal pudendal
    - penile
    - perineal

4. Neuroanatomy

The somatic system is composed of nerves responsible for motor and sensory function. The autonomic system is responsible for involuntary responses and control. We will review the thoracic, lumbar, and sacral portions of the somatic system and then the autonomic system.

Somatic System

Thoracic Nerves

The thoracic nerves of interest to the urologist are the intercostal nerves numbers 6 through 12 which run beneath the ribs within the costal groove and then travel between the internal oblique and transversus abdominus muscles to innervate many of the abdominal wall muscles. These nerves are responsible for motor and sensory function of these muscles and if injured, as can happen when a rib is resected during a flank incision, the result can be a bulge of the muscles in the area which that particular nerve supplies. From a clinical standpoint, it is important to be able to differentiate a flank bulge from a hernia, which is a correctable surgical complication.

Lumbar Plexus

A number of important nerves originate from the lumbar plexus (Table 8). The iliohypogastric nerve provides sensation for the lower abdominal wall and the pubic area and motor innervation to the lower abdominal wall. The ilioinguinal nerve has a primary sensory function and supplies the upper thigh, base of the penis and the upper scrotum. This nerve also travels in the inguinal canal and care must be taken not to damage it when operating in the inguinal area. The lateral femoral cutaneous nerve is responsible for sensation of the anterior and lateral portion of the upper leg. The genitofemoral nerve provides sensation to the cord, the scrotum, the anterior thigh, and motor function to the cremaster and the Dartos muscles. The femoral nerve provides sensation to the anteriomedial leg and motor function to the psoas muscle, the iliac and the knee extensors. The obturator nerve is responsible for thigh adduction and the sciatic nerve, which takes its origin from both the lumbar and the sciatic plexii, provides both sensation and motor function to the posterior thigh and lower leg (Netter 497, 498, 499, Hinman 4.11, 4.12).

Table 8

Lumbar Plexus

S = sensory
M = motor

Iliohypogastric	S M	-lower abdomen, pubis -lower abdominal wall
Ilioinguinal	S	-upper thigh, base of penis, upper scrotum travels in inguinal canal
Lateral femoral cutaneous	S	-anterior/lateral upper leg
Genitofemoral	S M	-sprematic cord, scrotum, anterior thigh -Cremaster and Dartos muscles
Femoral	S M	-anterior/medial leg -psoas, iliac, knee extensors
Obturator	M	-thigh adductors
Sciatic	S/M	-posterior thigh and lower leg

Clinical Cautions – Lumbar Plexus

A number of the nerves of the lumbar plexus can be injured during urologic surgery. The genitofemoral nerve lies directly atop the psoas muscle and can occasionally be mistaken for the psoas minor tendon and injured during a psoas hitch. If one is doing a psoas hitch it is important to recognize that a third of patients do not have a readily identifiable psoas minor tendon and care should be taken not to mistakingly hitch the bladder to the genitofemoral nerve. As noted earlier, the ilioinguinal nerve runs through the inguinal canal and can be inadvertently damaged during an inguinal dissection with loss of sensation to the upper thigh, base of the penis, and upper scrotum. The femoral nerve is hidden by the body of the psoas muscle proximally and can be injured by injudicious placement of retractors and lead to a loss of knee extension and anteromedial thigh sensation. The obturator nerve can be injured during a pelvic lymphadenectomy, which can lead to loss of the ability to adduct the thigh. It can also be stimulated by electricity during a transurethral resection of a bladder tumor, causing thigh adduction or a sudden medial kick. When this occurs unexpectedly an inadvertent bladder perforation can occur. Finally, the sciatic nerve passes posterior to the sacrospinous ligament and can be injured during a sacrospinous vault suspension or if a patient is placed in an exaggerated lithotomy position, in which case there may be tension and stretching of the sciatic nerve (Netter 496).

Sacral Plexus

The sciatic nerve, as noted above, originates both from lumbar and sacral roots. Also originating from the sacral roots is the posterior femoral cutaneous nerve whose perineal branch provides sensation for the perineum and posterior scrotum. The pudendal nerve is of much importance to urologists and has both sensory and motor functions. It gives off a perineal branch, a posterior scrotal branch, and a genital branch that becomes the dorsal nerve of either the penis or the clitoris. It is this branch that is responsible for penile and clitoral sensation. Keep in mind that the pudendal nerve like the internal pudendal artery leaves the pelvis and runs through Alcock's canal. Therefore, it is not encountered during routine pelvic surgery and in particular should not be encountered and damaged during a radical prostatectomy. That is the reason that even if the neurovascular bundles near the prostate are damaged, causing erectile dysfunction, penile sensation remains intact. The pudendal nerve also gives off a branch to the rhabdosphincter, which plays a role in urinary continence (Netter 410).

Autonomic System

The autonomic system is responsible for parasympathetic and sympathetic functions of various urologic organs. The pelvic nerves, or nervi erigente originate from the sacral plexus (Netter 410). These are parasympathetic nerves that go to the inferior hypogastric pelvic plexus where they combine with the sympathetic nerves and then give off the autonomic supply to the bladder, prostate and penis. More cephalad are the celiac and superior mesenteric plexii which are responsible for autonomic control of the adrenal glands, kidneys and upper ureters. Along the aorta a number of lumbar nerve roots that are largely sympathetic travel along and on the aorta and then coalesce just below the aortic bifurcation to form the superior hypogastric plexus. These largely sympathetic nerves are responsible for seminal emission and bladder neck closure. After a standard non-nerve sparing retroperitoneal lymph node dissection men may have loss of the ability to ejaculate because of damage to these nerves. From the superior hypogastric plexus bilateral sets of nerves called the hypogastric nerves travel to the inferior hypogastric plexus where they combine with the parasympathetic pelvic nerves (Netter 344, 416) (Table 9).

The inferior hypogastric or pelvic plexus lies lateral to the rectum with its midpoint at the tip of the seminal vesicles. There are multiple prostatic, rectal and vesical blood vessels that penetrate this plexus. These nerves are responsible for bladder and prostatic innervation and supply the neural component of the neurovascular bundles that run alongside the prostate until they continue within the corporal bodies of the penis as the cavernous nerves. These autonomic nerves are responsible for penile erection and detumescence. It is the neurovascular bundles that can be injured during a radical prostatectomy and this can lead to a loss of erectile function. If one looks at Netter's plate 410 you can clearly see how the somatic pudendal nerves run outside of the

Table 9

Autonomic

Celiac and Superior mesenteric plexus — -adrenal/kidney/upper ureter

Superior hypogastric plexus — -largely sympathetic -lumbar roots
-seminal emission
-bladder neck closure

→ continue as Hypogastric nerves (sympathetic)

→ combine with Pelvic nerves & Nervi Erigente (parasympathetic)

↓

Inferior hypogastric (pelvic) plexus -lateral to rectum

pelvis, and thus penile sensation is maintained after prostatectomy, whereas the autonomic neurovascular bundles travel alongside the prostate and can be damaged during radical prostatectomy, leading to erectile dysfunction.

5. Inguinal Canal and Femoral Triangle

Inguinal Canal

The inguinal canal contains the spermatic cord in males and the round ligament in females. There are three sides to the canal: anterior made up primarily by the external oblique, posterior made up of the transversus abdominus and transversalis fascia, and inferior made up of the inguinal ligament. Hesselbach's triangle is bordered by the medial margin of the inferior epigastric vessels, the lateral margin of the rectus muscle, and the inguinal ligament. When describing an inguinal hernia those that are lateral to Hesselbach's triangle are called indirect hernias, whereas those that come directly through the triangle are called direct hernias (Netter 259).

Femoral Triangle

The femoral triangle is bounded by the inguinal ligament at the base, the sartorius muscle laterally, the adductor longus muscle medially, and the floor is made up of the iliopsoas and pectineal muscles (Table 10). Within the femoral triangle from lateral to medial run the femoral nerve, femoral artery, and femoral vein. The femoral triangle is covered by fascia lata and there is an opening in the fascia lata, the fossa ovalis, through which the superficial vessels and the saphenous vein emerge. The node of Cabana is found at the junction of the saphenous vein and the superficial external pudendal vein and some feel this is important to identify when doing a node dissection for penile cancer. The fascia lata divides the deep and the superficial node groups (Netter 262, 500).

Table 10

Femoral Triangle

Base	- inguinal ligament
Lateral	- sartorius
Medial	- adductor longus
Floor	- iliopsoas and pectineal muscles

6. Adrenals

Adrenal Gland

The adrenal gland has a tripartite arterial supply. Superiorly the superior suprarenal artery is derived from the inferior phrenic artery. The middle suprarenal artery comes directly off of the abdominal aorta while the inferior suprarenal artery is derived from the renal artery. On the left side the adrenal vein empties into the left renal vein, whereas on the right the adrenal vein is a short vein that drains directly into the inferior vena cava. It enters the inferior vena cava almost posteriorly and can be the site of troublesome bleeding during a radical nephrectomy. The adrenal gland is separated into two distinct structures, both of which receive regulatory input from the nervous system. Nerves of the celiac plexus and the renal plexus innervate the adrenal glands. The adrenal medulla is at the center of the adrenal gland and is the body's main source of epinephrine and norepinephrine. The adrenal cortex, which surrounds the medulla, is separated into three zones: zona glomerulosa, zona fasciculata, and zona reticularis, which produce other important steroids. The adrenal gland lies within Gerota's fascia superior to the kidney (Netter 332, 347).

7. Kidney

Gerota's Fascia

Gerota's fascia is part of the intermediate stratum and the perinephric fat is within it. The anterior leaflet of Gerota's fascia is sometimes referred to as Toldt's fascia, while the posterior leaflet is sometimes referred to as Zuckerkandl's fascia. Laterally and superiorly the fascia is fused, while medially it is fused over the great vessels but contiguous with the contralateral side. Inferiorly the fascia is not fused, and a potential space exists. This is why renal bleeding tends to track inferiorly in the retroperitoneal space.

Kidneys

The kidneys lie in the retroperitoneum surrounded by perinephric fat and Gerota's fascia. The anterior relations are as follows: the right kidney has the adrenal just above and anterior to it as well as the liver, duodenum, and right colon. On the left side the adrenal, spleen, stomach, pancreas, jejunum, and left colon lie anterior to the kidney. Posterior to both the right and left kidneys lies the twelfth rib, diaphragm, transversus abdominus fascia, and quadratus lumborum and psoas muscles. The left kidney rests slightly higher than the right and will be anterior to the left eleventh rib as well (Table 11).

The renal pedicle is at the level of the first through third lumbar vertebrae. Anterior to posterior are the 1.) renal vein, 2.) artery and 3.) renal pelvis. The renal artery exits the aorta just below the take off of the superior mesenteric artery.

Renal Vasculature

While most people have one main renal artery, accessory arteries are not uncommon. Five segmental arteries come off of the main renal artery followed by interlobar arteries, arcuate arteries, interlobular arteries, and finally the afferent arteriole (Netter 335) (Table 12). The arteries are end arteries without cross communication. The posterior segmental artery is usually the first branch that comes off of the main renal artery prior to the hilum. The other segmental arteries are the apical, upper, middle, and lower arteries. The apical and lower arteries supply the uppermost and lowermost portions of the kidney, while the upper and middle arteries supply

Table 11

Kidneys - Anatomic Relations

	Anterior	
Right		Left
Adrenal		Adrenal
Liver		Spleen
Duodenum		Stomach
Colon		Pancreas
		Jejunum
		Colon
	Posterior	
Right	Right & Left	Left
	Rib 12, Diaphragm	Rib 11
	Transversus abdominus fascia	
	Quadratus lumborum, Psoas	

Table 12

Renal Vasculature

Main renal artery
Segmental arteries (5)
Interlobar arteries
Arcuate arteries
Interlobular arteries
Afferent arteriole

the majority of the anterior portion of the kidney. The posterior artery supplies much of the posterior portion. An avascular plane exists that separates the portion of renal parenchyma supplied by the anterior branches from that supplied by the posterior branch. This avascular plane is not at the mid-portion of the kidney but is, in fact, posterior to the convex border of the kidney. This plane is important if one is doing an anatrophic nephrolithotomy and seeks to bivalve the kidney with minimal bleeding. In today's era this is done less frequently (Netter 335, Hinman 12.34).

The venous structures in the kidney accompany the arteries. In contrast to the arteries there is cross-communication between the venous structures. The right renal vein is a relatively short vein which drains directly into the inferior vena cava. The left renal vein receives the adrenal and gonadal veins and then crosses anterior to the aorta and posterior to the superior mesenteric artery after which it drains into the inferior vena cava.

The cortex of the kidney is composed of nephrons, whereas the medulla is primarily composed of collecting ducts. Each individual nephron has an afferent arteriole which is a branch of an interlobular artery. The afferent arteriole enters the glomerulus, where filtration takes place. Whatever blood is left within the artery exits the glomerulus via the efferent arteriole. Whatever was filtered across the glomerular membrane travels through the proximal convoluted tubule, then the loop of Henle to the distal convoluted tubule, and then to the collecting duct (Netter 336). Multiple collecting ducts make up a pyramid, the tip of which is called a papilla. There are typically seven to nine papillae within a kidney and each is cupped by a minor calyx. On occasion one may see more than one papilla per minor calyx. The minor calyces are connected by necks, or infundibulae, to form two or three major calyces which coalesce to form the renal pelvis (Netter 334).

8. Ureter

The renal pelvis drains into the ureters which are generally 22-30 centimeters long. They run along the psoas muscle in the retroperitoneum where they are usually adherent to the posterior peritoneum. They cross the iliac vessels near the iliac bifurcation (Netter 341). In females they run behind the ovary, behind the uterine artery, near the cervix, and beneath a portion of the vaginal wall. All of these are sites where the ureter can be injured at the time of hysterectomy. In males the ureter runs behind the vas deferens. There are multiple arterial branches that supply the ureter. The upper ureter is supplied medially from the renal artery, the gonadal artery, and from direct branches off of the aorta. The lower ureter is supplied laterally from the iliac and vesical arteries and, in women, from branches off of the uterine artery. Once the arteries reach the ureter they run in longitudinal anastamosing plexii. The ureteral caliber is greatest in the abdominal portion where it is ten millimeters in diameter. There are three sites of narrowing: at the UPJ, over the iliacs, and at the ureterovesical junction. In these areas the ureteral diameter is from two to four millimeters.

9. Bladder

The bladder and urethra have both autonomic and somatic innervation. The parasympathetic system is the primary driver of normal bladder empting. The parasympathetic nerves are derived from the second to fourth sacral portion of the spinal cord and are sometimes called the pelvic nerves. The parasympathetic innervation travels via the inferior hypogastric plexus to the bladder body and stimulation of these nerves is responsible for bladder contraction. The sympathetic nerves originate from the tenth thoracic to the second lumbar portion of the spinal cord. They form part of the hypogastric nerve and the impulses travel via the inferior hypogastric plexus primarily to the trigone and bladder neck. The somatic innervation is primarily from S2 via the pudendal nerve to the external urethral sphincter (Hinman 13.35, 13.36, Netter 417) (Table 13).

The blood supply to the bladder is derived from the internal iliac artery via the superior and inferior vesical pedicles. The superior vesical pedicle is primarily supplied by the superior vesical artery. The superior vesical artery and the obliterated umbilical artery are derived from the same umbilical artery branch. Thus, if one can trace the obliterated umbilical artery down to its site of origin it is relatively easy to find the superior vesical artery and gain appropriate control over the superior vesical pedicle at the time of a cystectomy. The inferior vesical pedicle is supplied by the inferior vesical artery which usually comes directly off of the internal iliac artery, but may, in some cases, be a branch of the internal pudendal artery (Hinman 13.33, Netter 403).

In the adult the bladder is a pelvic organ. In children, it is an abdominal organ. Superiorly, the bladder is covered by peritoneum. In males, the rectum and Denonvillier's fascia are posterior. In females, the vagina is posterior. Anteriorly is a potential space called the space of Retzius. The detrusor muscle has three layers—outer longitudinal, middle circular and inner longitudinal. The trigone is made up of ureteric musculature that runs from the ureteral orifices to the bladder neck (Netter 365, 366).

Table 13

Bladder - Innervation

Sympathetic	**T** 10 - **L** 2	- hypogastric nerve (trigone, bladder neck)
Parasympathetic	**S** 2-4	- pelvic nerve (bladder body)
Somatic	**S** 2	- pudendal nerve (external sphincter)

10. Prostate

The average prostate weighs about 18 grams and is three to four centimeters long, four centimeters wide, and two centimeters deep. Anterior to the prostate lies the space of Retzius and the puboprostatic ligaments. The endopelvic fascia covers the prostate anterolaterally. Lateral to the prostate is fatty tissue, the levator ani and the neurovascular bundles. Posterior to the prostate is Denonvillier's fascia and the rectum. The bladder and seminal vesicals are superior and the urogenital diaphragm is inferior (Netter 384).

Transrectal ultrasound imaging has clarified the zonal anatomy of the prostate. The transition zone makes up 5%-10% of the normal volume of the prostate, is the area which gives rise to benign prostatic hyperplasia, and is where about 20% of prostate cancers originate. The central zone makes up 20% of the normal prostatic volume, surrounds the ejaculatory ducts, and is where a minority of prostate cancers arise. The peripheral zone makes up 75% of the normal volume of the prostate and is where the majority of prostate cancers arise.

The prostate is supplied by the prostatic branch of the inferior vesical artery. The prostatic branch gives off urethral and capsular branches. The urethral branches run perpendicular to the urethra near the bladder neck and then turn parallel to the urethra, and are what supply the "BPH adenoma." On the other hand, the capsular branches runs lateral to the prostate as part of the neurovascular bundle and give off various rami to the prostate. The venous return from the prostate is via the prostatic plexus, sometimes called Santorini's plexus. The prostatic plexus also receives inflow from the deep dorsal vein of the penis. It drains primarily to the internal iliac veins and communicates via Batson's plexus with the vertebral veins (Netter 403).

The prostate is innervated by the inferior hypogastric plexus. There is both sympathetic (hypogastric nerve) and parasympathetic (pelvic nerve) supply. The prostatic lymphatics drain to the internal iliac chain of lymph nodes.

11. Seminal Vesicals and Vasa Deferentia

The seminal vesicals are approximately five centimeters in length and fuse with the ampulla of the vas to form the ejaculatory ducts (Netter 384). Each vas deferens arises from the tail of the epididymis, runs posterior to the cord vessels, travels through the inguinal canal, passes through the internal ring and runs extraperitoneally, where it passes above the ureter and where the dilated terminal vas, the ampulla, fuses with the corresponding seminal vesical to form the ejaculatory duct. The ejaculatory duct then runs through the central zone of the prostate and empties into the prostatic urethra (Netter 390). The vesiculodeferential branch of the superior vesical artery supplies the vas deferens. The vas deferens is innervated mostly via sympathetic nerves from the inferior hypogastric plexus. Remember that the parasympathetic system is primarily responsible for erectile function while the sympathetic system is responsible for ejaculation. Thus, both the vasa deferentia and the seminal vesicles which play an important role during ejaculatory function are primarily subject to sympathetic control.

12. Urethra

Male

The male urethra is commonly divided into the posterior and anterior portions. The posterior portion is further divided into the prostatic and membranous urethra. The anterior portion is composed of the bulbar, penile, and glanular portions. The anterior urethra runs within the corpus spongiosum and there are multiple small glands that empty into it. The urethra has a dual blood supply. It is based on the internal pudendal artery that distally becomes the common penile artery and then gives off a number of branches. One important branch is the bulbourethral artery which directly supplies the corpus spongiosum. Another branch of the common penile artery is the dorsal artery which terminates at the glans. Because the corpus spongiosum and glans are intimately connected, blood flow from the glans then travels in a retrograde fashion through the corpus spongiosum. This is why the corpus spongiosum has what is called a dual blood supply: 1.) directly, in an antegrade fashion from the bulbourethral artery, and 2.) in a retrograde fashion via the glans from the dorsal penile artery. Therefore, during a urethroplasty you can cut across the entire corpus spongiosum and still expect blood flow in the distal portion (Netter 385, 403).

Female

The female urethra is approximately four centimeters long and has many small glands which distally are grouped to form Skene's glands that empty into the urethra and periurethral area. There is a rich plexus of veins and smooth muscle that helps provide resistance to increase the closure pressure and promote urinary continence (Netter 356).

13. Female Pelvic Floor

The female pelvic floor has three primary functions: 1.) prevent the abdominal contents from falling out; 2.) control the storage and evacuation of feces; and 3.) allow for conception and parturition. There are two components to the female pelvic floor: the viscerofascial layer which is made up of connective tissue and "fascia," and the muscular layer which is composed of the levator ani muscles. The components of the viscerofascial layer include structures such as the cardinal ligaments, the pubocervical fascia, and the prerectal fascia. It is important to remember that these "fascial layers" are not true fascia but instead are condensations of relatively loose areolar tissue. The pubovisceral muscles are made up of the components of the levator ani and run from the pubis to the coccyx in a sling-like configuration supporting the pelvic organs. The pubococcygeous runs from the pubis to the coccyx and as such connects relatively immobile structures—parts of the bony skeleton—and therefore has little contribution to overall pelvic floor support. The puborectalis runs from the pubis around the rectum and back to the pubis. It is attached to the lateral vaginal walls, penetrates the rectal walls, and does play an important role in pelvic floor support. The iliococcygeous, which runs from the ilium to the coccyx, is in more of a horizontal sheet configuration (Table 14). Much of the connection of the "fascial" layers to the pelvic side wall is via the arcus tendineus fascia pelvis (ATFP), a condensation of tissue on the ileum that runs from the pubis to the ischial spine (Netter 356).

14. External Genitalia

Penis

The penis is made up of the glans penis, the corpus spongiosum, and the paired corpora cavernosal bodies. The corpora cavernosal bodies are attached proximally via crura to the pubic arch. The distal three-quarters of each corporal body is closely apposed and distally evaginates into the glans. The corpus spongiosum encloses the urethra and terminates to join the glans (Netter 382). The corpora cavernosal bodies are enclosed within the tunica albuginea and are filled with erectile tissue made up of smooth muscle with intervening vascular spaces. They are divided by a septum, although distally there is communication between the two corporal bodies. This is why intracavernosal injections used for erectile dysfunction need only be injected into one corporal body to affect both corporal bodies. Buck's fascia surrounds the corporal bodies and the dorsal nerves, arteries, and vein lay under it. More superficially, a layer of loose areolar tissue, the Dartos fascia, surrounds Buck's fascia. The penile skin is the most superficial layer. The corpus spongiosum as well is enclosed by Buck's and Dartos fascia and there is minimal vascular communication between the corpora cavernosal and spongiosal bodies (Netter 381).

The arterial supply to the penis has a similar origin to that of the urethra. The internal pudendal artery becomes the penile artery terminally and then gives off the bulbourethral artery, the dorsal artery of the penis, and finally the cavernosal artery. One cavernosal artery on each side supplies blood to its respective corpora cavernosal body and is thus responsible for blood inflow to the penis leading to erection. There is also blood flow from the femoral artery via the external pudendal arteries to the superficial penile arteries and this is responsible for supplying the penile shaft skin (Netter 403).

There are three levels of venous return of blood from the penis. The superficial skin is drained via a superficial system where the superficial veins join to form a superficial dorsal vein that drains via the saphenous vein. The glans, the corpora spongiosum,

Table 14

Viscerofascial Layer	
Cardinal ligaments →	apex
Uterosacral ligaments →	apex
Pubocervical fascia →	bladder/pelvic side walls
Prerectal fascia →	rectum/pelvic side walls
Pubovisceral Muscles	
Levator ani – from pubis to coccyx – sling like	
Pubococcygeous	- connects immobile structures - little contribution to support
Puborectalis	- attached to lateral vaginal walls - penetrates rectal wall
Illeococcygeous	- horizontal sheet

and the distal two-thirds of the corpora cavernosal bodies drain via the intermediate system. Blood from the glans drains via the retrocoronal plexus into the deep dorsal vein. Blood from the corporal bodies drains via the circumflex veins into the deep dorsal vein. The deep dorsal vein then empties into the prostatic plexus. The deep system is responsible for draining the proximal one-third of the corpora cavernosal bodies and the bulbar portion of the spongiosum. The cavernosal veins drain to the internal pudendal veins, the bulbar veins drain to the prostatic plexus, and the crural veins drain to both the internal pudendal veins and the prostatic plexus (Hinman 16.31) (Table 15).

The penis is innervated by both somatic and autonomic nerves. The somatic nerves are responsible for sensory function. The dorsal nerve of the penis, a branch of the pudendal nerve which travels via Alcock's canal, is responsible for sensory function.

The autonomic system is responsible for normal erectile function. Both sympathetic and parasympathetic nerves from the inferior hypogastric plexus travel via the neurovascular bundle, lateral to the prostate, and then into the corporal bodies as the cavernous nerves.

Thus, one can see how, after a radical prostatectomy, where the neurovascular bundles are damaged, one might lose erectile function while maintaining sensory function, as the sensory nerves leave the pelvis via a different route and are not damaged during a radical prostatectomy.

Clitoris

The blood flow and innervation of the clitoris parallels that of the penis. Sensory function is via the clitoral branch of the pudendal nerve. These nerves run medial to the corporal bodies and then cross over to run on the lateral portion of the corporal bodies, terminating just short of the glans clitoris. On the other hand, clitoral engorgement is due to autonomic stimulation via the cavernous nerves from the inferior hypogastric plexus.

15. Testis and Scrotum

Testis

The normal testis is approximately 4-5 cm in length with a volume of 30 mL and is covered by the tunica albuginea. The arterial supply to the testis is via the testicular artery directly from the aorta and from a vasal artery from the superior vesical artery. The venous return is via the pampiniform plexus which coalesces to form the gonadal vein, which on the right side empties directly into the inferior vena cava and on the left side empties into the left renal vein (Netter 390).

Spermatogenesis takes place in the seminiferous tubules after which the spermatids travel via the rete testis to the efferent ductules and then via the convoluted epididymal duct to the vas deferens.

Scrotum

The layers of the scrotum are primarily derived from and continuous with the layers of the abdominal wall which are encountered as the testes descend into the scrotum. From inside out the layers include the tunica albuginea surrounding the testis, the visceral tunica vaginalis, the parietal tunica vaginalis, the internal spermatic fascia, the cremasteric muscle and fascia, the external spermatic fascia, the Dartos muscle and finally the scrotal skin (Netter 390).

Table 15

Penis

Arterial Supply

__Internal pudendal artery__

penile artery (via Alcock's canal)
- cavernosal arteries -corpora cavernosa
- bulbourethral – corpus spongiosum
- dorsal artery -cavernosal branches
  - circumflex
  - glans

femoral artery
- external pudendal arteries
- superficial penile arteries (supplies shaft skin)

Venous Return

__Superficial__ - superficial veins join
-superficial dorsal vein
⟶ saphenous vein

__Intermediate__ - glans, corpus spongiosum, distal 2/3 of corpora cavernosa
- retrocoronal plexus
- circumflex veins
  - deep dorsal vein
  - prostatic plexus

__Deep__ - proximal 1/3 of corpora cavernosa, bulb
- cavernous vein ⟶ internal pudendal
- bulbar vein ⟶ prostatic plexus
- crural vein ⟶ both of above

16. Questions

1. Which of the following structures is not typically encountered in the course of renal surgery through a flank incision?

A. Internal oblique muscle

B. Transversalis fascia

C. Rectus muscle

D. Thoracolumbar fascia

E. Transverses abdominus

2. Regarding Gerota's fascia, which of the following are true?

A. It is part of the inner stratum of retroperitoneal tissue

B. Inferiorly there is an open potential space

C. Perinephric fat is outside of it

D. Both A. and C.

E. None of the above

3. Which of the following is not typically a site of normal ureteral narrowing (where stones get caught)?

A. UPJ

B. Iliac vessels

C. Pelvic ureter

D. UVJ

4. Normal voiding is dependent on all of the following nerves except?

A. Pelvic

B. Hypogastric

C. Obturator

D. Pudendal

5. Which of the following is true about the prostate?

A. Most prostate cancer is from the transition zone

B. Most normal volume is in the peripheral zone

C. The central zone is primarily distal to the verumontanum

D. The primary blood supply is from the superior vesical artery

6. The adrenal glands receive blood supply from all of the following except?

A. Superior phrenic artery

B. Inferior phrenic artery

C. A direct branch from the aorta

D. A branch off of the renal artery

7. If one needs to ligate the hypogastric arteries for severe pelvic bleeding it should be done distal to which area?

A. Posterior division

B. Umbilical artery

C. Inferior vesical artery

D. Obturator artery

8. Which of the following nerves would one suspect was damaged if a patient lost the ability to adduct the thighs after pelvic surgery?

A. Ilioinguinal

B. Femoral

C. Obturator

D. Sciatic

9. Which of the following structures do not make up part of Hesselbach's triangle?

A. Inferior epigastric vessels

B. Lateral margin of the rectus muscle

C. Pectineal muscle

D. Inguinal ligament

10. In women the ureter is in close proximity to and can be damaged during gynecologic surgery on which of the following structures?

A. Ovary

B. Uterine artery

C. Cervix

D. Vaginal wall

E. All of the above

Answers

1. C.
The typical flank incision does not travel anteromedially to the border of the rectus. All other structures noted are traversed.

2. B.
It is part of the intermediate stratum and the perinephric fat is within it. B. is correct.

3. C.
Ureteral caliber is typically narrowest at the UPJ, over the illiacs and at the UVJ. There is no particular narrow point per se of the pelvic portion of the ureter.

4. C.
Obturator nerves allow for thigh adduction. Pelvic and hypogastric nerves carry the autonomic supply to the bladder and innervation to the external sphincter is via the pudendal.

5. B.
A., C. and D. are false—most cancer is in the peripheral zone, the central zone is proximal to the veru and the primary blood supply is from the inferior vesical artery.

6. A.
The adrenal has a tripartite blood supply and receives blood from all the options listed except the superior phrenic artery.

7. A.
The posterior division includes the gluteal artery which supplies the gluteus. Ligating proximal to this point may lead to pain in the buttocks.

8. C.
The obturator nerve is responsible for thigh adduction.

9. C.
Hesselbach's triangle is bordered medially by the rectus muscle, laterally by the inferior epigastrics and inferiorly by the inguinal ligament.

10. E.
All of these structures can be damaged during gynecological surgery.

Acknowledgement

Sarah McAchran, MD for reviewing and making suggestions to the manuscript.

Chapter 2: Pediatric Urology

Hiep Thieu Nguyen, MD, FAAP

Acknowledgment
Dr. Barry A. Kogan (Albany Medical College) kindly provided some of the figures.

Contents

1. Fetal Abnormalities

With the advent of routine prenatal ultrasonography (US), children with congenital anomalies of the genitourinary tract are now being detected prior to developing signs and symptoms such as urinary tract infection, abdominal mass, hematuria, kidney stones and pain. These children benefit from early diagnosis with the goal of preventing complications and to preserve renal function when possible. However, not all findings on prenatal US represent pathology; many have no clinical significance. The dilemma is to be able to differentiate which children require intervention from those who do not. Specific findings on prenatal US can help to make this differentiation.

US of the Fetal GU Tract

- Fetal kidneys
  * Ureteral bud formation at 5th week of gestation (wks.)

  * Urine formation at 5th-8th wks.
    - 5 cc/hr at 20th wks.
    - 50 cc/hr at 40th wks.

  * Can be visualized at 12th-13th wks.

  * Visualization of hydronephrosis at 12th-18th wks.

  * Distinct renal architecture at 20th wks.

  * Detailed examination is better in the 2nd and 3rd trimester

  * Renal measurements: 12 wks.-40 wks.
    - AP diameter: 0.8-2.6 cm
    - Transverse diameter: 0.9-2.6 cm
    - Length: 1.0-2.7 cm

- Fetal bladder:
  * Can be visualized at 14th wks.

  * Emptying of the fetal bladder can be seen at 15th wks.

  * Size:
    - 10 cc at 30th wks.
    - 50 cc at term

- Amniotic fluid:
  * Early = transudate of amnion

  * Later = fetal urine + lung fluid-swallowing

  * Amniotic fluid volume:
    - 380 cc at 20th wks.
    - 800 cc at 28th wks.
    - 800 cc at 40th wks.

  * Amniotic volume dependent on urine production at 16th wks.

  * Etiology of polyhydramnios (>1.5 L)
    - Esophageal obstruction
    - Multicystic kidney
    - Mesoblastic nephroma
    - Some obstructive processes

  * Etiology of oligohydramnios (<0.5 L)
    - Amnion nodosum
    - Amniotic fluid leak
    - Urinary tract obstruction

  * Consequences of oligohydramnios
    - Pulmonary hypoplasia
    - Potter's syndrome: flat nose, recessed chin, low set ears, bowed legs, small chest, tales equinovares, and hypoplastic hands
    - Limb deformities

- Genitalia:
  * Can be visualized by 24th wks.
  * In 40% of fetuses, the sex can be determined at this time point

Findings on Prenatal US That May Suggest GU Anomalies

- ***Hydronephrosis.*** Dilation of the renal pelvis (pelviectasis) and/or calyces (caliectasis) caused by obstruction or reflux.

- ***Renal pyramids.*** Echolucent structures within the kidney suggest normal renal development and are sometimes misinterpreted as dilated calyces.

- ***Echogenicity.*** Increased echogenicity similar to the appearance of the spleen or liver suggests the presence of renal parenchymal diseases such as dysplasia, severe obstruction or reflux, and inheritable cystic diseases.

- ***Parenchymal thinning.*** Decreased thickness of the renal parenchyma suggests the lost of functioning renal tissue caused by obstruction or reflux.

- ***Urothelial thickening.*** Increased thickness of the renal pelvis lining suggests the presence of variable dilation as seen with reflux or less often with obstruction.

- ***Duplication.*** Separation of the renal pelvic sinus echoes when no hydronephrosis is possibly associated with reflux or obstruction, such as in ectopic ureter or ureterocele.

- ***Renal cyst.*** Hypoechoic structures within the kidney are seen in multicystic dysplastic kidney (MCDK) or inheritable polycystic diseases.

- ***Intravesical cystic structures.*** Thin-walled cyst in the bladder suggests the diagnosis of an ureterocele.

- ***Urinoma***. A fluid collection around the kidney is seen in cases of severe obstruction.

- ***Bladder filling.*** Lack of bladder filling suggests poor urine production or bladder exstrophy, while lack of filling and emptying cycles suggests bladder outlet obstruction.

- ***Bladder wall thickness.*** Increased thickness of the bladder wall suggests the presence of bladder outlet obstruction or neurogenic dysfunction, but it must be interpreted in the context of bladder filling.

- ***Keyhole sign.*** Dilation of the posterior urethra suggests the presence of posterior urethral valves (Figure 1).

- ***Oligohydramnios.*** Markedly reduced amniotic fluid indicated by the absence of a pocket of fluid greater than 2 cm suggests poor urine output caused by obstruction and/or renal dysfunction.

Figure 1

Keyhole sign

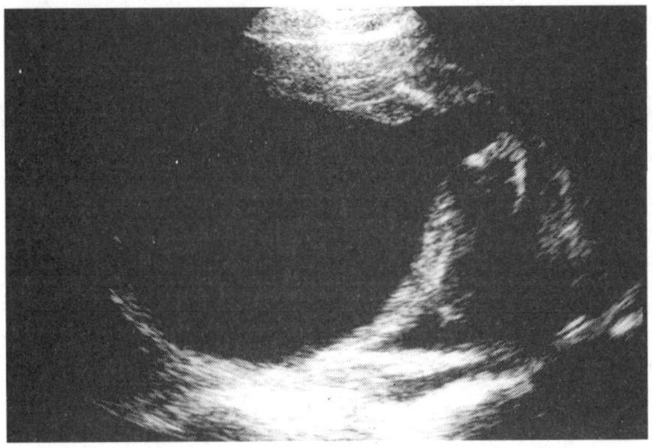

Keyhole sign observed on US suggesting the presence of posterior urethral valves.

Figure 2

Prenatal US demonstrating hydronephrosis

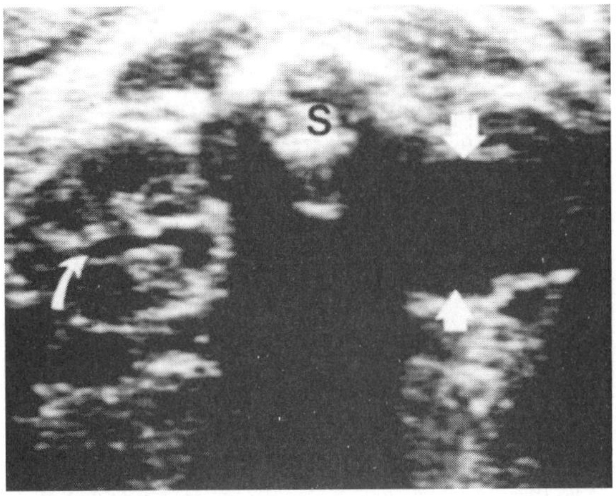

Prenatal US (cross-section) demonstrating hydronephrosis greater on the left than right. Measurement of the anterior-posterior diameter (between the white arrows) can be performed on this view of the kidneys.

Hydronephrosis is the most common abnormality detected on prenatal US. It is not a specific diagnosis but a finding.

• Defining pathologic hydronephrosis:

  * Anterior posterior diameter of the renal pelvis is the simplest and most sensitive parameter in defining pathologic hydronephrosis (Figure 2).

  * Dependent upon the gestation age

Date of Detection	**Degree**	**Pelvic Diameter**
2nd trimester	Mild	5-8mm
	Moderate	8-10mm
	Severe	>10mm
3rd trimester	Mild	<10mm
	Moderate	10-15mm
	Severe	>15mm

  * More likely to be pathological if there is:
    • Calyceal dilatation
    • Ureteral dilation
    • Chromosomal abnormalities
    • Multiple malformations
    • Oligohydramnios

  * Association with Down's syndrome is low (0.3%-3.3%)

• Differential diagnosis for hydronephrosis:

Transient/physiologic	50%-70%
UPJ obstruction	10%-30%
VUR	10%-40%
Megaureter	5%-15%
MCDK	2%-5%
PUV	1%-5%
Ureterocele, ectopic ureter, duplex system, urethral atresia, prune belly, PCKD, renal cysts	less common

• Fetal US appearance of the major diagnoses:

  * ***UPJ obstruction.*** Pelvi-calyceal dilatation without ureteral dilatation, usually unilateral.

  * ***UVJ obstruction.*** Dilatation of renal pelvis and ureter to the level of the bladder.

  * ***VUR.*** Variable degree of hydronephrosis or hydroureteronephrosis but there is no reliable findings to predict reflux on fetal US.

  * ***PUV.*** Bilateral hydroureteronephrosis with bladder wall thickening and keyhole sign is highly suggestive; however, variable findings are seen due to the wide spectrum of severity of the disease.

  * ***Ureterocele.*** Upper pole hydroureteronephrosis with a thin-walled cystic structure in the base of the bladder.

  * ***Ectopic ureter.*** Upper pole hydroureteronephrosis without an associated intravesical cystic structure.

  * ***MCDK.*** Non-reniform structure with multiple noncommunicating fluid-filled cystic spaces without a central large cyst and little renal parenchyma; most often confused with severe hydronephrosis.

  * ***Autosomal recessive polycystic kidney disease (ARPKD).*** Bilateral markedly enlarged and brightly echogenic kidneys.

  * ***Autosomal dominant polycystic kidney disease (ADPKD).*** Heterogeneous renal cysts in size and location.

  * ***Prune belly syndrome.*** Bilateral hydroureteronephrosis with an enlarged bladder, often confused with PUV.

Fetal Intervention

- Purpose:
  * Prevent pulmonary hypoplasia
  * Improve kidney function
  * Improve bladder function

- Types:
  * Early delivery
  * Open vesicostomy
  * Vesicoamniotic shunts—most common
  * Endoscopic relief of bladder outlet obstruction

- Indications:
  * Evidence of severe bladder outlet obstruction
  * Normal karyotype
  * No other systemic anomalies
  * Singleton and male fetus
  * Oligohydramnios
  * Noncystic kidneys
  * Favorable urinary indices by serial sampling over 3 days
    - Na <100
    - Cl <110
    - Osm <210
    - $\beta 2$ microglobulin <10-20
  * Informed consent

- Complications:
  * Shunt displacement
  * Preterm labor and prematurity
  * Chorioamnionitis
  * Iatrogenic gastroschisis
  * Urinary ascites
  * Limited improvement in bladder or kidney function

Postnatal Evaluation

- Immediate: renal/bladder (RUS) and voiding cystourethrogram (VCUG) within 1-2 weeks
  * Solitary kidney
  * Moderate or severe bilateral hydronephrosis
  * Ureterocele
  * Thick-walled bladder or keyhole sign

- Delayed:
  * Mild unilateral or bilateral hydronephrosis: RUS at 2-3 months; VCUG controversial
  * Moderate to severe unilateral hydronephrosis: RUS and VCUG at 1-2 months
  * Severe unilateral hydronephrosis: RUS, VCUG and intravenous pyelogram or MAG-3 renal scan at 1 month

- Antibiotic prophylaxis
  * If planning to get VCUG, then antibiotic prophylaxis should be given
  * Amoxicillin (25 mg/kg/day) or cephalosporin

2. Ureteropelvic Junction Obstruction

Definition

An impairment of urine flow from the renal pelvis into the proximal ureter, causing progressive dilatation of the renal pelvis and calyces and potential renal injury.

Etiology

- Primary:
  * Intrinsic obstruction (Figure 3)
    - Results from luminal narrowing of the UPJ with or without kinking
    - Usually characterized by excessive connective tissue and decreased smooth muscle content in the ureteral wall
    - Fixed obstruction
    - More commonly seen in infants and young children
  * Extrinsic obstruction (Figure 4)
    - Caused by compression of the ureter by anomalous (eg, lower pole) renal vasculature
    - Intermittent obstruction
    - More commonly found in older children and adults
- Secondary:
  * Due to marked VUR or PUV
  * Iatrogenic: postoperative
  * Uncommon

Epidemiology

- Incidence = 1 in 1500

Figure 3

IVP demonstrating UPJ obstruction

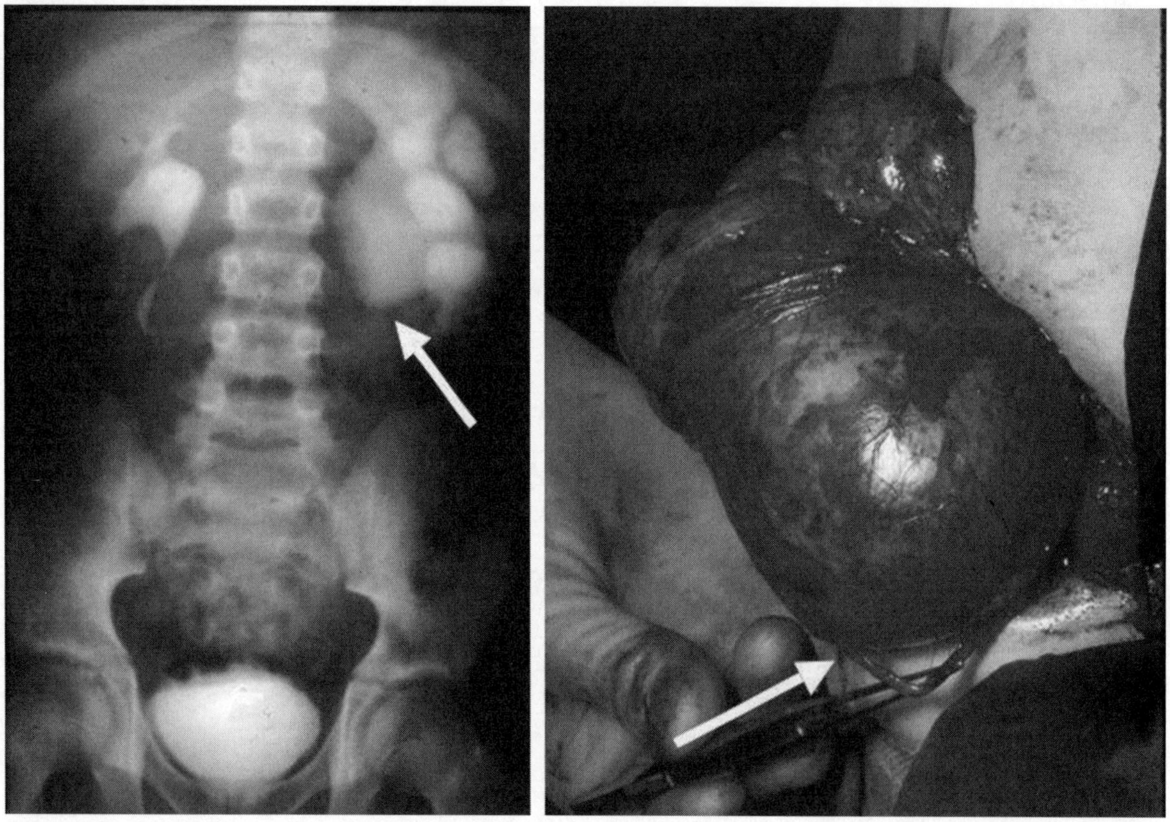

IVP demonstrating (left arrow) UPJ obstruction and intra-operative imaging demonstrating (right arrow) the corresponding primary intrinsic obstruction.

Figure 4

Primary extrinsic UPJ obstruction

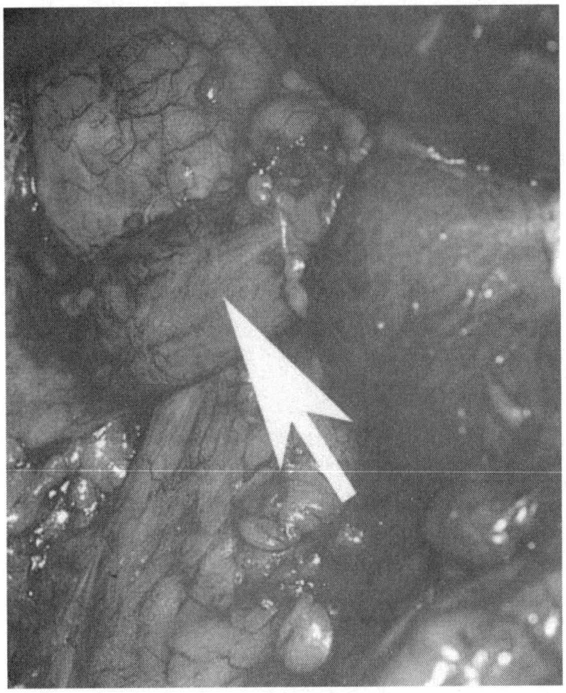

Intra-operative image of a primary extrinsic UPJ obstruction due to crossing vessels (arrow).

- Male to female ratio = 2:1
- Left to right ratio = 1.5:1
- Bilateral in 10%-40%
- Diagnosed most commonly by prenatal US
- Second most common cause of antenatal hydronephrosis
- Most common cause of obstructive uropathy in children

Associated Anomalies

- UPJ obstruction in the contralateral kidney (10%-40%)
- VUR (13%-42%)—usually low grade
- Renal dysplasia or MCDK (10%)
- Unilateral renal agenesis (5%)
- VATER syndrome (vertebral defects, imperforate anus, tracheoesophageal fistula and radial/renal dysplasia)—9%-21%

Symptoms

- Usually asymptomatic—diagnosed following evaluation of prenatal hydronephrosis
- Intermittent pain/vomiting (Dietl's crisis) in older children
- Palpable abdominal mass in young children
- Less common:
  * Urinary tract infection (UTI)
  * Hematuria or trauma
  * Stones
  * Failure to thrive or feeding difficulties
  * Hypertension
  * Incidental findings on US, CT, MRI or bone scan

Diagnosis

- US: standard imaging test to identify hydronephrosis
  * Does not diagnose obstruction or predict resolution
  * Possible correlation with clinically relevant obstruction:
    - Anterior posterior diameter of the renal pelvis (>15 mm)
    - Increase hydronephrosis on serial US examination
    - Increase in growth of the contralateral kidney on serial US examination
    - Resistive index (peak systolic velocity—lowest diastolic velocity) >0.75
- Diuretic radionuclide renography: assess differential function and assessment of washout from each kidney.

* Agents:
  • DTPA (99m Tc-diethylenetriaminpentaacetic acid): exclusively filtered by the glomeruli with an extraction fraction of 20%, providing an indirect means of measuring glomerular filtration rate (GFR)

  • MAG-3 (99m Tc-mercaptoacety triglycine): secreted by the proximal tubular cells with an extraction fraction of 50% and little background, providing an indirect means of measuring estimated renal plasma flow (ERPF)
* Not obstructed:
  • Symmetric uptake: differential renal function (DRF) >40%
  • Good washout: T 1/2 <10 minutes
* Obstructed:
  • Decrease in DRF on serial examination
  • Potential obstruction:
    * T 1/2 >30 minutes on one exam
    * Worsening T 1/2 on serial examination
  • False positive with immature kidney

• Radionuclide renography: assess differential renal function and scarring
  * Agents: DMSA (99m Tc-Dimercaptosuccinic acid) binds to functioning proximal tubular cells
  * Direct assessment of renal blood flow
  * More accurate than DTPA or MAG-3 in assessing renal function
  * Gold standard for evaluation of renal scarring

• Intravenous pyelogram
  * Less commonly used since radionuclide renography has become available
  * Beneficial when anatomy is very complex

• Pressure flow studies (Whitaker test)
  * Measurement of intrapelvic pressure during infusion of fluid into the renal pelvis
  * Calculate the decrease in pressure with time (pressure decay)
    • Not obstructed: rapid pressure decay
    • Obstructed: slow pressure decay
  * Pressure decay half-life reflects both efficiency of urine transport and relative compliance and volume of the collecting system

• Magnetic resonance imaging (MRI)
  * Able to define anatomy, calculate differential renal function and assess obstruction
  * Comparable to radionuclide renography
  * Disadvantages include cost, equipment limitation, sensitivity to patient motion and the need for sedation

• Cystoscopy with retrograde pyelogram
  * Infrequently performed as an isolated diagnostic modality
  * Risk of introducing infection
  * May be performed at the time of surgical repair to rule out concomitant distal ureteral obstruction

• Biochemical markers
  * Elevated N-acetyl-β-D-glucoasminidase (NAG) in the urine from the obstructed kidney
  * Elevated TGF-β1 in the urine from the bladder of patients with unilateral UPJ obstruction

Treatment

• Indication for surgical repair:
  * <40% function and poor washout parameters
  * Progressive hydronephrosis on serial US examination
  * Progressive loss of renal function on serial radionuclide renograms
  * Renal pelvic size >5 cm
  * Infection/stone

• Types of surgical repair:
  * Dismembered pyeloplasty (open surgical repair)
    • Most common and gold standard
    • Advantages:
      * Broad applicability including preservation of anomalous vessels
      * Excision of the pathologic UPJ and appropriate reposition of the UPJ
      * Ability to perform reduction pyeloplasty
    • >95% success rate
    • Stent/nephrostomy optional
    • Penrose drain is recommended when the approach is retroperitoneal
  * Endopyelotomy (endoscopic incision)
    • Can be performed antegrade or retrograde

- Contraindicated in patients with crossing vessels or with very large pelvis
- 80%-85% success rate
- Stenting is required
- May be good for postoperative obstruction

* Laparoscopic pyeloplasty
  - Reduced morbidity compared to open surgery especially in older children and young adults
  - Significant learning curve
  - Robotic assistance significantly reduces the difficulties associated with laparoscopic suturing
  - Success rate 90%-95%
  - Stent/nephrostomy optional

- Complications:
  * Early: uncommon
    - UTI
    - Prolonged urinary leakage from the Penrose drain; treat with stent
  * Late:
    - Lack of improvement in renal function or washout time
    - Worsening hydronephrosis
    - Pain or UTI
    - Worsening renal function

3. Ureterovesical Junction Obstruction (Obstructed Megaureter)

Definition

An impairment of urinary flow from the distal ureter into the bladder, resulting in dilation of the entire collecting system from the distal ureter to calyces.

Etiology

- Primary: due to a deficiency of smooth muscle in the ureterovesical ureter, resulting in an adynamic distal segment that impedes normal peristalsis of urine through the ureter (Figure 5)

Figure 5

Primary UVJ obstruction

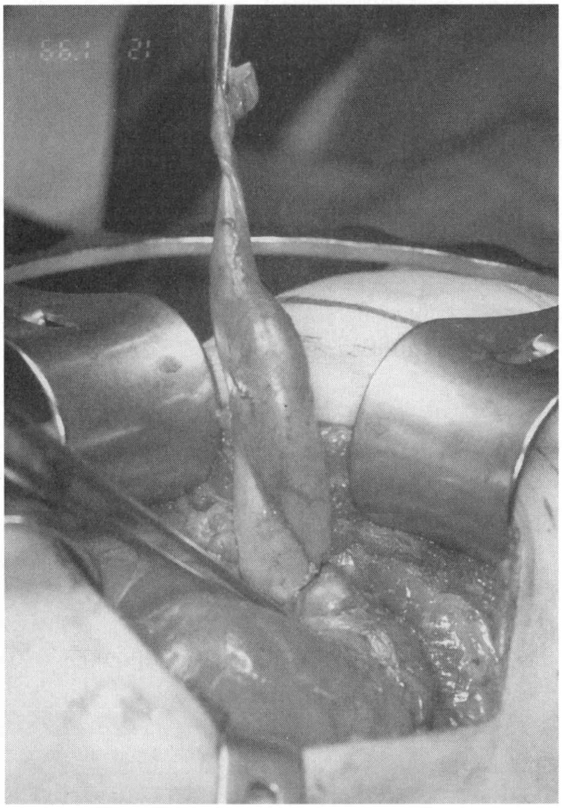

Intra operative image of a primary UVJ obstruction. Note the degree of dilatation in the proximal ureter but normal diameter at the distal segment.

• Secondary: due to extrinsic compression of the ureter by a thick bladder wall in pathological states such as posterior urethral valves or neurogenic bladder

Epidemiology

• Accounts for approximately 8% of children that presented with symptoms such as infection, hematuria or pain, and had hydroureteronephrosis on imaging studies

• Accounts for 23% of newborns with prenatally diagnosed hydronephrosis

• Third most common cause of antenatal hydronephrosis

• Male to female ratio = 2-4:1

• Left to right ratio = 1.6-4.5:1

• Bilaterally in 10%-25% of the cases

Associated Anomalies

• Contralateral renal anomalies (renal agenesis or MCDK)—9%

• Concomitant ipsilateral VUR (obstructed reflux megaureter)—2%

• Ureterocele and duplicated systems—uncommon

• Concomitant ipsilateral UPJ obstruction—rare

Symptoms

• Usually asymptomatic—diagnosed following evaluation of prenatal hydronephrosis

• Less common: UTI, stone and hematuria

Diagnosis

• US:
  * The presence of a dilated ureter distinguishes UVJ obstruction from UPJ obstruction (Figure 6)
  * Provides anatomic detail of the renal parenchyma, collecting system and the bladder
  * Baseline for the degree of hydroureteronephrosis for serial examination

• VCUG:
  * Need to rule out reflux as the etiology for the dilated ureter
  * Look for signs (such as thick-walled bladder or dilated posterior urethra) of secondary causes of UVJ obstruction such as neurogenic bladder and bladder outlet obstruction.

• Diuretic radionuclide renogram:
  * Evaluate function and washout
  * Need to define the region of interest around the distal ureter to accurately evaluate drainage from the ureter (Figure 7)
  * Defer study until after 3 months of age to allow for tubular maturation

• Less often used imaging modalities: IVP, MRI and pressure perfusion study

Figure 6

Dilated cystic structure

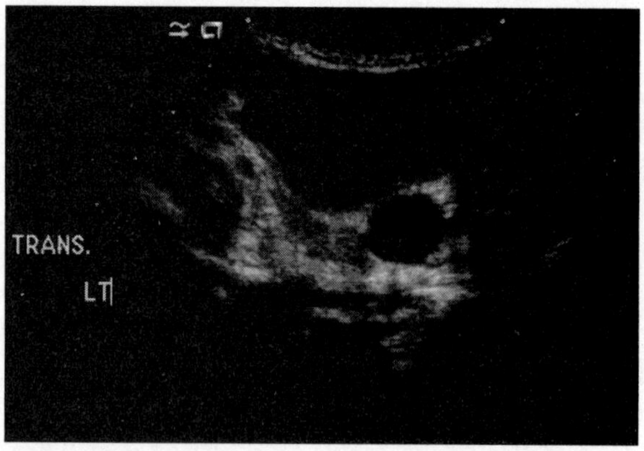

US demonstrating a dilated cystic structure behind the bladder, consistent with a dilated ureter.

Figure 7

MAG-3 scan

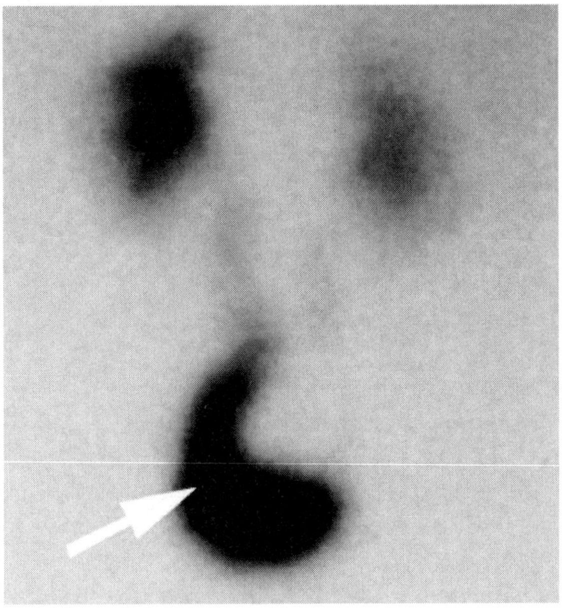

MAG-3 scan demonstrating a dilated left collecting system with much of dilatation occurring in the distal ureter (arrow).

- Cystoscopy with retrograde pyelogram
  * Infrequently performed as an isolated diagnostic modality
  * Risk of introducing infection
  * May be performed at the time of surgical repair

Treatment

- Depending on the mode of presentation
  * Asymptomatic—prenatal hydronephrosis
    - Natural history: most improve spontaneously
    - Significant risk for UTIs: need prophylactic antibiotic during the first six months to first year of life
  * Secondary UVJ obstruction
    - Correction of the underlying pathology

- Indication for surgical correction
  * Recurrent UTIs while on prophylaxis
  * Decrease in renal function
  * Progressive hydroureteronephrosis
  * Stones

- Types of surgical repair
  * Reimplantation of affected ureter (intravesical or extravesical)
    - Need a tunnel length to ureteral diameter ratio of 5:1
  * Ureteral tailoring may be needed to decrease the diameter of the ureter to allow for the appropriately sized tunnel to be created

  - Plication (Kalicinski or Starr)
    * Infolding of the ureteral wall
      * Advantages: preserves ureteral vascularity and reversible
      * Disadvantages: tissue bulk and spontaneous reopening of the infolding segment, resulting in VUR
    * Indicated for moderately dilated ureter
  - Excisional tapering (Figure 8)
    * Removal of lateral wall portion of the ureter with preservation of the medial blood supply to the ureter

Figure 8

Excisional technique of ureteral tapering

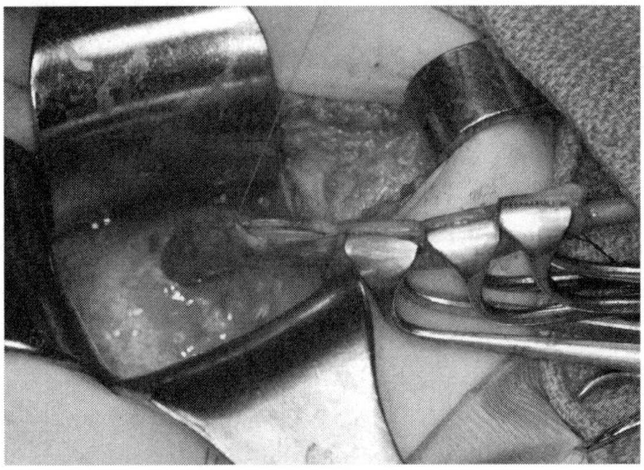

Intra operative image demonstrating the excisional technique of ureteral tapering.

  * Higher success rate
  * Indicated for ureters >1.75 cm in diameter or markedly thickened

- Complications:
  * Obstruction
    - Related to postoperative edema
      * Resolve with time (up to 8 wks.)
      * May require temporary diversion (stent or nephrostomy tube) if patients have symptoms (UTI or pain)
    - Related to ischemia of the distal ureter
      * Persistent obstruction
      * Required resection of the distal ureter and reimplantation
  * VUR
    - Mild cases resolve with time
    - When associated with UTI or persists, will need surgical correction
    - Need to rule out neurogenic or non-neurogenic bladder dysfunction as a contributory factor
    - May consider subureteric injection therapy, ureteral reimplantation or transureteroureterostomy

4. Ureteroceles

Definition

A cystic dilatation of the intravesical submucosal ureter, usually associated with an obstructed orifice that impairs urinary flow into the bladder (Figure 9). When associated with a duplicated system, the ureterocele is associated with the upper pole collecting system (Weigert-Meyer Law).

- ***Intravesical.*** The ureterocele is entirely contained in the bladder

- ***Extravesical.*** Any portion of the ureterocele extends into the bladder neck or urethra

- ***Stenotic.*** The narrowed opening of the ureterocele is found inside the bladder

- ***Sphincteric.*** The orifice of the ureterocele is distal to the bladder neck

- ***Sphincterostenotic.*** Combination of the above

- ***Cecoureterocele.*** A ureterocele that has an intravesical orifice but a submucosal extension that goes into the urethra

Etiology

Unknown, but it is hypothesized that it results either from an incomplete breakdown of the ureteral (Chwalla) membrane present at the time of the ureteral bud arising from the mesonephric duct or from a delay in the establishment of the lumen of the ureteral bud

Epidemiology

- Incidence: 1 in 500 to 1 in 4000

- Male to female ratio = 1:5-7

- Much more common in Caucasians

- Bilateral in 10%

Associated Anomalies

- Duplex system in 80% and single system in 20%
- VUR:
  * Ipsilateral lower pole—50%-70%
  * Contralateral renal unit—10%-30%
  * Ureterocele—uncommon, need to consider ectopic ureterocele with the orifice in the urethra allowing reflux into the ureterocele and its ureter

Symptoms

- Usually asymptomatic—diagnosed following evaluation of prenatal hydronephrosis

Figure 9

Ureterocele

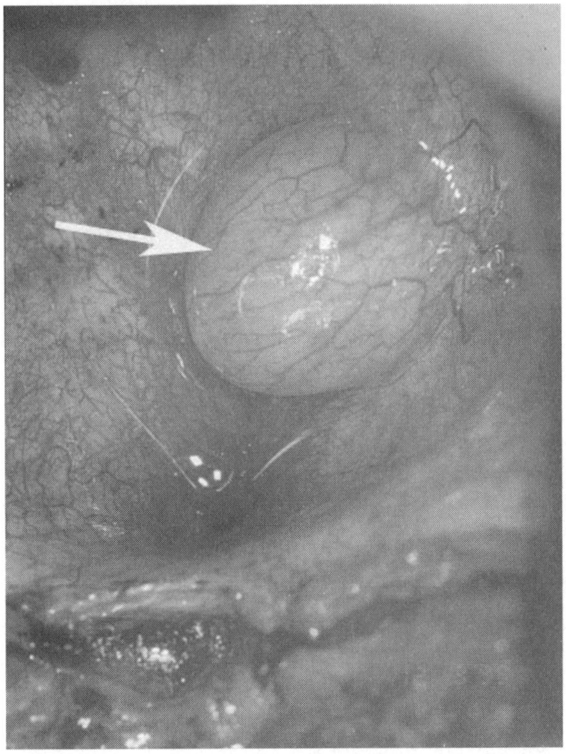

Intra operative image demonstrating a ureterocele (arrow)

- UTI and sepsis due to urinary stasis
- Abdominal mass due to obstruction of the upper collecting system and/or bladder
- Intralabial mass due to prolapse of the ureterocele into the introitus
- Voiding dysfunction (urgency and incontinence) associated with ureterocele
- Less commonly: hematuria, failure to thrive

Diagnosis

- US:
  * Identification of a thin-walled cystic mass within the bladder (Figure 10)
  * Pitfalls:
    - May be effaced and not visualized if the bladder is overdistended
    - May resemble the bladder if the bladder is empty
    - May be misidentified as a dilated or ectopic ureter

Figure 10

Cystic, thin-walled structure

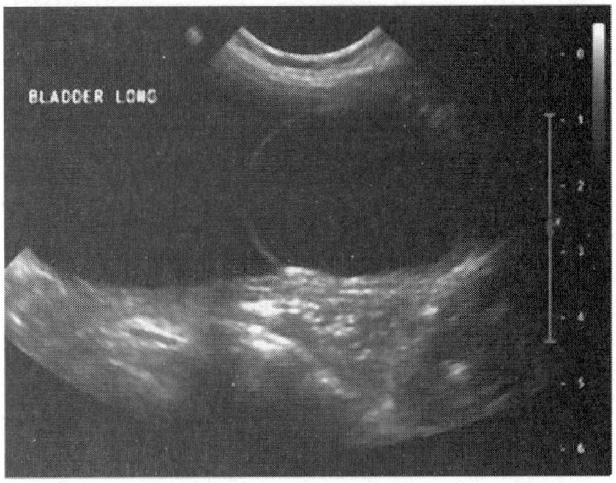

US demonstrating a cystic, thin-walled structure in the bladder consistent with a ureterocele

* Evaluation for a duplex system (renal parenchyma dividing central sinus echoes or different degrees of hydronephrosis between the upper and lower poles) (Figure 11)
* Identification of hydroureteronephrosis:
  • If in a duplex system, hydroureteronephrosis is typically seen in the upper pole.
  • If the ureterocele is not associated with upper pole hydronephrosis, consider nonobstructive ectopic ureterocele or ureterocele disproportion (atrophic upper pole).
  • Hydronephrosis associated with the lower pole is due to VUR.
* Assessment of the amount and quality of the parenchyma of the ipsilateral renal unit
* Evaluation of the contralateral kidney for associated anomalies

• VCUG:
  * Ureterocele appears as a smooth, broad-based filling defect located near the trigone

Figure 11

US demonstrating duplication of right collecting system

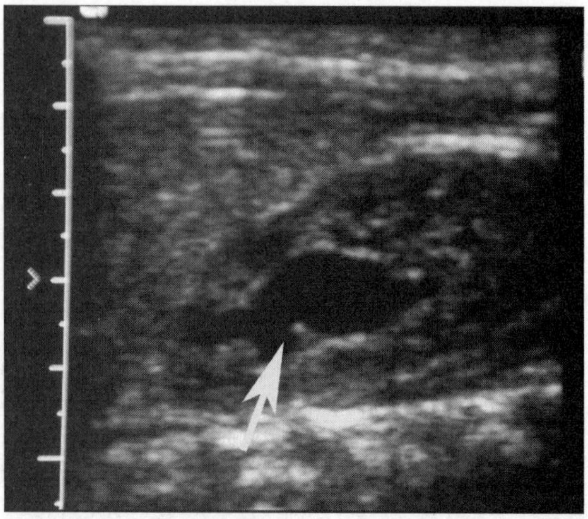

US demonstrating duplication of right collecting system, with moderate hydronephrosis in the upper pole (arrow) but no hydronephrosis in the lower pole

  * Images should be obtained in the early phases of filling, since the ureterocele may efface or evert into the ureter appearing to be a diverticulum later in filling.
  * Evaluate for reflux into ipsilateral and contralateral renal unit

• DMSA renal scan:
  * Evaluate the function of the associated renal unit to see if it is worth saving
  * Can also use DTPA or MAG-3 to get renal function as well as the degree of obstruction

• IVP:
  * Commonly the function of the renal moiety associated with the ureterocele (upper pole) is poor, resulting in delayed excretion of contrast or no excretion at all.
  * The associated renal moiety is deviated laterally from the spine due to the presence of hydronephrosis, pushing the lower pole laterally and inferiorly.
  * Due to the poor function of the upper pole, only the lower pole calyces are visualized, creating the "dropping lily" sign.
  * Due to the association with the dilated upper pole ureter, the lower pole ureter is laterally deviated, notched and travels in a serpiginous manner.
  * A "cobra head" sign is seen when contrast fills the ureterocele, creating a radiodense structure outlined by the radiolucent ureterocele wall.

• MRI, CT scan or cystoscopy: if anatomy is very complex

Treatment

• Goal:
  * Preserve renal function if possible
  * Minimize infection, obstruction and reflux
  * Maintenance of urinary continence

• Antibiotic prophylaxis: high risk of infection

• Surgical treatment:
  * Endoscopic management: Transurethral incision of ureterocele
    • Effective in relief of the obstruction

- Risk of developing reflux into the ureterocele system
- Minimal morbidity and outpatient procedure
- Effective for intravesical ureterocele but less effective for ectopic ureterocele
- Its role as the definitive treatment for ureterocele is very controversial; most likely will need secondary procedure
- Should be considered as first treatment of patients who present with urosepsis

* Open surgical repair
  - Options:
    * Heminephrectomy and upper pole ureterectomy with or without ureterocele excision
    * Ureteroureterostomy
    * Excision of the ureterocele with reimplantation
  - Definitive treatment but higher morbidity
  - Complications: recurrent reflux and UTIs
  - Controversial as to whether upper tract surgery is better than lower tract surgery

5. Renal Cystic Diseases

Definition

Microscopic or macroscopic fluid-filled sacs lined with epithelium.

- Located at various sites along the nephron

- May or may not communicate with the glomerulus, tubule, collecting duct or calyx

- Located diffusely throughout the kidney or only in one segment, in one kidney or both

Etiology

Most renal cystic conditions except for MCDK and benign multilocular cysts arise from nephrons or collecting ducts after they have formed.

- Genetic
  * Autosomal recessive polycystic kidney disease (ARPKD)
  * Autosomal dominant polycystic kidney disease (ADPKD)
  * Juvenile nephronophthisis (autosomal recessive)
  * Medullary cystic disease (autosomal dominant)
  * Congenital nephrosis (autosomal recessive)
  * Familial hypoplastic glomerulocystic disease (autosomal dominant)
  * Syndromes with cysts (such as tuberous sclerosis and von Hippel-Lindau disease)

- Nongenetic
  * Multicystic dysplastic kidney (MCDK)
  * Benign multilocular cyst (cystic nephroma)
  * Simple cysts
  * Medullary sponge kidney
  * Sporadic glomerulocystic kidney disease
  * Acquired renal cystic disease (such as end-stage renal disease ESRD and dialysis)
  * Calyceal diverticulum (pyelogenic cyst)

- Most common: simple renal cysts, MCDK, ADPKD and ARPKD (Table 1)

Table 1

Epidemiology, Diagnosis and Associated Anomalies

	Radiologic Findings	Associated Anomalies	Incidence
ARPKD	Large, homogenous, echogenic kidneys on US; functioning kidneys with radial streaking (sunburst pattern) on IVP	Hepatic fibrosis with biliary atresia	1:5000-40,000
ADPKD	Large kidneys with scattered macrocysts on US; may resemble ARPKD on US and IVP	Diverticulitis: liver, spleen and pancreatic cysts; intracranial aneurysms	1:500-1000
MCKD	Diffuses cysts of various size without a larger central cyst or visible communications between cysts on US; no function on DMSA or IVP	20%-40% with contralateral VUR; 3%-12% with contralateral UPJ obstruction; rare hypertension or malignancy	Most frequent cystic disease in newborn
Simple cysts	Cysts with normal renal parenchyma and kidney size on US or CT; no septation, irregular margins or calcifications; no enhancement on CT or MRI	None	Very common; increases with age

Symptoms

- Usually detected during routine prenatal US evaluation or from a family history
- For ARPKD, ADPKD and MCKD, may present with abdominal mass
- For ARPKD and ADPKD, may present hypertension, proteinuria or hematuria
- Usual age at clinical presentation for ARPKD is around the newborn period while for ADPKD is 3rd to 5th decades
- Large simple cysts can cause pyelocalyceal obstruction or hypertension

Treatment

- ARPKD: requires treatment for portal and systemic hypertension, congestive heart failure, and renal and hepatic failure
- ADPKD: requires treatment of systemic hypertension, UTIs, loin/back pain, renal failure
- MCKD: tends to regress spontaneously; surgical removal if fails to regress, or hypertension
- Simple cysts tend not to progress; surgical treatment (unroofing or percutaneous drainage) if patient has pain or hypertension

6. Posterior Urethral Valves

Definition

A membrane that arises from the verumontanum on the floor of the urethra, extending toward the bulbomembranous junction and attaching to the urethra throughout its circumference.

Has no active function but is a simple barrier to urine flow.

Etiology

It is hypothesized that the terminal ends of the Wolffian ducts mis-migrate and are integrated into the urethral wall abnormally, resulting in obliquely oriented ridges that act as one-way valves, impeding urine flow from the bladder.

Epidemiology

- Incidence: 1 in 5000-8000 males

- Accounts for up to 10% of obstructions diagnosed prenatally

Associated Anomalies: Due to the Consequences of PUV

- Lung-pulmonary hypoplasia

- Kidney:
  * Obstructive uropathy: reversible renal injury that improves with relief of obstruction; however, may recur with bladder dysfunction
  * Dysplasia:
    - Permanent level of injury that limits renal growth and may lead to progressive renal failure and hypertension
    - Associated with VUR (VURD syndrome); acts as pop-off mechanism protecting the contralateral kidney from the high bladder pressure
  * Tubular injury: resulting in inability to concentrate, which may lead to diabetes insipidus

- Ureters: poor contractility that leads to chronic hydroureteronephrosis in some cases

- Bladder: poor sensation, hypercontractility, low compliance with progression to myogenic failure, contributing to incontinence and incomplete emptying

Symptoms

- Newborns:
  * Detected on prenatal US
  * *In utero* findings include: oligohydranios, hydroureteronephrosis, echogenic kidneys, thickened bladder wall and dilated posterior urethra
  * Postnatal findings:
    - Respiratory distress due to pulmonary hypoplasia
    - Potter's facies and bowed/deformed limbs secondary to the oligohydramnios
    - Renal insufficiency resulting in failure to thrive, lethargy and poor feeding
    - Abdominal mass due to dilated bladder and hydroureteronephrosis
    - Ascites: urinary obstruction accounts for 40% of all cases of neonatal ascites

- Older children: present much later in life
  * UTI or voiding dysfunction (incontinence)
  * Renal insufficiency in 35% while ESRD in 10%

Diagnosis

- US: findings include hydroureteronephrosis, echogenic kidneys, thickened bladder wall and dilated posterior urethra (Figure 12)

- VCUG: Primary modality for diagnosis (Figure 13)
  * Dilated elongated posterior urethra with an elevated bladder neck
  * Thickened and trabeculated bladder
  * The valve structure is often visible
  * VUR—occurs in 50% of the cases

- Radionuclide renography: DMSA to evaluate renal function and MAG-3 if secondary UPJ or UVJ obstruction is suspected

- Cystoscopy: limited to those cases in which VCUG is equivocal

Figure 12

US demonstrating a thick-walled bladder

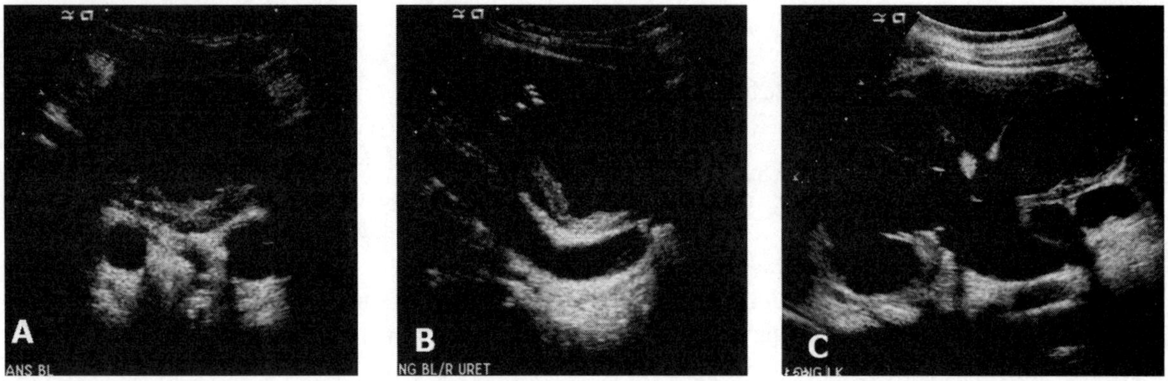

US demonstrating a thick-walled bladder A); dilated ureters B); and severe hydronephrosis with renal parenchymal thinning C). These findings are suggestive of bladder outlet obstruction such as PUV.

- Laboratory evaluation:
  - * Need to obtain serum creatinine, blood urea nitrogen and electrolytes
  - * Serum creatinine after 48 hours reflects newborn rather than maternal renal function
  - * Nadir serum creatinine >1.0 predicts high likelihood of developing ESRD
  - * Need to follow serum bicarbonate, sodium and potassium levels carefully due to the high incidence of salt loss and acidosis

Treatment

- Initial management:
  - * Urinary catheter drainage
  - * VCUG for diagnosis
  - * Follow electrolytes and creatinine until stabilized

- Endoscopic valve ablation:
  - * Disrupt the valves using Bugee electrode, cold knife, hooks, balloon catheters, valvulotomes or laser at the 5 and 7 o'clock position (occasionally at the 12 o'clock position)
  - * Complete resection leads to urethral and sphincter injuries (<5% with a limited resection)
  - * Often a catheter is left for drainage for 24 hours after the procedure

Figure 13

VCUG demonstrating characteristic findings of PUV

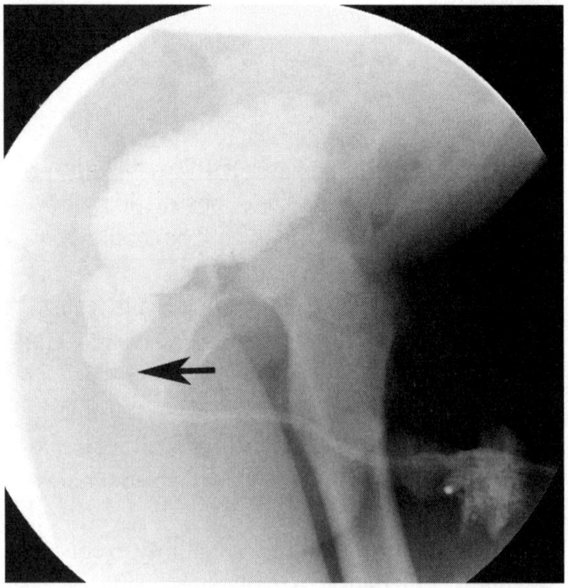

VCUG demonstrating characteristic findings of PUV including a dilated elongated posterior urethra with an elevated bladder neck, thickened and trabeculated bladder and the valve structure (arrow).

- Cutaneous vesicostomy
  * Indicated in infant too small for safe instrumentation or too ill
  * Does not cause permanent loss of bladder capacity

- Upper tract diversion
  * Ureterostomy or pyelostomy
  * Indicated in patients who fail to respond to bladder-level drainage (persistent infection or evidence of continued impairment of urinary drainage)
  * Will likely require further, more complicated reconstructive surgery
  * 80% of patients treated with upper tract diversion preserve their bladder capacity, while 69% preserve their bladder compliance

- Management of secondary VUR
  * 20%-32% resolve after valve ablation
  * If persists after valve ablation, need to make sure that bladder function is normalized and drainage is adequate
  * Antibiotic prophylaxis while awaiting spontaneous resolution
  * Reimplantation in a valve bladder has a high complication rate if the bladder is not well rehabilitated
  * High grade VUR associated with dysplastic renal units do not need to be removed unless patient has recurrent infection

- Management of nonrefluxing hydronephrosis
  * 49% resolve after valve ablation
  * If persists after valve ablation, need to make sure that bladder function is normalized and drainage is adequate
  * Most are due to chronic nonobstructive dilatation of collecting system and high urine output due to diabetes inspidus
  * Rare to have residual bladder outlet or UVJ obstruction

- Management of bladder dysfunction
  * Intrinsic bladder dysfunction may lead to deterioration of the upper urinary tract and incontinence (valve bladder syndrome)
  * Three urodynamic patterns identified (Table 2)

- These patterns of bladder dysfunction overlap in the majority of the patients and change with age

Table 2

Urodynamic Patterns

	Symptoms	More Common In	Treatment
Myogenic failure	Overflow incontinence, incomplete bladder emptying	Post-pubertal	Time and double voiding, α-blockers or intermittent catherization depending on severity
Detrusor hyperreflexia	Frequency and urge incontinence	Older children	Anticholinergics
Decreased compliance/ small capacity	Frequency and urge incontinence	Infants	Anticholinergics

- Management of renal dysfunction
  * Dysplasia: not treatable
  * Obstructive uropathy:
    - Provide low-pressure storage by treating bladder dysfunction
    - Provide adequate drainage of urine by regular emptying of the bladder with time/double voiding and/or nighttime catheter drainage
  * Prevent recurrent infection with management of VUR and nonrefluxing hydronephrosis
  * Control hypertension
  * High risk of renal failure during puberty due to the demands of rapid somatic growth
  * Predictors of poor renal function
    - Evidence of renal dysplasia on US
    - Age of presentation less than one year of age
    - Bilateral VUR
    - Nadir creatinine >1.0 during the first year of life
  * Renal transplant: good graft survival if bladder dysfunction is treated

7. Prune Belly Syndrome

Definition

Variable in severity, constellation of anomalies consisting primarily of deficiency of the abdominal wall musculature, bilateral undescended testis and urinary tract dilatation.

- Kidney:
  * Dilated with preserved calyceal anatomy; rarely UPJ obstruction
  * 50% with dysplasia

- Ureters:
  * Dilated, tortuous and redundant
  * Proximal portion more normal
  * 75% with VUR; rarely UVJ obstruction

- Bladder:
  * Massive, enlarged with pseudodiverticulum at the urachus
  * 25%-30% with a patent urachus
  * Large capacity with normal compliance and decreased sensation
  * 50% voids normally with normal voiding pressure, normal flow rates and low postvoid residuals.

- Urethra
  *Dilated prostatic urethra but no obstruction
  *Occasionally, urethral atresia or megalourethra

- Accessory sex organs:
  * Prostatic hypoplasia
  * Atretic, dilated or thickened vas and seminal vesicles
  * Epididymeal, efferent ductules and rete testis disjunction

- Testes: usually intra-abdominal

- Abdominal wall (Figure 14)
  * Skin, subcutaneous fat and a single fibrous layer on the peritoneum

  *Becomes less wrinkled and more pot-bellied as the child gets older

Figure 14

Prune belly syndrome

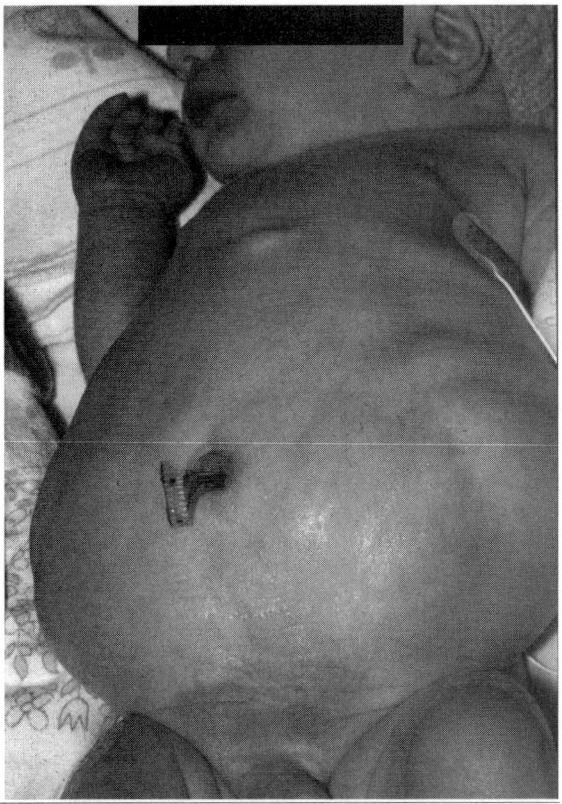

Typical abdominal finding in an infant with prune belly syndrome.

Etiology

- Most cases are sporadic with normal karyotype
- Association with Turner's syndrome, monosomy 16, trisomy 13 and trisomy 18
- Exact mechanism is not known; possible theories
  - * Early *in utero* posterior urethral obstruction
  - * Primary defect in the lateral plate mesoderm
  - * Intrinsic defect of the urinary tract leading to ureteral dilatation and fetal ascites
  - * Yolk sac defect

Epidemiology

- Incidence: 1 in 29,000-40,000
- 95% occurring in males; females have no genital abnormalities
- Higher incidence in twins, African Americans and children born to younger mothers
- Incidence decreasing, possibly due to prenatal diagnosis and elective termination

Associated Anomalies

- Cardiac: patent ductus arteriosus, ventricular septal defect, atrial septal defect and tetralogy of Fallot
- Pulmonary: lobar atelectasis, pulmonary hypoplasia, pneumothorax, pneumomediastinum
- Gastrointestinal: intestinal malrotation, intestinal atresia/stenosis, omphalocele, gastroschisis, Hirschsprung's disease, imperforated anus, hepatobiliary anomalies
- Orthopedics: pectus excavatum or carinatum, scoliosis, sacral agenesis, congenital hip subluxation or dislocation, genu valgum, talipes equinovarus, severe leg maldevelopment
- Splenic torsion and adrenal cystic dysplasia

Symptoms

- Prenatal diagnosis
  - * Similar US appearance to other causes of bladder outlet obstruction
  - * Irregular abdominal circumference may not be consistently seen until 30th wks.
- Renal insufficiency due to renal dysplasia and hypertension
- Recurrent pulmonary infection due to abdominal defect and associated pulmonary anomalies

Diagnosis

- VCUG to evaluate for reflux and rule out other causes of bladder outlet obstruction

- Radionuclide renogram: DMSA to evaluate renal function or MAG-3 to evaluate adequacy of urinary drainage

- Chest x-ray to evaluate for associated pulmonary anomalies

Treatment

- Management of associated pulmonary and cardiac issues

- Avoid urinary tract infection with circumcision, antibiotic prophylaxis and avoiding instrumentation

- Commonly observation is recommended since dilatation of the kidney, ureters and bladder most often improve with time

- Surgical intervention (supravesical diversion, cutaneous vesicostomy, reduction cystoplasty or ureteral reconstruction) is indicated if there is poor urinary drainage or recurrent infection

- Orchidopexy around 6 months of age

- Reconstruction of the abdominal wall for cosmesis and possible improvement in bladder, bowel and pulmonary function

8. Urinary Tract Infections

It is a common cause of fever in children and a more common cause of renal parenchymal damage. Many anomalies of the genitourinary tract predispose to UTI, but there are also many other host and bacterial factors. Recognition of these risk factors will allow for prompt diagnosis and prevention of recurrent infections.

Definition

- Difficult to distinguish between contamination, colonization and active infection

- Recurrent infection due to:
  * Unresolved bacteriuria during therapy
  * Bacterial persistence at an anatomic site
  * Reinfections

- Cystitis:
  * Infection localized to the bladder
  * Can lead to upper urinary tract infection

- Acute and focal pyelonephritis:
  * Infection localized to the renal parenchyma
  * Risks of renal scarring exponentially increase with the number of episodes
  * >17% of children with UTI acquire renal scarring

- Pyonephrosis:
  * Accumulation of purulent debris and sediment in the collecting system
  * High risks of developing urosepsis if instrumented
  * Need to rule out obstruction as an etiology

- Perinephric or renal abscess
  * Tissue necrosis leading to the formation of loculated areas filled with purulent debris
  * Less common since the development of broad-spectrum and powerful antimicrobials

- Renal scarring
  * Loss of functioning renal parenchyma due to focal ischemia and the release of bacteriocidal compounds
  * Leads to renal dysfunction/failure and hypertension (renin mediated)

Etiology and Associated Anomalies:

- Pathogenesis:
  * Ascending infection most common
  * Hematogenous spread (*S aureus*, *candida* and tuberculosis)
  * Lymphatic from rectal, colonic or periuterine areas
  * Direct from vesicovaginal or vesicointestinal fistula

- Bacterial factors:
  * Surface structures, pili and fimbriae
  * Most commonly caused by gram negative bacteria, especially *E coli*

- Host factors:
  * Age
  * Gender
  * Colonization (periurethral, preputial, vaginal and bowel)
  * Genetics (blood group antigens)
  * Prior renal scarring
  * Native immunity
  * Sexual activity
  * Genitourinary anomalies:
    - VUR and intrarenal reflux
    - Pregnancy
    - Neurogenic anomalies
    - UVJ, ureterocele and other cause of urinary obstruction
  * Iatrogenic: foreign bodies, catheters, IUD

- Surgically correctible causes of bacterial persistence in children:
  * Stones
  * Non-functioning renal units or segments
  * Ureteral stump after nephrectomy
  * Vesicointestinal or urethrorectal fistula
  * Vesicovaginal fistula
  * Necrotic papillae in papillary necrosis
  * Unilateral medullary sponge kidney
  * Urachal cyst
  * Urethral diverticulum

Epidemiology

- 51 per 100,000 children and 174 per 100,000 infants are hospitalized with UTI annually

- Accounts for 4.1%-7.5% of febrile illness

- Accounts for 2.4%-2.8% of physician visits for children

- Male to female ratio changes with age:

Age	**M/F Ratio**
Neonate	2.2 to 1
1-12 months	0.4 to 1
1-11 years	0.1 to 1
11-16 years	0.33 to 1

- Uncircumcised male at higher risk than circumcised male (10-20x)

Symptoms

- Infants: no reliable clinical symptom to rule in or out UTI as a source of infection

- Children less than 2 years of age: vague symptoms (fever, irritability, poor feeding, vomiting, diarrhea, abdominal distension or jaundice); none are reliable predictors of UTI

- Older children: signs better localized to the urinary tract (dysuria, incontinence, suprapubic, abdominal, or flank pain); many will still have non-specific symptoms

- Adolescents: signs better localized to the urinary tract; need to also consider concurrent sexually-transmitted diseases (Chlamydia and gonorrhea)

- Fever as a marker for pyelonephritis: sensitivity = 53%-84% and specificity = 44%-92%

Diagnosis

- Urinary specimens:
  - * Reliability depends upon method of collection (bag < voided < catherization < suprapubic bladder aspirate)
  - * Urinalysis:

Tests	Sensitivity (%)	Specificity (%)
Esterase	83 (67-94)	78 (64-92)
Nitrite	53 (15-82)	98 (90-100)
E or N	93 (90-100)	72 (58-91)
WBC	73 (32-100)	81 (45-98)
Bacteria	81 (16-99)	83 (11-100)
Any above	99.8 (99-100)	70 (60-92)

  - * Urine culture:

Collection	CFU	Prob. Infection (%)
Suprapubic	Gram neg. any	> 99
	Gram pos.	>1000
Catherization	$>10^5$	95
	$10^{4\text{-}5}$	Likely
	$10^{3\text{-}4}$	Repeat
	$<10^3$	Unlikely
Clean Catch		
Male	$>10^4$	Likely
Female	3 specimens: $>10^5$	95
	2 specimens: $>10^5$	90
	1 specimen: $>10^5$	80
	$5 \times 10^4 - 10^5$	Repeat
	$1-5 \times 10^4$ sympt.	Repeat
	$1-5 \times 10^4$ nonsympt.	Unlikely
	$<10^4$	Unlikely

  - * Radiologic exams:
    - US:
      - * Generalized enlarged kidneys (acute pyelonephritis) or focal hypoechoic or hyperechoic areas (focal pyelonephritis)
      - * Fluid levels, debris or air in the collecting system (pyonephrosis)
      - * Hydronephrosis if associated with obstruction or VUR
      - * Stones and other etiology for UTI
    - DMSA: defects correlating with areas of infection
      - * Gold standard for diagnosis of pyelonephritis
      - * Acute or chronic can be determined by serial exams
    - CT scan: areas of decreased perfusion correlating with areas of infection

Treatment

- Antibiotic therapy
  - * Intravenous antibiotics and hospitalization:
    - Infants less than one month of age
    - Urosepsis
    - Pyelonephritis in infants and younger children
    - Complicated by renal abscess or obstruction
  - * Oral antibiotics and outpatient management:
    - Uncomplicated UTI
    - Cystitis
    - Pyelonephritis in older children and adolescents
  - * Selection of antimicrobial agents:
    - Urinary tract sepsis
      - * 3rd generation cephalosporin with or without aminoglycoside
      - * Ticarcillin/clavulanate
      - * Imipenem or Meropenem
      - * Ampicillin with or without aminoglycosides
    - Acute uncomplicated pyelonephritis
      - * Fluoroquinolones (older patients)
      - * Amoxicillin/clavulanate
      - * 3rd generation cephalosporin
    - Acute uncomplicated UTI
      - * Trimethoprim-sulfamethoxazole (TMX-Sulfa)
      - * Penicillins
      - * Cephalosporin
      - * Nalidixic acid
      - * Fluoroquinolones
      - * Azithromycin
      - * Nitrofurantoin

* Risks for antimicrobial resistance:
  - Diabetes mellitus
  - Recent hospitalization
  - Recent antibiotic usage (particularly TMX-Sulfa)
  - Urinary tract malformations
  - Urethral catheters and other urinary tubes
  - Antimicrobial prophylaxis
* Prophylaxis:
  - Indications:
    * VUR
    * Lower urinary tract obstruction (UVJ obstruction, ectopic ureter or ureterocele)
    * Normal urinary tract but frequent reinfections
    * After acute UTI awaiting radiologic work-up
    * Urethral instrumentation
    * Immunocompromised host
    * Controversial: infants with UTI before 8-12 weeks of age and patients on clean intermittent catheterization with VUR

  - Agents:

Drug	**Daily Dosage**	**Age Limitations**
Nitrofurantoin	1-2 mg/kg	>1 month
TMX-Sulfa	TMX-1-2 mg/kg	>2 month
Cephalexin	2-3 mg/kg	
Amoxicillin	25 mg/kg	

- Follow-up imaging evaluation:
  * US: to evaluate for stones, hydronephrosis and other urinary tract pathology
  * VCUG or radionuclide cystogram (RNC)
    - To rule out reflux or bladder outlet obstruction
    - Performed when urine is sterile, bladder volume is normal, and bladder irritability is no longer present
    - Indicated in young infants, all males with 1st febrile UTI and school-age females with 1st febrile UTI
    - Not likely to be positive for VUR in adolescent females with febrile UTI or school-age females with cystitis
    - VCUG is preferable over RNC in cases in which risk of urinary abnormalities is high and urethral visualization is important
  * DMSA: to evaluate for function and scarring if there is a history of recurrent infection, high grade VUR or obstruction

9. Vesicoureteral Reflux

Definition

- Occurs when urine in the bladder flows retrograde into the upper urinary tracts

- Grading system

Grade	Reflux Into the Ureter	Reflux Into the Calices
I	+ distal segment only	- None
II	+ without tortuosity	+ without distention
III	+ with minimal tortuosity	+ with mild distention
IV	+ with moderate tortuosity	+ with moderate distention
V	+ with severe tortuosity	+ with severe distention

- In the absence of UTI, it does not cause scarring associated with pyelonephritis

- Can be associated with congenital renal dysplasia

- In the presence of UTI, can lead to renal scarring
  * Primarily at the poles and at the site of compound calyces
  * Incidence of scarring is related to the grade of the VUR
  * Young infants have the high risk of developing renal scarring
  * Less likely in older children and adolescents
  * Intrarenal reflux increases the risk of developing renal scarring (Figure 15)

Etiology

- Normal anatomy:
  * The ureter passes obliquely through the bladder wall with an appropriate submucosal tunnel length and opens onto the trigone of the bladder in a correct location.
  * VUR is prevented by the compression of the intravesical ureter against the bladder wall, which can only be accomplished with the appropriate ureterovesical junction (UVJ) anatomy.

- VUR:
  * Primary: maldevelopment or delayed maturity of the UVJ
  * Secondary: results from distortion of the UVJ by changes in the bladder secondary to other pathologies such as posterior urethral valves or neurogenic bladder

- Role of bladder dysfunction in promoting VUR

Figure 15

VCUG demonstrating intrarenal reflux

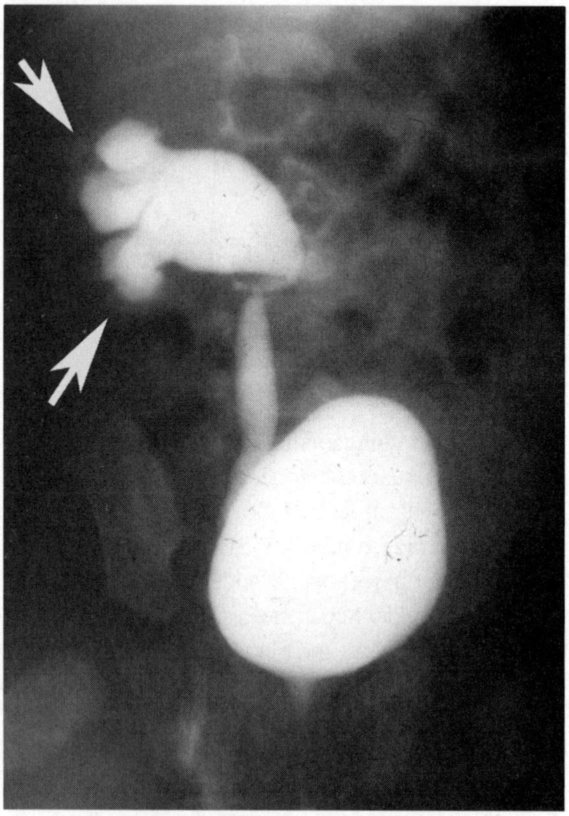

VCUG demonstrating intrarenal reflux (arrow).

Epidemiology

• Prevalence:
  * 0.4%-1.8% in the pediatric population
  * 30%-50% in children who present with a UTI
  * 70% in infants who present with a UTI
  * 25% in children with a history of prenatal hydronephrosis

• Genetic:
  * If a parent is affected, 50%-67% of the children will develop VUR
  * If a sibling is affected, 33%-50% of the siblings will develop VUR
  * 80% of identical twins concordant

• More common in Caucasians than African Americans

• Male to female ratio:
  * Infants = 3-4: 1
  * Older children = 1: 4-5

Associated Anomalies

• Renal abnormalities:
  * Dysplasia: incidence increases with high grade of VUR
  * Scarring: associated with increased episodes of UTI
  * MCDK and renal agenesis

• Primary and secondary UPJ obstruction:
  * Incidence of 9%-18%
  * Primarily with high grade VUR

• Ureteral duplication:
  * Commonly associated with complete ureteral duplication
  * Most often in the lower pole (Weigert-Meyer Law)

• Paraureteral diverticulum (Figure 16):
  * Distorts normal UVJ anatomy, leading to VUR
  * Does not significantly alter the resolution rate unless it is large in size

• Megacystis-megaureter association:
  * Massive bilateral VUR leads to dilatation of the bladder and ureters
  * May result in poor drainage and emptying

• Association with syndromes (VACTERL: vertebral, anal, cardiac, tracheo-esophageal, renal and limb abnormalities; CHARGE: coloboma, heart disease, atresia choanae, retarded development, genital hypoplasia and ear anomalies, and imperforated anus)

• Associated with pregnancy due to effects of maternal hormones on the smooth muscles in the urinary tract

Figure 16

VCUG demonstrating a right paraureteral diverticulum

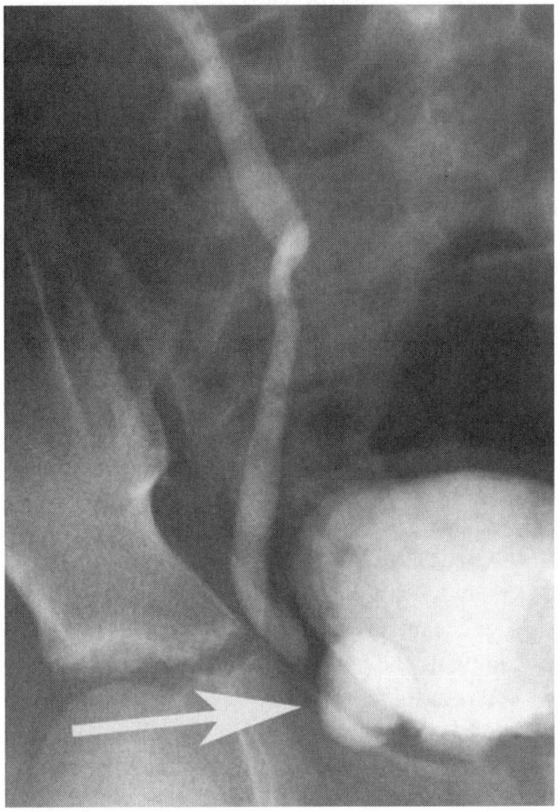

VCUG demonstrating a right paraureteral diverticulum (arrow) with VUR.

Symptoms

- Following evaluation for UTI, prenatal hydronephrosis or family history of reflux.

- Less common modes of presentation include hypertension, renal insufficiency/failure, incidental findings of a small or scarred kidney, or hydronephrosis observed on radiological imaging tests such as US, CT or MRI.

Diagnosis:

- VCUG or RNC:
  * Gold standard for diagnosing VUR
  * Also helps to identify other bladder and urethral anomalies that may cause 2nd VUR
  * VCUG provides better anatomic details and more complete grading of the VUR
  * RNC requires less radiation exposure and more sensitivity in detecting VUR but provides less anatomic details (Figure 17)
  * Obtain postvoid films to evaluate for concomitant UPJ obstruction

- US: cannot rule in or out the presence of VUR

- MSA renal scan to evaluate for renal scarring or dysplasia in high grade VUR (Figure 18)

Treatment

- Spontaneous resolution:
  * Dependent on grade:
    - Grade 1: >90%
    - Grade II: 60%-85%
    - Grade III: 50%
    - Grade IV: 25%-40%
    - Grade V: <20%
  * Dependent on age and sex:
    - Infants and young children have the highest chance of resolving
    - Males are more likely to resolve than females
  * Heavily influenced by bladder/bowel function

- Medical management:
  * First-line treatment with daily low-dose prophylaxis
  * Rationale for management:
    - Spontaneous resolution of VUR is common
    - Sterile reflux is benign
    - Extended use of prophylactic antibiotics is benign
    - Prevention of UTI will prevent progressive renal damage and hypertension
  * Antimicrobial prophylaxis may be discontinued in children greater than 7-8 years of age since the risk of renal scarring in these children is low

- Surgical management
  * Indications:
    - Breakthrough UTI on prophylactic antibiotic
    - Lack of compliance with medical management
    - Failure to resolve with time
    - High grade reflux with decreased renal function
    - New renal scar formation while on medical management
    - Parental preference
    - Rationale for management:
    - High grade reflux is less likely to resolve spontaneously
    - The success rate with surgical correction is high
  * Types:
    - Open surgery:
      * 98% success rate
      * Types:
        - Intravesical (Politano-Leabetter, Cohen, Glenn-Anderson)
        - Extravesical
          * Requires hospitalization and recovery time
    - Laparoscopic:
      * Mimics open surgical techniques
      * Reduces hospitalization and recovery time
    - Endoscopic:
      * Success rate dependent on the grade of reflux
      * No hospitalization required and short recovery time

* Complications:
  - Persistent reflux: need to rule out bladder dysfunction as a cause
  - Contralateral reflux:
    * Incidence: 5%-10%
    * Bilateral ureteral reimplantation for unilateral VUR is not needed unless there is a history of bilateral VUR
  - Obstruction:
    * Acute obstruction
      - Due to edema
      - Treatment with double J stent or nephrostomy tube
      - The majority will resolve without requiring additional surgery
    * Late obstruction due to ischemia or twisting of the ureter or stenosis of the orifice

Figure 17

RNC demonstrating right VUR

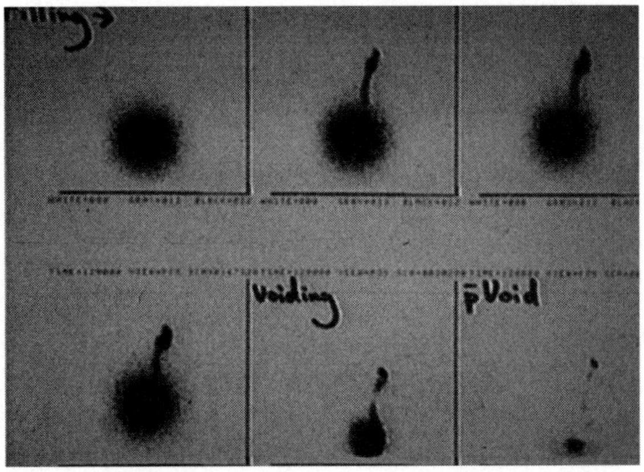

RNC demonstrating right VUR but cannot provide much other anatomic details compared to VCUG.

- Follow-up:
  * Reflux nephropathy:
  * 90% will have diminished GFR
  * 10% will develop ESRD
  * During pregnancy, associated with increased rates of pyelonephritis, toxemia, preterm delivery, fetal growth retardation, fetal loss and decreased maternal renal function
  * Hypertension: in 10% of children and 50% of adults with renal scarring

Figure 18

DMSA demonstrating kidneys

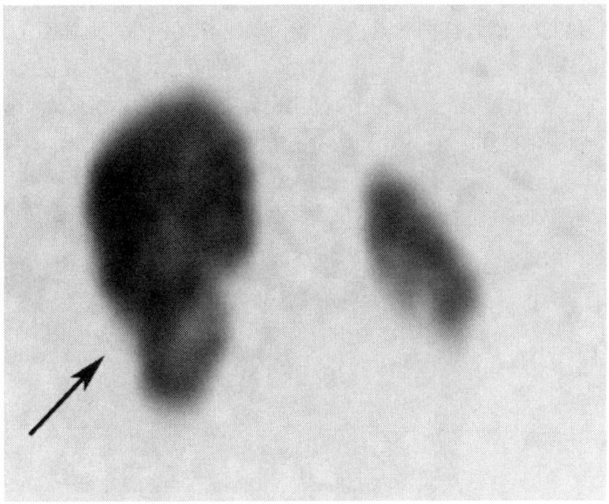

DMSA demonstrating a poor function, small right kidney and a left kidney with scarring (arrow) from a patient with VUR.

10. Further Reading

Book Chapters

Caldamone AA, Woodard JR. Prune belly syndrome. In: Wein AJ, Kavoussi LR, Novick AC, Partin AW, Peters CA, eds. *Campbell-Walsh Urology*. 9th ed. Philadelphia, PA: WB Saunders; 2007:3482-3496.

Carr MC, El-Ghoneimi A. Anomalies and surgery of the ureteropelvic junction in children. In: Wein AJ, Kavoussi LR, Novick AC, Partin AW, Peters CA, eds. *Campbell-Walsh Urology*. 9th ed. Philadelphia, PA: WB Saunders; 2007:3359-3383.

Casale AJ. Posterior urethral valves and other urethral anomalies. In: Wein AJ, Kavoussi LR, Novick AC, Partin AW, Peters CA, eds. *Campbell-Walsh Urology*. 9th ed. Philadelphia, PA: WB Saunders; 2007:3583-3603.

Glassberg KI. Renal dysgenesis and cystic disease of the kidney. In: Wein AJ, Kavoussi LR, Novick AC, Partin AW, Peters CA, eds. *Campbell-Walsh Urology*. 9th ed. Philadelphia, PA: WB Saunders; 2007:3305-3358.

Khoury A, Bagli DJ. Reflux and megaureter. In: Wein AJ, Kavoussi LR, Novick AC, Partin AW, Peters CA, eds. *Campbell-Walsh Urology*. 9th ed. Philadelphia, PA: WB Saunders; 2007:3423-3481.

Peters CA. Perinatal urology. In: Wein AJ, Kavoussi LR, Novick AC, Partin AW, Peters CA, eds. *Campbell-Walsh Urology*. 9th ed. Philadelphia, PA: WB Saunders; 2007:3176-3197.

Schlussel RN, Retik AB. Ectopic ureter, ureterocele and other anomalies of the ureter. In: Wein AJ, Kavoussi LR, Novick AC, Partin AW, Peters CA, eds. *Campbell-Walsh Urology*. 9th ed. Philadelphia, PA: WB Saunders; 2007:3383-3422.

Shortliffe LMD. Infection and inflammation of the pediatric genitourinary tract. In: Wein AJ, Kavoussi LR, Novick AC, Partin AW, Peters CA, eds. *Campbell-Walsh Urology*. 9th ed. Philadelphia, PA: WB Saunders; 2007:3232-3268.

Chapter 3: Pediatric Urological Oncology

Martin A. Koyle, MD, FAAP, FACS

Contents

1. Wilms' Tumor (WT)

Etiology

- This tumor is also called a **nephroblastoma**.
- First described by Max Wilms in 1889.
- Although surgery and then radiation (1915) were the predominant modalities utilized in therapy of this neoplasm for the first half of the 20th century, Farber's utilization of **actinomycin** ushered in the modern era of chemotherapy.
- The improved survival in **WT** reflects a success story of multimodal therapy and multicenter, cooperative studies.

Epidemiology

- **WT** is the **most common** GU tumor of children with an incidence of 8:1,000,000.
- More than 75% of the time, the age at diagnosis is **< 5 years**.
- The ratio of male to female occurrence is equal but the tumor is more common in blacks than Caucasians.
- In 5% of cases, this tumor is bilateral and may be multifocal in 12%.
- Although multicystic dysplastic kidney has been surmised to be a risk factor, the **National Wilms' Tumor Study (NWTS)** IV has suggested that >2000 prophylactic nephrectomies would be required in order to prevent a single case of WT.

Genetics

- Genetics are adding to our understanding of WT, in particular with the syndromic patients and those who are younger or with bilateral disease.
- In particular the following loci have proved to be of substantial importance:

  * **11p13 Loci**
  * **11p15 Loci**
  * **16q Loci**

- Genetic influences so far are found in only **10%** of all cases of sporadic WT.

Histopathology

- The pathology of WT reveals a **classic triphasic pattern** composed of **3 elements** in the favorable histology (**FH**) variant:

  * **Epithelial**
  * **Blastomal**
  * **Stromal**

- Despite being present in **only 5%** of specimens, the **anaplastic** or unfavorable histological variant (UH), this variant is associated with **>50% of the deaths.**
- Beckwith pointed out the importance of clusters of persistent nephrogenic blastemal cells termed **nephrogenic rests**.
- In clusters, they are histologically **identical** to WT and have been termed **nephroblastomatosis**.
- These entities are found in <1% of routine infant autopsies where WT is not found, but are found in **45%** of unilateral WT and **100%** of **bilateral cases**.

Clinical Presentation

- Usually, the clinical presentation is that of a healthy child with an abdominal mass.
- Hematuria is found in **<25%** and usually is microscopic only.
- Imaging has assumed an important role in the care of these patients and proper radiological evaluation is essential.
- Often an **ultrasound** will accompany the child and demonstrates a solid renal lesion.
- It is helpful if the ultrasonographer also evaluates the status of the renal veins and inferior vena cava.

- CT scan has allowed excellent evaluation of the contralateral kidney, liver and gross lymphadenopathy and also will include a baseline evaluation of the chest.

Surgical Staging

- In the United States, staging is traditionally surgical and done through a chevron transperitoneal incision, although it is now acceptable to address the pathology via a flank incision.

- In the past, the contralateral kidney in presumed unilateral disease was first inspected and palpated. With modern imaging, this is no longer mandatory.

- Ipsilateral nephrectomy is then performed with local lymph node sampling.

- If there is contiguous organ involvement, one should biopsy and close rather than attempting heroic surgery.

- In bilateral disease, chemotherapy can be initiated without a preliminary biopsy, but evaluation with biopsy and lymph staging might provide more information. NWTS staging has been based on surgical findings (Table 1).

- Surgery has an **associated 11% complication rate** with **hemorrhage** and **bowel obstruction being the two most common** complications reported.

- Rupture and/or tumor spillage increases the local recurrence rate by a factor of 6, and this along with the biopsy upstages the disease to III.

- It is recommended that presurgical downstaging with chemotherapy be employed if tumors are bilateral, unresectable, solitary kidney or have major vascular involvement.

- Adjuvant chemotherapy with **2-3 drug chemotherapy** is employed in all patients, and the role of radiation is being utilized less often, primarily in higher risk patients (Table 2).

Table 1

WT Staging

In America **(NWTS)** — surgical staging
In Europe **(SIOP)** — imaging
I - Confined tumor, total resection
II - Outside capsule (bx, spill), total resection
III - Incomplete resection, massive spill, + LN
IV - Distant mets (hematogenous)
V - Bilateral tumors

- Today, survival for FH disease stages I-III is >90% (Table 3).

- As with all pediatric cancer survivors, secondary tumors are more common, especially if patients have received chemotherapy and radiation.

- In patients who have received doxorubicin, at 20 years >20% of survivors will have developed congestive hear failure.

- Still, this agent (doxorubicin) in particular has been of particular importance in clear cell sarcoma of the kidney, a non-WT neoplasm.

- Utilizing it in treatment protocols has led to survival rates that approach those of WT.

- The same cannot be said for rhabdoid tumors of the kidney, a tumor with propensity to metastasize early to the brain and with a dismal prognosis (Figure 1).

Table 2

NWTS V Protocol

Stage	XRT	Chemo
I/II FH/UH	-	EE-4A
III/IV FH	+	DD-4A
II-IV, focal anaplasia	+	DD-4A
II-IV, diffuse anap.	+	Regimen 1
I-IV CCSK/rhabdoid	+	Regimen RTK

EE-4A = dactinomycin and vincristine
DD-4A = dactinomycin, vincristine and doxorubicin
Regimen 1 = dactinomycin, vincristine, doxorubicin, cyclophosphamide and etoposide
Regimen RTK = carboplatin, etoposide and cyclophosphamide

Table 3

NWTS III Outcomes

Stage	Histology	Survival (%)
I	FH	97
II	FH	92
III	FH	84
IV	FH	83
I-III	UH	68
IV	UH	55
All	FH	89
CCSK	--	75
Rhabdoid	--	26

FH = favorable histology
UH = unfavorable histology

Figure 1

Wilm's tumor algorithm NWTS-5

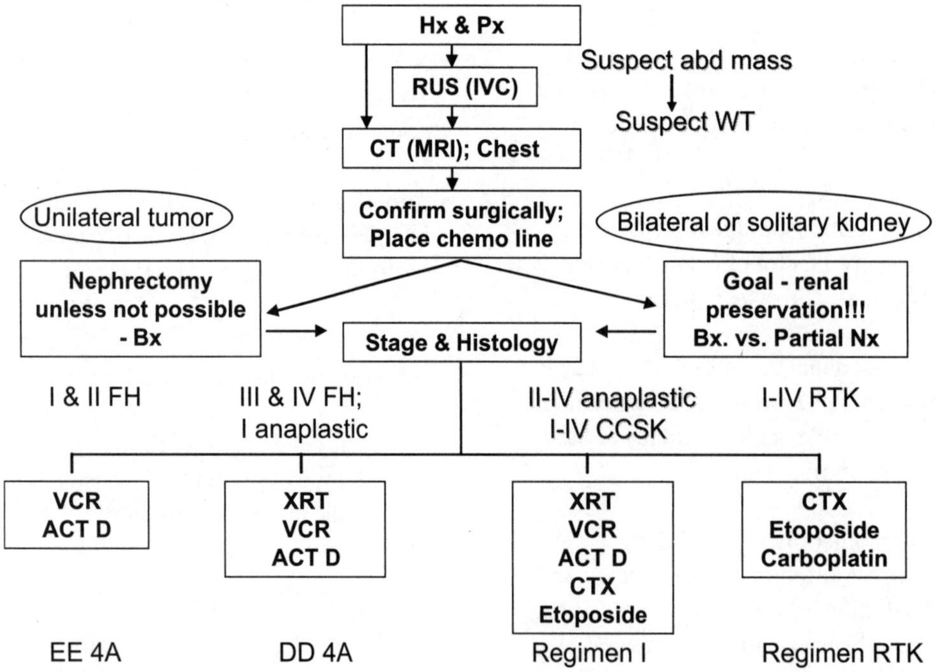

- Renal cell carcinoma is also found in children but interestingly is associated with a better survival rate, stage for stage. In children >10 years, incidence of WT and RCC is equal.

- Congenital mesoblastic nephroma is the most common renal neoplasm in infants <3 months and almost universally is associated with a benign course.

- Nephrectomy without chemotherapy is thus definitive in the bulk of patients with CMN.

2. Neuroblastoma

Etiology

- Neuroblastoma, like pheochromocytoma, is a tumor of **neural crest origin** that is from the cells that form the sympathetic nervous system.

- Most neuroblastomas tend to undergo spontaneous regression.

Epidemiology

- It is thought that this entity may occur as often as 1:200 live births, and thus the majority is not of any significance clinically.

- Indeed, attempts to screen for neuroblastoma utilizing VMA have led to a profound increase in diagnosis but no change in outcome.

Diagnostic Criteria

- Unlike in WT, these children appear sick and their tumors, when abdominal, cross the midline.

- Historically, calcifications were also found to occur more often than in WT. Sadly, >70% present with metastases at initial diagnosis.

- Unlike its sister lesion, pheochromocytoma, norepinephrine is not converted to epinephrine.

- Since VMA is the metabolite of both, it can serve as a urinary tumor marker.

- Imaging is similar to that performed for WT, although MIBG scanning can be used in equivocal cases.

- Bone marrow aspiration is performed in the diagnostic staging protocol, with positive aspirates being documented in 70%.

- As mentioned before, 70% of spot urine VMA assays will be positive, and 24 hour urines for all catecholamine are positive in almost all children with this tumor.

- Historically, the Evans Classification System has been replaced by the International Staging System (Table 4).

Table 4

International Neuroblastoma Staging System

1.	Localized tumor with complete resection
2a.	Localized tumor with/o complete gross resection; - L.N.
2b.	+ Ipsilateral and - contralateral L.N.
3.	Unresectable local tumor and/or + contralateral L.N.
4.	Distant + hematogenous or L.N. mets (excluding 4S)
4S.	Stage 1, 2a, or 2b tumor with spread to skin, liver, and/or B.M. (limited to <1 y/o)

- Prognostically, those with adrenal tumors do better than extra-adrenal, as do children who are <1 year of age.

- Prognosis is also worse when N-myc amplification is present, serum ferritin is elevated and when the DNA pattern is tetraploid.

- This is still a tumor, where surgical excision is of paramount importance to ultimate survival.

3. Rhabdomyosarcoma

Etiology

- This is the **most common soft tissue** sarcoma with up to one-third arising from genitourinary tract sites.

- It is derived from **mesenchymal origin** and demonstrates evidence of skeletal muscle differentiation.

Epidemiology

- There is a bimodal distribution with peaks in the first six years of life and then after puberty.

- Approximately 1:2,000,000 are diagnosed with this tumor annually, with males and females being affected equally.

- Genetically, abnormalities of the **2q37 locus** are thought to be important.

- Spread tends to be local followed by **lymphatic (20%)** and then **hematogenous (10%)**.

- The embryonal **(ERMS)** pathological variant predominates in **>90%** with alveolar and pleomorphic variants comprising the remainder.

Clinical Presentation

- The clinical presentation is dependent on the site of origin:

  * Bladder
  * Prostate
  * Vagina
  * Uterus
  * Perineum

- It is also dependent on the size of the tumor.

Imaging

- MRI is the best study to assess pelvic tumors.

- Due to costs and the necessity oftentimes for sedation, CT is used with greater frequency than MRI.

Treatment

- Surgery with biopsy of the lesion and assessment of local extension is the initial mode of therapy.
- This is followed by VAC based chemotherapy.
- VAC:

  * **Vincristine**
  * **Actinomycin D**
  * **Cyclophosphamide**
  * **+/- Ifosfamide**

- VAC is used with/without radiation with re-imaging and re-look surgeries, with the goal of primary organ preservation.
- The latter is possible in **two-thirds** of cases but the function of the preserved organ in the long run may be far less than hoped in the majority.

Staging

- Staging is now based on the **TNM system** rather than the Intergroup Rhabdomyosarcoma (IRS) system.
- IRS was based on surgical resectability (Table 5).
- Controversy still surrounds the management of small residual masses after therapy, especially if the pathology is mature rhabdomyoblasts.
- Survival overall has improved from **25% to >70%** over the last quarter century, **with >90% survival** in low stage, favorable histology patients (Table 6 and Figure 2).

Table 5

TMN-RMS

Stage	Site	T	Size	N	M
I	Non prost/bladder	T1-T2	a or b	0, 1, x	0
II	Blad/prost/others	T1-T2	a	0, x	0
III	Blad/prost/ others	T1-T2 T1-T2	a b	1 0,1, x	0 0
IV	All	T1-T2	a or b	0, 1	1

T1 = confined; T2 = extension
Size: a = <5 cm diam.; b = >5 cm diam.
Nodes: 0 = neg., 1 = pos., x = unknown
Mets: 0 = no distant mets, 1 = mets present

Table 6

Treatment Protocols and Outcomes

Clinical Group	IRS I	IRS II	IRS III
I – Favorable	81	85	93
II – Favorable	73	88	54
III – Favorable	70	79	89
I/II – Unfavorable	57	71	80
IV	26	27	27
Overall	55	63	71

Figure 2

Pelvic rhabdomyosarcoma algorithm

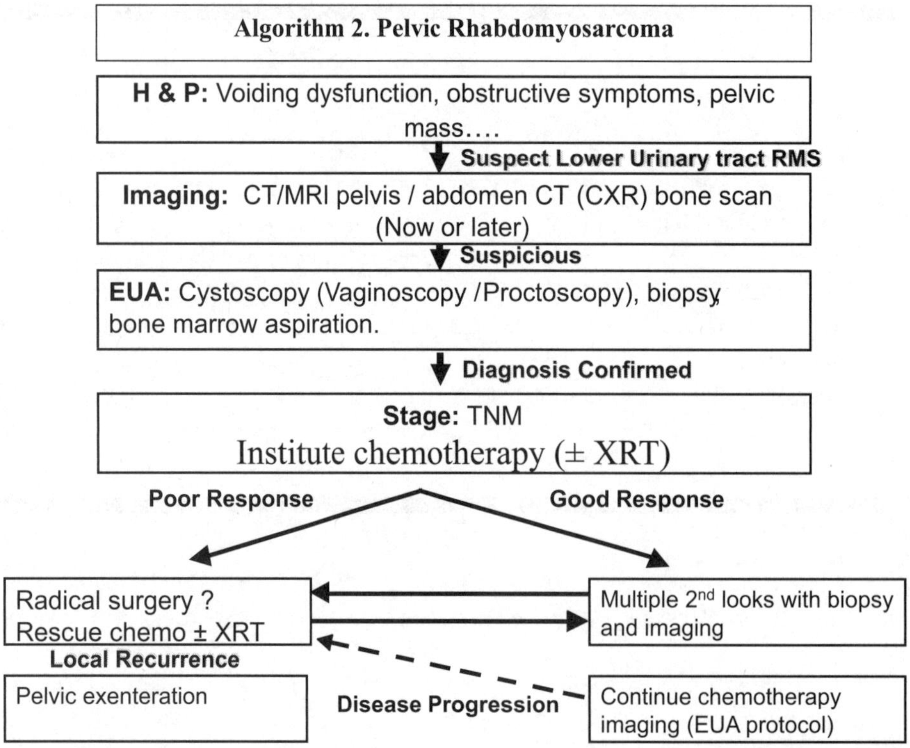

4. Testes Tumors

Etiology and Epidemiology

- Testes tumors in children occur in roughly 2-3:1,000,000 annually and represent 1%-2% of pediatric neoplasms.
- Whereas historically the majority of such tumors were thought to be yolk sac tumors (YST), recent data have lent doubt to this theory.
- **Teratoma is now thought to be the most common variant**, with YST incidence being similar to epidermoid cysts and testicular stromal tumors.
- The bulk of YST are localized, and unlike in adult germ cell neoplasms, hematogenous spread is greater than the lymphatic route.

Gene Markers

- Alpha-fetoprotein (AFP) is **elevated in >90%** of those diagnosed with YST, and beta hCG is not a useful marker to follow in prepubertal testicular neoplasms.
- It should be remembered that in infant males, AFP is elevated for up to 6-9 months postpartum.

Surgical and Medical Treatment

- Since 85% of tumors are confined, readical orchiectomy is usually curative.
- Routine lymph node dissection is not indicated.
- Platinum based chemotherapy is the mainstay of therapy for metastatic disease, with survival rates similar to those reported in the adult population.
- Teratoma should be suspected if an ultrasound of the testis reveals a heterogeneous lesion with internal echoes (calcification).
- In children <2 years, these tumors behave in a uniformly benign fashion.
- With a normal AFP, enucleation is possible and is the preferred treatment (Figure 3).
- Leydig cell tumors are the **most common stromal tumors** of the testis in children.
- They should be suspected by the classic clinical triad:

  * Precocious puberty
  * Testis mass (may be small though)
  * Elevated serum testosterone and urinary 17 ketosteroids

- These should be managed with enucleation whenever possible.

Premalignant Tumors

- Gonadoblastoma is an interesting pre-malignant tumor that occurs primarily in patients with disorders of sexual differentiation who have abnormal intra-abdominal gonads in patients with a **Y genotype.**
- More than **80%** of such patients are phenotypically female with a 46, XY chromosome makeup.
- The gonads are **streak in 22%**, dysgenetic in **18%** and indeterminate in the remaining majority.
- As many as one-third of these tumors are bilateral.
- As germ cell elements outgrow the stromal component after puberty, dysgerminoma **(malignant seminoma)** will develop in 10%-60%.
- Hence, prepubertal gonadectomy will prevent this tumor from developing.
- ERMS of the spermatic cord may present with lymph node involvement in almost one-third of patients.
- Still, routine lymph node dissection is not recommended.
- With chemotherapy alone, and no adjuvant radiation, survival rates exceed 90%.
- Lymphoma involves the testes in 4% of cases, while up to 25% of leukemia patients will have testicular disease.

Figure 3

Surgical flowchart for prepubertal testis tumors

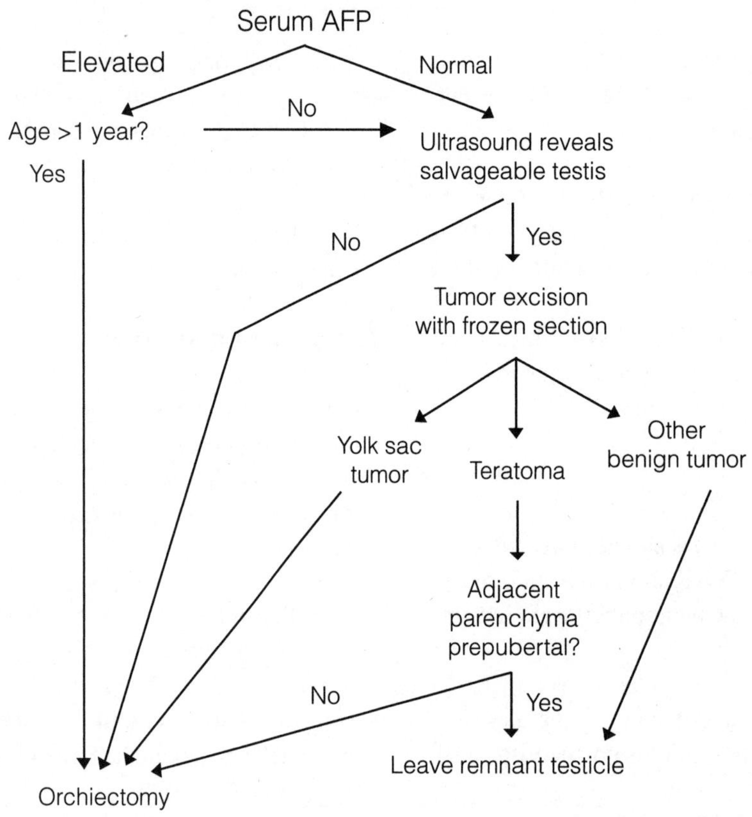

- Whereas routine biopsies were performed in the past, this is now done only if there is clinical evidence of testicular involvement.

- Further chemotherapy, gonadal radiation and even bone marrow transplant might be necessary in such scenarios.

Recent Issues

- Lastly, the issue of the undescended testis needs to be addressed.

- The more cephalad the testis prior to orchidopexy, the higher the likelihood of malignancy developing.

- Cancer might be developed in the contralateral descended gonad in up to 20% of instances.

- The risk of cancer developing overall is anywhere from 10-35 times that which occur in the patient with normally descended testes.

- Recent data has refuted our prior thoughts. It has now been shown that orchidopexy prior to puberty significantly reduces the risk of malignancy.

5. Conclusion

- Pediatric urological oncology represents an interesting constellation of entities that involve the urologist, oncologists and radiation therapists.
- Understanding of these tumors by each specialist and interaction with one another is of utmost importance in assuring that the patient receives the most appropriate therapy with the least potential for morbidity and the highest potential for quality, long-term survival.

6. References

Wilms' Tumor

1. Ritchey ML, Shamberger RC, Haase G, Horwitz J, Bergemann T, Breslow NE. Surgical complications after primary nephrectomy for Wilms' tumor: report from the National Wilms' Tumor Study Group. *J Am Coll Surg*. 2001; 192:63-68.
2. Green DM. Wilms' tumour. *Euro J Cancer.* 1997;33:409-418.
3. D'Angio GJ, Breslow N, Beckwith JB, et al. Treatment of Wilms' tumor. Results of the Third National Wilms' Tumor Study. *Cancer.* 1989;64:349-360.
4. Shamberger RC, Guthrie KA, Ritchey ML, et al. Surgery-related factors and local recurrence of Wilms tumor in National Wilms Tumor Study 4. *Ann Surg*. 1999; 229:292-297.
5. D'Angio GJ. Pre- or post-operative treatment for Wilms tumor? Who, what, when, where, how, why—and which. *Med Pediatr Oncol*. 2003; 41:545-549.

Neuroblastoma

1. Turkel SB, Itabashi HH. The natural history of neuroblastic cells in the fetal adrenal gland. *Am J Pathol*. 1974; 76: 225-244.
2. Peuchmaur M, d'Amore ES, Joshi VV, et al. Revision of the International Neuroblastoma Pathology Classification: confirmation of favorable and unfavorable prognostic subsets in ganglioneuroblastoma, nodular. *Cancer.* 2003;98:2274-2281.
3. O'Neil JA, Littman P, Blitzer P, Soper K, Chatten J, Shimada H. The role of surgery in localized neuroblastoma. *J Pediatr Surg*. 1985;20:708-712.

4. Matthay KK, Villablanca JG, Seeger RC, et al. Treatment of high-risk neuroblastoma with intensive chemotherapy, radiotherapy, autologous bone marrow transplantation, and 13-cis-retinoic acid. Children's Cancer Group. *N Engl J Med*. 1999;341: 1165-1173.

5. Nickerson HJ, Matthay KK, Seeger RC, et al. Favorable biology and outcome of stage IV-S neuroblastoma with supportive care or minimal therapy: a Children's Cancer Group study. *J Clin Oncol*. 2000;18: 477-486.

Rhabdomyosarcoma

1. Crist WM, Anderson JR, Meza JL, et al. Intergroup rhabdomyosarcoma study-IV: results for patients with nonmetastatic disease. *J Clin Oncol*. 2001;19:3091-3102.

2. Raney RB, Anderson JR, Barr FG, et al. Rhabdomyosarcoma and undifferentiated sarcoma in the first two decades of life: a selective review of intergroup rhabdomyosarcoma study group experience and rationale for Intergroup Rhabdomyosarcoma Study V. *J Pediatr Hematol Oncol*. 2001;23:215-220.

3. Ortega JA, Presence of well-differentiated rhabdomyoblasts at the end of therapy for pelvic rhabdomyosarcoma: implications for the outcome. *J Pediatr Hematol Oncol*. 2000;22:106-111.

4. Raney Jr, Heyn R, Hays DM, et al. Sequelae of treatment in 109 patients followed for 5 to 15 years after diagnosis of sarcoma of the bladder and prostate. A report from the Intergroup Rhabdomyosarcoma Study Committee. *Cancer*. 1993;71:2387-2394.

5. Ferrer FA. Bladder/prostate rhabdomyosarcoma: past, present and future. *J Urol*. 2006;176:1283-1291.

Testes Tumors

1. Pohl HG, Shukla AR, Metcalf PD, et al. Prepubertal testis tumors: actual prevalence rate of histological types. *J Urol*. 2004;172:2370-2372.

2. Olive D, Flamant F, Zucker JM, et al. Paraaortic lymphadenectomy is not necessary in the treatment of localized paratesticular rhabdomyosarcoma. *Cancer*. 1984;54:1283-1287.

3. Ross JH, Rybicki L, Kay R. Clinical behavior and a contemporary management algorithm for prepubertal testis tumors: a summary of the Prepubertal Testis Tumor Registry. Experience with testis sparing surgery for testicular teratoma. *J Urol*. 2002;168:1675-1679.

4. Shukla AR, Woodard C, Carr MC, et al. Experience with testis sparing surgery for testicular teratoma. *J Urol*. 2004;171:161-163.

5. Thomas JC, Stromal testis tumors in children: a report from the prepubertal testis tumor registry. *J Urol*. 2001;166:2338-2340.

6. Pettersson A, Richiardi L, Nordenskjold A, Kaijser M, Akre O. Age at surgery for undescended testis and risk of testicular cancer. *N Eng J Med*. 2007; 356:1835-1841

Chapter 4: Genital Abnormalities

Warren T. Snodgrass, MD

Contents

1. Intersexuality

Normal Sexual Differentiation

Internal and external genitalia are identical in both sexes until the 6th gestational week, when masculinization normally begins in males. This process is summarized in Figure 1.

The sex-determining region on the Y chromosome (SRY gene) initiates the active process by which the fetus is masculinized, by stimulating the indifferent gonadal primordia to develop a testis. Subsequent elaboration of testosterone by fetal Leydig cells and Müllerian inhibition substance by fetal Sertoli cells result in changes to internal ducts and external genitalia. MIS stimulates regression of the Müllerian ducts, leaving a vestigial appendix testis and prostatic utricle. Testosterone acts by local diffusion to effect development of the epididymis, vas deferens and seminal vesicle. External genitalia masculinize from androgen activity beginning in the 8th gestational week. Normally, systemic testosterone is converted by 5-alpha reductase II to dihydrotestosterone, to result in elongation of the genital tubercle and fusion of urethral folds to create a penis, fusion of labioscrotal folds into the scrotum and development of the prostate from the urogenital sinus. Both passive and active androgen actions are mediated by the androgen receptor. In the absence of androgenic stimulation, the internal and external genital primordia feminize, even without estrogen production.

Molecular Basis of Testicular Development

Genes known to influence development of the indifferent gonad from the urogenital ridge include:

- *WT1,* the Wilms' tumor gene

- *SF1,* steroidogenic factor 1

Genes involved in the transformation of the indifferent gonad into a testis include:

- *SRY,* the sex determining region found on the short arm of the Y chromosome

- *SOX 9,* SRYrelated OX genes

Those contributing to ovarian development include:

- *DAX 1,* dosage sensitive sex reversal region of X chromosome

Abnormalities in WT1 may explain the association between Wilms' tumor and genital abnormalities in WAGR and Denys-Drash syndromes. Mutations in SRY occur in up to 20% of gonadal dysgenesis cases in which 46,XY individuals have a female phenotype. Between 80% and 90% of 46,XX males have translocation of SRY from Y to an X chromosome.

Figure 1

Masculinization

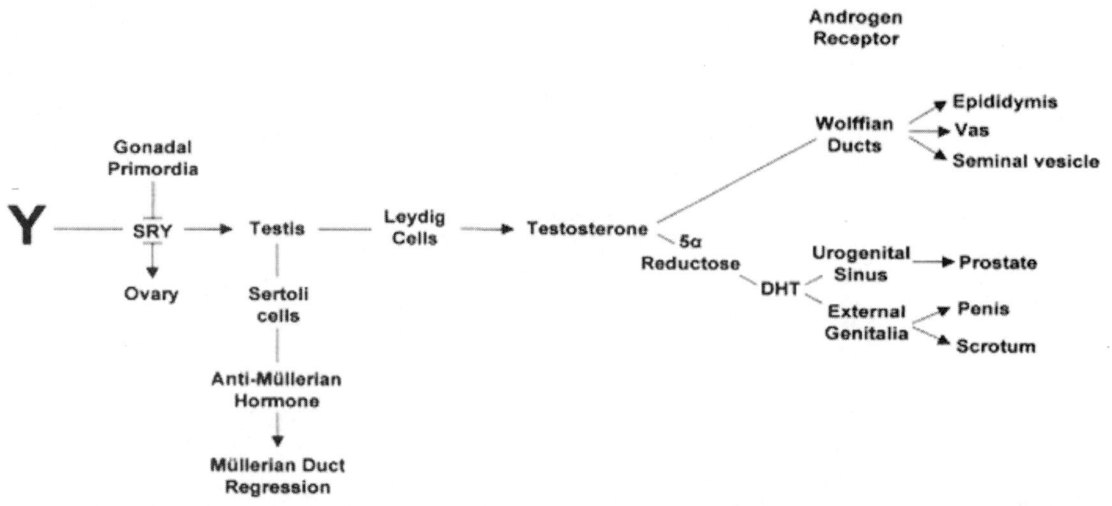

Figure 2

Traditional classification of intersex disorders

Gonadal Sex

Ovaries	*Ovary Testis*	*Streak Testis*	*Streaks*	*Testes*
46,xx	46,xx/46,xy 46,xx 46,xy	45,xo/46,xy	45,xo 46,xx 46,xy	46,xy
Female Pseudoherm	True Hermaphrodite	MGD	Gonadal Dysgenesis	Male Pseudoherm

Intersexuality: Gonadal Basis of Classification

The traditional classification of intersex disorders (Figure 2) is based upon gonadal histology, outlined above. Recently, new terminology was proposed to label intersexuality "disorders of sexual development" (DSD), and accordingly discontinue use of female pseudohermaphrodite (46,XX DSD), true hermaphrodite (ovatesticular DSD) and male pseudohermaphrodite (46,XY DSD).

Genital Ambiguity

Most often, DSD are suspected from an abnormal appearance of the external genitalia detected during the newborn examination. Generally, this can be considered inappropriate masculinization of a female, inadequate masculinization of a male or abnormal development due to dysmorphic gonads.

Examples of abnormal external genital phenotypes that should prompt consideration of DSD include:

- Clitoromegaly
- A "phallus" without palpable gonads
- An apparent female with palpable gonads
- Hypospadias with cryptorchidism

46,XX DSD

Female DSD may arise from exogenous exposure to androgens due to maternal ingestion or virilizing tumors, both of which are rare. Therefore, most 46,XX DSD results from endogenous androgen stimulation secondary to congenital adrenal hyperplasia (CAH).

CAH is an autosomal recessive defect in 1 of 3 enzymes needed for cortisol synthesis within the adrenal cortex, and is the most common overall etiology for DSD.

21 hydroxylase deficiency:

- 90% of CAH cases
- Diagnosed from elevated 17-hydroxyprogesterone and androstenedione
- Two-thirds salt wasting, due to impaired aldosterone production
- Variable genial ambiguity in females, but not in affected males

The condition is due to deficiency in CYP21, a pair of genes including the active CYP21B and inactive CYP21A on chromosome 6. Recombination between these homologous genes accounts for

Figure 3

Cortisol synthesis

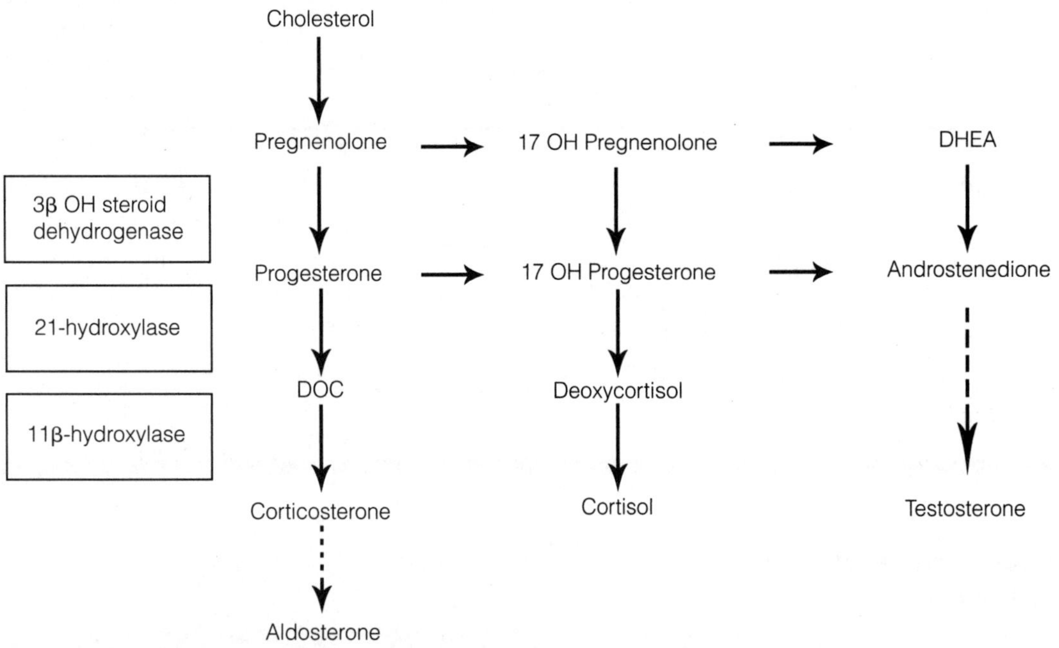

nearly all 21-hydroxylase deficiency cases. Variable reduction in 21-hydroxylase activity accounts for different degrees in genital ambiguity seen clinically, ranging from minimal clitoromegaly to severe masculinization with a completely formed phallus.

11-beta-hydroxylase Deficiency

- 9% of CAH cases

- Diagnosed by elevated 17-hydroxyprogesterone and deoxycorticosterone (DOC)

- Two-thirds eventually develop hypertension from salt retention, due to DOC

3-beta-hydroxysteroid Dehydrogenase Deficiency

- 1% of CAH cases

- Diagnosed by elevated 17-hydroxypregnenolone and dehydroepiandrosterone (DHEA)

- Severe salt wasting typical

- Ambiguity in males, due to impaired androstendione production

Evaluation of Suspected CAH

- Ambiguous genitalia: clitoromegaly, urogenital sinus, no palpable gonads

- Karyotype: 46,XX

- Pelvic ultrasonography: uterus

- Genitogram: urogenital sinus with vagina and cervix

- Hormone assays

Therapy for CAH

Medical. Cortisol and minerocorticoid replacement as indicated.

Surgical. Clitoroplasty/vaginoplasty.

46,XY DSD

In general, these disorders arise either from defective testosterone synthesis or, more commonly, from diminished response by target tissues to androgen stimulation. Any step in the process of masculinization depicted in Figure 1 potentially results in inadequate male development.

Defects in Androgen Production
The external genitalia vary from incompletely virilized to feminized, but often with palpable gonads. Müllerian ducts are normally suppressed by MIS from Sertoli cells, and typically these individuals are responsive to exogenous testosterone stimulation.

hCG/LH receptor defect of Leydig cells. Diagnosed by low serum testosterone despite normal to elevated LH.

Testosterone synthesis deficiencies. 5 enzymatic steps are involved in the conversion of cholesterol to testosterone, and defects in each has been associated with incomplete virilization.

5-alpha-Reductase II Deficiency
This autosomal recessive condition most often has been described among inbred populations in which the infant may be raised female but progressively masculinizes at puberty and assumes a male identity (penis at puberty).

The enzyme converts testosterone to dihydrotestosterone, which has greater affinity for the androgen receptor. Normal virilization of the external genitalia depends upon DHT.

- Elevated T:DHT ratio

- Ambiguous external genitalia (originally described as "pseudovaginal perineoscrotal hypospadias), suppressed Müllerian ducts from MIS

Androgen Insensitivity Syndrome

The androgen receptor (AR) is located on the long arm of the X chromosome. Most mutations involve the steroid-binding region so that the AR does not bind androgens, although additional factors appear to play a role in determining the ultimate phenotype in these cases, which ranges from partial to complete resistance to androgen activity.

Complete androgen insensitivity. Previously termed "testicular feminization," individuals are phenotypic females often diagnosed due to palpable gonads, sometimes presenting as hernias (1% of females with hernias) or from amenorrhea at puberty. MIS suppresses Müllerian ducts, although the finding of a rudimentary uterus in one-third of cases implies some activity of the AR is needed for complete MIS action. Similarly, a rudimentary epididymis and vas may be found. Retained testes have increased risk of malignancy, usually seminomas.

Partial androgen insensitivity. Ambiguous genitalia, with poor virilization at puberty in individuals raised as males. Atrial of testosterone therapy is usually recommended for penile stimulation; those with good responses are raised as males.

MIS Deficiency

This sex-linked autosomal recessive condition arises from gene mutations affecting either the production of MIS by Sertoli cells or its action on receptors to which MIS binds to induce apoptosis of Müllerian ducts. It is commonly referred to as *hernia uteri inguinalis*.

MIS deficiency is diagnosed by encountering fallopian tubes and a uterus during hernia surgery or exploration for undescended testes. Occasionally, both testes are found together within the hernia sac. The vas in an undescended testis runs within the wall of the uterus, making orchiopexy more difficult.

Ovatesticular DSD

True hermaphrodites have both ovarian and testicular tissue, either as distinct ovaries and testes or as ovatestes. There is geographic variability in the karyotype, which in Africa is usually 46,XX, while in Europe and North America is usually mosaic 46,XX/46,XYor 47,XXX/46,XY. A smaller number of patients in Europe, North America and Asia are 46,XY.

- Ambiguous genitalia that tends to be virilized

- Diagnosis depends upon demonstration of both ovarian and testicular tissue by gonadal biopsy

- Internal ducts vary according to ipsilateral gonadal histology, but there is usually a vagina

- Management includes removal of tissues discordant with assigned sex of rearing

- Fertility documented in females, but less certain in males, as there usually is a decrease in testosterone secretion requiring supplementation at puberty

Sex Chromosome DSD

Mixed Gonadal Dysgenesis

Classically, this term refers to patients with 1 testis and a streak gonad, the majority of whom are mosaic 45,X0/46,XY. The fact that 95% of boys found by prenatal amniocentesis with this karyotype have a normal phenotype demonstrates expression of mosaicism varies within tissues.

Patients have genital ambiguity related to the streak gonad, which has impaired testosterone and MIS secretion. Even the histologically normal, descended testis typically has diminished testosterone production at puberty.

- Ambiguous genitalia within a wide spectrum from predominantly feminized to masculinized

- Fallopian tube, unicornate uterus and vagina result from streak with impaired MIS secretion

- Streaks have increased risk for gonadoblastoma

Turner Syndrome

The karyotype typically is 45,XO and the absence of the 2nd sex chromosome is associated with:

- Female phenotype

- Bilateral streak gonads

- Short stature

- Sexual infantilism

- Somatic anomalies—typically webbed neck, widely spaced nipples, and increased incidence of aortic coarctation and renal anomalies, especially horseshoe kidney.

Those with pure 45,XO do not appear to be at risk for gonadal tumors, but a minority has Y chromosomal material which may lead to development of gonadoblastoma.

Mosaic Variants of Gonadal Dysgenesis

Mosaicism results in various karyotypes that include:

- 45.X/46,XX

- 45,X/47,XXX

- 45,X/46,XX/47,XXX

There is wide variation in gonads ranging from normal ovaries to streaks, and similarly somatic abnormalities are also less predictable.

Mosaicism also accounts for karyotypes with Y chromosomes.

- 45,X/46,XY (MGD)

- 45,X/ 47,XYY

- 45,X/46,XY/47,XYY

Gonads range from streaks to normal testes, accounting for variation in associated phenotype (female, ambiguous, male) and somatic abnormalities. Dysgenetic gonads with Y chromosome have greater risk for tumor development.

Pure Gonadal Dysgenesis

Patients with bilateral streak gonads have female phenotype and karyotype of either 46,XX or 46,XY. They are sexually infantile, but have normal stature and lack somatic abnormalities associated with absence of the 2nd sex chromosome mentioned above. Those with Y chromosome material are at increased risk for gonadal tumors.

Gonadoblastoma

Streaks and dysgenetic gonads associated with Y chromosome material are at an increased risk to develop gonadoblastoma, a tumor comprising germ cells, Sertoli cells and stroma. These may be detected at any age. Gonadoblastomas are benign, but premalignant with a propensity to transform into dysgerminomas. Removal of streaks and dysgenetic gonads associated with Y chromosomes is therefore advised following diagnosis.

2. Hypospadias

Etiology

The genital tubercle appears during the 4th week of gestation as anlage for development of either the clitoris or penis. Endodermal cells from the cloaca migrate along its ventral midline surface to create the urethral plate, while proliferating mesenchyme to either side establish urogenital folds. Subsequent phallic development is dependent upon androgenic stimulation during a critical time period from the 9th to 12th weeks. Testosterone produced by fetal Leydig cells within the testes is converted by 5-alpha-reductase II in the genital tubercle to dihydrotestosterone. DHT then binds to androgen receptors to initiate a cascade of downstream effects that currently are only partially understood. Androgen stimulation causes the genital tubercle to elongate and the urogenital (urethral) folds to migrate toward the midline and fuse, enclosing the urethral groove and thereby creating the urethra proximally to distally.

Hypospadias represents arrested penile development and is characterized by:

- Proximal opening of the urethral meatus
- Open glans wings
- Ventral deficiency of the prepuce (a dorsal hooded prepuce)
- Ventral penile curvature

Associated Anomalies

Hypospadias usually is an isolated defect. Arrested development of the penis thought to result in hypospadias occurs after 9 weeks, which is well after renal formation. Therefore it is not necessary to image the urinary tract even in boys with proximal hypospadias. An enlarged prostatic utricle may occur with proximal hypospadias, but its clinical significance is almost always limited to intraoperative difficulty in catheter placement and so VCUG to visualize the utricle is unnecessary.

Reasons for Surgical Intervention

- The proximal meatus, even when distally located, may be associated with a deflected, spraying stream difficult to aim
- The minority with severe ventral curvature may not be able to have sexual intercourse
- To correct the abnormal appearance of the penis and foreskin

Timing of Surgery

- >3 months of age for full-term, otherwise healthy infants
- Preferably before 18 months, when genital awareness begins

Preoperative Hormonal Stimulation

- No randomized study compares outcomes in patients with vs. without preoperative hormonal stimulation
- Proponents claim improved vascularity of skin to be used for flaps and increased size of the glans, usually in proximal cases
- Intramuscular or topical testosterone is used according to surgeon preference

Surgical Repair

Routine Steps Include:

- ***Orthoplasty.*** Straightening ventral curvature. Degloving penile skin often resolves suspected curvature, leaving ~15% of distal, but over 50% of proximal cases with persistent ventral bending. Curvature <30° most often is corrected by midline dorsal plication, whereas that >30° may prompt ventral lengthening by corporotomy with dermal grafting of the resultant defect

- *Urethroplasty.* Most cases today involve tubularization of the urethral plate, usually with dorsal midline relaxing incision to widen the plate. Augmentation of the urethral plate can be accomplished with prepucial skin flaps for urethroplasty, or the plate can be excised and replaced with flaps or grafts, in 1 or 2 stage repairs

- *Glansplasty.* Glans wings are approximated over the neourethra, taking care not to make the new meatus too small, which would result in meatal stenosis

- *Skin closure.* Traditionally by circumcision, but can also be done with foreskin reconstruction to create a natural appearance

When the scrotum extends lateral and superior to the penis, usually in proximal hypospadias, and/or has a deep cleft, scrotoplasty to correct these abnormalities can be done at the time of hypospadias repair, since the genital tubercle giving rise to the penis has a different blood supply than the labioscrotal folds that form the scrotum.

Complications

Fistula. This is the most common complication following urethroplasty. Steps to reduce its occurrence include subepithelial, layered closure of the neourethra, turning all epithelium into the lumen, and barrier layers such as dartos and/or tunica vaginalis flaps interposed between the neourethra and skin stitches. A fistula occurring at the coronal margin often requires reoperative distal urethroplasty and glansplasty for correction, whereas those more proximally usually can be closed and covered with a barrier tissue layer.

Meatal stenosis. Although stenosis may occur from ischemia with flaps, in tubularization procedures it more likely is iatrogenic, indicating the urethral plate was not incised deeply enough or was tubularized too far distally.

Urethral stricture. Most commonly seen with tubularized flaps or grafts, especially at the proximal anastomosis to the native urethra. Treatment depends upon stricture length and method of prior urethroplasty. DIVU may be effective for strictures less than 1 cm after onlay flap or tubularized plate repairs. DIVU is not effective after tubularized flap or graft procedures, when the stricture is >1 cm, or after prior DIVU.

Diverticulum. Prepuce and penile skin are elastic tissues and, when incorporated into the neourethra, can distend, especially if the meatus offers some resistance to flow. Produces a characteristic ballooning with voiding and post-void dribbling.

Dehiscence. The repair can partially or completely dehisce, sometimes from tension on the wound or use of fast absorbing sutures, such as chromic catgut.

Most complications require additional surgery for correction. The presence of any complication should prompt concern as there may be additional problems. For example, a fistula can occur alone or in association with meatal stenosis and/or a diverticulum. Typically, secondary repairs are delayed at least 6 months to allow tissues to heal from prior surgery.

3. Cryptorchidism

Incidence

- 3% term infant boys

- 0.8% 1-year-old boys

Normal descent occurs at approximately the 28th week, and so preterm infants have a higher incidence of cryptorchidism at birth. The presumed stimulus for postnatal descent is the testosterone surge that occurs from 6-12 weeks, briefly elevating testosterone levels to near pubertal values. Therefore, postnatal descent occurs by 4 months and surgery for undescended testis can be performed at any time subsequently. Data from testicular biopsies indicates initially normal germ cell counts in cryptorchid testes, but after 1 year of age the counts diminish, which provides an additional incentive to proceed with early correction.

Etiology

- Occurs in various syndromes

- Occurs with defects in the hypothalamic–pituitary–testis axis, most notably in Prader Willi syndrome

- 3.5x increase if another family member is affected

- Cause for sporadic UDT—the most common manifestation—remains unclear

Reasons for Therapy

Fertility
- Approximately 7% of normal men are subfertile

- Approximately 10% of men with unilateral UDT are subfertile

- Approximately 33% of men with bilateral UDT are subfertile

Malignancy. Tumors are estimated to develop in 0.5%-1% of cryptorchid testes during teenage or adult years. There is no increased risk for tumors in the contralateral, normally descended testis. Orchiopexy before puberty reduces cancer risk. Untreated UDTs that form tumors most often develop seminoma, whereas tumors in testes after orchiopexy are most often non-seminomas (due to reduction in seminoma risk).

Cosmesis. Patients may be disturbed, especially at puberty, by the appearance of an empty hemiscrotum.

Differential Diagnosis

Retractile testis. A normally descended testis pulled intermittently into the superficial pouch outside the external ring by cremasteric muscular contraction. Typically, history is negative for UDT at birth (probably reflecting influence of maternal hormones and the postnatal testosterone surge), and on physical examination the testis can be brought into the scrotum and will remain in location unless the cremasteric muscle is stimulated.

Nubbin. A nonpalpable testis can indicate either the presence of a viable testis (usually intraabdominal, but sometimes extraabdominal), or a nubbin representing the testicular remnant from presumed intrauterine torsion during descent. The majority of nubbins are within the scrotum and most often associated with compensatory hypertrophy of the contralateral descended testis (2 cm or larger).

Diagnostic Tests

Imaging studies. No test is sufficiently accurate to detect an intraabdominal testis. Occasionally, ultrasound may be used in an obese child to detect a nonpalpable but extraabdominal testis.

Laboratory tests. None are necessary for boys with palpable testes. The occasional boy with bilateral nonpalpable testes may benefit from testing to determine the presence of at least 1 viable testis before exploration. FSH, LH and testosterone are obtained, and FSH >3x normal with low testosterone indicates anorchia. Those with FSH, LH <3x normal can undergo hCG stimulation testing to detect a rise in testosterone, indicating a testis. MIS can also be measured, with any value most likely indicating presence of a testis.

Treatment Options

hCG. Not used as primary therapy to prompt descent in the United States, sometimes considered to distinguish a retractile from undescended testis.

Orchiopexy. Routine steps include: transection of gubernaculum; dissection of hernia sac; placement into subdartos pouch.

Additional maneuvers to gain length. Intraabdominal dissection to free peritoneum from the testicular vessels up to pelvic inlet.

Prentiss maneuver. Opening transversalis fascia to move the testis medially under the inferior epigastric vessels.

Fowler-Stevens. Transection of the internal spermatic vessels, relying upon collaterals from vasal vessels to nourish the testis. Usually performed well proximally from the testis. Procedures can be done in 1 stage or 2, with the latter consisting of a 1st stage vessel clipping followed by orchiopexy several months later after collaterals are well-established. FS orchiopexy should not be performed after the hernia sac has been removed and the vessels extensively dissected.

Staged orchiopexy. A testis that does not reach the scrotum despite high dissection can be placed at the distal point it then reaches, followed by a secondary procedure at least 6 months later to displace it further into the scrotum. These secondary procedures are more difficult, due to scarring from the first operation, but usually are successful in bringing the testis to the scrotum.

Complications

Atrophy. Volume loss can occur with seemingly uneventful orchiopexy, or more commonly after vessel ligation for either 1 or 2 stage Fowler-Stevens orchiopexy.

Retraction. Ideally the testis is placed in the scrotum without tension, but remaining tension or scar contracture occasionally result in proximal displacement.

Association of Intersex With Hypospadias and UDT

Congenital adrenal hyperplasia. Any virilized newborn with bilateral nonpalpable testes should be considered to be a female with CAH regardless of the extent of phallic development.

Mixed gonadal dysgenesis. Typically presents as hypospadias with 1 undescended testis.

Ovatesticular DSD. True hermaphrodites may present with hypospadias and UDT.

A karyotype should be obtained in boys with UDT and any penile anomaly.

4. Testicular Torsion

Prenatal and in Newborns

Extravaginal Torsion

Testicular descent occurs around 28 weeks, and during this process torsion can occur before the testicle becomes fixed within the scrotum. Unlike torsion in older children, this twisting involves the entire spermatic cord and may extend back into the abdomen.

Nubbins

The most common presentation of prenatal torsion is unilateral nonpalpable testis, which must be distinguished from cryptorchidism with a viable testis in the abdomen. The fact that the vast majority of these testicular remnants (nubbins) are found within the scrotum indicates prenatal torsion usually occurs after the testis has descended. Twisting of the cord to within the abdomen results in apparent blind-ending vas and vessels above the internal ring when laparoscopy is performed, but if the scrotum is explored a nubbin usually is found. There is an 8% incidence of finding germ cells within these remnants, prompting concern regarding their removal for presumed potential risk of malignancy.

Postnatal Torsion

Occasionally, torsion occurs shortly before or after birth, and is detected by presence or development of a palpable mass and discoloration of the hemiscrotum. These findings indicate response to ischemia and so urgent exploration would not be expected to salvage the testis, although there have been anecdotal reports of salvage. Because testicular salvage is not likely, the risk of anesthesia is increased in newborns, and propensity for contralateral torsion is less than in intravaginal torsion in older children, traditionally surgery has not been recommended to pex the contralateral side. However, concern for contralateral torsion, which results in anorchia and may not be detected until there is evidence of necrosis, today leads many pediatric urologists to promptly explore these patients to remove the ipsilateral testis and pex the other.

Imaging

As with intravaginal torsion in older patients, lack of arterial flow within the testis indicates torsion, but Doppler ultrasound to demonstrate intratesticular arterial blood flow is challenging in newborns, and lack of experience with the test by general radiologists may reduce reliability of reported findings.

Differential Diagnosis

Rarely, testis tumors will be detected in newborns as a mass, including yolk sac tumors, teratomas, and juvenile granulose cell tumors or other stromal tumors. Of these, only yolk sac tumors are malignant.

Surgery

The possible finding of a tumor has led to recommendations that surgery for suspected torsion in newborns be performed through an inguinal incision. However, since tumors are very uncommon and usually benign, a scrotal incision can also be considered. The contralateral testis is exposed and fixed to scrotal dartos with 3 stitches using fine permanent suture.

In Children and Teens

Intravaginal Torsion

Twisting of the testis suspended within the tunica vaginalis may occur anytime after the neonatal period, most commonly in teens during puberty.

Presentation. Children often do not present until there is visible evidence of scrotal reaction to a necrotic testis. Typical complaints in older boys and teens are abrupt onset of ipsilateral testicular pain with variable nausea and vomiting. Sometimes there is a history of prior brief episodes of similar pain that resolved spontaneously. If the patient presents within a few hours of onset, examination should demonstrate no scrotal edema or erythema. The involved testis may be found riding high in comparison to the other side, and lying transversely.

Therapy. Surgery to remove the necrotic appendix is rarely indicated, as the inflammation and associated symptoms will resolve within several days without intervention. Exploration is needed only when testicular torsion cannot be excluded. Patients with torsed appendices can be managed with anti-inflammatory medications and warm baths for symptomatic relief.

Imaging. Doppler ultrasound shows greatly diminished or absent arterial blood flow within the testis compared to the contralateral side, but as discussed below is not needed and may delay therapy when the diagnosis is clear from history and physical exam.

Therapy. Urgent scrotal exploration is performed to reduce ipsilateral torsion and pex the contralateral side. Orchiopexy involves 3 point fixation—medially, laterally and ventrally—to secure the tunica albuginea of the testis to scrotal dartos using fine permanent sutures. Obviously, necrotic testes are removed. When testis viability is in doubt, the testis is detorsed and set aside to reperfuse while the other side is pexed and then reexamined. A small incision can be made into the tunica albuginea to evaluate return of blood flow. Testes with questionable return of flow are often preserved but may be noted in follow-up to have diminished volume.

Torsion of Testicular Appendix

Testicular/Epididymal Appendices

These structures are vestigial remnants of Müllerian and Wolffian ducts, respectively. Each has small vessels providing blood flow, and torsion results in ischemic necrosis of the appendix.

Presentation. Young children typically present with signs of scrotal reaction, including edema and erythema. Older children and teens may complain of an onset of pain and present before there is visible reaction to the ischemic necrosis. A "blue dot" sign representing the discolored ischemic appendix may be observed through the scrotal wall. Patients with torsed appendixes typically have less severe pain than those with testicular ischemia, and are comfortable at rest but bothered by movement of the inflamed hemiscrotum.

Imaging. Doppler ultrasound demonstrates preserved arterial blood flow within the testis, typically with increased flow around the testis and inflammatory enlargement of the ipsilateral epididymis. The radiologist may diagnose *acute epididymitis* based upon the appearance of the epididymis, but this should not be confused with infection of the epididymis.

The Acute Scrotum

Differential Diagnosis

Testicular torsion, torsion of appendix testis or epididymis, and acute epididymitis can each present with pain and/or signs of scrotal inflammation Figure 4 and Tables 1-2. Other considerations include: hydroceles, insect bites to the scrotum, idiopathic scrotal edema or Schönlein-Henoch purpura (which can be associated with scrotal pain and edema).

Torsion of an appendix testis is the most common finding in children with acute scrotum, while epididymitis is very uncommon and most often distinguished by fever and UTI. The acute scrotum creates considerable angst for emergency room physicians, urologists and radiologists fearful of legal ramifications from missing testicular torsion. The most important finding is the presence or absence of scrotal reaction, as this indicates response to prior ischemic necrosis in the case of torsed appendix or testicular torsion. The absence of such reaction implies acute onset and potential ability to salvage a torsed testis, and so patients with significant pain but without scrotal reaction should have emergent scrotal exploration without delays for imaging. Those males with obvious scrotal reaction may benefit from imaging primarily to distinguish a torsed appendix from a missed testicular torsion, as the latter will need surgery to pex the contralateral side. The rare child with epididymitis typically pre-

Table 1

Differential Diagnosis: Testicular Torsion and Torsed Appendix

Testicular Torsion	Torsed Appendix
• Acute onset of pain, nausea and vomiting	• Gradual onset of pain
• No scrotal reaction; high riding, transverse testis	• Scrotal reaction with edema, erythema
• UA normal	• UA normal
• US: decreased/absent intratesticular arterial flow	• US: intratesticular arterial flow, "epididymitis"

Table 2

Epididymitis
Gradual onset of pain
Fever, scrotal edema/erythema
UA infected
US: increased testicular/paratesticular flow. Inflammatory enlargement of epididymis

Figure 4

Painful testis

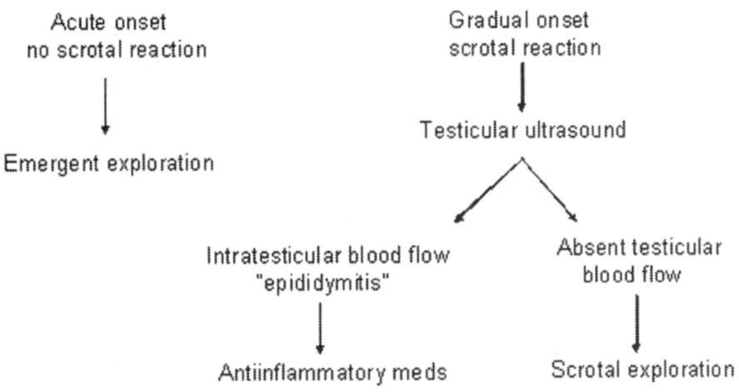

sents with a febrile UTI, which should be treated with appropriate antibiotics and then subsequently evaluated with renal ultrasonography and VCUG.

5. Hernias and Hydroceles

Etiology

During testicular descent, peritoneum coating the ventral surface of the testis accompanies it to the scrotum, leaving a communication to the abdomen that subsequently closes. Persistence or later reopening of the sac results in hernia or hydrocele, which by definition are indirect, extending lateral to the inferior epigastric vessels down the inguinal canal. Weakness of the floor of the canal medial to the inferior epigastrics, creating direct hernia that occurs in adults, is rare in children.

Definitions

Hydrocele. When the processus vaginalis in the groin closes, some fluid typically is trapped around the testis.

Communicating hydrocele. The processus vaginalis remains open sufficiently to allow intraperitoneal fluid down the groin to intermittently distend the tunica vaginalis.

Cord hydrocele. The neck of the tunica vaginalis is closed, but the processus vaginalis remains open, allowing fluid to distend a sac above the testicle.

Hernia. Intraabdominal contents, such as bowel or omentum, extend down the processus vaginalis.

Diagnosis

Patients typically present with painless enlargement of the hemiscrotum and/or groin. Hydroceles are stable in size, whereas communicating hydroceles and hernias may vary with increases and decreases in intraabdominal pressure, exhibiting increased size when the child is active and reduced size during rest.

Physical examination demonstrates the enlarged but nontender hemiscrotum. Fluids within a hydrocele will transilluminate. When a hernia is suspected but not seen on examination, the child can be stood up and/or stimulated to try to increase abdominal pressure to distend the sac.

Imaging

Although rarely needed, ultrasound confirms fluid or bowel within a sac. KUB may show loops of bowel within the scrotum.

Therapy

Hydroceles in infants resolve spontaneously. Occasionally, an infant is referred with extremely large, tense hydroceles that distend the scrotum and obscure the penis. In these cases, the processus vaginalis is either closed or quite small, or else the fluid would drain back in the abdomen when the child is resting. Despite their appearance, these large hydroceles also do not require intervention and resolve within 1-2 years of life.

Communicating hydroceles. Infants with fluctuating hydroceles can also be managed expectantly, anticipating spontaneous closure of the processus vaginalis within 1-2 years. Communicating hydroceles in older boys may also close without surgery, although it is routine to operate those detected after the first 2 years of life.

Hernias. When the bowel is within the sac, surgery is planned for the near future because of risk for incarceration.

Surgery

Unlike adult hydroceles, pediatric hydroceles and hernias are approached through inguinal incisions, not the scrotum.

The purpose of surgery is to close the neck of the patent processus vaginalis near the internal ring. The sac around the testis does not require removal, and such excision may increase risk for injury to the vas.

Despite closure of the sac and the internal ring and drainage of fluid from around the testicle, sometimes fluid, possibly lymphatic in origin, reaccumulates within the tunica vaginalis and creates concern if the sac remains open. However, this fluid will spontaneously reabsorb over a period of a few months.

Management of the contralateral side with unilateral presentation remains controversial. Despite negative history and physical exam, there is the possibility the processus vaginalis is either currently open or will re-open in the future. This risk decreases over time, prompting some to recommend bilateral groin surgery in infants within the 1-2 years of life. Others use laparoscopy through the ipsilateral sac to distend or visualize the contralateral side, but an apparently open internal ring does not necessarily correlate with the development of a clinical hernia or hydrocele. At the very least, families should be alerted to the possibility of metachronous hernia/hydrocele whenever unilateral surgery is performed.

Hernias in Females

Girls may present with distention of the groin or labia, indicating a hernia.

A gonad palpated within the hernia most often is an ovary.

1% of female hernias are found to represent males with complete androgen resistance, and the gonad within the sac is a testis. This may be suspected during office examination if a Q-tip passed into the introitus indicates an obviously short vagina.

6. Adolescent Varicocele

Incidence

- Occasionally diagnosed in prepubertal boys
- Most often detected during routine school or sports physicals in teenagers
- Approximately 20% of teens have varicoceles, which is similar to reported adult incidence

Presentation

- Most varicoceles in adolescents are asymptomatic
- Occasionally a teen will note fullness, a mass or testicular discomfort with exertion
- Most are Grade III (grossly visible)
- The ipsilateral testis may be diminished in volume

Treatment

The incidence of varicocele exceeds the incidence of male infertility, meaning therapy for all detected cases would result in overtreatment, while no intervention might represent undertreatment. Since no test currently predicts future fertility related to varicocele, the following recommendations are based upon consensus:

- Surgical correction for ipsilateral volume loss >10%-20%
- Surgical correction for symptomatic varicoceles
- Surgical correction for bilateral varicoceles
- Observation for varicoceles without testicular hypotrophy
- Option for surgery for Grade III varicoceles if parents prefer intervention

Catch-up growth is often observed when varicoceles associated with testicular hypotrophy are corrected in teens before completion of pubertal development.

Complications

Hydrocele. Incidence up to 15%, especially with ligation of lymphatics and the internal spermatic artery. Usually noted more than 6 months postoperatively; most resolving spontaneously or with simple aspiration and drainage, although some require scrotal hydrocelectomy.

Recurrent varicocele. Reported more common with testicular artery-sparing procedures.

7. Epispadias/Exstrophy

Epispadias

- This rare condition occurs either alone or in association with exstrophy

- Males with distal epispadias involving the glans are usually continent, while those with penopubic epispadias usually have stress incontinence from an incompetent bladder neck. The penis is also short, especially with increasing width of the symphysis pubis separation

- Females with epispadias are incontinent, although they can provide a misleading history of episodic leakage rather than continuous dribbling that might be expected from the associated bladder neck anomaly

Bladder Exstrophy

- Almost always associated with epispadias, but otherwise are isolated anomalies in most cases. The diagnosis is obvious by inspection, and KUB shows the typical separation of the symphysis pubis

- Vesicoureteral reflux develops following bladder closure, and there is an increased risk if inguinal hernias

Cloacal Exstrophy

- In this condition, the cecum does not tubularize, but is open in the lower abdominal midline. On either side is an open hemibladder exstrophy, superiorly ileum typically prolapses, and distally a small hindgut is encountered under the abdominal wall. In males, the penis is completely separated into 2 components with corpora cavernosa and a hemiglans

- Renal anomalies, including hypoplasia, pelvic kidney and reflux, are common

- There is a high incidence of associated anomalies, including cardiac defects, myelomeningocele, short gut syndrome due to inadequate small bowel length and limb malformations.

Management Principles

Isolated epispadias in males is corrected in the 1st 6 months of age, and closure of the penopubic urethral defect may improve bladder volume over time in both epispadias and bladder exstrophy. Bladder neck surgery in either condition typically is deferred until the bladder has a volume of at least 60 cc and is usually done between ages 3-6 years. Antibiotic prophylaxis is used for vesicoureteral reflux.

Bladder exstrophy is closed soon after birth. If possible, surgery in the first 24 hours is preferred by many to allow approximation of the pubis symphysis without osteotomies, relying upon maternal relaxin effects to bring the pubis together. There has been much discussion in recent years regarding relative merits of traditional staged epispadias/exstrophy repair vs. "complete primary repair." With either approach, more than one operation is required and relative benefits of one vs. the other remain uncertain.

Cloacal exstrophy repair begins with tubularization of the cecal plate, reduction of ileal prolapse and colostomy using the end of the hindgut. The bladder halves can be simultaneously closed or sewn together in the midline to create an isolated bladder exstrophy to be repaired at a later date. Males have been managed with genital reconstruction or sex reassignment, depending in part on the size and separation of penile components. The greatest initial problem in these children is short gut syndrome, requiring hyperalimentation in the majority.

8. References

1. Joseph D. Intersex, Parts I and II. *AUA Update Series*, Lessons 5 and 6. Volume XXII; 2003.

2. Hughes IA, Houk C, Ahmed SF, Lee PA. Consensus statement on management of intersex disorders. *J Pediatric Urol*. 2006;2:148-162.

3. Snodgrass W, Mitchell ME. New concepts regarding chordee and the urethral plate in hypospadias surgery. *AUA Update Series*. Lesson 27. Volume XVIII; 1999.

4. Snodgrass WT, Nguyen MT. Current technique of tubularized incised plate hypospadias repair. *Urology*. 2002;60:157-162.

5. Snodgrass WT, Koyle MA, Baskin LB, Caldamone AA. Foreskin preservation in penile surgery. *J Urol*. 2006;176:711-717.

6. Manzoni G, Bracka A, Palminteri E, Marrocco G. Hypospadias surgery: when, what and by whom? *BJU Int*. 2004 ;94:1188-1195.

7. Husmann DA, Rathbun SR. Long term follow-up of visual internal urethrotomy for management of short (<1cm) penile urethral strictures following hypospadias repair. *J Urol*. 2006;176:1738-1741.

8. Smith GHH, ed. Orchiopexy: tips and techniques. *Dialogues in Pediatric Urology*. April 2005;(26):5.

9. Jordan GH, Brady JD. Laparoscopic techniques for the management of the impalpable undescended testicle: parts I and II. *AUA Update Series*. Lessons 30 and 31. Volume XX; 2001.

10. Kaefer M, Diamond D, Hendren WH, et al. The incidence of intersexuality in children with cryptorchidism and hypospadias: stratification based on gonadal palpability and meatal position. *J Urology*. 1999;162:1003-1007.

11. Wenzler DL, Bloom DA, Park JM. What is the rate of spontaneous testicular descent in infants with cryptorchidism? *J Urol*. 2004;171:849-851.

12. Miller KD, Coughlin MT, Lee PA. Fertility after unilateral cryptorchidism. *Horm Res*. 2001;55:249-253.

13. Lee PA, Coughlin MT. Fertility after bilateral cryptorchidism. *Horm Res*. 2001;55:28-32.

14. Wood HM, Elder JS. Cryptorchidism and testicular cancer: separating fact from fiction. *J Urol*. 2009;181:452-461.

15. Yerkes EB, Robertson FM, Gitlin J, et al. Management of perinatal torsion. *J Urol*. 2005;174:1579 1582.

16. Eaton SH, Cendron MA, et al. Intermittent tes ticular torsion. *J Urol*. 2005;174:1532-1535.

17. Belman AB, Rushton HG. Is the vanished testis always a scrotal event? *BJU Int*. 2001;87:480-483.

18. Baker LA, Sigman D, Mathews R. AN analysis of clinical outcomes using color Doppler ultrasonography for testicular torsion. *Pediatrics*. 2000;105:604-607.

19. Johnson CW, Fisch H, Hensle TW. The adolescent varicocele. *AUA Update Series*. Lesson. 33. Volume XXIII; 2004.

Chapter 5: Essentials of Uroradiology

Fergus V. Coakley, MD

Contents

All figures for this chapter appear starting on page 132

1. Imaging Modalities for Uroradiology

Overview

Imaging is integral to the modern practice of urology, as it is used for diagnosis, therapeutic guidance and follow-up of a wide variety of urological conditions. The range of imaging modalities that are available includes: plain radiographs, intravenous urography, fluoroscopy, ultrasound, CT, MRI, nuclear medicine and interventional radiology procedures. Optimal use of imaging in urologic practice requires matching the appropriate modality to the clinical setting and question. The purpose of this chapter is to provide an overview of uroradiology with an emphasis on clinical applications, in order to allow an informed use of the available modalities in an expeditious fashion that optimizes patient care while also providing a strong foundation in uroradiology for urology residents reaching the end of their training. From the latter viewpoint, it is important to know not only the primary indications for the various imaging modalities, but also those diagnoses that have distinctive features on a given modality; both of these aspects are summarized in Table 1. It should be noted that this chapter provides an overview of critical aspects of uroradiology, but should not be regarded as a comprehensive review.

CT Technique and Terminology

Basics of CT and CT Density

CT is the backbone of uroradiology, having virtually replaced IVU for the evaluation of urinary calculi and being critical for the detection and characterization of adrenal, renal and upper tract masses, and other urologic diseases. As such, a basic understanding of CT technique and terminology is helpful. In CT, an x-ray source (tube) rotates around the patient. The x-ray beam passes through the patient and strikes a detector system. A computer collects the signal from the detector system, and uses the large amount of data collected to form axial images of the patient, where the density of each picture element (or pixel, generally 512 x 512 pixels per slice) is proportional to the attenuation of the corresponding volume of tissue (voxel). Tissue that highly attenuates the x-ray beam (eg, bone or urinary stones) is white, while tissue that causes less attenuation of the x-ray beam is relatively black (eg, fat or air). The attenuation of a given tissue type is measured using Hounsfield Units (HU), a scale that runs from -1000 to +1000. The scale is anchored by the attenuation of air (set as -1000 Hounsfield units) and pure water (set as 0 Hounsfield units). In general, simple fluid, such as in renal cysts, has a density -20 to +20 HU. High density or hemorrhagic cysts contain fluid of higher attenuation, typically 60-100 HU. Macroscopic fat, as in a renal angiomyolipoma or an adrenal myelolipoma, is of lower density, typically -40 to -100 HU.

Conventional, Spiral and Multidetector CT

CT was invented in 1972 by Godfrey Hounsfield in his laboratory at EMI in England, with initial clinical installations in 1974. The first CT scanner required several hours to acquire the data for a single slice, and took several days to reconstruct the corresponding image. Data acquisition and image reconstruction became progressively faster during the 1970s and 1980s, although the speed of the scanners remained limited by the need for "stop-start" slice-by-slice acquisition. That is, in conventional CT, an axial slice is generated by rotating an x-ray tube and detector array in a 360° circle around the patient. After a 360° rotation, the rotating gantry reverses direction to prevent disruption of the tethered cables that transfer the data from the detector array to the computer. Such sequential slice acquisition limits the speed of conventional CT, prevents volumetric data acquisition, results in slice misregistration (due to inconsistent patient breath holding from slice to slice), and limits temporal resolution so that multiphase volumetric scanning is not possible. The development of spiral (or helical) CT in the late 1980s represented a technologic breakthrough. In spiral CT, data is carried from the rotating gantry to the computer by slip rings, which allow continuous gantry rotation and data transfer. Scanning can be performed while the patient is moved slowly but continuously through the gantry. The ability to continuously scan allows for "non-stop" volumetric data acquisition. Data are gathered on a 3-dimensional volume in a spiral fashion. Images are reconstructed from the data volume. Physical and clinical performance studies of spiral CT were first reported in 1989, and these scanners rapidly entered clinical practice. Spiral CT was an important technological advance, but many limitations and compromises remained. The rotational speed of the gantry was generally 1 rotation per second, and clinical results suggested that a pitch (ratio of longitudinal distance

Table 1

Primary Indications and Diagnoses with Particularly Distinctive Features on Each Modality for the Major Imaging Modalities Relevant to Uroradiology.

Modality/Procedure	Primary Indication	Distinctive ("Spot") Diagnoses
Plain radiography	Follow-up of urinary stone disease (non-contrast CT generally preferable at baseline)	Staghorn calculus Nephrocalcinosis (cortical vs. medullary) Emphysematous pyelonephritis Oxalosis Horseshoe kidney
Intravenous urogrpahy	Largely replaced by non-contrast CT for flank pain	Congenital ureteropelvic junction obstruction Cobra-head of ureterocele
Retrograde pyelography	Suspected upper tract TCC	Goblet sign of ureteral transitional cell carcinoma Fibroepithelial polyp
Cystography	Bladder leak/rupture	Blader leak (intra- vs. extraperitoneal) Pinecone appearance of spastic neurogenic bladder
Voiding cystourethrography	Bladder outlet obstruction	Posterior urethral valves Reflux
Retrograde urethrography	Bladder outlet obstruction	Urethral stricture Urethral tear
Ultrasound	Upper tract pathology Testicular mass	Angiomyolipoma Testicular cancer Tubular ectasia of rete testis
CT	Upper tract pathology	Adrenal mass with macroscopic fat — myelolipoma Adrenal mass with venous invasion —adrenocortical carcinoma Renal mass with macroscopic fat — angiomyolipoma Renal mass with venous invasion — renal cell carcinoma Lucent filling defect — Transitional cell carcinoma, hematoma, fungus-ball
MRI	Problem-solving, contrast allergy or renal impairment[a]	As for CT, plus; "Light bulb" bright adrenal mass on T2W image — pheochromocytoma

[a]The appropriate use of MRI in renal impairment is currently evolving due to the recent association of gadolinium with nephrogenic systemic fibrosis.

moved by the table-top during 1 gantry rotation to beam collimation) greater than 2 was undesirable. As a result, either large volumes could be covered or thin sections acquired, but not both. The next major advance was the development of systems with more than one row of detectors, allowing the x-ray beam to pass through a thicker slab of tissue, while preserving high spatial resolution. The earliest multidetector CT system had 2 detector rows, and in 1998 a scanner with 4 detector rows became commercially available. Modern multislice (or multidetector) CT using up to 64 detector rows essentially abolishes the remaining obstacles to rapid isotropic (same resolution in x, y and z directions) volumetric imaging by utilizing multiple side-by-side detectors simultaneously. Such multislice CT systems can reconstruct a 512 by 512 matrix image from millions of data points in less than a second. An entire body cavity (brain, chest, or abdomen) can be scanned in 5-10 seconds using the most advanced multislice CT systems. Faster imaging with modern scanners is due not only to multiple detector rows but also to increased gantry rotational speed. Many commercial scanners are now capable of a complete gantry rotation in 0.5 seconds or less.

Phases of Enhancement at CT

After the peripheral intravenous administration of iodinated contrast, the contrast material follows the venous drainage to the right heart, and then passes through the lungs to the left heart, from where it is ejected into the systemic circulation. Within the abdomen and pelvis, the first structures to show enhancement are the arteries. Strong arterial enhancement is seen beginning approximately 20 seconds after the commencement of the intravenous contrast bolus (typically a volume of 100-150 cc is injected at a rate of 2-5 cc per second). This is the arteriographic or early arterial phase of enhancement. From a urologic perspective, the next tissue of interest to demonstrate enhancement is the renal cortex, with strong cortical enhancement seen at 40-45 seconds after the initiation of the contrast bolus. This is the corticomedullary or late arterial phase of enhancement. At approximately 80-100 seconds after the start of the bolus, the cortex and the medulla are both well-enhanced, and this is the nephrographic phase. Finally, contrast is excreted by the kidneys and begins to opacify the collecting systems and bladder. Such opacification is seen over a relatively long time period, beginning approximately 2 minutes after the start of the contrast bolus, and persisting for a variable period of time thereafter, on the order of hours. Upper tract opacification images obtained during this late or delayed period (known as the *excretory phase*), and images acquired during this time period form the basis of CT urography (CTU). Of note, CTU may be performed with technical modifications aimed at optimizing distention and opacification of the collecting system, such as hydration, diuretic administration and changes in position, although such modifications remain under investigation and are not essential for the term CT urography to be appropriate. Images obtained without the administration of intravenous contrast may be referred to as non-contrast, non-enhanced or pre-contrast images. Strictly, such images are not acquired during a "phase of enhancement," although the term non-contrast phase is frequently employed in daily practice. Using such terminology, 5 enhancement phases of urologic interest can be identified (Figure 1):

- *Non-contrast phase*. This is the optimal set of images for detection of calcification, particularly the detection of urinary calculi. These images also provide a baseline for the assessment of enhancement.

- *Arteriographic or early arterial phase*. These images are primarily acquired for the evaluation of arterial pathology, such as fibromuscular dysplasia.

- *Late arterial or corticomedullary phase*. These images also provide good evaluation of arterial pathology and, in addition, occasionally allow for improved detection of renal masses that demonstrate very rapid enhancement, either wholly or in part. Renal cell carcinomas are sometimes hypervascular and better detected in this phase (Figure 2).

- *Nephrographic phase*. This is the standard phase with the assessment of the abdominal and pelvic viscera, including the urinary tract. While hypervascular masses are occasionally better seen during the corticomedullary phase, overall more renal masses are visible in the nephrographic phase than the corticomedullary phase (Figure 3).

- *Excretory phase*. This is the optimal phase for evaluation of the collecting system. In general, both the non-contrast and excretory phase images are required from the diaphragm to the symphysis pubis, in order to provide complete visualization of the entire urinary tract.

Split Bolus Protocol

Based on the discussion above, there are 5 different phases during which the urinary tract can be imaged during a CT examination. The obvious question is which of these phases are critical in routine practice, as in the evaluation of a patient with hematuria. The non-contrast phase is vital for the detection of stones, and also very useful as a baseline for enhancement. Early arterial phase images are generally not critical unless highly selective visualization of the arterial system is of particular interest (late arterial phase images also provide good evaluation of arterial pathology). The corticomedullary or late arterial phase images are of a somewhat questionable utility, but provide arterial evaluation and also will occasionally better demonstrate a hypervascular renal cell carcinoma that might be missed on the nephrographic phase. As such, it is our institutional practice to routinely acquire such images. The nephrographic phase is the standard phase for evaluation of the abdominal and pelvic viscera, and is also routinely acquired. Finally, evaluation of the collecting system is obviously critical in a patient with hematuria, and these images are also routinely acquired.

The need to acquire images in 4 distinct phases of enhancement (non-contrast, corticomedullary, nephrographic and excretory) raises a number of practical problems, including a relatively large radiation dose to the patient and the need to acquire, store and analyze a large number of images. In addition, such a protocol places greater demand on the scanner itself, ultimately reducing the useful lifespan of the expensive x-ray tubes. For such reasons, several institutions have adopted a technical modification known as the split bolus protocol, that is essentially a "trick" that allows for a reduced number of images (Figure 4). In the split bolus protocol, the non-contrast images are acquired in the usual fashion. Then a small amount of the bolus, eg, 40 cc, is administered. Nothing is done for the subsequent 4-5 minutes, when the remaining major part of the bolus, eg, 110 cc, is administered. Corticomedullary and nephrographic phases are then acquired based on a time delay from the start of the main bolus. The trick of this technique is that simultaneous with the corticomedullary and nephrographic phase images, excretory phase images are also required, because the contrast administered for the "mini bolus" of 40 cc has already passed into the collecting systems. The need for a separate acquisition of excretory phase images is thus obviated.

Safe Use of Intravascular Iodinated Contrast

Nephrotoxicity

Renal impairment is 1 of the major side effects of intravenous iodinated contrast administration. The true frequency of contrast nephropathy is difficult to establish, because there are no standard diagnostic criteria, but it is clear that the primary risk factor is baseline renal impairment, especially with coexistent diabetes. Routine creatinine testing prior to contrast administration is generally not considered necessary in all patients; the major indications are age over 70 years and diabetes. The decision to proceed with contrast administration in patients with a creatinine greater than 1.5 mg/dL should *always* be a matter of clinical judgment, based on the individual circumstances of the patient and following consultation between the radiologist and requesting physician. If contrast administration is considered essential, the following options should be considered.

- *Oral acetylcysteine*. A frequently cited study claimed a 9-fold reduction in contrast-induced nephropathy in chronic renal insufficiency patients receiving 600 mg acetylcysteine (Mucomyst®) orally twice daily on the day before and the day of a contrast-enhanced study, when compared to controls.

- *Sodium bicarbonate infusion*. A recent trial of patients with a baseline creatinine of at least 1.1 mg/dL study found a significant reduction (P=0.02) in the frequency of nephrotoxicity (defined as an increase of 25% or more in serum creatinine within 2 days of contrast) in those randomized to sodium bicarbonate infusion (1 of 60) compared to sodium chloride (8 of 59). Patients received 154 mEq/L of either sodium chloride or sodium bicarbonate, as a bolus of 3 mL/kg per hour for 1 hour before iopamidol contrast, followed by an infusion of 1 mL/kg per hour for 6 hours after the procedure. The advantage of this regime is that it can be implemented rapidly, facilitating the early scanning of patients from the Emergency Department, for example.

- *Hydration*. Intravenous hydration can be achieved with 1/2 normal saline at 75-100 cc/hr for 12 hours before and 12 hours after contrast administration.

- Decrease total amount of contrast administered.

- Increase the amount of time between contrast-enhanced studies.

- Discontinue other nephrotoxic drugs.

While these options may be helpful, it should be remembered that contrast nephropathy is uncommon and usually transient. A critical diagnostic study should *not* be delayed because of excessive concern regarding possible contrast nephropathy. In addition, it should be noted that there is little data on the combined use of these approaches, although the clinical setting may dictate which regimen is more practical in a patient with elevated creatinine. For example, the 2-day acetylcysteine regimen may be simplest to administer prior to an elective outpatient study, while a 1-hour infusion of sodium bicarbonate may be more appropriate before an unplanned emergency study.

Prior Contrast Reaction

Premedication is generally reserved for patients with a history of a significant prior contrast reaction. The risk of a repeat reaction in a patient with a history of prior severe reaction is 18.5%, even with non-ionic contrast media. The use of premedication to prevent reactions to intravascular non-ionic contrast media is controversial. The most supportive study states premedication reduces the incidence of all reactions by approximately 60%, but it is unclear whether the statistical power and methodology of the study allows extrapolation of this risk reduction to patients developing moderate and severe reactions, ie, those of most concern. Corticosteroids are the critical component of any premedication regime, and should be given at least 6 hours before the test. For simplicity, an oral regime is recommended, such as 50 mg prednisone or 32 mg methylprednisolone (Medrol®), 300 mg cimetidine (Tagamet®) or 150 mg ranitidine (Zantac®), and 50 mg diphenhydramine (Benadryl®) all given 12 and 2 hours before the study.

Safe Use of Intravascular Gadolinium

Gadolinium-containing chelates perform essentially the same function at MRI as iodinated intravascular contrast media do at CT. Unlike iodinated contrast, gadolinium was traditionally considered extremely safe, with very minor risks of contrast reaction and nephrotoxicity. As such, renal impairment was often quoted as 1 of the primary reasons for performing MRI. This situation changed rather dramatically in 2006, when reports began to emerge that high-dose gadolinium studies in patients with severe renal impairment were associated with the development of nephrogenic systemic fibrosis (NSF). NSF is a chronic condition in which patients experience swelling and tightening of the skin that develops over a period of days to several weeks. NSF was first observed in 1997 and described in 2000, and has only been seen in individuals with renal impairment. In many cases, the thickening of the skin inhibits joint movement, and in severe cases, affected patients may be unable to walk. NSF can also affect the liver, lungs, muscles and heart. There is no specific treatment, although restoration or improvement of renal function may help. At first, NSF was thought to be perhaps an extremely rare complication, seen only with high-dose studies and certain formulations of gadolinium. While information on this topic continuous to emerge, it now appears that NSF can develop after any type of gadolinium and the condition may develop even after standard doses of gadolinium in as many as 3%-5 % of patients with severe renal impairment who receive gadolinium. While the situation remains in flux, it seems clear that gadolinium administration in patients with renal failure will require much greater caution in the future, and assessment of renal function prior to contrast-enhanced MRI will be required with much greater frequency than before. That said, it would be unfortunate if an important diagnostic study was delayed or not performed because of an overabundance of caution, and the appropriate use of contrast-enhanced MRI in any given situation will require close consultation between referring physicians, nephrologists and radiologists.

2. Adrenal Masses

Normal Appearances

The normal adrenal glands are small, measuring approximately 4 x 2 x 0.5 cm and weighing 3-6 grams each. They have a V- or Y-shaped appearance, because each has a medial and lateral limb. The adrenal glands are of a fixed anatomic relationship to vessels, which can be useful for localization, particularly when other anatomy is distorted, such as after nephrectomy (Figure 5). The right adrenal gland lies posterior to the upper inferior vena cava, while the left lies posterior to the splenic vessels. No strict definition of an adrenal mass or enlargement has been established, but, in general, a nodule is considered present if there is a focal contour deformity, and enlargement is generally considered present if the thickness of the adrenal gland exceeds 7-10 mm. The adrenal glands have 2 layers, an outer cortex and inner medulla. The cortex makes up about 10% of the adrenal gland, and is derived from the urogenital ridge. The cortex secretes various steroid hormones, including aldosterone, corticosteroids and trace amount of sex hormones. Remembering that steroid hormones are based on the backbone of the cholesterol molecule helps to explain why adrenal adenomas (benign tumors of the adrenal cortex) are lipid-rich. This lipid richness can be exploited at imaging to help characterize adrenal adenomas, since it results in low density at non-enhanced CT and signal loss on opposed phase gradient echo MR imaging. The inner medulla makes up approximately 90% of the adrenal gland, and has a separate embryological origin, being derived from the neural crest. The medulla secretes catecholamine, primarily epinephrine and norepinephrine.

Overview of Adrenal Masses

Various classification terms for adrenal masses exist, such as benign or malignant, functional or non-functional. A more practical classification is presented in Table 2, which is based on the frequency with which adrenal masses are encountered in clinical practice. While this table is not comprehensive, it easily covers 99% of the adrenal masses seen in clinical practice. Each of the entities in Table 2 is discussed in more detail below, but it should be noted that the non-functional adenoma is by far the most common adrenal mass seen on a day-to-day basis.

Table 2

Practical Classification of Adrenal Masses

Common	Non-Functional adenoma Metastasis
Uncommon	Myelolipoma Pheochromocytoma Functional adenoma
Very Rare	Adrenocortical carcinoma Adrenal cyst

Non-functional Adrenal Adenoma

Non-functional adrenal adenomas are very common, as indicated by autopsy frequency of 3% for adenomas of 3 mm or greater in size and 1% for adrenal adenomas of 5 mm or greater in size. Given the current resolution of CT and MRI, the latter figure of 1% is likely a fair reflection of the frequency with which patients may be expected to have an incidental adrenal adenoma during imaging with these modalities. Of note, the frequency of non-functional adrenal adenomas increases with age, being 5% for patients over 60 years. In general, non-functional adrenal adenomas are believed to be of little to no clinical significance. Various associations have been proposed, such as with hypertension and diabetes, although it is conceivable that such associations are spurious and simply reflect closer examination of the adrenal glands in such patients. More recently, there has been some interest in the finding that perhaps 5%-25% of patients with traditionally defined non-functional adrenal adenomas may in fact have subclinical hormonal dysfunction, although the true relevance of this finding remains to be established.

At imaging, adrenal adenomas are typically small, well-defined and homogenous. In addition, because of their high lipid content, they are of low density on non-enhanced CT and demonstrate signal loss at opposed phase gradient echo MR imaging. Finally, it is an empirical observation that they demonstrate rapid wash out of intravenous contrast. Based on these considerations, there are 2 time points at which CT density measurements may be used to characterize adrenal adenomas, the non-contrast images and delayed phase images (Figure 6). With respect to non-contrast CT images, 0, 10 and 18 Hounsfield units have all been proposed as potential attenuation thresholds, below which an adrenal mass can be confidently characterized as an adrenal adenoma (Table 3). In general, it is safe to use a threshold of 18 Hounsfield units, particularly if other secondary characteristics, such as small size and homogeneity, are also present. With respect to delayed phase CT thresholds, the situation is somewhat more complex, since presumably there will be dependency both on the time delay and the volume and concentration of contrast administered. That said, a density of under 52 Hounsfield units or a wash-out of greater than 60% at 15 minutes both appear to be useful criteria (Table 4). It is particularly noteworthy that contrast wash-out appears to be a feature of adrenal adenomas, even if they are not lipid rich, and may therefore help characterize some adrenal masses as adenomas that could not be so classified using only non-enhanced CT image density (Figure 7). Opposed phase gradient echo MR imaging, is a special type of T-1 weighted sequence that is sensitive to the presence of microscopic fat. 2 sets of images are acquired, 1 in phase and 1 out of phase (opposed phase). Voxels that contain pure fat or pure water have the same intensity on both in and out of phase images. Voxels that contain a mixture of fat and water demonstrate signal loss. This gives rise to a distinctive "etching" or "India ink" artifact on opposed phased imaging. Because the boundaries of muscles and organs that are surrounded by fat contain voxels that represent mixed fat and water, they turn black on the opposed phase image. If the parenchyma (as opposed to the boundary) of an adrenal mass demonstrates clear cut darkening on opposed phased imaging, then a diagnosis of adrenal adenoma can be made with confidence (Figure 8). A quantitative study at Memorial Sloan-Kettering Cancer Center (MSKCC) showed that a signal loss on opposed vs. in-phase imaging of greater than 45% was 80% sensitive and 100% specific in the diagnosis of adrenal adenoma. While such quantitative criteria can be used, a qualitative study at Massachusetts General Hospital showed that simple visual evaluation of clear cut signal loss was also highly accurate, and just as good as quantitative evaluation.

Table 3

Sensitivity and Specificity of Different Attenuation Thresholds for the Characterization of Adrenal Adenomas at Non-enhanced CT

Cut-off	Sensitivity	Specificity	n
<0 HU	47	100	66
<10 HU	79	96	66
<18 HU	85	100	61

Table 4

Sensitivity and Specificity of Different Attenuation and Washout Thresholds for the Characterization of Adrenal Adenomas at Delayed Contrast-enhanced CT

Delay	Cut-off	Sensitivity	Specificity	n
60 min	<30 HU	95	100	51
15 min	<37 HU	96	96	76
10 min	<52 HU	92	95	135
15 min	>60% washout	86	92	71[a]

[a]Only lipid-poor (>10 HU on NECT) adenomas included.

Functional Adrenal Adenomas

These are rare tumors that present clinically with hormonal features related to excess corticosteroids (Cushing's syndrome), mineralocorticoid (Conn's syndrome) or sex hormones (various adrenogenital syndromes). With respect to imaging, non-functional and functional adrenal adenomas are indistinguishable and clinical or biochemical correlation is critical. 3 other points should be remembered when imaging suspected functional adenomas:

- Cushing's syndrome, when not due to exogenous steroids, is usually secondary to a pituitary tumor producing excess ACTH that then induces adrenal hyperplasia. Accordingly, imaging abnormalities of the adrenal glands in Cushing's syndrome, even unifocal enlargement, often reflect secondary hyperplasia rather than an autonomous primary functional nodule tumor of the adrenal gland (Figure 9).

- Conn's syndrome, or primary hyperaldosteronism, is increasingly diagnosed with better testing and found in 5%-13% of patients with hypertension. It is due with approximately equal frequency to either idiopathic bilateral adrenal hyperplasia or an aldosterone producing adrenal adenoma (aldosteronoma).

- When evaluating patients with Conn's syndrome, even a small unifocal nodule is likely to be an aldosteronoma (Figure 10). Adrenalectomy is usually indicated for such a finding. In the absence of a clear cut unilateral nodule, or if CT findings are equivocal, adrenal vein sampling can be undertaken in an attempt to determine if there is a lateralized source of excess aldosterone from the adrenal glands.

Adrenal Metastases

Metastases to the adrenal glands are found in 27% of cancer patients at autopsy, with common primary sites including breast, lung, melanoma and renal cell carcinoma. In particular, it should be noted that renal cell carcinoma can involve the adrenal gland not just by direct upward invasion, but also by hematogeneous spread. Thus, it is possible to have a renal cell carcinoma on one side of the body, and have hematogenous metastases to the adrenal on the contralateral side (Figure 11). Overall, given the frequency of adrenal adenomas in the general population, it is clear that the primary consideration to an adrenal mass in a cancer patient is incidental adenoma vs. metastasis. Overall, approximately 44% of adrenal masses in cancer patients are metastatic, although this number will clearly vary with the nature and stage of the primary malignancy.

The imaging findings of adrenal metastases are variable. They may be small and homogenous, mimicking adenomas (except that they are not of low density on noncontrast CT), or large and irregular (Figure 12). They may be unilateral or bilateral (note that even if bilateral, adrenal insufficiency is extremely rare). Metastases to the adrenal glands hardly ever invade the adrenal vein, which is a finding seen almost exclusively with primary adrenocortical carcinoma. At MR imaging, adrenal metastases are of variable T2 signal intensity, so that while high T2 signal intensity may favor a diagnosis of metastases, low T2 signal intensity can be seen with both metastases and adenomas. Adrenal metastases are usually hypermetabolic on PET scans, and this may be a useful test for an indeterminate adrenal mass in an oncologic patient (Figure 13).

Adrenal Myelolipoma

Adrenal myelolipomas are rare sporadic benign tumors of the adrenal gland containing fat and bone marrow (myelo) elements, with an autopsy frequency of 1-2 per thousand. Hemorrhage has been reported, and the occasional finding of calcification within these masses may be related to prior subclinical episodes of bleeding. At imaging, the fat elements of the tumor result in a characteristic finding of macroscopic fat in an adrenal mass (Figure 14). This appearance is virtually diagnostic of myelolipoma. While case reports of macroscopic fat in adrenal adenomas and carcinomas have been described, examination of these cases show that in general, only a tiny speck of fat was present in an otherwise non-fatty mass, and real life confusion between myelolipoma and these other entities is unlikely.

Pheochromocytoma

Pheochromocytoma are functional tumors of medullary origin that secrete excess catecholamine[3], resulting in the characteristic syndrome of episodic hypertension. Approximately 1 in 200 cases of hypertension are due to pheochromocytoma. These tumors are characterized by the so called 10% rule, because approximately 10% of these tumors are malignant, 10% are multiple, 10% occur outside the adrenal gland, and 10% are familial pheochromocytomas.

At imaging, pheochromocytomas are typically 2 to 5 cm, well-defined ovoid masses of high T2 signal intensity (Figure 15). The latter finding has been referred to as the "light bulb" sign, although in practice, this is not a frequently encountered finding. More commonly, these tumors are prone to internal hemorrhage, necrosis, and sometimes calcification and these latter findings can be useful in suggesting the diagnosis (Figure 16). Overall, pheochromocytomas have quite a variable imaging appearance, and clinical correlation is often critical in suggesting the correct diagnosis. That said, it is possible for a pheochromocytoma to be unsuspected clinically, raising the question as to the likelihood of catecholamine crisis if such patients were inadvertently given intravenous contrast or underwent biopsy. Limited studies suggest that intravascular contrast is unlikely to precipitate a catecholamine crisis even in an unblocked pheochromocytoma, but that biopsy is quite likely to result in such an event. If pheochromocytoma is a consideration for an adrenal mass, it may be worth while to perform an MIBG scan, which has a sensitivity of 76-100% and near 100% positive predictive value for the diagnosis of pheochromocytoma (Figure 17).

Adrenocortical Carcinoma

Primary adrenocortical carcinoma is an extremely rare malignancy, with an incidence of 1 per million per year. The imaging findings are those of a large irregular heterogeneous mass, often with necrosis or calcification. These findings, while certainly suggestive of malignancy, do potentially overlap with those of a large atypical adenoma, pheochromocytoma or metastasis. 2 imaging findings that might be helpful in suggesting the correct diagnosis are venous invasion (Figure 18) (an adrenal mass with venous invasion to be considered an adrenocortical carcinoma until proven otherwise) and metastases (35% of patients have metastatic spread at diagnosis).

Adrenal Cysts

Adrenal cysts are rare, with an estimated frequency of 1-2 per 10,000 with a female predominance. Adrenal cysts are classified as:

- Endothelial – 45% —benign simple cyst
- Hemorrhagic – 40%—these are important because very occasionally they are malignant (Figure 19)
- Paracystic – 10%—they are usually echinococcal (hydatid disease)
- Epithelial – 5% —benign simple cyst

Because of the occasional occurrence of malignancy within an adrenal cyst, 1 traditional approach to these lesions has been to recommend surgical resection in all cases. This is probably somewhat aggressive and conservative management may be appropriate for those adrenal cysts with a clearly benign simple appearance, that is thin-wall (under 3 mm), small (under 6 cm), with lesions of homogeneous fluid density (-20 to +20 Hounsfield units), with or without thin hairline calcifications or septa. If the cystic mass is not clearly simple, then invasive resection or biopsy may be appropriate.

Practical Imaging Approach to an Adrenal Mass

When an adrenal mass is encountered at imaging, a logical stepwise approach will usually result in a noninvasive diagnosis.

Are distinctive imaging findings present? This is usually not the case, but the finding of macroscopic fat (myelolipoma), fluid (adrenal cyst) or venous invasion (adrenocortical carcinoma) leads rapidly to specific diagnosis; however, keep in mind that adrenal cysts are occasionally malignant and should be examined for complex features.

Does the patient have a known primary extra-adrenal malignancy? If the answer is yes, then the primary differential consideration is between an incidental adenoma and a metastasis. CT, possibly with delayed images, or in- and out-of-phase imaging will usually lead to the diagnosis of adenoma, if this is the pathology present. Remember, however, that the inability to make a diagnosis of adenoma based on the absence of low density at CT or the absence of sufficient signal loss at out of phase MR imaging does not indicate the mass is a metastasis, since lipid-poor adenoma is still a consideration. In such a scenario, biopsy or PET scanning may be helpful, assuming the that the distinction is not academic, such as in a patient with widely disseminated metastatic disease.

Does the patient have clinical or biochemical signs of an endocrinopathy, namely Conn's syndrome, Cushing's syndrome, adrenogenital syndrome or catecholamine excess? Such findings will lead to a diagnosis of functional adenoma (but remembering that adrenal nodularity in the setting of Cushing's syndrome may reflect hyperplasia rather than an autonomous functional adenoma), pheochromocytoma or, sometimes, adrenocortical carcinoma (since this tumor can be functional).

If none of the above questions have a positive answer, the mass is truly incidental, and the vast majority of these are non-functional adenomas.

Occasionally, an incidental mass will be an adrenocortical carcinoma and appropriate workup for this consideration should be undertaken. 1 question that arises from the approach outlined above is whether an adrenal "incidentaloma" can ever be a metastasis from an occult primary malignancy. An important study from MD Anderson Cancer Center strongly suggests that the answer to this question, for all practical purposes, is no. In a review of 1639 patients with metastatic disease of unknown primary origin, 95 (5.8%) of the patients had adrenal metastases. Only 4 (0.2%) of these patients had the adrenals as the only site of metastatic disease. In these 4 patients, all the tumors were over 6 cm, and the tumors were bilateral in 3 patients. The conclusion of this study is that a small solitary incidental adrenal mass is highly unlikely to be the initial manifestation of an occult primary malignancy.

3. Renal Masses

Overview

Contrast-enhanced CT is the gold standard for the detection of renal masses. Using this modality as the standard of reference, IVP is markedly limited in the detection of renal masses, particularly at smaller sizes, and even ultrasound demonstrates substantial limitations. It should be noted that detection and characterization are different, though often related, imaging endpoints, and there are times when CT may need to be supplemented by other modalities, such as ultrasound or MRI to fully characterize a CT-detected renal mass. From a practical standpoint, renal masses can be classified as solid, cystic or indeterminate (Table 5). Given that the distinction of solid from cystic is a critical first step in classifying renal masses, it is important to note the following points.

Table 5

Practical classification of renal masses

Solid	Non (macroscopic) fat-containing (renal cell carcinoma – rarely, fat poor angiomyolipoma, oncocytoma, lymphoma, metastases to the kidney or upper tract transitional cell carcinoma) (Macroscopic) fat containing (angiomyolipoma)
Cystic	Benign simple cyst (Bosniak 1) Benign (appearing) high density cyst (Bosniak 2) Benign (appearing) mildly complex cyst (Bosniak 2) Possibly malignant moderately complex cyst (Bosniak 3) Probably malignant markedly complex cyst (Bosniak 4)
Indeterminate	Too small to characterize Unclear if solid or cystic Bosniak 2F cyst Unclear if fat-containing or not

Benign Simple Cysts

Irrespective of modality, benign simple cysts are ovoid lesions with thin-to-imperceptible walls that demonstrate a sharp parenchymal interface. At ultrasound, simple cysts are anechoic with posterior acoustic enhancement. At CT, simple cysts are of uniform fluid attenuation (-20 to +20 HU) and non-enhancing. At MR imaging, simple cysts are of low T1 signal intensity, extremely high T2 signal intensity (comparable to fluid in the spinal canal, gall bladder or bowel loops) and non-enhancing after the administration of gadolinium (Figure 20). More complex cysts are characterized by the presence of proteinaceous fluid, walls, septa, calcification or nodules. For practical purposes, the identification of walls or septa in a lesion implies that it is cystic.

Enhancement

Enhancement of a lesion refers to a demonstrable uptake of intravascular contrast (which could be at ultrasound, CT or MRI) and indicates that a lesion is solid, since solid tissue includes blood vessels and will contain the contrast agent, while cysts do not have blood vessels fluid and do not contain the contrast agent. At CT, enhancement is generally defined as an increase in attenuation of 10 Hounsfield units or more when compared with the non-contrast baseline. At MRI, enhancement is defined as an increase in signal intensity of 15% or more when compared to the baseline. While these thresholds are empirically established, it is important not to relax these criteria, because papillary renal cell carcinomas can be of limited vascularity and enhancement, and even a small increase in attenuation or intensity may be the only indicator of their true solid nature (Figure 21). In cases of equivocal enhancement, ultrasound can usually distinguish solid from cystic masses.

De-enhancement

De-enhancement is a newer concept, but is simply the converse and logical phenomenon of enhancement. De-enhancement refers to a decrease in the presence of contrast within a solid lesion when delayed post-contrast images are compared to early post-contrast images ("what goes up, must come down"), and reported studies suggest a drop in CT density of 15 HU on delayed images is indicative of a solid lesion. De-enhancement can be helpful in 2 settings: first, when a suspected renal mass is detected on a post-contrast study and delayed images are obtained, but no pre-contrast images are available; second, when a lesion is not well seen on non-contrast images, precluding confident placement of a region of interest for evaluation of enhancement (Figures 22 and 23).

Pseudo-enhancement

Pseudo-enhancement is another phenomenon that has been described in recent years. This refers to an artifactual increase in density that can be seen in small (10-15 mm or less) cysts after contrast administration at CT, irrespective of the thickness of the slices acquired. The basis of this phenomenon is not completely understood, but conceptually the problem can be considered "bleeding" of high density from adjacent renal parenchyma into the measurement performed on the small cyst. Artifactual increases of density of up to 28 HU have been described due to pseudo-enhancement (Figure 24), and could potentially result in a mischaracterization of a small cyst as a solid lesion.

Subtraction Images

The term "subtraction images" may be encountered when discussing the presence or absence of enhancement at MRI. This refers to the process of electronically subtracting the pre-gadolinium images from post-gadolinium images, such that, at least in theory, the resulting images should only show enhancing structures in varying shades of gray, with non-enhancing tissue appearing black. This technique is sometimes useful when a lesion is of high signal intensity before gadolinium is administered, since it is then visually difficult to determine if the lesion has become even brighter after gadolinium administration (Figure 25). The technique does require good registration of the pre- and post-gadolinium images, since otherwise subtraction will not be successful, and objective criteria for enhancement on subtraction images (what "shade of gray" is solid?) have not been defined and the assessment of enhancement is therefore subjective.

Characterization of Solid Renal Masses

Solid renal masses can be subdivided into those that do not contain macroscopic fat and those that do. This is a critical distinction, because the characterization of solid renal masses can be summarized by 2 rules:

- A solid renal mass that does not contain macroscopic fat is a renal cell carcinoma, until proven otherwise. There are a small number of other solid, non-fat containing renal masses (that are usually distinguishable based on clinical or radiological features); these are fat-poor angiomyolipoma, oncocytoma, renal transitional cell carcinoma, renal lymphoma and metastasis to the kidney.

- A solid renal mass that contains macroscopic fat is an angiomyolipoma.

Macroscopic fat is best assessed on CT, and this determination can often be made by the naked eye, looking for density within the renal mass that is similar to nearby subcutaneous or perinephric fat (Figure 26). Sometimes, a small amount of fat will be difficult to establish visually, but the presence of a CT attenuation value under -20 HU is generally indicative of adipose tissue. Small amounts of fat may require thin section, non-contrast images for optical detection (Figure 27). At MRI, macroscopic fat can be identified because it will be of the same signal intensity as nearby subcutaneous or perinephric fat on all sequences, and will also demonstrate suppression of signal intensity with fat saturation techniques (Figure 28). At ultrasound, fat is classically very echogenic (Figure 29), although this is not a reliable sign, because renal cell cancers can sometimes be quite echogenic as well.

Renal Cell Carcinoma

The typical renal cell carcinoma is a solid well-circumscribed mass of variable size within the renal parenchyma that does not contain macroscopic fat and demonstrates enhancement with contrast (Figure 30). Occasionally, renal cell carcinomas have an infiltrative appearance (Figure 31). Up to 61% of renal cell carcinomas are now found incidentally at imaging performed for other reasons. The incidence of renal cell carcinoma is rising but it may well be that this reflects the increasing use of imaging in the population, resulting in the detection of more small renal cell carcinomas of questionable clinical importance. For example, the clinical frequency of renal cell carcinoma in patients over 70 is 0.3%, but renal cell carcinomas are found at gross inspection in 1.5% of autopsies and at microscopy in 22% of autopsies. Furthermore, in multivariate analysis of patient outcome, the mode of presentation (incidental versus symptomatic) is an independent significant predictor, in addition to tumor size and tumor histology. These data suggest that renal cell carcinoma is analogous to prostate cancer, in that indolent or microscopic disease that is unlikely to threaten the long-term health or survival of the patient is common and that overdiagnosis of subclinical disease is a real entity. That said, when a renal cell carcinoma is diagnosed in an individual patient, it is clearly incumbent to offer appropriate therapy.

In North America, renal cell carcinoma is frequently staged using the Robson system (Table 6). Inspection of this table shows that 2 critical local observations from an imaging viewpoint are venous invasion and locoregional nodal metastases. Venous invasion can be seen in up to 23% of renal cell carcinomas, with invasion into the inferior vena cava in up to 10% of cases. Venous invasion can be identified at

Table 6

Robson Staging System for Renal Cell Carcinoma

Stage	Description
I	Organ confined (intracapsular)
II	Invasion of perirenal fat only
III	A: Venous invasion B: Local nodal metastases C: Both
IV	Distant metastases

ultrasound, CT, MRI or conventional venography. In most cases, modern spiral CT performed with multi-phase imaging and multi-planar reformation can adequately demonstrate the presence and extent of tumor thrombus, particularly extension into the right heart which may necessitate cardio-thoracic surgical involvement at the time of resection (Figure 32). In problematic cases, both MRI and conventional venography are somewhat more accurate, although MRI has the advantage of the being less invasive. Locoregional adenopathy (defined in the usual fashion as a short axis greater than 1 cm) can be seen in approximately 25% of patients with renal cell carcinoma, but about half the time pathology shows no metastatic disease in the nodes, suggesting nodal enlargement in renal cell carcinoma is often reactive in nature.

Fat-poor Angiomyolipoma

An estimated 5% of angiomyolipomas have insufficient fat to be demonstrably fat-containing at imaging. These masses mimic renal cell carcinoma, and occasionally a resection will be performed for a presumed renal cell carcinoma and the final pathology demonstrates fat-poor angiomyolipoma (Figure 33). Arguably, this remains appropriate management, since the preoperative probability of such a lesion being a renal cell carcinoma is extremely high and it is difficult to see how surgery could be avoided. That said, there is increasing interest in better characterization of small, solid, non-fatty renal masses, since it is increasingly recognized that many of these lesions turn out to be fat-poor angiomyolipomas or oncocytomas, and a variety of secondary signs of fat-poor angiomyolipoma have been studied:

Enhancement characteristics: Fat poor angiomyolipomas demonstrate more uniform and prolonged enhancement than renal cell carcinomas, but the existing data would suggest such findings are not sufficiently accurate to allow confident non-surgical management, although conceivably might be used to justify surveillance in a patient with multiple comorbidities.

Histogram pixel analysis: CT histogram analysis, in which the CT densities of the individual pixels within a region of interest are displayed as a histogram of number of pixels vs. attenuation, has been reported as helpful in the demonstration of very small quantities of fat within fat-poor angiomyolipomas (Figure 34). This remains to be validated in larger studies.

Ultrasound features: The relatively characteristic marked echogenicity of angiomyolipomas on ultrasound (Figure 29) is only partially due to fat content, and may be related to the vascular or muscular component. This suggests that marked echogenicity might be useful even in fat-poor angiomyolipomas, but unfortunately too much overlap exists with echogenic renal cell carcinomas for this to be useful. That said, some findings may be helpful; for example, shadowing is seen only with angiomyolipomas, while hypoechoic rings and intratumoral cysts are seen only in renal cell carcinoma. Unfortunately, these findings are seen in only a minority of cases, and are therefore not particularly helpful.

Opposed phase MRI: It has been suggested that opposed phase MRI might be helpful to detect small amounts of fat in angiomyolipomas, but this is a dangerous suggestion because microscopic fat can be present in clear cell renal carcinomas and these tumors can show significant signal loss on opposed phase MRI. (Remember that the clear cell variant of renal cell carcinoma is so called because of the presence of intracellular *lipid* and or glycogen.)

Oncocytoma

Oncocytoma is a rare benign tumor that appears as a solid, non-fat-containing renal mass. The tumors mimic renal cell carcinoma not only radiologically, but also histopathologically—to the point where some pathologists believe oncocytoma is not a distinct benign tumor, but rather a low grade variant of renal cell carcinoma. 2 radiological features have been described and are said to be distinctive, namely the presence of a central stellate scar or of a "spoke wheel" pattern on angiography (Figure 35). In reality, it is unlikely that detection of either feature would be sufficiently compelling to obviate surgery.

Renal Transitional Cell Carcinoma

Most upper tract transitional cell carcinomas can be identified based on clinical or imaging findings. Clinically, the majority of these patients will have a history of bladder cancer, and transitional cell carcinoma should be a leading consideration for any upper tract abnormality in a patient with such a history. Radiologically, upper tract transitional cell carcinoma is often primarily located in the pelvicaliceal system (Figure 36), rather than the renal parenchyma, and also may result in pelvicaliceal dilatation due to obstruction. That said, occasionally, an upper tract transitional cell carcinoma will exist largely or entirely within the renal parenchyma (Figure 37), in which case the distinction from renal cell carcinoma may be difficult. It should be noted that a renal mass with pelvicaliceal invasion is suggestive of a transitional cell carcinoma, but that this feature can also be seen with renal cell carcinoma (while pelvicaliceal invasion is reported histopathologically in up to 14% of renal cell carcinomas, it is rarely seen at imaging).

Renal Lymphoma

At autopsy, 30%-60% of lymphoma patients demonstrate renal involvement, although renal involvement is seen in only 3%-8% of lymphoma patients undergoing CT. Primary lymphoma of the kidneys is rare, and most patients with lymphomatous involvement of the kidneys will also have extra renal disease, which serves as a useful imaging clue to the correct diagnosis (Figure 38). Certain patterns of varying distinctiveness may be seen when the kidneys are involved. In particular, multiple small masses, renal invasion by spread from the retroperitoneum, diffuse infiltration of the kidneys, perinephric encasement, or a single homogeneous mass (the latter may mimic renal cell carcinoma) have all been described. Perinephric encasement is probably the most suggestive pattern with respect to the specific diagnosis of lymphoma, although it is not the most common (Figure 39).

Metastasis to the Kidney

At autopsy, 2%-20% of patients dying of cancer have metastases to the kidney, with common primary sites being lung, breast, stomach, pancreas, colon and melanoma. In practice, metastases to the kidney are rarely recognized at CT, and when seen, usually occur in the setting of widely disseminated disease (Figure 40). For example, in one series, the kidneys were the sole site of involvement in only 3 of 27 patients with metastases to the kidney. Metastases to the kidney are often small and multifocal or perinephric in distribution. Unifocal involvement can occur, in which case the findings may mimic renal cell carcinoma, and this pattern is said to be more common in patients with colorectal cancer.

Cystic Renal Masses (Bosniak Classification)

Benign simple cyst (Bosniak category 1)
Benign simple cysts are very common, occurring in 30% of patients over 50 years. The accuracy of imaging approaches 100% when all of the well-known morphologic features are present. These include an ovoid uniocular lesion with a thin-to-imperceptible wall that is well-circumscribed with a sharp parenchymal interface. At CT, the lesion is of uniform fluid density (-20 to +20 H) (Figure 20).

Benign high density cyst (Bosniak category 2)
These are benign cysts that meet all of the criteria for a benign simple cyst, except that the cyst fluid is greater than 20 HU in density (often the range of 50-90 HU), and this is believed to reflect hemorrhagic or proteinaceous content. At ultrasound, such internal hemorrhage or protein may be recognized by low level echogenicity within the cystic lesion, while at MRI, hemorrhagic or proteinaceous content may result in high T1 signal intensity that does not suppress with fat saturation (Figure 41). Such lesions can still be classified as benign, provided non-contrast images are present to confirm that the lesion is truly non-enhancing.

Benign mildly complex cyst (Bosniak category 2)
This is the second type of Bosniak category 2 cyst, and this designation is appropriate for a cyst that otherwise has the features of a simple cyst but contains hairline-thin septa or fine curvilinear calcification (Figure 42).

Possibly malignant complex cyst (Bosniak category 3)
Features that constitute signs of possible malignancy include thick or irregular walls or septa, irregular thick calcification or non-enhancing nodules (Figure 43). The risk of malignancy in a Bosniak 3

cyst is approximately 50%, and accordingly these lesions are generally managed by resection.

Malignant complex cysts (Bosniak category 4)
Features that result in a Bosniak 4 categorization for a cystic lesion include irregular enhancing thick wall, enhancing or large nodules, or the presence of solid components (Figure 44). Most Bosniak 4 lesions are cystic renal cell carcinomas, although occasionally an upper tract transitional cell carcinoma may be predominantly cystic. It should be noted that cavitary necrosis does not truly constitute a cystic lesion, and when such cases are excluded, approximately 3.5% of renal cell carcinomas are cystic.

Bosniak Classification of Renal Cysts: FAQs

Can Bosniak 2 lesions be malignant, despite having a benign appearance?
There are 2 types of Bosniak 2 cysts, the high density cyst and the mildly complex cyst. 1 case report described renal cell cancer in a high density cyst, but the focus of malignancy was microscopic and on the cyst wall. Given the frequency of microscopic renal cell carcinoma at autopsy, it is arguable that this was a coincidence, and certainly this single case report is hardly sufficient evidence to change the traditional approach to high density cysts. A few case reports have described cancer in mildly complex Bosniak 2 cysts, though there is only 1 good series. In this series, 23 cystic renal cancers were resected and their preoperative Bosniak appearance examined. The study claims that 1 of the lesions was a mildly complex (Bosniak 2) cyst, although the legitimacy of this characterization is difficult to confirm, since images were not provided in the publication. Again, this seems insufficient evidence to change the common assumption that mildly complex cysts are benign.

What are Bosniak category 2F lesions?
The distinction of Bosniak 2 from Bosniak 3 lesions is critical, because the former will be dismissed as benign, while the latter will likely undergo resection because of the high risk of malignancy. As such, any reader making a Bosniak 2 assignment clearly requires a high degree of confidence in this categorization, but there are times where cysts have some degree of complexity that introduces doubt and uncertainty. In such cases, there is the additional classification of Bosniak 2F (F stands for follow-up), which Bosniak himself has described as "a group of cystic lesions that are not complex enough to be characterized as category 3 but that are more complex than category 2 lesions." The features that result in a Bosniak 2F categorization are an increased number of hairline thin septa, minimal thickening of septa or wall, minimal enhancement of hairline thin septa or wall, thick or nodular calcification, or high density cysts over 3 cm. The problem with these characteristics, as acknowledged by Bosniak himself, is that they are largely subjective. Nonetheless, when a mildly complex cyst is seen that is on the borderline between Bosniak 2 and 3, an assignment of Bosniak 2F maybe useful, since surveillance may result in a more confident diagnosis at follow up imaging. The good news is that most such lesions appear to be benign, and in 1 retrospective study of 42 cases, with a mean follow-up of 6 years, only 1 cystic renal cell carcinoma was ultimately diagnosed.

Is there a scientific (ie, not medicolegal) basis for suggesting follow-up of renal masses?
While this question may also be relevant to solid renal masses, it follows logically from discussion of Bosniak 2F lesions. Unfortunately, while follow-up is often suggested as an appropriate method of distinguishing benign from malignant renal lesions, the scientific basis for this approach is somewhat limited. For example, the growth rate of oncocytomas does not differ significantly from that of Fuhrman grade 1 renal cell carcinomas. More disturbingly, it has been shown that small presumed renal cell carcinomas can remain relatively stable in size over several years, and then grow quite dramatically.

Is the Bosniak system objective?
While the Bosniak system is widely used, it is not clear that it is sufficiently objective and reproducible. In an interesting study where 70 cystic masses were classified by 3 readers, major discrepancies (ie, Bosniak category 1 or 2 vs. 3 or 4) were seen in 11 (16%) of cases. The authors of this study suggested that interobserver variation in distinguishing Bosniak 2 and 3 lesions may present difficulties in recommending surgical vs. conservative management.

Do cystic renal cell carcinomas matter?
While cystic renal cell carcinomas tend to be of lower grade and stage than control groups of matched solid renal carcinomas, there is still an appreciable mortality associated with these cancers, and appropriate treatment is still indicated. In 1 study, there was an 82% 4-year, disease-specific survival for cystic renal cell carcinoma.

Indeterminate Renal Masses

Too Small To Characterize ("TSTC"): Hypodense lesions under 1-1.5 cm in the kidney are very common, and too small to characterize using density measurement. Such measurements are unreliable in small lesions, due to both partial voluming in the Z axis and also the phenomenon of pseudo-enhancement. The available evidence suggests that the vast majority of such lesions are small cysts and they can generally be dismissed, unless there is a visual concern or possibly a clinical concern, such as a high-risk patient with prior renal cell carcinoma or von Hippel-Lindau disease.

Unclear if the lesion is solid or cystic: Occasionally, the criteria described above for distinguishing solid and cystic masses may conflict within or between modalities. This is uncommon, and the situation can usually be resolved by additional imaging, although management should be tailored to each patient.

Bosniak 2F Lesion: These are cysts in which sufficient complexity is present to result in some disquiet in assigning a Bosniak 2 categorization, but the lesion is not considered sufficiently complex to merit resection. As noted above, these lesions can be followed, although the logic for this approach is debatable.

Unclear if fat containing or not: This is probably the least common type of indeterminate renal lesion, but occasionally a solid mass will be seen with some fat at the periphery, and it may be unclear whether this is tumoral fat (indicating angiomyolipoma) or entrapped fat adjacent to a renal cell carcinoma (Figure 45). Alternatively, a tiny speck of fat within a large solid lesion may be considered insufficient for a confident diagnosis of angiomyolipoma. Again, management should be tailored to the individual patient, but with the general caution that it is probably safer to remove an indeterminate lesion than to miss a potential cancer.

Angiomyolipoma

Angiomyolipomas are rare, benign, hamartomous tumors of the kidney that are composed of blood vessels ("angio"), smooth muscle ("myo") and fat ("lipo"). Most are sporadic, but some are associated with tuberous sclerosis. The latter is a particular consideration if the tumors are multiple or associated with other manifestations, such as pulmonary lymphangio-leiomyomatosis. The "lipo" component of angiomyolipomas is critical for imaging characterization, since it is estimated that 95% contain demonstrable fat, and so the imaging rule is "a solid renal mass that contains *macroscopic* fat is an angiomyolipoma." The typical angiomyolipoma is a well-defined mass in the renal cortex, measuring up to 5 cm that is composed largely of fat density adipose tissue (Figure 26). The lesions are often exophytic, in which case the finding of a parenchymal notch or a vascular pedicle extending from the kidney into the lesion can help confirm that it is of renal origin, and therefore an exophytic angiomyolipoma (Figure 46). 2 obvious questions arise with respect to angiomyolipoma. First, can renal cell carcinoma contain fat? If so, can fat-containing renal cell carcinoma be mistaken for angiomyolipoma? Renal cell carcinomas can, on very rare occasions, contain macroscopic fat. 3 mechanisms have been described, namely entrapment of adjacent fat (either perinephric fat, sinus fat or even tumorous fat in an adjacent angiomyolipoma), bone marrow formation in osseous metaplasia within the tumor or fat-producing necrosis. From a practical point of view, all these mechanisms are likely to be associated with an obvious heterogeneous or necrotic tumor mass, so in real life it is highly unlikely that a fat-containing renal cell carcinoma would truly mimic an angiomyolipoma.

4. Renal Calcification and Urinary Stones

Overview

Renal calcification is usually focal and within the pelvicaliceal system, due to stone formation (nephrolithiasis), but occasionally diffuse calcification can be seen in the parenchyma (nephrocalcinosis). These topics will be discussed separately.

Nephrolithiasis

Imaging of Flan Pain

Non-enhanced CT is much more sensitive for urinary stones than intravenous urography, and has largely replaced IVU in patients with suspected ureteral colic (Figure 47). The sensitivity of non-enhanced spiral CT for depicting a renal or ureteral stone is 94%-98%, while that of US is approximately 20% and IVU is 52%-59%. Non-enhanced CT is also useful for identifying causes of flank pain other than nephrolithiasis, such as appendicitis and diverticulitis. In a study of 93 patients referred for clinically suspected renal colic, a change in treatment plan was made in 57 patients (61%) based on findings at non-enhanced CT. In theory, 90%-95% of stones are sufficiently radiopaque to be visible by plain radiography. In practice, the plain radiograph is very limited in the evaluation of renal colic, because multiple radiodensities can mimic stones (eg, gallstones, costochondral cacifications, bone islands and fecal densities) and because stones may be easily missed (eg, radiolucent stones and stones obscured by bowel content or bone). Ultrasound can be used to identify obstruction in a patient with flank pain, but the endpoint is demonstration of hydronephrosis rather than direct visualization of a stone (although sometimes an obstructing calculus may be seen high in the ureter through the acoustic window for the kidney, or in the distal ureter through the bladder). Bowel and bone limit acoustic access to the rest of the ureter in the retroperitoneum. The main drawback of US is that not all obstructed kidneys have dilated pelvicaliceal systems, either because dilatation has not yet developed, the upper tract has decompressed by forniceal rupture or the upper tract is noncompliant. In addition, the diuretic effect of intravenous contrast likely explains why dilatation is occasionally absent at ultrasound but present at IVU. The reported false negative rate for ultrasound in acute flank pain ranges from 6%-38%. Traditionally, IVU has been the standard of reference for renal colic evaluation, because it combines both functional and anatomic assessment, and because direct opacification of the urinary system facilitates identification of radiolucent stones. The main disadvantages of IVU are the need to administer IV contrast and the duration of the study, which can be particularly prolonged when delayed films are required in high-grade obstruction. However, while IVU reliably demonstrates obstruction, the cause is not always clearly shown. In a series of 46 patients with calculous ureteral obstruction, the stone was not visible at IVP in 6 (13%). The 6 missed stones were confirmed by retrograde pyelography, ureteroscopy or spontaneous passage. In 2 other series, obstructing stones were missed by IVU in 12 of 28 and 6 of 11 patients. The emergence of non-enhanced CT probably accounts for the apparent drop in IVU sensitivity for stone identification. In the past, an IVU showing mild hydroureteronephrosis but no stone was often reported as "possible recent stone passage." It is possible that many of these cases were due to small urographically occult stones.

Stone Characterization by Imaging

Imaging features that reflect stone composition and formation include morphology, internal structure and density.

Stone morphology: Most stones are small and round, which is relatively nonspecific. Pure calcium oxalate stones are often homogenous, dense and smooth. Mixed calcium oxalate stones may be irregular in shape, inhomogeneous and may have dendritic projections. Staghorn calculi are so called because they develop in the pelvicaliceal system, and in advanced cases have a branching configuration that resembles the antlers of a stag. Staghorn calculi are typically composed of magnesium ammonium phosphate (struvite), which forms in urine that has abnormally high pH (above 7.2). This high pH usually develops because of recurrent urinary tract infection with Gram-positive microorganisms, such as *Proteus mirabilis*. However, large urate acid and cystine stones can also have a staghorn configuration, and staghorn calculi in children or young adults with no history of infection are frequently composed of cystine. Radiographically, struvite stones are relatively low density.

Low-density struvite stones may not be appreciated on plain radiographs, but can be readily detected by US or CT. IVP or retrograde pyelography may also be used to demonstrate the typical branching appearance of staghorn calculi. Faceted stones are usually multiple and have arisen in a small cavity, such as a renal pelvis above an ureteropelvic junction obstruction or in a caliceal diverticulum, where the stones are minimally mobile but in contact with each other. Lithotripsy may be inappropriate for such stones, because residual small fragments may not pass.

Internal structure: Most stones are homogeneously dense. Struvite stones may have a laminated appearance, with alternating dense and relative lucent layers.

Density: In the IVP era, stones were traditionally divided into radiopaque (calcium and struvite stones) and radiolucent (pure cystine, urate, and matrix or mucoprotein stones). This division was not precise, because so-called lucent stones could become secondarily calcified and become at least partially opaque. More importantly, the distinction between radiopaque and radiolucent stones has become obsolete in the CT era. Due to the exquisite sensitivity of CT to even small amounts of calcium, all stones appear opaque (ie, white) on CT. The only common exception to this statement is the occurrence of indinavir stones in HIV patients (indinavir is a protease inhibitor that is poorly soluble in urine, and may form obstructive stone-like precipitates after excretion into the collecting system). These "lucent" stones may still be detectable due to secondary calcification or to signs of ureteral obstruction in the setting of an HIV patient with flank pain (Figure 48).

Differentiation of Stones from Phleboliths

A problem with non-enhanced CT is that stones, particularly in the pelvis near the ureterovesical junction, must be differentiated from phleboliths. The soft tissue rim around the stone is presumed to be the edematous ureteral wall. In a study of CT in 442 patients, of whom 136 had ureteral calculi, it was found that a thin rim of soft tissue surrounding a calcification (the "soft tissue rim sign," Figure 49) was seen in 105 of 136 ureteral calculi and in only 20 of 259 phleboliths. The converse sign, the "comet tail sign," where a thin linear soft tissue structure is seen leading up to a calculus without an associated rim of soft tissue around the calculus (Figure 50), is often described as a characteristic of a phlebolith rather than a ureteral stone. However, the comet tail sign is neither sensitive nor specific for phleboliths and, when observed in patients with ureteral obstruction, was shown to actually represent a ureteral calculus in 50%-67% of cases. Use of a computer workstation or PACS, which allows dynamic scrolling of axial CT images as well as 3-dimensional reformations, is also useful to define the path of a ureter and determine whether a calcification is within or external to a ureter. In the rare case when a CT examination is equivocal for location of a calcification, intravenous contrast material may be administered to opacify the renal collecting system, allowing more precise depiction of the ureter relative to the calcification.

Prognosis of Ureterolithiasis

Both the size and location of ureteral stones are predictive of whether the ureteral stones will pass with conservative medical management, or whether surgical intervention will be required. At CT, a stone which is 4 mm or smaller in axial diameter will have a greater than 75% likelihood of passing with conservative management, while stones 9 mm or larger are less than 50% likely to pass without intervention. Similarly, stones which are identified in the mid-ureter or more distally have a greater than 60% likelihood of passing without need for invasive intervention, while more proximal stones are less than 50% likely to pass without intervention.

Nephrocalcinosis

Nephrocalcinosis refers to radiologically demonstrable, diffuse fine parenchymal (noncalyceal) renal calcification. The calcification may be predominantly medullary or cortical. Common causes of medullary nephrocalcinosis (Figure 51) are hyperparathyroidism, renal tubular acidosis and medullary sponge kidney. The most common cause of cortical nephrocalcinosis is chronic glomerulonephritis (Figure 52). Other causes include acute cortical necrosis, Alport syndrome and renal transplant rejection. Diffuse renal calcification can occur in children with oxalosis, resulting in a characteristic radiological appearance (Figure 53).

5. Renal Infection and Infarction

Pyelonephritis

Pyelonephritis generally results from ascending infection, and vesicoureteral reflux is seen in 30%-50% of affected children. Common organisms are *E coli*, *P mirabolis* and *Klebsiella*. Hematogenous infection is less common and usually produces microabscess, often with negative urine cultures. Imaging findings are quite variable, and are related to the degree and duration of infection. IVU is normal in about 75% of cases. Findings characteristic of pyelonephritis include a decreased or delayed nephrogram which may be patchy or striated, enlargement of the involved kidney (due to edema), and pelvicalyceal effacement due to compression by the edematous parenchyma. Ultrasound is usually normal. Nonspecific findings that may be seen include renal enlargement, focal wedge-shaped decreased echogenicity and loss of pyramidal visualization. Focal decreased perfusion may be seen with Doppler techniques. CT findings extend from striation due to scattered areas of wedge-shaped decreased perfusion, through renal enlargement and even abscess formation. There may be fascial thickening and blurring of the perinephric fat. CT is the most sensitive imaging modality for the evaluation of pyelonephritis and its complications (Figure 54).

Emphysematous Pyelonephritis

Emphysematous pyelonephritis refers to pyelonephritis with gas formation, and is usually due to infection by a gas forming organism (*E coli*, most commonly) in diabetics or immunocompromised patients. Imaging (particularly CT) shows air in the kidney, perirenal space or collecting system (Figure 55). Emphysematous pyelonephritis is a life-threatening condition with a mortality approaching 50%. Treatment is nephrectomy.

Xanthogranulomatous Pyelonephritis

Xanthogranulomatous pyelonephritis is a rare, chronic renal inflammatory disease characterized by destruction and replacement of renal parenchyma with lipid-laden macrophages, which are also known as xanthoma or foam cells. Most patients have a history of obstructing stones, often staghorn, complicated by multiple urinary tract infections. The condition is most common in middle-aged women, although any age and sex can be affected. Clinical features are nonspecific, and include fever, malaise, flank pain and weight loss. Ultimately, chronic inflammatory changes extend outside the kidney into neighboring tissues, including the psoas muscle, diaphragm, bowel and lung. Renal involvement by the inflammatory process may be diffuse or focal. Features that suggest the diagnosis of xanthogranulomatous pyelonephritis at imaging include (Figure 56):

- Presence of a staghorn calculus
- Obstructive hydronephrosis with calyceal dilatation and decreased renal function. Irregularity of the calices may be present, due to superimposed papillary necrosis
- Replacement of the renal parenchyma by multiple small abscess cavities
- Marked perinephric inflammatory changes

Distinction from renal malignancy may be difficult in the rare focal form of xanthogranulomatous pyelonephritis. Treatment is nephrectomy, and partial nephrectomy can be done for the focal type.

Fungal Infection

Fungal infection of the kidney is usually an opportunistic infection in diabetic or immunocompromised patients, or patients with indwelling catheters. The most common organism is *Candida albicans* or other candidal species. Candidal infection of the kidneys may occur as the result of systemic or primary renal candidiasis. Primary renal candidiasis is most commonly seen in diabetic women. Pathologically, fungi which are filtered by the glomeruli become lodged in the distal tubules, where they proliferate and produce microabscesses. Papillary necrosis ensues as the fungi infiltrate the tips of the renal papillae. The fungi are then extruded into the renal collecting system, resulting in fungus balls (mycetomas). The fungus balls may cause obstruction, resulting in hydronephrosis, pain and even renal failure, if severe and long-standing. Fungal infection of the kidneys can be diagnosed through demonstrating fungal hyphae in urine.

On imaging, fungus balls are seen as multiple small filling defects in the collecting systems (Figure 57). Other findings include diminished excretion of contrast, papillary necrosis and hydronephrosis. CT is the preferred imaging modality for evaluating fungal balls and for fungal pyelonephritis in general. It can accurately depict morphologic lesions, functional abnormalities in contrast uptake and excretion, as well as associated complications, such as perinephric abscess. Treatment includes systemic anti-fungal therapy. Instrumentation of the urinary tract with direct removal of the fungus balls may be helpful as adjuvant therapy.

Renal Infarction

Renal infarction may result from embolic or thrombotic disease. Thrombotic disease usually affects the larger vessels, including the main renal artery, while emboli may affect vessels of various sizes. Renal artery emboli usually come from the heart, and typically result in the sudden onset of flank pain, hematuria, proteinuria, fever and leukocytosis. In contrast, patients with thrombotic disease usually present with hypertension or renal insufficiency. Thrombotic disease usually results from atherosclerosis, though blunt abdominal trauma may cause intimal tears with subsequent dissection and thrombosis. Excretory urography shows absent enhancement of the affected renal segment. On ultrasound, the infarcted area may be visibly enlarged and hypoechoic. Doppler may show absent intrarenal arterial signal, or a tardus-parvus waveform if there is incomplete occlusion or collateral supply. Subtle renal infarcts are best demonstrated on CT, where they appear as wedge-shaped, cortically based, hypodense areas (Figure 58). Renal swelling may also be seen. The rim sign may be present if the entire kidney is involved. That is, the entire kidney is non-enhancing except for the outer 2-4 mm of cortex, which is perfused by capsular branches. Nuclear imaging shows a photopenic area corresponding to the region of ischemia or infarction. Arteriography provides the definitive diagnosis, showing abrupt termination of vessels or filling defects. Cortical atrophy and irregular scarring are seen as late sequelae. In the case of end-stage renal artery thrombosis, a small kidney with a smooth contour is seen unless multiple small infarcts had independently occurred. Treatment of renal ischemia consists of anticoagulation, intraarterial thrombolytic therapy and surgical revascularization.

6. Renal Trauma

Overview

Renal injury occurs in 8%-10% of abdominal trauma patients, particularly those with blunt (rather than penetrating) trauma. From a clinical perspective, the management of renal injury is increasingly conservative, with a higher threshold for surgical intervention. From a radiological perspective, contrast-enhanced CT is the preferred imaging option, although 1-shot IVU and ultrasound are alternatives (Figures 59 and 60), particularly in an unstable patient with multiple other injuries where transfer to a CT scanner may be too risky or time-consuming. Renal trauma is graded based on the imaging appearances using the American Association for the Surgery of Trauma System (Table 7).

CT Appearances

Since the American Association for the Surgery of Trauma grading system is heavily dependent on imaging, it is important to have a good understanding of CT terminology and distinctions in renal trauma (Figures 61-63).

Subcapsular hematoma appears as a well-defined, high-density fluid collection adjacent to the kidney, which is often crescentic or elliptical in shape and may deform the kidney. A subcapsular hematoma is well-defined peripherally and may deform the kidney.

Perinephric hematoma, unlike subcapsular hematoma, is ill-defined peripherally, not associated with renal deformation and may be associated with a visible laceration.

Renal contusion appears as an ill-defined area of reduced enhancement and excretion.

Renal infarction appears as a well-defined and wedge-shaped area of absent enhancement.

Active hemorrhage is characterized by linear or flame-like intense contrast enhancement within a

Table 7

American Association for the Surgery of Trauma System for Grading Renal Trauma

Grade	American Association for the Surgery of Trauma System (Moore et al - J Trauma 1989; 29: 1664-6)
I	Hematuria with normal imaging studies Contusion Nonexpanding subcapsular hematoma
II	Nonexpanding perinephric hematoma confined to retroperitoneum Superficial laceration <1 cm deep without collecting system injury
III	Renal laceration >1 cm deep without collecting system injury
IV	Renal laceration into the collecting system Main renal artery or vein injury with contained hemorrhage Segmental infarction without associated laceration Expanding subcapsular hematoma compressing kidney
V	Shattered or devascularized kidney Ureteropelvic avulsion Complete laceration or thrombus of the main renal artery or vein

laceration or hematoma during the early phase of enhancement, with later washout.

Urinary extravasation is also characterized by extraluminal contrast, but unlike active hemorrhage, the contrast accumulates progressively over a multiphase CT study, rather than being primarily transient and in the arterial phase. In addition, a urinary leak is generally contiguous with the upper track at some point.

Pseudoaneurysm appears as an intense focus of contrast in a laceration or hematoma during the early phase of enhancement, but, unlike active hemorrhage, the area of enhancement is focal and rounded rather than linear or flame-like.

Renal laceration appears as a jagged or linear parenchymal disruption which may contain fresh or clotted blood.

Traumatic Renal Devascularization

A devascularized kidney after trauma is a grade 5 injury. CT findings of a non-enhancing kidney are distinctive (Figure 64). These patients often have little to no hematuria or hematoma, and the devascularization is usually the result of a partial dissecting tear with thrombus in the renal artery. Successful surgical salvage is rare, but perhaps worth attempting if the other kidney is absent or injured. Nephrectomy may be appropriate for an unstable patient, or for the development of hypertension as a delayed complication.

Indications for Surgery

Probably the only absolute indication for surgery after renal trauma is life-threatening renal hemorrhage. Relative indications include: the presence of extensively devitalized tissue (greater than 50% of the renal parenchyma), urinary extravasation that cannot be controlled by stenting or nephrostomy, and arterial thrombosis. 87% of urinary leaks can be managed without surgery. Intermediate grade injuries can also usually be handled without surgery, and aggressive monitoring, percutaneous drainage and angiographic embolization can help reduce the laparotomy rate to about 10%.

7. Ureteral Disease

Congenital Ureteropelvic Junction Obstruction

Congenital ureteropelvic junction obstruction is the most common congenital anomaly of the urinary tract, and 10%-40% of cases are bilateral. The disorder is due to functional narrowing of the ureteropelvic junction, producing variable degrees of hydronephrosis that may be intermittent. The condition may be due to intrinsic abnormal motility of the ureteropelvic junction or a crossing anomalous vessel, and some controversy exists as to the relative frequency of these etiologies (although it should be noted that these mechanisms are not mutually exclusive, and, for example, a congenital anomalous crossing vessel might cause disordered motility as a pressure effect on the developing ureteropelvic junction). Congenital ureteropelvic junction obstruction may present as an abdominal mass (ie, the hydronephrotic kidney) in the neonate. The disorder is being increasingly discovered prenatally, due to the increasing use of obstetric ultrasound. In many cases, the abnormality is clinically silent until adulthood when symptoms of flank pain, fever or, rarely, hypertension cause the patient to seek medical attention.

At imaging, the condition results in hydronephrosis with a non-dilated ureter, in the absence of a detectable stone or stricture at the ureteropelvic junction (Figure 65). Milder or intermittent forms may be difficult to distinguish from a prominent extrarenal pelvis, and imaging during acute symptoms or the use of a diuretic renogram may then be helpful. Conversely, with longstanding or very high grade obstruction, an essentially nonfunctioning kidney may be present. CT or MR angiography may be used to depict an associated crossing vessel.

Ureteral Carcinoma

Ureteral carcinoma is a rare malignancy and accounts for only about 1% of all urinary tract tumors. Most are transitional cell carcinomas. At IVU or CT urography, ureteral carcinomas are typically seen as a solitary non-calcified filling defect in the upper tract, often with upstream dilatation. The ureter below the filling defect is often dilated for a short distance, presumably because it is "held open" by the firm tumor. This results in the classic "goblet" sign (Figure 66). CT or MRI may be helpful in demonstrating periureteral extension or more distant spread of disease. Most patients have a history of bladder transitional cell carcinoma, and any upper tract filling defect in a patient with this history should be considered recurrent transitional cell carcinoma until proven otherwise (Figure 67).

Ureteral Fibroepithelial Polyp

Ureteral fibroepithelial polyp is a rare, benign ureteral tumor composed of a fibrovascular core covered by transitional epithelium. Flank pain and hematuria are the most common presenting symptoms. Ultrasound demonstrates a variable degree of hydronephrosis. On IVU, fibroepithelial polyps appear as a pedunculated filling defect of varying length. Polyps of up to 13 cm in length have been described, and the finding of a long linear filling defect in the ureter should suggest the diagnosis (Figure 68). Polyps are usually solitary, but may be multiple, and typically smooth, cylindrical and mobile. Fibroepithelial polyps are most common in the upper third of the ureter, and in the 20-40-year-old age group.

8. Bladder Disease

Bladder Cancer

Overview

Bladder cancer is relatively uncommon, but does account for 2% of cancer deaths. 90% of bladder cancers are transitional cell cancers, and these are associated with smoking, aniline dyes and increasing age. 8% are squamous cell carcinomas, for which the risk factors are stone and chronic inflammation. 2% are adenocarcinomas, and these are associated with congenital anomalies and chronic inflammation. With respect to the latter, it should be noted that a bladder mass arising in the midline anteriorly should raise the possibility of urachal adenocarcinoma (Figure 69).

Imaging

The imaging appearances of bladder cancer are somewhat variable, with low grade tumors appearing as polypoid papillary masses within the bladder lumen (Figure 70), while higher grade tumors tend to result in more focal infiltrative wall thickening (Figure 71). Surface calcification or encrustation on polypoid masses is occasionally seen, and is relatively distinctive (Figure 70). The detection rate of bladder cancer by imaging, whether ultrasound, IVU or CT, is approximately 70%-90%. All modalities can miss smaller or flat tumors, and consequently cystoscopy remains the standard of reference for the detection of bladder cancer.

Staging

For simplicity, bladder cancer staging can be divided into tumors that are superficial, invasive (into the bladder muscle layer, perivesical fat or regional nodes) or metastatic (Table 8). Staging is important because it allows prediction of prognosis and treatment planning. Examination of Table 7 shows that the critical imaging features that might be amenable to imaging detection are muscle invasion, perivesical fat invasion, and lymph node metastasis. Unfortunately, published results show that evaluation of these features is of relative limited accuracy for all modalities, although there are times when unequivocal radiological findings may be present (Figure 72). It should be noted that not every soft density mass seen in the bladder at CT is a bladder cancer, and the radiological differential includes

Table 8

Simplified Staging System for Bladder Cancer, Highlighting the Important Findings that May be Detected by Imaging (muscle layer invasion, extension into perivesical fat, adenopathy and distant metastases)

Stage	%	Survival	Main Rx options
Superficial	70%	82%–100% at 5 years	TURBT, fulguration, ± intravesical Rx
Invasive	10% 10% 5%	Muscle layer: 63%–83% at 5 years Perivesical fat: 45%–55% at 5 years Regional nodes: 25% at 5 years	Radical cystectomy, radiotherapy (if nonsurgical)
Metastatic	5%	5% at 2 years	Chemotherapy, RT, palliative surgery

hematoma, pheochromocytoma and leiomyoma (Figure 73).

Bladder Rupture

Traumatic bladder rupture may be extraperitoneal (50%-71%), intraperitoneal (25%-43%), or combined extra- and intraperitoneal (7%-14%). Extraperitoneal rupture is generally due to perforation by a bony fragment (pelvic fractures are seen in 89%-100% of cases) or an avulsion tear at the fixation points of the puboprostatic ligaments. It usually occurs close to the bladder base anterolaterally. Intraperitoneal rupture is typically a "burst" injury where a blow to the abdomen perforates the dome of a full bladder. At conventional or CT cystography, extraperitoneal rupture results in flame-shaped, starburst or feather-like perivesical contrast extravasation while intraperitoneal rupture results in intraperitoneal pools of contrast that outline bowel loops (Figures 74-75). The distinction of the 2 types of bladder rupture is important, because 85% of extraperitoneal ruptures will heal with catheterization alone, while most intraperitoneal ruptures require surgical repair.

Neurogenic Bladder

Neurogenic bladder refers to bladder dysfunction secondary to disturbance of the complex neurological pathways that regulate bladder filling and emptying. Conditions which can cause neurogenic bladder include: cerebrovascular disease, multiple sclerosis, Parkinson disease, motoneuron disease, spinal cord injury, spina bifida, diabetes, pelvic surgery or intervertebral disc herniation. Modern assessment of neurogenic bladder may require urodynamic and electrophysiological assessment for complete evaluation. A variety of detailed classifications have been developed to describe neurogenic bladder; however, from the imaging viewpoint, there are essentially 2 recognizable types—the spastic bladder and the atonic bladder.

Spastic neurogenic bladder results in urination, is involuntary and frequent, and a true sensation of fullness is lacking. At imaging, the bladder is small and trabeculated with a typical "pine cone" or "Christmas tree" appearance (Figure 76).

Atonic (or flaccid) neurogenic bladder typically results in retention with overflow incontinence. At imaging, the bladder is large, capacious and smooth (Figure 77). Radiological distinction from a bladder that is physiologically large can sometimes be difficult, but coexistent fecal loading of the large bowel may help suggest an underlying neurological problem.

9. Prostatic Disease

Zonal Anatomy

Awareness of the often poorly understood zonal anatomy of the prostate is important for interpreting imaging of both benign prostatic hyperplasia (a disease of the central gland) and prostate cancer (mainly a disease of the peripheral zone). The simplest conceptual approach to the zonal anatomy of the prostate is the 2-compartment model, where the prostate is likened to a cone containing a scoop of ice cream. The "cone" is the peripheral zone, and makes up 70% of the prostate gland by volume in young men. The ducts of the peripheral zone glands drain to the distal prostatic urethra. The "scoop of ice cream" is the central zone, and makes up 25% of the prostate gland volume in young men. The ejaculatory ducts traverse the central zone, and the ducts of the central zone drain to the region of the verumontanum clustered around the entry of the ejaculatory ducts. The final 5% of the prostate consists of the transition zone, which is composed of 2 small bulges of tissue that surround the vesumontanum in a horseshoe-like fashion. This 2-compartment model is deficient anteriorly, where the peripheral zone is interrupted by the anterior fibromuscular stroma, a band of smooth muscle mixed with fibrous tissue that forms a thick shield over the anterior aspect of the gland. As a result, the peripheral zone lies predominantly lateral and posterior to the central zone.

Confusion regarding the zonal anatomy of the prostate arises because the zonal anatomy changes with age (Figure 78). The transition zone is the portion of the prostate that develops benign prostatic hyperplasia. As a result, the transition zone becomes progressively bigger with age and compresses the surrounding central zone. The latter becomes the surgical pseudocapsule. 1 approach to incorporate and simplify this age-related complexity is to refer to the transition and central zones collectively as the central gland. Using this terminology, the prostate is composed of the peripheral zone and central gland, such that the central gland is composed mainly of central zone tissue in young men and mainly of transition zone tissue in older men. Given that prostate cancer is largely a disease of older men, in the population that comes to MRI, it is reasonable to regard the terms "central gland" and "transition zone" as essentially synonymous.

Benign Prostatic Hyperplasia

Imaging can be used in benign prostatic hyperplasia to detect hydronephrosis, determine the post-void residual urinary volume and determine the size of the prostate prior to treatment. These observations can all be well-evaluated using ultrasound. Findings on IVU that may be caused by prostatic enlargement and bladder outlet obstruction include: a horizontal orientation to the normally downward course of the distal ureter (so-called "J-hooking"), hydroureteronephrosis, ureteral tortuosity, bladder trabeculation, diverticula, elevation of the bladder base and an increased post-void residual urinary volume (Figure 79). At cross-sectional imaging (ultrasound, CT, or MRI), benign prostatic hyperplasia results in a heterogeneous nodular appearance to the transition zone of the prostate, sometimes with small focal calcifications. The prostate may become extremely large and protrude into the bladder base, although there is only a loose relationship between symptoms of outlet obstruction and prostate volume.

Prostate Cancer

Prostate cancer is the second most common fatal malignancy in men. The greatest dilemma in the care of prostate cancer patients is the limited ability of all available methods (including imaging) to predict tumor behavior, and allow informed treatment stratification that aligns active surveillance with indolent tumors and definitive treatment (by surgery or radiation) with aggressive tumors. As such, the use of imaging in the evaluation of prostate cancer is a subject of controversy, with the exception of CT or bone scintigraphy for the detection of metastatic disease (Figures 80-81). Typically, prostate cancer appears as a focus of reduced echogenicity in the peripheral zone of the prostate at transrectal ultrasound, sometimes with increased vascularity at Doppler interrogation (Figure 82). Transrectal ultrasound is undoubtedly useful in the localization of the prostate for needle biopsies, but appears of limited accuracy in the localization or staging of tumor, even with the addition of Doppler techniques. At endorectal MRI, prostate cancer is typically seen as an ovoid or crescentic subcapsular focus of reduced T2 signal intensity (Figure 83). In single institutional studies, endorectal MRI has shown considerable promise in the diagnosis, staging and post-treatment surveillance of prostate cancer, particularly when combined with the newer techniques of spectroscopic, perfusion and diffusion imaging, but the results of multi-institutional studies have been somewhat disappointing. Some of the controversy with respect to the role of imaging in local evaluation of prostate cancer arises from the variability of published results, which raises concerns about interobserver variability and lack of reproducibility. For example, the reported staging accuracy of transrectal ultrasound ranges from 58%-90%, and the reported staging accuracy of endorectal MRI ranges from 54%-90%. Nodal evaluation is equally limited, with very variable published results.

10. Urethral Disease

Urethral Stricture

Inflammation and trauma are the leading causes of acquired urethral strictures, including prior gonorrhea and catheterization. Post-traumatic strictures result from partial or complete urethral rupture, usually as a result of pelvic fracture. Imaging plays a major role in the diagnostic evaluation of urethral stricture. The study of choice is a combination of retrograde urethrogram (which distends the anterior urethra) and voiding cystourethrogram (which distends the posterior urethra). In addition to distending different portions of the urethra, such a combined approach allows better evaluation of the upper end of a stricture, may reveal a stricture obscured by obliquity on the retrograde urethrogram and allows assessment of upstream dilatation (indicating functionally significant narrowing) (Figure 84). High-frequency ultrasound can also be used for evaluation of the stricture length (Figure 85), particularly as an adjunct to surgical planning.

Urethral Disruption

The prostatic urethra, membranous urethra and urogenital diaphragm form a unit during trauma, so the usual site of disruption is the bulbomembranous junction. Posterior urethral trauma occurs in 10%-15% of pelvic fractures, almost always in men. Retrograde urethrography is the most common imaging test used to evaluate posterior urethral trauma, and is indicated in a man with a pelvic fracture who has gross hematuria, blood at the meatus, perineal swelling, an impalpable prostate or an inability to urinate. The radiographic findings can be used to classify the urethral injury as types I, II and III. In type V, the urethra is intact, but is stretched and narrowed due to elevation of the bladder by hematoma. In type II, there is a tear at the prostatomembranous junction (previously described as the "classic" injury), and contrast extravasates into the true pelvis above the urogenital diaphragm. In type III, the urethra is torn below the urogenital diaphragm and contrast extravasates into the perineum and scrotum. Type II or III injuries may be subclassified as partial or complete. A tear is indicated by the extravasation of contrast (Figure 86). If the bladder also fills with contrast, the tear is partial (30%), but if the bladder does not fill, the tear is complete (70%). If the urethrogram is normal, the catheter should be advanced into the bladder and a cystogram performed to evaluate for possible bladder rupture. While urethrography has been the traditional modality used to evaluate urethral injuries, the length of urethral injury and extent of associated soft tissue damage can be difficult to evaluate. MRI can be used to complement conventional urethrography in this setting. By accurately defining the pelvic anatomy, it provides valuable information to guide the surgical plan and determine whether a transperineal or suprapubic approach should be used.

Urethral Diverticulum

Urethral diverticula occur in as many as 1%-6% of all women. They typically arise from the posterior wall of the urethra, bulging into the vagina or vaginal introitus. Occasionally, they arise laterally or anteriorly. The origin is unknown. Most are probably acquired, though some may be congenital. Possible causes include: infection and obstruction of periurethral glands, trauma from childbirth or repeated catheterization. Symptoms are often nonspecific, consisting of urgency, frequency, dysuria, dyspareunia, recurrent urinary tract infection, dribbling and incontinence. Careful examination may demonstrate a palpable tender suburethral mass. Occasionally, pus may be expressed from such a mass, or it may contain a palpable store or even a hard nodule, due to complicating carcinoma. Urethral diverticula in women may be difficult to visualize radiographically. They may be visible on a voiding cystourethrogram, but only if they fill and distend with contrast. If the diagnosis is strongly suspected clinically, then special techniques to generate high pressure in the urethra should be used to force contrast into the diverticulum. This can be achieved by occluding the meatal opening with a finger during voiding, or by using a special double-balloon catheter technique that essentially seals the urethra at both ends and forces contrast into the diverticulum from a hole in the catheter between the balloons (Figure 87). Transvaginal sonography and MRI have also been used to image urethral diverticula in women, particularly when standard imaging has failed to demonstrate a suspected diverticulum (Figure 88).

11. Testicular Masses

Testicular Cancer

Testicular cancer accounts for 1% of all malignancies in men, and is the most common cancer between the ages of 15-34 years. Most testicular cancers present as a palpable painless testicular mass that is hypoechoic at ultrasound (Figure 89). If performed, MRI demonstrates a mass which is relatively iso-intense to the surrounding normal testicular parenchyma on T1-weighted images and hypo-intense on T2-weighted images, and which shows brisk and early enhancement after intravenous gadolinium. This combination of findings in a young man is virtually diagnostic of testicular cancer, and warrants surgical exploration and radical orchiectomy. Percutaneous biopsy is rarely performed for preoperative confirmation, because it may cause malignant spread along the needle tract, and because the probability of malignancy exceeds 90%.

Simple Testicular Cysts

Simple testicular cysts are recognized with increasing frequency due to increasing use of ultrasound and improvements in ultrasound technology. There are 2 types: cysts of the tunica albuginea and intratesticular cysts. Tunica albuginea cysts may be incidental findings, or present with pain, swelling and a firm, pinhead-sized mass. The incidence is said to increase with age. The etiology is unknown; they may be due to post-inflammatory cystic dilatation of individual ductules. At ultrasound, they are small, subcapsular, sharply demarcated, uni- or multi-locular cysts, with no solid portions and no disturbance of the adjacent parenchyma. Intratesticular cysts represent incidental findings,and are usually impalpable. They are typically solitary and adjacent to the rete testis. Intratesticular cysts may contain spermatozoa and are frequently associated with spermatoceles, suggesting they may be due to post-inflammatory or post-traumatic obstruction of the testicular tubule system. In practice, difficulties arise when a very small cyst cannot be definitely characterized, or when a cyst deep in the testis raises concern of a small cystic teratoma. Such lesions may require imaging surveillance.

Tubular Ectasia of the Rete Testis

Tubular ectasia of the rete testis is a benign condition, often bilateral, which is usually seen in elderly men. It is commonly associated with epididymal abnormalities (spermatoceles, epididymal cysts and epididymitis). Ultrasound shows numerous small tubular cystic structures within the rete testis (Figure 90) —a characteristic finding. MRI shows non-enhancing serpiginous tubular structures of low T1 and high T2 signal intensity in the vicinity of the rete testis. No specific treatment is required.

Epidermoid Cyst

Epidermoid cysts account for less than 1% of all testicular neoplasms. The tumor consists histologically of cystic cavities which contain desquamated keratinized epithelium and are lined by stratified squamous epithelium. Skin appendages, such as sebaceous glands and hair follicles, do not occur. Price defined the following criteria for the pathological diagnosis of testicular epidermoid cyst:

- The lesion is within the testicular parenchyma
- The cyst contains keratinized debris or amorphous material with cleft-like spaces
- The cyst wall consists of fibrous tissue with an inner lining of squamous epithelium
- Teratomatous elements are not present in either the cyst wall or the adjacent parenchyma
- The cyst wall is discrete and separate from the tunica albuginea

Epidermoid cysts present as a painless, palpable, firm solitary mass. Bilateral epidermoid cysts are very rare. At ultrasound, epidermoid cysts are well circumscribed ovoid lesions with variable echogenicity. The cyst wall may be hypo- or hyperechoic. The cyst content may be anechoic, uniformly hypoechoic, heterogeneously hypoechoic, or consist of concentric rings of hypo- and hyperechogenicity. The latter can give rise to a typical "target" or "onion" appearance. This laminated appearance should suggest the diagnosis. Calcification of the cyst wall or cyst content can occur. These lesions may represent a benign monodermal form of teratoma. However, carcinoma *in situ* is not found in adjacent seminiferous tubules, unlike typical teratoma. They are considered benign tumors which can be safely treated by local excision, with organ preservation.

Dermoid Cyst

These differ histologically from epidermoid cysts in that they contain skin appendages. They are rare tumors of the testis, though the rarity may be partially due to misclassification of these tumors as epidermoid cysts, or to classification of the tumors as benign monodermal mature teratomas. They present as painless testicular masses. No case of metastasis arising from a testicular tumor regarded as being a dermoid cyst has been well-documented, and these cysts can be considered benign, differentiated teratomas. To our knowledge, imaging features have not been specifically described. Based on the histological similarity, overlap with the imaging findings of epidermoid cysts appears likely.

Leydig Cell Tumor

Leydig cell tumors arise from the Leydig cells of the testicular stroma. They are the most common of the non-germ cell testicular tumors, and account for 2%-3% of all testicular neoplasms. The age distribution is bimodal, occurring in children between 5-10 years and in adults between 30-35 years. Only 5%-10% of Leydig cell tumors are malignant, and most of these occur in the elderly. Both testes are involved in 5%-9% of patients. The tumors may secrete estrogens, androgens, progesterone or corticosteroids, and consequently 30%-40% of patients have an endocrinopathy. Patients may present with gynecomastia or precocious puberty, without a palpable testicular mass. Leydig cell tumors appear at ultrasound as well-demarcated, homogeneous hypoechoic masses, a nonspecific appearance indistinguishable from germ cell cancer. A hyperechoic pattern has been described in 2 cases. The tumors are usually small and slow-growing. Orchiectomy is the treatment of choice, although partial orchiectomy has been described in a case of bilateral tumor. The prognosis is good, except for malignant Leydig cell tumors, which are generally unresponsive to treatment.

Sertoli Cell Tumor

Sertoli cell tumors arise from the testicular stroma, like Leydig cell tumors. They usually occur in childhood. Even in this population they are rare; Sertoli cell tumors accounted for less than 4% of a series of 556 pediatric testicular tumors. They typically present as a unilateral testicular mass under 1 year of age, though bilateral cases have been described. Echogenicity is variable, but the dense collagenous stroma of the tumor may result in a hyperechoic pattern. Endocrinopathy is rare, but can result in gynecomastia, virilization or feminization. 10% of adult cases are malignant, but pediatric cases are nearly always benign and adequately treated by simple orchiectomy. Large cell, calcifying Sertoli cell tumor is a subtype characterized microscopically by the presence of large Sertoli cell with abundant eosinophilic cytoplasm, and macroscopically by the presence of calcifications of various sizes. This results in a characteristic sonographic picture of multiple nodular calcifications of varying sizes, in otherwise normal appearing testes. The calcifications are macroscopic, and are not to be confused with testicular microlithiasis. This tumor type constitutes 1 of the components of Carney's complex, and should alert the physician to the possibility of cardiac myxomas in the patient and family members.

Adenomatoid Tumor

Adenomatoid tumors usually occur in the epididymis, but can occur in the testis and are said to account for up to 5% of testicular tumors. They are thought to arise from mesothelial cells. They arise from the tunica albuginea and therefore are always found in the periphery of the testis. Most present as a slow-growing mass in the third to fifth decade. On imaging they appear as well-circumscribed masses which are of variable echogenicity, but generally iso- to hyperechoic. This appearance should prompt intraoperative frozen section biopsy, since if the diagnosis is confirmed radical orchiectomy can be averted

Testicular Mass Due to Disseminated Malignancy

Lymphoma and leukemia are the most common extratesticular malignancies to cause testicular involvement. Lymphoma accounts for 1%-7% of all testicular tumors, and is a frequent cause of testicular enlargement in men over 50 years (Figure 91). The testis is usually involved secondary to systemic disease, it is sometimes a site of post-chemotherapy recurrence, and rarely is the primary organ. Involvement is bilateral, either simultaneous or successive, in 50% of cases. Leukemic infiltration is usually seen in children, and the testis is the most common site of relapse of acute leukemia. About 50% of patients have bilateral involvement. Gray-scale sonography of both lymphomatous and leukemic testicular involvement typically shows diffuse or multifocal decreased echogenicity, which can be more subtle and ill-defined than the typical well-circumscribed hypoechoic mass of primary testicular malignancy. Lymphomatous and leukemic testicular involvement is generally hypervascular on color Doppler sonography, irrespective of tumor size or extent. This is in contrast to primary tumors, which are usually hypovascular on color Doppler when under 1.6 cm, and hypervascular when over 1.6 cm. These findings may help suggest the diagnosis in the appropriate clinical setting.

Nonlymphomatous metastases to the testes are rare, and usually incidental autopsy findings. Reported autopsy rates vary from 0.02%-2.5%. A more recent autopsy study of 1715 solid extratesticular malignancies showed metastases to the testes in 16 (0.9%). Of these, only 6 (38%) were macroscopically evident. The common primary sites are lung, prostate, stomach and large bowel—accounting for 75% of cases (Figure 92). Rare but reported primary tumors are melanoma, renal cell carcinoma, pancreatic carcinoma, adrenocortical carcinoma, transitional cell carcinoma and cholangiocarcinoma. Neuroblastoma and Wilm's tumor are possible primary sites in children. Imaging findings of metastases to the testes have not been specifically described.

Neuroblastoma

Neuroblastoma is a primitive neuroectodermal tumor arising from the sympathetic nervous system. It may occur anywhere in the neck, thorax, abdomen or pelvis, with approximately one-third occurring in the adrenal glands. Neuroblastoma is the second most common solid tumor of childhood. There is a slight male predominance, and incidence is increased in neurofibromatosis. 25% occur in the first year of life, and up to 60% occur in the first 2 years of life. The usual presentation is an incidentally discovered abdominal mass, often by a parent. Plain radiographs are often helpful in diagnosis as at least half of these tumors contain calcium, which is usually stippled but may be linear or ring-shaped (Figure 93). This is in distinction to Wilms' tumor, which rarely calcifies (5% or less). Other plain film findings include paravertebral widening bony destruction or widening of the interpedicular distances. Ultrasound can usually distinguish neuroblastoma from other solid abdominal masses. IVU has some value in differentiating neuroblastoma from Wilms' tumor when this distinction is unclear. Neuroblastoma classically displaces the kidney without distorting the renal collecting system, while the collecting system is usually deformed by Wilms' tumor. In addition, the kidney may appear displaced laterally with neuroblastoma. CT is the imaging procedure of choice in evaluating patients with neuroblastoma (Figure 94). CT is able to depict the full extent of the lesion, including vascular encasement and metastases. Up to 85% of tumors are calcified on CT. While helpful, the role of MRI in the evaluation of patients with neroblastoma has yet to be determined (Figure 95).

Nephroblastoma (Wilms' tumor)

Wilms' tumor is the most common renal neoplasm in children with a peak incidence at 2 years of age. Nearly 50% of cases occur prior to 3 years of age and 75% before 5 years of age (the tumor is rare in newborns). Patients present with an abdominal mass (90%), hypertension (50%), pain and/or gross hematuria. The tumor is bilateral in 5%-10% of cases. Bilateral tumors are virtually always associated with nephroblastomatosis. Nephroblastomatosis is the presence of multiple or diffuse nephrogenic rests, embryonal tumors that result from abnormal renal histogenesis and are precursor of Wilms' tumor. It is characterized by the presence of multiple, well-defined round or ovoid foci in the periphery of the renal cortex (Figure 96). The tumor may spread to paraaortic and renal hilar nodes, lung, bones (less common) and liver. Hepatic or pulmonary metastases are found in 30% of patients at presentation. The lesion may also invade vascular structures. Syndromes associated with an increased incidence of Wilms' include: Beckwith-Wiedemann syndrome, hemihypertrophy, sporadic aniridia, Drash syndrome and chromosome 11 deletion.

Radiological evaluation demonstrates an intrarenal mass, and the initial study is generally an abdominal ultrasound (Figure 97). The tumor can appear evenly echogenic, but more echolucent areas representing necrosis may be seen. US can also be used to evaluate the renal vein or inferior vena cava for tumor extension. When a tumor is identified within the inferior vena cava, the proximal extent of the thrombus must be established prior to operation. Cardiac extension of such a tumor thrombus may produce few or no signs, but it can, on rare occasion, be responsible for sudden death following manipulation and embolization of the tumor at laparotomy. CT of the abdomen usually shows the tumor to be a large, complex renal mass, which is typically sharply marginated (Figure 98).

Renal Ectopia

As the fetal kidneys ascend from their pelvic position to meet the adrenal glands, each kidney acquires blood supply from the neighboring vessels. The initial supply from the external and internal iliac vessels is lost during this process, and blood supply directly from the aorta is acquired in the 8th week of development. Any abnormality in acquiring such blood supply or an abnormality of the spine may prevent cephalic migration from occurring. This will result in a renal ectopia or an abnormal position of the kidney. The findings on urography depend on the degree of renal function in the pelvic kidney and the presence of associated abnormalities. On sonography, the reniform mass will be present in the pelvis with a characteristic pattern of renal sinus echoes. A functioning mass of renal parenchyma can be usually identified on CT. Ectopic kidneys are more susceptible to infection, obstruction, blunt trauma and inadvertent intraoperative injury. The most common renal ectopia is the pelvic kidney (Figure 99), which is often associated with conditions like ureteropelvic junction obstruction, reflux, infection and urolithasis. Vascular supply to the kidney is from a low-lying renal artery either from the aorta or iliac vessels. Multiple renal vessels are common. Bilateral pelvic kidneys are rare. Due to its characteristic central sinus complex and corticomedullary differentiation, it is easily distinguished from a primary pelvic tumor on ultrasound. Crossed renal ectopia is the term used when both kidneys lie on the same side and can be fused or nonfused, fused being more common (Figure 100). The vascular supply is often anomalous and varying degrees of malrotation are seen. Thoracic kidney is an uncommon anomaly where the kidney lies above the diaphragm, having herniated through the foramen of Bochdalek. Vessels may come off from the high abdominal or thoracic aorta.

Horseshoe Kidney

Horseshoe kidney is a congenital anomaly in which the kidneys are connected by an isthmus, usually in the lower poles. The band of parenchymal tissue has its own blood supply. In some cases, the connecting band consists purely of fibrous tissue. It is thought to occur due to an abnormal position of the umbilical artery which disturbs the normal cephalad migration of the kidneys, so that it stops at the inferior mesenteric artery. The blood supply is usually from multiple arteries including the aorta, the inferior vena cava, the common external and internal iliac arteries and the inferior mesenteric artery. The isthmus is usually in front of the aorta and inferior vena cava. Horseshoe kidney is the most common congenital anomaly of renal form, occurring in 1 in 400 births with a 2:1 male predominance, without clear evidence of hereditary transmission. One-third of patients remain asymptomatic, while the remainder may have calculi (75% metabolic, 25% struvite), infection or obstruction. One-third may have an associated ureteropelvic junction obstruction. Patients are also more prone to injury from blunt abdominal trauma. There is an increased incidence of malignancy in horseshoe kidneys. On intravenous urography, the kidneys are malrotated with the lower poles rotated medially (Figure 101). The pelves are rotated anteriorly, with the lower calyces projected more medially than the ureter. The diagnosis may be difficult to make on ultrasound. Both CT (Figure 102) and MRI demonstrate the positional abnormality of the kidneys and the connecting band.

Reflux

Vesicoureteral reflux is the retrograde passage of urine from the bladder into the ureter. This is abnormal, because the normal vesicoureteral reflux junction acts as a 1-way valve, allowing the normal antegrade passage of urine into the bladder, but preventing flow in the reverse direction. Vesicoureteral reflux may be primary or secondary. Primary vesicoureteral reflux is common in childhood, and is believed to be due to a developmental deficiency in the muscle layer of the ureterotrigonal region. Familial cases have been described. Other congenital causes of vesicoureteral reflux include: complete ureteral duplication (reflux typically occurs into the ureter of the lower pole moiety), ectopic ureter, prune belly syndrome and congenital (Hutch) periureteral diverticulum. Acquired causes include bladder wall edema or fibrosis, prostatectomy, bladder neck incision and ureteral reimplantation. Vesicoureteral reflux is a potentially serious condition, because it may lead to renal damage by allowing reflux of infected urine from the bladder to the kidney, which results in pyelonephritis, or by allowing transmission of bladder voiding pressures to the kidneys, causing hydronephrosis. Resulting renal disease is known as reflux nephropathy. Patients may present with pyelonephritis, cystitis or uremic symptoms. Asymptomatic pyelonephritis may be discovered as an incidental finding on routine urinalysis. The incidence of vesicoureteral reflux in healthy children is under 1%, but is 20%-50% in children with urinary tract infection.

The definitive test for the diagnosis of reflux is conventional contrast cystogram (Figure 103). Films are taken during bladder filling, during voiding and after voiding. An international grading system has come into general use for the assessment of the severity of reflux, which allows objective comparison of therapeutic modalities. In grade I reflux, contrast refluxes into the ureter only, opacifying part or all of the ureter. In grade II reflux, contrast reaches the renal pelvis, which is not dilated. In grade III reflux, contrast reaches the renal pelvis, with mild dilatation of the ureter and pelvicaliceal system. In grade IV reflux, there is moderate pelviureteroectasis, with obliteration of the forniceal angles but preservation of the papillary impressions. In grade V reflux, there is moderate-to-severe pelviureteroectasis, with near complete or complete obliteration of the papillary impressions. (Reflux may also be demonstrated by voiding radionuclide cystography; it is sometimes detected by ultrasound.) Vesicoureteral reflux may be unilateral, bilateral or intermittent. Children with lower grades of primary vesicoureteral reflux can often be successfully managed with medical treatment, with spontaneous resolution as they grow up. Other children may require surgery.

Ureterocele

Ureterocele is a dilatation of the distal end of the ureter where it enters the bladder. It may be uni- or bilateral. This is usually thought to be caused by narrowing of the ureteral orifice. The back pressure causes the bulging of the lower ureter into the bladder. This is commonly associated with duplex kidneys, in which case this is always associated with the upper element of the duplex. It can be seen, however, at the lower end of a singleton ureter (orthotopic ureterocele). Ureterocele is the primary consideration for a filling defect in the pediatric bladder, and the diagnosis can be easily confirmed by ultrasound (Figure 104). Ureteroceles may be detected as an incidental "cobra-head" appearance of the distal ureter at IVU (Figure 105). These vary in size with ureteral peristalsis. When small they may not be clearly visible, unless observed for a period of time when ureteral peristalsis will cause distension of the distal ureter and the ureterocele within the bladder. When renal function is good, these can also be demonstrated by excretory urography as a thin-walled structure within the bladder. When large and poorly functioning, they can be seen as a negative filling defect on micturating cystourethrography but can easily be masked by the dense contrast during this examination.

Posterior Urethral Valves

Posterior urethral valves are anomalous developmental mucosal folds in the prostatic urethra, and are the embryological equivalent of the hymen in females. Posterior urethral valves are the most common cause of urethral obstruction in children, with an incidence of 1 in 5000-8000 male births. The clinical presentation of posterior urethral valves is highly variable, and related to the degree of obstruction. Severe cases may cause intrauterine or postnatal death. Antenatal ultrasound may suggest the diagnosis by demonstrating bilateral hydroureteronephrosis, an enlarged bladder and oligohydramnios. After birth, children may present with mild-to-severe symptoms of outflow obstruction. The urinary stream is often poor and dribbling. Hydronephrotic kidneys may be palpable, as may the enlarged bladder. Occasionally, the only clinical feature may be failure to thrive. Urinary tract infections may occur, as may renal impairment or failure. Voiding cystourethrography is the definitive radiographic study (Figure 106). The posterior urethra is elongated and dilated, with a prominent bladder neck. The valves may be seen as linear radiolucent defects. Typically, retrograde urethrography is normal, because the retrograde flow compresses the valves against the urethral wall. In posterior urethral valves, the dilated prostatic urethra has a cylindrical outline with a rounded inferior margin, whereas in bladder neck dysfunction, the dilated urethra has a triangular configuration with a sharp inferior beak. However, endoscopy may be required for definitive distinction between these 2 conditions.

13. References

Imaging Modalities for Uroradiology

1. Cohan RH, Sherman LS, Korobkin M, Bass JC, Francis IR. Renal masses: assessment of corticomedullary-phase and nephrographic-phase CT scans. *Radiology*. 1995;196:445-451.

2. Chow LC, Sommer FG. Multidetector CT urography with abdominal compression and three-dimensional reconstruction. *Am J Roentgenol*. 2001;177:849-855.

3. B. Tippins, William E. Torres, Bruce R. Baumgartner, Deborah A. Are Screening Serum Creatinine Levels Necessary prior to Outpatient CT Examinations? *Radiology*. 2000;216:481-484.

4. American College of Radiology. *Manual on Contrast Media*. Edition 4.1, 1998 (revised 2001).

5. Tepel M, van der Giet M, Schwarzfeld C, Laufer U, Liermann D, Zidek W. Prevention of radiographic-contrast-agent-induced reductions in renal function by acetylcysteine. *N Engl J Med*. 2000;343:180-184.

6. Solomon R, Werner C, Mann D, et al. Effects of saline, mannitol, and furosemide to prevent acute decreases in renal function induced by radiocontrast agents. *N Engl J Med*. 1994;331:1416-1420.

7. Merten GJ, Burgess WP, Gray LV, et al. Prevention of contrast-induced nephropathy with sodium bicarbonate: a randomized controlled trial. *JAMA*. 2004;291:2328-2334.

8. Siegle RL, Halvorsen RA, Dillon J, et al. The use of iohexol in patients with previous reactions to ionic contrast material. A multicenter clinical trial. *Inv Radiol*. 1991;26:411-416.

9. Dawson P, Sidhu PS. Is there a role for corticosteroid prophylaxis in patients at increased risk of adverse reactions to intravascular contrast agents? *Clin Radiol*. 1993;48:225-226.

10. Katayama H, Yamaguchi K, Kozuka T, Takashima T, Seez P, Matsuura K. Adverse reactions to ionic and nonionic contrast media. A report from the Japanese Committee on the Safety of Contrast Media. *Radiology*. 1990;175:621-628.

11. Lasser EC, Berry CC, Mishkin MM, et al. Pretreatment with corticosteroids to prevent adverse reactions to nonionic contrast media. *AJR*. 1994;162:523-526.

12. Public Health Advisory—Gadolinium-containing Contrast Agents for Magnetic Resonance Imaging (MRI): Omniscan, OptiMARK, Magnevist, ProHance, and MultiHance. Available at http://www.fda.gov/Drugs/DrugSafety/PostmarketDrugSafetyInformationforPatientsand-Providers/ucm142882.htm. Accessed June 7, 2009..

13. Public Health Advisory—Update on Magnetic Resonance Imaging (MRI) Contrast Agents Containing Gadolinium and Nephrogenic Fibrosing Dermopathy. Available at http://www.fda.gov/Drugs/DrugSafety/PublicHealthAdvisories/ucm124344.htm. Accessed June 7, 2009.

14. Sadowski EA, Bennett LK, Chan MR, et al. Nephrogenic Systemic Fibrosis: Risk Factors and Incidence Estimation. *Radiology*. 2007;243(1):148-157.

15. Broome DR, Girguis MS, Baron PW, Cottrell AC, Kjellin I, Kirk GA. Gadodiamide-associated nephrogenic systemic fibrosis: why radiologists should be concerned. AJR *Am J Roentgenol*. 2007;188:586-592.

Adrenal Masses

1. Lee MJ, Hahn PF, Papanicolaou N, et al. Benign and malignant adrenal masses: CT distinction with attenuation coefficients, size, and observer analysis. *Radiology*. 1991;179:415-418.

2. Korobkin M, Brodeur FJ, Yutzy GG, et al. Differentiation of adrenal adenomas from nonadenomas using CT attenuation values. AJR *Am J Roentgenol*. 1996;166:531-536.

3. Korobkin M, Brodeur FJ, Francis IR, Quint LE, Dunnick NR, Goodsitt M. Delayed enhanced CT for differentiation of benign from malignant adrenal masses. *Radiology*. 1996;200:737-742.

4. Korobkin M, Brodeur FJ, Francis IR, Quint LE, Dunnick NR, Londy F. CT time-attenuation washout curves of adrenal adenomas and nonadenomas. *Am J Roentgenol*. 1998;170:747-752.

5. Szolar DH, Kammerhuber FH. Adrenal adenomas and nonadenomas: assessment of washout at delayed contrast-enhanced CT. *Radiology*. 1998; 207:369-375.

6. Caoili EM, Korobkin M, Francis IR, Cohan RH, Platt JF, Dunnick NR, Raghupathi KI. Adrenal masses: characterization with combined unenhanced and delayed enhanced CT. *Radiology*. 2002;222:629-633.

7. Mayo-Smith WW, Lee MJ, McNicholas MM, Hahn PF, Boland GW, Saini S. Characterization of adrenal masses (< 5 cm) by use of chemical shift MR imaging: observer performance versus quantitative measures. *Am J Roentgenol*. 1995;165:91-95.

8. Schwartz LH, Panicek DM, Koutcher JA, et al. Adrenal masses in patients with malignancy: prospective comparison of echo-planar, fast spin-echo, and chemical shift MR imaging. *Radiology*. 1995;197:421-425.

9. Young WF Jr. Minireview: Primary Aldosteronism - Changing Concepts in Diagnosis and Treatment. *Endocrinology*. 2003;144:2208-2213

10. Berkman WA, Bernardino ME, Sewell CW, Price RB, Sones PJ Jr. The computed tomography-guided adrenal biopsy. An alternative to surgery in adrenal mass diagnosis. *Cancer*. 1984;53:2098-2103.

11. Gollub MJ, Bosniak MA, Schlossberg P, Chachoua A. Extension of a secondary adrenal neoplasm into the inferior vena cava. *Abdom Imaging*. 1994;19:359-360.

12. Mukherjee JJ, Peppercorn PD, Reznek RH, et al. Pheochromocytoma: effect of nonionic contrast medium in CT on circulating catecholamine levels. *Radiology* 1997;202:227-231.

13. Casola G, Nicolet V, vanSonnenberg E, et al. Unsuspected pheochromocytoma: risk of blood-pressure alterations during percutaneous adrenal biopsy. *Radiology*. 1986;159:733-755.

14. Ferrozzi F, Bova D. CT and MR demonstration of fat within an adrenal cortical carcinoma. *Abdom Imaging*. 1995;20:272-274.

15. Schlund JF, Kenney PJ, Brown ED, Ascher SM, Brown JJ, Semelka RC. Adrenocortical carcinoma: MR imaging appearance with current techniques. *JMRI*.1995;5:171-174.

16. Lumachi F, Tregnaghi A, Zucchetta P, et al. Sensitivity and positive predictive value of CT, MRI and 123I-MIBG scintigraphy in localizing pheochromocytomas: a prospective study. *Nucl Med Commun*. 2006;27:583-587.

17. Koizumi M, Endo K, Sakahara H, Nakashima T, Nakano Y, Nakao K, Torizuka K. Computed tomography and 131I-MIBG scintigraphy in the diagnosis of pheochromocytoma. *Acta Radiol Diagn (Stockh)*. 1986;27:305-309.

18. Lee JE, Evans DB, Hickey RC, Sherman SI, Gagel RF, Abbruzzese MC, Abbruzzese JL. Unknown primary cancer presenting as an adrenal mass: frequency and implications for diagnostic evaluation of adrenal incidentalomas. *Surgery*. 1998;124:1115-1122.

19. Warshauer DM, McCarthy SM, Street L, et al. Detection of renal masses: sensitivities and specificities of excretory urography/linear tomography, US, and CT. *Radiology*. 1988;169:363-365.

20. Birnbaum BA, Jacobs JE, Ramchandani P. Multiphasic renal CT: comparison of renal mass enhancement during the corticomedullary and nephrographic phases. *Radiology*. 1996;200:753-758.

21. Davidson AJ, Hartman DS, Choyke PL, Wagner BJ. Radiologic assessment of renal masses: implications for patient care. *Radiology*. 1997;202:297-305.

22. Macari M, Bosniak MA. Delayed CT to evaluate renal masses incidentally discovered at contrast-enhanced CT: demonstration of vascularity with deenhancement. *Radiology*. 1999;213:674-680.

23. Ho VB, Allen SF, Hood MN, Choyke PL. Renal Masses: Quantitative Assessment of Enhancement with Dynamic MR Imaging. *Radiology*. 2002;224:695-700.

Renal Masses

1. Macari M, Bosniak MA. Delayed CT to evaluate renal masses incidentally discovered at contrast-enhanced CT: demonstration of vascularity with deenhancement. *Radiology*. 1999;213:674-680.

2. Birnbaum BA, Maki DD, Chakraborty DP, Jacobs JE, Babb JS. Renal cyst pseudoenhancement: evaluation with an anthropomorphic body CT phantom. *Radiology*. 2002;225:83-90.

3. Jayson M, Sanders H. Increased incidence of serendipitously discovered renal cell carcinoma. *Urology*. 1998;51:203-205.

4. Stanley, RJ. Inherent dangers in radiologic screening. *Am J Roentgenol*. 2001;177:989-992.

5. Lee CT, Katz J, Fearn PA, Russo P. Mode of presentation of renal cell carcinoma provides prognostic information. *Urol Oncol*. 2002;7:135-140.

6. Robson CJ, Churchill BM, Anderson W. The results of radical nephrectomy for renal cell carcinoma. *J Urol*. 1969;101:297-301.

7. Tongaonkar HB, Dandekar NP, Dalal AV, Kulkarni JN, Kamat MR. Renal cell carcinoma extending to the renal vein and inferior vena cava: results of surgical treatment and prognostic factors. *J Surg Oncol*. 1995;59:94-100.

8. Kallman DA, King BF, Hattery RR, et al. Renal vein and inferior vena cava tumor thrombus in renal cell carcinoma: CT, US, MRI and venacavography. *J Comput Assist Tomogr*. 1992;16:240-247.

9. Studer UE, Scherz S, Scheidegger J, et al. Enlargement of regional lymph nodes in renal cell carcinoma is often not due to metastases. *J Urol*. 1990;144:243-245.

10. Kim JK, Park SY, Shon JH, Cho KS. Angiomyolipoma with minimal fat: differentiation from renal cell carcinoma at biphasic helical CT. *Radiology*. 2004;230:677-684.

11. Paivansalo M, Lahde S, Hyvarinen S, Kallioinen M, Jalovaara P. Renal angiomyolipoma. Ultrasonographic, CT, angiographic, and histologic correlation. *Acta Radiol*. 1991;32:239-243.

12. Siegel CL, Middleton WD, Teefey SA, McClennan BL. Angiomyolipoma and renal cell carcinoma: US differentiation. *Radiology*. 1996;198:789-793.

13. Outwater EK, Bhatia M, Siegelman ES, Burke MA, Mitchell DG. Lipid in renal clear cell carcinoma: detection on opposed-phase gradient-echo MR images. *Radiology*. 1997;205:103-107.

14. Newhouse JH, Wagner BJ. Renal oncocytomas. *Abdom Imaging*. 1998;23:249-255.

15. Urban BA, Buckley J, Soyer P, Scherrer A, Fishman EK. CT appearance of transitional cell carcinoma of the renal pelvis: Part 1. Early-stage disease. *Am J Roentgenol*. 1997;169:157-161.

16. Urban BA, Buckley J, Soyer P, Scherrer A, Fishman EK. CT appearance of transitional cell carcinoma of the renal pelvis: Part 2. Advanced-stage disease. *Am J Roentgenol*. 1997;169:163-168.

17. Uzzo RG, Cherullo EE, Myles J, Novick AC. Renal cell carcinoma invading the urinary collecting system: implications for staging. *J Urol*. 2002;167:2392-2396.

18. Palapattu GS, Pantuck AJ, Dorey F, Said JW, Figlin RA, Belldegrun AS. Collecting system invasion in renal cell carcinoma: impact on prognosis and future staging strategies. *J Urol*. 2003;170:768-772.

19. Urban BA, Fishman EK. Renal lymphoma: CT patterns with emphasis on helical CT. *Radiographics*. 2000;20:197-212.

20. Choyke PL, White EM, Zeman RK, Jaffe MH, Clark LR. Renal metastases: clinicopathologic and radiologic correlation. *Radiology*. 1987;162:359-363.

21. Helenon O, Merran S, Paraf F, et al. Unusual fat-containing tumors of the kidney: a diagnostic dilemma. *Radiographics*. 1997;17:129-144.

22. Tada S, Yamagishi J, Kobayashi H, Hata Y, Kobari T. The incidence of simple renal cyst by computed tomography. *Clin Radiol*. 1983;34:437-439.

23. Davidson AJ, Hartman DS, Choyke PL, Wagner BJ. Radiologic assessment of renal masses: implications for patient care. *Radiology*. 1997;202:297-305.

24. Curry NS, Bissada NK. Radiologic evaluation of small and indeterminant renal masses. *Urol Clin North Am*. 1997;24:493-505.

25. Davidson AJ, Hartman DS, Choyke PL, Wagner BJ. Radiologic assessment of renal masses: implications for patient care. *Radiology*. 1997; 202:297-305.

26. Rosenberg ER, Korobkin M, Foster W, Silverman PM, Bowie JD, Dunnick NR. The significance of septations in a renal cyst. *Am J Roentgenol*. 1985;144:593-595.

27. Wolf JS Jr. Evaluation and management of solid and cystic renal masses. *J Urol*. 1998;159:1120-1133.

28. Curry NS, Cochran ST, Bissada NK. Cystic renal masses: accurate Bosniak classification requires adequate renal CT. *Am J Roentgenol*. 2000; 175:339-342.

29. Davidson AJ, Hartman DS, Choyke PL, Wagner BJ. Radiologic assessment of renal masses: implications for patient care. *Radiology*. 1997; 202:297-305.

30. Rosenberg ER, Korobkin M, Foster W, Silverman PM, Bowie JD, Dunnick NR. The significance of septations in a renal cyst. *Am J Roentgenol*. 1985;144:593-595.

31. Onishi T, Oishi Y, Goto H, Tomita M, Abe K, Sugaya S. Cyst-associated renal cell carcinoma: clinicopathologic characteristics and evaluation of prognosis in 27 cases. *Int J Urol*. 2001;8:268-274.

32. Hartman DS, Weatherby E 3rd, Laskin WB, Brody JM, Corse W, Baluch JD. Cystic renal cell carcinoma: CT findings simulating a benign hyperdense cyst. *Am J Roentgenol*. 1992;159:1235-1237.

33. Koga S, Nishikido M, Inuzuka S, Sakamoto I, Hayashi T, Hayashi K, Saito Y, Kanetake H. An evaluation of Bosniak's radiological classification of cystic renal masses. *BJU Int*. 2000;86:607-609.

34. Israel GM, Bosniak MA. Follow-up CT of moderately complex cystic lesions of the kidney (Bosniak category IIF). *Am J Roentgenol.* 2003; 181:627-633.

35. Bosniak MA, Birnbaum BA, Krinsky GA, Waisman J. Small renal parenchymal neoplasms: further observations on growth. *Radiology.* 1995; 197:589-597.

36. Rendon RA, Stanietzky N, Panzarella T, Robinette M, Klotz LH, Thurston W, Jewett MA. The natural history of small renal masses. *J Urol.* 2000;164:1143-1147.

37. Siegel CL, McFarland EG, Brink JA, Fisher AJ, Humphrey P, Heiken JP. CT of cystic renal masses: analysis of diagnostic performance and interobserver variation. *Am J Roentgenol.* 1997;169:813-818.

38. Han KR, Janzen NK, McWhorter VC, et al. Cystic renal cell carcinoma: biology and clinical behavior. *Urol Oncol.* 2004;22:410-414.

Renal Calcification and Urinary Stones

1. Abramson S, Walders N, Applegate KE, Gilkeson RC, Robbin MR. Impact in the emergency department of unenhanced CT on diagnostic confidence and therapeutic efficacy in patients with suspected renal colic: a prospective survey. 2000 ARRS President's Award. American Roentgen Ray Society. *Am J Roentgenol.* 2000;175:1689-1695.

2. Thornbury JR, Parker TW. Ureteral calculi. *Semin Roentgenol.* 1982;17:133-138.

3. Svedstrom E, Alanen A, Nurmi N. Radiologic diagnosis of renal colic: The role of plain films, excretory urography, and sonography. *Eur J Radiol.*1990;11:180-183.

4. Laing FC, Jeffrey RB, Wing VW. Ultrasound versus excretory urography in evaluating acute flank pain. *Radiology.* 1985;154:613-616.

5. Juul N, Brons J, Torp-Pedersen S, Fredfeldt KE. Ultrasound versus intravenous urography in the evaluation of patients with suspected obstructing urinary calculi. *Scand J Urol Nephrol.* 1991; supple 137:45-47.

6. Rodgers PM, Bates JA, Irving HC. Intrarenal Doppler ultrasound studies in normal and acutely obstructed kidneys. *Brit J Radiol.* 1992;65:207-212.

7. Niall O, Russell J, MacGregor R, Duncan H, Mullins J. A comparison of noncontrast computerized tomography with excretory urography in the assessment of acute flank pain. *J Urol.* 1999;161:534-537.

8. Smith RC, Rosenfield AT, Choe KA, et al. Acute flank pain: Comparison of non contrast-enhanced CT and intravenous urography. *Radiology.* 1995;194:789.

9. Coll DM, Varanelli MJ, Smith RC. Relationship of spontaneous passage of ureteral calculi to stone size and location as revealed by unenhanced helical CT. *Am J Roentgenol.* 2002;178:101-103.

10. Fielding JR, Silverman SG, Samuel S, Zou KH, Loughlin KR. Unenhanced helical CT of ureteral stones: a replacement for excretory urography in planning treatment. *Am J Roentgenol.* 1998;171:1051-1053.

11. Sourtzis S, Thibeau JF, Damry N, Raslan A, Vandendris M, Bellemans M. Radiologic investigation of renal colic: unenhanced helical CT compared with excretory urography. *Am J Roentgenol.* 1999;172:1491-1494.

12. Smith RC, Verga M, McCarthy S, Rosenfield AT. Diagnosis of acute flank pain: value of unenhanced helical CT. *Am J Roentgenol.* 1996; 166:97-101.

13. Reiter WJ, Schon-Pernerstorfer H, Dorfinger K, Hofbauer J, Marberger M. Frequency of urolithiasis in individuals seropositive for human immunodeficiency virus treated with indinavir is higher than previously assumed. *J Urol*. 1999;161:1082-1084.

14. Schwartz BF, Schenkman N, Armenakas NA, Stoller ML. Imaging characteristics of indinavir calculi. *J Urol*. 1999;161:1085-1087.

15. Bruce GR, Munch LC, Hoven AD, et al. Urolithiasis associated with the protease inhibitor indinavir. *Urology*. 1997;50:513-518.

16. Blake SP, McNicholas MM, Raptopoulos V. Nonopaque crystal deposition causing ureteric obstruction in patients with HIV undergoing indinavir therapy. *Am J Roentgenol*. 1998;171:717-720.

17. Leroy AJ. Diagnosis and treatment of nephrolithiasis: Current perspectives. *Am J Roentgenol*. 1994;163:1309-1313.

18. Amis ES, Newhouse JH. Urinary stone disease. In Amises, Newhouse JH (eds): *Essentials of Uroradiology*. Boston, MA: Little Brown; 1991: 213-231.

19. Heneghan JP, Dalrymple NC, Verga M, Rosenfield AT, Smith RC. Soft-tissue "rim" sign in the diagnosis of ureteral calculi with use of unenhanced helical CT. *Radiology*. 1997;202:709-711.

20. Guest AR, Cohan RH, Korobkin M, et al. Assessment of the clinical utility of the rim and comet-tail signs in differentiating ureteral stones from phleboliths. *Am J Roentgenol*. 2001;177:1285-1291.

Renal Infection and Infarction

1. Morehouse HT, Weiner SN, Hoffman JC. Imaging in inflammatory disease of the kidney. *Am. J. Roentgenol*. 1984;143:135-141.

2. Piccirillo M, Rigsby C, Rosenfield AT. Contemporary imaging of renal inflammatory disease. *Infect Dis Clin North Am*. 1987;1:927-964.

3. Browne RF, Zwirewich C, Torreggiani WC. Imaging of urinary tract infection in the adult. *Eur Radiol*. 2004;14:E168-E183.

4. Grayson DE, Abbott RM, Levy AD, Sherman PM. Emphysematous infections of the abdomen and pelvis: a pictorial review. *Radiographics*. 2002;22:543-561.

5. Roy C, Pfleger DD, Tuchmann CM, Lang HH, Saussine CC, Jacqmin D. Emphysematous pyelitis: findings in five patients. *Radiology*. 2001;218:647-650.

6. Joseph RC, Amendola MA, Artze ME, et al. Genitourinary tract gas: imaging evaluation. *Radiographics*. 1996;16:295-308.

7. Wan YL, Lee TY, Bullard MJ, Tsai CC. Acute gas-producing bacterial renal infection: correlation between imaging findings and clinical outcome. *Radiology*. 1996;198:433-438.

8. Zorzos I, Moutzouris V, Korakianitis G, Katsou G. Analysis of 39 cases of xanthogranulomatous pyelonephritis with emphasis on CT findings. *Scand J Urol Nephrol*. 2003;37:342-347.

9. Goldman SM, Hartman DS, Fishman EK, Finizio JP, Gatewood OM, Siegelman SS. CT of xanthogranulomatous pyelonephritis: radiologic-pathologic correlation. *Am J Roentgenol*. 1984;142:963-969.

10. Hayes WS, Hartman DS, Sesterbenn IA. From the Archives of the AFIP. Xanthogranulomatous pyelonephritis. *Radiographics*. 1991;11:485-498.

11. Erden A, Fitoz S, Karagulle T, Tukel S, Akyar S. Radiological findings in the diagnosis of genitourinary candidiasis. *Pediatr Radiol.* 2000;30:875-877.

12. Morris BS, Chudgar PD, Manejwala O. Primary renal candidiasis: fungal mycetomas in the kidney. *Australas Radiol.* 2002;46:57-59.

13. Dembner AG, Pfister RC. Fungal infection of the urinary tract: demonstration by antegrade pyelography and drainage by percutaneous nephrostomy. *Am. J. Roentgenol.* 1977;129:415-418.

14. Kale H, Narlawar RS, Rathod K. Renal fungal ball: an unusual sonographic finding. *J Clin Ultrasound.* 2002;30:178-180.

15. Suzer O, Shirkhoda A, Jafri SZ, Madrazo BL, Bis KG, Mastromatteo JF. CT features of renal infarction. *Eur J Radiol.* 2002;44:59-64.

16. Harris RD, Dorros S. Computed tomographic diagnosis of renal infarction. *Urology.* 1981;17:287-289.

17. Glazer GM, Francis IR, Brady TM, Teng SS. Computed tomography of renal infarction: clinical and experimental observations. *Am J Roentgenol.* 1983;140:721-727.

18. Harris RD, Dorros S, Scheible FW. Appearance of renal infarction on computed tomography. *Comput Radiol.* 1983;7:181-187.

19. Kamel IR, Berkowitz JF. Assessment of the cortical rim sign in posttraumatic renal infarction. *J Comput Assist Tomogr.* 1996;20:803-806.

20. Wong WS, Moss AA, Federle MP, Cochran ST, London SS. Renal infarction: CT diagnosis and correlation between CT findings and etiologies. *Radiology.* 1984;150:201-205.

21. Yucel C, Ozdemir H, Akpek S, Gurel K, Kapucu LO, Arac M. Renal infarct: contrast-enhanced power Doppler sonographic findings. *J Clin Ultrasound.* 2001;29:237-242.

Renal Trauma

1. Moore EE, Shackford SR, Pachter HL, et al. Organ injury scaling: spleen, liver, and kidney. *J Trauma.* 1989;29:1664-1666.

2. Haas CA, Dinchman KH, Nasrallah PF, Spirnak JP. Traumatic renal artery occlusion: a 15-year review. *J Trauma.* 1998;45:557-561.

3. Knudson MM, Harrison PB, Hoyt DB, et al. Outcome after major renovascular injuries: a Western trauma association multicenter report. *J Trauma.* 2000;49:1116-1122.

4. Bertini JE, Flechner SM, Miller P. The natural history of traumatic branch renal artery injury. *J Urol.* 1986;135:228-230.

5. Boone TB, Gilling PJ, Husmann DA. Ureteropelvic junction disruption following blunt abdominal trauma. *J Urol.* 1993; 150:33-36.

6. Bretan PN, McAninch JW, Federle MP. Computerized tomographic staging of renal trauma: 85 consecutive cases. *J Urol.* 1986;136:561-565.

7. Carroll PR, McAninch JW, Klosterman P. Renovascular trauma: risk assessment, surgical management, and outcome. *J Trauma.* 1990;30:547-552.

8. Cass AS, Luxenberg M, Gleich P. Clinical indications for radiographic evaluation of blunt renal trauma. *J Urol.* 1986;136:370-371.

9. Corr P, Hacking G. Embolization in traumatic intrarenal vascular injuries. *Clin Radiol.* 1991;43:262-264.

10. Dinkel HP, Danuser H, Triller J. Blunt renal trauma: minimally invasive management with microcatheter embolization experience in nine patients. *Radiology.* 2002;223:723-730.

11. Federle MP, Kaiser JA, McAninch JW. The role of computed tomography in renal trauma. *Radiology.* 1981;141:455-460.

12. Hagiwara A, Sakaki S, Goto H. The role of interventional radiology in the management of blunt renal injury: a practical protocol. *J Trauma*. 2001;51:526-531.

13. Harris AC, Zwirewich CV, Lyburn ID. Ct findings in blunt renal trauma. *Radiographics*. 2001;21:S201-S214.

14. Jeffrey RB, Cardoza JD, Olcott EW: Detection of active intraabdominal arterial hemorrhage: value of dynamic contrast-enhanced CT. *Am J Roentgenol*. 1991;156:725-729.

15. Kamel IR, Berkowitz JF. Assessment of the cortical rim sign in posttraumatic renal infarction. *J Comput Assist Tomogr*. 1996;20:803-806.

16. Kawashima A, Sandler CM, Corriere JN: Ureteropelvic junction injuries secondary to blunt abdominal trauma. *Radiology*. 1997;205:487-492.

17. Kenney PJ, Panicek DM, Witanowski LS. Computed tomography of ureteral disruption. *J Comput Assist Tomogr*. 1987;11:480-484.

18. Lane MJ, Katz DS, Shah RA. Active arterial contrast extravasation on helical CT of the abdomen, pelvis, and chest. *Am J Roentgenol*. 1998; 171:679-685.

19. McAndrew JD, Corriere JN. Radiographic evaluation of renal trauma: evaluation of 1103 consecutive patients. *Br J Urol*. 1994;73:352-354.

20. McAninch JW, Federle MP. Evaluation of renal injuries with computerized tomography. *J Urol*. 1982;128:456-460.

21. McGahan JP, Richards JR, Jones CD. Use of ultrasonography in the patient with acute renal trauma. *J Ultrasound Med*. 1999;18:207-213; quiz 215-216.

22. Morey AF, McAninch JW, Tiller BK. Single shot intraoperative excretory urography for the immediate evaluation of renal trauma. *J Urol*. 1999; 161: 1088-92.

23. Moudouni SM, Patard JJ, Manunta A: A conservative approach to major blunt renal lacerations with urinary extravasation and devitalized renal segments. *BJU Int*. 2001; 87: 290-4.

24. Nicolaisen GS, McAninch JW, Marshall GA: Renal trauma: re-evaluation of the indications for radiographic assessment. *J Urol*. 1985; 133: 183-7].

25. Santucci RA, McAninch JM: Grade IV renal injuries: evaluation, treatment, and outcome. *World J Surg*. 2001; 25: 1565-72.

Ureteral Disease

1. Lawler LP, Jarret TW, Corl FM, Fishman EK. Adult ureteropelvic junction obstruction: insights with three-dimensional multi-detector row CT. *Radiographics*. 2005;25:121-134.

2. Khaira HS, Platt JF, Cohan RH, Wolf JS, Faerber GJ. Helical computed tomography for identification of crossing vessels in ureteropelvic junction obstruction-comparison with operative findings. *Urology*. 2003;62:35-39.

3. Mitsumori A, Yasui K, Akaki S, et al. Evaluation of crossing vessels in patients with ureteropelvic junction obstruction by means of helical CT. *Radiographics*. 2000;20:1383-1393.

4. Dyer RB, Chen MY, Zagoria RJ. Classic signs in uroradiology. *Radiographics*. 2004;24:S247-S280.

5. Fritz GA, Schoellnast H, Deutschmann HA, Quehenberger F, Tillich M. Multiphasic multidetector-row CT (MDCT) in detection and staging of transitional cell carcinomas of the upper urinary tract. *Eur Radiol*. 2006;16:1244-1252.

6. Gonzalez Resina R, Rodriguez Corchero J, Campoy Martinez P, et al. Transitional cell carcinoma of the upper urinary tract: spectrum of imaging findings. *Radiographics*. 2005;25:1609-1627.

7. Baron RL, McClennan BL, Lee JK, Lawson TL. Computed tomography of transitional-cell carcinoma of the renal pelvis and ureter. *Radiology*. 1982;144:125-130.

8. Harvin HJ. Ureteral fibroepithelial polyp on MDCT urography. *Am J Roentgenol*. 2006;187:W434-W435.

9. Bellin MF, Springer O, Mourey-Gerosa I, et al. CT diagnosis of ureteral fibroepithelial polyps. *Eur Radiol*. 2002;12:125-128.

10. Stukart RA, van Haga JJ, Bruijnes E. Fibroepithelial ureteral polyps. *Urol Int*. 1984;39:336-338.

Bladder Disease

1. Caskurlu T, Tasci AL, Sevin G, Cek M, Carbone A, Gezeroglu H. The role of trans-rectal echography (TRE) in the evaluation and staging of bladder tumors: comparison with suprapubic echography and computerized axial tomography. *Arch Ital Urol Androl*. 1998;70:1-6.

2. Ravi R, Rao RC, Ahlawat R, Berry M. Carcinoma bladder: comparative evaluation of urinary cytology, excretory urography and ultrasonography. *Indian J Cancer*. 1990;27:55-61.

3. Voges GE, Tauschke E, Stockle M, Alken P, Hohenfellner R. Computerized tomography: an unreliable method for accurate staging of bladder tumors in patients who are candidates for radical cystectomy. *J Urol*. 1989;142:972-974.

4. Amendola MA, Glazer GM, Grossman HB, Aisen AM, Francis IR. Staging of bladder carcinoma: MRI-CT-surgical correlation. *Am J Roentgenol*. 1986;146:1179-1183.

5. Fisher MR, Hricak H, Tanagho EA. Urinary bladder MR imaging. Part II. Neoplasm. *Radiology*. 1985;157:471-477.

Prostatic Disease

1. Coakley FV, Hricak H. Radiologic anatomy of the prostate gland: A clinical approach. *Radiologic Clinics of North America*. 2000;38:15-30.

2. Scheckowitz EM, Resnick MI. Imaging of the prostate. Benign prostatic hyperplasia. *Urol Clin North Am*. 1995;22:321-332.

3. Grossfeld GD, Coakley FV. Benign prostatic hyperplasia: clinical overview and value of diagnostic imaging. *Radiol Clin North Am*. 2000;38:31-47.

4. Boczko J, Messing E, Dogra V. Transrectal sonography in prostate evaluation. *Radiol Clin North Am*. 2006;44:679-687.

5. Littrup PJ, Bailey SE. Prostate cancer: the role of transrectal ultrasound and its impact on cancer detection and management. *Radiol Clin North Am*. 2000;38:87-113.

6. McClennan BL. Diagnostic imaging evaluation of benign prostatic hyperplasia. *Urol Clin North Am*. 1990;17:517-536.

7. Rajesh A, Coakley FV. MR imaging and MR spectroscopic imaging of prostate cancer. *Magn Reson Imaging Clin N Am*. 2004;12:557-79.

8. Coakley FV, Qayyum A, Kurhanewicz J. Magnetic resonance imaging and spectroscopic imaging of prostate cancer. *J Urol*. 2003;170:S69-S75.

Urethral Disease

1. Sung DJ, Kim YH, Cho SB, et al. Obliterative urethral stricture: MR urethrography versus conventional retrograde urethrography with voiding cystourethrography. *Radiology*. 2006;240:842-848.

2. Kawashima A, Sandler CM, Wasserman NF, LeRoy AJ, King BF Jr, Goldman SM. Imaging of urethral disease: a pictorial review. *Radiographics*. 2004;24:S195-S216.

3. Gallentine ML, Morey AF. Imaging of the male urethra for stricture disease. *Urol Clin North Am*. 2002;29:361-372.

4. Kim B, Hricak H, Tanagho EA. Diagnosis of urethral diverticula in women: value of MR imaging. *Am J Roentgenol*. 1993;161:809-815.

5. Neitlich JD, Foster HE Jr, Glickman MG, Smith RC. Detection of urethral diverticula in women: comparison of a high resolution fast spin echo technique with double balloon urethrography. *J Urol*. 1998;159:408-410.

6. Hricak H, Secaf E, Buckley DW, Brown JJ, Tanagho EA, McAninch JW. Female urethra: MR imaging. *Radiology*. 1991;178:527-535.

7. Jacoby K, Rowbotham RK. Double balloon positive pressure urethrography is a more sensitive test than voiding cystourethrography for diagnosing urethral diverticulum in women. *J Urol*. 1999;162:2066-2069.

8. Ryu J, Kim B. MR imaging of the male and female urethra. *Radiographics*. 2001;21:1169-1185.

9. Choudhary S, Singh P, Sundar E, Kumar S, Sahai A. A comparison of sonourethrography and retrograde urethrography in evaluation of anterior urethral strictures. *Clin Radiol*. 2004;59:736-742.

10. McAninch JW, Laing FC, Jeffrey RB Jr. Sonourethrography in the evaluation of urethral strictures: a preliminary report. *J Urol*. 1988;139: 294-297.

11. Golomb J, Leibovitch I, Mor Y, Morag B, Ramon J. Comparison of voiding cystourethrography and double-balloon urethrography in the diagnosis of complex female urethral diverticula. *Eur Radiol*. 2003;13:536-542.

12. Heidenreich A, Derschum W, Bonfig R, Wilbert DM. Ultrasound in the evaluation of urethral stricture disease: a prospective study in 175 patients. *Br J Urol*. 1994;74:93-98.

13. Gupta N, Dubey D, Mandhani A, Srivastava A, Kapoor R, Kumar A. Urethral stricture assessment: a prospective study evaluating urethral ultrasonography and conventional radiological studies. *BJU Int*. 2006;98:149-153.

14. Narumi Y, Hricak H, Armenakas NA, Dixon CM, McAninch JW. MR imaging of traumatic posterior urethral injury. *Radiology*. 1993;188:439-443.

15. Dixon CM, Hricak H, McAninch JW. Magnetic resonance imaging of traumatic posterior urethral defects and pelvic crush injuries. *J Urol*. 1992;148:1162-1165.

Testicular Masses

1. Silverberg E. Cancer in young adults (ages 15 to 34). *CA*. 1982;32:32-42.

2. Bree RL, Hoang DT. Scrotal ultrasound. *Rad Clin N Am*. 1996;34:1183-1205.

3. Hricak H, Hamm B, Kim B. *Imaging of the Scrotum: Textbook and Atlas*. New York, NY: Raven Press; 1995: 49-93.

4. Yalowitz BR, Eble JN, Wilks DC. Spermatozoa-containing simple cysts of the rete testis. *J Urol*. 1989;142:1572-1573.

5. Brown DL, Benson CB, Doherty FJ, et al. Cystic testicular mass caused by dilated rete testis: sonographic findings in 31 cases. *AJR*. 1992; 158:1257-1259.

6. Tartar VM, Trambert MA, Balsara ZN, et al. Tubular ectasia of the testis: sonographic and MR imaging appearance. *AJR*. 1993;160:539-542.

7. Thomas RD, Dewbury KC. Ultrasound appearance of the rete testis. *Clin Radiol*. 1993;47:121-124.

8. Price EB. Epidermoid cysts of the testis: A clinical and pathological analysis of 69 cases from the testicular tumour registry. *J Urol*. 1969;102:708.

9. Sanderson AJ, Birch BR, Dewbury KC. Case report: Multiple epidermoid cysts of the testes - the ultrasound appearances. *Clin Rad*. 1995;50:414-415.

10. Maxwell AJ, Mamtora H. Sonographic appearance of epidermoid cyst of the testis. *J Clin* Ultrasound. 1990;18:188-190.

11. Malvica RP. Epidermoid cyst of the testicle: An unusual sonographic finding. *AJR*. 1993;160:1047-1048.

12. Meiches MD, Nurenburg MD. Sonographic appearance of a calcified simple epidermoid cyst of the testis. *J Clin Ultrasound*. 1991;19:498-500.

13. Bahnson RR, Slasky BS, Ernstoff MD, et al. Sonographic characteristics of epidermoid cyst of the testicle. *Uroradiology*. 1990;35:508.

14. Cohen EL, Mandel E, Goodman JD, et al. Epidermoid cyst of the testicle: ultrasonographic characteristics. *Urology*. 1984;24:79-81.

15. Heidenreich A, Engelman UH, Vietsch HV, et al. Organ preserving surgery in testicular epidermoid cysts. *J Urol*. 1995;153:1147-1150.

16. Kressel K, Schnell D, Thon WF, et al. Benign testicular tumors: a case for testis preservation? *Eur Urol*. 1988;15:200-204.

17. Burt AD, Cooper G, MacKay C, et al. Dermoid cyst of the testis. *Scot Med J*. 1987;32:146-148.

18. Avery GR, Peakman DJ, Young JR. Unusual hyperechoic ultrasound appearance of testicular Leydig cell tumour. *Clin Radiol*. 1991;43:260-261.

19. Brosman SA. Testicular tumors in prepubertal children. *Urology*. 1979;13:581-588.

20. Liu P, Thorner P. Sonographic appearance of Sertoli cell tumour: with pathologic correlation. *Pediatr Radiol*. 1993;23:127-128.

21. Noszian IM, Balon R, Eitelberger FG, et al. Bilateral testicular large-cell calcifying Setoli cell tumor and recurrent cardiac myxoma in a patient with Carney's complex. *Pediatr Radiol*. 1995;25:S236-S237.

22. Mackay B, Bennington JL, Skoglund RW. The adenomatoid tumor: fine structural evidence for a mesothelial origin. *Cancer*. 1971;27:109-115.

23. Feuer A, Dewire DM, Foley WD. Ultrasonographic characteristics of testcular adenomatoid tumors. *J Urol*. 1996;155:174-175.

24. Horstman WG, Sands JP, Hooper DG. Adenomatoid tumor of the testicle. *Urology*. 1992; 40: 359-361.

25. Wheeler JE. Testicular tumors. In: Hill GS, Ed. *Uropathology*. New York, NY: Churchill Livingstone; 1989:1085-1088.

26. Ritzen EM. Testicular relapse of acute lymphoblastic leukemia (ALL). *J Reprod Immunol*. 1990;18:117-121.

27. Musmanno MC, White JM. Scrotal ultrasonography as an adjunct to testis biopsy in leukemia. *Urology*. 1990;35:239-241.

28. Mazzu D, Jeffrey RB, Ralls PW. Lymphoma and leukemia involving the testicles: findings on gray-scale and color Doppler sonography. *AJR*. 1995;164:645-647.

29. Horstman WG, Melson CL, Middleton WD, et al. Testicular tumors: findings with color Doppler US. *Radiology*. 1992;185:733-737.

30. Hanash KA, Carney JA, Kelalis PP. Metastatic tumors to the testicles: routes of metastasis. *J Urol*. 1969;102:465-468.

31. Tiltman AJ. Metastatic tumours in the testis. *Histopathology*. 1979;3:31-37.

32. Grignon DJ,Shum DT, Hayman WP. Metastatic tumours of the testes. *Can J Surg*. 1986;29:359-361.

Pediatric Uroradiology

1. Kirks DR, Merten DF, Grossman H, Bowie JD. Diagnostic imaging of pediatric abdominal masses: an overview. *Radiol Clin North Am*. 1981; 19:527-45.

2. Alexander F. Neuroblastoma. *Urol Clin North Am*. 2000;27:383-92.

3. Lonergan GJ, Schwab CM, Suarez ES, Carlson CL. Neuroblastoma, ganglioneuroblastoma, and ganglioneuroma: radiologic-pathologic correlation. *Radiographics*. 2002;22:911-34.

4. Mehta K, Haller JO, Legasto AC. Imaging neuroblastoma in children. *Crit Rev Comput Tomogr*. 2003;44:47-61.

5. Hugosson C, Nyman R, Jorulf H, McDonald P, Rifai A, Kofide A, Jacobsson B. Imaging of abdominal neuroblastoma in children. *Acta Radiol*. 1999;40:534-542.

6. Riccabona M. Imaging of renal tumours in infancy and childhood. *Eur Radiol*. 2003;13:L116-L129.

7. Goske MJ, Mitchell C, Reslan WA. Imaging of patients with Wilms' tumor. *Semin Urol Oncol*. 1999;17:11-20.

8. Bellin MF, Maidenberg M, Raveau V, et al. MR imaging of adult Wilms' tumor: correlation with US, CT, and pathology. *Urol Radiol*. 1990;12:148-150.

9. Montgomery P, Kuhn JP, Berger PE, Fisher J. Multifocal nephroblastomatosis: clinical significance and imaging. *Pediatr Radiol*. 1984;14:392-395.

10. Fernbach SK, Feinstein KA, Donaldson JS, Baum ES. Nephroblastomatosis: comparison of CT with US and urography. *Radiology*. 1988;166:153-156.

11. Birmole BJ, Borwankar SS, Vaidya AS, Kulkarni BK. Crossed renal ectopia. *J Postgrad Med*. 1993;39:149-151.

12. McCarthy S, Rosenfield AT. Ultrasonography in crossed renal ectopia. *J Ultrasound Med*. 1984;3:107-112.

13. Strauss S, Dushnitsky T, Peer A, Manor H, Libson E, Lebensart PD. Sonographic features of horseshoe kidney: review of 34 patients. *J Ultrasound Med*. 2000;19:27-31.

14. Siegfried MS, Rochester D. Computed tomography appearance of fused (horseshoe) kidney. *J Comput Tomogr*. 1983;7:301-304.

15. Fazio L, Razvi H, Chin JL. Malignancy in horseshoe kidneys: review and discussion of surgical implications. *Can J Urol*. 2003;10:1899-1904.

16. Dacher JN, Hitzel A, Avni FE, Vera P. Imaging strategies in pediatric urinary tract infection. *Eur Radiol*. 2005;15:1283-1288.

17. Riccabona M, Fotter R. Urinary tract infection in infants and children: an update with special regard to the changing role of reflux. *Eur Radiol*. 2004;14:L78-L88.

18. Agrawalla S, Pearce R, Goodman TR. How to perform the perfect voiding cystourethrogram. *Pediatr Radiol*. 2004;34:114-119.

19. Jequier S, Jequier JC. Reliability of voiding cystourethrography to detect reflux. *Am J Roentgenol*. 1989;153:807-810.

20. Kroovand RL. Ureterocele. *Urol Clin North Am*. 1983;10:445-449.

21. Nussbaum AR, Dorst JP, Jeffs RD, Gearhart JP, Sanders RC. Ectopic ureter and ureterocele: their varied sonographic manifestations. *Radiology*. 1986;159:227-235.

22. Griffin J, Jennings C, MacErlean D. Ultrasonic evaluation of simple and ectopic ureteroceles. *Clin Radiol*. 1983;34:55-57.

23. Macpherson RI, Leithiser RE, Gordon L, Turner WR. Posterior urethral valves: an update and review. *Radiographics*. 1986;6:753-759.

14. Figures

Figure 1A

Noncontrast CT image

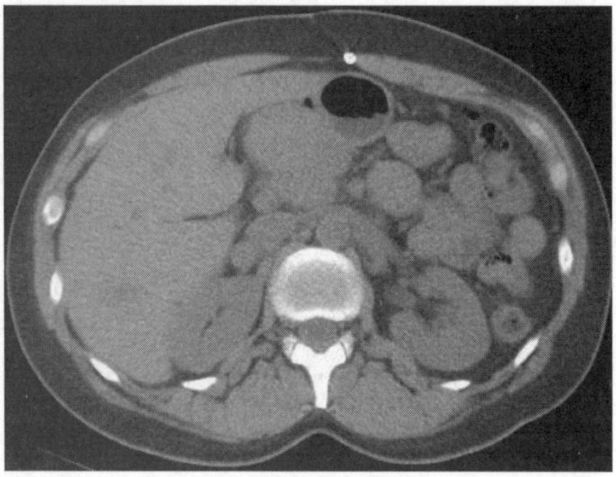

These images are used for detection of urinary stones and other calcifications, and also serve as a baseline for assessment of enhancement when compared to post-contrast images.

Figure 1B

Arteriographic (early arterial phase) CT image

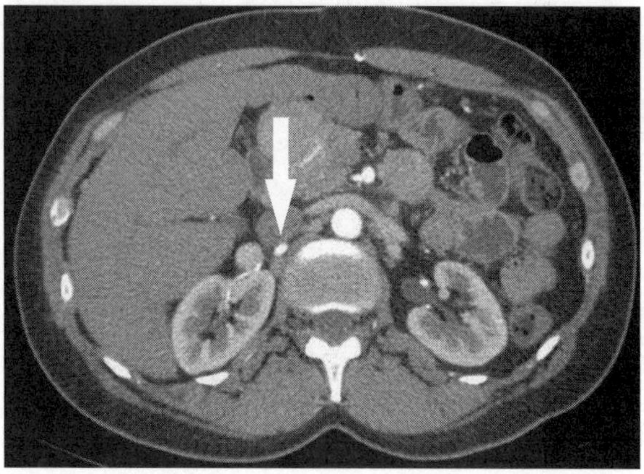

In this phase, contrast is predominantly within the arterial system, as seen in the well-opacified right renal artery (arrow) in this patient.

Figure 1C

Corticomedullary or late arterial phase CT image

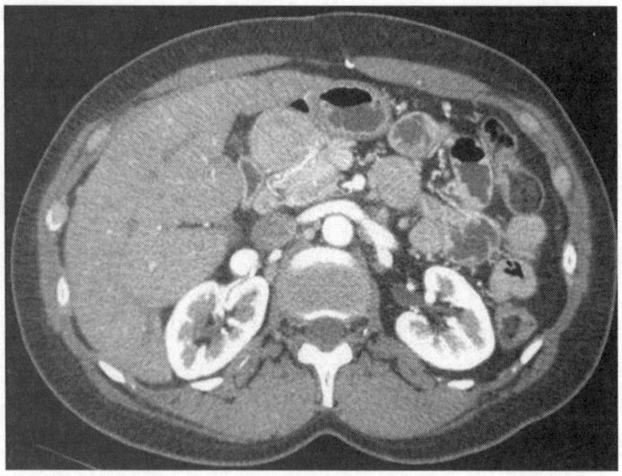

In this phase, the cortex shows marked enhancement, while the medulla remains relatively unenhanced. Arterial opacification remains prominent.

Figure 1D

Nephrographic phase CT image

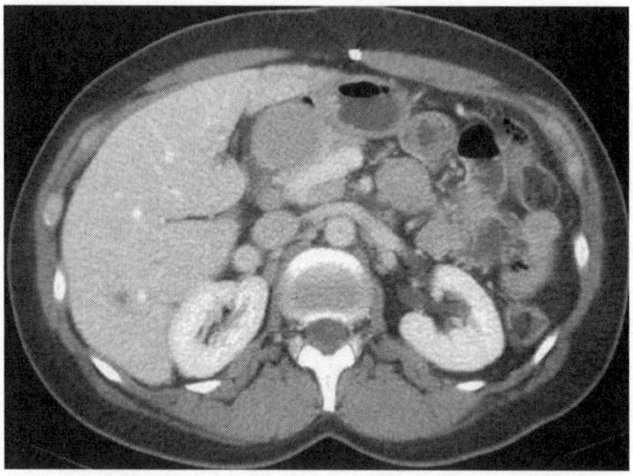

In this phase, the cortex and medulla are isodense. This is the standard phase for the assessment for the abdominal viscera.

Figure 1E

Excretory phase CT image

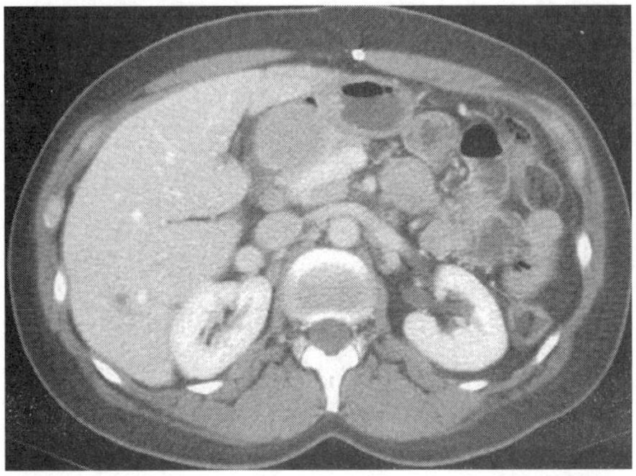

These images are obtained several minutes after the injection of intravenous contrast, and excreted contrast is seen within the collecting systems, as in the left renal pelvis (arrow) of this patient.

Figure 2A

Corticomedullary phase image

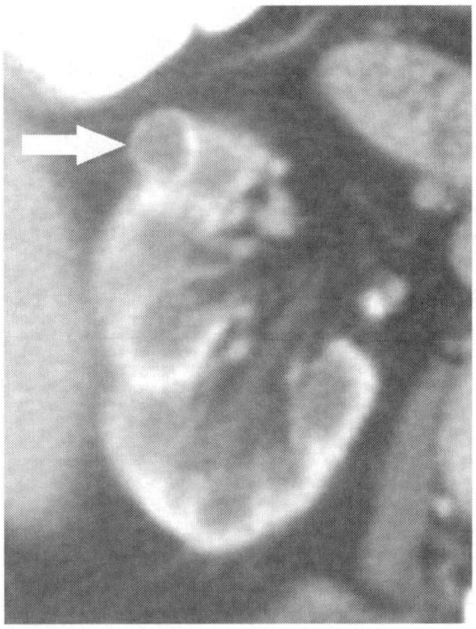

Shows a small renal cell carcinoma (arrow) with a hypervascular rim.

Figure 2B

Nephrographic phase CT image in the same patient

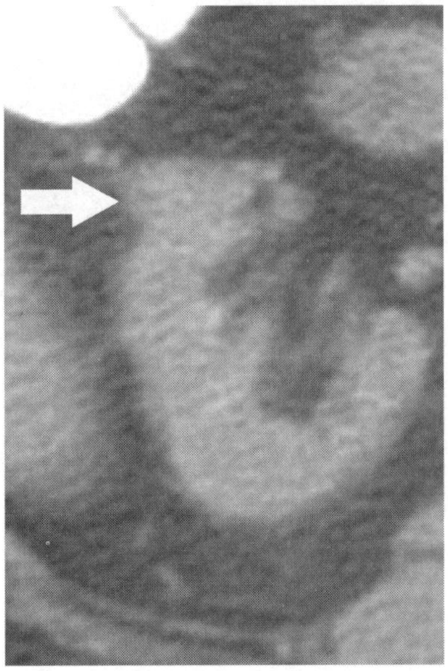

The carcinoma is less appreciable, being visible simply as a contour deformity (arrow). While it is uncommon, a wholly or partially hypervascular renal cell carcinoma is occasionally better seen during the corticomedullary than the nephrographic phase, as in this case.

Figure 3A

Axial CT image in the cortico-medullary phase

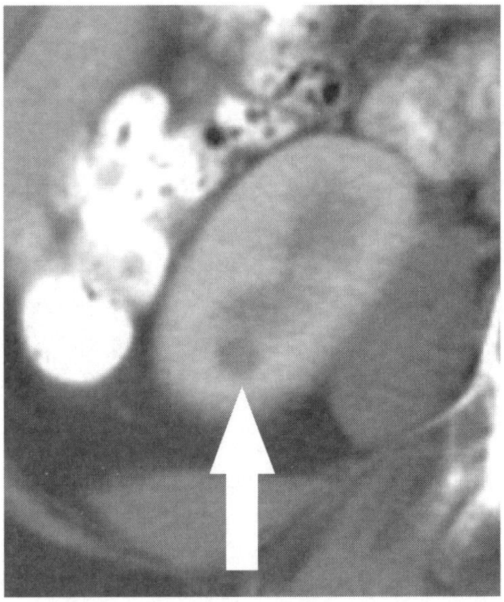

Shows a barely appreciable hypodense lesion (arrow).

Figure 3B

3B Axial CT image in the nephrographic phase

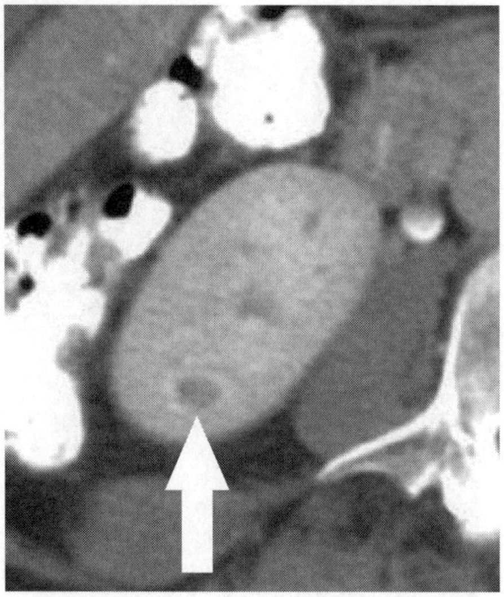

Shows the small hypodense lesion to be more appreciable. In general, renal lesions are better detected on the nephrographic phase than the corticomedullary phase as in this case.

Figure 4A

Schematic illustration demonstrating the traditional approach to a renal protocol CT

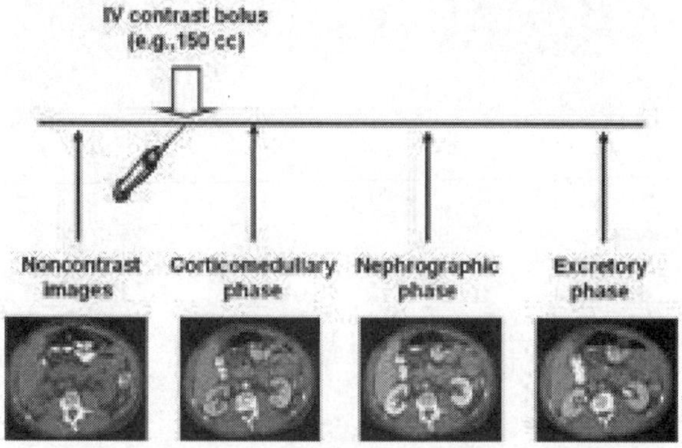

Noncontrast images are acquired followed by administration of intravenous contrast bolus. Subsequently, corticomedullary, nephrographic, and excretory phase images are sequentially acquired.

Figure 4B

Schematic illustration demonstration of the split bolus protocol

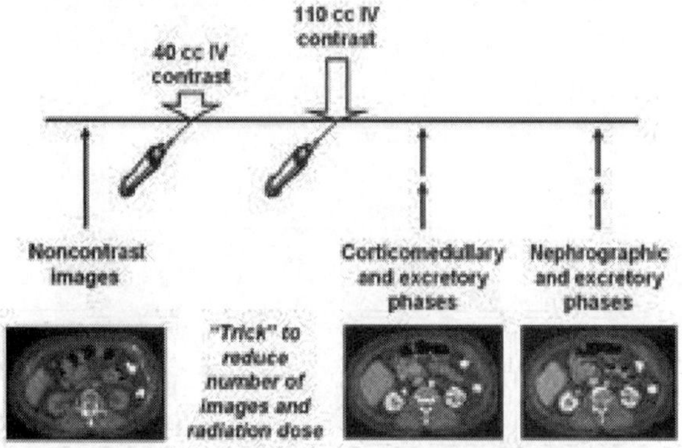

As in the standard protocol, non-contrast images are acquired. Then a small component of the contrast bolus is administered. No images are acquired for the subsequent 4-5 minutes, when the remaining portion of the bolus is administered. Corticomedullary and nephrographic phase images are acquired after the major of the part of the bolus. These images also include an excretory phase, due to excretion of the initially administered smaller part of the contrast bolus. The use of such a split bolus protocol is essentially a trick that reduces the number of images and radiation dose.

Figure 5

Axial contrast-enhanced CT image demonstrating the normal vascular relationships of the adrenal glands

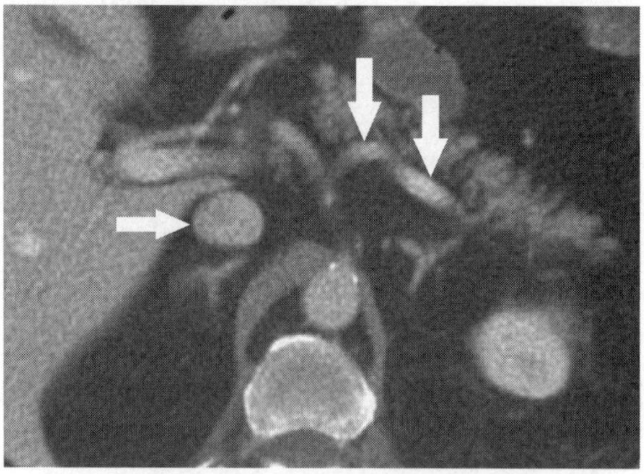

Such images are useful in localizing the adrenal glands in difficult cases or when the anatomy is distorted. Both adrenal glands are seen as V- or Y-shaped structures, the right adrenal gland lying posterior to the inferior vena cava (horizontal arrow) and the left adrenal gland seen posterior to the splenic vessels (vertical arrows).

Figure 6a

Axial non-contrast CT image of a left adrenal adenoma (arrow)

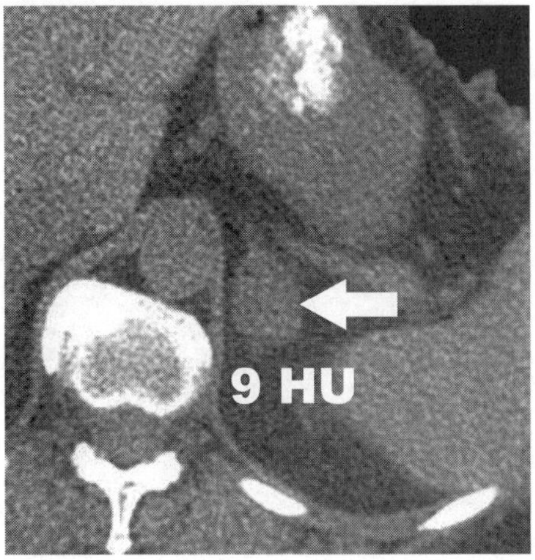

The low density (9 Hounsfield units) of the lesion confirms that it is an adenoma.

Figure 6b

Axial contrast-enhanced CT image in the nephrographic phase

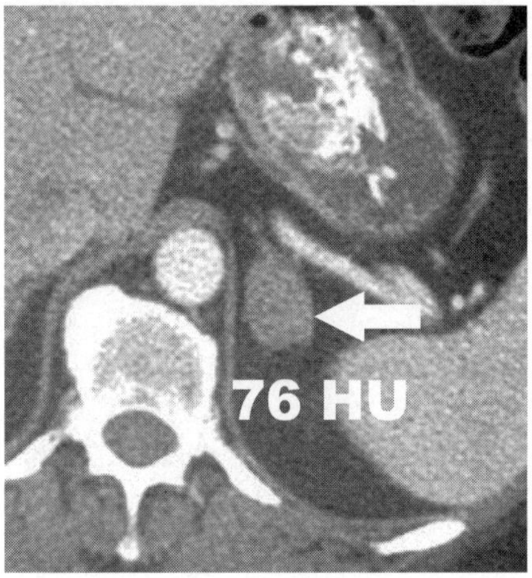

Shows the adenoma (arrow) enhanced, rising to a density of 76 Hounsfield units. In this phase of enhancement, the CT density measurements of adenomas overlap of those of non-adenomas, and do not help in the distinction of these two pathologies.

Figure 6c

15-minute delayed post-contrast-enhanced image

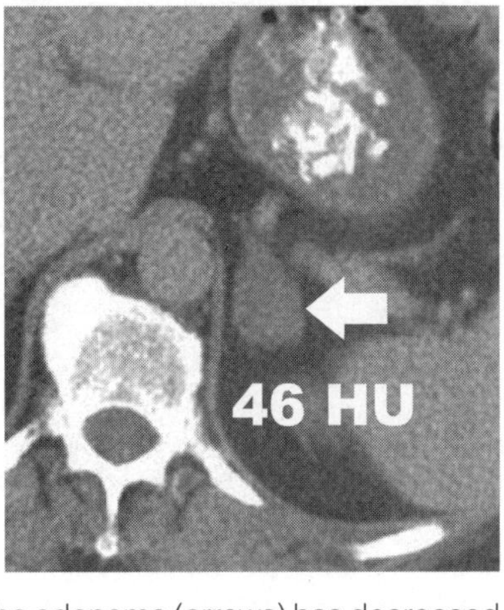

Shows the adenoma (arrows) has decreased in density to 46 Hounsfield units. Such a decrease in density is typical of adenomas, and other adrenal masses such as metastases to the adrenal glands will typically not deenhance to this extend. A density of under 52 Housfield units at 15 minutes is suggestive of an adenoma, as in this case (46 Hounsfield units).

Figure 7A

Non-contrast axial CT image

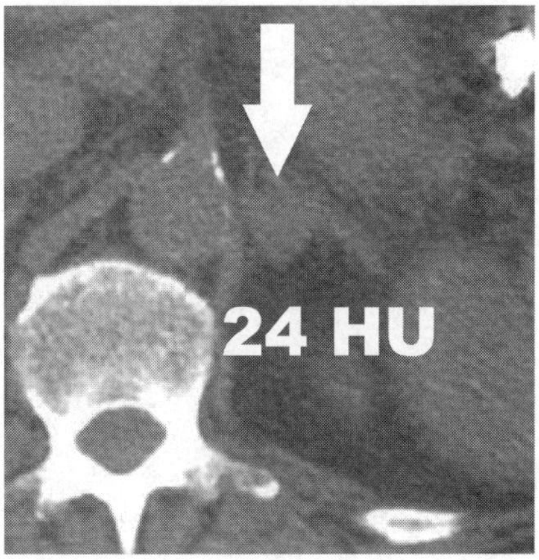

Shows a left adrenal nodule (arrow) that is not of low enough density to be classified as an adenoma.

Figure 7B

Axial post-contrast CT enhanced image

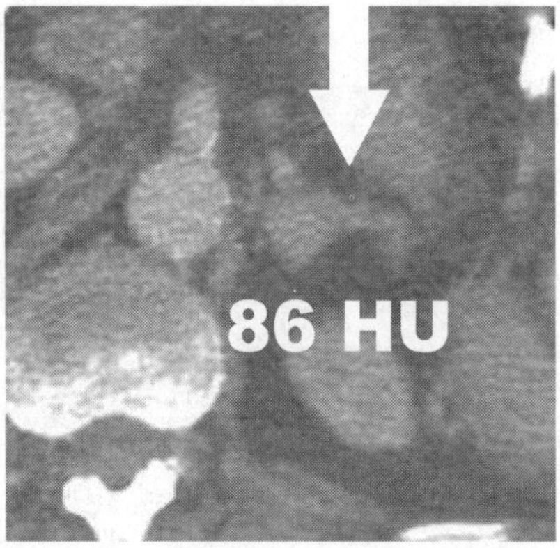

Shows the nodule (arrow) enhancing to a density of 86 Hounsfield units.

Figure 7C

15-minute delayed post-contrast image

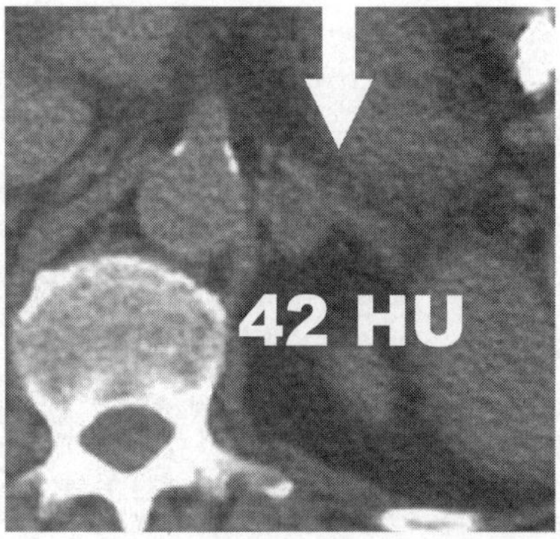

Shows the nodule has decreased to a density of 42 Hounsfield units. Such a decrease in density is indicative of an adenoma, despite the fact that the lesion was not of sufficiently low density on non-contrast images. The wash-out phenomenon can be used to characterize adenomas that cannot be so characterized on non-contrast images (presumably because they are lipid poor).

Figure 8A

Coronal in-phase gradient echo T1-weighted MR image of a right adrenal mass (arrow)

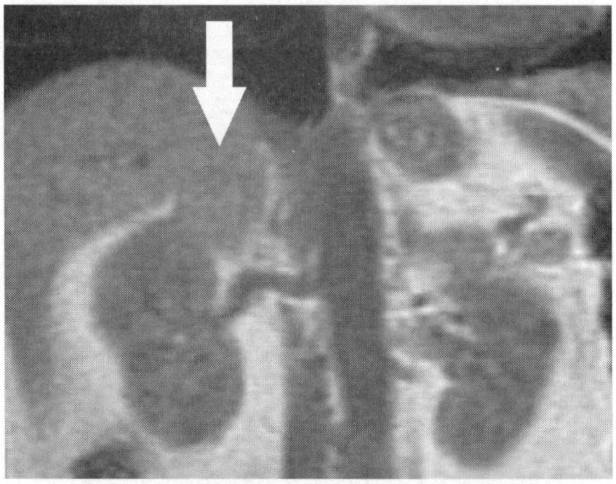

Figure 8B

Coronal opposed-phase gradient echo T1-weighted image

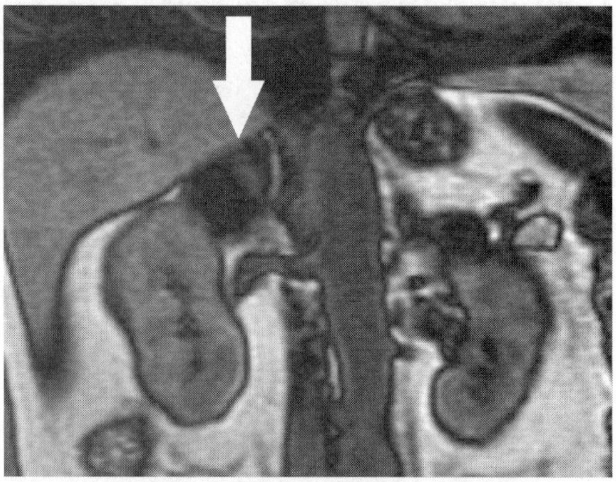

Demonstrates marked signal loss in the mass (arrow), consistent with an adenoma. Such signal loss is characteristic of tissue that contains a substantial amount of microscopic fat, as in adrenal adenomas that are lipid-rich due to their derivation from the adrenal cortex. The characteristic India ink or etching artifact seen at the boundary of the viscera on opposed-phase imaging is distinctive of this sequence, and due to signal loss in boundary voxels that are mixtures of fat (in the retroperitoneum) and water (in the visceral organ).

Figure 9

Axial contrast-enhanced CT image in a patient with Cushing's syndrome

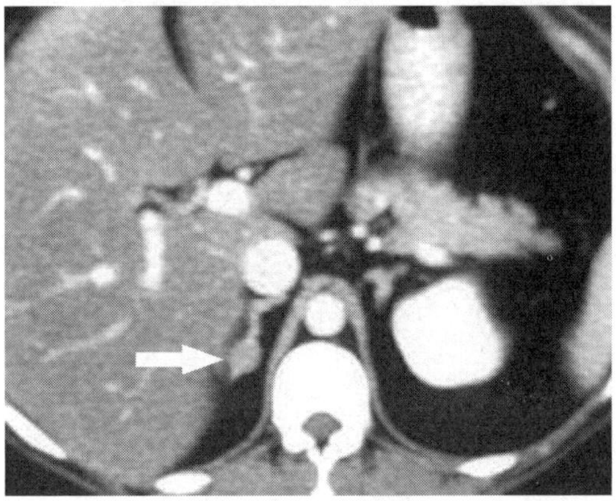

Shows a small unifocal right adrenal nodule (arrow). In the setting of Cushing's syndrome, such a nodule is more likely a focus of hyperplasia induced by excessive ACTH from the pituitary gland.

Figure 10

Figure 10 Axial contrast-enhanced CT image in a patient with Conn's syndrome

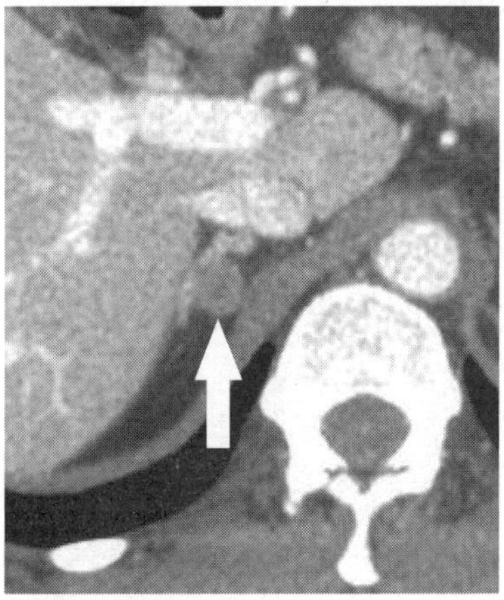

In a patient with Conn's syndrome, even a very small unifocal adrenal nodule (arrow) is likely to be a functional adenoma producing excessive aldosterone (aldostronoma).

Figure 11

Coronal reformatted post-contrast CT image in a patient with a renal cell carcinoma in the upper pole of the left kidney

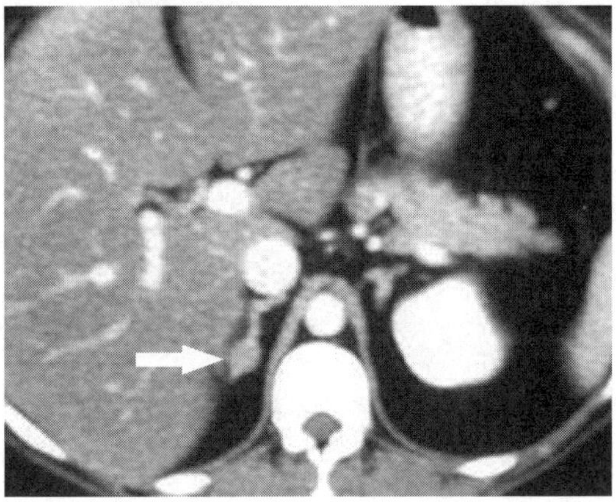

A metastasis (arrow) is visible in the right adrenal gland.

Figure 12A

Axial contrast-enhanced CT image

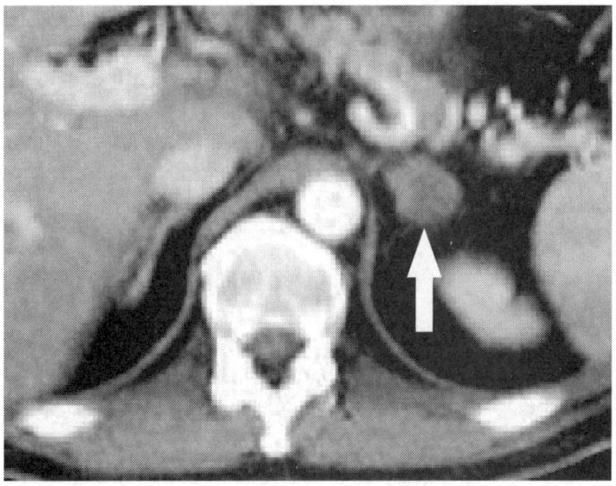

Shows a relatively small uniform adrenal metastases (arrow).

Figure 12B

Axial contrast-enhanced CT image in a different patient showing large heterogeneous bilateral adrenal metastases (arrows)

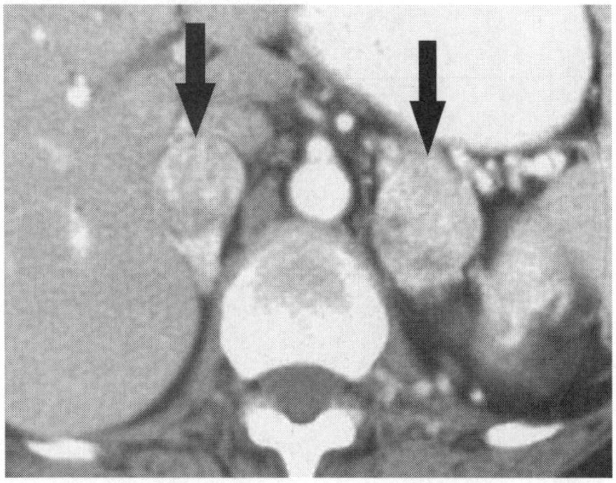

Adrenal metastases have a variable appearance.

Figure 13A

Axial contrast-enhanced CT image showing a small non-specific adrenal nodule (arrow) in a patient with lung cancer.

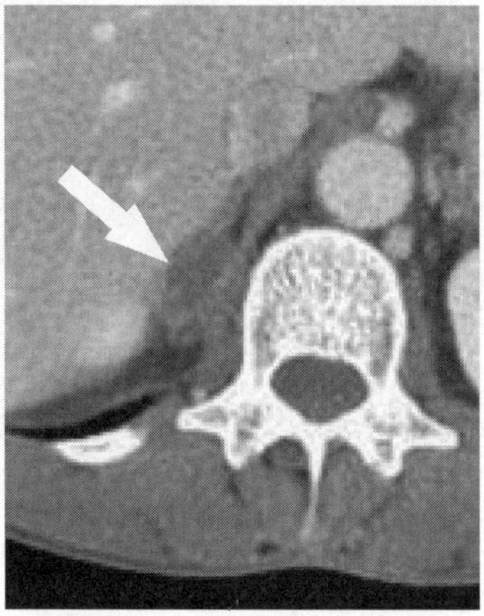

Figure 13B

Axial PET image

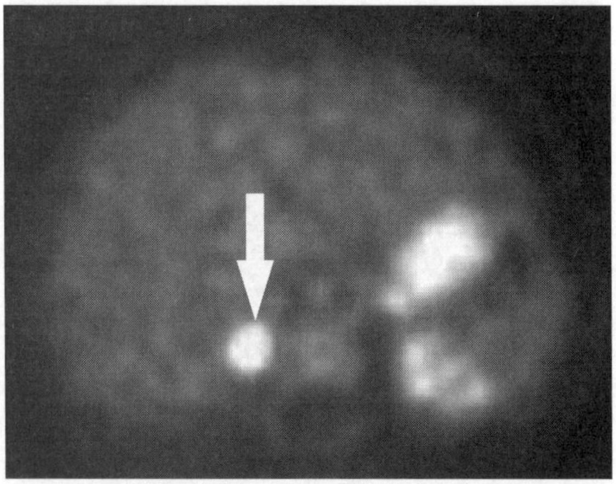

Shows intense uptake within the adrenal nodule (arrow), consistent with a metastatic deposit.

Figure 14

Axial contrast-enhanced CT image in a patient with a left adrenal myelolipoma (arrow)

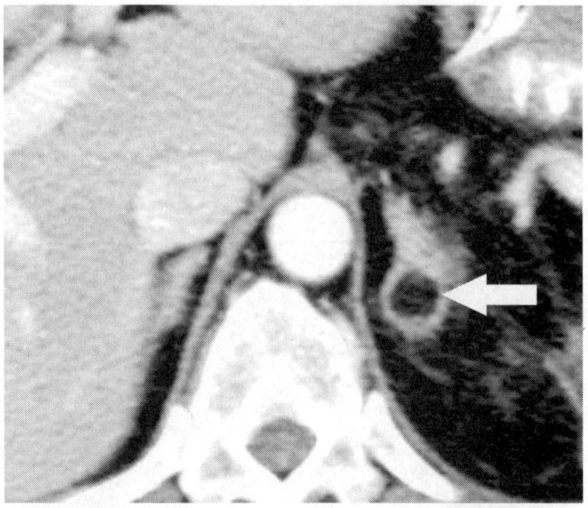

The nodule is clearly of macropscopic fat density, being similar in CT appearance to the adjacent retroperitoneal fat.

Figure 15

Axial T2-weighted image showing a right adrenal pheochromocytoma (arrow)

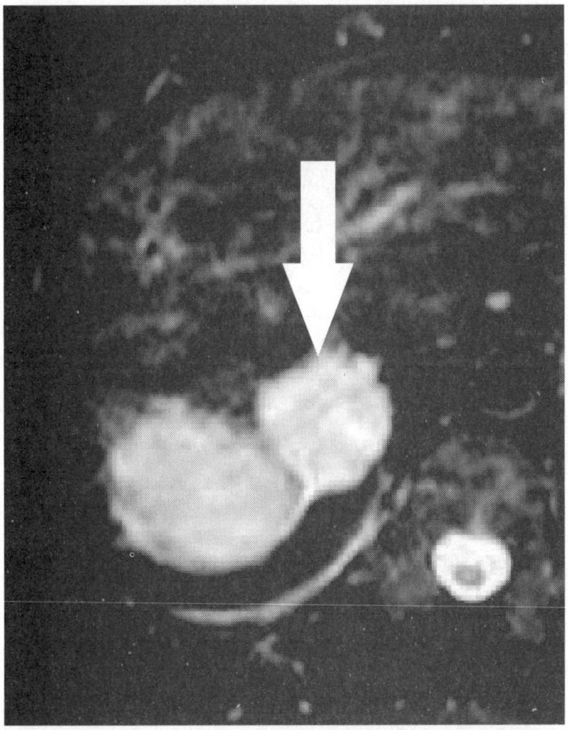

Note that the lesion is of extremely high T2 signal, approaching that of cerebrospinal fluid. This "lightbulb" sign is said to be characteristic of pheochromocytoma, although in practice it is infrequently observed.

Figure 16

Axial T2-weighted MRI image in a patient with a left adrenal pheochromocytoma

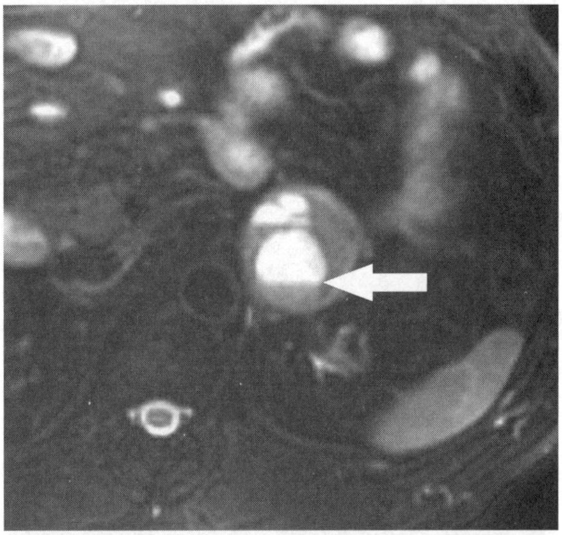

Internal cystic change and hemorrhage is a useful sign that an adrenal mass may be a pheochromocytoma. Note the fluid level (arrow) in this lesion, due to cyst formation with internal hemorrhage.

Figure 17A

Axial T1-weighted post-contrast MRI image showing a relatively non-specific heterogeneously enhancing left adrenal mass (arrow)

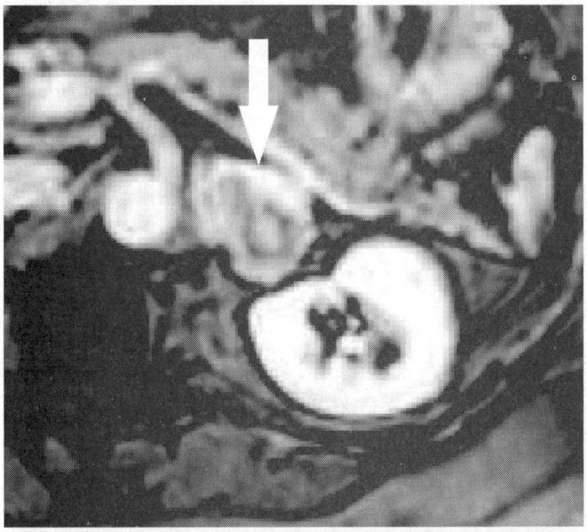

Figure 17B

Coronal image from a MIBG scan in the same patient

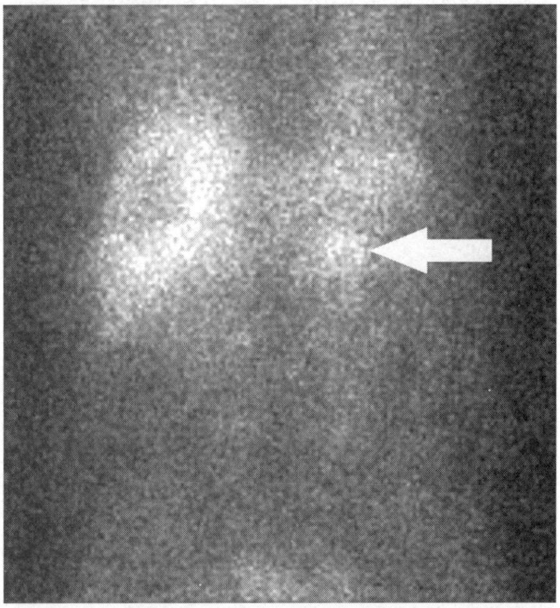

Shows increased uptake within the adrenal lesion (arrow), confirming it is a pheochromocytoma.

Figure 18

Coronal T2-weighted MRI image showing a large heterogeneous mass superior to the left kidney

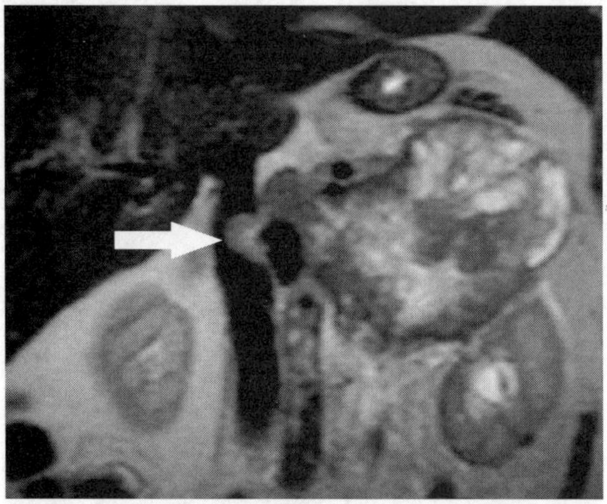

Tumor invasion (arrow) is seen into the inferior vena cava. The finding of venous invasion in association with an adrenal mass is strongly suggestive of an adrenocortical carcinoma, as in this case.

Figure 19B

Axial T2-weighted image showing a mass has marked internal complexity

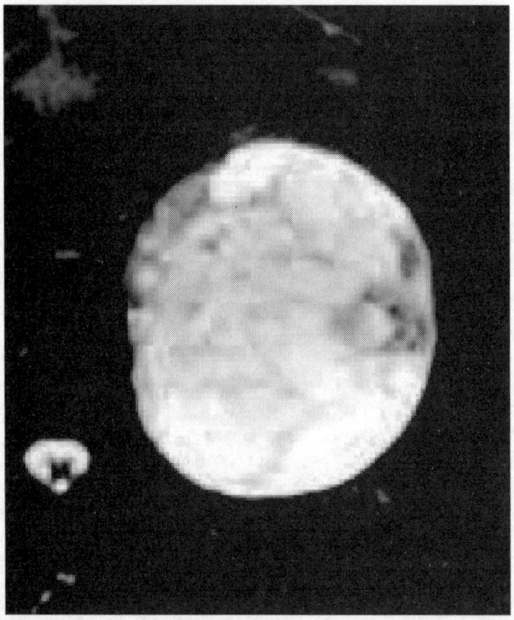

This lesion was resected and the final pathology demonstrated a benign hemorrhagic adrenal pseudocyst. Resection is an appropriate management for such lesions, because a small number of these hemorrhagic masses harbor malignancy.

Figure 19A

Coronal reformat CT image showing a large cystic lesion superior to the left kidney

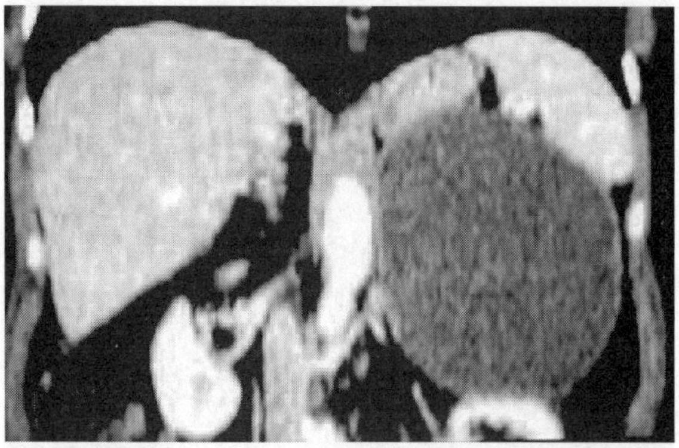

Figure 20A

Ultrasound image demonstrating a well-circumscribed anechoic lesion (arrow) in the lower pole of the right kidney with posterior acoustic enhancement

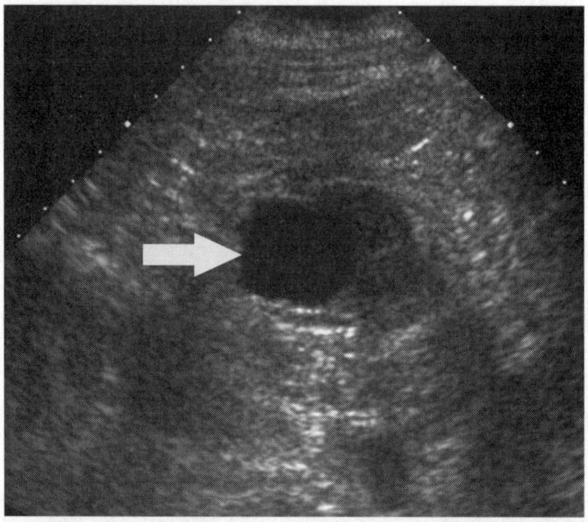

This is a typical simple cyst.

Figure 20B

Axial contrast-enhanced CT image

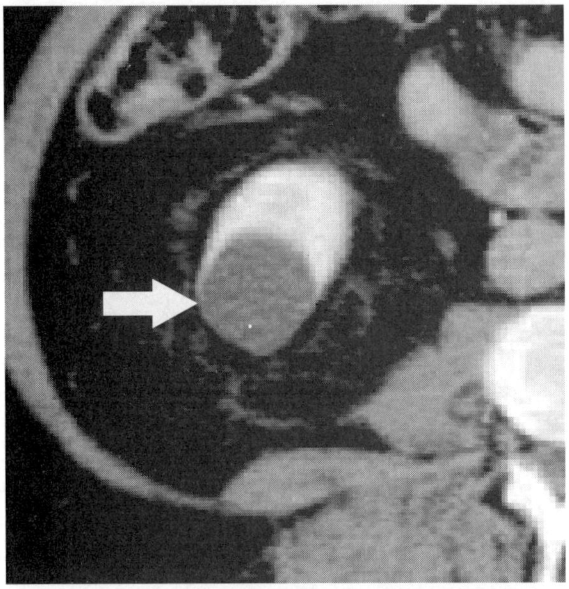

Shows the lesion (arrow) is of uniform water density (8 Hounsfield units) with a imperceptible wall and a well-circumscribed interface with the adjacent renal parenchyma.

Figure 20C

Coronal T2-weighted MRI image

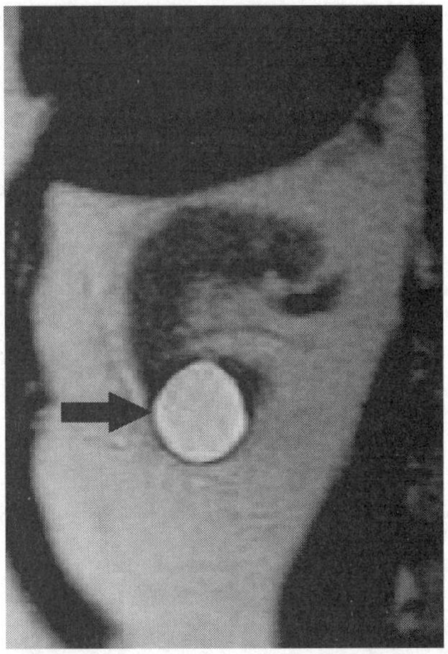

Shows the lesion (arrow) is of extremely high T2 signal intensity, consistent with fluid content.

Figure 20D

Axial post-contrast T1-weighted image

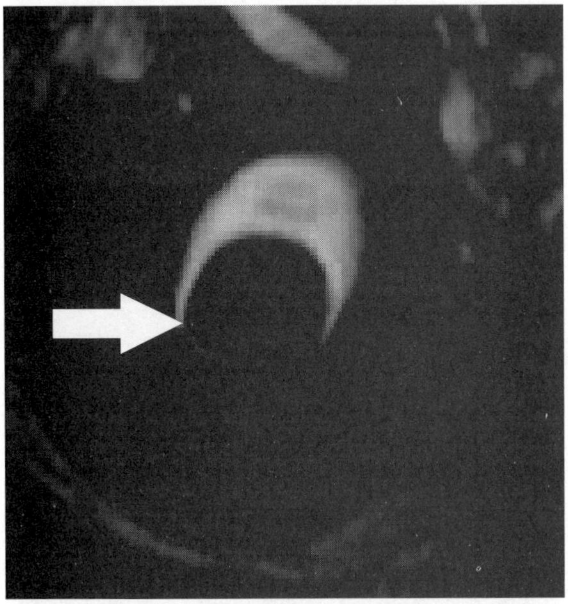

Confirms the lesion (arrow) is non-enhancing and cystic.

Figure 21A

Axial non-contrast image

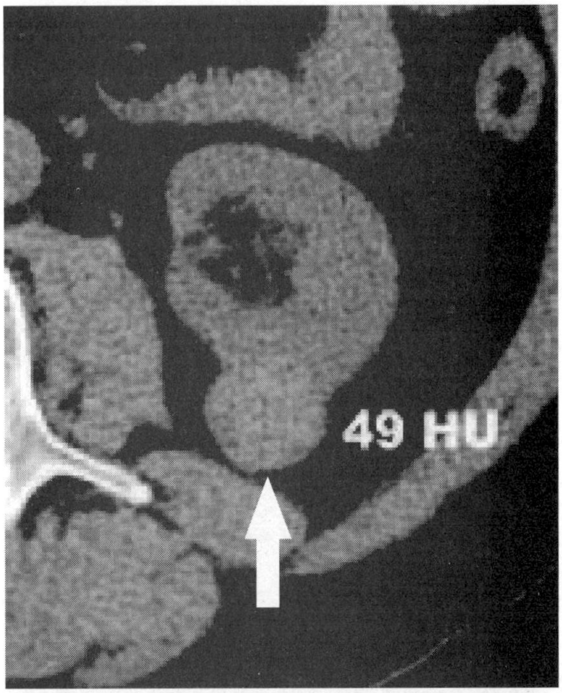

Shows a non-specific lesion (arrow) arising from the posterior aspect of the left kidney. The lesion is of intermediate density (49 Hounsfield units).

Figure 21B

Axial contrast-enhanced CT image

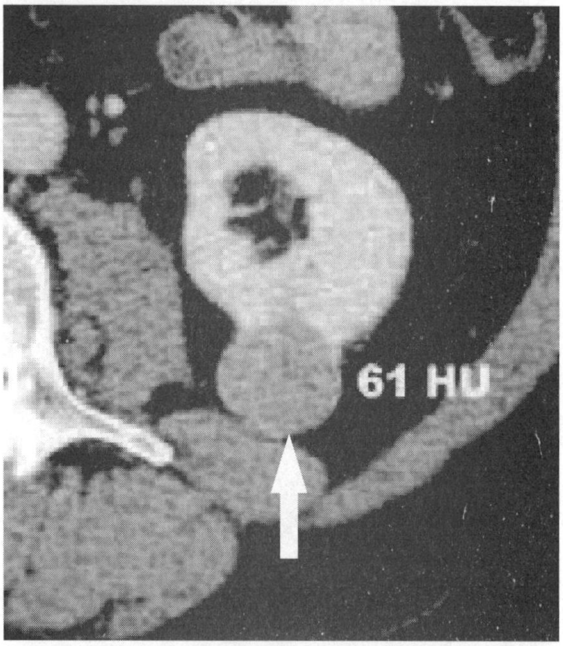

Shows the lesion (arrow) increases in density to 61 Hounsfield units. A diagnosis of papillary renal cell carcinoma was confirmed at surgery. An increase in density of over 10 Hounsfield units is indicative of enhancement, and suggests the lesion is solid. In particular, papillary renal cell carcinoma can demonstrate minimal enhancement, as in this case. In cases of doubtful enhancements by CT, ultrasound may be helpful to document the solid vs. cystic nature of a mass.

Figure 22A

Axial contrast-enhanced CT image

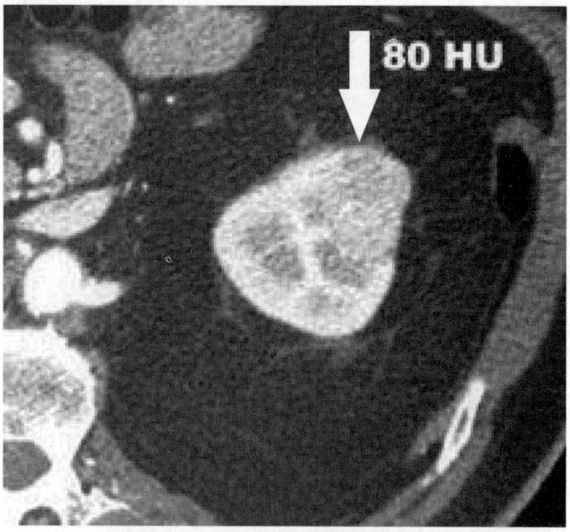

Shows a mass (arrow) in the left kidney. Non-contrast images were not obtained in this case, so based on this image alone, it is not possible to determine whether this is high density cysts or a solid mass.

Figure 22B

Delayed contrast-enhanced CT image

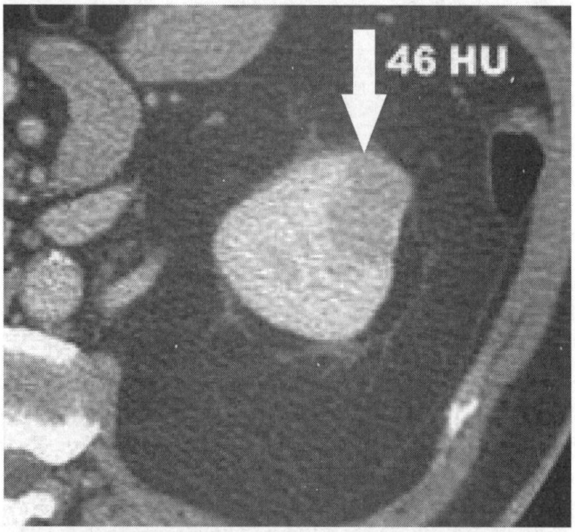

Shows the mass (arrow) has decreased in density to 46 Hounsfield units. This de-enhancement confirms that the lesion is solid, and resection documented the presence of a renal cell carcinoma.

Figure 23A

Axial contrast-enhanced CT image

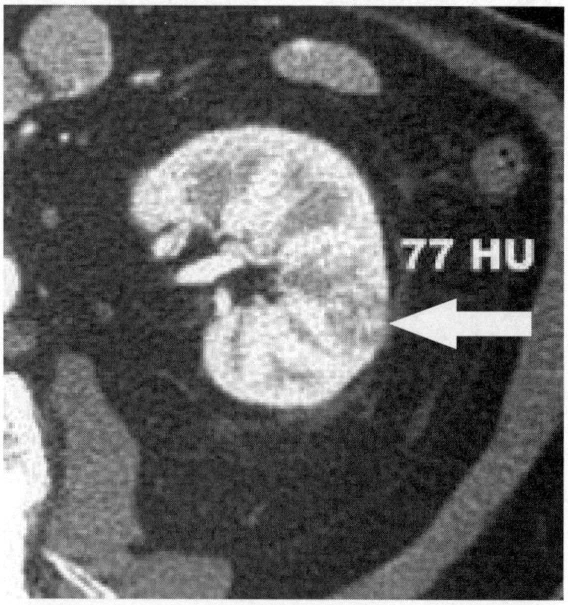

Shows a small high density lesion (arrow) in the left kidney.

Figure 23B

Corresponding axial non-contrast CT image

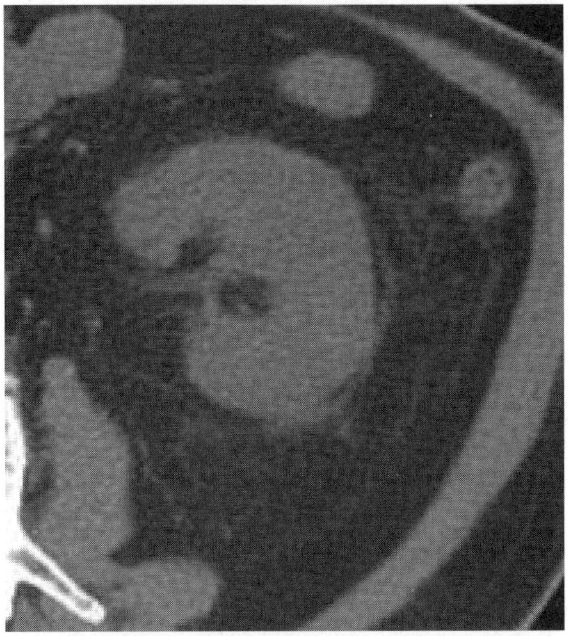

Shows that the lesion is difficult to localize, precluding confident placement of a region of interest to confirm enhancement.

Figure 23C

Delayed contrast-enhanced CT image

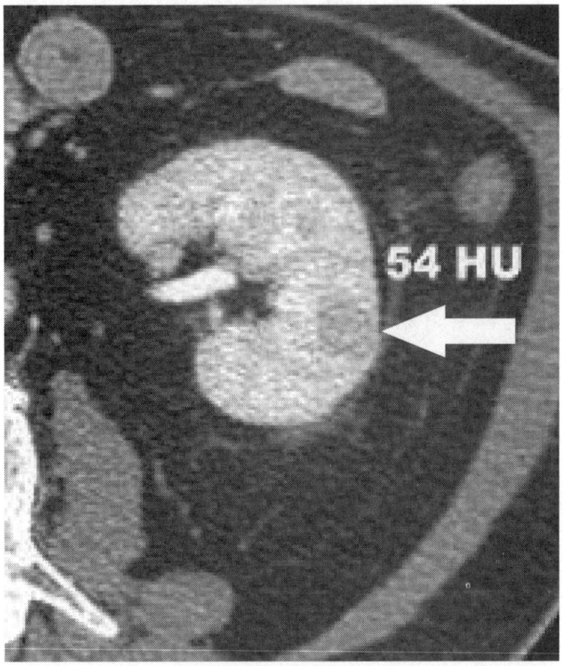

Shows the lesion (arrow) has decreased in density to 54 Hounsfield units. Resection confirms that this was a solid renal cell carcinoma. De-enhancement can be useful to confirm the solid nature of a lesion that is not visible on non-contrast images.

Figure 24A

Axial non-contrast-enhanced CT image

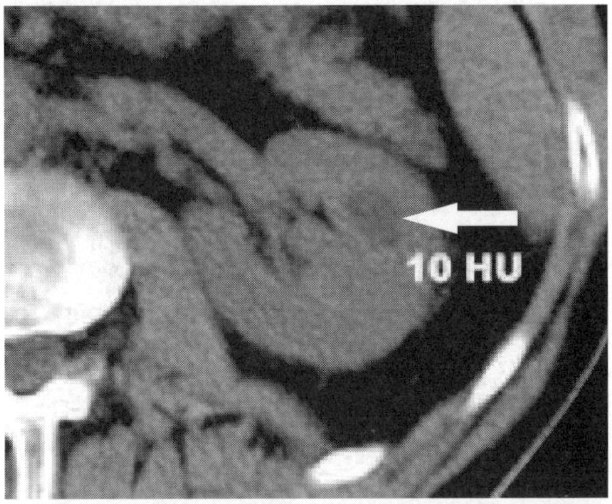

Shows a small hypodense lesion (arrow) in the left kidney.

Figure 24B

Axial contrast-enhanced CT image

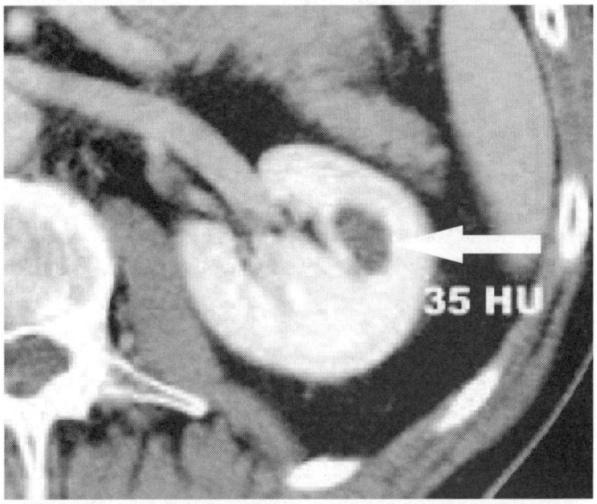

Shows the lesion (arrow) has increased from 10 Hounsfield units to 35 Hounsfield units. However, MRI confirmed that this lesion was a cyst, and the increase in CT density was artifactual. Such spurious increases in CT density can be seen in small cysts at CT, and is known as pseudoenhancement.

Figure 25A

Axial T1-weighted MR image showing a lesion (arrow) of high T1 signal in the left kidney

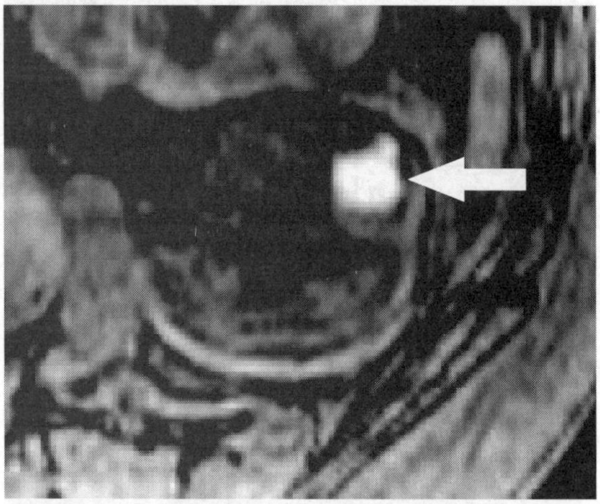

Figure 25B

Axial post-contrast MRI image

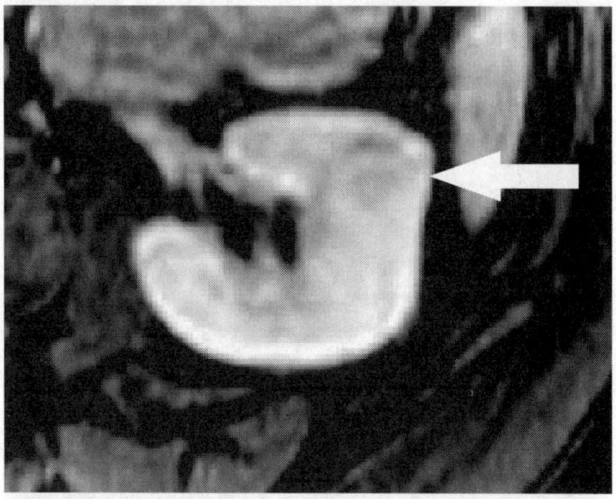

Shows the lesion is now isointense to the adjacent to the renal parenchyma. It is difficult to assess visually whether the lesion (arrow) has increased in signal intensity or not.

Figure 25C

Subtraction image generated by electronically subtracting the pre-contrast image from the post-contrast image

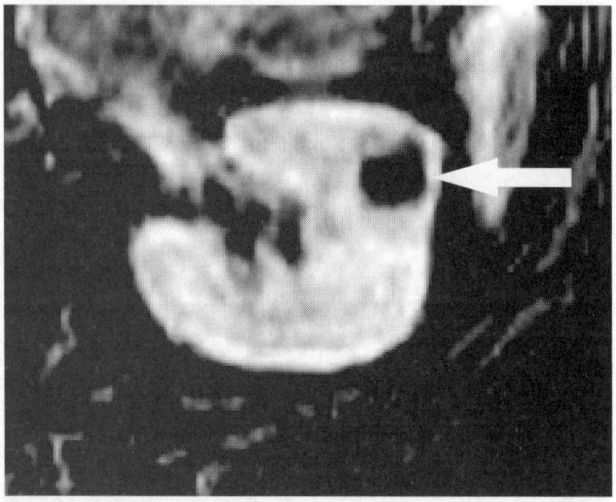

Shows that the lesion (arrow) is non-enhancing (black). Subtraction images can be helpful in the assessment of enhancement, particularly when the lesion is of high T1 signal intensity prior to gadolinium administration. In such a setting, it is difficult to visually appreciate whether there is further increase in T1 signal after contrast.

Figure 26

Axial contrast-enhanced CT image

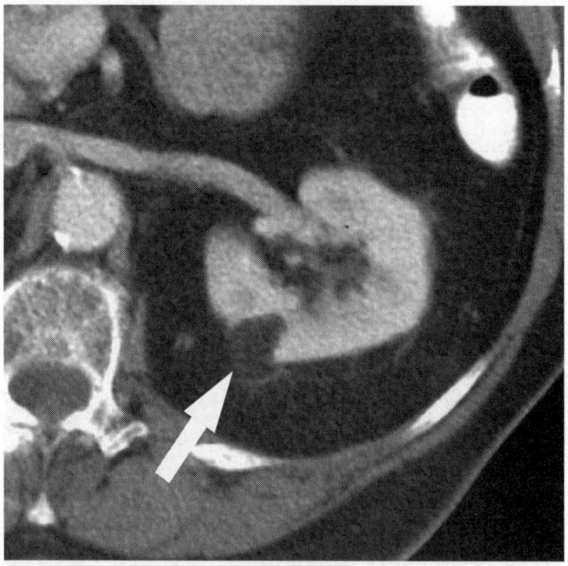

Shows a typical angiomyolipoma (arrow) arising from the left kidney. The mass is clearly of similar CT density to the adjacent retroperitoneal fat. For all practical purposes, a renal mass that contains macroscopic fat is an angiomyolipoma.

Figure 27A

Axial contrast-enhanced 7mm thick CT image

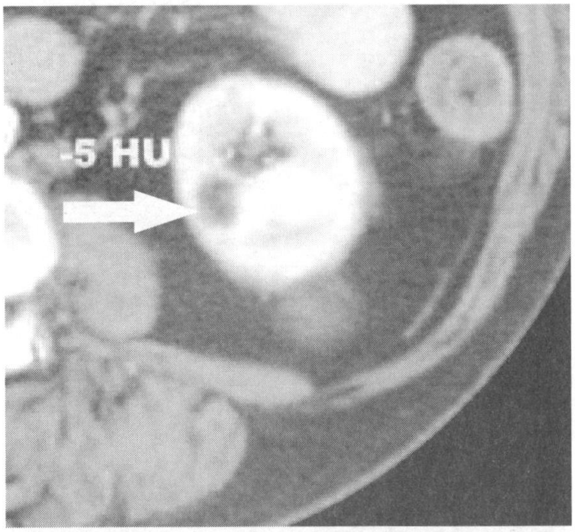

Shows a hypodense lesion (arrow) in the left kidney that is not of sufficiently low density (-5 Hounsfield units) to confirm the presence of macroscopic fat.

Figure 27B

Axial 2.5mm thick non-contrast CT image

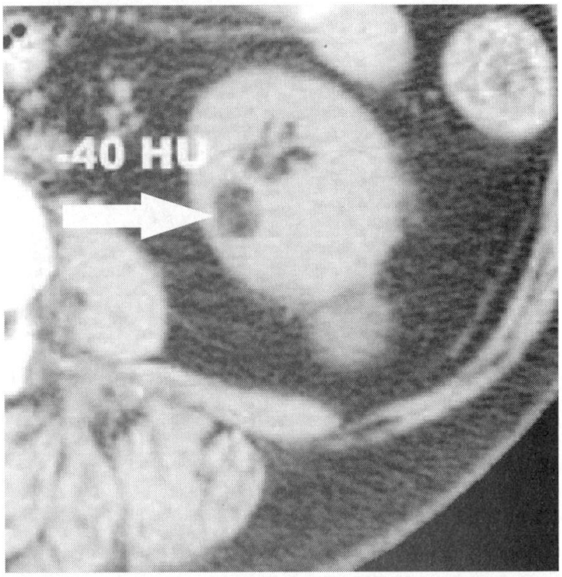

Shows that the lesion (arrow) is of fat density (-40 Hounsfield units), confirming the presence of macroscopic fat and the diagnosis of angiomyolipoma.

Figure 28A

Axial T1-weighted MR image

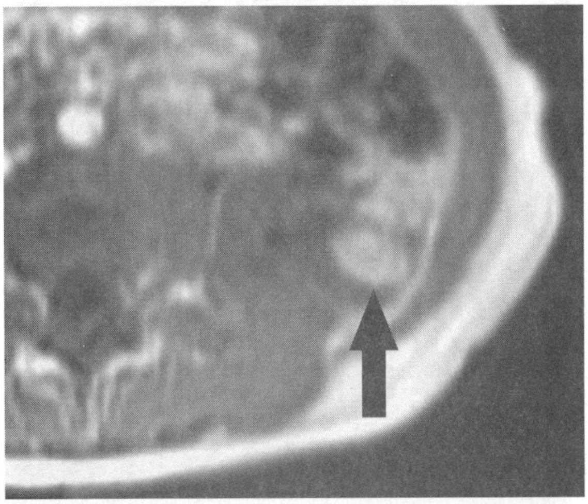

Shows a lesion (arrow) of high T1 signal intensity in the left kidney.

Figure 28B

Axial fat saturated T1-weighted MRI image.

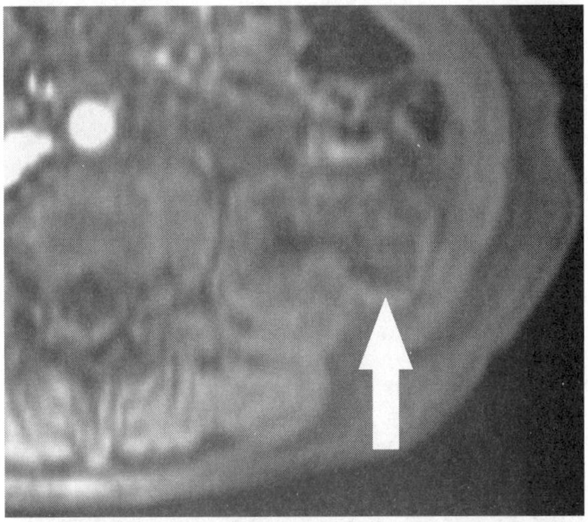

Shows that the lesion (arrow) has lost signal intensity, confirming it contains macroscopic fat and is therefore an angiomyolipoma.

Figure 29

Ultrasound image

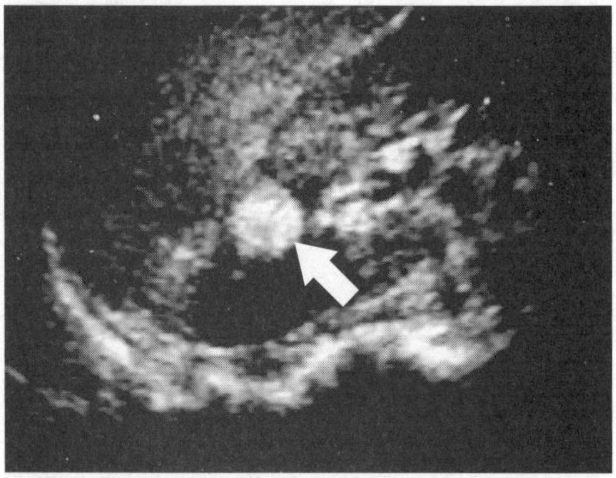

Shows the typical marked echogenicity of an angiomyolipoma (arrow) in the upper pole of the right kidney.

Figure 30A

Axial non-contrast CT image

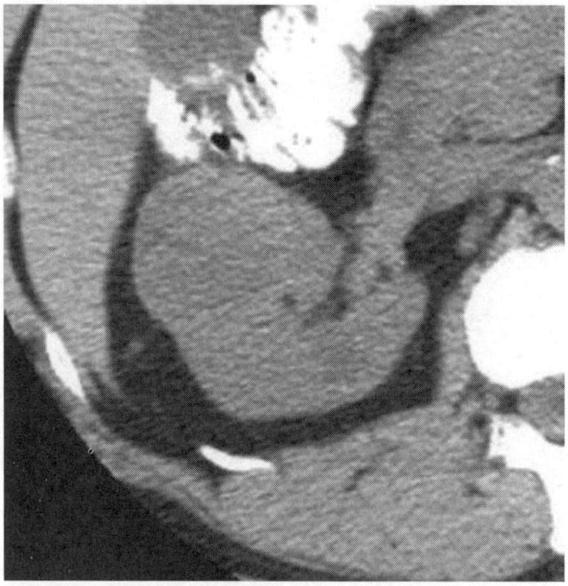

Shows a contour bulge in the right kidney, without visible macroscopic fat.

Figure 30B

Axial contrast-enhanced CT image

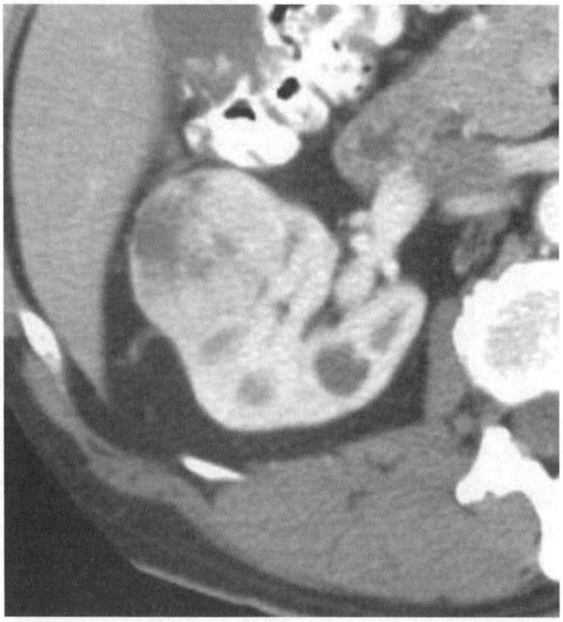

Shows a heterogeneously enhancing mass in the right kidney. The appearance is typical of a renal cell carcinoma, and density measurements are not required to confirm enhancement because the visual appearances are so distinctive.

Figure 31

Axial contrast-enhanced CT image

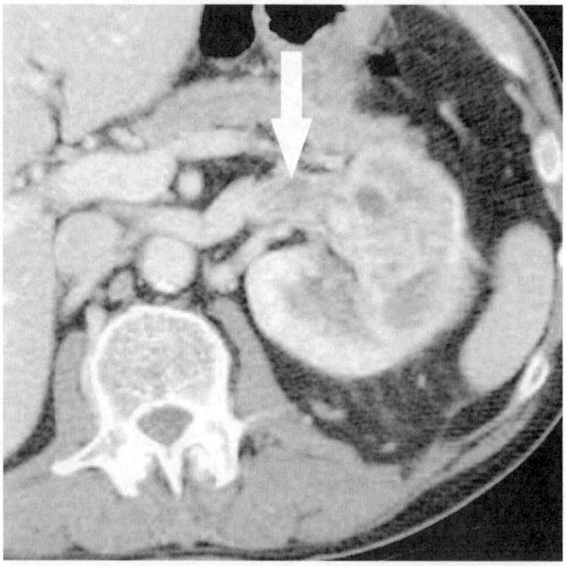

Shows an infiltrative mass in the left kidney, associated with left renal vein invasion (arrow). While renal cell carcinoma is usually well-circumscribed, it is occasionally more infiltrative, as in this case.

Figure 32

Coronal reformative CT image

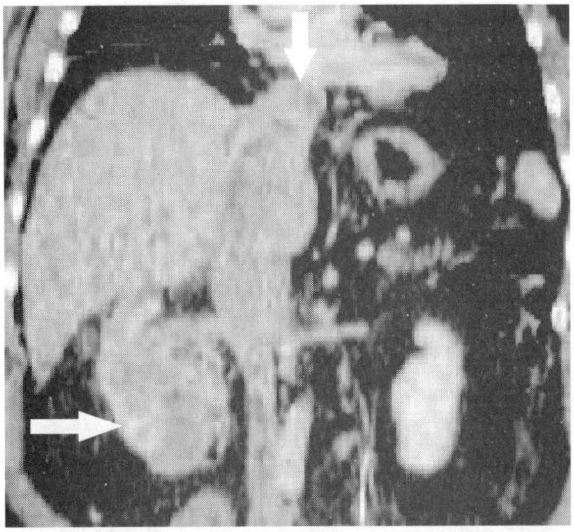

Shows almost complete replacement of the right kidney by a mass (horizontal arrow) with tumor thrombus extending into and expanding the inferior vena cava, reaching with the upper end of the tumor thrombus (vertical arrow) being at the level of the diaphragm.

Figure 33

Axial contrast-enhanced CT image

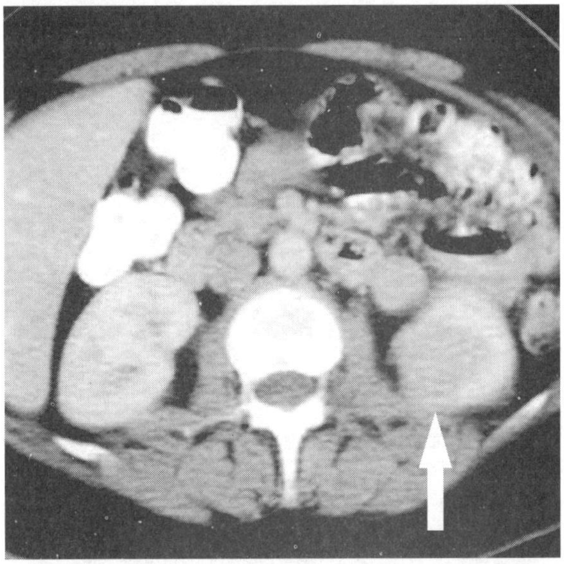

Shows a uniformly enhancing mass (arrow) in the left kidney, without macroscopically visible fat. Resection documented that this lesion was a fat poor angiomyolipoma, although the presumptive preoperative diagnosis was a renal cell carcinoma based on the imaging appearance.

Figure 34A

Axial contrast-enhanced CT image

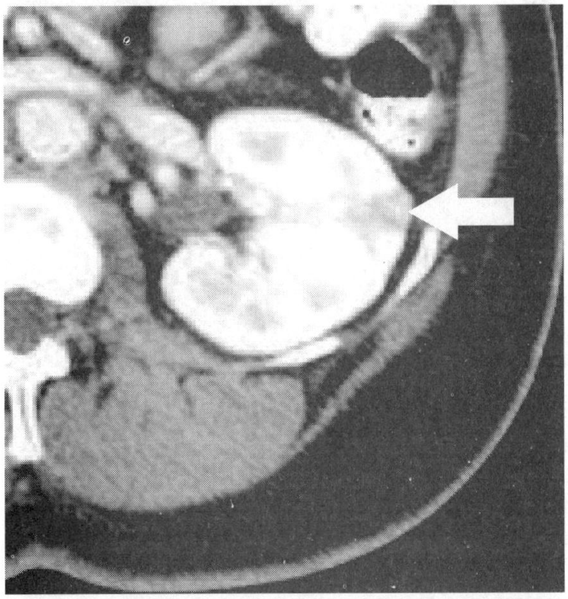

Shows a small nonspecific lesion (arrow) in the left kidney.

Figure 34B

Axial non-contrast-enhanced CT image

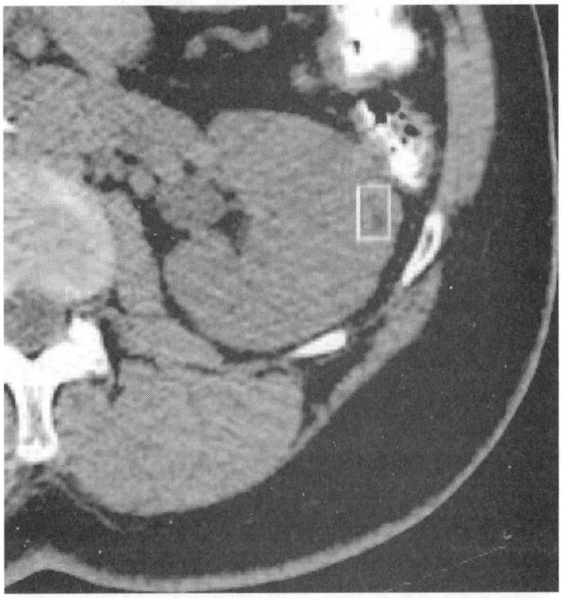

Does not show appreciable macroscopic fat in the lesion. Histogram analysis was performed on the region of interest indicated by the white rectangle.

Figure 34C

Histogram analysis from the region of interest in Figure 34B

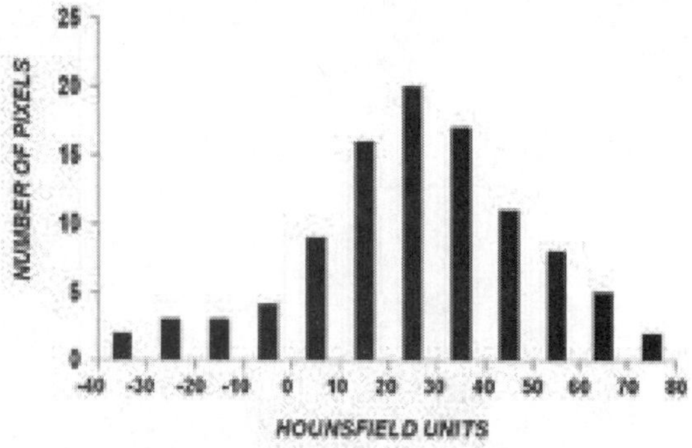

Shows that several voxels have a density under -20 Hounsfield units. A final diagnosis of fat-poor angiomyolipoma was established. While the use of histogram analysis was helpful in this case, the criteria for establishing the diagnosis of a fat-poor angiomyolipoma using this analytical approach has not been well-established.

Figure 35A

Axial contrast-enhanced CT image

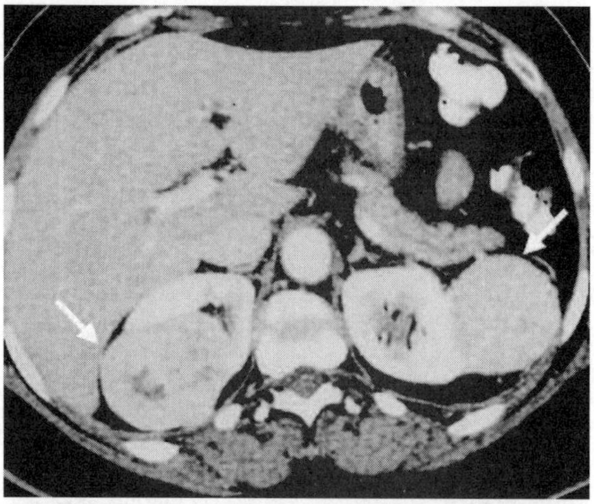

Shows bilateral oncocytomas (arrows). The lesion in the right kidney has a central stellate scar, but this finding is not seen in the lesion in the left kidney. While a central stellate scar may suggest the diagnosis of oncocytoma, it is difficult to distinguish such a central scar from cavitary necrosis in a renal cell carcinoma.

Figure 35B

Arteriogram (in a different patient) showing the typical spoke-wheel appearance of an oncocytoma in the right kidney

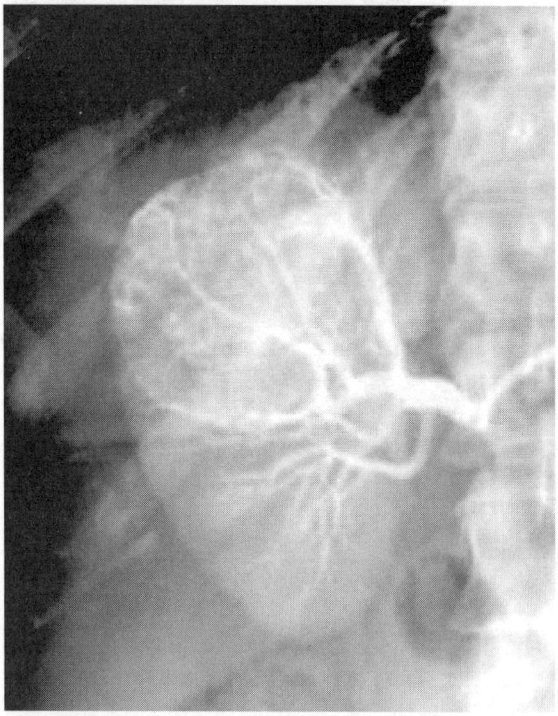

While such an appearance is suggestive, it is difficult to see how the findings could be considered sufficiently convincing to obviate the need for surgical confirmation.

Figure 36

Axial contrast-enhanced CT image

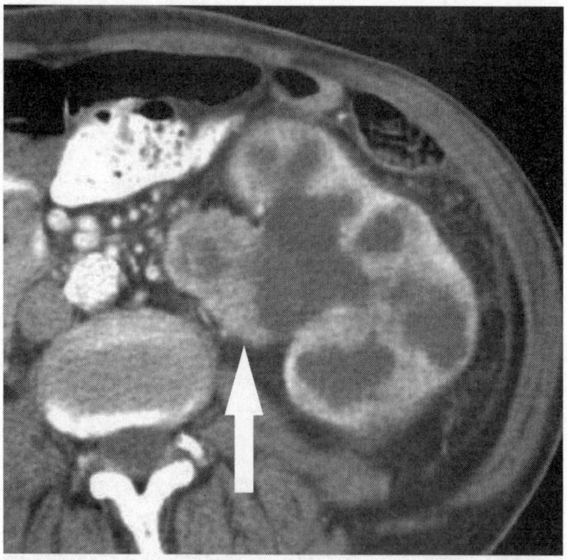

Shows upper tract transitional cell carcinoma in the left kidney. Infiltrative tumor is seen along the wall of the pelvis (arrow), with similar infiltrative tumors seen within the dilated cavities.

Figure 37

Axial contrast-enhanced CT image

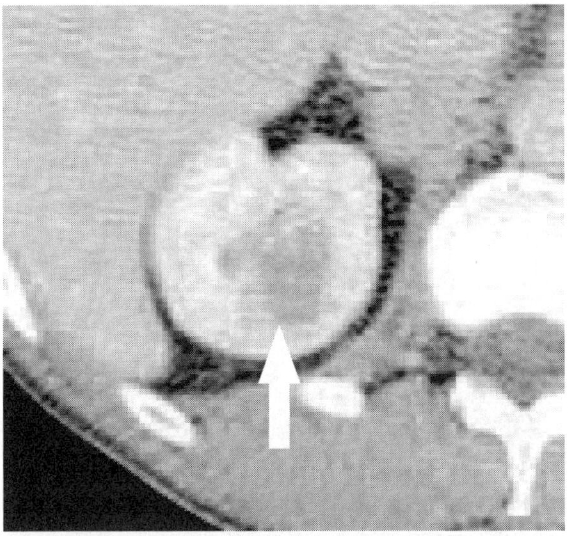

Shows an intraparenchymal hypodense mass within the right mass (arrow) within the right kidney. This was a proven transitional cell carcinoma, although the radiologic appearances overlap with that of renal cell carcinoma.

Figure 38

Axial contrast-enhanced CT image

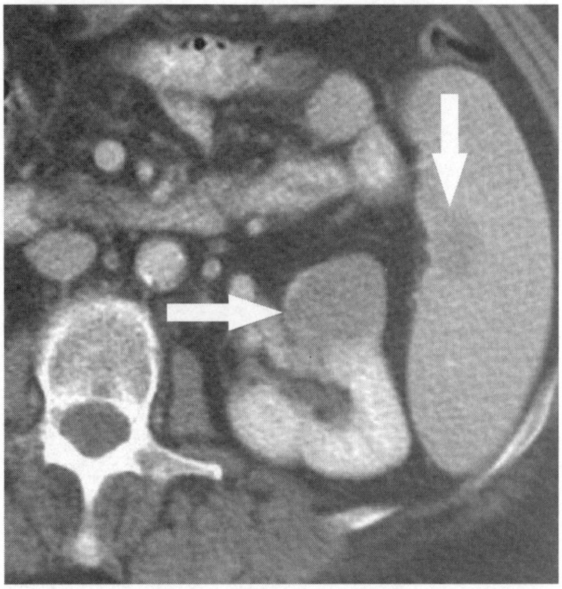

Shows a unifocal mass (horizontal arrow) in the left kidney. The appearance is suggestive of a renal cell carcinoma, but an additional hypodense mass (vertical arrow) is present in the spleen. The final diagnosis was renal lymphoma. The presence of extra renal disease can be a useful clue to the diagnosis of lymphoma.

Figure 39

Axial contrast-enhanced CT image

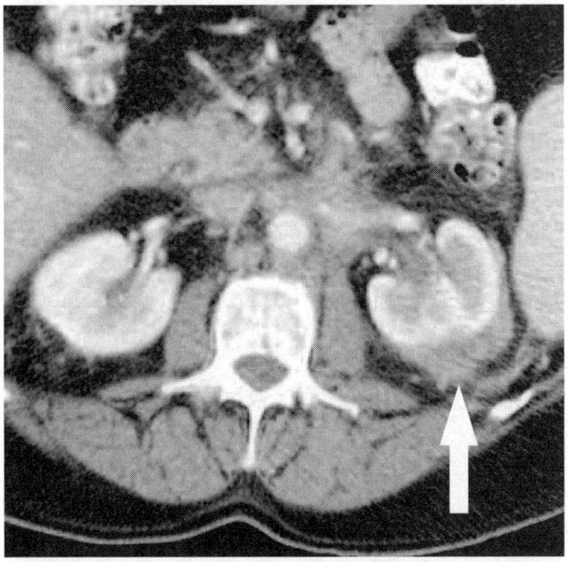

Shows infiltrative soft perinephric soft tissue encasing the left kidney, and also similar infiltrative soft tissue in the left periaortic space and surrounding the left renal artery. Perinephric encasement is typical of lymphomatous involvement of the kidneys, although it is not the commonest pattern.

Figure 40

Axial contrast-enhanced CT image in a patient with widely disseminated metastatic breast cancer

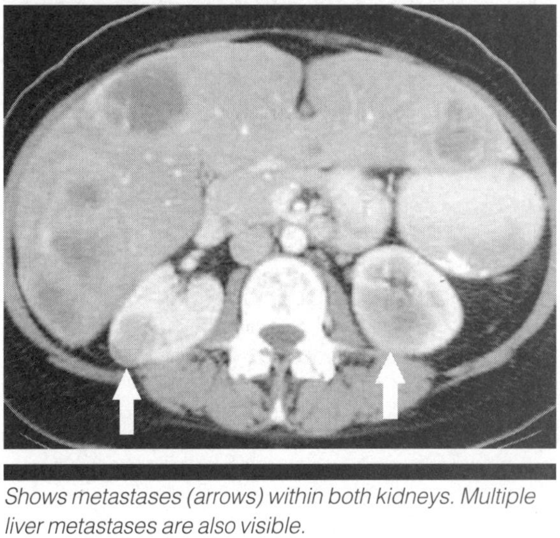

Shows metastases (arrows) within both kidneys. Multiple liver metastases are also visible.

Figure 41A

Axial non-contrast CT image

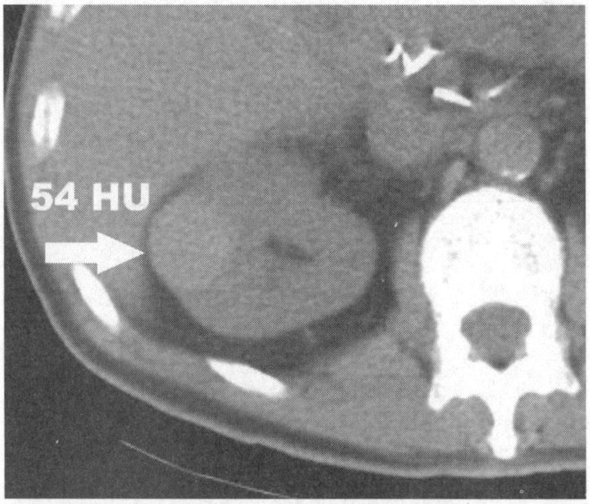

Shows a lesion (arrow) of intermediate density (54 Hounsfield units) in the right kidney.

Figure 41B

Axial contrast-enhanced CT image

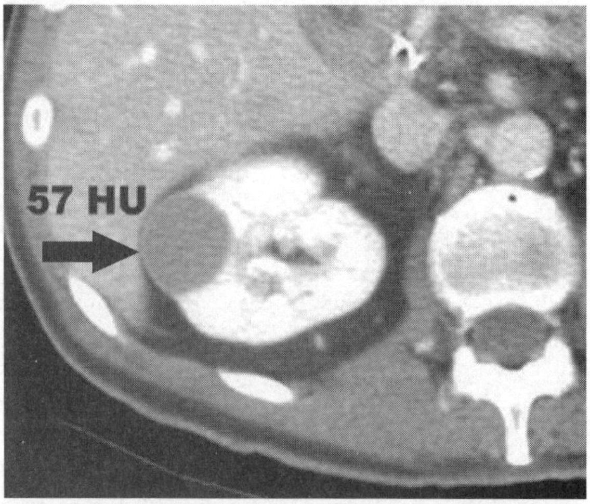

Shows that the lesion (arrow) is non-enhancing (the observed increase in 3 Hounsfield units from 54 to 57 does not constitute enhancement). The lesion is also of uniform density and well-circumscribed, and is characteristic of a hyperdense Bosniak II cyst.

Figure 42

Axial contrast-enhanced CT image

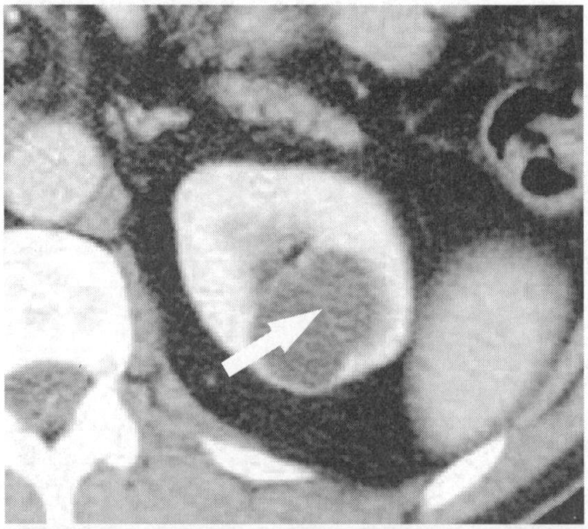

Shows a cystic lesion in the left kidney that contains a very thin septum (arrow). This is a mildly complex Bosniak II cyst. Such mildly complex features are benign.

Figure 43

Axial contrast-enhanced CT image

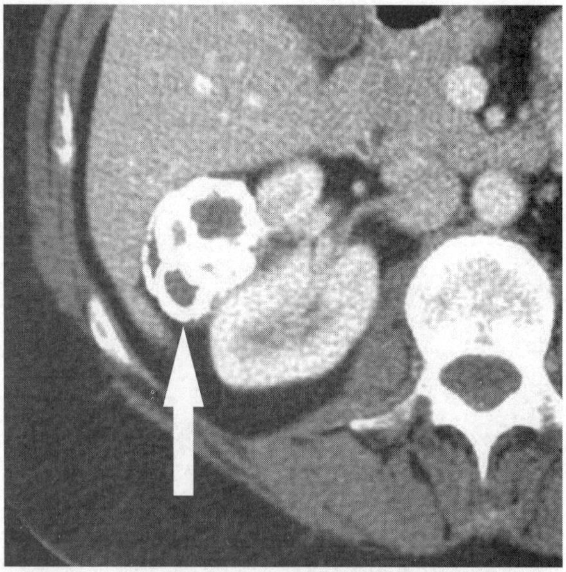

Shows a heavily and thickly calcified cystic mass (arrow) in the right kidney. Thickly calcified walls and septa are indicative of a Bosniak III lesion, and such lesions have approximately 50% chance of malignancy. This lesion was resected and found to be a calcified cystic renal cell carcinoma.

Figure 44

Axial contrast-enhanced CT image

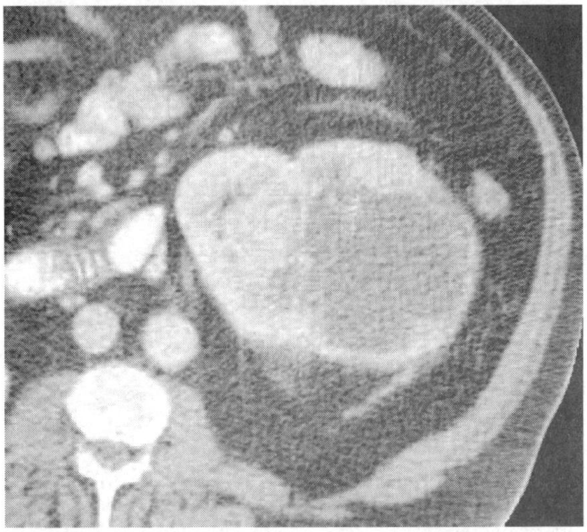

Shows a markedly complex cyst in the left kidney, with a thickly enhancing and nodular wall. Such markedly complex features of those of a Bosniak IV cyst, and this lesion were found to be a cystic renal cell carcinoma at resection.

Figure 45

Axial contrast-enhanced CT image

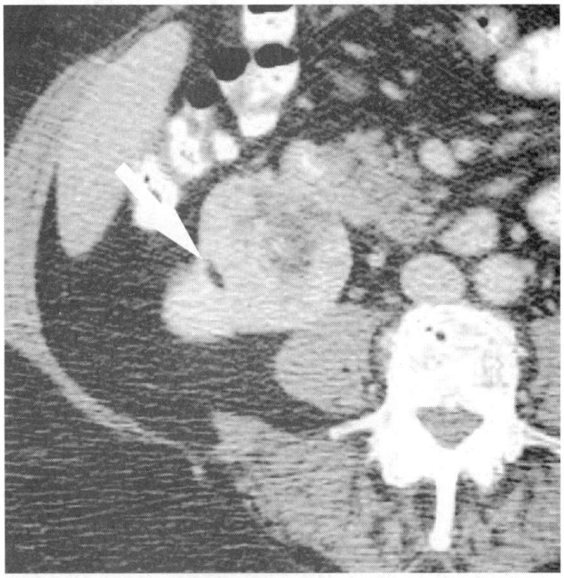

Shows a heterogeneously-enhancing mass in the right kidney. A small sliver of fat (arrow) is seen at the periphery of the lesion. While it is difficult to know whether this fat is within the mass or represents entrapped fat peripherally, the primary consideration should remain renal cell carcinoma, and this diagnosis was confirmed surgically.

Figure 46

Axial contrast-enhanced CT image

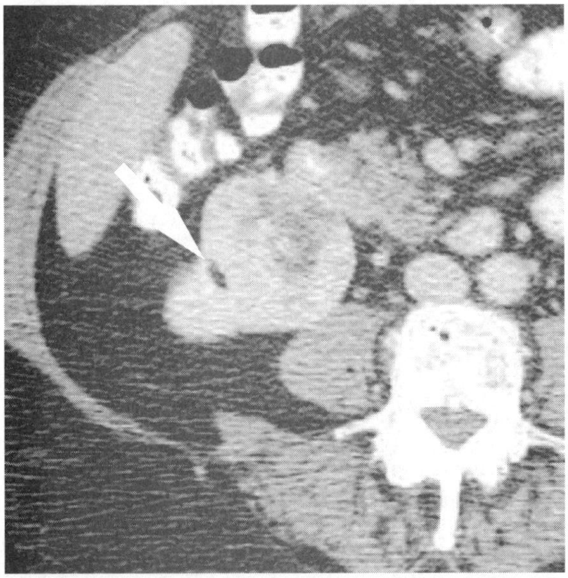

Shows a fat density mass arising from the left kidney. The mass is largely exophytic, but a parenchymal notch is visible in the kidney, as a vascular pedicle (arrow), hoping to confirm the diagnosis of an exophytic angiomyolipoma.

Figure 47

Coronal reformatted non-contrast CT image

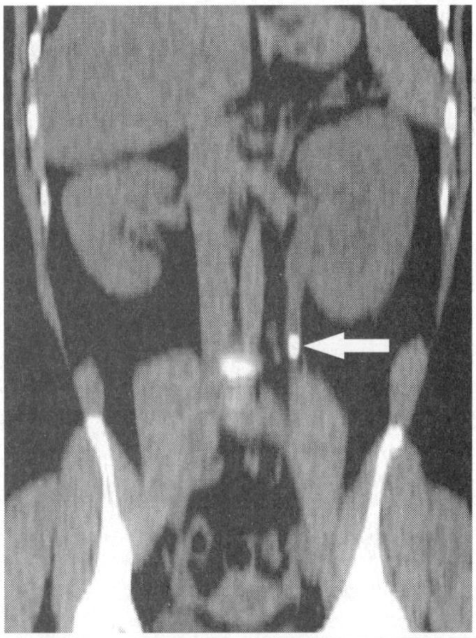

Shows left hydroureteronephrosis that can be traced to the level of an obstructing stone (arrow) in the upper to mid left ureter. Non-contrast CT as demonstrated excellent accuracy in the diagnosis of obstructive calculi, and has essentially replaced IVU in the evaluation of suspected renal colic.

Figure 48

Coronal reformatted non-contrast CT images in a patient with HIV infection receiving indinavir (Crixivan)

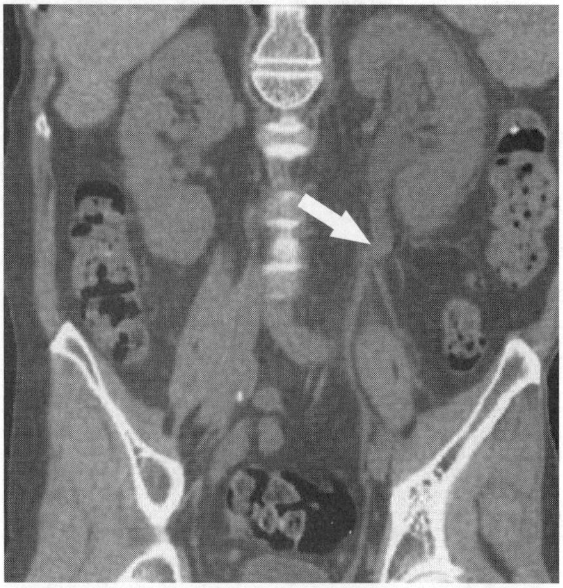

Left hydroureteronephrosis can be traced at the level of upper to mid-left ureter (arrow) but there is no visible stone at the point of transition from dilated to non-dilated ureter. For practical purposes, indinavir stones are the only urethral calculi that are radiolucent at CT, although secondary signs may help establish the diagnosis, as in this case.

Figure 49

CT image

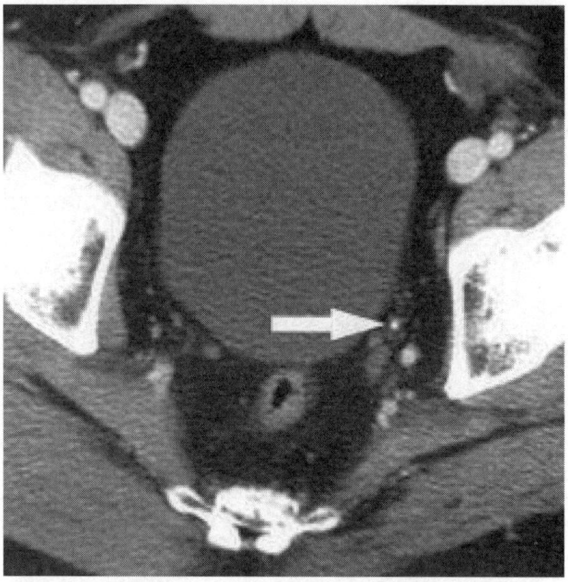

Shows a small stone (arrow) in the distal left ureter. A thin surrounding rim of tissue is visible, representing edematous ureteral wall. This so-called ureteral rim sign helps differentiating a ureteral calculus from a phlebolith.

Figure 50

Non-enhanced CT image

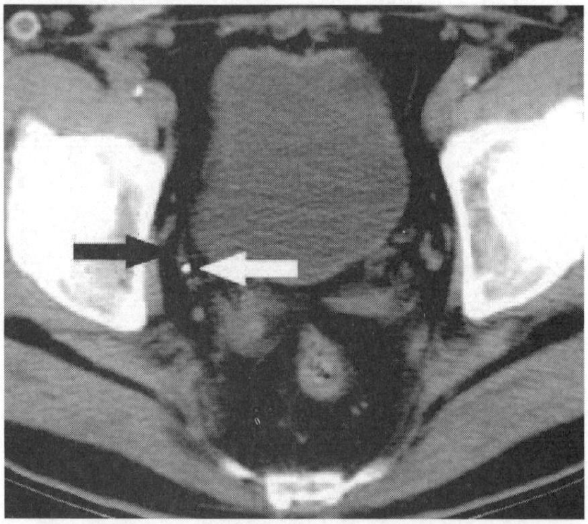

Shows a pelvic phlebolith (white arrow). A linear strand of tissue (black arrow) is seen extending from the phlebolith. This tissue strand is believed to represent the atretic vessel within which the phlebolith formed, and this so-called "comet-tail" sign is another finding that may help distinguish stones and phleboliths.

Figure 51

Bilateral nephrocalcinosis in a patient with medullary sponge kidney

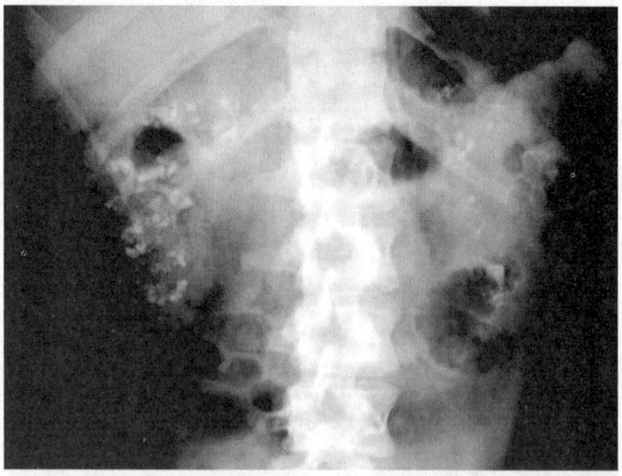

Note that the calcifications are relatively coarse and correspond to the locations of the medullary pyramids, where the calcifications form.

Figure 52

Plain abdominal radiograph demonstrating bilateral cortical nephrocalcinosis, with a thin rim of calcification visible around the periphery of the kidneys

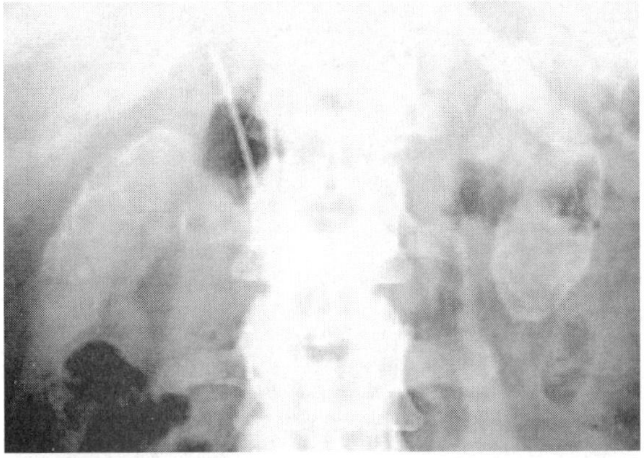

Such an appearance is most commonly due to chronic glomerulonephritis.

Figure 53

Plain abdominal radiograph in a child

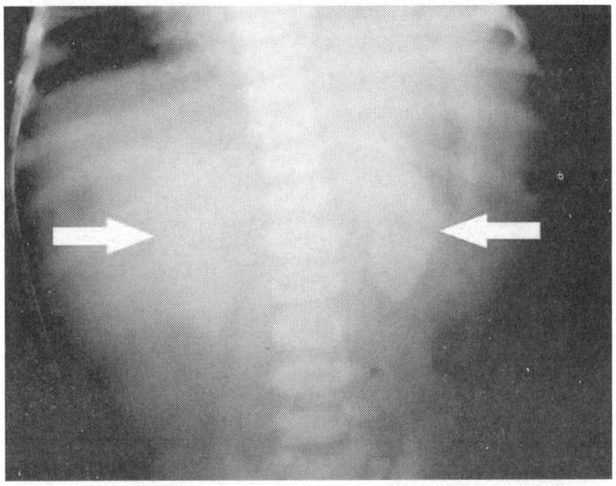

Demonstrates the characteristic nephrocalcinosis (arrows) seen in children with primary hyperoxaluria (oxalosis).

Figure 54A

Axial contrast-enhanced CT image

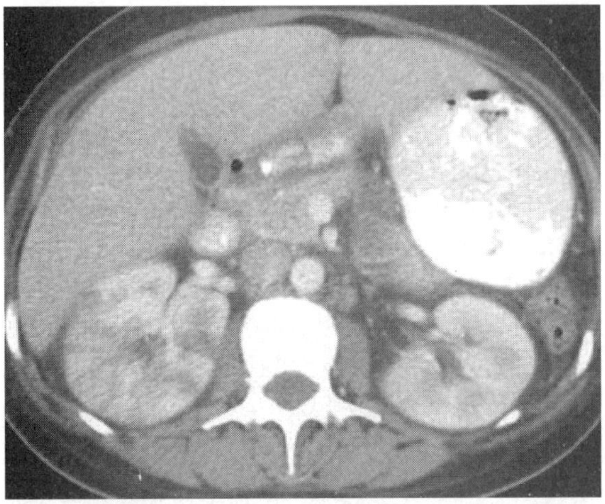

Shows wedge-shaped striations in the right kidney, due to pyelonephritis.

Figure 54B

Axial contrast-enhanced CT image in a different patient

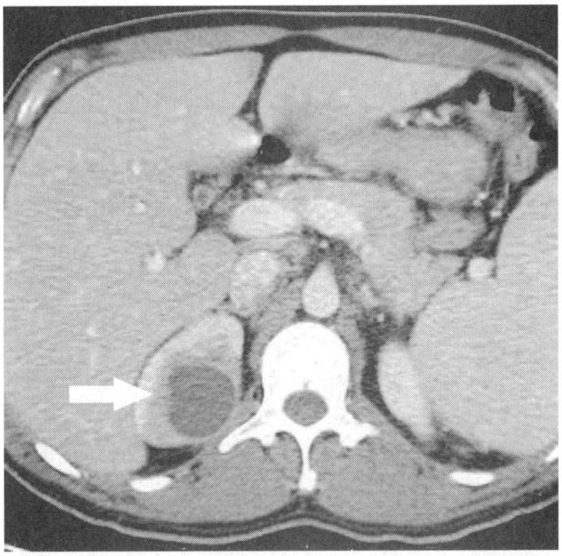

Shows formation of an abscess (arrow) in addition to the clinical scenario of sepsis; this lesion can be distinguished from a simple cyst by the presence of a peripheral irregular rim of low density edematous renal parenchyma.

Figure 55

Plain abdominal radiograph

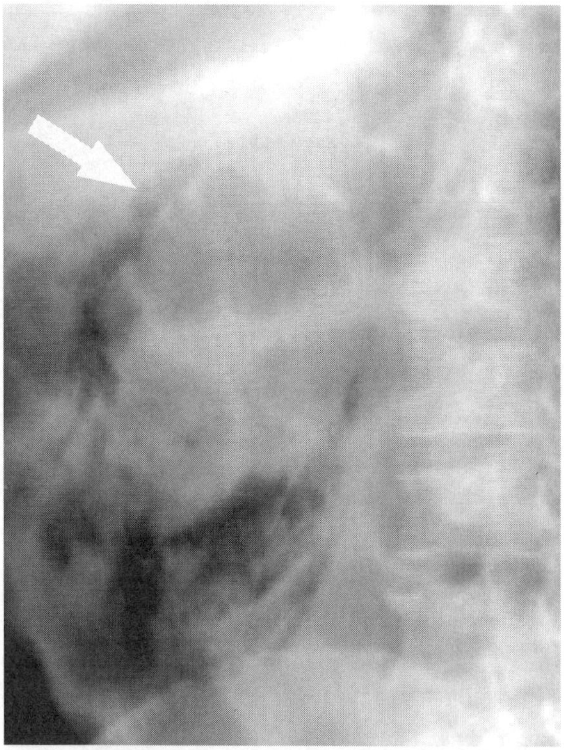

Shows air (arrow) surrounding the right kidney due to emphysematous pyelonephritis.

Figure 56

Axial contrast-enhanced CT image

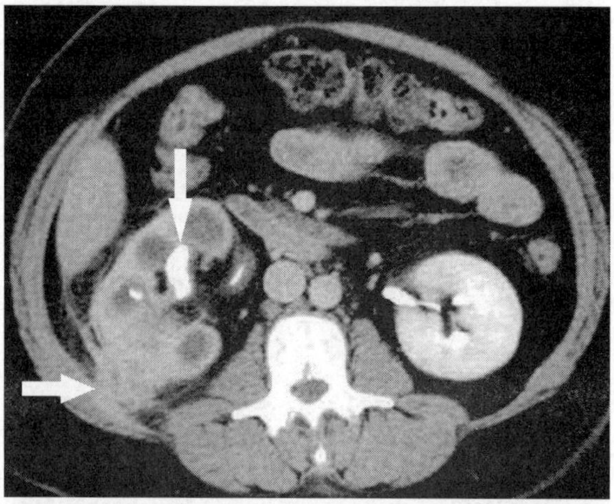

Shows the typical appearances of xanthogranulomatous pyelonephritis in the right kidney. The kidney shows caliceal dilatation due to the presence of a staghorn calculus (vertical arrow) and reduced enhancement in the kidney. In addition, inflammatory changes (horizontal arrows) can be seen in the perinephric space extending to the posterior abdominal wall.

Figure 57

Axial contrast-enhanced CT image in a patient with fungal pyelonephritis

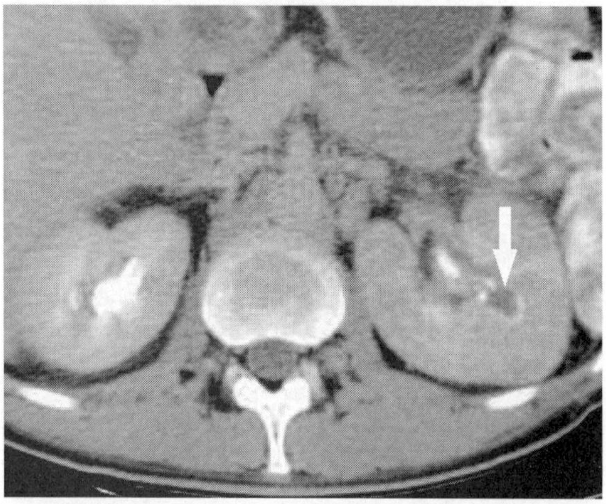

A lucent filling defect (arrow) is seen in a left-sided calyx, due to a fungus ball. The differential for such a lucent filling defect in the upper tract include hematoma and transitional cell carcinoma.

Figure 58

Axial contrast-enhanced CT image in a patient with systemic lupus erythematosus

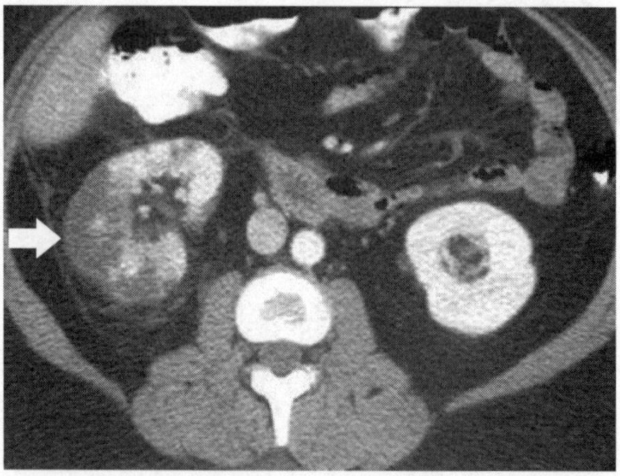

Wedge-shaped areas (arrow) of irregular hypodensity are seen in the right kidney, consistent with renal infarcts.

Figure 59

One-shot IVU in a patient after a motor vehicle accident

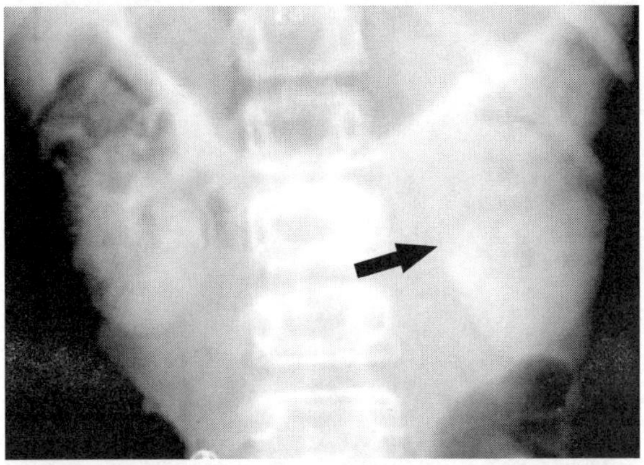

The nephrogram of the left upper kidney is virtually absent above a visible fracture line (arrow).

Figure 60

Ultrasound image showing a post-traumatic perinephric hematoma (between arrows)

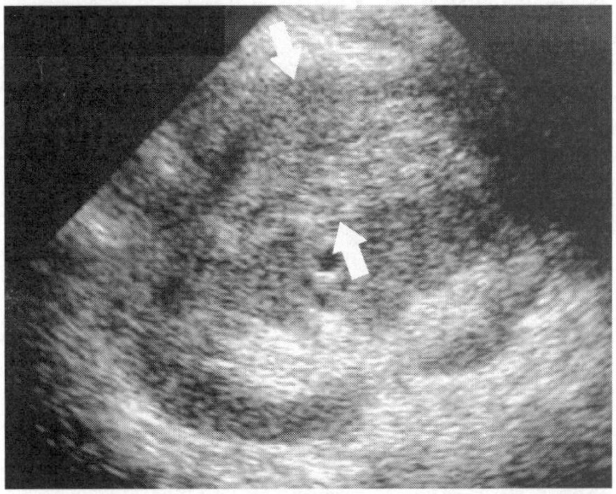

Figure 61A

Axial contrast-enhanced CT image

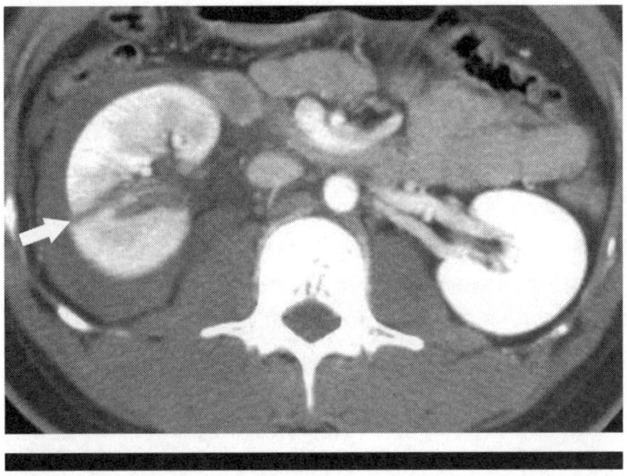

Shows a post-traumatic fracture (arrow) in the right kidney. Ill-defined low density surrounding the right kidney with an irregular outer margin is consistent with associated perinephric hematoma.

Figure 61B

Axial contrast-enhanced CT image in a different patient

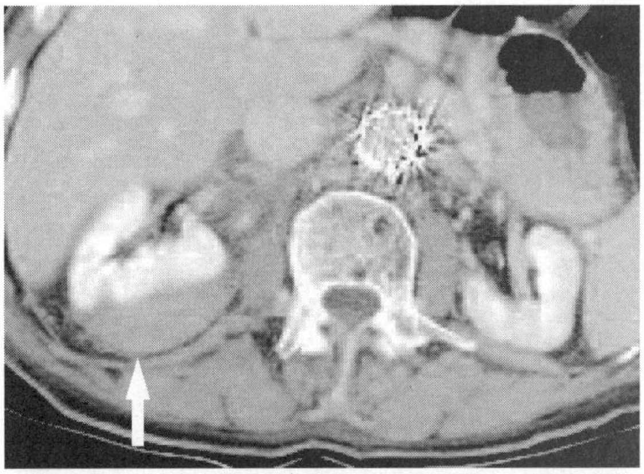

Shows a subcapular hematoma (arrow) in the right kidney. Note that the subcapular hematoma has a smooth outer margin and deforms the underlying kidney.

Figure 62A

Axial contrast-enhanced CT image

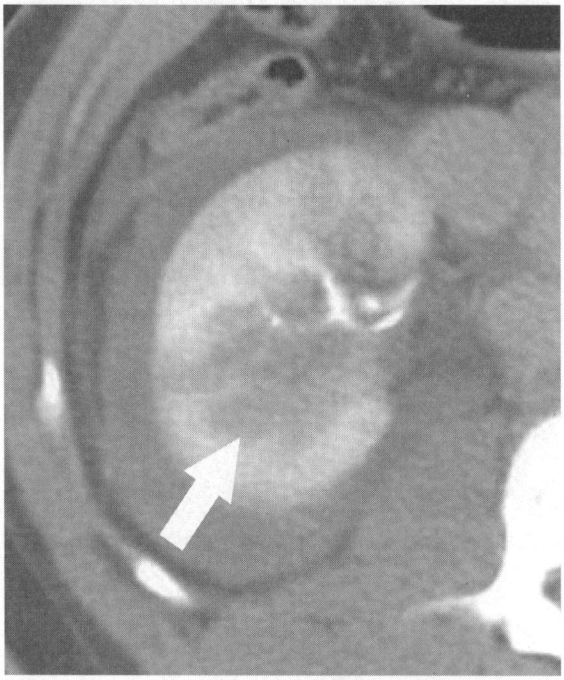

Shows a ill-defined hypodense area (arrow) in the right kidney, consistent with a contusion.

Figure 62B

Axial contrast-enhanced CT image

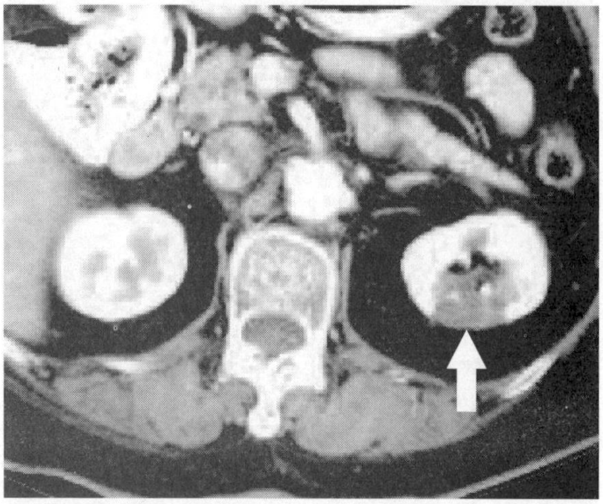

Showing a wedge-shaped area of non-enhancement (arrow) in the left kidney, consistent with infarction.

Figure 63A

Photomontage showing the appearance of active extravasation on early and late post-contrast CT images after trauma

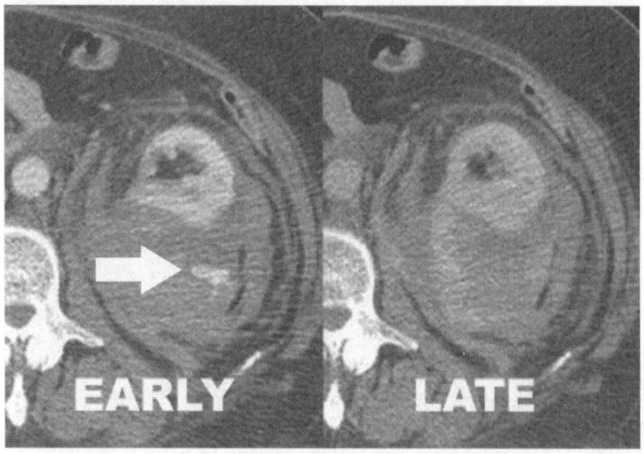

The active extravasation is seen as an irregular focus of brisk enhancement (arrow) within a large perinephric hematoma. The extravasated contrast has dispersed on the later image.

Figure 63B

Photomontage showing the appearance of urinary extravasation on early and late post-contrast images

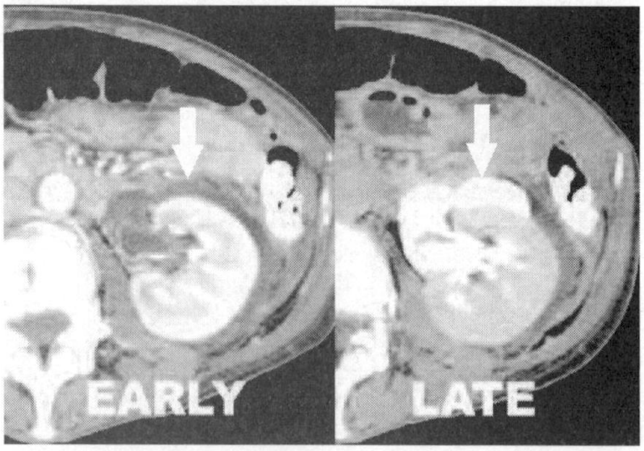

The extravasation appears as a non-specific collection of fluid (arrow) on the early image. On the delayed phase image, extravasated contrast (arrow) is seen anterior to the left kidney, and also is contiguous with the left renal pelvis.

Figure 63C

Photo montage showing the appearances of a pseudo-aneurysm on early and late post-contrast images

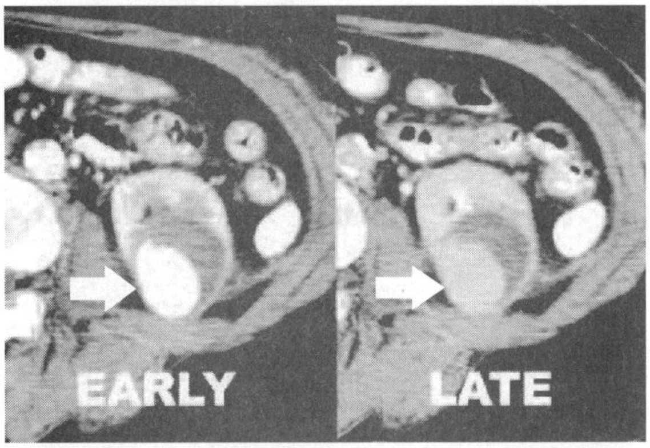

The pseudoaneurysm is seen as a focus of intense rounded smooth enhancement (arrow) on the early image, which gradually fades on the delayed phase image (arrow).

Figure 64

Axial contrast-enhanced CT image

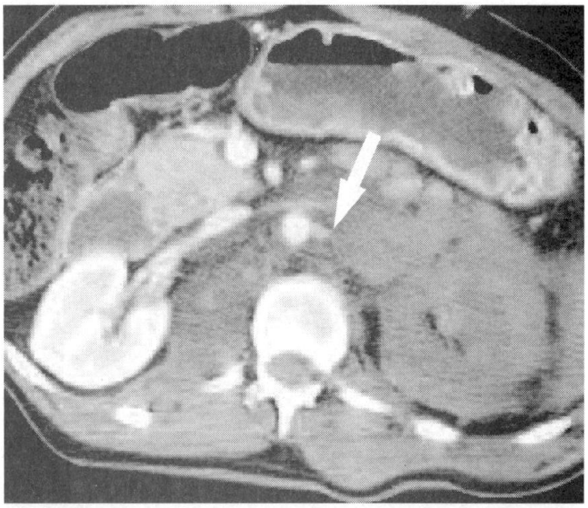

Shows a devascularized left kidney in a patient after a motor vehicle accident. Note that the left renal artery has a blind-ending (arrow). This is likely due to an occlusive intimal tear, the commonest etiology of devascularization after trauma.

Figure 65A

MAG3 renogram in a patient with right ureteropelvic junction obstruction

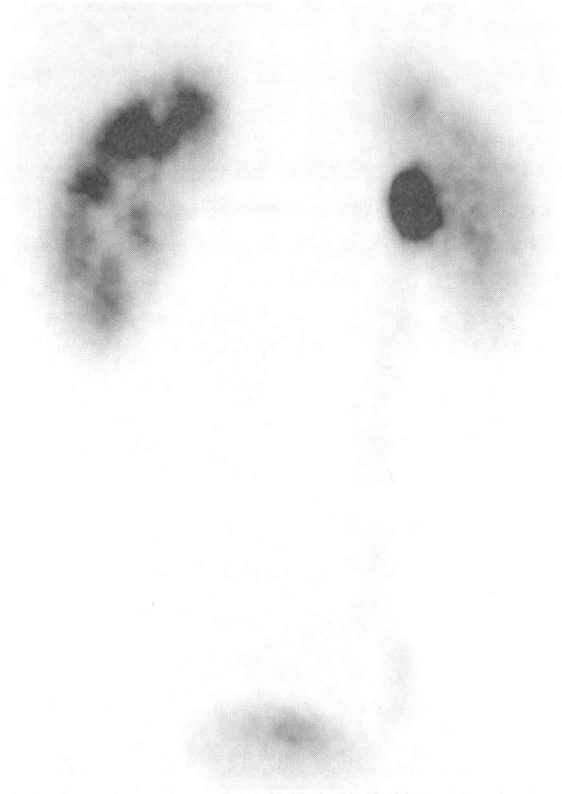

Shows retention of the isotope within the right kidney without visible excreted activity within the right renal pelvis.

Figure 65B

Retrograde pyelogram showing marked right hydronephrosis to the level of the ureteropelvic junction, below which the ureter is of normal caliber

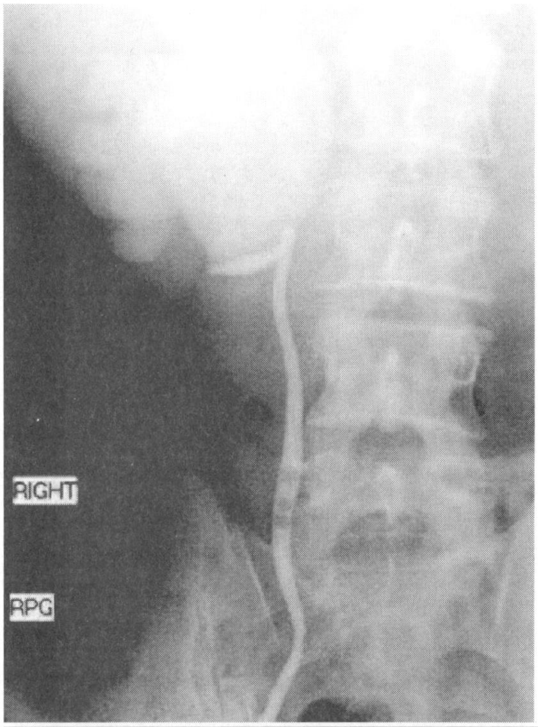

The appearance is typical of ureteropelvic junction obstruction. Lucent filling defects within the right mid ureter are due to air bubbles.

Figure 65C

Coronal reformatted CT image in the same patient

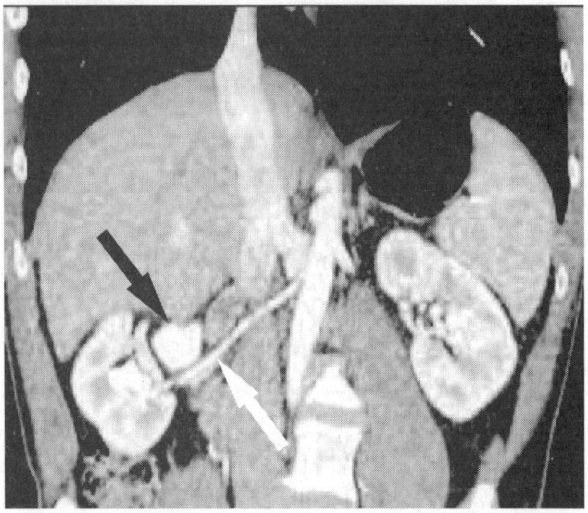

Shows contrast within the dilated pelvis (black arrow) and an underlying crossing anomalous left renal artery (white arrow).

Figure 66

Retrograde pyelogram showing a lucent filling defect (arrow) in the left ureter

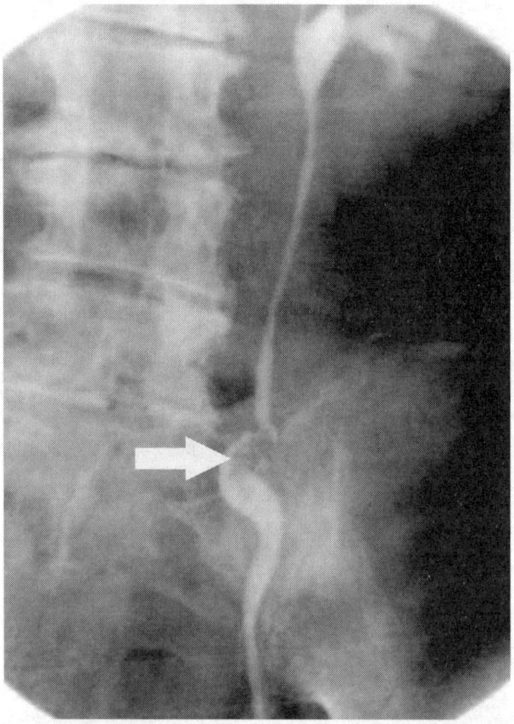

Note that the ureter below the filling defect is slightly dilated. This "goblet" side is relatively characteristic of ureteral transitional cell carcinoma, because the stiff tumor holds open the ureter.

Figure 67

Axial contrast-enhanced CT image in a 84-year-old man with a history of bladder cancer

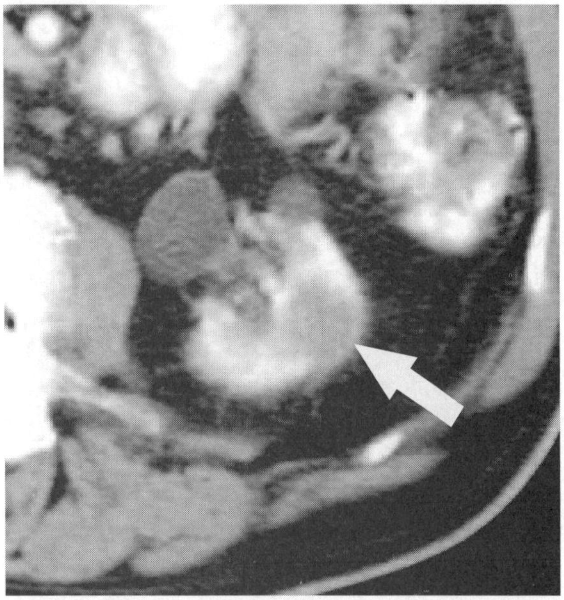

A hypodense mass (arrow) in the left kidney was found to be a transitional cell carcinoma at resection. Transitional cell carcinoma should be considered in the differential for a solid renal mass in a patient with a history of bladder cancer.

Figure 68A

Axial contrast-enhanced CT image in a 56-year-old women with a 5-year history of reccurrent hematuria

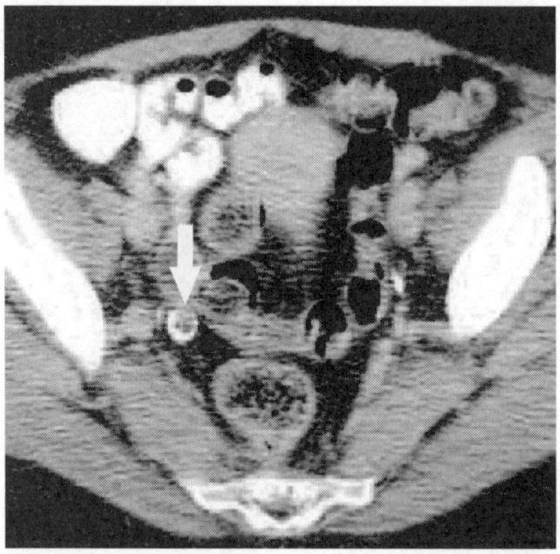

Shows a lucent filling defect in the distal right ureter (arrow).

Figure 68B

Coronal reformatted CT image

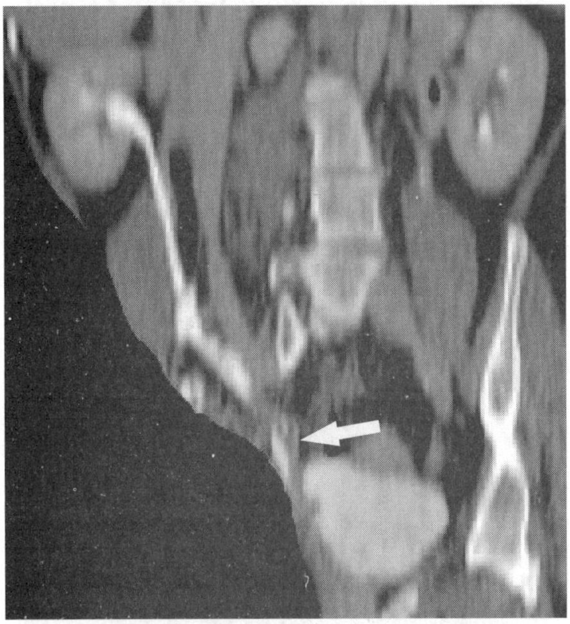

Demonstrates that the filling defect (arrow) has a linear configuration in the distal ureter. Final histopathology confirmed the diagnosis of a fibroepithelial polyp.

Figure 69

Axial contrast-enhanced CT image in a patient with a urachal adenocarcinoma

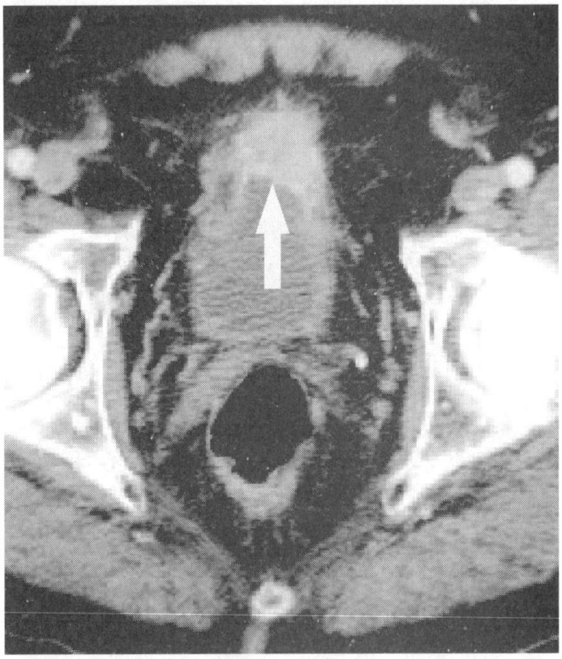

The finding of a midline anterior bladder mass (arrow) should raise consideration of a urachal cancer.

Figure 70

Axial contrast-enhanced CT image

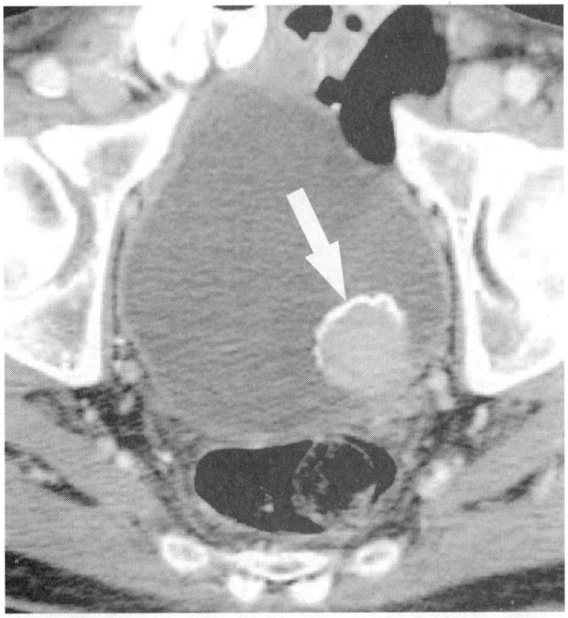

Shows a polypoid filling defect in the bladder with surface calcification (arrow). This appearance is typical of transitional cell carcinoma.

Figure 71

Sagittal T2 weighted post-gadolinium image

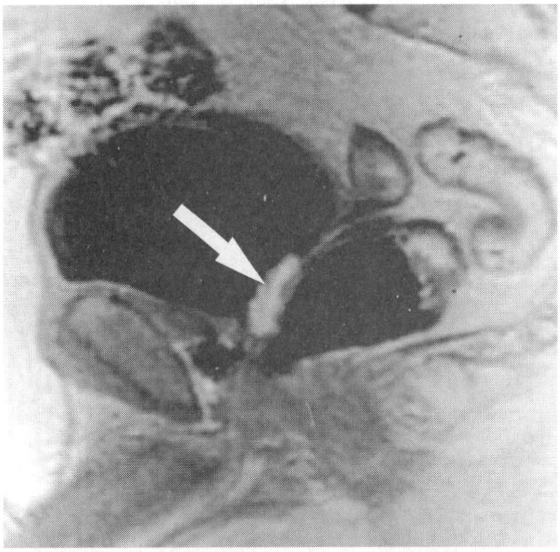

Shows an infiltrative enhancing lesion in the (arrow) posterior wall of the bladder. Such an infiltrative appearance is typical of higher grade transitional cell carcinoma.

Figure 72A

Coronal T2 weighted MRI image

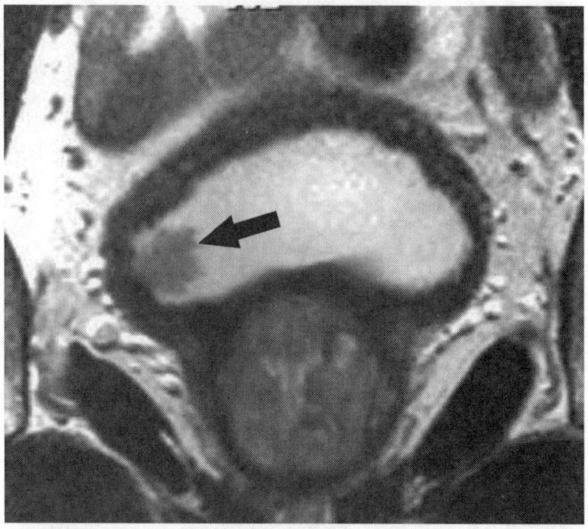

Shows a polypoid transitional cell carcinoma (arrow) in the bladder. The muscular wall of the bladder can be seen as a low signal layer deep to the tumor, and there is no sign of tumor extension into this muscle layer.

Figure 72B

Axial contrast-enhanced CT image in a patient with an infiltrative transitional cell carcinoma encasing most of the bladder wall

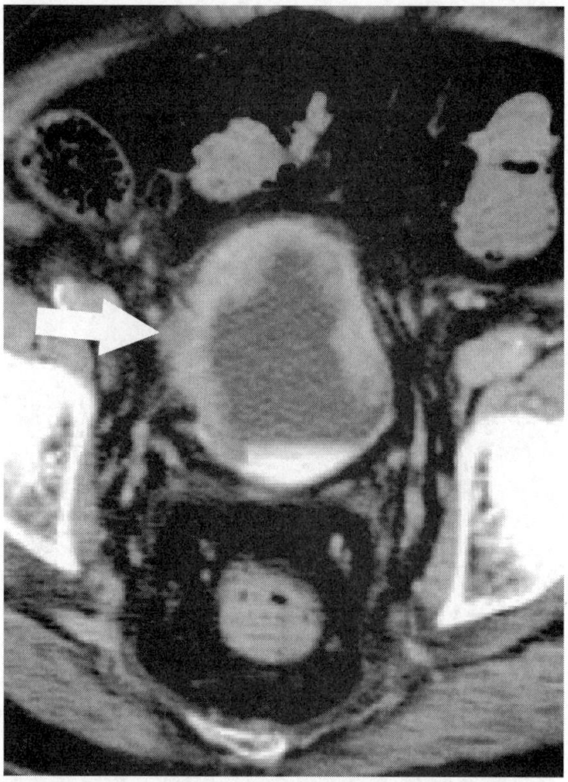

A focus of extravesicalextension (arrow) is visible.

Figure 72C

Axial contrast-enhanced CT image in a patient with an infiltrative transitional cell carcinoma of the bladder

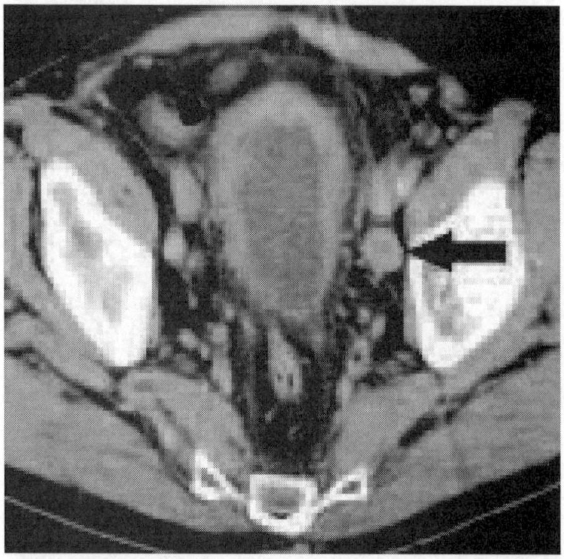

Metastatic adenopathy (arrow) is visible abutting the left pelvic side wall.

Figure 73A

Photomontage showing the appearance of hematoma within the bladder on prone and supine post-contrast CT images

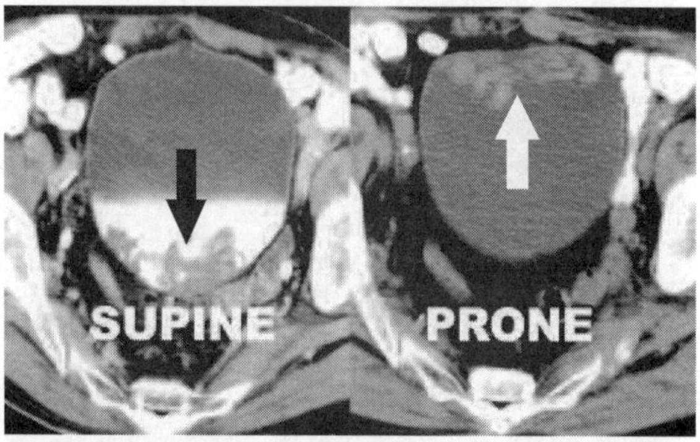

Note that the hematoma (arrow) changes position between prone and supine scans.

Figure 73B

Axial T2-weighted MRI image in a patient with a pheochromocytoma (arrow) of the bladder wall.

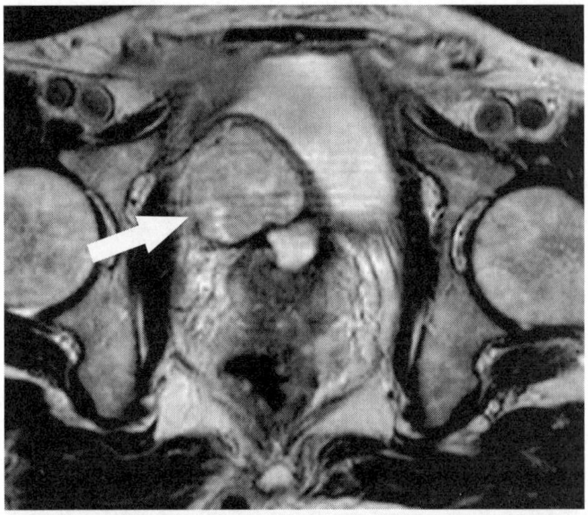

Figure 73C

Axial T2-weighted MRI image in a patient with a leiomyoma (arrow) of the bladder wall.

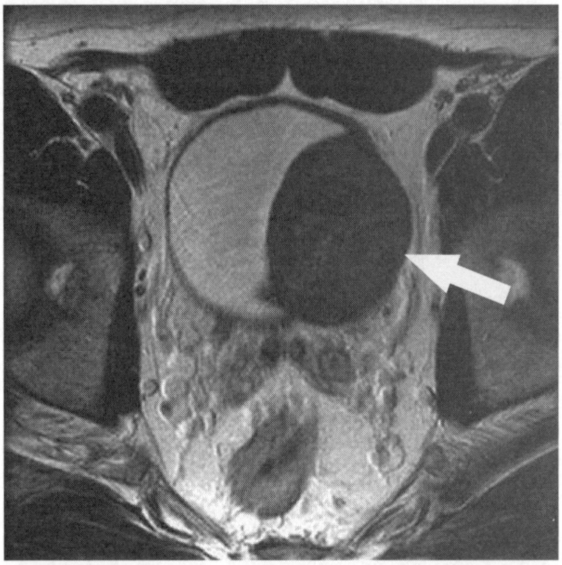

The finding of low T2 intensity would be unusual for a malignant mass, and other diagnosis should be considered.

Figure 74A

Cystogram in a patient after a motor vehicle accident

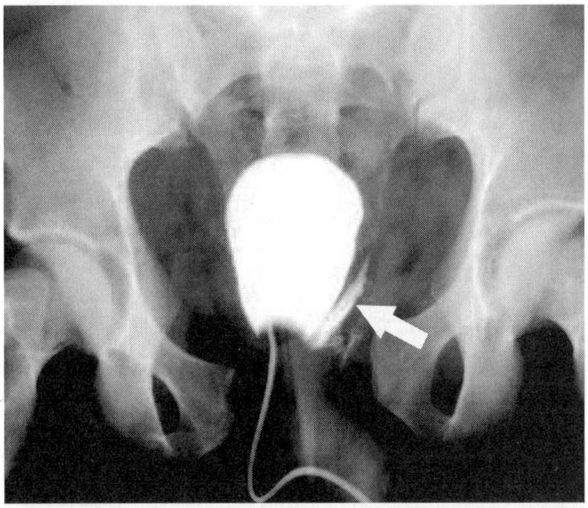

The typical flame shaped appearance (arrow) of extraperitoneal extravasation is evident, consistent with extraperitoneal bladder rupture. Note there is also wide post-traumatic diastasis of the symphysis pubis.

Figure 74B

Cystogram demonstrating the typical appearance of intraperitoneal bladder rupture, with extravasated contrast outlining bowel loops

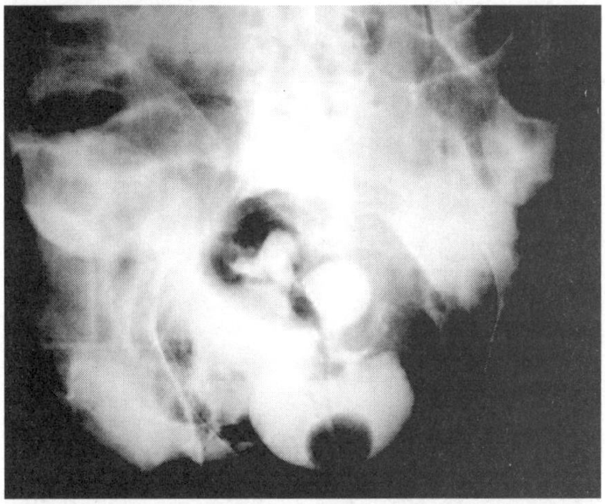

Figure 75A

CT cystogram showing perivesical contrast extravasation (arrow) due to extraperitoneal bladder rupture

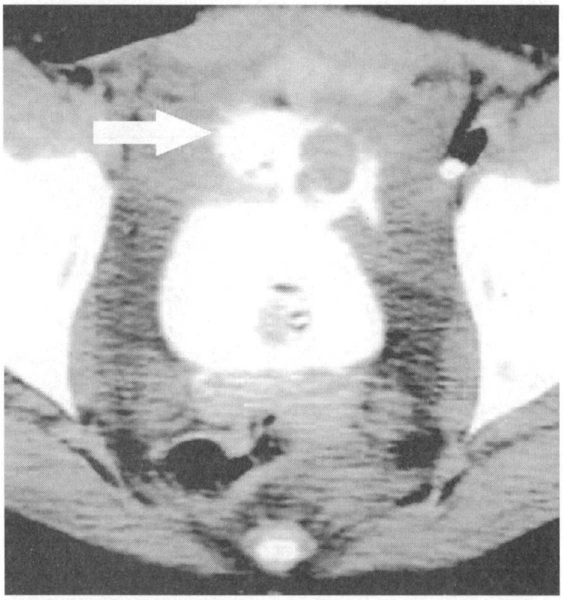

Figure 75B

Axial CT cystogram image showing extravasated contrast outlining bowel loops within the pelvis and lower abdomen due to intraperitoneal bladder rupture

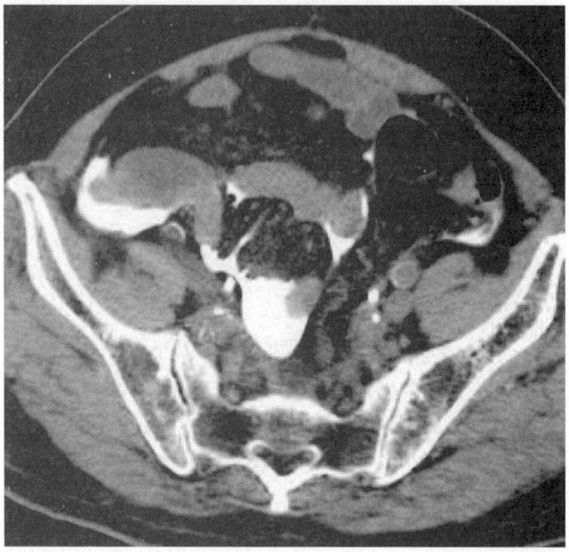

Figure 76

Cystogram showing the typical "pine cone" or "Christmas tree" appearance of a spastic neurogenic bladder

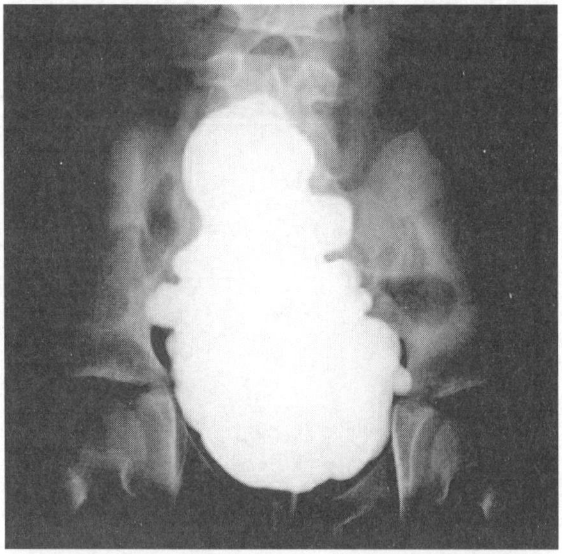

In this case, the findings were due to sacral agenesis.

Figure 77

Axial contrast-enhanced CT image in a patient with a flaccid neurogenic bladder

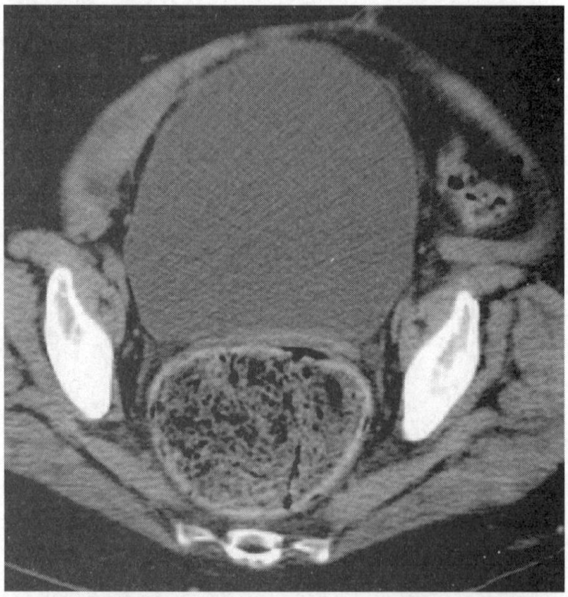

The bladder seemed to be of large volume, although the distinction from physiologic distention is difficult. However, note fecal loading within the rectum. This coexistent finding should raise consideration of neurological problems.

Figure 78A

Coronal T2-weighted MR image of the prostate in a healthy 26-year-old man

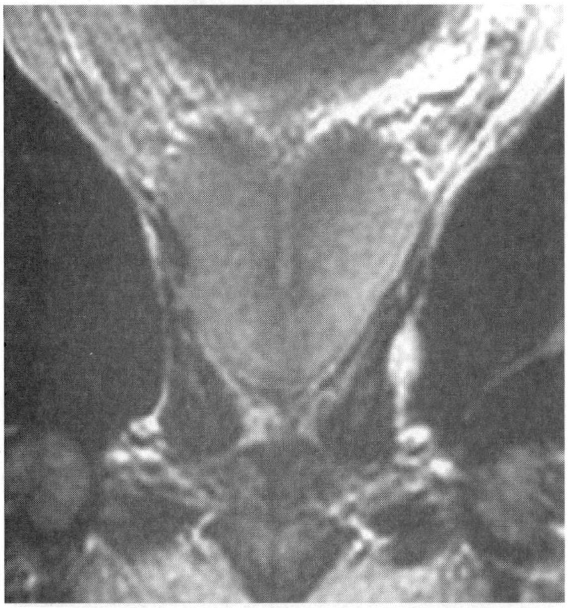

The prostate is small, of uniform intermediate T2 signal intensity, and lacks visible zonal differentiation.

Figure 78B

Coronal T2-weighted MR image of the prostate in a healthy 50-year-old man

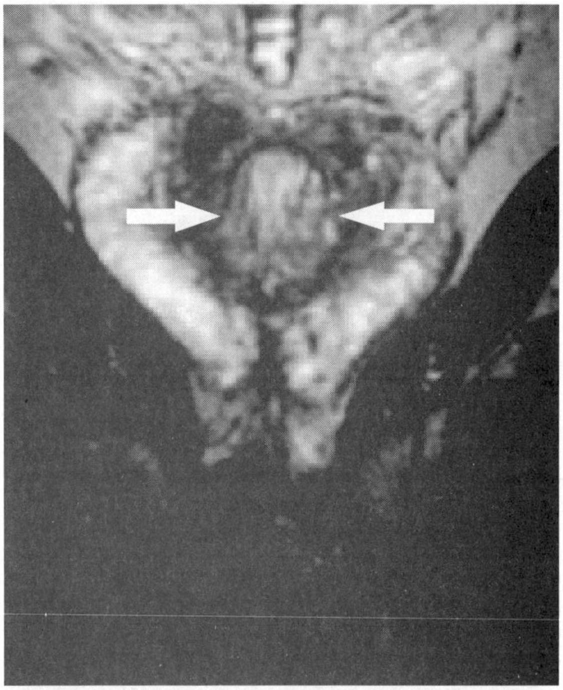

The prostate is of intermediate size due to early changes of benign prostatic hyperplasia, and the hyperplastic transition zone (arrows) can be seen as a central globular structure, surrounded by the compressed central zone.

Figure 78C

Coronal T2-weighted MR image of the prostate in a healthy 78-year-old man

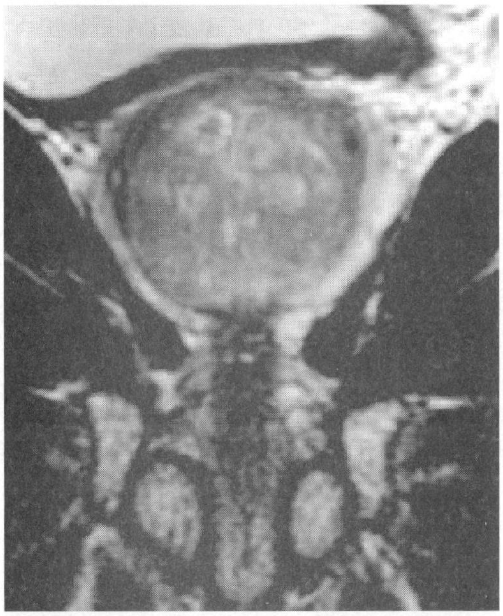

The prostate is enlarged due to marked hyperplastic changes in the transition zone. The peripheral zone is compressed to a rim of thin tissue and the central zone is barely visible as thin "pseudocapsule" between the transition and peripheral zones.

Figure 79

IVU in a patient with marked benign prostatic hyperplasia

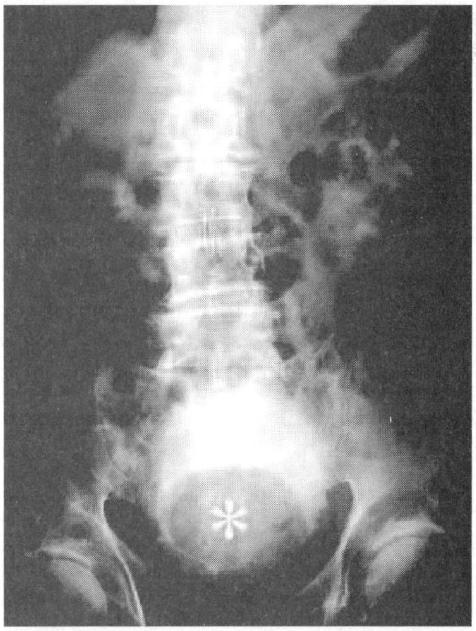

Shows a large filling defect (asterisk) indenting and lifting the bladder base. This filling defect is the markedly large prostate. Note the bladder is also trabeculated.

Figure 80A

Axial contrast-enhanced CT image in a patient with metastatic prostate cancer, demonstrating adenopathy (arrow) along the pelvic side wall and external iliac chains

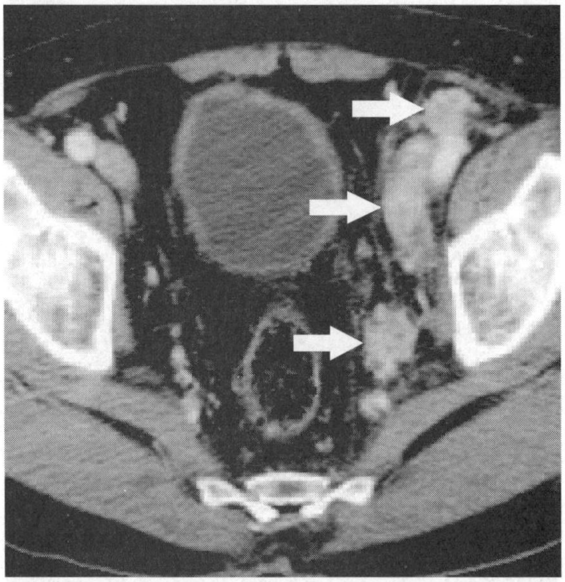

Figure 80B

Axial contrast-enhanced CT image in the same patient at a higher level demonstrating retroperitoneal adenopathy (arrow) due to metastatic prostate cancer

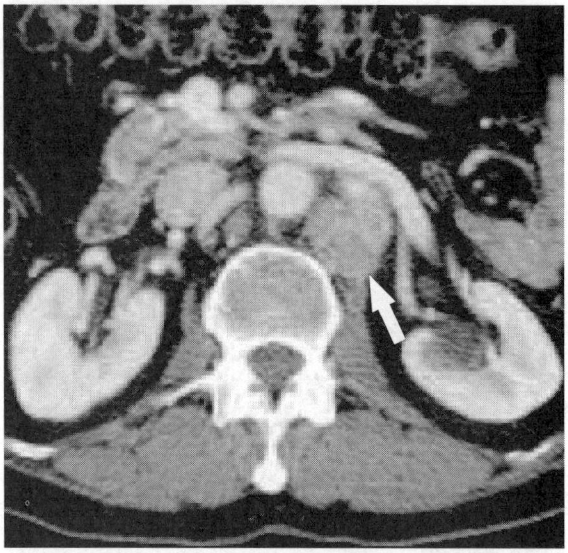

Figure 81

Bone scan showing the typical appearances of widely metastatic prostate cancer with multifocal areas of increased uptake in the pelvis and spine

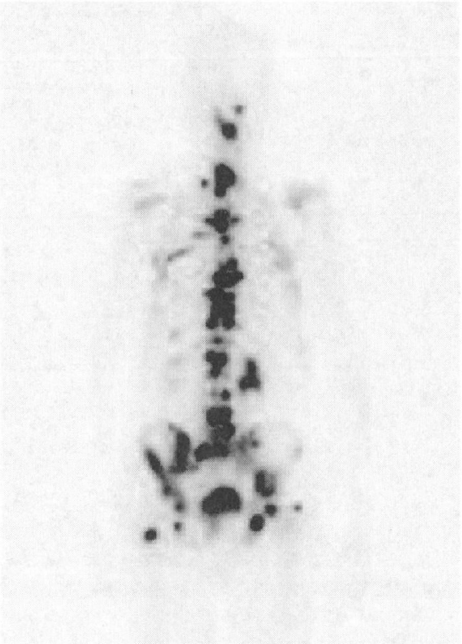

Figure 82A

Transrectal ultrasound showing a hypoechoic area (arrow) in the left peripheral zone of the prostate due to prostate cancer

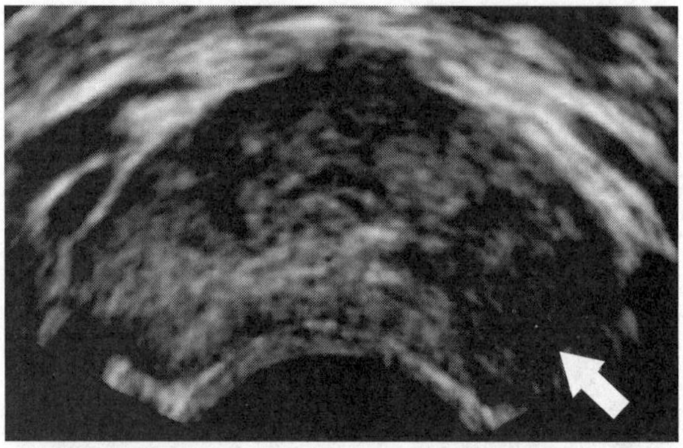

Figure 82B

The addition of Doppler interrogation shows increased vascularity within the lesion (arrow), again typical of prostate carcinoma

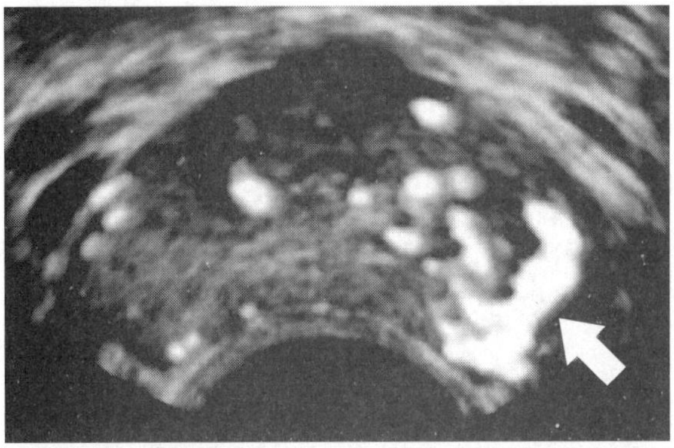

Figure 83

Axial T2-weighted MRI image in a patient with prostate cancer

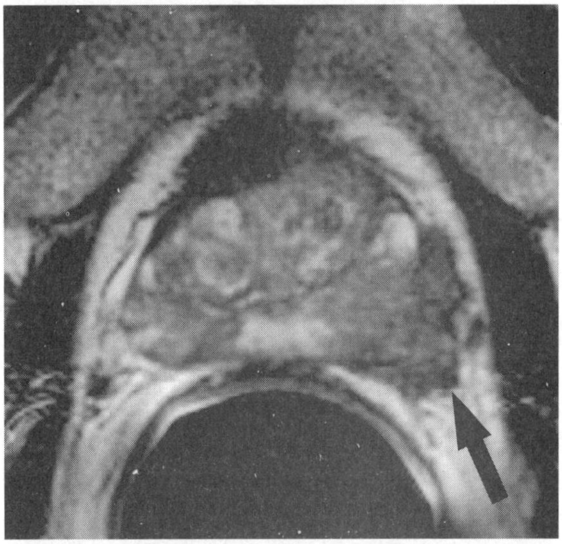

Shows a large irregular focus of low T2 signal intensity in the left peripheral zone of the prostate. The lesion has an irregular interface with the adjacent periprostatic fat and extracapsular extension is evident (arrow).

Figure 84A

Retrograde urethrogram in a patient with a stricture of the bulbar urethra

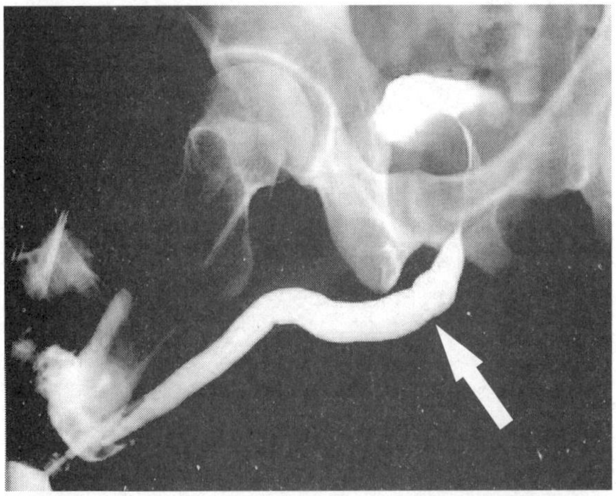

The stricture (arrow) is not well appreciated due to obliquity.

Figure 84B

Voiding cystourethrogram in the same patient

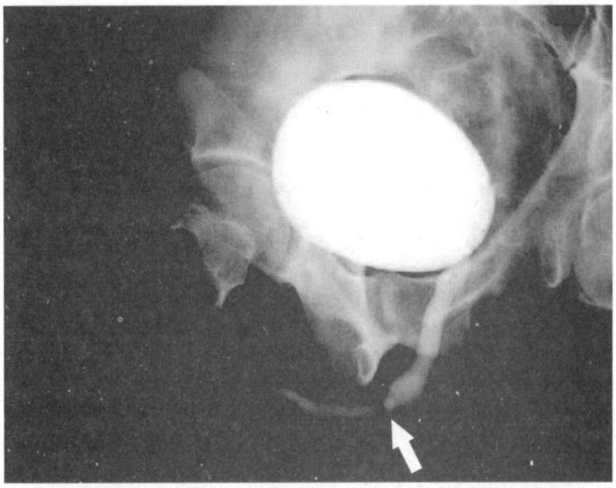

This image better delineates the stricture (arrow), and also documents upstream dilatation of the urethra, confirming functionally significant obstruction.

Figure 85

High frequency ultrasound image of the urethra showing irregular wall thickening (arrow) of a urethral stricture

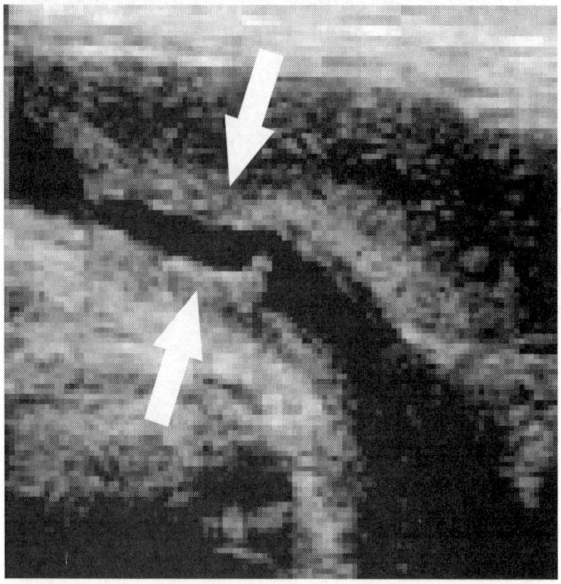

Figure 86

Retrograde urethrogram in a patient with traumatic urethral disruption

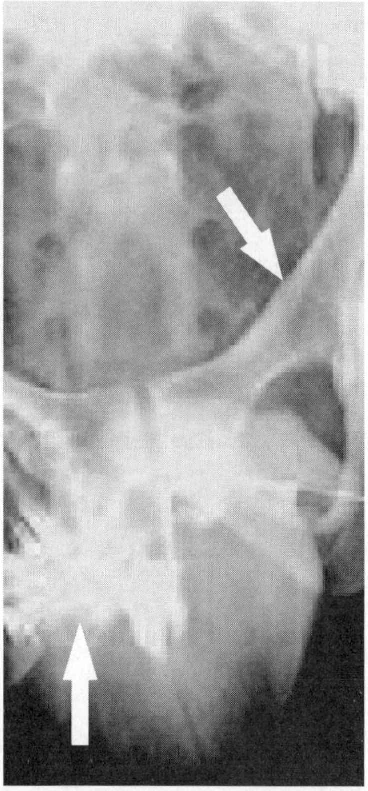

Extravasated contrast is evident (vertical arrow) within the soft tissues of the pelvis. A fracture line can also be seen in the left superior pubic ramus (oblique arrow).

Figure 87

Cystogram performed with a double balloon technique shows a large urethral diverticulum (arrow)

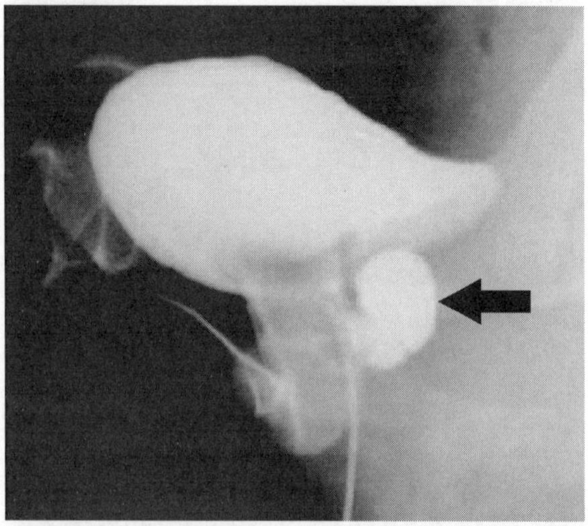

Figure 88

Axial T2-weighted MRI image showing a urethral diverticulum (arrow)

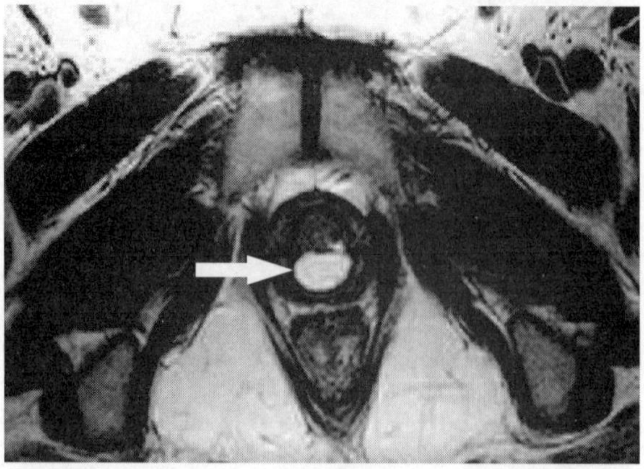

Figure 89

Ultrasound image shows a large heterogeneously hypoechoic mass (between arrows) in the upper pole of the testes due to testicular cancer

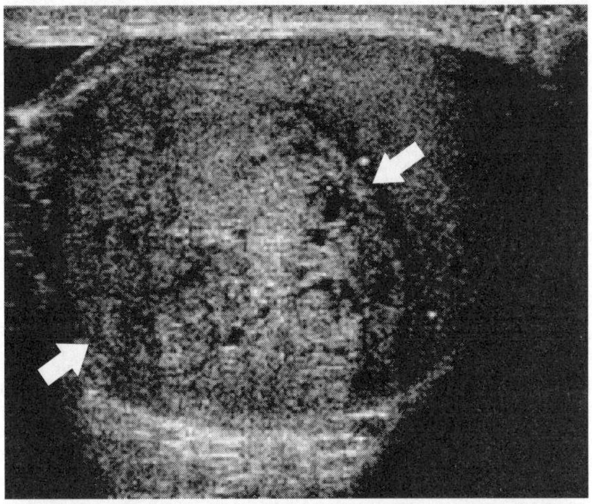

Figure 90

Testicular ultrasound showing the typical appearance of tubular ectasia of the rete testis (arrow)

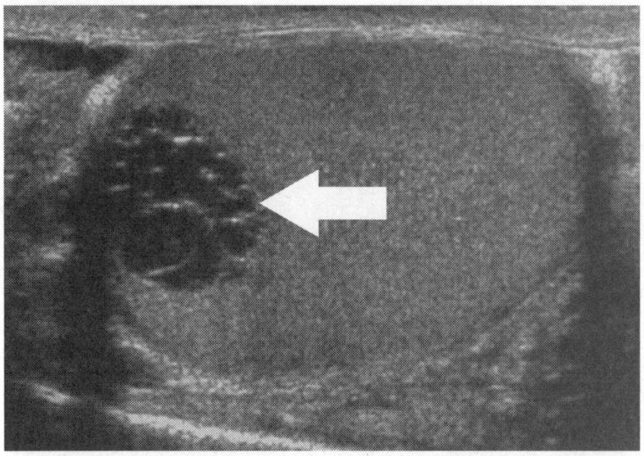

Figure 91

Photomontage of bilateral testicular ultrasound with Doppler showing a hypervascular mass (arrow) in 1 testis

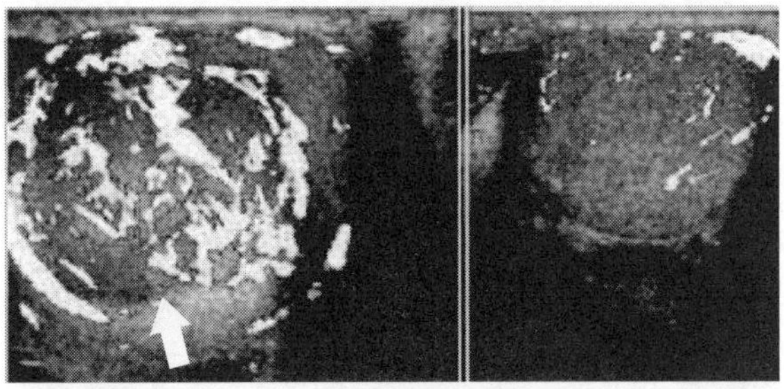

This mass was due to lymphomatous spread in an elderly male patient.

Figure 92

Testicular ultrasound showing a heterogeneous and enlarged testis

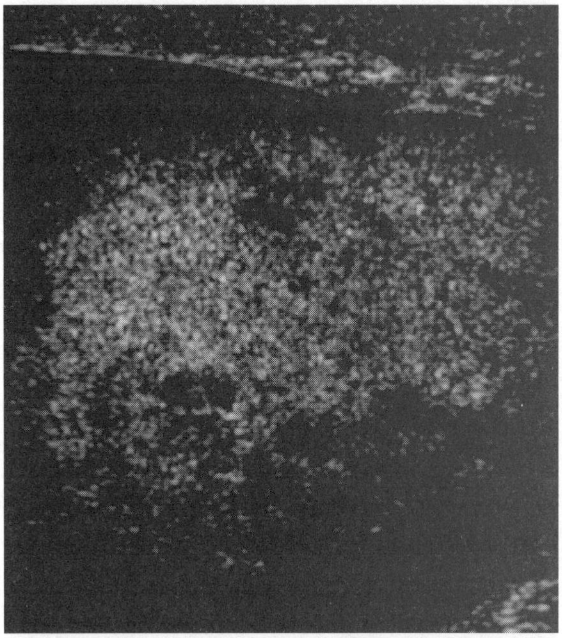

In this case, it was due to metastatic prostate cancer.

Figure 93

IVU demonstrating the typical stippled calcification of neuroblastoma

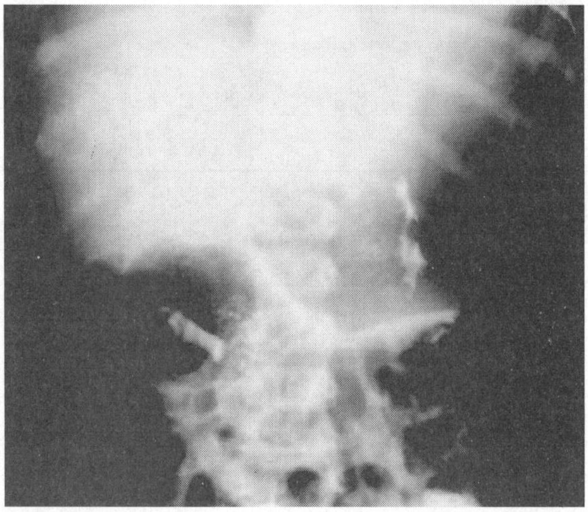

Figure 94

Axial contrast-enhanced CT image

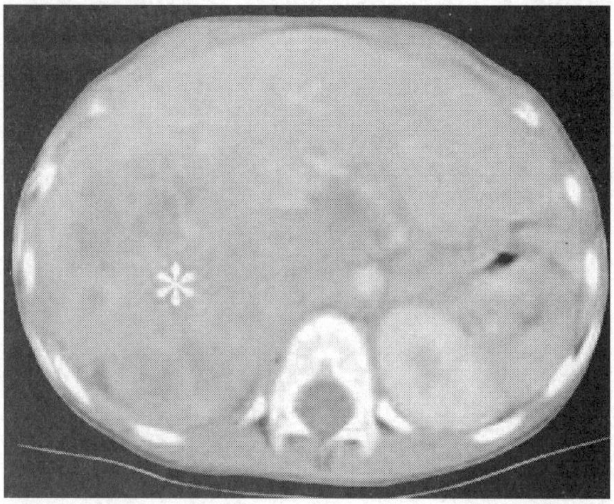

Shows a large heterogeneous mass (asterisk) above the right kidney, with leftward displacement of the aorta and obliteration of the inferior vena cava. This was a proven neuroblastoma.

Figure 95

Coronal T1-weighted post-contrast MRI image

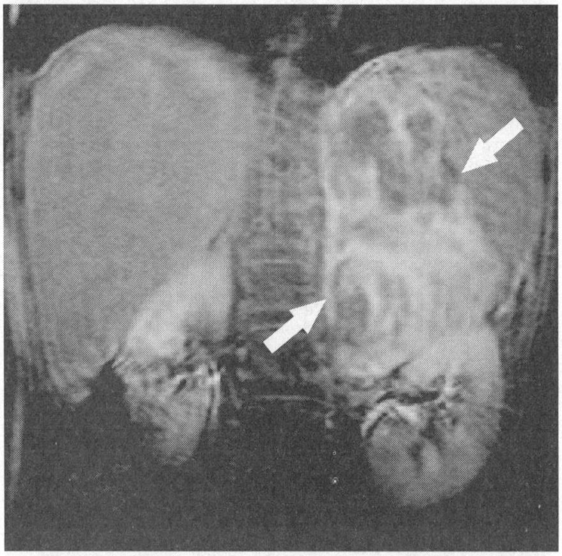

Shows a heterogeneously enhancing neuroblastoma (between arrows) above the left kidney.

Figure 96

Axial contrast-enhanced CT image of nephroblastomatosis in a 9-month-old boy

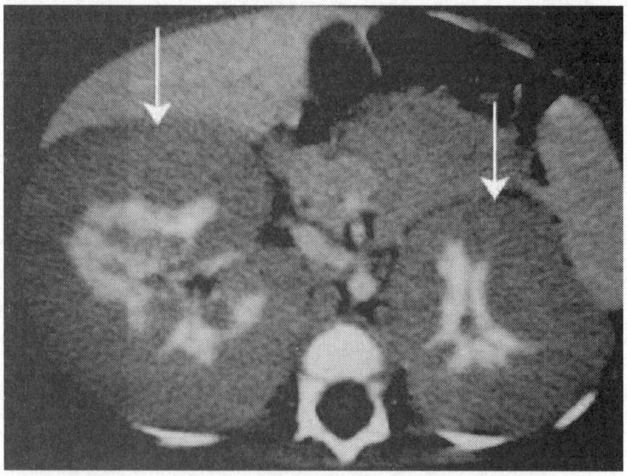

Shows bilaterally enlarged kidneys due to presence of cortical hypodense, non-enhancing, soft tissue mass (arrows). Note distorted remaining renal parenchyma centrally.

Figure 97

Ultrasound image showing a Wilm's Tumor (between calipers) in the kidney

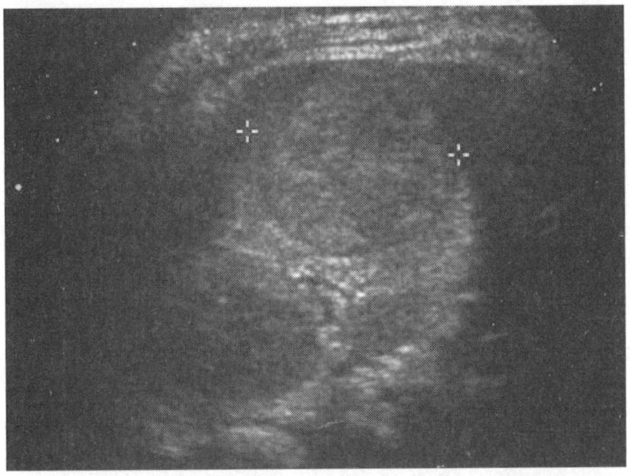

Figure 98

Axial contrast-enhanced CT image showing a Wilm's tumor (arrow) in the right kidney

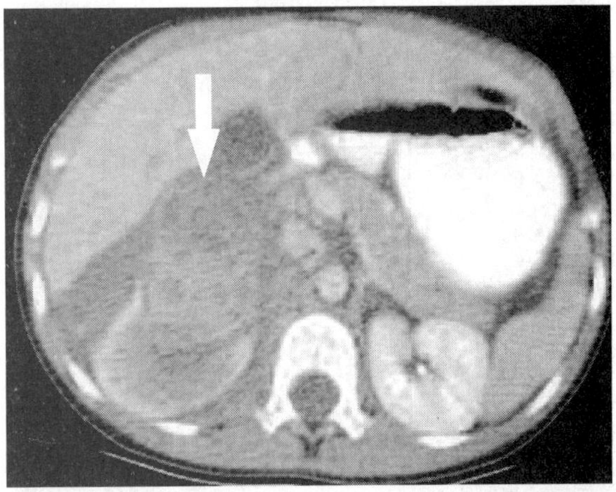

Figure 99

Axial contrast-enhanced CT image showing a pelvic kidney (arrow) anterior to the sacrum

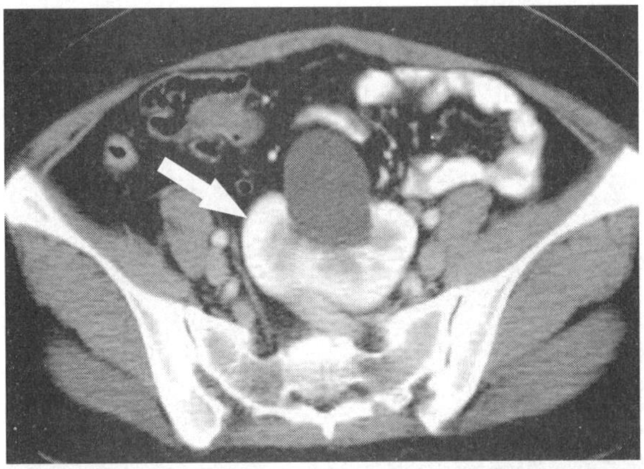

Figure 100

Coronal T2-weighted MRI image of crossed unfused ectopia

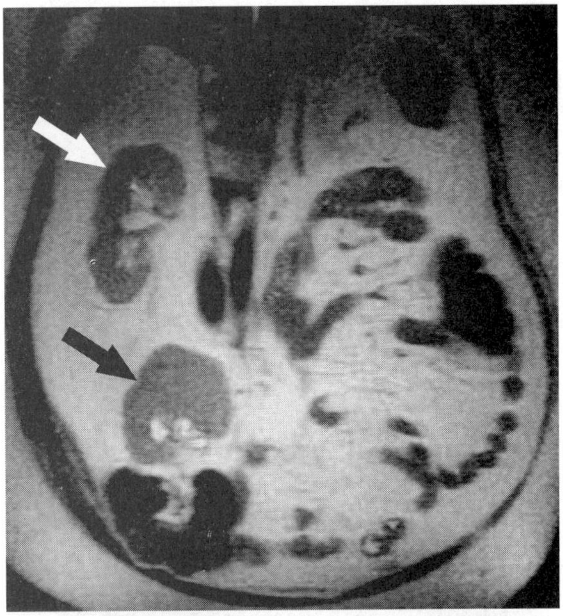

Note that the right kidney (white arrow) is located normally while the left kidney (black arrow) is located abnormally in the right lower quadrant.

Figure 101

IVU of horseshoe kidney, showing the pelvicaliceal systems to be malrotated with medial deviation inferiorly

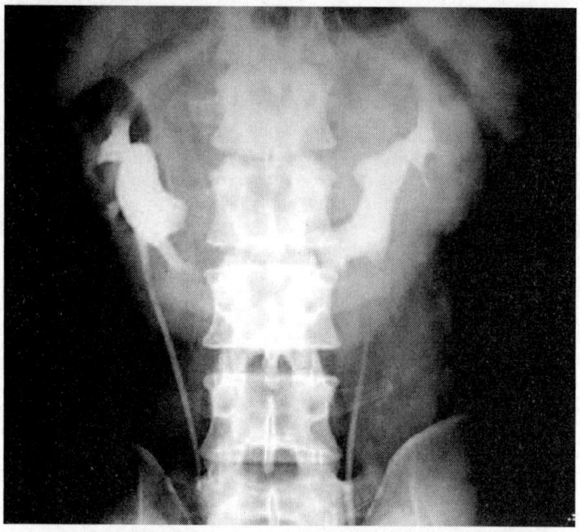

Figure 102

Coronal reformat CT image showing a horseshoe kidney

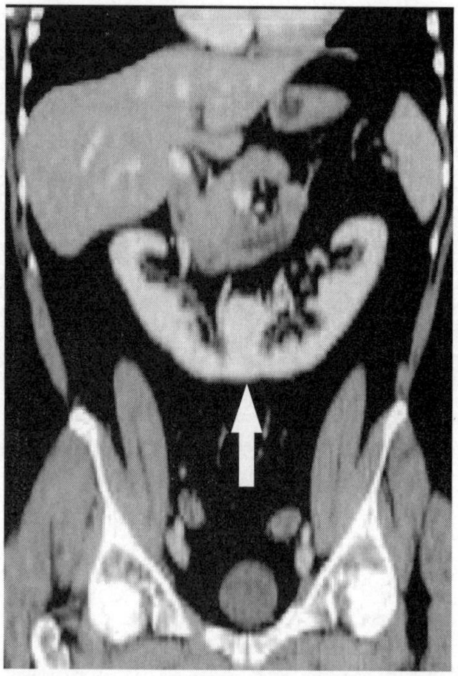

The bridging tissue (arrow) between the lower folds of both kidneys is clearly documented.

Figure 103

Voiding cystourethrogram showing marked bilateral vesicoureteral reflux

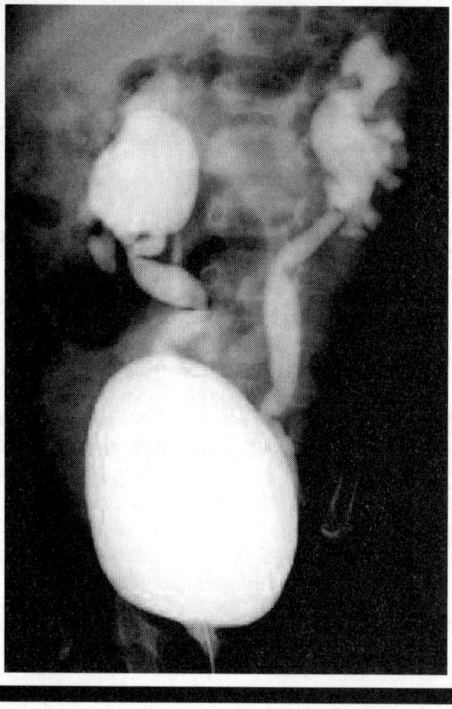

Figure 104A

Cystogram showing a filling defect (arrow) in the bladder of a child.

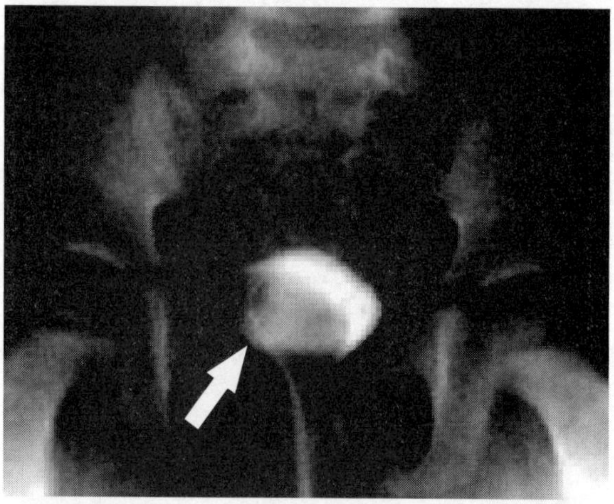

Figure 104B

Ultrasound image confirms that the lesion (arrow) is fluid-containing, consistent with a ureterocele

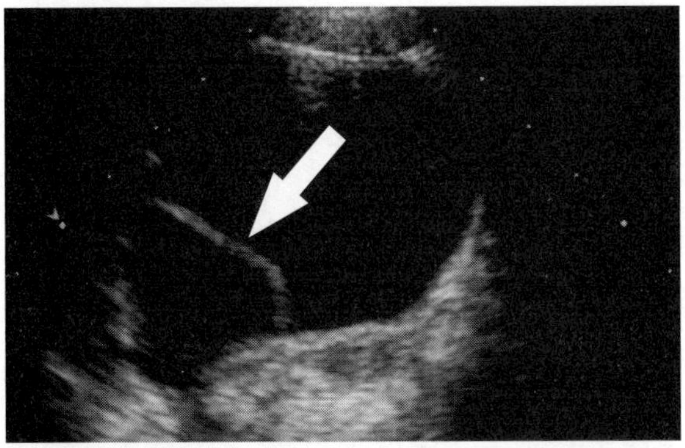

A ureterocele is the primary consideration for a filling defect in the bladder of a child.

Figure 105

IVP showing the typical cobra-head appearance (arrow) of the distal right ureter due to a ureterocele

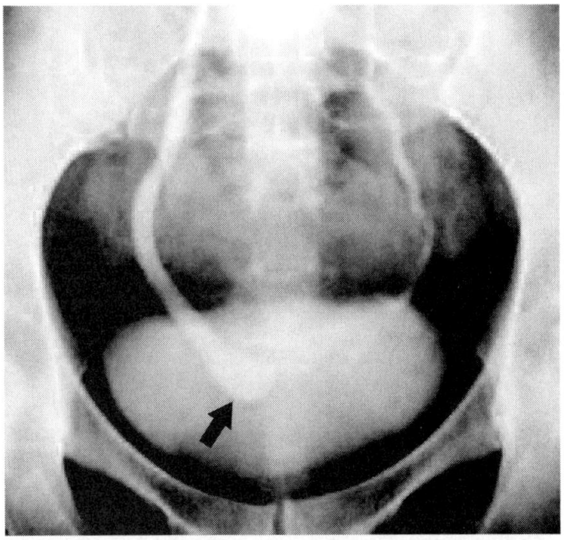

Figure 106

Voiding cystourethrogram in a patient with posterior urethral valves

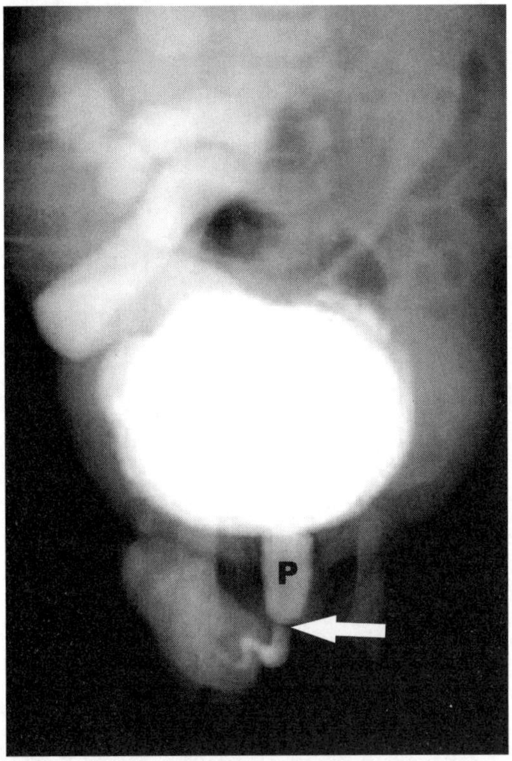

Note that the prostatic urethra (P) is dilated and elongated, with a horizontal filling defect (arrow) inferiorly due to the valve leaflets.

Chapter 6: Urologic Pathology

Jo Ellen Krueger, MD

Contents

1. Cytology of the Urogenital Tract

1. Types of Epithelial Cells Encountered

Transitional epithelium (urothelium)—bladder, ureters, proximal urethra

Squamous cells—bladder trigone (40% of women), distal urethra

Glandular cells—caused by foci of glandular metaplasia in the GU tract

2. Use of Cytology

A. Diagnosis and follow-up of patients with neoplasms of the urinary tract

B. Screening of high risk patients (eg, chemical industry workers)

C. **Sampling Techniques:**
   1. Voided urine—catheterization can dislodge clusters of cells and induce mild atypia
   2. Washings and Brushings
      a. produce abundant well-preserved cells for evaluation
      b. risk of false positive as instrumentation may result in "papillary" clusters as well as red blood cells

D. **Cytology of Normal Cells**
   1. Transitional cells
      a. Superficial transitional cells—form the majority of cells in specimens
         - Vary greatly in size and shape, but generally are large, flat, polygonal cells with abundant thin (transparent) cytoplasm
      b. Deep transitional cells—tend to have a smaller size and a denser cytoplasm
      c. **Cytoplasm**: cyanophilic (**blue**) and **vacuolated**
      d. **Nuclei**: tend to have **one or two round/oval nuclei** with **smooth contours**, finely granular chromatin ("salt and pepper"), and well-defined nuclear membranes
      e. N:C ratio may be high, but never exceeds 1:2
      f. Nucleoli are inconspicuous or absent in normal cells
      g. Multinucleation (as in >2, <50) and small red nucleoli can be seen after catheterization, as a reactive change
      h. In voided urines, transitional cells are shed singly; in washings/brushings, the cells tend to be aggregated in sheets. If there are no fibrovascular cores, however, these sheets do not represent papillary clusters
      i. Increased numbers of transitional cells can be seen with:
         - instrumentation/catheterization
         - calculi
         - inflammatory and neoplastic conditions
   2. Squamous Cells
      a. Normally seen in voided urine as a contaminant from the distal urethra/vagina/vulva; also may be seen arising from the bladder trigone in 40% of women and in men on estrogen therapy for prostate cancer
      b. Also increased in cases of chronic irritation and inflammation
   3. Columnar cells
      a. Due to glandular metaplasia in the bladder and ureters (in men, may also originate from the prostate or seminal vesicles after prostatic massage)
      b. Prostate cells
         - Form small aggregates that maintain a "ball-like" or glandular configuration
         - Cells are small and may be columnar or round with slightly pink cytoplasm; cytoplasm also is often foamy or vacuolated
         - Nucleus: single, small, round or oval, with finely granular chromatin
      c. Seminal vesicle cells
         - Usually smaller than transitional cells and are almost always degenerated
         - Nuclei are enlarged and hyperchromatic with little or no chromatin structure ("glassy" appearance)
         - Cytoplasm contains golden-yellow lipochrome pigment and vacuoles

3. Inflammatory and Other Non-neoplastic Conditions

A. Reactive transitional cells
1. Nuclei become enlarged and hyperchromatic with prominent nucleoli, but maintain their smooth borders and low N:C ratio
2. Binucleation/multinucleation common

B. Bacterial/fungal/parasitic infections
1. Usually associated with lots of neutrophils, red cells, and lymphocytes in the urine (a few lymphocytes and some scattered red cells can be seen in normal people)
2. The usual suspects in these situations include:
   a. Bacteria—especially gram negative rods
   b. *Candida*—see budding yeast and pseudohyphae
   c. *Trichomonas*—most common parasite in the United States; in Egypt, look for *Schistosomiasis*
3. Remember: if you see a lot of bugs and yeast, but no inflammation, the most likely explanation is contamination of the specimen

C. Viral infections
1. HSV: look for multinucleated transitional cells with "ground glass" nuclei and large eosinophilic intranuclear inclusions surrounded by a halo
2. CMV: classically associated with an enlarged nucleus which contains a single irregular blue-ish "bird's eye" inclusion
3. Polyoma virus:
   - seen most often in immunocompromised hosts
   - has been associated with interstitial nephritis and obstruction of the ureteral lumen and may be important in renal transplantation
   - **"decoy cells"**: huge cells with large nuclei having interrupted nuclear membranes and **glassy basophilic inclusions** that push chromatin to the edges
   - because of their high N:C ratio, cells may mimic carcinoma (hence the name "decoy cells") but the key to their benign nature is the glassy chromatin pattern and the relative paucity of affected cells

4. Tumors of the Urinary Bladder

A. **Transitional cell papillomas**—virtually impossible to detect by cytology unless a cell block is used. Which is never. So just forget about it

B. **Low-grade transitional cell carcinoma**
1. Papillary fragments or cell clusters
2. Cells have a high N:C ratio
3. Nuclei vary in size and shape, but often appear indented or grooved
4. Variability of nuclear staining within a given group
5. These findings are most significant in a voided urine sample (since similar features can be induced by instrumentation)
6. Transitional carcinoma cells are usually larger than normal transitional cells, and have eccentric nuclei, but chromatin is still fairly evenly distributed
7. Nucleoli are absent or small

C. **High-grade transitional cell carcinoma and carcinoma in situ**
1. Large numbers of poorly cohesive cells that shed singly or in small clusters
2. High N:C ratio
3. Nuclei are large, hyperchromatic, pleomorphic, with prominent red nucleoli
4. Chromatin is coarsely clumped
5. Look at the background to distinguish between TCC and CIS: a "dirty" background with cellular debris and numerous neutrophils suggests invasion, while a "clean" background suggests that the tumor may still be in situ

D. **Squamous cell carcinoma**
1. Represents 5% of bladder tumors, and is associated with chronic inflammatory conditions (calculi, diverticulum, cord bladder, schistosomiasis)
2. Urine specimens show abundant keratinized cells ("hard" peach/pink cytoplasm) with large hyperchromatic nuclei, and often have a "dirty" background because the lesions are usually advanced (invasive)

E. Adenocarcinoma

1. Represent less than 5% of bladder tumors
2. If arising in the dome, often originate from urachal remnants, whereas those in the bladder base are derived from islands of glandular metaplasia
3. Tend to shed as small clusters (balls) rather than as single cells
4. Cytoplasm is often vacuolated and nuclei have prominent nucleoli
5. Poorly differentiated adenocarcinoma can be indistinguishable from high-grade TCC
6. Whenever the diagnosis of adenocarcinoma is made, must rule out metastatic disease (esp. from colon)

5. Effects of Therapy

A. TURP: see nuclear enlargement and dying cells for days or weeks post-procedure

B. Irradiation/chemotherapy: cellular enlargement and hyperchromasia—see larger nuclei but N:C ratio is typically preserved (one key to the reactive nature of these cells). Also: should see degenerative changes, with poorly preserved ("smudged") chromatin

C. BCG treatment: granulomas; lymphocytes and histiocytes in the background; cellular enlargement/nuclear hyperchromasia

2. Renal Tumors I: Pediatric Renal Tumors

1. Wilms' Tumor (Nephroblastoma)

A. General

1. Comprises >80% of renal tumors in childhood
2. Occurs most frequently in children 2-4 years of age; extremely uncommon in children <6 months and >6 years
3. Slight preponderance of females; bilateral in 4.4% of cases
4. May be associated with other congenital anomalies:
   a. WAGR syndrome
   b. Beckwith-Wiedemann syndrome—5% of patients develop Wilms' tumor
   c. Denys-Drash syndrome
5. Clinical presentation:
   a. Large abdominal mass that may cross the midline
   b. Hematuria, abdominal pain, intestinal obstruction, hypertension
   c. Laboratory: may have increased erythropoeitin level without polycythemia
   d. Radiology: calcification uncommon (in contrast to neuroblastoma)

B. Gross Pathology

1. Usually large (>5 cm, >500 g)
2. Cut surface is typically solid, soft, and gray or pink, resembling brain tissue
3. Foci of hemorrhage and necrosis are often present
4. Cysts are common
5. May appear well circumscribed

C. Pertinent Histopathologic Definitions

1. Nephrogenic rests: foci of persistent nephrogenic cells resembling those of the developing kidney
   a. **Perilobar nephrogenic rests**—located at the edge of the lobe
      - have well-defined smooth borders and show a predominance of blastema
      - often are numerous or diffuse
      - may be present in approximately 1% of infants < 3 months of age
   b. **Intralobar nephrogenic rests**—located in the cortex or medulla within the renal lobe where they mingle irregularly with the renal parenchyma
      - show a predominance of stroma

- usually are single
- almost never seen except with Wilms' tumor

c. **Nephroblastomatosis:** the diffuse or multifocal presence of nephrogenic rests, or multicentric or bilateral Wilms' tumor

2. Nephrogenic rests are present in approximately 41% of patients with unilateral Wilms' tumor, but are present in 95% of patients with bilateral Wilms' tumor. Therefore, careful examination of the grossly uninvolved renal tissue is important, since the presence of nephrogenic rests indicates a greater probability of synchronous or metachronous bilaterality

D. Microscopic Pathology

1. Wilms' tumors are typically composed of three elements:
   a. **Blastema:** consists of sheets of randomly arranged, densely packed small cells with darkly staining nuclei, frequent mitotic figures, and inconspicuous cytoplasm, resembling other "small blue cell tumors" of childhood
   b. **Epithelial component:** consists of small tubules or cysts lined by primitive columnar or cuboidal cells
      - may form structures resembling glomeruli, or may display mucinous, squamous, neural, or endocrine differentiation
      - predominantly cystic Wilms' tumors that contain blastema and other Wilms' tumor tissues in the septa, are designated cystic partially differentiated nephroblastoma

   c. **Stromal component:** may differentiate along the lines of any type of soft tissue
      - myxoid and fibroblastic stroma types are the most common.
      - smooth muscle, skeletal muscle, fat, cartilage, bone,and neural components may also be present
2. Anaplasia
   a. Defined as the combination of cells with **very large hyperchromatic nuclei** and **multipolar mitotic figures**
   b. The enlarged nuclei must be at least three times the size of typical blastema nuclei in both axes, and hyperchromasia must be obvious
   c. **Hyperdiploid** mitotic figures must be present
   d. **Mitotic figures** should be **enlarged** as well
   e. **Anaplasia is significant, as it predicts resistance to treatment**

F. Clinical Behavior and Prognosis

1. Most important prognostic indicator is stage
2. Other prognostically significant features:
   a. Age <2 years
   b. Size (weight)
   c. Anaplasia (bad)
   d. Extensive tubular differentiation (good)
   e. Extensive skeletal muscle differentiation (good)
   f. Mucin production (bad)
   g. DNA ploidy
3. Most common metastatic sites: peritoneum, liver,and lung (metastasis to bone is rare, in contrast to neuroblastoma)
4. Now 90% long-term survival using three modalities (surgery, chemotherapy, radiation therapy)
5. Patients with anaplastic features in the tumors tend to be more resistant to treatment: they are often older than 2 years of age, and typically present with more advanced disease

2. Mesoblastic Nephroma

A. General

1. Most common renal neoplasm in the infants <3 months; uncommon after 6 months
2. May be associated with polyhydramnios and prematurity
3. Usually presents with abdominal mass

B. Gross Pathology

1. Typically large with a firm, gray-white, trabeculated (whorled) cut surface
2. Often unencapsulated; may extend into surrounding tissues

C. Microscopic Pathology

1. Classical mesoblastic nephroma
   a. Moderately cellular proliferation of thick interlacing bundles of spindle cells with elongated nuclei that usually infiltrate renal and perirenal tissues

b. Entrapment of glomeruli and renal tubules is common
c. Mitotic figures are rare (0-1 per 10 hpf)
2. Cellular mesoblastic nephroma:
a. Densely cellular proliferation of polygonal cells with pushing borders
b. Mitotic figures in the range of 8-30 per 10 hpf
c. Cysts are common in this pattern

D. Clinical Behavior and Prognosis

1. Good prognosis: surgical resection is almost invariably curative
2. Adverse prognostic indicators:
a. Age >3 months
b. Incomplete resection
c. Cellular histological pattern

3. Clear Cell Sarcoma

A. General

1. Highly malignant neoplasm comprising 6% of pediatric renal tumors
2. Most diagnosed in patients between 12 and 36 months of age
3. 66% of patients are male
4. Propensity to metastasize to bone is marked: it is at least 10 times more likely to metastasize to bone than other pediatric renal tumors—in fact, it was originally known as "bone-metastasizing renal tumor of childhood"

B. Gross Pathology

1. Variable appearance: homogeneous gray and lobular, or variegated with firm, gray whorled tissue and light pink soft areas; 30% have cystic areas
2. Most appear to be well circumscribed
3. Often weighs more than 500 g
4. Almost always unilateral

C. Microscopic Pathology

1. Monotonous sheet of cells with pale (but not truly clear) cytoplasm
2. At higher magnification, cells appear to be arranged in cords separated by vascular septa having a "chicken wire" pattern
3. Neoplastic cells have pale or vacuolated cytoplasm and indistinct borders
4. Nuclei contain finely dispersed chromatin and small nucleoli
5. One helpful feature is the infiltrative border between the clear cell sarcoma and the surrounding renal parenchyma

D. Clinical Behavior and Prognosis

1. Death rate has been reduced to 30%-40% by modern chemotherapy
2. May have late recurrences, so outcome is ultimately iffy

4. Rhabdoid Tumor of Kidney

A. General

1. The most malignant renal neoplasm of childhood, this tumor usually metastasizes widely and causes death within 12 months of diagnosis
2. Patients are typically <1 year, rarely older than 3 years of age
3. Male > female (1.5:1)
4. May be associated with atypical teratoid tumors of CNS and paraneoplastic hypercalcemia
5. EM shows characteristic concentric whorls of microfilaments in the cytoplasm

B. Gross Pathology

1. No evidence of encapsulation (in contrast to Wilms' tumor or clear cell sarcoma)
2. Often located medially in the kidney, and the renal sinus and pelvis are almost always infiltrated
3. Yellow-gray or light tan friable ("mushy") tumors with hemorrhage, necrosis

C. Microscopic Pathology

1. Diffuse "sheet-like" growth pattern
2. Neoplastic cells are large and polygonal with abundant eosinophilic cytoplasm—superficially resemble skeletal muscle cells, but do not stain for desmin
3. Round nuclei with prominent membranes and large nucleoli
4. Cytoplasm often contains an eosinophilic globular inclusion that displaces the nucleus
5. Infiltrative borders
6. Vascular invasion common

D. Clinical Behavior and Prognosis

Extremely malignant, aggressive behavior: 75% of patients die within 12 months of diagnosis

3. Renal Tumors II: Renal Cell Carcinoma

1. Epidemiology

A. Comprises 80%-90% of adult primary renal tumors, 3% of all adult malignancies
1. Approximately 23,000 new cases/year in the United States
2. Peak incidence in sixth and seventh decades; rarely seen in children
3. Male > female (2:1)

B. Etiology and Pathogenesis

1. Originally thought to arise from heterotopic adrenal rests within the kidney (hence: "hypernephroma")
2. Now known to have several distinct cytogenetic abnormalities, 90% of which involve loss of the tumor suppressor genes at 3p25
3. Other etiologic agents/risk factors
   a. Smoking—major risk factor, accounting for up to 30% of tumors
   b. Obesity—particularly in women; accounts for approximately 25% of tumors
   c. Long term phenacetin and acetaminophen exposure as well as exposure to other chemicals (petroleum products, industrial chemicals, cadmium)
   d. Kidney stones
   e. In most cases, the carcinogenic influence is not known

C. Signs and Symptoms

1. "Classic" triad of symptoms: hematuria, pain, and a flank mass (only seen in 10% of patients)
2. Other symptoms include:
   a. **Abdominal pain, weight loss, anorexia**
   b. **Fever** of unknown origin
   c. **Elevation of the ESR**
   d. Sudden appearance of a scrotal mass, usually left-sided—due to obstruction of testicular vein by tumor
   e. **Hypochromic anemia**—secondary to bone marrow suppression, not hematuria
   f. Liver changes (**Stauffer's syndrome**)—elevated alkaline phosphatase, ALT, AST with hepatosplenomegaly, coagulopathy, and elevated alpha-globulin concentrations
   g. Systemic amyloidosis
   h. **Paraneoplastic syndromes:**
      - hypercalcemia of malignancy (pseudohyperparathyroidism)

- erythrocytosis—secondary to erythropoeitin production by tumor
- hypertension—secondary to renin production by the tumor
- gynecomastia—secondary to prolactin or gonadotropin production by tumor.
    i. RCC is also notorious for presenting as **metastatic tumor with unknown primary**—and to complicate matters, is one of the "great mimickers"

2. Associations and Syndromes

A. von Hippel-Lindau Disease—autosomal dominant: 3p25 mutation

1. Central nervous system and retinal hemangioblastoma
2. Epididymal cystadenomas
3. Pheochromocytomas
4. Cysts of the pancreas and kidney
5. Renal cell carcinoma (30%-50% of patients develop tumors: often bilateral and multiple, with an earlier age at presentation)

B. Tuberous Sclerosis

1. Hamartomas of brain, retina, skin, kidney, heart, bone, and lung
2. Renal cysts
    a. Angiomyolipomas
    b. Renal cell carcinomas (often bilateral)

C. Autosomal Dominant Polycystic Kidney Disease—association with RCC is controversial

D. Acquired Renal Cystic Disease—strong association with RCC

E. Familial RCC—uncertain whether these are hereditary, coincidence, or reflect shared exposure to carcinogens

3. Clear Cell Renal Cell Carcinoma

A. Most common form of RCC—represents approximately **70% of RCC tumors**

B. Genetics

1. Loss of genetic material (thought to be a tumor suppressor gene) on the short arm of chromosome 3 (3p) is the most frequent and consistent abnormality
2. May also see gain of 5q
3. c-myc activation may also play a role

C. Gross Pathology

1. Classically demonstrates a variegated cut surface with golden-yellow regions alternating with areas of hemorrhage, necrosis, and cyst degeneration
2. Usually well circumscribed with bulging borders
3. May have central stellate area of edematous gray connective tissue
4. May be multicentric in 14% of cases, and bilateral in 1% of cases

D. Microscopic Pathology

1. Cells have abundant clear cytoplasm (result of artifact in which the cytoplasmic lipid/glycogen is lost during fixation, leaving behind clear "holes" where the lipid was)
2. Some cells may have granular eosinophilic cytoplasm as well—and these cells may even predominate. But as long as there are clear cells present, the tumor is classified as a clear cell RCC
3. Growth pattern: nests, tubules, cysts. Often the tubular and cystic patterns demonstrate central hemorrhage—so-called "blood lakes"
4. Delicate interconnecting vasculature ("chicken wire vasculature")
5. Nuclei of the clear cells are central and round, ranging from small and hyperchromatic with indistinct nucleoli to large and pleomorphic with prominent nucleoli
6. **Sarcomatoid growth pattern** may be seen in 5% of tumors, and carries a worse prognosis
7. Variants: multilocular cystic renal cell carcinoma
    a. Grossly appears to be a multilocular cyst

   b. Histologically, the septa demonstrate focal areas of clear cells, and clear cells often line the cysts
   c. Better prognosis, as these have a very low potential for recurrence or metastasis

E. Differential Diagnosis
1. TCC of the renal pelvis (with clear cell change)
   a. *Check the vascular pattern for "chicken wire vasculature" of RCC*
   b. *Positive staining for cytokeratin or CEA suggest urothelial origin*
2. Cystic nephroma is hard to distinguish from multilocular cystic RCC
   a. *Check fibrous septa of cysts to see if clear cells are there: at this point, the presence of clear cells—no matter how few—is interpreted as indicative of RCC*
3. Wilms' tumor (in children and adolescents)
   a. *Look for blastema and stromal components for dx of Wilms'*
4. Xanthogranulomatous pyelonephritis
   a. *Often confused with RCC because patients present with flank mass and kidney demonstrates tumor-like mass of yellow tissue. In addition, the presence of foamy histiocytes may be misconstrued as a population of clear cells*
   b. *Check for chicken-wire vasculature (lacking in XGPN)*
   c. *Check cytoplasm: foamy (XGPN) vs. clear (RCC)*
5. Malakoplakia
   a. *Grossly looks like a large yellow mass infiltrating the perinephric fat*
   b. *Histologically the large eosinophilic histiocytes (van Hansemann cells) may mimic eosinophilic cells of RCC*
   c. *Check for Michaelis-Gutmann bodies (spherical blue things in the cytoplasm)*
6. Leiomyosarcoma
   a. *May be confused with sarcomatoid RCC*
   b. *When you see a "sarcoma" (spindle cell neoplasm) in the kidney, you have to hunt carefully for areas that look more typical for RCC—remember:* ***a sarcomatoid RCC is far more common than a primary sarcoma***

4. Chromophil (Papillary) Renal Cell Carcinoma

A. Second most common type of RCC—**represents 10%-15% of RCC tumors**

B. Used to be called papillary, but people started subdividing as "tubulopapillary" and "solid" variants, etc. So was designated "chromophil" RCC in the Mainz classification to emphasize that the dx is not made on architecture alone

C. Uncertain if chromophil RCC carries a better or worse prognosis than clear cell RCC, but there is a 16% 10-year mortality

D. Sarcomatoid variant probably has same poor prognostic implication as it does in clear cell RCC

E. Genetics
1. Typically associated with trisomy (or tetrasomy) 17 and 7 and loss of Y chromosome
2. Loss of 3p and gain of 5q (as seen in clear cell RCC) are NOT found in chromophil RCC

F. Gross Pathology
1. Typically light-tan, well circumscribed
2. Cut surface may have a granular "friable" appearance, reflecting papillary architecture
3. Dense fibrous pseudocapsule

G. Microscopic Pathology
1. Typically have predominantly papillary or tubulopapillary architecture
2. Papillae consist of delicate fibrovascular cores covered by a single layer of neoplastic cells.
3. Papillae may be expanded by numerous foamy histiocytes
4. Nuclei tend to be round, regular, small and low-grade

5. Chromophobe Renal Cell Carcinoma

A. Comprises approximately **5% of RCC** tumors

B. Affects men and women equally

C. May have a better prognosis than clear cell RCC

D. Genetics
1. Loss of multiple chromosomes is common: 1,2,10,13,6,21 and 17 (90% of cases)
2. Loss of 3p (as in clear cell RCC) is NOT seen
3. Trisomy/tetrasomy 17, 17 and loss of Y (as is seen in chromophil RCC) is NOT seen

E. Gross Pathology: solitary, solid beige or light brown, circumscribed

F. Microscopic Pathology
1. Two recognized histologic variants: typical and eosinophilic
2. Typical pattern:
   a. Usually solid growth pattern, but may show some tubules
   b. Cells are large and polygonal with abundant pale/flocculent (frothy) cytoplasm
   c. Cytoplasm appears to condense at the edges, so the **cytoplasmic membranes are very thick and distinct**
   d. Nuclei are small and centrally located with small to medium-sized nucleoli
   f. Mitotic figures are infrequent or rare
   g. **Hale's colloidal iron stain** is positive (stains chromophobe cells vivid blue); as opposed to a negative reaction in clear cell RCC
3. Eosinophilic pattern
   a. Cells have abundant brightly eosinophilic cytoplasm
   b. May see a slight "halo" around the nuclei
   c. Hale's colloidal iron stain is positive
   ** this is important because on H&E, eosinophilic variant of chromophobe RCC looks just like oncocytoma, and the distinction between the two may depend upon a Hale's colloidal iron stain: the chromophobe RCC will be positive, while the oncocytoma will be negative*

6. Collecting Duct Carcinoma (Bellini Duct Carcinoma)

A. Represents about 1% of renal tumors

B. Gross Pathology
1. Tumor often arises in the medullary region with extension into the cortex or hilar tissues
2. Gray-white cut surfaces with central necrosis and infiltrative borders

C. Microscopic Pathology
1. Consists of irregular duct-like structures, nests and cords of cells in an abundant loose slightly basophilic stroma
2. Nuclei are pleomorphic with thick nuclear membranes
3. "Hobnail" (tombstone?) appearance of the cells lining the duct lumens is helpful feature

D. Differential diagnosis
1. TCC—vimentin negative (CDC is vimentin positive)
2. other types of RCC—Ulex europaeus negative (CDC is Ulex europaeus positive)

7. The Fuhrman Grading System for Renal Cell Carcinoma (Table 1)

A. **The entire tumor receives the grade of its worst component, regardless of extent**

Table 1

Fuhrman Grading System for Renal Cell Carcinoma

Grade	Nuclear Size	Nuclear Shape	Chromatin	Nucleoli
1	<10 micrometers	Round	Dense	Inconspicuous
2	15 micrometers	Round	Finely granular	Small, not visible with 10X objective
3	20 micrometers	Round/oval	Coarsely granular	Prominent
4	>20 micrometers	Pleomorphic, multilobated	Open, hyperchromatic	Macronucleoli

B. Note that mitotic figures are NOT a part of this system; however, the finding of >1 mitosis/10 hpf may be indicative of worse prognosis

C. 5-year survival rates: 86% for grade 1; 24% for grade 4

D. Sarcomatoid histology is also significant: patients with even small foci of sarcomatoid carcinoma have a much worse prognosis than patients without

8. Spread and Outcome

A. **Treatment:** Surgery is the principal therapy for RCC

B. Clinically occult RCC may present at distant sites with unknown primary, or may recur years after an apparently successful radical nephrectomy

C. **Clinical course** is notoriously unpredictable
   1. Metastases to bone are fairly common—especially to scapula
   2. Overall, T1 and T2 patients have 10-yr survival of up to 80%
   3. Patients with metastatic dz at dx generally die within 5 years
   4. Occasional cases of spontaneous regression have been reported

4. Renal Tumors III: Beyond Renal Cell Carcinoma

I. Epithelial Tumors

A. Oncocytoma
   1. Originates from the renal cortex
   2. Generally discovered incidentally during radiologic examination of the kidneys for other reasons
   3. At one time oncocytomas were thought to be "granular cell" RCC but these tumors have distinctive properties that set them apart from RCCs:
      a. Staining characteristics
      b. Benign course
      c. Males > females (2:1)
      d. Age > 50 years
   4. Classically associated with a "spoke-and-wheel" appearance on radiographs
   5. Gross pathology:
      a. Classically described as **mahogany brown with a central stellate scar** (contrasting with bright golden-yellow appearance of RCC)
      b. Hemorrhage and necrosis are rare (as opposed to RCC)—in fact, the presence of gross necrosis or hemorrhage militates against a diagnosis of oncocytoma
      d. Bilaterality/multicentricity noted in 3.6% of cases
      e. Rare: oncocytomatosis—numerous tumors of cortex
   6. Microscopic pathology:
      a. Cells are arranged in **diffuse sheets or as cellular "islands"** in a background of loose edematous connective tissue **("archipelaginous architecture")**
      b. **Cytoplasm is intensely eosinophilic** and finely granular
      c. **Nuclei are characteristically round with inconspicuous nucleoli,** although occasional bizarre nuclei can be seen.
      d. **Mitotic figures are absent or rare**
      e. Features warranting a designation of **atypical oncocytoma**:
         - Microscopic vascular invasion
         - Microscopic extension into the perirenal fat

      f. Features impermissible in a renal oncocytoma
         - Mitotic figures
         - Papillary architecture
         - Clear or spindle cells
         - Positive colloidal iron stain

- Chromophobe-type vesicles seen by electron microscopy
- Gross vascular invasion
- Gross extension into the perirenal fat

7. Ultrastructural (EM) features:
   a. **Cytoplasm is filled with mitochondria**
   b. Chromophobe RCC has cytoplasm filled with round/oval vesicles by EM
   c. Clear cell RCC has cytoplasm filled with vacuoles and lots of rough ER by EM
8. Differential diagnosis: Eosinophilic variant of chromophobe RCC
   a. **Hale's colloidal iron stain is negative in oncocytoma** and is positive in a chromophobe RCC
   b. EM shows mitochondria in an oncocytoma and reveals perinuclear vesicles/vacuoles in a chromophobe RCC.
9. Treatment and Prognosis:
   a. As the tumor is usually indistinguishable from RCC, the treatment is generally **nephrectomy**
   b. Clinically oncocytoma is distinguished from chromophobe RCC because of its **benign course**. (A few reports have suggested that some of these tumors may metastasize; however, since the diagnosis of "metastatic oncocytoma" was based upon H&E features alone, one cannot rule out the possibility that these cases may actually represent metastatic chromophobe RCC. No typical oncocytoma has ever metastasized.)

B. Medullary Carcinoma

1. Recently described in a report from the AFIP
2. May represent the "aggressive end" of collecting duct carcinoma
3. Seen most commonly in younger patients with sickle cell disease
4. Gross: ill-defined mass in medulla; hemorrhage and necrosis
5. Micro: variable compositions of pleomorphic cells
6. Mean survival after resection: 15 weeks

C. Renal Cortical Adenoma

1. This remains a disputed entity, since metastases have been recorded from many small (<3.0 cm) renal cortical tumors. "All cancers start out small."
2. Small renal cortical tumors are frequently found at autopsy or nephrectomy, but are more frequent in kidneys "scarred" by pyelonephritis or renal vascular disease
3. Best candidates for RCAs are <1.0 cm, well-demarcated and typically subcapsular. Cut surface is usually yellow or gray
4. Micro: bland, closely-packed cells forming tubules and papillary structures. Nuclei are uniform and mitoses infrequent. The interface with normal kidney should be sharply defined, without stromal reaction or inflammation. *Any clear cell neoplasm in the renal cortex, no matter how small or how bland, should be considered a carcinoma*
5. Prognosis: impossible to predict biologic behavior of these lesions; if they truly are "adenomas," they will not metastasize or invade

2. Mesenchymal Tumors

A. Angiomyolipoma

1. Benign tumor composed of fat, muscle and thick-walled blood vessels
2. Probably more of a hamartoma than a true neoplasm
3. Occurs in two distinct settings:
   a. Those associated with **tuberous sclerosis***
      - Approximately 50% of patients with TS develop these tumors
      - Tend to be asymptomatic, multiple, bilateral, and small
      - Strong female predominance

   b. Those not associated with tuberous sclerosis (**sporadic**)
      - Tumors tend to be large, symptomatic, and solitary
4. Gross pathology:
   a. Range in size from 1-20 cm (average: 9 cm)
   b. Typically **golden-yellow**, but color depends on proportion of fat/muscle/vessel
   c. Well demarcated but not encapsulated; may show local invasion
   d. Cut surface may resemble a lipoma
5. Microscopic pathology:
   a. Contains **varying amounts of smooth muscle, fat, and thick-walled vessels**
   b. Frequent finding is **radial arrays of smooth muscle around the vessels**

c. **Blood vessels are abnormal, with thick walls like arteries, but eccentric small lumens.** Lack elastic tissue so rupture easily
d. **Nuclear pleomorphism** may be pronounced but has no prognostic significance
e. **Mitotic figures** may be present—**no prognostic significance**
f. May see **local invasion** and **vascular invasion** of the vena cava—**no prognostic significance**
g. May see "metastatic" lesions in lymph nodes and spleen, but these should not be misinterpreted as sarcoma
h. **The smooth muscle cells react with HMB-45** (typically a melanoma marker), which helps distinguish this neoplasm from other "spindle cell" neoplasms of the kidney

6. Differential diagnosis:
   a. Lipoma
   b. Leiomyoma
7. Clinical behavior and treatment:
   a. Hemorrhage is the most common serious complication (more likely if size >4 cm)
   b. **Surgical intervention recommended for tumors >4 cm**
   c. These tumors **do not metastasize**, even with "atypical" features. Presence of angiomyolipoma outside the kidney represents multicentric disease

B. Leiomyosarcoma

1. Most common primary renal sarcoma, but not nearly as common as sarcomatoid RCC
2. Usually in patients > 40 years; women > men (2:1)
3. Gross pathology:
   a. Firm solid tumor with well-circumscribed margins
   b. **Whorled cut surface** but may have **hemorrhage and necrosis**
   c. May arise from renal capsule or renal vein
   d. Renal and perirenal infiltration are common
4. Microscopic pathology:
   a. **Spindle-cell neoplasm** with fascicular growth
   b. **Necrosis, nuclear pleomorphism, and mitoses are common**
5. Differential diagnosis:
   a. **Leiomyoma**
   The presence of necrosis, nuclear pleomorphism, and more-than-rare mitotic figures should suggest malignant dx (LMS)
   b. **Sarcomatoid RCC**
   Sample areas for more typical RCC features. Do a keratin stain: positive in RCC; negative in LMS

5. Adrenal Gland

1. Normal Histology

A. The adrenal gland is composed of two endocrine organs: the **cortex** (derived from mesoderm) and the **medulla** (derived from neuroectoderm)

B. **Cortex** is divided into three layers, all of which respond to ACTH stimulation:
  1. Zona glomerulosa (outer layer)—aldosterone production
  2. Zona fasciculata (middle layer)—glucocorticoid production
  3. Zona reticularis (inner layer)—sex hormones

C. **Medulla** contains two cell types
  1. Pheochromocytes
     a. Contain epinephrine and norepinephrine
     b. Large polygonal cells with poorly defined cell borders
     c. Abundant cytoplasm is usually granular and faintly blue
  2. Sustentacular cells—"supporting" cells that surround the nests of pheochromocytes

2. Lesions of the Adrenal Cortex

A. Congenital Adrenal Hyperplasia
  1. Autosomal recessive defect in the biosynthesis of cortisol
  2. Responsible for the large majority of cases of adrenogenital syndrome developing in the first year of life (although may occasionally have initial presentation in adulthood)
  3. Various enzyme deficiencies may result in CAH, but most common ones are:
     a. 21-hydroxylase deficiency (>90% of cases): virilization and salt wasting.
     b. 11-beta hydroxylase deficiency (5% of cases): virilization and hypertension
  4. Pathologic change is the same, regardless of the defect, and consists of diffuse cortical hyperplasia, especially of zona reticularis

B. Acquired Adrenal Hyperplasia
  1. Defined as adrenal gland weight > 6g
  2. Always bilateral
  3. Microscopically: increased thickness of zona reticularis and fasciculata with lipid depletion of the fasciculata cells
  4. May have nodular or diffuse pattern
     a. Diffuse pattern
        - **ACTH-dependent ("pituitary dependent")** because typically results from excessive ACTH production by pituitary or other neoplasm
     b. Nodular pattern
        - **ACTH-independent ("adrenal dependent")**
        - may represent progression of diffuse pattern
        - includes **primary pigmented nodular adrenal cortical hyperplasia**, as seen with Carney's syndrome

C. Adrenocortical Adenoma
  1. Often incidental findings; can be found in any age group
  2. Gross findings:
     a. Usually solitary lesions, well-encapsulated
     b. Cut surface is solid, homogeneous yellow
     c. By definition, generally <5 cm or <50 g
  3. Microscopic findings:
     a. Recapitulate the zona glomerulosa and zona fasciculata
     b. Bizarre nuclei may be seen, but mitoses are exceptionally rare or absent
     c. May contain foci of myelolipoma (see below)
  4. Variations on the theme:
     a. **"aldosterone-omas"**—golden-yellow color; contain "spironolactone bodies"
     b. **"black adenomas"**—dark brown due to the presence of lipofuscin pigment; generally nonfunctioning, but may occasionally be associated with primary aldosteronism or Cushing's syndrome
     c. **adrenocortical oncocytomas**: highly eosinophilic cytoplasm due to numerous mitochondria
  5. Immunohistochemical profile:
     a. Keratin (+) > vimentin (+) (as opposed to adrenocortical carcinoma)
     b. EMA (-) (as opposed to renal cell carcinoma)

D. Adrenocortical Carcinoma

1. Clinical characteristics:
   a. Males and females affected equally
   b. Average age is 50 yrs
   c. 50% accompanied by hormonal manifestations
2. Gross findings:
   a. Weight usually >100g
   b. Cut surface frequently demonstrates necrosis and hemorrhage
3. Histologic findings:
   a. Giant cells with abundant cytoplasm and bizarre nuclei may be present
   b. Potential criteria of malignancy:
      - nuclear grade III or IV
      - **mitoses >5/50 HPF**
      - Atypical mitoses
      - Paucity or absence of clear cells
      - Diffuse architecture
      - Necrosis
      - Capsular or vascular invasion
      - **Spindled tumor cells**
   c. **However, nothing short of detecting metastases firmly discriminates benign from malignant**
4. Immunohistochemical profile:
   a. Vimentin (+) > keratin (+) (as opposed to adrenocortical adenoma)
   b. EMA (-), CEA (-), B72.3 (-) (as opposed to renal cell carcinoma)
5. **Differential diagnosis** includes **adenoma** (distinction based on size, weight, mitotic activity, and spindling of tumor cells) and **renal cell carcinoma** (check for gland formation and presence of abundant cytoplasmic glycogen, and do immunohistochemical stains)
6. Generally demonstrates hematogenous spread to retroperitoneum, kidney, liver (60%), lymph nodes (40%), peritoneum, bone, etc.
7. Prognosis: 50% 2-year survival rate; 20%-35% 5-year-survival rate

3. Lesions of the Adrenal Medulla

A. Neuroblastoma

1. Clinical characteristics
   a. Patients are almost always <4 yrs of age (median age 21 months) who present with abdominal mass
   b. May be associated with Beckwith-Wiedeman syndrome, neurofibromatosis, or as complication of fetal hydantoin syndrome
   c. 70% occur in the retroperitoneum, the majority of which involve the adrenal gland
2. Gross findings:
   a. Large soft, gray, relatively well-circumscribed
   b. Hemorrhage, necrosis, and **calcifications** are common
3. Microscopic findings:
   a. "Small round blue cell tumor" with very little evidence of differentiation
   b. Classically characteristic feature is the presence of **Homer-Wright rosettes**: collections of tumor cells arranged around a central area filled with pink fibrillary material (which represents tangled neuritis). There is no central lumen
4. Immunohistochemistry: positive for neuroendocrine markers like **NSE, neurofilament, chromogranin, synaptophysin**
5. Clinical staging of neuroblastoma:
   Stage I: Tumor confined to the organ or structure of origin
   Stage II: Tumors extending in continuity beyond the organ or structure of origin, but not crossing the midline; regional lymph nodes in the ipsilateral side may be involved
   Stage III: Tumors extending in continuity beyond the midline; regional lymph nodes may be involved bilaterally
   Stage IV: Remote disease involving the skeleton, organs, soft tissues, distant lymph node groups, or other structures
   Stage IV-S: Patients who would otherwise be stage I or II but who have remote disease confined to one or more of the following sites: liver, skin, or bone marrow (but no bony metastases by radiographic skeletal survey)

6. Prognostic factors in neuroblastoma:
   a. Shimada classification looks at the quality of the stroma, the degree of differentiation within the neuroblasts, the age of the patient, and the MKI (mitotic-karyorrhectic index) to come up with "favorable" and "unfavorable" histology subgroups
   b. N-myc amplification, loss of chromosome 1p, and extra copies of 17q are significantly associated with unfavorable outcome
7. Clinical course:
   a. May occasionally undergo maturation and spontaneous regression
   b. May locally invade surrounding tissues: intraspinal extension and kidney
   c. May metastasize, most commonly to
      - liver **(Pepper's syndrome)**
      - skeletal system, especially skull and orbit (Hutchison's syndrome)
      - lymph node
      - ovary
8. Treatment: surgical excision, multi-agent chemotherapy, bone marrow transplant
9. Prognosis: 30% 3-year survival

B. Ganglioneuroblastoma

(malignant ganglioneuroma)

1. Clinical characteristics: found most commonly in young children but may present in early adulthood; usually occur in retroperitoneum
2. Gross findings: more homogeneous with firmer consistency than neuroblastoma
3. Microscopic findings:
   a. **Intermediate degree of differentiation between neuroblastoma and ganglioneuromas**
   b. Neurophil (pink fibrillary matrix) is much more apparent
   c. Two microscopic varieties:
      - **Imperfect** (better prognosis) and **composite** (worse prognosis)

C. Ganglioneuroma

1. Clinical characteristics:
   a. Invariably **benign**
   b. Only rarely in adrenal, usually in **retroperitoneum or posterior mediastinum**
   c. Almost always associated with catecholamine synthesis
2. Gross: large encapsulated masses of gray-white firm tissue
3. Microscopic findings: looks like neurofibroma (fibrous tissue and schwann cells), but has **abnormal but mature ganglion cells (multinucleated).**

D. Adrenal Medullary Hyperplasia

1. Clinical characteristics:
   a. Can cause symptoms akin to pheochromocytoma and can actually give rise to benign/malignant pheochromocytoma
   b. May be associated with von Recklinghausen's disease, MEN-IIb (Gorlin's syndrome) and somatostatin-rich duodenal carcinoid
2. Gross findings: **always bilateral**
3. Microscopic findings: **nodular or diffuse pattern**

E. Pheochromocytoma

1. Clinical characteristics:
   a. Classic triad of sweating attacks, headaches, and tachycardia
   b. Hypertension may be intermittent or sustained.
   c. Increased **urine vanillylmandelic acid** (VMA) and metanephrines in up to 90% of cases
   d. **"10% tumor"**: 10% bilateral, 10% in children, 10% extra-adrenal, 10% malignant
   e. May secrete
      - **Epinephrine**
      - **Norepinephrine** (if extra-adrenal, only secrete norepinephrine since adrenal cortex is necessary for methylation of norepinephrine to epinephrine.)
      - ACTH (occasionally), which can result in Cushing's syndrome
      - Parathormone (occasionally), which can result in hypercalcemia
   f. Extra-adrenal sites: retroperitoneum, mediastinum, bladder
   g. May be associated with neurofibromatosis, renal artery stenosis, other paragangliomas, adrenal cortical tumors, or Von Hippel-Lindau disease
   h. Familial cases may be seen as a component of MEN IIa (Sipple's syndrome) or MEN IIb (Gorlin's syndrome)

2. Gross findings: encapsulated, yellow-white to red-brown, soft
3. Microscopic findings:
   a. Tumor cells are arranged in well-defined nests (***"zellballen"***) bound by delicate spindled S-100 sustentacular cells
   b. Cells vary in size and shape considerably and have finely granular cytoplasm
   c. Huge/hyperchromatic nuclei do not indicate malignancy; in fact, **the only reliable evidence of malignancy is metastases**
4. Hematogenous spread is common, usually to bone (ribs, spine)
5. Treatment: surgical excision
6. Prognosis: excellent (if benign); otherwise die within a year (if malignant)

4. Miscellaneous Adrenal Lesions

A. Adrenal Hemorrhage

1. Especially common in infants during the first few weeks of life
2. May be caused by neuroblastoma, hypoxia, septicemia, decreased platelets, DIC, etc.
3. Waterhouse-Friedrichsen syndrome: acute bilateral hemorrhagic infarcts of the adrenal cortex, most commonly secondary to meningococcal or pseudomonal septicemia (DIC-related)

B. Adrenal Cytomegaly

1. Usually detected in infancy—part of Beckwith-Wiedeman syndrome
2. Consists of giant cells with large hyperchromatic nuclei containing pseudoinclusions

C. Tuberculosis

1. One of the classic causes of Addison's disease
2. Glands are enlarged, calcified, and obliterated by granulomatous inflammation

D. Myelolipoma

1. Usually incidental findings in obese adults with otherwise normally functioning bone marrow. Typically hormonally inactive
2. Consist of mature adipose tissue with active bone marrow elements

6. Renal Cystic Diseases

1. Renal Dysplasia

A. A dysplastic **kidney is a kidney with aberrant differentiation of the nephron.** It is *not:*
   1. Premalignant (ie, "dysplasia" does not suggest "neoplasia")
   2. A hypoplastic kidney (which is small but normally developed)
   3. A polycystic kidney (which is cystic, but doesn't contain dysplastic elements)

B. Two Theories of Dysplasia

1. Urinary tract obstruction in utero—may or may not play a role
2. Fundamental defect in the inducer tissue (ureteric bud) or responding tissue (metanephric blastema): in other words, **the ureteric bud is inhibited from branching** as it normally should, **or the metanephric blastema fails to respond** to the organizing influence of the ureteric bud

C. Multicystic and Aplastic Dysplasia

1. **Clinical presentation:**
   a. Multicystic dysplasia is the most common cause of a renal mass in a child
   b. Usually unilateral, but bilateral disease can occur (Potter's syndrome), in which case death generally occurs in infancy due to pulmonary hypoplasia
2. **Gross appearance:** highly variable appearance, ranging from the large multicystic kidney to the small aplastic kidney
3. **Histological appearance:** also very variable, with two characteristic elements:
   a. Primitive or dysplastic ducts—lined by columnar epithelium and surrounded by a collar of spindle cells
   b. Fetal or immature appearing cartilage—thought to be derived from the **metanephric blastema**
   c. Renal cortex is usually thinned; may contain immature nephrons
4. **Variations on the theme:**
   a. Focal Dysplasia
      - Tend to present in infancy with renal insufficiency and small reniform kidneys with normal ureters and pelves

- Biopsy shows a focal form of dysplasia characterized by an admixture of normal nephrons and aberrantly formed nephrons usually with microcysts and cartilage or dysplastic ducts
- The renal prognosis is bleak, and the infant usually develops progressive renal failures as it grows

b. Segmental Dysplasia
- Occurs only in kidneys with duplication of the collecting system (duplex kidney)
- The upper pole is affected, and histologically shows the same range of aberrant nephrogenesis encountered in aplastic and multicystic dysplasia

c. Dysplasia associated with lower tract obstruction
- Bilateral renal dysplasia may be associated with **urethral stenosis, posterior urethral valves**, or **bladder neck obstruction**
- Gross appearance: kidneys are typically reniform, may be large or small, but show distinct corticomedullary differentiation
- The bladder is either hypertrophic or greatly dilated, and the ureters are dilated and tortuous
- There may be a severe degree of dysplasia with scant nephronic elements or only a peripheral zone of dysplastic elements with normal deeper nephrons

d. Hereditary renal adysplasia and urogenital adysplasia
- Renal agenesis, aplastic dysplasia, and multicystic dysplasia are the most severe forms of metanephric kidney maldevelopment, and are usually sporadic unless associated with multiple malformation syndromes
- Rarely may be hereditary in an **autosomal dominant** fashion (hereditary renal adysplasia)

2. Polycystic Kidney Diseases

A. Infantile Polycystic Kidney Disease

1. Clinical features:
   a. **Autosomal recessive** (Potter type I)
   b. Four types: perinatal, neonatal, infantile, and juvenile
   c. **Most cases result in stillbirth or early neonatal death.**
   d. Affected neonates have massively enlarged, diffusely cystic kidneys that produce abdominal distension and compress thoracic organs; death usually ensues due to pulmonary hypoplasia
   e. If the kidneys are nonfunctional, Potter's phenotype may develop
   f. May be accompanied by a liver lesion that looks like congenital hepatic fibrosis.
2. Gross: cysts **extend through the renal parenchyma in "rays" oriented perpendicular to the cortex** imparting a **spongy** quality.
3. Histology:
   a. Cysts consist of **dilated collecting ducts** lined with uniform cuboidal cells
   b. Nephrons between the collecting ducts appear normal
   c. In older patients, cysts may be less prominent with more interstitial scarring and glomerulosclerosis, resulting in a superficial resemblance to APKD

B. Adult Polycystic Kidney Disease

1. General:
   a. **Autosomal dominant (Potter type II)**
   b. Most common cystic renal disease, and 3rd or 4th leading cause of renal failure
   c. Most common genetically transmitted disease (1: 500-1,000): the principal gene has been localized to **chromosome 16** (90% of cases); a gene on **chromosome 4** has also recently been implicated
2. Clinical Features:
   a. Most present in **4th to 6th** decade with 100% penetrance at the age of 80
   b. 25% of patients lack a family history
   c. **Chronic flank pain** is the most common complaint followed by hematuria and acute flank pain (due to hemorrhage into a cyst)
3. Complications:
   a. **Hypertension** from compression of the intrarenal vasculature by expanding cysts
   b. **Perinephric abscess** (60% mortality rate) following UTI
   c. **Berry aneurysms** of the Circle of Willis (5%-15% of cases)

d. **Kidney stones** (10% of cases)
e. **Renal cell carcinomas** (1%-5% of cases)

4. Gross features: Cysts progressively enlarge in size and number, resulting in **massive renal enlargement,** although the **normal reniform shape** is preserved
5. Histologic features: fairly nondescript
   a. Most of the cysts are lined with a single layer of flattened to cuboidal epithelium
   b. Remaining parenchyma may show interstitial inflammation, glomerulosclerosis

3. Cysts (Without Dysplasia) in Hereditary Syndromes

A. Medullary Cystic Disease/ Juvenile Nephronophthisis

1. Hereditary tubulointerstitial disease that is usually classified as a cystic disease because 75% of cases are accompanied by medullary cysts
2. Clinical features: affected individuals present with:
   a. **Polyuria** and **polydipsia** due to salt wasting
   b. **Anemia** disproportionately severe for the level of renal insufficiency
   c. **Growth retardation**
3. Four types have been described:
   a. **Familial juvenile nephronophthisis**—autosomal recessive; presents in infancy/childhood
   b. **Renal-retinal disease**—autosomal recessive; presents in adulthood
   c. **Medullary cystic disease**—autosomal dominant (15% of cases); presents in adulthood
   d. **Sporadic medullary cystic disease**—nonfamilial (15% of cases)
4. Gross appearance:
   a. The kidneys are usually **small due to cortical atrophy**
   b. Cysts measure up to 1 cm and congregate at the corticomedullary junction
5. Microscopic features:
   a. Nonspecific: chronic inflammation, tubular atrophy, interstitial fibrosis
   b. Prominent lymphoid infiltrate is usually present
   c. Cyst formation seems to remain fairly stable, but the interstitial inflammation progresses, resulting in glomerulosclerosis and renal failure.

B. Von Hippel-Lindau Disease

1. Autosomal dominant disorder with:
   a. Retinal/cerebellar/spinal **hemangioblastomas**
   b. **Pheochromocytoma**
   c. **Epididymal** and **pancreatic cystadenomas**
   d. **Multiple** and **bilateral renal cysts** (70% of patients)
   e. **Renal cell carcinoma**, often bilateral and multiple (50% of patients)
2. Microscopic features: renal cysts are lined by single or multiple layers of clear cells, mimicking low-grade renal cell carcinoma

C. Tuberous Sclerosis

1. Autosomal dominant disorder characterized by:
   a. Mental retardation
   b. Epilepsy
   c. Angiofibromas
   d. Cardiac rhabdomyomas
   e. Renal angiomyolipomas
   f. Renal cysts—actually uncommon, but can (particularly in children) become quite large, mimicking APKD
2. Microscopic features: the cysts are lined by large eosinophilic cells with large hyperchromatic nuclei
3. Complications: renal cell carcinoma may develop, but far less likely than in Von Hippel-Lindau disease

4. Miscellaneous Conditions

A. Acquired Cystic Kidney Disease

1. Development of multiple and bilateral renal cysts in patients whose chronic renal failure cannot be attributed to a hereditary cystic disease
2. Clinical features
   a. Bilateral and asymptomatic in its early stages
   b. Cysts are present in 8% of patients at the time dialysis is started and increase in incidence, number, and size proportional to the duration of dialysis
3. Gross features:
   a. The cysts initially form in the proximal tubules of end-stage kidneys
   b. Most cysts are less than 0.5 cm but may enlarge to 2-3 cm in diameter

c. Initially the cysts are cortical, but in advanced cases medullary cysts form and the entire kidney may be replaced by cysts and resemble a smaller version of APKD

4. Histology: the cysts are lined with flattened, cuboidal, or columnar epithelium and may contain a proteinaceous to hemorrhagic fluid
5. Complications: intrarenal and retroperitoneal hemorrhage, cyst infection, and renal cell carcinoma

B. Medullary Sponge Kidneys

1. Characterized by cysts in the papillary collecting ducts of one or more renal pyramids
2. Clinical features:
   a. Usually **bilateral** and more common in **males**
   b. Usually detected radiographically in adults being evaluated for **nephrolithiasis**
   c. Patients tend to have **normal renal function**
3. Gross: kidneys are not enlarged
4. Histology:
   a. **Papillary collecting ducts** are dilated and lined with cuboidal/flattened epithelium
   b. Can be distinguished from medullary cystic disease and IPKD by patient age and by cyst locations: in medullary cystic disease, the cysts are located at the corticomedullary junction, while in the juvenile form of IPKD the cysts are in the cortex and medulla and do not congregate at the papilla

C. Simple Cortical Cysts

1. Most common cystic renal lesion
2. Rare before the age of 40, and increase in frequency with increasing age
3. Gross: in older patients, may be multiple and large
4. Histology: lined with a flattened layer of cells, or may lack an epithelial lining

D. Multilocular Cyst

1. Uncommon nonfamilial lesion felt to be a benign neoplasm related to the cystic partially-differentiated Wilm's tumor (aka, multilocular cystic nephroma or differentiated nephroblastoma)
2. Peak presentation is biphasic: seen in children (often females) <2 years of age and in patients 40-70 years of age
3. Radiology: avascular mass causing calyceal distortion
4. Diagnostic criteria:
   a. Unilateral, solitary, and multilocular
   b. **Cyst does not communicate with the renal pelvis or between locules**
   c. Septations consist of fibrous tissue only (no parenchyma)
   d. Residual renal tissue is normal
5. Gross features
   a. Typically large, well-circumscribed mass that protrudes into the pelvis
   b. Fibrous pseudocapsule and delicate fibrous trabeculae
   c. No calcification, hemorrhage, or necrosis
6. Histologic features: locules separated by a variably cellular connective tissue and lined by cuboidal or flattened epithelium

7. Penis and Scrotum I: Non-neoplastic Lesions

1. Normal Anatomy and Histology

A. Penis: composed of paired corpora cavernosa and a single corpus spongiosum
1. The two cavernous bodies lie on the dorsum of the penis and are surrounded by a double layer of dense fibrous connective tissue called **Buck's fascia** (tunica albuginea)
2. The corpus spongiosum lies in the ventral aspect of the penis and surrounds the urethra in its center
3. The glans represents the distal expansion of the corpus spongiosum

B. Foreskin
1. Nonkeratinizing squamous epithelium in uncircumcised males; keratinizing squamous epithelium in circumcised males. Composed of five layers:
   a. Epidermis
   b. Dermis
   c. Dartos
   d. Lamina propria
   e. Squamous mucosa
2. Dermis contains sweat glands and sebaceous glands but no hair follicles.

C. Scrotum
1. Composed of three major layers:
   a. Skin
   b. Dartos muscle
   c. Fascia (external spermatic, cremasteric, and internal spermatic)
2. Dermis contains hair follicles as well as apocrine, eccrine, and sebaceous glands
3. Left side is usually lower due to the longer length of the left spermatic cord

2. Non-neoplastic Diseases of the Penis

A. Inflammatory Processes
1. Phimosis may demonstrate chronic inflammation, fibrosis, edema, vascular congestion; or may be histologically normal
2. Plasma cell balanitis (Zoon's balanitis or balanitis circumscripta plasmacellularis)
   a. Benign disorder, etiology unknown
   b. Affects **only uncircumcised males**
   c. Gross: Presents as a **single large (>2 cm) bright red moist patch** on the glans or inner prepuce. Biopsy is mandatory because the clinical appearance mimics erythroplasia of Queyrat/Bowen's disease as well as candidal balanitis
   d. Histology:
      - Distinct upper dermal **band-like infiltrate** containing...you guessed it!...a bunch of **plasma cells**
      - dermis also contains a lot of dilated capillaries
      - overlying epidermis may be thin or partially absent
      - keratinocytes appear "diamond-like" or rhomboid-shaped and are separated by clear spaces (intracellular edema)
3. Balanitis xerotica obliterans (BXO):
   a. Male equivalent to lichen sclerosus et atrophicus in females
   b. Usually affects **older men**
   c. Gross:
      - well-defined white patch on the glans penis or prepuce that envelopes or involves the urethral meatus
      - Lesion may be firm in long-standing cases, due to underlying fibrosis
   d. Histology: three layers
      - **Epidermis**, which is atrophic and hyperkeratotic
      - Beneath the thinned epidermis is a **homogenized collagen layer**
      - Beneath the collagen layer is a **band-like lymphoplasmacytic infiltrate**
   e. Etiology: usually idiopathic but may be associated with carcinoma
   f. Treatment: laser therapy, circumcision, steroids, antifungal agents, and retinoids
4. Reiter's syndrome:
   a. Characterized by the triad of arthritis, urethritis, and conjunctivitis
   b. Most patients also have mucocutaneous lesions as well
   c. Clinical:
      - Male patients in third or fourth decade
      - **Endemic form**: sexually transmitted – follows urethritis
      - **Epidemic form**: secondary to enteric infections (may also have urethritis)

d. Causative agents include:
- ***Chlamydia trachomatis*** (most common agent in sexually transmitted cases)
- *Ureaplasma urealyticum*
- *Shigella flexneri*
- *Salmonella* species
- *Campylobacter* species
- *Yersinia enterocolitica*
- *Neisseria gonnorhea*

e. Genetic susceptibility: 60%-80% of patients are **HLA-B27 positive**

f. Genital involvement:
- **Balanitis circinata**
  i. more common form (85%)
  ii. painless lesion beginning as small red papules that enlarge centrifugally to form a circular or ringlike configuration.
- **Keratodermia blennorrhagica**
  i. predominantly cutaneous form affecting the palms and soles
  ii. characterized by erythematous macules that enlarge to form hyperkeratotic papules with red halos
  iii. clinically and histologically similar to psoriasis

g. Histology:
- epidermis becomes thickened with broad rete pegs
- hyperkeratosis, parakeratosis
- neutrophilic aggregates in the uppermost layer of the epidermis

5. Peyronie's disease:

a. Clinical features
- Affects men between the ages of 20 and 80 years (mean = 53 years)
- Present with **painful erection accompanied by distortion, bending, or constriction of the erect penis**
- Time course varies from a few months to a few years
- Usually have **palpable plaques or nodules** on the dorsal surface of the erect penis; examination of the flaccid penis may be unremarkable

b. Histology:
- fibrosis of the tunica albuginea without involvement of the corpora cavernosa; fibrosis may have a "proliferative" look similar to fibromatosis
- Calcification and ossification (os penis) may occur, especially in older men.
- Early lesions demonstrate perivascular inflammation in the loose connective tissue between the tunica albuginea and the sinusoids of the corpora cavernosa

c. Clinical course and treatment:
- Disease resolves spontaneously in less than one-third of patients
- Disease progression occurs in up to 40% of patients
- The disease remains stable in the remainder
- Treatment includes surgical excision of the plaques, radiotherapy, and steroid injections

B. Infections

1. Gonorrhea:

a. Agent: ***Neisseria gonorrhea*** (**Gram-negative** "biscuit-shaped" **diplococci**)

b. Gonorrhea means "flow of semen" referring to the exudate of gonorrheal urethritis

c. Clinical: profuse purulent or scant "gleet" urethral discharge with burning micturition

d. Transmission: sexual

e. Chief complication: urethral stricture

f. Mimicked by—and often accompanied by—chlamydial infection, so need lab tests to distinguish

g. Treatment: antibiotics

2. Syphilis:

a. Agent: ***Treponema pallidum***

b. **Gram-negative spirochete**

c. Three clinical stages:
- **Primary**: tiny papule on the penis, usually at site of trauma that progresses to the ulcerated chancre, a round painless ulcer with sharp margins and a clean indurated base. With or without therapy, the primary chancre heals within 6-8 weeks
- **Secondary**: the spirochetal organisms proliferate in the lymphatic system and blood for 6 weeks to 6 months, producing symmetric skin lesions and generalized lymphadenopathy

- **Tertiary**: characterized by granulomas ("gummas"); may also demonstrate CNS involvement in this stage

d. Histologic findings:
   - **Primary stage**:
     i. Spirochetal organisms can be identified in scrapings from the chancre (usually seen best using dark-field microscopy)
     ii. histologically, the characteristic change is a dense lymphoplasmacytic infiltrate around vessels (esp. plasma cells)
     iii. antibody test: negative
   - **Secondary stage**: organisms may or may not be visualized by special stains (Warthin-Starry stain) on tissue, or by dark-field microscopy (scrapings)
     i. antibody test: positive
   - **Tertiary stage**: granulomatous inflammation (gummas) with "hard" granulomas that eventually demonstrate central caseous necrosis.

e. Therapy: dependent on stage; consists of antibiotic treatment.

3. Herpes Simplex:
   a. Agent: **Herpes simplex virus, type 2**
   b. Clinical: pain, itching, urethral discharge, dysuria, and tender lymphadenopathy
   c. Histology:
      - vesicles with adjacent **multinucleated giant cells containing characteristic intranuclear inclusions**

   d. Treatment: acyclovir and phosphonoformate trisodi decrease duration and intensity of primary and recurrent episodes, but are not curative

4. Candidiasis:
   a. Agent: ***Candida albicans***
   b. Causes balanitis or balanoposthitis, characterized by bright red patches of inflammation with numerous minute pustules and erosions
   c. Most commonly found in **uncircumcised males**
   d. Predisposing conditions: Diabetes mellitus, antibiotic treatment, and immunosuppression
   e. Diagnosis confirmed by **KOH prep**
   f. Treatment: antifungal agents

5. Molluscum contagiosum:
   a. Agent: **Molluscum contagiosum virus** (a pox virus)
   b. Incubation: 2-7 weeks
   c. Clinical: multiple discrete dome-shaped 3-6 mm papules with central umbilications through which milky-white fluid may be expressed under pressure
   d. Affects all age groups
   e. Histology:
      - **cup-shaped invagination** of acantholytic epidermis into the dermis
      - cytoplasmic inclusions ("molluscum bodies" or "Henderson-Patterson bodies") are identifiable within the stratum malphigii. The inclusions progressively enlarge as cells reach the surface, and also change from being eosinophilic to being basophilic and granular as they enlarge and displace the nucleus

   g. Treatment: podophyllin or silver nitrate or laser vaporization

3. Non-neoplastic Disease of the Scrotum

A. Fournier's Gangrene

1. Idiopathic form of necrotizing fasciitis of the subcutaneous tissue and skeletal muscle of the genitals and perineum, especially the scrotum
2. Lesions begin as reddish plaques with necrosis and are accompanied by severe systemic symptoms including pain and fever
3. Causative agents are most commonly **staphylococcal or streptococcal species**, which may or may not be mixed with gram-negative bacilli and anaerobic bacteria
4. Predisposing factors include: diabetes, immunosuppression, alcoholism, recent surgical intervention, trauma, and morbid obesity
5. This is a serious, life-threatening condition requiring surgical intervention, and broad spectrum antibiotics

B. Idiopathic Scrotal Calcinosis

1. Occurs in two settings:
   a. calcification of preexisting epidermal or pilar cysts
   b. calcification of dermal connective tissue in the absence of cysts (idiopathic)
2. Usually young men, present with multiple long-standing firm-to-hard nodules measuring up to 3 cm in diameter

3. Overlying skin is generally intact, although it may ulcerate and extrude cheesy material
4. Histology: lesions are located in the dermis and are characterized by globules of cyanophilic (bluish) calcific material with or without accompanying granulomatous inflammation
5. Treatment: surgery if symptomatic

C. Epidermal Cyst
1. Common in the scrotum
2. Single or multiple rubbery nodules filled with gray-white cheesy material
3. Histologically, they are lined by keratinizing squamous epithelium

8. Penis and Scrotum II: Tumors and Tumor-like Lesions

1. Condyloma acuminatum

A. Etiologic agent: human papilloma virus

B. Clinical features: usually sexually transmitted; variable incubation period

C. Gross features: flat, warty or papillary lesions, typically involving glans or urethral meatus

D. Histologic Features
1. Proliferation of squamous epithelium with papillomatous architecture (warty) showing orderly epithelial maturation
2. Hyperkeratosis (thickened keratin layer), parakeratosis (pyknotic nuclei within the keratin layer), and koilocytes (raisin-oid cells within a clear "halo") are characteristic features
3. Penile condylomas are usually cytologically benign, although treatment with podophyllin or lasers may cause marked cytologic atypia – a history of prior treatment is therefore always appreciated
4. Viral strains 6 and 11 are common in typical condyloma without dysplasia, while strains 16, 18, 31 and 33 are more common in the dysplastic forms of condyloma

E. **Prognosis and Treatment:** may spontaneously regress in 50% of cases, but are otherwise treated with podophyllin or laser

2. Premalignant Lesions

A. Erythroplasia of Queyrat
1. Clinical: usually uncircumcised men in 5th-6th decades
2. Gross features: **bright red, glistening, velvety plaque** on the **glans and the prepuce**; may also involve urethral meatus, frenulum, or neck of the penis
3. Histologic features: squamous carcinoma in situ (full thickness involvement by neoplastic cells with loss of maturation, etc.)
4. Prognosis: 10% of patients progress to invasive squamous cell carcinoma, and 2% develop distant metastases

5. Differential diagnosis (clinical): Zoon's balanitis, drug eruptions, psoriasis, lichen planus, and other inflammatory processes

B. Bowen's Disease

1. This is essentially the same lesion as erythroplasia of Queyrat, in the sense that it represents squamous cell carcinoma in situ; however, unlike erythroplasia of Queyrat, Bowen's disease does not have the velvety red patch, and it more often involves the shaft of the penis rather than the glans/prepuce area
2. Clinical: presents slightly earlier than erythroplasia of Queyrat (4th-5th decades)
3. Gross features: sharply demarcated **hyperkeratotic plaque**, usually on **shaft** of penis
4. Histologic features:
   a. squamous cell carcinoma in situ
   b. hyperkeratosis is more common than in erythroplasia
5. Prognosis: approximately 5%-10% progress to invasive squamous cell carcinoma

C. Bowenoid Papulosis

1. Clinical: multiple papules in young men that histologically resemble squamous cell carcinoma in situ
2. Gross: usually occur on penile shaft; papules range from 0.2 to 1.0 cm; sometimes coalesce to form plaques like condyloma acuminata
3. Histologic features:
   a. Hyperkeratosis, parakeratosis, and papillomatosis
   b. May show a little more maturation evident in the epithelium than is seen in Bowen's or Erythroplasia, but you may still see mitotic figures in the upper layers of the epithelium
4. Prognosis: spontaneous regression occasionally occurs

3. Malignant Neoplasms of the Penis

A. General Features

1. Cancer of the penis is uncommon, affecting approximately 1/100,000 men in North America; other areas (Haiti, Uganda, Brazil, etc.) have a much higher rate of penile carcinoma (10%-12%)
2. 95% of penile carcinomas are squamous cell type

B. Squamous Cell Carcinoma

1. Predisposing factors:
   a. **Lack of circumcision** combined with **poor hygiene**
   b. **Phimosis**: smegma may play a role in both phimosis and SCCA of penis
   c. **Viral** (human papilloma virus infection) – questionable.
2. Clinical features: men >40 years; blacks > whites (2:1).
3. Gross features:
   a. May be exophytic and fungating or ulcerated and infiltrative
   b. typical location is glans penis or prepuce; rare sites include shaft and urethral meatus
4. Histologic features:
   a. Well-differentiated SCCA shows finger-like downward invasion with extensive keratin formation and prominent intercellular bridges
   b. Poorly-differentiated SCCA form little or no keratin, have numerous mitotic figures and marked nuclear pleomorphism
   c. Moderately-differentiated SCCA lies somewhere between the two extremes
   d. In general: exophytic/papillary lesions tend to be well-differentiated, while the ulcerating/infiltrative lesions are moderately- to poorly-differentiated
5. Clinical behavior:
   a. Locally invasive, destroying the prepuce and penile shaft
   b. Metastases can go to ipsilateral or contralateral inguinal lymph nodes
   c. Hematogenous spread is uncommon, despite the rich vascularity of the corpora cavernosum
6. Staging: The most commonly used systems are the Jackson system and the AJCC system
7. Treatment and prognosis:
   a. Grade and stage are the best predictors of clinical behavior, with **stage being the most important factor**
   b. Well-differentiated tumors typically present earlier, involve the prepuce, and have a better long-term survival (80%), while poorly-differentiated tumors tend to present later, involve the shaft, and are more often associated with inguinal or distant metastases

C. Squamous Cell Carcinoma: Variations on the Theme

1. Verrucous Carcinoma:
   a. **Clinical**: accounts for 5%-16% of penile malignancies
   b. **Gross**: large, fungating, exophytic/warty mass arising in coronal sulcus with spread to glans and prepuce
   c. **Histologic features**:
      - well-differentiated squamous cell carcinoma with broad pushing borders rather than the finger-like infiltrative borders of a typical squamous cell carcinoma
      - cytologic atypia is minimal and mitotic figures are rare
   d. **Behavior**: locally invasive but typically does not metastasize; may recur if inadequately excised
   e. **Differential diagnosis**: condyloma acuminatum (giant condyloma of Buschke and Löwenstein) and the more typical form of SCCA. (Actually, some people feel that the giant condyloma of B and L may be the same entity as verrucous carcinoma; however, verrucous carcinoma typically is not associated with HPV, whereas the giant condyloma is.)
   f. **Treatment**: radical or partial penectomy reduces the risk of recurrence to 33%, so this is the recommended treatment. (80% recurrence with local excision.)
   Importantly: radiation should be avoided as it may induce dedifferentiation into a highly aggressive spindle cell squamous carcinoma
2. Spindle cell (sarcomatoid) squamous cell carcinoma:
   a. Rarely reported on the penis
   b. Gross: often forms polypoid mass
   c. Histologic features: spindle cell neoplasm with focal squamous differentiation
   d. Behavior: aggressive clinical course

D. Malignant Melanoma

1. Less than 100 reported cases
2. Usually in white males, 5th-6th decades
3. Gross: black, brown, or blue variegated papules with irregular borders and irregular pigmentation
4. Histologic features:
   a. Nests of melanocytes at the dermal-epidermal junction
   b. Atypical melanocytes may "migrate" to the upper layers of the epidermis
   c. Infiltrative component shows prominent nucleoli and none of the maturation that is often seen in nevi

4. Malignant Lesions of the Scrotum

A. Squamous Cell Carcinoma

1. Scrotal squamous cell carcinoma was the first cancer linked to occupational exposure: Potts first described the higher frequency among men exposed to high levels of dust and soot (chimney sweeps, cotton factory workers)—hence, scrotal SCCA was at one time called "Pott's cancer" or "chimney sweep's cancer"
2. The offending agent has subsequently been identified as 3'4'-benzpyrene
3. SCCA is the most common malignant neoplasm of the scrotum, but is still much less common than SCCA of the penis
4. Clinical: slow-growing warty lesion, usually single, located on anterolateral aspect of scrotum; with time the lesions ulcerate and may be associated with rolled edges and purulent exudate; usually affects men in 6th-7th decades; left > right (probably related to carcinogen exposure); 50% have inguinal metastases at the time of presentation
5. Histologic features: Looks like SCCA of the penis
6. Staging: Lowe's system is the most common staging system used
7. Treatment and Prognosis: poor prognosis (30%-52% survival at 5 years)

B. Paget's Disease

1. Essentially represents an adenocarcinoma in situ
2. Clinical: 6th-7th decades, fairly rare, but **most cases are associated with an underlying carcinoma** (especially bladder, urethra, or prostate)
3. Gross: scaly eczematous lesion
4. Histologic features:

a. Intraepithelial proliferation of atypical cells with vacuolated cytoplasm and large vesicular nuclei
b. Atypical cells tend to cluster at the tips of the rete pegs
c. **Intracytoplasmic mucin vacuoles (highlighted by PAS or mucicarcmine)**
d. Hyperkeratosis, parakeratosis, and papillomatosis are common

5. Differential diagnosis: SCCA and melanoma (just do mucin stain to clinch the dx of Paget's)

C. Leiomyosarcoma

1. Sarcoma of the scrotum is very unusual, but the most common form is leiomyosarcoma
2. Tumor arises from the Dartos muscle; less than 20 cases have been described

9. Bladder I: Non-neoplastic Lesions

1. Normal Histology

A. **Urothelium**: 5-7 cells thick, with umbrella, intermediate, and basal cells. The urothelium renews approximately once per year

B. **Lamina propria**: loose fibrovascular tissue with highly variable, delicate smooth muscle fibers (muscularis mucosae)

C. **Muscularis**: several layers of muscle tissue

D. **Urachus**: central lumen lined by epithelium; surrounded by fibrous tissue and smooth muscle

2. Normal/ Metaplastic Lesions

A. Von Brunn's Nests

1. Well-circumscribed nests of benign urothelial cells in the lamina propria without obvious attachment to the overlying epithelium
2. Thought to be a "normal" feature of the bladder mucosa, most commonly in trigone

B. Cystitis Cystica

1. Essentially von Brunn's nests which have undergone central cystic degeneration
2. Usually seen as a pearly submucosal cyst

C. Cystitis Glandularis

1. Found in 71% of bladders, usually microscopic but may be grossly apparent as raised, red nodular lesions; particularly common in the trigone
2. Typical type: similar to cystitis cystica except have:
   a. **Cuboidal or columnar epithelium**
   b. **One or more surrounding layers of urothelial cells**
3. Intestinal type: Less frequently there is a:
   a. **Tall columnar** epithelial lining with obvious **mucin production and goblet cells**
   b. **No surrounding layer of urothelium**
4. In patients with long-standing chronic inflammation like in-dwelling catheters, paraplegics, and people with stones, the intestinal type can become diffuse, and is termed "intestinal metaplasia"

5. The intestinal type—when diffuse (ie, intestinal metaplasia)—is associated with an **increased risk of bladder adenocarcinoma**

D. Squamous Metaplasia

1. Nonkeratinizing: stratified squamous epithelium usually at the trigone and bladder neck
   a. Seen in 85% of reproductive age women and 75% of menopausal women
   b. May also be seen in men receiving estrogen therapy for prostate cancer
   c. No clinical significance, other than the fact that patients may have urinary urgency and frequency ("pseudomembranous trigonitis")
2. Keratinizing (leukoplakia): stratified squamous epithelium with keratin layer on top; looks like a flat gray-white plaque, and typically involves anterior wall.
   a. 20% of patients will have **synchronous bladder cancer**
   b. 20% of patients **will develop bladder** cancer at a later date
   c. **Commonly precedes squamous cell carcinoma in areas where schistosomiasis is endemic**

E. Nephrogenic Metaplasia (Nephrogenic Adenoma)

1. In adults, more common in males (2:1); in children, more common in females
2. 75% occur in the bladder, but usually does not involve the anterior wall
3. Clinical features: typically solitary and may be associated with previous GU surgery (60%), calculi (15%), trauma (10%), renal transplant (8%)
4. Histologic features: small simple tubules lined by a single layer of bland cuboidal to low-columnar cells ("hobnail" cells) with clear or eosinophilic cytoplasm
   a. May also have cystic, polypoid, papillary, and diffuse patterns.
   b. No mitoses or atypia.
5. Differential diagnosis: Prostate ca, TCC, and clear cell adenocarcinoma

3. Cystitis

A. Nonspecific Cystitis

1. Polypoid (papillary) cystitis:
   a. Characterized by **chronic inflammation and edema** of the lamina propria
   b. Most often seen with **indwelling catheters (80%)** and **fistulas**
   c. Urothelium is usually normal thickness with umbrella cells present
2. Follicular cystitis:
   a. Characterized by **lymphoid follicles** in lamina propria, typically with germinal centers
   b. Often occur in patients with **bladder cancer (40%)** and in patients with **urinary tract infections (35%)**
3. Giant cell cystitis:
   a. Characterized by **atypical mesenchymal cells** with enlarged multinucleated nuclei in the lamina propria
4. Hemorrhagic cystitis:
   a. Characterized by **congested vasculature and hemorrhage** in the lamina propria
   b. Etiologies include: **chemical toxins** (cyclophosphamide, busulfan, thiotepa, aniline dyes, and insecticides), **radiation**, viral infection, and idiopathic

B. Specific Forms of Cystitis

1. Eosinophilic cystitis:
   a. Characterized by dense infiltrate of **eosinophils** in the lamina propria and muscularis
   b. Often seen in patients with **invasive TCC**
   c. May be seen in patients with **transurethral resection or biopsy**
   d. Rarely may represent **allergic** cystitis
2. Interstitial cystitis (Hunner's ulcer):
   a. May or may not be associated with an "ulcer"
   b. Grossly appears as hemorrhagic spots or linear cracks
   c. Characterized by **lymphoplasmacytic infiltrate** in lamina
   d. May see **increased mast cells**
   e. **No microscopic findings are pathognomonic**: must use clinical correlation
   f. Typically seen in females (90%) ages 30-50
   e. Etiology unknown (but it is **not bacterial**)

3. Post-surgical necrobiotic granulomas:
   a. Characterized by **granulomas with serpiginous borders** and **central acellular eosinophilic material**
   b. Typically seen after surgery (hence the name)
4. BCG granulomas:
   a. See loss of urothelium and marked chronic inflammation in the lamina propria
   b. **Epithelioid granulomas** may be seen which **lack central necrosis**
   c. Typically seen after BCG treatment (again, hence the name)
5. Radiation cystitis:
   a. See loss of urothelium with the remaining urothelial cells showing **nuclear atypia**, **smudgy chromatin**, but normal **N/C ratio**
   b. Blood vessels become hyalinized
   c. Cytoplasm becomes very vacuolated
   d. Typically seen 3-6 weeks post-radiation.
6. Reaction to topical chemotherapy:
   a. Induces denudation of the urothelium; similar changes to radiation including nuclear pleomorphism and hyperchromasia

C. Infectious Cystitis

1. Bacterial cystitis: most common cause of cystitis, usually due to coliform bacteria
   a. Histology: ulcerated urothelium with neutrophils in lamina propria
2. Encrusted cystitis: may arise when **urea-splitting bacteria alkalinize the urine** and **inorganic salts are deposited** in the damaged mucosa
   a. Most commonly seen in **women**
   b. Histology: lesions are covered by a coat of fibrin (pink stuff) mixed with calcified necrotic debris (dark purple stuff) and inflammatory cells
3. Emphysematous cystitis: usually occurs in women and diabetics, with the causative agents being *E coli* or *Aerobacter aerogenes*.
   a. Histology: **empty cavities lined with flattened cells** and surrounded by **thin septa**
4. Malakoplakia: occurs due to **impairment of mononuclear cells in killing phagocytosed bacteria** (*E coli* but also *Proteus vulgaris*, *Aerobacter aerogenes*, and *Klebsiella pneumoniae*); more common in women
   a. Gross: multiple, soft yellow plaques
   b. Histology: accumulation of histiocytes with eosinophilic cytoplasm **(von Hansemann histiocytes)** in the superficial lamina propria beneath an intact urothelium
   c. The histiocytes contain laminated calcified cytoplasmic inclusions **(Michaelis-Goodman bodies)** with a bulls-eye appearance
   d. **Must see M-G bodies for diagnosis**
5. Tuberculous cystitis: almost always follows renal infection by ***M tuberculosis***
   a. Histology: **granulomatous inflammation with epithelioid histiocytes and multinucleated giant cells surrounding caseous necrosis**
6. Schistosomiasis: usually due to ***Schistosoma haematobium***
   a. May be characterized by polyps, ulcers, squamous metaplasia, chronic inflammation, and the presence of ova in the lamina propria
   b. Ulcers are more common in the chronic stage when there are a large number of eggs

4. Miscellaneous Lesions

A. Exstrophy

1. Normal bladder surface is quickly inflamed and ulcerated, and undergoes squamous and intestinal metaplasia
2. Untreated patients have an increased risk of cancer, but surgical closure prevents this

B. Diverticula

1. Saccular evaginations of the bladder mucosa
2. Usually seen in males with outlet obstruction (prostatic hyperplasia)
3. May be associated with squamous or intestinal metaplasia
4. There is an increased risk of carcinoma arising within these diverticula

C. Amyloidosis

1. When it occurs in the bladder, it is usually primary rather than systemic
2. Adults generally affected, men = women
3. Typically present with hematuria
4. Histologically characterized by deposition of eosinophilic "glassy" material in lamina and muscularis propria (Congo red positive with "apple-green" birefringence)

D. Patent Urachus

1. Microscopic remnants of the urachus are common
2. Remember: urachus connects bladder and the allantois
3. The discontinuous epithelium-lined duct can give rise to cysts, sinuses, or neoplasms, particularly adenocarcinomas mimicking colonic type

E. Endometriosis

1. Typically seen in menstruating women
2. Most women will have a history of previous pelvic surgery (50%)
3. Bladder is the most common site of urinary tract involvement, although only 1% of patients with endometriosis will have bladder involvement
4. See endometrial glands, stroma, and hemosiderin-laden macrophages

10. Bladder II: Tumors of the Urinary Bladder

1. Benign Epithelial Neoplasms

A. Urothelial Papilloma

1. Comprises 2%-3% of papillary urothelial tumors
2. Small, usually unifocal, and consist of delicate fibrovascular stalks covered by cytologically and architecturally normal urothelium
3. Tend to occur in younger patients (<50 yrs)
4. Often recur (73%) and may be associated with later development of invasive TCC in 10% of patients
5. Some experts have advocated including the exophytic papilloma in the "papillary urothelial neoplasm of low malignant potential" (along with grade I TCCs), although that is not currently a widespread practice

B. Inverted Urothelial Papilloma

1. Uncertain etiology: some authors consider it a neoplasm, others feel it is reactive (à la cystitis glandularis/cystitis cystica)
2. Most commonly occurs in middle-aged men presenting with hematuria or irritative symptoms
3. Most are small, single, and appear as smooth domed masses at the trigone
4. Microscopic:
   a. **Trabecular** type:
      - anastomosing cords or sheets of urothelium arising from the overlying mucosal surface
      - in some cases gland-like spaces may be present, but the secretions are PAS+ and not mucicarmine+ (ie, not true glandular spaces)

   b. **Glandular** type:
      - nests of urothelium with pseudoglandular (urothelial lining) or glandular (goblet cell lining) differentiation
      - in this case, the secretions are mucicarmine + (true mucin secretion)
5. Can see nonkeratinizing squamous metaplasia, but if there is keratinization, look for cancer
6. Generally show little or no cytological atypia: a little bit is OK, but lots of atypia with numerous mitoses would favor a dx of invasive cancer.

2. Malignant Epithelial Neoplasms

A. Urothelial Carcinoma

1. Epidemiology:
   a. **Whites > blacks; males > females**
   b. Median age: 65 years
2. Etiology and pathogenesis: risk factors include
   a. **Tobacco smoke**: 33% of TCCs occur in cigarette smokers
      - cigarettes >> pipes and cigars >> smokeless tobacco (essentially no increased risk)
      - cigarette smokers have 2-4x increased risk, which decreases gradually once they quit smoking
      - thought to be related to nitrosamines and 2-naphthylamine
   b. **Occupational exposure**: 33% of cases
      - especially: dye industry (benzidine and 2-naphthylamine)
   c. **Phenacetin**: significant risk only when high cumulative doses (2 kg) are reached
   d. **Cyclophosphamide**:
      - 10.7% increased risk at 12 years; latency of 65-141 months
      - thought to be due to accumulation of acrolein (degradation product)
      - majority of tumors are TCC, but can also result in squamous cell carcinoma, adenocarcinoma, and leiomyosarcoma
   e. **Radiation**: risk of TCC is increased 2-4x in women who have received pelvic radiation for cervical cancer
   f. **Cytogenetics**:
      - commonly reported abnormalities: loss of Y, loss of chromosome 9, and trisomy 7
      - loss of Y chromosome has been correlated with a worse prognosis
      - can be useful for following low-grade TCCs, as the most common abnormality in these tumors is loss of 9
      - thought to be a tumor suppressor gene on long arm of 9, which is lost in up to 50% of TCCs (9q-)
   g. **Heredity**: does not play a big role in TCC
3. Clinical features: 90% present with painless hematuria
4. Diagnosis:
   a. **Urine cytology**: good for following high-risk population, but not good for a screening procedure
   b. **Cystoscopy and biopsy**: currently the primary diagnostic tool
   c. **Cystograms and excretory urography**: it is important to screen for upper tract disease as the cause of the presenting symptom (hematuria) and to exclude synchronous upper tract cancer in patients with bladder TCC
5. Urothelial carcinoma in situ:
   a. CIS is usually associated with prior or synchronous bladder tumors
   b. The diagnosis is based more upon **the presence of severe cytological atypia, not necessarily full-thickness urothelial involvement**
      - Characterized by large pleomorphic cells with prominent nucleoli and numerous (atypical) mitoses
      - Cells have a random orientation, giving overall "disorganized" appearance to the mucosa
      - There is often striking discohesion resulting in extensive loss of the epithelial cells ("denuding cystitis")—which is why cytology can be so helpful in these lesions
      - May or may not be associated with marked superficial chronic inflammation
      - Commonly involve the prostatic urethra (67%), prostate gland (up to 40%) and ureters (up to 57%)
      - Typically see a loss of blood group antigens (A, B, and H)
   c. Prognosis: 32%-83% of patients with TCIS will develop invasive cancer, and up to 34% already have microinvasion elsewhere at the time of dx
6. Papillary and nonpapillary urothelial carcinoma:
   a. **Papillary TCC**:
      - Gross:
        i. usually solitary **exophytic** lesions involving the **lateral and posterior walls** of the bladder; rarely involve the dome
        ii. commonly present with painless hematuria
      - Microscopic:
        i. Generally characterized by papillae with delicate fibrovascular cores
        ii. **Grade I**: thickened epithelium (>7 cell layers) but very little cytological atypia; rare or absent mitotic figures

iii. **Grade II**: greater degree of nuclear pleomorphism and some disruption of the normal architecture, but should still be able to distinguish a papillary architecture; number of cell layers may be increased, decreased, or normal

iv. **Grade III**: severe nuclear atypia; cellular discohesion, loss of normal architecture; frequent mitotic figures

- 80% of TCCs are noninvasive at the time of dx
- The majority of invasive papillary TCCs are grade II or III
- A consensus classification in 1998 suggested regrouping tumors into "tumors of uncertain malignant potential," "low-grade," and "high-grade." The jury is still out on the utility of such a scheme, but Table 2 presents the general breakdown (FYI)

b. **Nonpapillary TCC**:

- May be polypoid, sessile, ulcerated, and infiltrative
- Most invasive TCCs are grade III and consist of cohesive nests of cells with large hyperchromatic nuclei, moderate amount of cytoplasm, and sometimes demonstrating peripheral palisading
- Typically see angular nuclei with grooving, high mitotic rate
- The invasive nests stir up a desmoplastic reaction (fibrotic) which can be helpful in diagnosing early lesions
- **Squamous differentiation** occurs in up to 20% and is significant in that it portends a worse prognosis: the diagnosis must be based upon the presence of keratin pearls and/or intercellular bridges (ie, it can't just "look" squamoid)
- **Glandular differentiation** is defined as the presence of true glandular spaces (not just cells with mucin in them)
- **Sarcomatoid variant**: contains epithelial (TCC-ish) and spindle-cell components → tends to occur in older patients (60s-70s) and is highly malignant (25% survival at 2 years)

7. Critical pathologic staging rests upon the **presence or absence of muscularis propria invasion**

B. Squamous Cell Carcinoma

1. Clinical features:

a. In areas where schistosomiasis is endemic, SCCA accounts for up to 73% of bladder cancers, but **in the United States and UK, this tumor comprises only 3%-6% of all bladder cancers**

b. Typically seen in males (M:F = 1.7:1); with a mean age of 65.5 years.

Table 2

Histological Grading Categories for Papillary Urothelial Tumors

WHO	Pauwels	WHO/ISUP
Papilloma	Papilloma	Papillary urothelial neoplasm of low malignant potential (PUNLMP)
Grade 1	Grade 1	Papillary urothelial neoplasm of low malignant potential (PUNLMP)
Grade 2	Grade 2a Grade 2b	Urothelial carcinoma, low grade Urothelial carcinoma, high grade
Grade 3	Grade 3	Urothelial carcinoma, high grade

c. Presenting complaint: hematuria or irritative symptoms

d. Many will have advanced disease at the time of dx

2. Etiology and pathogenesis:

a. **Schistosomiasis**: Three types (*S mansoni*, *S japonicum*, and *S haematobium*) but only *S haematobium* causes bladder cancer

b. **Chronic bladder irritation** (catheters, urinary retention, recurrent infections, stones)

c. Bladder **diverticula**

3. Gross: bulky necrotic masses that usually fill the bladder

4. Histology: **The diagnosis of squamous carcinoma of the bladder is reserved for those tumors with pure squamous histology** (ie, if there is any urothelial ca—even if it is only in situ—the dx should be TCC with squamous differentiation)

5. Grading: assessed according to the degree of keratinization (lots = well-differentiated; none = poorly-differentiated)

6. Staging: same system as is used for TCC

7. Prognosis: prognosis remains poor (13.5% survival at 5 years; 5.3% survival at 10 years) with death usually due to local recurrence rather than metastasis

C. Adenocarcinoma

1. Primary adenocarcinoma of the bladder accounts for less than 1% of all bladder tumors and generally falls into two groups:

a. Those occurring in the urachus

b. Those occurring in the bladder proper

2. Urachal adenocarcinomas:

a. Diagnosis requires

- location in the **dome** with primary involvement of the muscle or deeper structures
- presence of a suprapelvic mass,
- tumor growth in the bladder wall extending into the space of Retzius
- **sharp demarcation between tumor and adjacent normal urothelium**
- Absence of cystitis cystica/glandularis elsewhere in the bladder
- Presence of urachal remnants

b. Urachal adenoca. typically occur in adult males, mean age 50.6 years

c. Thought to occur due to intestinal metaplasia of the urachal remnant

d. Generally form **discrete masses in the dome of the bladder** and **appear to be centered in the wall of the bladder** rather than based in the mucosa

e. Microscopic: usually colloid carcinoma (cells floating in mucin) but may have signet ring or columnar morphology

f. Staging: same as used for TCC

g. Treatment and natural history: partial or radical cystectomy with en bloc resection of urachal remnant and umbilicus

h. Survival is poor: 37% and 17% at 5 and 10 years, respectively

4. Nonurachal adenocarcinomas:

a. Clinical features

- Accounts for the **majority of bladder adenocarcinomas**
- Males > females; mean age 59.4 years
- Hematuria is the most common presenting complaint
- Up to 40% of patients will have metastatic dz at the time of dx

b. Etiology and pathogenesis

- Most cases **arise from intestinal metaplasia** of the urothelium
- Most commonly occur in patients with **nonfunctioning bladder, chronic irritation, obstruction, and cystocele**
- **Cystitis glandularis** is present in 14%-67% of patients
- May also occur in the setting of exstrophy

c. Histology: generally divided into 6 categories

- Adenocarcinoma NOS
- Enteric (looks like intestinal adenoca)
- Signet ring
- Mucinous (colloid—cells floating in mucin)
- Clear cell
- Mixed—two or more of the above patterns

d. Grading: no currently accepted grading standard

e. Staging: use the same system as TCC

f. Treatment and natural history:

- Radical cystectomy/cystoprostatectomy with pelvic lymph node dissection is the recommended treatment

- Chemo and radiation play uncertain roles
- Poor prognosis overall: 5- and 10-year survivals are 17% and 11%, respectively

D. Small Cell Carcinoma

1. <1% of bladder tumors
2. Males > females; 60-70 years old
3. Hematuria is the common presenting symptoms
4. Paraneoplastic syndromes are rare
5. Gross: highly variable
6. Histology: sheets of small round blue cells with numerous mitoses, crush artifact, nuclear molding, and necrosis
7. Unlike other bladder tumors: if there is an element of small cell ca and some TCC, the lesion is designated "small cell ca with focal areas of TCC" (rather than TCC with small cell differentiation)
8. Will stain for neuroendocrine markers (NSE, chromogranin, and synaptophysin)
9. Prognosis: poor

3. Paraganglioma

A. Clinical Features

1. Found equally in males and females
2. Thought to arise from the paraganglionic tissue within the bladder wall
3. Hematuria is the common presenting complaint, but the classic scenario is paroxysmal hypertension with micturition

B. Histology

1. Intramural lesions with predilection for the trigone, anterior wall, and dome
2. Generally pink-tan or yellowish, well-circumscribed, lobulated appearance
3. Histology: nesting growth pattern (zellballen)—sort of like pheochromocytoma
4. Mitotic figures are rare, and necrosis is absent
5. No definite pathologic feature that predicts benign or malignant course

C. **Treatment and natural history:** may recur if not completely excised; metastases occurred in <15% of cases (only 2 cases showed distant mets)

4. Benign Mesenchymal Neoplasms

A. Leiomyoma

1. More common in women
2. Obstructive symptoms are most common (ball-and-valve effect of tumor)
3. Gross: submucosal mass
4. Micro: spindle cell proliferation with cigar-shaped nuclei and no mitoses

B. Postoperative Spindle-cell Nodule

1. More of a reactive process than a tumor
2. Clinical history of surgery within past 120 days at the site where the lesions arose
3. Gross: friable nodular mass
4. Micro: interlacing fascicles of spindle cells; high mitotic rate; minimal nuclear atypia, though.
5. Treatment: resolve spontaneously

C. Inflammatory pseudotumor

1. More of a reactive process than a tumor
2. Clinical: no history of recent surgery; females > males; age 20-50 years
3. Hematuria is the most common presenting complaint
4. Gross: solitary nodule forming polypoid lesion
5. Micro: spindle cells in a myxoid matrix with prominent vasculature; mitoses common; lots of eosinophils
6. DDx: Leiomyosarcoma

5. Malignant Soft Tissue Neoplasms

A. Rhabdomyosarcoma

1. Rare in adults, more common in children (boys > girls)
2. Clinical: generally present with obstruction and hematuria
3. Gross: forms polypoid masses (sarcoma botryoides)

4. Trigone is the most common place
5. Histologically, most are embryonal (small round blue cell tumor with focal strap cells)

B. Leiomyosarcoma
1. The most common sarcoma arising in the bladder
2. Mean age 52 years; several have occurred following cyclophosphamide treatment
3. Often lobulated grossly, with or without ulceration
4. Micro: spindle cells with cigar-shaped nuclei, numerous mitoses
5. Differential dx: spindle cell variant of TCC (sarcomatoid carcinoma)
   a. Check for areas that look like typical TCC (epithelial component)
   b. Do stains: LMS will stain for actin and desmin (muscle markers); sarcomatoid carcinoma will stain for cytokeratin (epithelial marker)

11. Prostate I: Non-neoplastic Lesions of the Prostate

1. Normal Histology

A. Ducts
1. Elongated branching, tubular structures with a ruffled, undulating luminal surface
2. Some of the larger ducts may be lined by transitional epithelium (so TCC can arise within the prostate)

B. Acini: small, rounded simpler glands with lobular arrangement around the ducts

C. Cell Types
1. Epithelial:
   a. **Columnar secretory epithelial cells** line the smaller ducts and the acini
      • Have abundant clear cytoplasm
      • Stain for PSA and PAP
   b. **Basal cells** are the second layer of cells located between the secretory cells and the basement membrane
      • scant cytoplasm, small round nuclei
      • Stain for cytokeratin, NOT for PSA and PAP
2. Stromal
3. Neuroendocrine: The prostate has the highest number of endocrine-paracrine cells of any GU organ

D. Seminal Vesicles
1. Form large complex glands with papillary tufts
2. Look for "monster cells" (highly pleomorphic and enlarged) and lipofuscin (golden-brown pigment)

2. Prostatic Hyperplasia

A. Can first be seen at 20-30 yrs; increases steadily after age 40

B. Clinical
1. Typically results in smoothly enlarged prostate
2. Symptoms due to obstruction (urgency, frequency, nocturia, etc.)
3. Etiology: unknown, but most likely related to androgen stimulation with estrogen synergism

C. Histologic Features

1. Both glands and stroma can become hyperplastic
2. Hyperplastic glands typically are large with complex papillary infoldings
3. Cytologically benign, with two cell layers, bland nuclei, and abundant pale cytoplasm.
4. Will often see corpora amylacea (bright pink laminated concretions) in these areas
5. Also often associated with chronic lymphocytic infiltrate—very nonspecific finding.

3. Infarcts

A. 20%-25% of BPH specimens have infarcts

B. Grossly appear mottled and yellowish with hemorrhagic rim

C. Microscopically, demonstrate "zoning" effect

1. Central **coagulative necrosis**
2. Surrounded by **hemorrhage and inflammation** with reactive glands
3. Surrounded by a zone in which the glands show **squamous metaplasia**

4. Prostatitis

A. Acute Bacterial Prostatitis

1. Clinically associated with UTIs, increased numbers of inflammatory cells in the prostatic secretions, and growth of bacterial organisms from prostatic secretions
2. Majority are caused by gram-negative organisms (*E coli*)
3. Micro: sheets of neutrophils in and around the acini

B. Chronic Bacterial Prostatitis

1. Clinically characterized by recurrent UTIs caused by the same pathogens.
2. Mostly caused by gram-negative organisms; NOT by chlamydia or trichomonas (contrary to popular belief)
3. Micro: Lymphocytic inflammation around the acini with neutrophils in the lumina
4. Chronic prostatitis is generally a clinical—rather than a histologic—diagnosis, since the features we use to dx chronic prostatitis are quite similar to the inflammatory changes seen in BPH; however, if the patient has an elevated PSA and has a marked lymphocytic infiltrate with luminal neutrophils, we will comment on the findings since they may explain his elevated PSA

C. Nonbacterial Prostatitis

1. Inflammatory condition of unknown cause
2. Most common prostatitis syndrome
3. Diagnosis is based upon negative cultures and a negative history of UTIs

D. Granulomatous Prostatitis

1. Mycobacterial:
   a. May occur in patients with **systemic TB** (3%-12%), but now is more commonly seen with **BCG treatment** for TCC
   b. Most cases of tuberculous prostatitis arise from **hematogenous spread**
   c. Histologically, the features of BCG prostatitis are indistinguishable from those of tuberculous prostatitis:
      - **Small noncaseating granulomas** that are **well-demarcated** from the surrounding stroma
      - Some larger granulomas **may show central caseation** (consists of grummous fine granular debris, as opposed to coagulative necrosis which is amorphous fibrinoid material with ghost-like outlines of vessels, cells, etc.)
   d. Treatment: BCG granulomas resolve on their own; TB needs treatment
2. Malakoplakia:
   a. As in malakoplakia of the bladder, this reflects an inability to digest bacteria following phagocytosis
   b. Symptoms include urinary retention, urgency, frequency, etc.
   c. Clinically can mimic cancer because causes an indurated prostate on exam and may appear as a hypoechoic lesion on transrectal ultrasound
   d. Histologically: **von Hansemann histiocytes + Michaelis-Gutmann bodies** (see bladder section for more details)

3. Nonspecific granulomatous prostatitis:
   a. Most commonly diagnosed granulomatous prostatitis
   b. Etiology is thought to be due to **inflammatory reaction** to bacterial toxins, cell debris, and secretions spilling into the stroma **from blocked ducts**
   c. Major significance is that it **can mimic carcinoma** on rectal exam, ultrasound, and give an elevated PSA
   d. Histologically, the **granulomas are less well-formed**, and are associated with **dense stromal inflammatory infiltrate** with scattered giant cells
   e. Have **more mixed inflammatory infiltrate** than is seen in infectious granulomatous prostatitis (plasma cells, neutrophils, lymphocytes)
   f. **Associated with ruptured acini** (as opposed to infectious, which will have intact acini)
   g. Treatment: warm sitz baths, fluids,and antibiotics if a UTI is documented
4. Postsurgical granulomas:
   a. Appears to be a **reaction to cauterized tissue**
   b. Can occur anywhere from 9 days to 52 months post-TURP
   c. Histologically have the same appearance as post-surgical granulomas elsewhere:
      - **serpiginous border** (geographic pattern)
      - **central fibrinoid necrosis**
      - surrounded by palisaded histiocytes
   d. Treatment: None

5. Basal Cell Hyperplasia

A. May occur in association with BPH or atrophy

B. Histologically, the glands are small and angular, and appear blue at low power due to the multilayering of basal cells that have scant cytoplasm

C. Hyperplasia ranges from a few layers to solid nests; may occasionally show cribriform architecture

D. Typically have bland cytologic features (no nucleoli, etc.)

E. Can do keratin immunostains to confirm cell type.

6. Clear Cell Cribriform Hyperplasia

A. Recently described benign lesion that may be confused with PIN or adenocarcinoma

B. Composed of numerous cribriform glands separated from one another by a modest amount of stroma in a pattern of nodular hyperplasia

C. The epithelial cells have distinctive clear cytoplasm and small bland nuclei with inconspicuous or small nucleoli

D. Often surrounded by a striking basal cell layer

E. Cribriform "bridges" are delicate and demonstrate "streaming" of the nuclei, rather than rigid perpendicular alignment

7. Atrophy

A. Can give rise to firm gland with hypoechoic lesions on transrectal ultrasound

B. Histologically characterized by **well-formed glands** with very **basophilic appearance** due to scanty cytoplasm rather than nuclear enlargement (as is seen in PIN)—[in contrast, adenocarcinomas have abundant cytoplasm]

C. Glands are often **angulated** and surround a central dilated duct (adenocarcinoma has small round glands that do not maintain lobular architecture)

8. Squamous Metaplasia

A. Common adjacent to infarcts or following antiandrogen therapy and in neonates (response to maternal hormones)

B. In general, the cells lack reactivity to prostatic markers (PSA, PAP)

12. Prostate II: Tumors of the Prostate

1. Polyps of the Prostatic Urethra

A. Clinical presentation: hematuria

B. Several types have been described, including:
  1. **Prostatic type**
    a. Gross: small (1 cm)
    b. Micro:
      - delicate papillae/glands with pale epithelium identical to normal prostate
      - PSA and PAP positive
    c. Behavior: benign; almost never recur
  2. **Adenomatoid type** (a.k.a., nephrogenic adenoma)
      - benign, but recurrence is common
  3. **Adenomatous type** (villous adenoma)
    a. may be forerunner to endometrioid carcinoma of prostatic urethra
    b. Micro:
      - resembles hyperplastic endometrium with bright eosinophilic cytoplasm and crowded blue nuclei.
      - PSA and PAP positive

2. Prostatic Intraepithelial Neoplasia (PIN)

A. Generally accepted as the probable precursor lesion for many cases of prostatic carcinoma

B. Divided into **low grade** (mild dysplasia/grade 1) and **high grade** (moderate dysplasia/grade 2 and severe dysplasia/grade 3)

C. High-grade PIN is a marker for cancer

D. Micro
  1. On low power, glands appear large but very **basophilic** (blue), due to larger nuclei, higher N:C ration, nuclear crowding and pseudostratification
  2. Gland architecture remains **complex**—as in BPH
  3. Basal cells are present, if only focally
  4. **Nucleoli** are prominent in high-grade PIN

E. Low-grade PIN is not diagnosed

3. Prostatatic Adenocarcinoma

A. Clinical
  1. Most common cancer in adult men; **second leading cause of cancer-related death** in males
  2. Microscopic foci of cancer may begin in the 30s; present in 70% of men by age 70
  3. Metastases most commonly occur to **bone** (osteoblastic), **lung**, and **pelvic (obturator) lymph nodes**

B. Gross Features
  1. **80%** occur in the **peripheral zone**; 10%-20% occur in the transition zone
  2. Often difficult to detect grossly: said to have yellow color, but more often appear gray-white

C. Microscopic Features
  1. Main criteria include
    a. **Small uniform glands**
    b. **Single layer** of epithelium (no basal cell layer)
    c. **No lobular organization** to the glands
    d. Prominent **nucleoli**
  2. Helpful clues are the presence of sharp **crystalloids** and/or **blue mucin** in the gland lumina
  3. Neoplastic glands like to track along the nerves
  4. The **Gleason system** classifies prostate cancer into 5 grades based upon low-power **architectural** features. Because studies demonstrated that prostate cancer behaves more like an **average** of its most common architectural grades, the two predominant grades are given and then added to give a Gleason's score:

Primary (most prevalent) grade +
Secondary (2nd most prevalent) grade =
Gleason score

Figure 1

Gleason grading system for prostatic adenocarcinoma

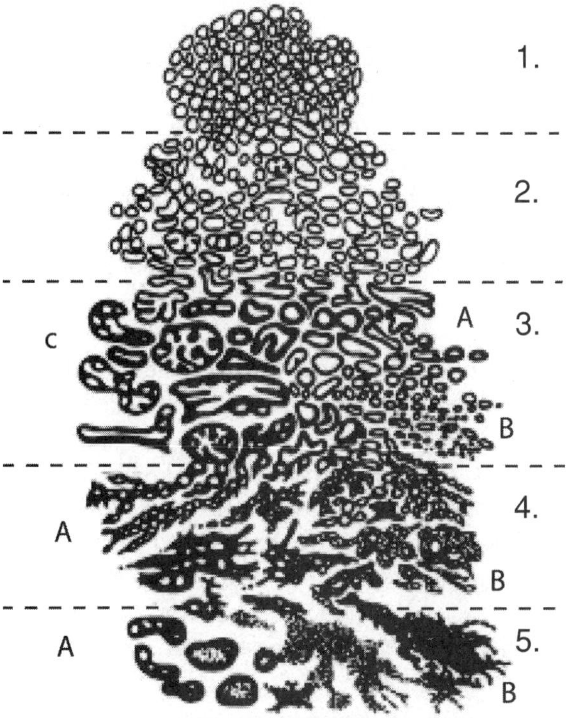

D. The Gleason Grading System (Figure 1)

1. Grade 1:
   - **circumscribed nodules** of **uniform, single, separate**, closely-packed glands
   - usually have benign nuclei; may occasionally have nucleoli (remember: Gleason's grades are based on architectural—not cytologic—features)
   - glands tend to be larger than those seen in the higher-grade
   - cells usually have abundant eosinophilic cytoplasm
   - virtually never seen on needle biopsy
   - usually found in the transition zone
2. Grade 2:
   - again, a **nodular pattern** of tumor; however, the edge of the tumor nodule may show **minimal extension of glands into the surrounding non-neoplastic prostate**
   - glands are more loosely arranged and not quite as uniform as in grade 1
   - as in grade 1, the glands are still larger than grade 3 and up
   - cells have abundant eosinophilic cytoplasm
   - rarely seen in needle biopsy because the lower grade adenocarcinomas (Gleason's scores 2-4) are generally located in the transition zone.
3. Grade 3:
   - tumor **infiltrates** in and among the non-neoplastic prostate.
   - glands have marked variation in size and shape
   - glands tend to be smaller than in grade 1 or 2.
   - in contrast to pattern 4, the glands in Gleason pattern 3 are **discrete units**. (If one can mentally draw a circle around well-formed individual glands, then it is a Gleason pattern 3.)
   - smoothly circumscribed nodules of tumor with cribriform architecture are also considered grade 3. (Do not confuse with clear cell cribriform hyperplasia.)
4. Grade 4:
   - The main distinction between grade 3 and grade 4 is **fusion of the glands**: the glands are no longer single and separate as seen in patterns 1-3; they are fused and ill-defined, even at low power.
   - **lumina are lost** (ie, glands are being poorly formed)
   - **raggedly infiltrating borders** of glands form chains or masses.
   - the **hypernephroid variant** is automatically grade 4 (characterized by clear cells with dot-like nuclei)
   - the **mucinous variant** is automatically classified as grade 4 (cells floating in a sea of mucin)
5. Grade 5:
   - **no gland formation** is evident
   - tumor infiltrates as **solid mass or single cells**
   - the **signet ring cell type** and **comedocarcinoma pattern** (cribriform pattern with central necrosis) are both automatically classified as grade 5.

E. Other Variations on the Adenocarcinoma Theme

1. Sarcomatoid carcinoma/carcinosarcoma
   a. Adenoca; having a **malignant spindle-cell component**

b. Usually seen **post-radiation** therapy (50% of cases)

c. **Highly aggressive** tumors

2. "Endometrioid" adenoca. of the prostatic urethra

a. Typically an **exophytic papillary mass** in the vicinity of the prostatic utricle

b. PSA and PAP positive

c. Microscopically demonstrates a **papillary or cribriform arrangement** of complex glands with tall columnar tumor cells

d. **Usually Gleason grade 3 or 4**, but may be considered a grade 5 if comedonecrosis is present

3. Mucinous variant:

a. **Tumor cells floating in a sea of mucin**

b. Extracellular **mucin** must comprise **at least 25% of the tumor**

c. **Gleason grade 4**

4. Signet ring cell variant:

a. Tumor cells contain **intracytoplasmic** mucin droplets that compress the nucleus against the cell membrane

b. **At least 25%** of the tumor must be composed of cells having this morphology

c. **Gleason grade 5**

5. Small cell variant:

a. Tumor composed of **sheets of cells** with **small nuclei** containing **finely-stippled chromatin**

b. **Nucleoli are inconspicuous** and **cytoplasm is scant**

c. Nuclear molding is often identified

d. **PSA and PAP stains are negative**

e. **Highly aggressive** lesions often present with metastatic disease to solid organs

f. Serum PSA may only be slightly elevated

g. 50% are associated with typical adenocarcinomatous component

h. **Gleason grade 5**

4. Transitional Cell Carcinoma of the Prostate

A. Primary TCC of the prostate is very rare: arises in the prostatic ducts

B. Secondary TCC is fairly common, representing spread from a bladder primary

1. May be due to direct spread along urothelium or invasion from outside in.
2. Micro: looks like TCIS extending along ducts into acini
3. Invasion of prostatic stroma is a poor prognostic indicator

C. Differential diagnosis: prostatic adenocarcinoma

1. TCC usually does not form glands (adeno. grades 1-4 do form glands)
2. TCC is PSA negative (adeno. is PSA positive)
3. TCC has "uglier" nuclei with angulations, etc. (adeno. nuclei tend to be round with or without round nucleoli)

5. Squamous Cell Carcinoma of the Prostate

A. Very rare in North America

B. Seen in association with schistosomiasis

C. Squamous metaplasia may occur in adenocarcinomas treated with radiation or hormones (particularly estrogens)

6. Treatment Effects

A. Hormone Therapy

1. Changes in the normal prostate include

a. **Atrophy** with a decrease in number and size of glands

b. **Basal cell hyperplasia**

c. **Transitional cell metaplasia**

d. **Lymphocytic infiltrate**

2. Changes in tumor cells include:
   a. **Small hyperchromatic nuclei**
   b. **Inconspicuous nucleoli**
   c. **Abundant clear cytoplasm**
   d. Occasionally only single cells will remain that look like histiocytes
3. Bizarre stromal cells may be present

B. Radiation Therapy

1. Changes in the normal prostate include
   a. Marked **atrophy** of normal glands
   b. **Nuclei** may become **enlarged and pleomorphic**
2. Changes in tumor cells are variable, but **Gleason score often increases** after treatment (although **prognosis does not change**)

13. Testis I: Non-neoplastic Disorders

I. Cryptorchidism

A. True Cryptorchidism

1. Causes include:
   a. Anatomical anomalies of the gubernaculum,
   b. Hormonal dysfunction (hypogonadotropic hypogonadism)
   c. Mechanical impairment (short spermatic cord, underdeveloped vaginal process)
   d. Dysgenesis (primary testicular anomaly)
   e. Heredity
2. Decreased spermatogenesis in cryptorchid testes may be multifactorial:
   a. Transient hypogonadotropic hypogonadism
   b. Primary testicular anomaly
   c. Injury caused by increased temperature
3. **Histology**:
   a. Atrophic and sclerotic seminiferous tubules with thickened basement membranes
   b. Tubules with Sertoli cells and spermatogonia only
   c. Mixed tubular atrophy with relative Leydig cell hyperplasia
   d. Hypoplastic rete testis

B. Congenital Anomalies Associated With Cryptorchidism

1. Cryptorchidism may be associated with Klinefelter's, Noonan's, Kallmann's, Prader-Willi, and prune belly syndromes
2. Undescended testes may also be seen in trisomies 13, 18, 21, and the Aarskog-Scott and Rubinstein-Taybi syndromes
3. Most cryptorchid patients have persistent processus vaginalis and inguinal hernia
4. Other urologic anomalies (10.5% of patients) include:
   a. Hypospadias
   b. Complete duplication of urinary tract
   c. Kidney malrotation
   d. Nonobstructive ureteral dilatation
   e. Posterior urethral valves
   f. Sperm excretory duct anomalies, including:
      - Ductal fusion anomalies (25%)—fusion of epididymis to testis or vas deferens, usually with intraabdominal or high scrotal cryptorchidism

- Ductal suspension anomalies (59%)—caput epididymis attached to testis while corpus and cauda are separated by mesentery
- Anomalies associated with absent or vanishing testes (16%)

C. Complications of Cryptorchidism

1. Testicular cancer:
   a. Risk of testicular cancer is 5%-10% higher in cryptorchid than in noncryptorchid patients
   b. 10% of patients with testicular cancer have cryptorchid testes
   c. Most frequent tumor in cryptorchid testis is seminoma
2. Infertility: more commonly seen in bilateral cryptorchidism, although orchiopexy performed <4 years of age seems to preserve fertility

2. Infertility

A. Basic Definitions

1. Spermatogenic arrest: rare because germ cell maturation usually does not arrest at the level of a defined germ cell type (therefore, "irregular hypospermatogenesis" is more often appropriate in cases where the germ cell arrest occurs at varying degrees of maturation)
2. Spermatocytic arrest (meiotic arrest): incidence varies from 12%-30%
3. "Disorganization of the seminiferous epithelium": a relatively worthless diagnosis that has not been supported by any light microscopic or ultrastructural evaluation. Just what is disorganized epithelium?
4. Tubular blockage: when at least 50% of the tubules lack central lumens; found in 28% of infertile men, so may represent a real lesion (likely some variant of germ-cell sloughing)

B. Common Lesions Seen on Testicular Biopsies

1. Sertoli cell-only syndrome:
   a. Seminiferous epithelium consists only of Sertoli cells and rare spermatogonia
   b. Adult Sertoli cells have characteristically pale, triangular nuclei with irregular indented outlines
   c. Clinical: normal external genitalia, well-developed secondary male characteristics, azoospermia, elevated FSH, normal or elevated LH, and normal or slightly low testosterone
   d. Histology: characteristic **"windswept"** appearance to the seminiferous tubules
2. Tubular hyalinization:
   a. Nonspecific catch-all category in which azoospermic patients demonstrate diffuse hyalinization of seminiferous tubules
   b. Because hyalinization is the end-stage of atrophy, the causes of tubular hyalinization are numerous, and include: dysgenesis, hormonal deficit, ischemia, obstruction, inflammation, physical or chemical agents, and autoimmunity
3. Diffuse lesions in spermatogenesis:
   a. **Lesions in the basal compartment of the seminiferous tubules** include all infertile testes with normal numbers of spermatogonia per tubular profile, but decreased numbers of other types of germ cells (a.k.a., "immature germ cell sloughing"). Diagnosis is based on finding >4% of ejaculated cells are spermatogonia
   b. **Lesions in the adluminal compartment of the seminiferous tubules** are classified according to the most abundant type of sloughed germ cell: young spermatids, later primary spermatocytes, and early primary spermatocytes
      Etiology of adluminal defects is most likely obstruction:
      - Rete testis obstruction—usually due to varicocele
      - Seminiferous tubule obstruction—usually dysgenetic or post-orchitic
   c. **Lesions in the basal and adluminal compartments of the seminiferous tubules** are the most frequent findings on testicular biopsy and can be classified into two major groups:
      - Hypospermatogenesis: defined as reduced numbers of both spermatogonia and primary spermatocytes with **primary spermatocytes outnumbering spermatogonia**

i. may be **pure** (proportionate decrease in all types of germ cells) or be **associated with primary spermatocyte sloughing**

ii. Etiology: hormonal dysfunction, congenital germ cell deficiency, Sertoli cell dysfunction, Leydig cell dysfunction, androgen insensitivity, exposure to chemical or physical agents, and vascular malfunction

iii. Usually patients have deficits in FSH, LH, or hyperprolactinemia, or adrenal/thyroid dysfunction

- Spermatogonia maturation arrest: defined as fewer than 17 spermatogonia per tubular profile, with fewer primary spermatocytes than spermatogonia

  i. spermatids are absent

  ii. most frequent causes include: **cryptorchidism, alcoholism** or exposure to other toxic substances, chemotherapy, and hypogonadotropic hypogonadism

C. Infertility Associated With Chromosomal Anomalies

1. Klinefelter's syndrome:

   a. Abnormal number of X chromosomes with primary gonadal insufficiency

   b. Frequency: 1/1000 – 1/4000 surviving newborns; **1/100 patients in mental institutions**, and 3.4/100 infertile men

   c. Karyotype: **47XXY** (80%); remaining 20% have chromosomal mosaicism with at least two X chromosomes

   d. Most common clinical findings are:
      - **Eunuchoid phenotype with increased stature** (disproportionate lengthening of the lower extremities)
      - **Incomplete virilization**
      - **Gynecomastia**, often bilateral
      - **Mental retardation**

   e. External genitalia are normally developed with small to normal testes

   f. Histology: classically **see small hyalinized seminiferous tubules with pseudoadenomatous clusters of Leydig cells** (the Leydig cells only appear to be increased due to the decreased testicular volume)

   g. Increased incidence of **extragonadal germ cell tumors**, while testicular germ cell tumors are rare
      - Most occur in the mediastinum (70%) followed by the pineal gland, CNS, and retroperitoneum
      - Most frequent types: teratoma and choriocarcinoma; embryonal and seminomas are rare

   h. Often associated with panhypopituitarism or incomplete hypopituitarism

2. 46 XX males:

   a. **Clinical features similar to Klinefelter's** (small testes, azoospermia, normal or small penis, gynecomastia, and minimal secondary sex characteristics) but **stature is normal and intelligence is normal**

   b. Incidence: 1/9000 live births

   c. These patients have **hypergonadotropic hypogonadism** with elevated levels of FSH and LH, and normal or low testosterone

   d. Biopsy reveals decreased numbers of germ cells with or without Sertoli cell-only pattern. Leydig cells are not quite as "hyperplastic" as in Klinefelter's

   e. Etiology is controversial… and I'll leave it at that

3. 47 XYY syndrome:

   a. Patients tend to be tall and may display psychopathic personalities

   b. Incidence: 1.5/1000 live births; 3/100 men in mental institutions and prisons

   c. Normal external genitalia and secondary sex characteristics, but decreased fertility

   d. Biopsy reveals **mixed tubular atrophy** (Sertoli cell-only tubules admixed with hypospermatogenic tubules)

   e. Serum testosterone levels are normal, as are LH levels

5. Down's syndrome (trisomy 21)

   a. Patients usually have cryptorchidism, small testes, and hypoplasia of the penis and scrotum

   b. Adults have azoospermia or oligospermia secondary to a primary testicular deficiency

   c. FSH and LH levels are elevated while testosterone is normal or low

6. Prader-Willi syndrome (chromosome 15p11-12):

   a. Characterized by hypogonadism, obesity, muscular hypotonia, mental and physical retardation, and acromicria

b. Incidence: 1/25,000 live births (60% more common in males)
c. FSH, LH, testosterone, and estradiol levels are low
d. Penis and testes are hypoplastic and most patients have cryptorchidism
e. Biopsy of adults with this syndrome demonstrates infantile morphology

D. **Infertility Resulting From Physical and Chemical Agents**
1. Occupational exposure: carbon disulfide (production of rayon); dibromochloropropane (soil fumigant); lead (inorganic); oral contraceptive manufacture; radiation; heat, etc.
2. Cancer therapy: radiotherapy (especially prepubertal), chemotherapy (cyclophosphamide, procarbazine), surgery

3. Inflammation and Infection

A. **Orchitis**
1. Viral—usually due to **mumps virus** and **Coxsackie B virus**. Mumps orchidoepididymitis:
   a. Complicates 14%-35% of adult mumps cases, and is bilateral in 20%-25%
   b. Epididymal involvement alone is rare
   c. Clinical symptoms appear 4-6 days after parotiditis symptoms, but may also occur without parotid involvement
   d. Histology: multifocal acute inflammation of interstitium and seminiferous tubules
   e. With time, testes shrink, and bilateral involvement usually results in infertility
   f. Incidence is low in childhood
2. Bacterial—usually associated with ***E coli*** epididymitis
   a. Histology: **tubules covered up with intense acute inflammation** with or without **abscess formation** (usually seen with *E coli*, strep, staph, Pneumococci, *Salmonella enteritidis*, and *Actinomyces israelii*)
   b. Complications: testicular infarct, scrotal pyocele and chronic draining scrotal sinus
3. Granulomatous—
   a. **Tuberculosis**:
   - The incidence of tuberculous orchoepididymitis has recently increased with the advent of AIDS
   - Usually associated with involvement of the GU tract elsewhere, especially prostate involvement (which, in turn, is usually secondary to renal tuberculosis)
   - In children, involvement of the testis usually represents hematogenous spread from pulmonary infection
   - Tuberculous orchoepididymitis occurs predominantly in adults (72% are > 35 years, 18% are > 65 years of age)
   - Symptoms: scrotal pain and testicular enlargement; fever and constitutional symptoms may be infrequent or absent altogether
   - Histology: caseating and noncaseating granulomas with acid-fast bacilli

   b. **Syphilis**
   - Syphilitic orchitis may be congenital or acquired
   - In congenital, both testes are enlarged at birth (secondary syphilis); in adults, acquired syphilitic orchitis represents tertiary stage of disease.
   - Early in disease, painless testicular enlargement occurs
   - Histology: early lesions consist of predominantly plasmacytic inflammation beginning in the mediastinum testis and testicular septa, and later extending into the seminiferous tubules
     i. tubules slough their epithelium and become sclerotic
     ii. vessels demonstrate endarteritis obliterans
     iii. small gummas may be present
   - Gummatous orchitis is characterized by the presence of one or multiple well-delineated gray-yellow necrotic lesions that histologically show ghosts of seminiferous tubules with inflammatory infiltrate of lymphocytes, plasma cells, and a few giant cells
   - Special stains (Warthin-Starry) may demonstrate spirochetes

   c. **Sarcoidosis**
   - Preferentially affects young black adults
   - GU involvement is unusual but typically asymptomatic
   - Testicular sarcoidosis is usually unilateral and nodular

- Histology: noncaseating granulomas—but diagnosis of exclusion so must do bug stains
- Important differential diagnosis is seminoma, which may show an intense sarcoid-like reaction; also: spermatocytic granulomas may look like sarcoid

B. Malakoplakia

1. Testicular involvement occurs in 12% of cases of malakoplakia of the GU tract
2. Grossly: testis enlarged with yellow-brown parenchyma, often with abscesses
3. Histology: as always, look for von Hansemann histiocytes and Michaelis-Gutmann bodies

4. Testicular Infarcts

A. Torsion of the spermatic cord is the most frequent cause of testicular infarct

B. Trauma and lesions of the spermatic cord may also result in infarction

C. Clinical symptoms mimic testicular tumor

D. Histology: "ghost-like" appearance of parenchyma—outlines of tubules and supporting structures, but has a generalized "washed-out" or diffusely eosinophilic appearance (coagulative necrosis)

14. Testis II: Germ Cell Tumors

1. General

A. 95% of testicular tumors are of germ cell derivation, and usually occur in young men

B. Rarely, supporting and interstitial cells can give rise to sex-cord stromal tumors and hamartomatous lesions

C. Staging of germ cell tumors remains controversial, but is roughly divided into:

1. Early localized stage (confined to testis)
2. Early dissemination (retroperitoneal lymph nodes metastases)
3. Advanced dissemination (supradiaphragmatic metastases)

D. Patterns of Metastases

1. Testicular neoplasms generally metastasize to the retroperitoneal lymph nodes first
2. Tumors may metastasize via lymphatics (seminomas), hematogenously (choriocarcinoma), or both (embryonal).

E. Epidemiology

1. Occur almost exclusively in young men (peak age = 30 yrs), with the one exception being spermatocytic seminoma
2. Incidence is highest among Caucasian males; higher frequency in upper socioeconomic class.
3. Risk factors:
   a. **Cryptorchidism** (3.5-5X increased risk)
      - if unilateral, the contralateral testis is also at increased risk but not to as great a degree as the actual cryptorchid testis
      - 2%-8% of patients with cryptorchid testes intratubular germ cell neoplasia of the "unclassified type" (IGCNU), and at least 50% of those men go on to develop germ cell tumors within 5 years

   b. **Prior testicular germ cell tumor** (5-10x increased risk)
      - 2%-5% of patients with one germ cell tumor will develop a tumor in the contralateral testis (especially if the second testis has biopsy-proven IGCNU)
      - 50% develops within 3-5 years of the first tumor, but delays of over 10 years have been reported

- The second tumor may have the same or different histology from the first tumor
- Chemotherapy given for the first tumor decreases the risk of tumor development in the second testis

c. **Family history (first degree relative)** (5.5X increased risk)
- these patients also have a greater incidence of bilateral tumors (8%-14% frequency vs. 2%-5% frequency in patients without a family history of germ cell tumors)

d. Gonadal dysgenesis with a Y chromosome (50X increased risk)
- Especially 46XY gonadal dysgenesis (Swyer's syndrome), mixed gonadal dysgenesis, and dysgenetic male pseudohermaphroditism
- 25%-30% of these patients develop gonadoblastoma
- gonadectomy is recommended in any patient with these syndromes since invasive tumors can develop in childhood

e. **Androgen insensitivity syndrome** (15x increased risk)
- 5%-10% of patients with androgen insensitivity also develop germ cell tumors so prophylactic gonadectomy should be performed by puberty (22% risk of germ cell tumor in patients >30 yrs)

4. Alcohol and tobacco use, prior vasectomy, and radiation do NOT increase the risk of germ cell tumors

2. Intratubular Germ Cell Neoplasia

A. All forms of testicular germ cell tumor—except for spermatocytic seminoma—arise from a common precursor known as "intratubular germ cell neoplasia of the unclassified type" (IGCNU) [conceptual equivalent of carcinoma in situ]

B. Begins as a basilar proliferation of seminoma-like cells with clear cytoplasm and enlarged hyperchromatic nuclei containing one or two prominent nucleoli

C. By all forms of examination—light microscopic, ultrastructural, cytogenetic, etc.—the cells of IGCNU are identical to seminoma cells which suggests that IGCNU and seminoma are the precursor lesions to the other forms of germ cell tumors. However, cells of IGCNU can also differentiate along other pathways to produce embryonal, chorio, or yolk sac tumors, either when they are still intratubular (in situ) or at the time of invasion

D. Gross: testis may be unremarkable or may be atrophic and fibrotic

E. Micro: proliferation of malignant germ cells, which may be undifferentiated or may resemble specific neoplastic types (embryonal, etc.)
1. neoplastic cells usually appear at the basilar aspect of the tubules
2. clear cytoplasm, large cells, prominent nucleoli, and hyperchromatic nuclei
3. Often spread to rete testis in a "pagetoid" fashion, intermixing with and usually "lifting up" non-neoplastic epithelium
4. when the cells fill and distend the tubules, the term intratubular seminoma is used rather than "IGCNU"
5. The cells are PLAP (placental alkaline phosphatase) positive

F. Prognosis: 50% proceed to invasive germ cell tumors within 5 years

3. Classic Seminoma

A. Most common form of pure testicular germ cell tumor, accounting for approximately 50% of germ cell tumors

B. Clinical Features
1. Average age is 40 years (10 years later than other germ cell neoplasms)
2. Present with painless testicular mass
3. Gynecomastia may occur as a result of elevated HCG (usually seen in tumors with syncytiotrophoblast cells)
4. 30% have metastases at the time of diagnosis

C. Laboratory Values

1. AFP normal
2. HCG elevated in 10%-20% of stage I patients, and in >25% of patients with disseminated disease
3. Levels of HCG > 40 IU/L are poor prognostic indicator

D. Pathologic Findings

1. Gross: tan or cream-colored, multinodular tumor with bulging cut surface
2. Micro:
   a. Cells are large with **clear or lightly eosinophilic cytoplasm** and **well-defined cytoplasmic membranes**; vesicular nuclei generally contain one or two prominent **nucleoli**
   b. Sheetlike growth pattern interrupted with **branching fibrous septa containing inflammatory (lymphocytic) infiltrate**
   c. Mitoses may be numerous → used to be interpreted as "anaplastic" feature if there were >3/hpf, but now that term is no longer used (no prognostic difference)
   d. Septa may render a nesting or "cord-like" appearance to the tumor at low power
   e. Syncytiotrophoblasts (large, multinucleated cells) may be scattered through some tumors, and usually correlate with elevated HCG levels
   d. With time, many seminomas develop foci of scarring or may become edematous with the formation of microcysts
   e. Often proliferates within the tubules, so can see associated "intratubular seminoma" in adjacent testicular parenchyma
   f. Intratubular spread into the rete testis occurs in pagetoid fashion
3. Special studies:
   a. Cells are PAS positive (glycogen in the cytoplasm) and PLAP positive
   b. Epithelial membrane antigen (EMA) is negative
   c. AFP negative

E. Treatment and Prognosis

1. Early seminoma (stage I or II): orchiectomy and radiation to para-aortic and paracaval nodes; cure rate >95% for stage I
2. Most patients with nonbulky retroperitoneal disease are also cured (87%)
3. Chemotherapy is recommended for patients with "bulky" retroperitoneal disease (defined as mets >5-10 cm in diameter) → cure rate is still high in this group (80%)
4. Prominent lymphocytic reaction in the tumor is good prognostic feature

4. Spermatocytic Seminoma

A. Clinical Features

1. Represents 1%-2% of testicular germ cell tumors
2. Occurs only in the testis, usually on the right side
3. Not associated with cryptorchidism
4. Average age is 52-58 years (vs. 40 yrs for classic seminoma)
5. Whites >> African-Americans and Asians
6. All serum markers (AFP, HCG, LD) are negative

B. Pathologic Features

1. Multinodular fleshy white tumor with mucoid and cystic areas, +/- hemorrhage
2. Paratesticular extension may uncommonly occur
3. Histologically: cord-like or nested growth pattern with edematous cystic areas
4. A lymphocytic infiltrate is usually not seen
5. Three major cell types:
   a. **Small, lymphocyte-like cell** (6-8 micrometers)
      - smudged, degenerated appearance with minimal cytoplasm
   b. **Intermediate-size cell** (15-20 micrometers)
      - round nucleus with granular or filamentous (spireme) chromatin and scant cytoplasm
   c. **Giant cells** (50-100 micrometers)
      - may be multinucleated or uninucleate, and often have spireme chromatin as well

C. Special Studies

1. PAS negative because the cells lack glycogen in their cytoplasm
2. AFP/PLAP/etc. are usually negative

D. Treatment and Prognosis

1. Only one credible case of a metastasizing spermatocytic seminoma (other cases are most likely misdiagnosed testicular lymphomas)
2. Orchiectomy alone is generally curable
3. Adjuvant therapy is not warranted, and may even be harmful.

E. Differential Diagnosis: classic seminoma

5. Embryonal Carcinoma

A. Usually identified as a component of mixed germ cell tumors (87%) rather than in pure form

B. Clinical Features

1. Average age: 30 years; extremely rare in childhood
2. Mets are clinically evident in 40% of patients at the time of diagnosis, and an additional 20%-30% of patients will have evidence of metastatic disease at staging

C. Laboratory Values: AFP usually not elevated in pure embryonal carcinoma, but may be elevated if there is an element yolk sac tumor; HCG may be elevated in 60% of cases (again, correlates with the presence of syncytiotrophoblasts in the tumor); LDH and PLAP can also be elevated

D. Pathologic Features

1. Poorly circumscribed gray-white tumor with hemorrhage and necrosis
2. Three major histologic patterns:
   a. **solid**—diffuse sheet-like growth
   b. **tubular/glandular**—forms well-defined glands with cleft-like or round lumina
   c. **papillary**—may or may not have fibrovascular cores
3. Prominent areas of coagulative necrosis
4. In situ component usually looks like comedocarcinoma, with central necrosis of the tumor cells within the tubules; the necrotic areas can be calcified → "hematoxylin-staining bodies"
5. Cells have abundant eosinophilic cytoplasm and pleomorphic nuclei with prominent nucleoli
6. Cell borders are ill-defined (as opposed to seminoma) and the nuclei often look like they are abutting each other or "piling up"
7. A minor amount of undifferentiated stroma is considered reasonable; too much stroma, however, and you have to think about a mixed germ cell tumor with embryonal and teratomatous component
8. Some tumors may have small foci of yolk sac tumor, but the neoplastic cell in embryonal carcinoma can actually differentiate into yolk sac —which explains why pure embryonal carcinomas are so unusual

E. Special Studies

1. AFP positivity generally indicates a yolk-sac component—only a small percentage of pure embryonal carcinomas will be positive for AFP
2. PLAP positivity occurs in 86%-97% of tumors, but is patchy and weaker than that seen in seminomas
3. Strong cytokeratin staining
4. EMA is negative

F. Differential Diagnosis: yolk sac tumor; choriocarcinoma; seminoma; lymphoma

G. Treatment and Prognosis

1. Stage I disease: 40% relapse, but most can be salvaged with chemotherapy
   a. Treatment: orchiectomy +/- lymph node dissection vs. careful surveillance
   b. Survival of 97%
2. Stage II disease with nonbulky retroperitoneal involvement
   a. Treatment: orchiectomy and lymph node dissection +/- adjuvant therapy
   b. >95% survival
3. Stage II disease with bulky disease or more advanced stage
   a. Treatment: as above, only with chemotherapy added
   b. Survival is 70%-80%
4. Prognostic factors in patients with nonseminomatous germ cell tumors: tumor stage, extent of tumor marker elevation, age of patient (older is worse), the presence of choriocarcinoma, and the proliferative index by flow cytometry

6. Yolk Sac Tumor

A. Clinical Features

1. Most common tumor in prepubertal children (average age = 18 months)
2. Postpubertal tumors occur at average age of 25-30 years
3. Childhood yolk sac tumors are not associated with cryptorchidism
4. Present with painless testicular mass
5. Evidence of metastases is very rare at diagnosis

B. Laboratory Values: significantly elevated AFP (hundreds to thousands of ng/ml) as opposed to minor elevations that may be seen in embryonal or teratoma

C. Pathologic Features

1. Children: solid gray-white tumor nodules with myxoid or gelatinous cut surface
2. Adults: heterogeneous appearance with hemorrhage and necrosis, b/c usually part of a mixed germ cell tumor (MGCT)
3. Eleven patterns have been described but the most common are:
   a. Microcystic (honeycomb, reticular, vacuolated)—most common—intracellular vacuoles create attenuated lengths of cytoplasm that imparts a "spiderweb"-like appearance; often seen in conjunction with the myxomatous and solid patterns
   b. Endodermal sinus (perivascular): consists of a central vessel rimmed by fibrous tissue which is, in turn, surrounded by malignant epithelium (**Schiller-Duval bodies** or **glomeruloid bodies**)
   c. Myxomatous—stellate or spindle cells dispersed in a myxomatous stroma that stains very palely with H&E; often seen in conjunction with microcystic pattern
   d. Solid: may resemble seminoma because the cells have pale cytoplasm and well-defined borders; however, yolk sac won't have the fibrovascular stroma with the lymphoid infiltrates
      - other solid patterns may resemble blastema (small round blue cells in solid sheets), but these areas generally are admixed with more typical areas of yolk sac tumor
4. A general feature of yolk sac tumor is the deposition of extracellular basement membrane (92% of cases), which consist of eosinophilic bands of matrix deposited between the neoplastic cells
5. Another helpful (but not diagnostic) feature is the presence of hyaline globules that are PAS positive, and may occasionally be AFP positive

D. Special Studies

1. Majority are positive for AFP with a patchy staining pattern
2. Cytokeratin is positive in virtually all cases
3. 40%-80% may be positive for PLAP
4. Most are negative for EMA

E. Differential Diagnosis

1. Solid pattern must be distinguished from seminoma
2. Distinction from embryonal may be of lesser significance, since embryonal often transforms into yolk sac

F. Treatment and Prognosis:

1. Adults: treated like embryonal (see previous section for guidelines)
2. Children: 80% are stage I, and are treated by orchiectomy with close surveillance (no retroperitoneal lymph node dissection); 5-year survival = 91%
3. Presence of metastatic yolk sac tumor bodes poorly for prognosis, as the metastatic lesions are typically resistant to chemotherapy

7. Teratoma

A. Clinical Features

1. Children:
   a. **Second most common form of testicular germ cell tumor in children** (yolk sac is the most common), accounting for 14%-18% of cases
   b. Mean age = **20 months**; >4 yrs is unusual
   c. Associated with a variety of congenital anomalies:
      - hemihypertrophy
      - spina bifida
      - retrocaval ureter
      - hernia

2. Adults: usually occurs as component of a MGCT and are present in more than half of all MGCT and over 25% of all nonseminomatous germ cell tumors
3. Metastatic potential increases with adult population even when the histology is of a pure mature teratoma (probably because the tumor developed along the IGCNU → seminoma → teratoma → mature teratoma pathway)

B. Pathologic Features

1. Mature teratoma often contains multiple cysts, generally under 1 cm in diameter
2. Gray white cartilaginous areas may also be present
3. Fleshy or hemorrhagic regions generally correlate with immature foci or may be nonteratomatous components
4. Histologically, teratomas consist of a variety of somatic-type tissues, most commonly including cartilage, smooth and skeletal muscle, neuroglia, enteric type glands, squamous or respiratory epithelium, and urothelial islands—all of which are considered "mature" elements, even in the presence of atypia
5. Immature elements:
   a. **Neuroepithelium**—small hyperchromatic cells arranged in tubules or rosettes
   b. **Blastema**—nodular collections of oval cells with scant cytoplasm and hyperchromatic nuclei with or without tubules (so may kind of resemble Wilm's tumor)
   c. **Embryonic tubules**—lined by cuboidal cells with scant inconspicuous cytoplasm
   d. **Low-grade myxomatous mesenchyme**—immature stroma often arranged concentrically around islands of epithelium, resembling developing smooth muscle in the embryonic GI or respiratory systems
6. Current recommendations are to assess the amount of immature elements in a given tumor, but thus far "grading" the degree of immaturity (just as with grading the degree of atypia in a mature teratoma) does not have prognostic significance
7. Malignancy may arise within a teratoma, although the phrase "malignant transformation" may be somewhat misleading since it implies that teratomas are not, by themselves, malignant
   a. An overtly malignant component in a teratoma may have an immature or mature appearance, ie, invasive adenocarcinoma of GI type, squamous cell carcinoma and undifferentiated carcinoma are examples of mature types; PNET, embryonal rhabdomyosarcoma, or Wilm's tumor-like elements would be "immature" types
   b. diagnosis pretty much depends on finding overgrowth of the remainder of the teratoma by the malignant elements (carcinoma, sarcoma, etc.)
   c. the prognostic significance of an overtly malignant element in teratoma is still uncertain

C. Special Studies

1. Staining is usually as would be expected for the given somatic types of cells (cytokeratin positive in squamous epithelium, etc.)
2. AFP may be present within enteric or respiratory-type epithelium; thus, pure teratoma may be associated clinically with mildly elevated AFP levels

D. Differential Diagnosis

1. Dermoid and epidermoid cysts (benign) must be distinguished from mature teratoma (malignant)
   a. Dermoid cyst: epidermal-lined cyst with adnexal structures in the wall
   b. Epidermoid cyst: epidermal-lined cyst lined with keratinizing squamous epithelium but lacking associated adnexal structures
2. These cysts show no atypia, are not associated with immature elements, and are generally not associated with IGCNU

E. Treatment and Prognosis

1. Prepubertal patients are cured by orchiectomy
2. Postpubertal patients with mature teratoma have a guarded prognosis – 70% survival (with or without seminomatous component)
3. Patients may die of metastatic disease having nonteratomatous components

8. Choriocarcinoma

A. Clinical Features

1. Uncommon component of mixed germ cell tumors (15% of cases)
2. Pure choriocarcinoma is extremely rare (0.3% of testicular tumors)
3. Most patients present with symptoms of metastatic disease, unlike the other tumors in which a palpable testicular mass is the most common presenting complaint
4. Testicular tumor may remain occult even after the metastasis has been identified
5. Metastases particularly like the lung, brain, and GI tract, and spread hematogenously
6. Patient age: 2nd to 3rd decades

B. Laboratory Values: markedly elevated HCG → secondary hormonal manifestations such as gynecomastia and thyrotoxicosis (because HCG cross-reacts with TSH)

C. Pathologic Features

1. Testis may show hemorrhagic nodule or have residual scarring from regression of the original lesion
2. Histologically: classical combination of syncytiotrophoblasts (multinucleated cells with smudged, degenerate-appearing nuclei) admixed with cytotrophoblasts (mononuclear cells with pale-staining cytoplasm)
3. Usually has hemorrhage surrounding the tumor and the central portion of the neoplasm is invariably necrotic

D. Special Studies

1. HCG stains are strongly positive in the syncytiotrophoblasts and less so in the cytotrophoblasts
2. Cytokeratin is positive as well
3. AFP staining may be seen in 50% of tumors

E. Treatment and Prognosis: Has a fairly aggressive course, although patients may achieve substantial tumor-free survival with chemotherapy

9. Mixed Germ Cell Tumors

A. Classified as nonseminomatous tumors even if seminoma is one of the components

B. Comprise 30% of all germ cell tumors, and 69% of all nonseminomatous germ cell tumors of the testis

C. Clinical Features:

1. Patients have the same features as those with nonseminomatous germ cell tumor, and most present with a testicular mass
2. Average age: 28 years (slightly younger than pure seminomas)
3. AFP and HCG may be elevated in 60% and 55%, respectively, of these patients

D. Gross Features: MGCT often have variegated cut surface with hemorrhagic and necrotic areas

E. Histologic Features: areas demonstrate embryonal, seminomatous, teratomatous, yolk sac or choriocarcinomatous differentiation

F. Treatment and Prognosis: MGCT patients are managed like nonseminomatous patients

10. Regression of Germ Cell Tumor

A. Primary germ cell tumors were, at one time, thought to arise in the retroperitoneum; however, increasing evidence seems to suggest that most likely these retroperitoneal tumors represent metastatic spread of primary testicular lesions that have regressed by the time of diagnosis

B. Examination of the testis generally reveals a scar-like focus where the tumor once was

C. Choriocarcinoma is particularly likely to produce metastatic spread in the face of a "burned-out" testicular tumor, although regression may be seen in any of the germ cell types

15. Testis III: Non-germ Cell Tumors

1. Leydig Cell Tumor

A. Sex-cord stromal tumor that comprises 1%-3% of testicular tumors; some seen in association with Klinefelter's and with cryptorchid testes

B. 3% are bilateral

C. May produce endocrine symptoms due to increased production of androgens and/or estrogens

D. Presenting complaint in **adults**: testicular mass and gynecomastia

E. Presenting complaint in **children**: precocious pseudopuberty ("pseudo" because they get growth of pubic hair and penis but no spermatocytic maturation in the non-neoplastic testis)—symptoms typically regress with tumor removal

F. Gross Features: Solid brown nodules within the testicular parenchyma; average size 3.0 cm

G. Microscopic Features
1. Tumor cells have well-defined outlines and abundant eosinophilic cytoplasm
2. May have numerous eosinophilic crystalloids (crystals of Reinke)
3. Tumor cells may have marked pleomorphism with giant atypical forms
4. Growth pattern is generally solid

H. Clinical Behavior: 10% are malignant—malignancy may be suggested by high mitotic rate, necrosis, large size (avg. 7.5 cm), and blood vessel invasion

I. Treatment: orchiectomy (+ lymph node dissection if suspect malignant tumor)

2. Sertoli Cell Lesions

A. Sertoli Cell Hyperplasia
1. Seen in 50% of patients with cryptorchid testes but may also be seen in normal testes
2. Frequency decreases with age
3. May be a manifestation of abnormal sexual maturation

B. Sertoli Cell Adenomas
1. Often seen in patients with testicular feminization
2. Microscopic features: composed of elongated tubules lined by Sertoli-like cells

C. Sertoli Cell Tumors
1. May arise in the normal testes and are associated with gynecomastia in 30% of cases
2. Gross: well-circumscribed gray-white nodules with firm and focally cystic areas
3. Microscopic features: tubules lined by Sertoli-like cells.
   a. solid areas may be confused histologically with seminomas
   b. positive staining for vimentin, keratin, alpha-1-antitrypsin, and neuron-specific enolase
   - **10% malignant** with metastatic involvement of paraaortic and iliac lymph nodes (suspect with high mitotic rate, pleomorphic cells, large tumor size, and necrosis)
   - Treatment: orchiectomy (+ excision of metastatic lesions, as indicated)
   - Adjuvant chemo and radiation has been helpful in malignant tumors

3. Other Testicular Tumors

A. Lymphoma
1. 5% of all testicular lesions, but is the most common testicular tumor in elderly patients
2. 50% of patients with bilateral testicular masses will have lymphoma
3. Most cases are large noncleaved or immunoblastic B-cell lymphomas
4. Most patients have systemic disease by the time they develop testicular involvement, and the prognosis is poor
5. Treatment: orchiectomy for stage I and II disease
6. Micro: tubules are normal but the interstitium is infiltrated by sheets of lymphocytes (small round blue cells) → LCA positive if in doubt

B. Leukemia
1. Not uncommonly seen in children, particularly at the first site of relapse following bone marrow remission
2. Microscopic rate of involvement is approximately 20%

3. Radiation may help control testicular involvement, but most patients will go on to develop bone marrow relapse

C. Carcinoid Tumors

1. May be seen as a component of a germ cell tumor, as a primary neoplasm arising from autochthonous neuroendocrine cells, or as a metastasis from a GI primary
2. Rarely occur in children
3. Gross: firm, yellow-brown nodules
4. Micro: ribbon and festoon-like growth pattern of argyrophil or argentaffin cells
5. Most cured by orchiectomy
6. Usually NOT associated with carcinoid syndrome

16. Testicular Adnexae

1. Epididymal Tumors

A. Adenomatoid Tumor

1. Most common neoplasm of the epididymis
2. Presents in patients in 3rd or 4th decades
3. Clinically presents as a mass, sometimes associated with pain
4. Gross: small, firm, grayish white nodule +/- small cysts
5. Micro: unencapsulated lesion that may involve adjacent testis
   a. Proliferation of cells ranging from cuboidal to flattened, which form solid cords with an epithelial appearance admixed with channels having dilated lumina-like vascular structures
   b. may have abundant smooth muscle, desmoplastic response, or be infiltrated by inflammatory cells
   c. Special stains; (+) for keratin and EMA but negative for CEA and factor VIII related antigen
6. May also arise in the spermatic cord, ejaculatory duct, fallopian tubes, and uterus
7. Felt to arise from mesothelial cells
8. Often seen in association with chronic inflammation and fibrosis, so may represent a peculiar form of nodular mesothelial hyperplasia
9. DDX: epithelioid hemangioma (Factor VIII related antigen positive)
10. Behavior: benign

B. Mesothelioma

1. Arises from tunica vaginalis
2. Most cases are malignant; may occasionally be associated with asbestos exposure
3. Behave aggressively with potential for late recurrence and metastasis

C. Papillary Cystadenoma

1. May be seen as part of the von Hippel-Lindau syndrome, in which circumstances these tumors are more likely to be bilateral
2. Gross: measures 1-5 cm and is well circumscribed, either cystic or solid
3. Micro: papillary infoldings lined by columnar cells with abundant clear cytoplasm
4. Special stains: positive for soybean agglutinin
5. DDX: renal cell carcinoma (which is negative for soybean agglutinin)

D. Carcinoma: extremely rare; usually adenocarcinoma or undifferentiated; very poor prognosis

2. Rete Testis: Adenocarcinoma

A. Very rare

B. May be difficult to distinguish from malignant mesothelioma of the tunica vaginalis

C. Diagnostic Criteria

1. Involvement centered on hilum of testis
2. Lack of direct extension through the parietal tunica
3. Transitions from the tumor to normal rete testis epithelium
4. No evidence of teratoma
5. Lack of any other primary tumor

17. References

Bostwick DG, Eble JN, eds. *Urologic Surgical Pathology*. St. Louis, MO: Mosby; 1997.

Murphy WM, Grignon DJ, Perlman EJ. *AFIP Atlas of Tumor Pathology (Fourth Series, Fascicle 1): Tumors of the Kidney, Bladder, and Related Urinary Structures*. Washington, DC: AFIP/ARP Press; 2004.

Chapter 7: Renal Physiology and Pathophysiology

Una J. Lee, MD
Hadley M. Wood, MD
Daniel A. Shoskes, MD, FRCS(C)

Contents

1. Objectives

- The objective of this chapter is to help urologists pass board and recertification examinations
- Given the complexity of renal physiology and pathophysiology, a review of this topic can be overwhelming
- Recognizing this fact, I have provided a chapter in outline form, to be a concise and rapid overview of renal physiology

2. Basic Renal Anatomy

Arteries are end arteries. Veins communicate.

- Blood enters the kidney through the renal arteries, and divides into progressively smaller arteries:

  * ***Interlobar artery***

  * ***Arcuate artery***

  * ***Interlobular artery***

- Until it enters the glomerular capillary through the ***afferent arteriole***

Basic unit of the kidney is the nephron.

- Blood enters the glomerular capillary through the afferent arteriole
- The ***glomerulus*** is a tuft of capillaries interposed between two arterioles (afferent and efferent); located in the renal cortex
- Blood exits the glomerular capillary through the ***efferent arteriole***
- Figure 1 shows renal architecture demonstrating processes of filtration, reabsorption, secretion and excretion in the nephron

Figure 1

Renal architecture demonstrating processes of filtration, reabsorption, secretion and excretion in the nephron

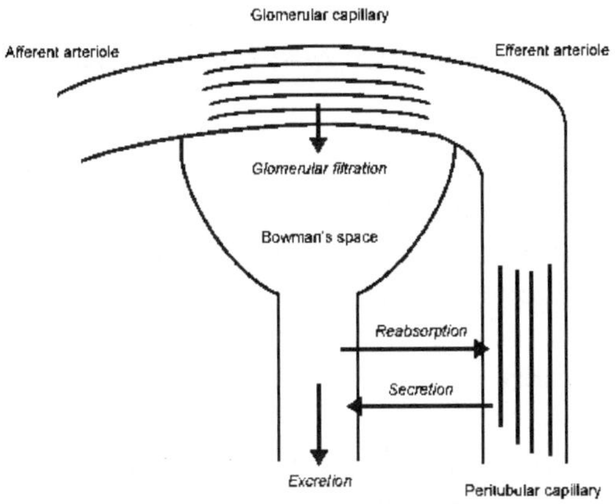

Adapted from Costanzo LS. BRS Physiology. *3rd ed. Baltimore, MD: Williams & Wilkins; 2003:171.*

3. Renal Hemodynamic Definitions

Renal Blood Flow (RBF)

- 20%-25% of cardiac output
- Blood to kidneys per minute (1200 mL/min)
- Directly proportional to the pressure difference between the renal artery and the renal vein, and inversely proportional to the resistance of the renal vasculature

Renal Plasma Flow (RPF)

- Plasma flow to kidneys per minute (670 mL/min)
- Varies with hematocrit (RPF=RBF x [1-Hct])
- Clearance of para-aminohippuric acid (PAH) is used to measure effective RPF. PAH can also be used to measure RBF

Glomerular Filtration Rate (GFR)

- Volume of plasma filtered per minute by the glomeruli (125 mL/min males, 100 mL/min females). Note the units!

Filtration Fraction (FF)

- Filtration of RPF filtered across the glomerular capillaries
- GFR:RPF (about .18-.22)
- Thus, ***about 20% of the RPF is filtered.*** The remaining 80% leaves the glomerular capillaries by efferent arterioles and becomes the peritubuar capillary circulation
- See Table 1 for effect of afferent and efferent arteriole constriction on RPF, GFR and filtration fraction

Table 1

Effect of Renal Plasma Flow on Filtration Fraction

Effect	RPF	GFR	FF (=GFR/RPF)
Afferent arteriole constriction	↓	↓	Remains constant (no change)
Efferent arteriole constriction	↓	↑	↑

Glomerular Filtration Rate (GFR): Reflects Overall Renal Function

- Important function of the kidney is the process of glomerular filtration.
- ***Balance of hydrostatic and oncotic pressures.***
- ***Hydrostatic pressure controlled by relative tonicity of pre-and postglomerular arterioles.***
- Hyper-renin state will maintain GFR by postglomerular arteriolar constriction.
- GFR may be approximated by creatinine clearance, since creatinine is filtered, not resorbed and minimally secreted.
- Estimates of GFR with blood urea nitrogen (BUN) and serum [creatinine]
- When GFR decreases, both BUN and serum (creatinine) increase
- In prerenal azotemia (hypovolemia), BUN in creases more than serum creatinine and there is a resultant increased BUN/creatinine ratio (>20:1)
- ACE inhibitors cause vasodilation of both the afferent and efferent arterioles, however, proportionally more dilation of the efferent arteriole. This results in a drop in glomerular hydrostatic pressure and decreased GFR

Clearance

- Indicates the volume of plasma cleared of a substance per unit time
- Units of clearance are mL/min and mL/24hr
- Clearance = [urine concentration x (urine volume/time)] / plasma concentration
- ***Most widely used estimate of GFR is the 24- hour creatinine clearance (CrCl)***
  - * CrCl overestimates GFR by 10%-20% due to tubular secretion of creatinine
  - * See Figure 2 for Cockcroft-Gault formula for CrCl calculation

Figure 2

Cockcroft-Gault formula for creatinine clearance

$$\text{CrCl (mL/min)} = \frac{([140 - \text{age}] \times ([\text{Ideal body weight in kg}])}{(\text{Plasma creatinine } [\text{mg/dL} \times 72])} \times 0.85 \text{ (women)}$$

$$\text{CrCl (mL/min)} = \frac{\text{urine Cr \% urine vol}}{\text{Serum creatinine}}$$

(total creatinine should be 1 mg/kg/hr)

4. Control of Vascular Tone

- Vascular tone is the net result of vasoconstrictive and vasodilatory forces, which is essential in maintaining RBF, GFR, tubular renal function and systemic blood pressure

Vasoconstrictors

- Endothelin (most potent vasoconstrictor)
- Angiotensin II
- Atrial natriuretic peptide (ANP)
- Vasopressin
- Norepinephrine

Vasodilators

- Prostaglandins (PGE-2)
- Acetylcholine
- Serotonin/bradykinin (NO mediated)
- Glucocorticoids
- *Nitric oxide (potent vasodilator)*
- ***Carbon monoxide (potent vasodilator)***

Renin-Angiotensin System

- Mechanism
  1. Macula densa cells sense decreased BP → rennin is secreted
  2. Angioteninogen cleaved to angiotensin I
  3. Angiotensin I cleaved by angiotensin-converting enzyme (ACE) (from lung) to angiotensin II

- ***Overall action of angiotensin II: increases intravascular volume and increases BP via:***

  * Potent vasoconstriction (efferent arteriole constriction)

  * Release of aldosterone from adrenal cortex

  * Release of ADH from posterior pituitary

  * Stimulates the hypothalamus to increase thirst

- Maintain appropriate water, acid and electrolyte balance using passive and active mechanisms
- Reabsorb selectively up to 99% of the glomerular filtrate
- Respond to endocrine signals to make necessary changes to the fluid prior to excretion (eg, excrete more acid, conserve more water)
- See Figure 3 for diagram of renal tubular organization

Proximal Tubule

- Reabsorbs 100% of glucose and amino acids, 90% of bicarbonate and 80%-90% of inorganic phosphate and water
- ***Solutes active, water passive:*** water reabsorption in the proximal convoluted tubule is a passive process, driven by the reabsorption of other solutes and the subsequent osmotic gradient that develops between the lumen and intercellular space
- ***Na reabsorption*** through Na^+-H^+ and Na^+-solute active transporters

Figure 3

Renal tubular organization

Osmolality gradient in loop of Henle allows concentration of urine in the collecting duct

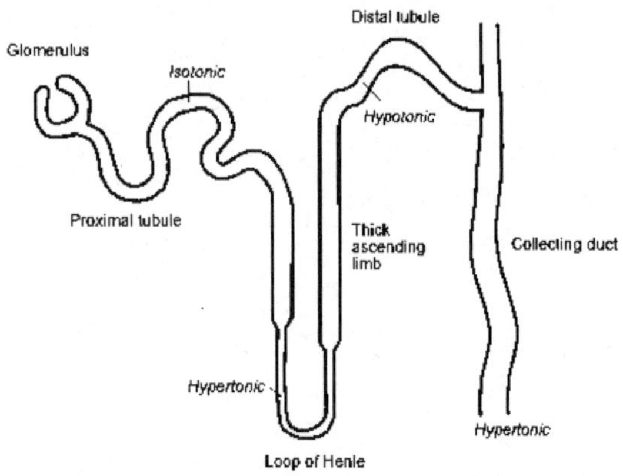

- Majority of sodium, chloride and water is reabsorbed in the proximal tubule driven by active forces
- HCO_3 generated in cell and absorbed with Na^+
- Secretes ammonia, which acts as a buffer for secreted H^+

Loop of Henle

- Early water and urea permeability, filtrate becomes hypertonic
- Later Na^+-Cl permeability
- Final, Na^+-Cl actively transported, filtrate hypotonic
- ***Creates high interstitial osmolality (highly hypertonic) which permits maximal urinary concentration***

Thick Ascending Limb

- ***The "diluting" segment***
- Active transport of NH_4 and Na
- Aldosterone and ADH augment Na^+ reabsorption
- PGE-2 reduces Na^+ reabsorption

Collecting Duct

- Provides final touches to Na^+, HCO_3- and K^+
- Na absorbed, K^+ secreted (stimulated by aldosterone)
- H^+ secreted based on blood pH
- NH_3–secreted into lumen and can trap H^+ to make NH_4
- Reabsorption of water is regulated by vasopressin (ADH)

- ADH acts on receptors located on the basolateral membrane of the principal cells of the collecting ducts. Induces migration and insertion of water permeable protein channels to the luminal membrane

- If ADH is present, permeable to water and water is drawn by hypertonic medulla

- Osmolality of medulla can reach 1200 mOsm

Countercurrent Multiplier

- ***Ultimate goal is to produce high osmolality in the medulla which is later used for urinary concentration***

  * Loop structure generates a longitudinal gradient

  * ***Thin ascending limb contains active sodium transporters and is water permeable***

  * Thick ascending limb has solute pump and is water impermeable

  * Collecting duct is water permeable in the presence of circulating ADH

6. Diuretic Effects

Thiazide Diuretics

- HCTZ, chlorthalidone, metolazone

- ***Mechanism: inhibit Na^+ and Cl reabsorption in distal convoluted tubule, reducing the diluting capacity of the nephron***

- Reduce GFR and RBF

- ***Decreases urinary calcium***

- In diabetes insipidus, they have an antidiuretic effect

- Hyponatremia may occur with thiazide diuretics

Loop Diuretics

- Furosemide, ethacrinic acid, bumetanide

- ***Mechanism: inhibit Na/K/Cl cotransporter on the luminal membrane of the thick ascending portion of loop of Henle***

- Increased diuresis and ***increased excretion of Na, K, Cl, Ca and Mg***

- ***Reduce medullary solute content and impair urinary concentrating and diluting capacity***

7. Disorders of Water and Sodium

Primary Goals

- Maintain blood pressure
- Excrete wastes

Mechanisms

- Thirst
- ADH
- Aldosterone

8. Tubular Handling of Water

Osmolality

- POsm = 2 x plasma [Na] + [glucose]/18 + [BUN]/2.8
- The osmolality of plasma is tightly regulated around a mean of 290 mOsm/kg (± 5mosm/kg)
- Therefore, kidney is able to adjust the rate of water excretion over a wide range, generating dilute urine when water is abundant and a concentrated urine when water is scarce

Osmolality Changes

- Loop of Henle creates an osmolality gradient in the medullary interstitium
- Collecting duct traverses medulla: urine concentrated by osmotic water removal when duct wall made permeable by ADH

Response to Water Loss

- In response to increased plasma osmolality or decreased arterial circulating volume:
  * Increased thirst and increased water intake
  * Increased ADH and decreased water excretion
    - Leads to water retention

How Water Disorders Develop

- For any electrolyte disorder, you need 2 components:
  1. Something must change the concentration (eg, loss of sodium through an NG tube); and
  2. Something must interfere with the normal physiologic response

9. Electrolyte Disorders

Hyponatremia and Hypernatremia Evaluation and Treatment

- ***2 key factors are volume status and urinary sodium that will lead you to the diagnosis***

  1. Determine the volume (water) status of the patient
  2. Determine why the normal compensatory mechanisms have failed
  3. Therapy is directed at both the cause of the condition and the water imbalance itself

Hyponatremia

- ***Water excess relative to extracellular sodium that has not been handled by normal compensatory mechanisms of thirst suppression and decreased ADH***
- Serum sodium >125 mmol/L→ Mild hyponatremia is usually asymptomatic
- Serum sodium <120 mEq/L→ With more severe acute hyponatremia, nausea, headache, confusion, agitation, and incontinence may develop. Seizures, coma, respiratory arrest, and death can occur with profound acute hyponatremia
- Difficult to distinguish between volume depletion and euvolemic hyponatremia on clinical examination. In these cases, measurement of ***the urine sodium concentration can be helpful***
- A low urine sodium concentration suggests decreased effective arterial volume, whereas in SIADH, the urine sodium is usually greater than 30 mmol/L
- ***Central pontine myelinolysis*** can be caused by rapid correction of hyponatremia

Sodium Deficit

- Hypovolemic patient has a sodium deficit greater than their water deficit
- Sodium deficit = *volume of distribution* x body weight (kg) x (125–plasma [Na])
- *Volume of distribution* for men=0.5 and women=0.6

Hypernatremia

- Disorder of urine concentration with inadequate water intake
- Water balance is altered, and total body sodium can be high, normal or low
- In contrast to hyponatremia, which usually results from a defect in renal water handling, the ***primary defect in hypernatremia is impaired water intake***
- More commonly, hypernatremia results from inadequate fluid intake in the setting of increased free water losses
- Geriatric patients are at increased risk because renal concentrating ability and thirst decline with age, although the osmoreceptors' response to hypernatremia is maintained
- In acute hypernatremia, the water deficit can be replaced relatively rapidly
- In chronic hypernatremia (>24 to 48 hours duration), plasma sodium should be decreased by 1 to 2 mmol/L/hour until symptoms resolve and then the rate of correction slowed so that the sodium is normalized over the ensuing 24 to 48 hours
- Free water deficit=0.6 x body weight in kg x [(plasma sodium/140) -1]

Secretion of Acid

- Active Na-H pump
- Glomerular filtration of buffers
- HCO_3, HPO_4
- Ammonia (NH_3) secreted in tubule combines to form nondiffusible NH_4 (ammonium ion)

10. Acid-Base Disorders

- Normal arterial blood pH ranges from 7.37 to 7.43, maintained by lungs (PCO_2) and kidneys (HCO_3)
- Sudden changes tempered by buffers in blood
  * First, check the pH for acidosis or alkalosis. See Figure 4, acid-base evaluation flowchart
  * Second, check the pCO_2 to determine if it's a primary respiratory disorder (versus metabolic)
    - Metabolic acidosis—a primary process that causes [HCO_3] to fall
    - Metabolic alkalosis—a primary process that causes [HCO_3] to rise
    - Respiratory acidosis—a primary process that causes pCO_2 to rise
    - Respiratory acidosis—a primary process that causes pCO_2 to fall
  * Third, check compensation formulas for coexisting (mixed acid-base) disorders
    - If compensation not appropriate, suspect mixed disorder
  * ***When you see a metabolic acidosis, always calculate the anion gap*** (Na-[Cl+HCO_3]) looking for "extra" anions (normal is 10-12)

Simple Acid-Base Disorders

- ***Metabolic Acidosis***
  * Expected $pCO_2 = 1.5 \times [HCO_3-] + 8 \pm 2$ (Winter's formula)
- ***Metabolic Alkalosis***
  * Expected pCO_2 = 6 mm Hg per 10 mEq/L in HCO_3
- ***Respiratory Acidosis***
  * Acute Expected HCO_3 =1 mEq/L for each 10 mm pCO_2

Figure 4

Acid-base evaluation algorithm

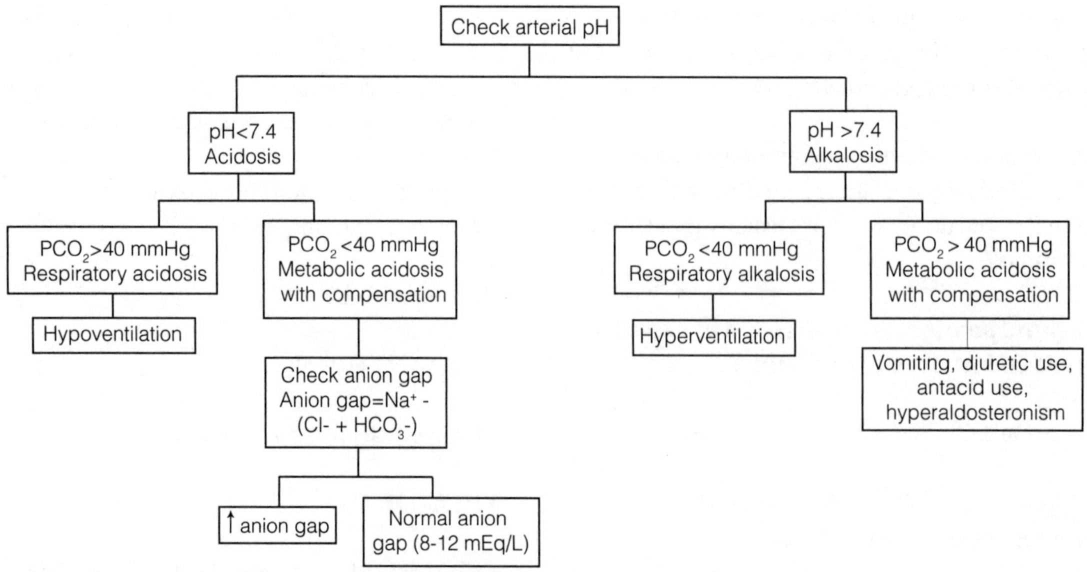

* Chronic Expected HCO_3 =3.5mEq/L for each 10 mm Hg pCO_2

- *Respiratory Alkalosis*

  * Acute Expected HCO_3 =2 mEq/L for each 10 mm Hg pCO_2

  * Chronic Expected HCO_3- =5 mEq/L for each 10 mm Hg pCO_2

Metabolic Disorders

- When normal metabolism is impaired, acid forms (eg, poor blood supply stops oxidative metabolism and lactic acid forms)

- Metabolic disorder has a raised H^+ level with a normal pCO_2. To maintain the equilibrium, the high H^+ would cause a reciprocal fall in the HCO_3-. However, in practice respiratory compensation occurs and lowers the pCO_2, which reduces both the H^+ and the HCO_3- (ie, metabolic acidosis lowers the bicarbonate level and respiratory compensation lowers it further).

- See Table 2 for summary of metabolic disorders and Table 3 for summary of acid-base primary disorders and compensatory responses

Primary Disorder

- pH = 7.18, pCO_2 = 14, HCO_3 = 14, Na = 140, Cl = 104

  * pH is low → therefore acidosis

  * Bicarb is low → therefore metabolic acidosis

  * pCO_2 is low→ expected compensation

  * Predicted pCO_2 compensation is 1.5*4+8 = 14

  * Anion gap 140-(104+14) = 22 → (elevated anion gap)

- Therefore, anion gap metabolic acidosis with appropriate compensation

Respiratory Disorders

- *Respiratory acidosis*

Table 2

Summary of Metabolic Disorders

Metabolic Acidosis	Metabolic Alkalosis
With elevated anion gap	*Chloride-responsive*
Ketoacidosis (diabetes, chronic alcoholism)	Vomiting or nasogastric drainage
Lactic acidosis	Surreptitious laxative abuse
Renal failure	Diuretics
Intoxication	Posthypercapnic states
With normal anion gap	*Chloride-resistant*
GI alkali loss (diarrhea, ileostomy, colostomy)	Severe Mg or K deficiency
Renal tubular acidosis	Diuretics (thiazides or loop diuretics)
Interstitial renal disease	Hypermineralocorticoidism
Ureterosigmoidostomy, ureteroileal conduit	Licorice, chewing tobacco
Acetazolamide therapy	Inherited disorders
Ingestion of ammonium chloride	

Table 3

Summary of Acid-base Primary Disorders and Compensatory Responses

	pH	PCO_2	$[HCO_3^-]$	Compensatory Response
Metabolic acidosis	↓	↓	↓ (primary disorder)	Hyperventilation
Metabolic alkalosis	↑	↑	↑ (primary disorder)	Hypoventilation
Respiratory acidosis	↓	↑(primary disorder)	↑	Renal $[HCO_3^-]$ reabsorption
Respiratory alkalosis	↑	↓(primary disorder)	↓	Renal $[HCO_3^-]$ secretion

* When breathing is inadequate, carbon dioxide (a respiratory acid) accumulates. The extra CO_2 molecules combine with water to form carbonic acid ($H2CO_3$) which contributes to an acidic pH

* Due to insufficient respiration, so consider central, mechanical and obstructive causes.

* Headache and drowsiness lead to coma and death

* Pure respiratory acidosis (high pCO2) causes molecules of CO2 and water to form carbonic acid which ionizes to increase both HCO3- and H+. The H+ changes slightly due to buffering of H+ by hemoglobin. At this raised pCO2, the kidney compensates by eliminating H+. To maintain chemical equilibrium the HCO3- rises further (ie, respiratory acidosis raises the bicarbonate level and metabolic compensation raises it further)

• *Respiratory alkalosis*

* Due to hyperventilation

* Resulting from anxiety, fever, pain, septicemia, iatrogenic (ventilator settings)

* May have tetany, parasthesia

Mixed Disorder

• pH = 7.42, pCO_2 = 65, HCO_3 = 41, Na 143, K 3.1, Cl 88

* pH is normal

* Bicarb is 17 too high → metabolic alkalosis

* pCO_2 should be 1.7*6+40 = 50.2

* Measured pCO_2 is 65

* Too much pCO_2 retained so also has respiratory acidosis

11. Disorders of Potassium

- Mostly intracellular
- Serum levels do not reflect total body content in disease states
- K^+ driven into cells by insulin, bicarbonate, beta-agonists
- Changes in dietary intake handled by intracellular stores and urinary excretion
- Excretion promoted by aldosterone, high distal Na^+ load, chronic acidosis

Hypokalemia

- ***Usually increased loss (GI, urine) or intracellular shift***
- ***Alkylosis = Low K^+***
- ***Iatrogenic causes common***
- ***Diuretics, laxatives, amphotericin, theophylline, postobstructive diuresis***
- Metabolic causes include: hyperaldosterone states, Cushing syndrome
- Tachycardia, heart block, ***ST depression***
- Treat underlying cause, replace K^+ (40 mEq/hr IV)
- Magnesium depletion promotes potassium wasting; important to correct Mg if repleting K^+

EKG Changes in Hypokalemia

- The EKG in hypokalemia may appear normal or may have only subtle findings immediately before clinically significant dysrhythmias
  * Ventricular dysrhythmia
  * Prolongation of QT interval
  * ST-segment depression
  * T-wave flattening
  * *Appearance of U waves*

Hyperkalemia

- ***Usually reflects decreased renal excretion or shift out of cells (acidosis)***
- GI bleed or hemolysis will often exacerbate
- ***Most common causes include: renal failure, drugs (K^+ sparing diuretics, ACE inhibitors, beta blockers), chronic acidosis (RTA type 4) and hyperaldosteronism***
- Usually asymptomatic until cardiac changes
  * Short QT, peaked T waves, ventricular arrhythmia
- Mild increase→ reverse predisposing cause
- Moderate→ use binding agents (Kayexalate®)
- Severe→ give calcium/insulin/glucose drip; dialysis

EKG Changes in Hyperkalemia

- EKG changes have a sequential progression of effects, which roughly correlate with the potassium level
- EKG findings:
  * ***Early changes of hyperkalemia include peaked T waves, shortened QT interval and ST segment depression***
  * These changes are followed by bundle branch blocks causing ***a widening of the QRS complex, increases in the PR interval and decreased amplitude of the P wave***
  * These changes reverse with appropriate treatment

Treatment of Hyperkalemia

- Institute treatment based on clinical severity of hyperkalemia
- Direct treatment at stabilizing the myocardium, shifting potassium from the extracellular environment to the intracellular compartment, and promoting the renal excretion and GI loss of potassium

  * **Calcium gluconate**

    - Used to reduce the risk of ventricular fibrillation caused by hyperkalemia
    - Does not lower potassium, only reduces effect on cardiac rhythm
    - Acts quickly and can be lifesaving, thus they are the first-line treatment for severe hyperkalemia when the ECG shows significant abnormalities (eg, widening of QRS interval, loss of P wave, cardiac arrhythmias)
    - Not indicated when the ECG shows only peaked T waves
    - Calcium gluconate dose: 10 mL of 10% sol IV over 2 min

  * ***Sodium Bicarbonate***

    - Bicarbonate ion neutralizes hydrogen ions and raises urinary and blood pH

Table 4

Clinical Manifestations of Electrolyte Abnormalities

Electrolyte	Low Serum Concentration	High Serum Concentration
Na^+	Nausea, malaise, headache, lethargy, obtundation, disorientation, stupor, seizures, coma	Lethargy, weakness, irritability, twitching, seizures, coma
Cl^-	Due to metabolic alkalosis	Due to nonanion gap acidosis
K^+	Muscle weakness, ileus, cramps, parathesias, ST segment depression, U waves, flattened T waves	Muscle weakness or paralysis, cardiac conduction abnormality, peaked T waves, widened QRS, arrhythmias
Ca^{2+}	Tetany/neuromuscular irritability, fatigue, anxiety, depression, papilledema, seizures	Fatigue, weakness, anorexia, depression, abdominal pain, constipation, nephrolithiasis, renal tubular dysfunction (decreased concentrating ability), and acute and chronic renal insufficiency
Mg^{2+}	Weakness, anorexia, tetany, delirium, coma	Neuromuscular toxicity: somnolence, loss of deep tendon reflexes, muscle paralysis, delirium, cardiopulmonary arrest
PO_4^{2-}	Bone loss, metabolic encephalopathy, muscle dysfunction	Tumor lysis syndrome, rhabdomyolysis, renal failure

- Onset of action within minutes, lasts approximately 15-30 minutes

- Dose: 1 mEq/kg slow IV push or continuous IV drip; not to exceed 50-100 mEq. Use 8.4% solution in adults and children, 4.2% solution in infants

* *Glucose and insulin*

  - Glucose and insulin temporarily shift K^+ into cells; effects occur within first 30 min of administration

  - Administer glucose along with insulin to prevent hypoglycemia

  - Adult dose: 5-10 U regular insulin and 1-2 amps D50W IV bolus

* *Sodium polystyrene sulfonate (Kayexalate)*

  - Exchanges Na^+ for K^+ and binds it in gut, primarily in large intestine, decreasing total body potassium

  - Onset of action after PO ranges from 2-12 hours

  - Adult dose: 25-50 g mixed with 100 mL of 20% sorbitol PO/PR. Multiple doses may be necessary

* *Dialysis*

  - Immediate onset of action.

  - Requires dialysis access

Tubular Handling of Calcium

- Only 1%-3% of Ca^{2+} that is filtered by the kidney is excreted

- The majority of Ca^{2+} reabsorption occurs passively along the proximal tubule and the thick ascending limb of Henle's loop

- Fine tuning of Ca^{2+} reabsorption takes place along the distal convoluted tubule and the connecting tubule, where the remaining 15% of filtered Ca^{2+} is transcellularly reabsorbed

Role of Vitamin D and PTH in Calcium Homeostasis

- *Vitamin D* is involved in normal bone mineralization by maintaining normal serum calcium and phosphorus levels through ***increased intestinal absorption of calcium and phosphorus and increased renal absorption of calcium***

- *PTH* maintains normal serum calcium and phosphorus ***by increasing bone resorption, increasing renal reabsorption of calcium and excretion of phosphorus, and stimulating calcitriol production***

- ***Increased PTH→ increase urinary phosphate excretion by reducing proximal tubule reabsorption of phosphate***

Response to Hypocalcemia

- Increased intestinal reabsorption of calcium

- Increased PTH

  * Decreased renal calcium excretion

  * Increased bone resorption

12. Renal Tubular Acidosis

- A family of syndromes of metabolic acidosis resulting from defects in tubular H^+ secretion and urinary acidification. See Table 5 for a summary of RTA types.

RTA Type 1

- ***Most common form***
- ***Failure of H^+ secretion in the distal nephron***
- ***Stones usually calcium phosphate.***
  * High urine pH, Ca^{2+} and low urine citrate
- Hyperchloremic metabolic acidosis with high urinary pH
- ***Diagnose by urine pH>5.5***, if no metabolic acidosis, provoke with ammonium chloride test
- ***Treat by oral alkalinization and citrate***, monitor for low potassium during therapy

RTA Type 2

- ***Failure of bicarbonate reabsorption in the proximal tubule***
- More common in ***children***
- ***Normal citrate, no stones***
- Growth retardation, metabolic bone disease (think of Charles Dickens' Tiny Tim character)
- ***Treat with $NaHCO_3$***

RTA Type 4

- ***Impaired cation exchange in the distal tubule with reduced secretion of H^+ and K^+***

Table 5

Summary of Types of Renal Tubular Acidosis

	Type 1	Type 2	Type 4
Location	Distal	Proximal	Distal
Problem	Impaired distal acidification	Reduced proximal bile reabsorption same features but can acidify urine	Aldosterone deficiency or resistance
Serum K^+	↓	↓	↑
Urinary pH	↑ >6.0 (inappropriate)	↓	↓
Management	K^+, bicarb	K^+, bicarb	Mineralcorticoids, low K^+ diets
Notes	Hypo K, hyper Cl, nonanion gap metabolic acidosis 75% of these patients get stones	HCO_3 wasting from inability to absorb	Hyper K, hyper Cl

- *Hyperkalemia (only RTA type with high K^+)*
- Often have azotemia and hypertension
- *Treatment aimed to reduce potassium*

13. Effects of Urinary Diversion

- *Dependent on bowel segment, length used, time of exposure, solute concentration, renal function, urine pH*

Stomach

- *Hypochloremic, hypokalemic metabolic alkalosis*
- More significant problem if patient has exiting renal insufficiency
- Treatment includes: proton pump blockers and acidification with dilute hydrochloric acid

Jejunum

- *Hyponatremic, hypochloremic, hyperkalemic metabolic acidosis*
- Rehydrate with NaCl and $NaHCO_3$
- *Sodium chloride replacement and thiazides are treatments of choice*

Ileum and Colon Diversions

- *Hyperchloremic metabolic acidosis*
- Predisposed by impaired renal function
- Ammonium absorption with chloride is exchanged for Na and HCO_3
- Inability to secrete acid as ammonium depletes buffers
- Treat with Na bicarbonate and/or nicotinic acid (chloride transport inhibitor)
- *Urea and creatinine are reabsorbed by both the ileum and colon*
    - * Therefore, serum concentrations of urea and creatinine are less accurate measures of renal function after urinary diversion
    - * Affects bone metabolism through a decrease in calcium reabsorption and impaired Vitamin D metabolism

- The resulting ***chronic acidosis may produce osteoporosis or osteomalacia***

Consequences of Malabsorption

- The ***ileum*** is the site of ***Vitamin B_{12} and of bile acid absorption***

- Resection of up to 60 cm of ileum in patients who retain their terminal ileum and ileocecal valve is ***generally well tolerated***

- If more than 100 cm of ileum is resected, fat-soluble Vitamin (A, D, E and K) malabsorption results

- Vitamin B_{12} deficiency results in anemia and neurological degeneration

- Oxalate absorption is increased, because the unabsorbed fat saponifies with calcium, which is no longer available to form a chelate with oxalate. This raises serum and urinary oxalate levels and urinary stones may result

14. Postobstructive Diuresis

- Requires bilateral obstruction or obstruction of solitary unit

- Mechanisms

  * Na leak, urea ***osmotic diuretic, loss of concentrating ability*** from urea washout in medulla

- Mild form can be corrected by oral intake

- Severe cases require partial IV replacement and electrolyte monitoring

15. References

1. Vikas B, Le T, Chandwani R, Ozturk A. *First Aid for the USLME Step 1 2006*. New York, NY: McGraw-Hill; 2006.

2. Burkhard FC, Kessler TM, Mills R, Studer UE. Continent urinary diversion. *Crit Rev Oncol Hematol*. 2006 Mar;57(3):255-64. Epub 2005 Dec 1.

3. Costanzo LS. Renal and acid-base physiology. In: *BRS Physiology*. 3rd ed. Baltimore, MD: Williams & Wilkins; 2003:161-213.

4. Fall PJ. Hyponatremia and hypernatremia. A systematic approach to causes and their correction. *Postgrad Med*. 2000 May1;107(5):75-82.

5. Field M, Pollock C, Harris D. *The Renal System: Basic Science and Clinical Conditions*. New York, NY: Harcourt Publishers; 2001.

6. Fried LF, Palevsky PM. Hyponatremia and hypernatremia. *Med Clin North Am*. 1997 May;81(3):585-609.

7. Garth D, et al. Hyperkalemia. *Emedicine.com*. April 25, 2006.

8. Levy David A. *Urology Pearls of Wisdom*. Boston, MA: Boston Medical Publishing; 2001.

9. Mandal AK. Hypokalemia and hyperkalemia. *Med Clin North Am*. 1997 May; 81(3): 611-39

10. Mattu A, Brady WJ, Robinson DA. Electrocardiographic manifestations of hyperkalemia. *Am J Emerg Med*. 2000 Oct;18(6):721-9.

11. Mensenkamp AR, Hoenderop JG, Bindels RJ. Recent advances in renal tubular calcium reabsorption. *Curr Opin Nephrol Hypertens*. 2006 Sep;15(5):524-9.

12. Shayman JA. Renal pathophysiology. In: Shayman JA, ed. *Lippincott's Pathophysiology Series*. Philadelphia, PA: JB Lippincott Co; 1995.

13. Shoskes DA, McMahon A. Renal physiology and pathophysiology. In: Wein AJ, Kavoussi LR, Novick AC, et al, eds. *Campbell-Walsh Urology*. 9th ed. Philadelphia, PA: Elsevier; 2007:1129-1155.

14. Verive M, D Jaimovich, et al. Hypokalemia. *Emedicine.com*. March 30, 2006.

16. Questions

1. Which of the following is true about sodium and the kidney?

A. By definition, hypernatremia is always associated with elevated total body sodium content

B. Normal compensation for hyponatremia is decreased ADH secretion and thirst suppression

C. Abnormal elevation of serum lipids can lead to a measured false elevation of serum sodium

D. If asymptomatic hyponatremia does not improve within 24 hours, intravenous hypertonic saline should be started

E. In therapy of symptomatic hyponatremia, the goal should be a normal serum sodium of 135 meq/L within 48 hours

2. Which of the following is NOT true about potassium?

A. ACE inhibitors may be a cause of hypokalemia

B. Potassium is primarily an intracellular ion

C. Acidosis drives potassium out of the cell into the circulation

D. A high sodium load in the distal tubule promotes potassium excretion

E. The upper limit for safe intravenous potassium infusion is 40 meq/hr

3. Which of the following is true about acidosis?

A. Increasing the blood HCO_3 level increases the anion gap

B. Direct bicarbonate loss from the kidney would lead to metabolic acidosis and a normal anion gap

C. Lactic acidosis usually presents as a non-anion gap metabolic acidosis

D. Appropriate respiratory compensation for a metabolic acidosis is decreased respiration with an increased PCO_2

E. It is not possible to have both a respiratory and metabolic acidosis at the same time

4. All of the following can increase total GFR except:

A. Increased RBF

B. Increased intraglomerular (hydraulic) pressure

C. Increased glomerular permeability

D. Increased efferent arteriolar resistance

E. Increased functioning nephron number

Answers

1. B.
The physiologic response to hyponatremia is decreased ADH secretion and thirst suppression.

2. A.
ACE inhibitors may cause hyperkalemia.

3. B.
Direct bicarbonate loss is "measured" in the anion gap and therefore leads to metabolic acidosis with a normal anion gap.

4. C.
Glomerular permeability is already maximal under normal conditions for water and small solutes, so GFR will not increase significantly with increased glomerular permeabililty. Rather, one sees increased filtration of larger substances such as albumin.

Chapter 8: Renovascular Disease

Hadley M. Wood, MD
Una J. Lee, MD
Daniel A. Shoskes, MD FRCS(C)

Contents

1. Definitions

A. Hypertension

1. Definition

Table 1

Blood Pressure (BP) Classification	Systolic BP mm Hg	Diastolic BP mm Hg
Normal	<120	And <80
"Prehypertension"*	120-139	Or 80-89
Stage I hypertension	140-159	Or 90-99
Stage II hypertension	≥160	Or ≥100

** "Prehypertension" should be treated aggressively in diabetics and those with kidney disease to a goal of 130/80*

2. Incidence

a. Age 60-69, 50%; age >70, 75%

b. Lifetime risk: 86%-90% female; 81%-83% male

3. Scope of Problem

a. 30% adults unaware of BP

b. >40% with hypertension are not on treatment

c. Two-thirds of patients with hypertension are not being controlled to <140/90 mm Hg

d. End-stage renal disease (ESRD) is on the rise; diabetes and hypertension are the most common causes of ESRD

B. Renovascular Hypertension (RVH)

1. Renal Duplex Criteria

a. Renal artery peak systolic velocity >1.8 m/s, >60% stenosis, or no Doppler signal

2. Angiographic/Magnetic Resonance (MR)/ Computed Tomography (CT) Criteria

a. No clear-cut definition

b. Some say 75% stenosis, while others quote 50% stenosis (Vasbinder, 2001)

3. Incidence: Poorly Characterized

a. <1-3% of all hypertensive patients have RVH 18%-20% among patients undergoing cardiac angiography

b. 35%-50% among patients undergoing angiography for aortic occlusive disease (Olin, 1990)

C. Ischemic Nephropathy

1. Renal failure due to hemodynamically significant atherosclerotic renal artery stenosis and related renal parenchymal disease.

2. Estimates of 8%-10% of new cases of ESRD caused by ischemic nephropathy (Novick, 2006)

2. Pathophysiology

Figure 1

Hypertension, kidney disease, and renal artery demonstrate significant overlap

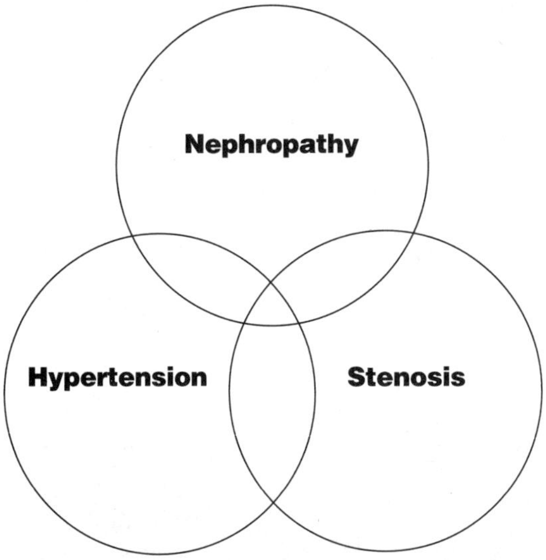

B. Mechanism of Ischemic Nephropathy (Figure 1)

1. Critical stenosis necessary

2. Injury is initially reversible, but then progresses to permanent damage

3. At end-stage, interstitial fibrosis and ischemic nephropathy result

4. Glomerulosclerosis and atheroembolism seen on biopsy (Figure 2 and Figure 3) suggests that kidney is unlikely to be salvaged with revascularization, and 5-year survival (predominantly from cardio- and cerebrovascular events) drops to only around 50% (Krishnamurti, 1999)

C. Unilateral RVD

1. Equivalent to the "2-kidney-1-clip" model, whereby increased BP is accompanied by increased plasma renin activity (PRA)

a. Nonstenotic kidney is subjected to higher perfusion pressures leading to pressure naturesis (excretion of sodium, lowering pressure) causing increased aldosterone and renovascular vasoconstriction

A. RVD Associated With:

1. Ischemic nephropathy

2. Hypertension

Figure 2

Relationship between renal artery stenosis and renal blood flow

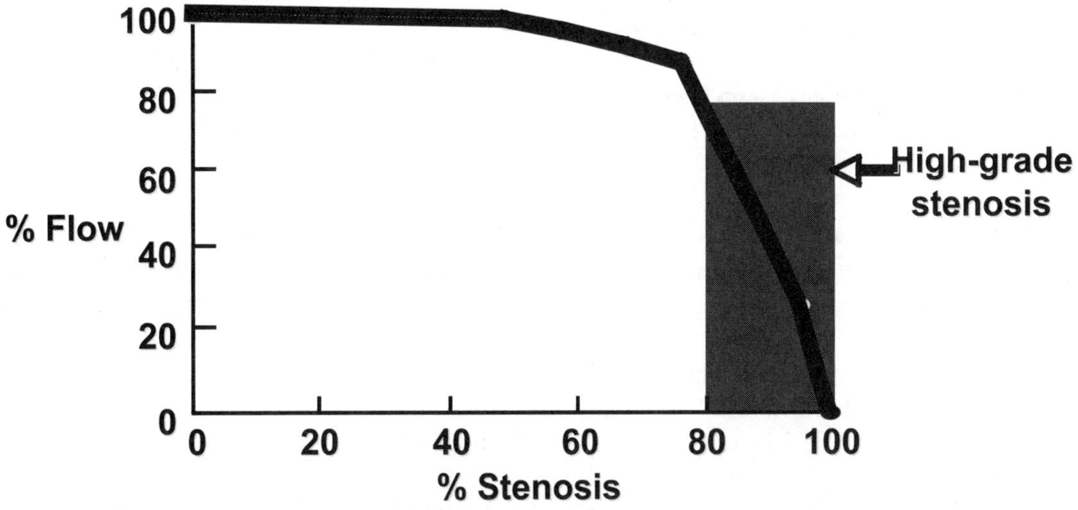

Figure 3

Renal histopathology in ischemic nephropathy

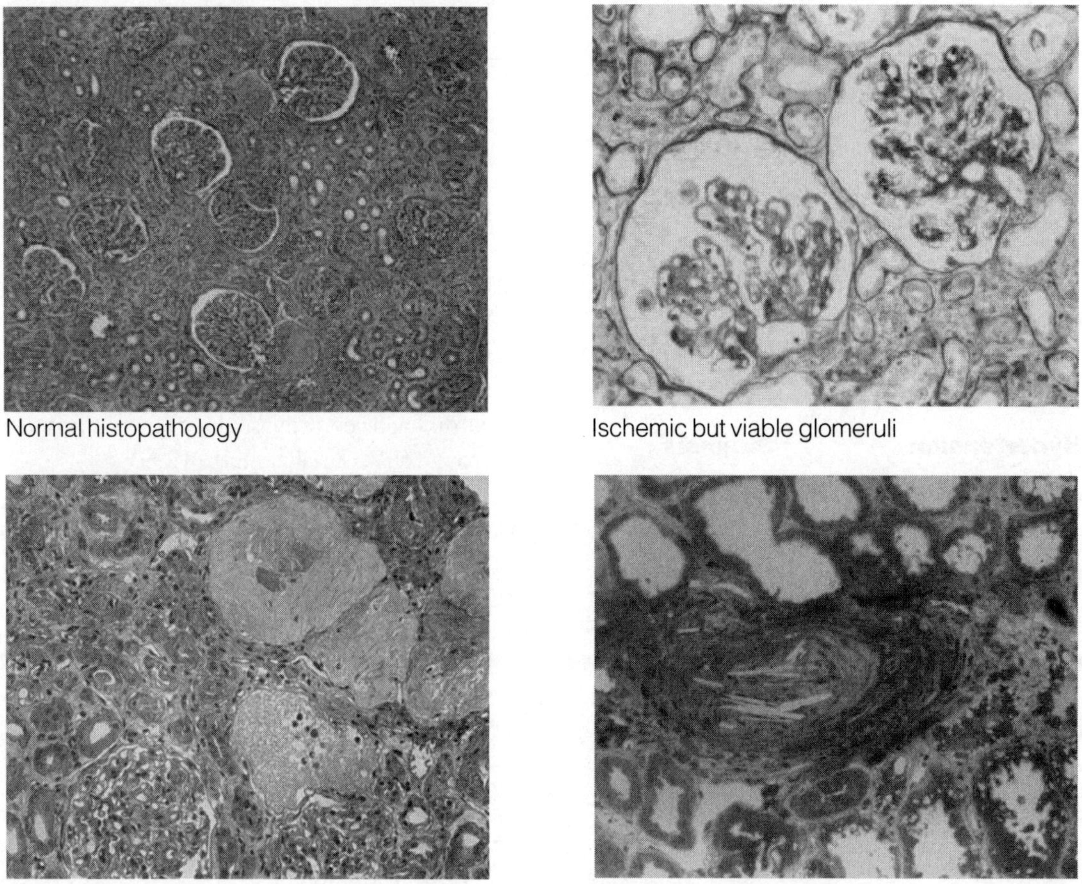

Normal histopathology | Ischemic but viable glomeruli | Glomerulosclerosis | Atheroembolism

b. Subsequent decrease in perfusion pressure to the stenotic kidney causes release of renin

D. Bilateral RVD, or Solitary Kidney RVD

1. Equivalent to the "1-kidney-1-clip" model, whereby PRA remains normal, and BP is non-responsive to angiotensin blockade

a. In the absence of a normally perfused kidney, excessive sodium cannot be excreted in response to higher perfusion pressures.

b. Sodium and water retention occur, leading to volume expansion, which is the primary mechanism of elevated BP in this model (Figure 4)

E. Renin – Increased by:

1. Reduced sodium delivery to distal tubule
2. Hypoperfusion of juxtaglomerular cells
3. Beta-adrenergic stimulation
4. Prostaglandin E2 (PGE2) & prostacyclin (PGI2)

F. Angiotensin II (ATII) – Powerful Effector of Multiple Actions Downstream, Including:

1. Efferent arteriolar vasoconstriction
2. Peripheral vasoconstriction
3. Renal sodium retention

Figure 4

Goldblatt (1930s) demonstrated that reduced perfusion to the kidney can cause increased arterial blood pressure

Two-kidney hypertension | One-kidney hypertension

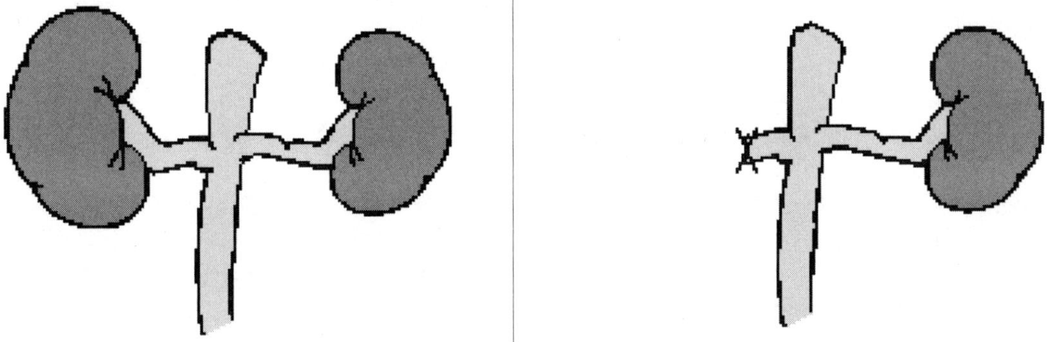

Blood pressure	Renin	Volume
↑	High	Normal

ARB/ACE inhibitors help

Blood pressure	Renin	Volume
↑	Normal	High

Only help when Na depleted

4. Aldosterone secretion

5. Vascular hypertrophy/remodeling (ATI receptor mediated)

6. Sympathetic activation

7. Left ventricular hypertrophy

G. The RAS System Generates an Appropriate Response to Hypovolemia or Hypotension, but a Pathologic Cycle in RVD

H. Difficult to Determine Whether a Hypertensive Patient Will Respond to Renal Revascularization or Stenting

1. A lot of overlap with essential hypertension, diabetes, obesity, and smoking, which are common sources of irreversible renal disease.

2. Data suggest renovascular hypertension is associated with increased sympathetic input, manifested by greater variability in BP throughout the day. This can be documented with 24-hour ambulatory BP monitoring)

3. May demonstrate higher nocturnal BP than essential hypertensives

4. May demonstrate hypokalemia and hyponatremia

5. More likely to have reduced glomerular filtration rate (GFR)

3. Classification of Lesions

A. Atherosclerotic (70%-90%)

1. Usually involves ostium and proximal one-third of main renal artery

2. Systemic disease

3. Progression common, with 18% occlusion rate over 5 years

B. Fibromuscular Disease (10%-30%)

1. Primarily localizes to distal ½ of renal artery or branched renal vessels

2. Typically affects women 15-50 years of age

3. Classified by arterial layer – intima, media, or adventitia, which lesion predominates

a. Medial Fibroplasia (Figure 6)

- Most common
- Women 25-50
- Commonly bilateral
- Progression less common
- "String of beads" appearance on angiography
- Middle to distal portion of artery
- Associated with Erlers-Danlos IV

b. Perimedial fibroplasia (Figure 7)

Women aged 15-30

Figure 5

Renin-angiotensin system (RAS) primarily responsible for observations of Goldblatt

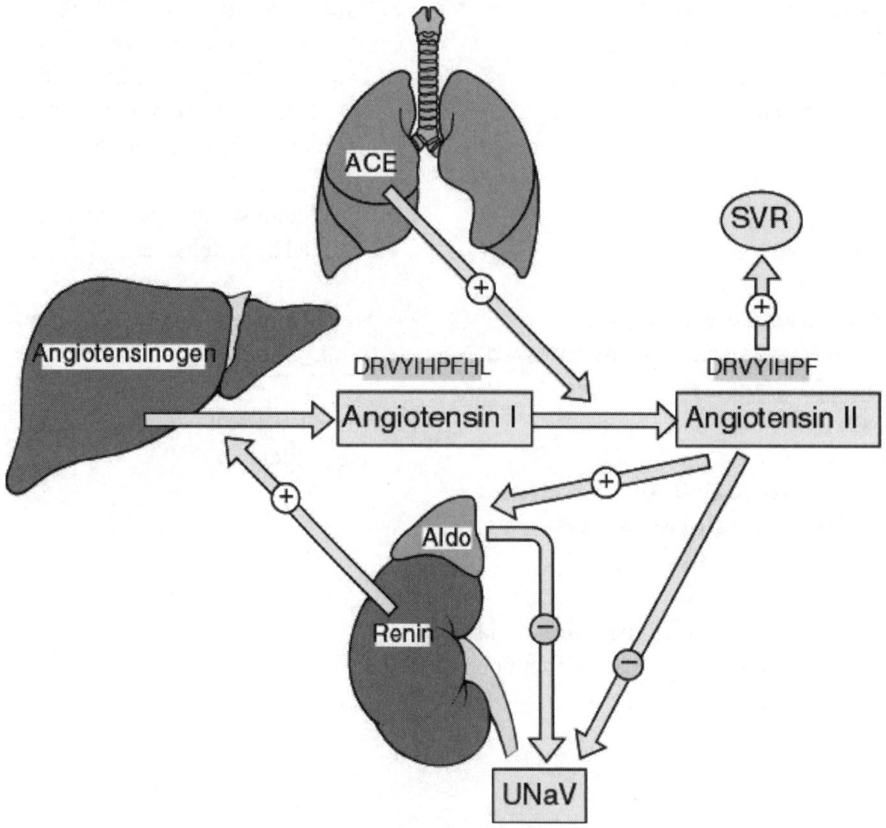

Figure 6

Atherosclerotic renovascular disease

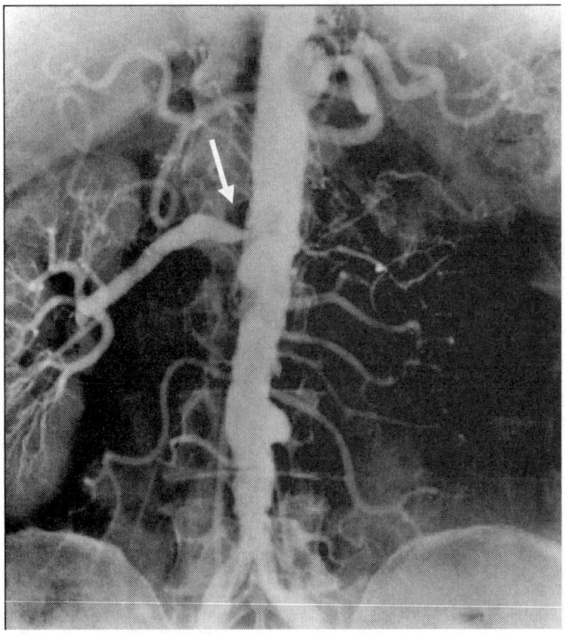

High-grade stenosis in solitary kidney

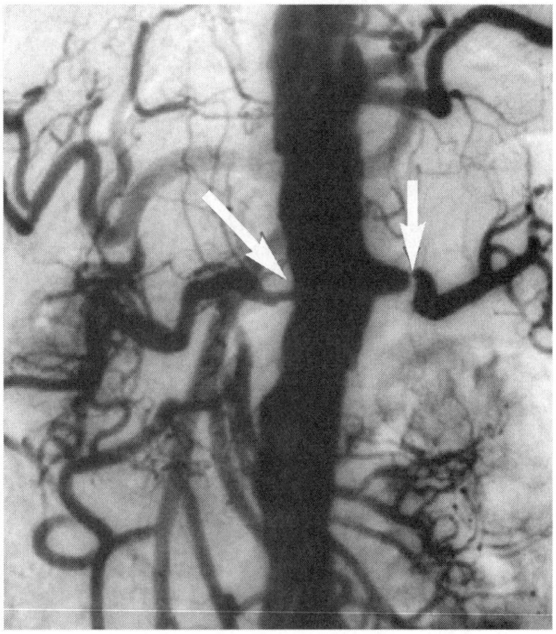

High-grade bilateral stenosis

Collateral circulation common

Progression common

Homogenous collar of elastic tissue at junction of media and adventitia

More focal than medial hyperplasia, but there may be multiple constricted areas

c. Intimal fibroplasia (Figure 8)

Focal, concentric, long stenosis

Appearance of vasculitis, distinguished by lack of markers of inflammation and isolation to renal vessels only

Children and adolescents

Collagen inside elastic membrane

May dissect

Progression common

d. Adventitial (periarterial or fibromuscular)

Rarest

Children and adolescents

Frequently progressive

Sharply demarcated areas of stenosis

Figure 7

Medial fibroplasia

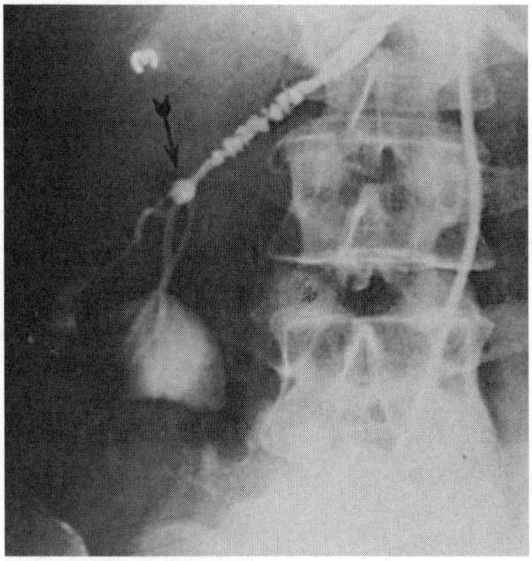

- Most common fibrous
- Women 25-50
- Commonly bilateral
- "String of beads"
- Involves distal two-thirds and "branches"
- Progression less common

Figure 8

Perimedial fibroplasia

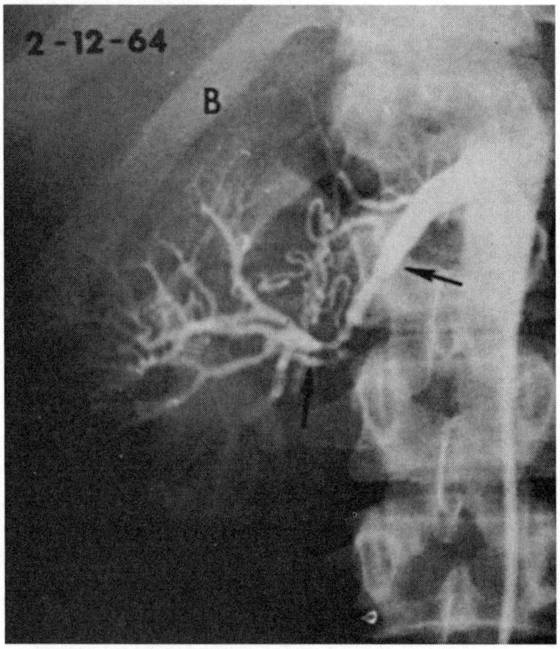

- Women aged 15-30
- Collateral circulation common
- Tight stenosis and progression common

Figure 9

Intimal fibroplasia

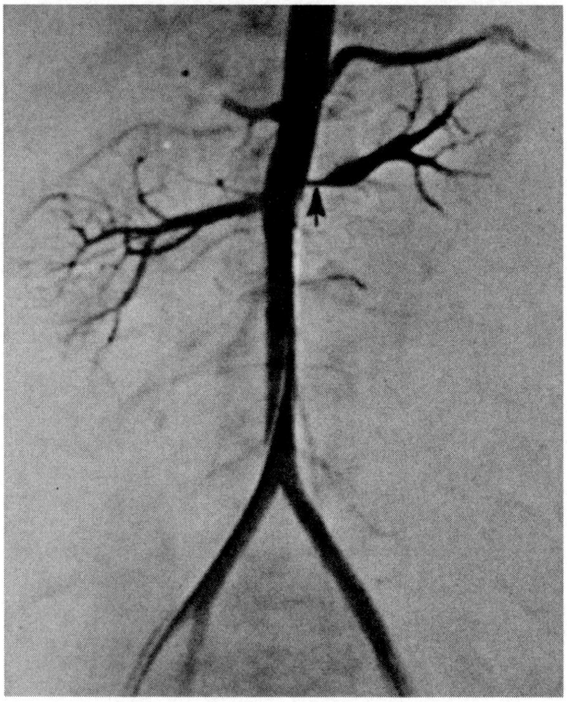

- Children and adolescents
- Collagen inside elastic membrane
- May dissect
- Progression common

4. Clinical Evaluation

A. When to Consider Evaluation for RVH (Chobanian, 2003.) (Figure 10)

1. Onset of hypertension <30 yo or >55 yo

2. Abdominal bruit, especially if a diastolic component is present

3. Accelerated hypertension/malignant crisis

4. Hypertension that had been easy to control becomes resistant

5. Recurrent flash pulmonary edema

6. Azotemia of uncertain etiology (especially if no proteinuria)

7. Acute renal failure precipitated by ace inhibitor (ACEI) or angiotensin receptor blocker (ARB)

8. Lack of family history

9. Disseminated atherosclerotic disease

10. Renal size disparity

Figure 10

RVH diagnostic algorithm

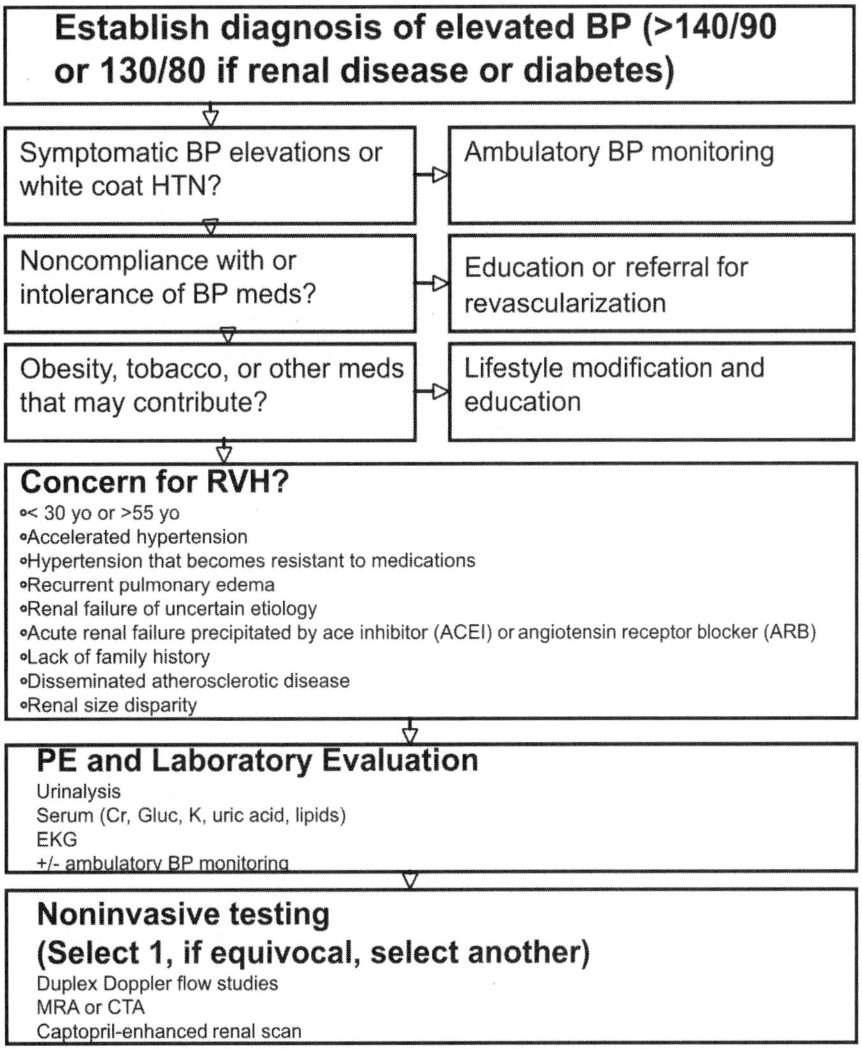

B. Screening

1. Recommendations from Seventh Report of the Joint National Committee on Prevention, Detection, Evaluation, and Treatment of High Blood Pressure

a. Urinalysis, serum studies (Cr, glucose, K, uric acid, lipids) and electrocardiogram (EKG), +/- ambulatory BP monitoring

b. Recommended noninvasive options include: Captopril-enhanced renal scan, duplex Doppler flow studies, and magnetic angiography

c. "While renal artery angiography remains the gold standard for identifying the anatomy of the renal artery, it is not recommended for diagnosis alone because of the risk associated with the procedure. At the time of intervention, an arteriogram will be performed using limited contrast to confirm the stenosis and identify the anatomy of the renal artery."

2. Noninvasive tests—How Good are They?

a. ACE-enhanced renal scan

- Limited value for anatomy but excellent functional study and can help predict response to surgery
- Poorer sensitivity and specificity than MR or CT

b. Duplex ultrasound (U/S)

- Diastolic blood flow velocity is measured by resistive index (RI) and suggests small vessel disease and parenchymal damage.
- If RI >0.80, revascularization unlikely to improve renal function
- Sensitivity 80%-90%; specificity 80%-90%

c. 3D contrast-enhanced MR arteriogram

- Poor visualization of distal arteries, but sensitivity and specificity of >90% for proximal arterial segments; thus better for atherosclerotic lesions vs. fibromuscular dysplasia
- Sensitivity 88%-100%; specificity 75%-100%
- Uses gadolinium – non-nephrotoxic

d. Spiral CT Arteriogram

- Sensitivity 94%-100%; specificity 92%-99%
- Contrast media—risk of nephrotoxicity

3. Invasive Tests—How Good are They?

a. Angiography

- Significant inter-observer variability in determining what is a "clinically significant" lesion

b. Selective renal vein sampling for renin:

- If renal vein (RV) renin lateralizes to one kidney, the likelihood of favorable blood pressure improvement after revascularization is >90%, but if RV renin fails to lateralize, the likelihood of benefit is still near 50%

5. Medical and Surgical Management

A. Medical

1. Most patients are already on multiple-drug therapy when they are referred

2. Select medical management based on risk of ischemic nephropathy and lesion progression

   a. Medial fibroplasia and atherosclerotic (without ischemic nephropathy) best for medical management

3. ATII and aldosterone play a direct role in end organ damage to kidney, peripheral vessels and heart, therefore, drug treatment can be targeted at interrupting this cycle—ARBs, ACE-I, and beta blockade important first line drugs

   a. If goal BPs can be achieved with ARB/ACEI, outcomes are comparable to surgical revascularization

4. Aggressive lifestyle modification and health management necessary: smoking cessation, lipid management, diabetes control

5. Possible regression of atherosclerotic disease with aggressive lipid management and smoking cessation

B. Surgical: PRTA, Stenting, Revascularization

1. Reserved for Situations Where:

   a. BP not controlled with meds, or patient does not tolerate meds

Figure 11

RVD treatment algorithm: medical and surgical management

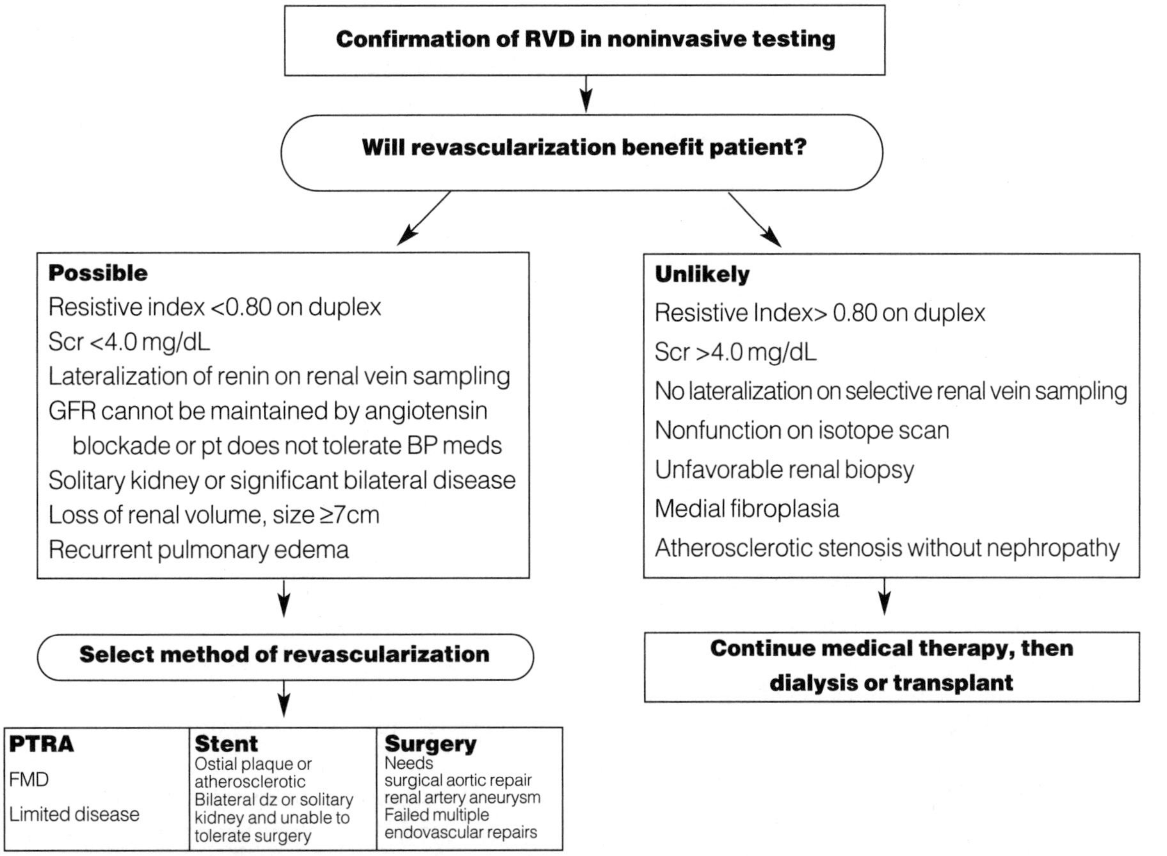

b. ARBs/ACE-I significantly reduce GFR (by >30% or increased Cr by >0.5mg/dL) by loss of compensatory filtration pressure

c. Significant bilateral, or solitary kidney, renal stenosis

d. Recurrent, difficult to control, congestive heart failure

e. Loss of renal volume over time, but kidney size still at least 7 cm

f. Function on isotope scan

g. Favorable renal biopsy

h. Collateral circulation

i. SCr< 4.0 mg/dL

2. Percutaneous Transluminal Renal Artery Angioplasty (PTRA)

a. Poor outcome for ostial atherosclerotic lesions (29%)

b. Little benefit over medical treatment alone in prospective trials for atherosclerotic RVD

c. First-line approach with fibromuscular dysplasia

d. Restenosis rates 7%-27% except for atherosclerotic lesions (near 50% restenosis rate)

3. Stenting

a. Better outcomes for ostial lesions vs. PTRA alone (75%)

b. Expected improvements in BPs in well-selected patients about 25/10 mm Hg

c. CORAL trial (Cardiovascular Outcomes in Renal Artery Lesions)—compares medical management with and without stenting; accrual underway.

d. Restenosis rates 10%-15%, coated stents may perform better

e. Post-stent acute decline in renal function in 10%-20% of patients likely from cholesterol atheroembolism

f. For patients with significant bilateral disease or solitary kidneys, stenting associated with non-significant improvements in GFR, nearly 10% restensosis, 5% dissection, but significant decreases in BP

4. Surgical Revascularization

a. Major indications:

- Patients undergoing surgical aortic repair
- Patients with renal artery aneurysm–risk of rupture: absent/incomplete calcification, >2 cm diameter, expanding, hypertension, pregnancy
- Multiple failed endovascular repairs

b. In most series of patients with impaired renal function before revascularization, little or no recovery of GFR follows either surgical or endovascular restoration of blood flow

c. Signs of reversibility

- Progressive occlusion
- Collaterals
- Retrograde arterial filling
- Size >7 cm
- Cr < 4.0
- Preservation of glomeruli on biopsy

c. Technical success 89%-97%

d. Hypertension control for patients with fibromuscular dysplasia undergoing surgical repair:

cured = 33%-63%;
improved = 24%-57%;
failure to improve = 3%-33%

e. Retrospective studies suggest similar moderate and long-term outcomes between endovascular and open revascularization

f. Graft thrombosis rate ~4%, perioperative mortality ~3% (Fergany, 1995)

g. Surgical approaches (Figure 10)

- Hepatorenal
- Splenorenal
- Ileorenal
- Arteriotomy
- Aortorenal
- Thoracic aorta—renal

Figure 12

Techniques for surgical revascularization in ARAS

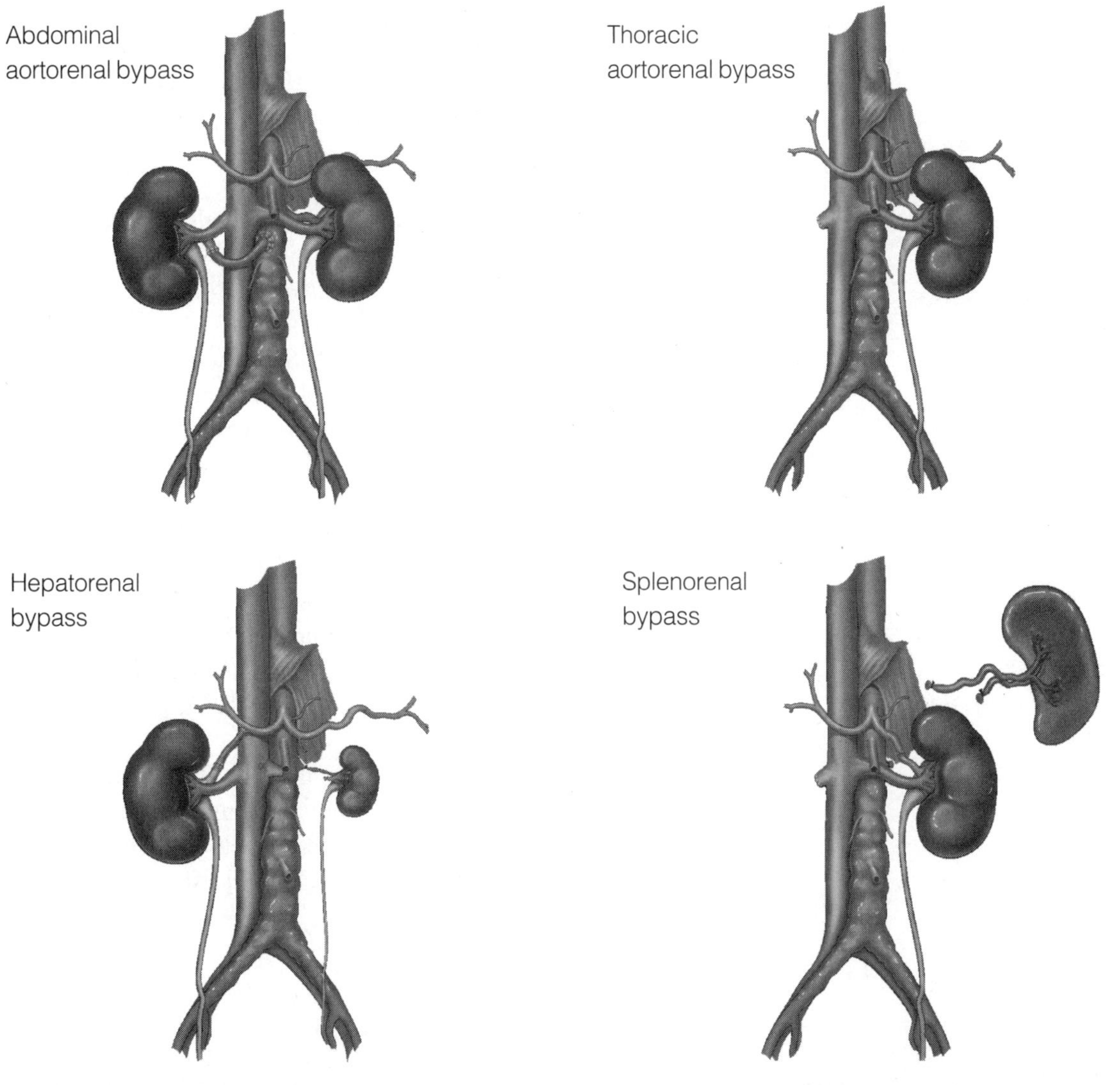

5. Other Surgical Interventions

a. Nephrectomy if small and nonfunctioning

b. Autotransplantation an option in young patients with complicated anatomy (Sevmis, 2006)

6. Further Reading

Anderson CA, Hansen KJ, Benjamin ME, Keith DR, Craven TE, Dean RH. Renal artery fibromuscular dysplasia: results of current surgical therapy. *J Vasc Surg*. 1995;22:207-216.

Anderson GH, Blakemen N, Streeten DH. The effect of age on prevalence of secondary forms of hypertension in 4429 consecutively referred patients. *J Hypertens*. 1994;12:609-615.

Atkinson AB, Davies DL, Leckie B, et al. Hyponatremic hypertensive syndrome with renal artery occlusion corrected by captopril. *Lancet*.1979;2:606-609.

Basso N, Tarragno NA. History about the discovery of the renin-angiotensin system. *Hypertension*. 2001;38:1246-1249.

Berglund G. Secondary hypertension in the community. In: Birkenhager WH, Reid JL, eds. *Handbook of Hypertension*. Amsterdam, Netherlands: Elsevier; 1985:249-254.

Brunner HR, Kirshmann JD, Sealey JE, Laragh JH. Hypertension of renal origin: evidence for two different mechanisms. *Science*. 1971;188:1316-1317.

Chabova V, Schirger A, Stanson AW, McKusick M, Textor SC. Outcomes of atherosclerotic renal artery stenosis managed without revascularization. *Mayo Clin Proc*. 2000;75:437-444.

Chobanian AV, Bakris GL, Black HR, et al and the National High Blood Pressure Education Program Coordinating Committee. Seventh Report of the Joint National Committee on Prevention, Detection: Evaluation, and Treatment of High Blood Pressure. *Hypertension*. 2003;42;1206-1252.

DeForrest JM, Knappenberger RC, Antonaccio MJ, Ferrone RA, Creekmore JS. Angiotensin II is a necessary component for the development of hypertension in the two-kidney, one-clip rat. *Am J Cardiol*. 1982;49:1515-1517.

EdwardsMS, Craven TE, Burke GL, RH Dean, Hansen KJ. Renovascular Disease and the Risk ofAdverse Coronary Events in the Elderly: A Prospective, Population-Based Study. *Arch Intern Med*. 2005;165:207-213.

Fergany A, Kolettis P, Novick AC. The contemporary role of extra-anatomical surgical renal revascularization in patients with atherosclerotic renal artery disease. *J Urol*. 1995;153(6):1798-1802.

Forbes JM, Hewitson TD, Becker GJ, Jones CL. Simultaneous blockade of endothelin A and B receptors in ischemic acute renal failure is detrimental to long-term kidney function. *Kidney Int*. 2001;59: 1333-1341.

Galaria II, Surowiec SM, Rhodes JM, et al. Percutaneous and open renal revascularizations have equivalent long-term functional outcomes. *Ann Vasc Surgery*. 2005;19(2):218-228.

Gavras H, Brunner HR, Thurston H, Laragh JH. Reciprocation of renin dependency with sodium volume dependency in renal hypertension. *Science*. 1975;188:1316-1317.

Gavras H, Brunner HR, Vaughan ED, Laragh JH. Angiotensin-sodiuminteraction in blood pressure maintenance of renal hypertensive and normotensive rats. Science. 1973;180:1369-1370.

Goldblatt H, Lynch J, Hanzal RE, Summerville WW. Studies on experimental hypertension, I: The production of persistent elevation of systolic blood pressure bymeans of renal ischemia. *J Exp Med*. 1934;59:347-379.

Iantorno M, Pola R, Schinzari F, et al. Association between altered circadian blood pressure profile and cardiac end-organ damage in patients with renovascular hypertension. *Cardiology*. 2003;100:114-119.

Isles CG, Robertson S, Hill D. Management of renovascular disease: a review of renal artery stenting in ten studies. *QJM*. 1999;92:159-167.

Kashyap VS, Sepulveda RN, Bena JF, et al. The management of renal artery atherosclerosis for renal savage: Does stenting help? *J Vasc Surg*. 2007; 45(1):101-108.

Kennedy DJ, Colyer WR, Brewster PS, et al. Renal insufficiency as a predictor of adverse events and mortality after renal artery stent placement. *Am J Kidney Dis*. 2003;14:926-935.

Krishnamurthi V, Novick AC, Myles JL. Atheroembolic disease: effect onmorbidity and survival after-revascularization for atherosclerotic renal artery stenosis. *J Urol*. 1999;161:1093-1096.

Leiner T, de Haan MW, Nelemans PH, van Engelshoven JMA, Vasbinder GBC. Contemporary imaging techniques for the diagnosis of renal artery stenosis. *Eur Radiol*. 2005;15:2219-2229.

Leung DA, Hagspiel KD, Angle JF, Spinsoa DH, Matsumoto AH, Butty S. MR angiography of the renal arteries. *Radiol Clin North Am*. 202;40: 847-865.

Martinez AG, Novick AC, Hayes JM. Surgical treatment of renal artery stenosis after failed percutaneous transluminal angioplasty. *J Urol*. 1990; 144:1094-1096.

Mounier-Vehier C, Cocketeaux B, Haulon S, et al. Changes in renal blood flow reserve after angioplasty of renal artery stensosis in hypertensive patients. *Kidney Int*. 2004;65:245-250.

Novick AC, Ziegelbaum M, Vidt DG, Gifford RW Jr, Pohl MA, Goormastic M. Trends in surgical revascularization for renal artery disease: ten years' experience. *JAMA*. 1987;257:498-501.

Olin JW, Melia M, Young JR, Graor R, Risius B. Prevalence of atherosclerotic RAS in patients with atherosclerosis elsewhere. *Am J Med*. 1990; 88:46N-51N.

Plouin PF, Chatellier G, Darne B, Raynaud A. Blood pressure outcome of angioplasty in atherosclerotic renal artery stenosis: a randomized trial. *Hypertension*. 1998;31:822-829.

Postma CT, Joosten FB, Rosenbusch G, Thien T. Magnetic resonance angiography has a high reliability in the detection of renal artery stenosis. *Am J Hypertens*. 1997;10:957-963.

Radermacher J, Chavan A, Bleck J, et al. Use of Doppler ultrasonography to predict the outcome of therapy for renal-artery stenosis. *N Engl J Med*. 2001;344:410-417.

Rihal CD, Textor SC, Breen JF, McKusick MA, Grill DE, Hallett JW, Holmes DR. Incidental renal artery stenosis among a prospective cohort of hypertensive patients undergoing coronary angiography. *Mayo Clin Proc*. 2002;77:309-1316.

Rossi GP, Cesari M, Chiesura-Corona M, Miotto D, Semplicini A, Pessina AC. Renal vein renin measurements accurately identify renovascular hypertension caused by total occlusion of the renal artery. *J Hypertens*. 2002;20:975-984.

Safian RD, Textor SC. Renal artery stenosis. *N Engl J Med*. 2001;344:431-442.

Sevmis S, Karakayali H, Boyvat F, Aytekin C, Haberal M. Renal autotransplantation for the treatment of complex renovascular hypertension. *Transplant Proc*. 2006;38(10):3412-3415.

Slovut DP, Olin JW. Fibromuscular dysplasia. *N Engl J Med*. 2004;350:1862-1871.

Stanley JC. Surgical treatment of renovascular hypertension. *Am J Surg*. 1997;174:102-110.

Strong CG, Junt JC, Sheps SG, Tucker RM, Beratz PE. Renal venous renin activity: enhancement of sensitivity of lateralization by sodium depletion. *Am J Cardiol*. 1971:27:602-611.

Textor SC, Wilcox CS. Renal artery stenosis: a common, treatable cause of renal failure? *Ann Rev Med*. 2001;52:421-422.

Tollefson DFJ, Emst CB. Natural history of atherosclerotic renal artery stensosis associated with aortic disease. *J Vasc Surg*. 1991;14:327-331.

Uzzo RG, Novick AC, Goormastic M, Mascha E, Pohl M. Medical versus surgicalmanagement of atherosclerotic renal artery stenosis. *Transplant Proc*. 2002;34:723-725.

Van de Ven PJ, Kaatee R, et al. Arterial stenting and balloon angioplasty in ostial atherosclerotic renovascular disease: a randomized trial. *Lancet*. 1999;144:1094-1096.

Van Jaarsveld BC, Krijnen P, Pieterman H, et al for the Dutch Renal Artery Stenosis Intervention Cooperative Study Group. The effect of balloon angioplasty on hypertension in atherosclerotic renal-artery stenosis. *N Engl J Med*. 2000;34:1007-1014.

Van Jaarsveld BC, Pieterman H, Can Dijk LC, et al. Inter-observer variability in the angiographic assessment of renal artery stenosis. DRASTIC study group. Dutch Renal Artery Stenosis Intervention Cooperative. *J Hypertens*. 1999;17:1731-1736.

Vasbinder GB, Nelemans PJ, Kessels AG, Kroon AA, De Leeuw PW, van Engelshoven JM. Diagnostic tests for renal artery stenosis in patients suspected of having renovascular hypertension: ameta-analysis. *Ann Intern Med*. 2001;135:401-411.

Webster J, Marshall F, Abdalla M, et al. Randomised comparison of percutaneous angioplasty vs. continued medical therapy for hypertensive patients with atheromatous renal artery stenosis. *J Hum Hypertens*. 1998;12:329-335.

Working Group on Renovascular Hypertension. Detection, evaluation, and treatment of renovascular hypertension. Final Report. *Arch Intern Med*. 1987;147:820-829.

Zoccali C, Mallamaci F, Finocchiaro P. Atherosclerotic renal artery stenosis: epidemiology, cardiovascular outcomes, and clinical prediction rules. *J Am Soc Nephrol*. 2002;13:S179-S183.

7. Questions

1. Which of the following is more likely to be associated with renovascular hypertension?

A. Positive family history

B. Mild hypertension

C. Age of onset of 22 for hypertension

D. BP well controlled with a diuretic alone

E. Kidneys equal size by ultrasound

2. Which of the following does NOT increase the risk of renal artery aneurysm rupture?

A. Pregnancy

B. 1.5 cm diameter

C. Incomplete calcification

D. Size increased from 3 months ago

E. Untreated hypertension

3. Which of the following increases the likelihood that renal revascularization for ischemic nephropathy will improve renal function?

A. Unilateral disease

B. Use of a drug eluting stent

C. Kidney size < 7 cm

D. Cr >5.0 mg/dL

E. Retrograde arterial filling on angiogram

Answers

1. C.

2. B.

3. E.

Chapter 9: Renal Transplantation

Daniel A. Shoskes, MD, FRCS(C)
Alain Duclos, MD

Contents

1. Introduction

A. Renal transplantation is usually the preferred form of renal replacement therapy, as it significantly improves life expectancy

- Relative risk of mortality

*All dialysis patients	1.00
*Patients on waiting list	0.4
*Cadaveric kidney transplant	0.32
*Living kidney transplant	0.21

B. The surgical procedure and its associated medical management (immunosuppression) are cost effective if the transplanted organ lasts more than 2 years

C. The immunosuppressive agents used to prevent transplant rejection introduce complications on their own:

- Infections
- Cancer
- Diabetes
- Hypertension
- Coronary artery disease

2. Basic Transplantation Immunology

A. The immune system has evolved mechanisms to recognize potential threats:

- Recognition of determinants that do not belong to the host (self vs. nonself theory)
- Recognition of situation associated with potential threats such as inflammation, to the host (safe vs. danger theory)

B. Based on animal skin grafts, the laws of transplantation were discovered

- Isografts (tissue from the same individual or from an identical twin) succeed
- Xenografts (tissue from different species) fail immediately
- Allografts (different individual from within the same species) fail over variable time

C. The immune system has evolved 2 distinct ways to recognize and to respond to danger that may threaten the host:

- Innate immunity
  - * Recognizes inflammation and tissue destruction
  - * Can recognize and target specific structures on certain organisms (bacteria, tumor cells)
  - * Not associated with immune memory: the next encounter with the same organisms will not be more rapid or more effective
  - * Cells and mechanisms:
    - Macrophages
    - Monocytes
    - Polymorphonuclear cells (PMN)
    - Complement
    - NK (natural killer) cells
- Acquired immunity
  - * Recognizes and responds to specific targets (antigens)
  - * Activation generates effector cells (cytotoxic T-lymphocytes and plasma cells) together with memory cells
  - * Associated with long-lasting memory: the next encounter with similar organisms will be faster and more effective

* Consist of:
    • T-cells, B-cells (cellular arm)
    • Antibodies (humoral arm)

D. Antigen Recognition

• Antigen recognition is central to the generation of both specific effector and memory cells

• By T-cells
  * Larger molecule (antigen) must be broken down into smaller peptide fragments that T-cells can recognize specifically and then respond to:

    • The receptor at the surface of the T-cells is called the T-cell receptor (TCR) (Figure 1)

    • The peptides must be displayed by specialized antigen-presenting cells (APCs)

• The APCs will also express other molecules required for T-cell activation (so-called "second-signal")

• After successful antigen recognition:
  * Clonal proliferation of T-cells and generation of memory cells
  * Cytotoxic T lymphocytes (usually CD8 molecule on their surface) can kill target cells via cell-surface acting molecules (perforins)
  * Helper T lymphocytes (usually bearing the CD4 molecule on their surface) secrete cytokines required for both CD8 T cells and B-cells activation

• By B cells
  * Receptor is a surface immunoglobulin (sIg)
  * sIg, unlike the TCR, can "see" the whole antigen by recognizing its tertiary structure
  * There is no need for antigen processing for recognition
  * Cytokines from helper T-cells are required for B-cell activation, together with antigen recognition by the B-cells
  *After successful antigen recognition

• Clonal proliferation of B-cells and generation of memory cells

Figure 1

T-cell – APC interaction

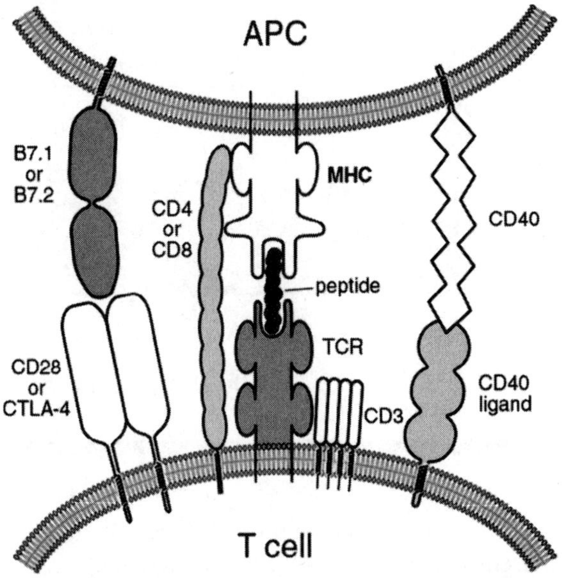

• Plasma cell generation: terminally differentiated cells that produce large quantity of antigen-specific antibody

E. Human Leukocyte Antigens (HLA)

• Group of genes on chromosome 6 also known as the human major histocompatibility complex (MHC) (Figure 2)

• Highly polymorphic

• Class I
  * The major antigens are HLA-A, B and C and are made of more than 1200 alleles
  * They display intracellular peptides and interact with CD8 T-cells

• Class II
  * The major antigens are HLA-DP, DQ and DR and are made of more than 700 alleles
  * MHC class II display extracellular peptides and interact with CD4 T-cells

• APCs are further divided into professional (dendritic cells, macrophages and B-cells) or nonprofessional (fibroblasts, vascular endothelial cells)

Figure 2

Polymorphism of HLA locus

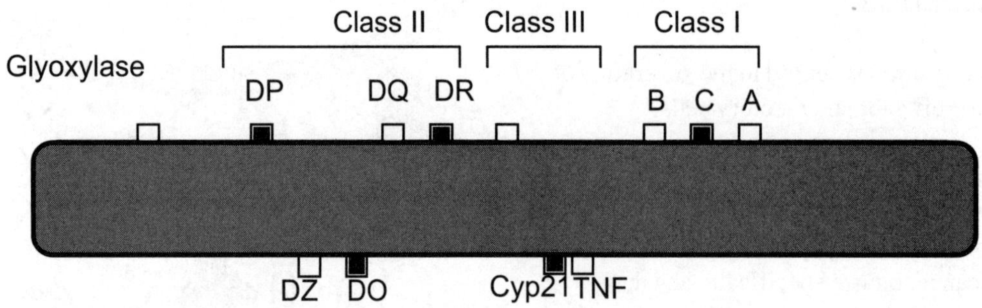

Short arm of chromosome 6: HLA complex

depending on whether or not they need activation to present antigen. In area of tissue injury, more cells can function as APCs

F. T-cell Education

- The TCR is randomly generated, including potentially auto-reacting cells

- Mechanisms are in place to limit the presence of such autoreactive cells

- In the thymus
  - * There is positive selection for T-cells expressing a TCR that binds to self MHC (so they can all function properly)
  - * There is negative selection for T-cells expressing a TCR that very tightly binds to self MHC (would auto-react)

- In periphery
  - * The thymus can obviously not display every antigen present in the organism: other mechanisms must be present to prevent autoimmune cells
  - * When a T-cell recognizes an auto antigen without a second signal, it is turned off (anergy) or dies (deletion)

G. Immune Cell Activation

- Macrophages, monocytes and dendritic
  - * Professional APCs (see above)
  - * They are among the first cells to respond to injury by localizing to sites of trauma
  - * They release chemoattractant molecules and increase the level of responsiveness of the immune system through cytokines such as tumor necrosis factor (TNF) and interleukin-1 (IL-1)

- After CD4 T-cells recognize antigen, they release IL-2 and interferon-gamma (INF gamma), leading to clonal expansion and activation of both B- and T- cells

- T-cell activation will generate antigen specific cytotoxic T lymphocytes which can kill foreign cells

- Activated B-cells become plasma cells (antibody factories) and memory B-cells (for more rapid response to the same antigen later on)

- Molecular mechanisms for CD4 T-cell activation
  - * Proper CD4-MHC engagement together with second signal (CD28) will lead to increased intracellular ionized calcium from both intracellular and extracellular stores. The CD3 complex, associated to the TCR, is central to those early events.

* The increase in intracellular calcium will cause activation of calcineurin, a calcium-dependent phosphatase (calcineurin)
* The activated calcineurin will then dephosphorylate a transcription factor (NFAT: Nuclear Factor of Activated T-cells) sequestered in the cytoplasm, exposing its nuclear translocation signal, allowing its export to the nucleus of the cell
* NFAT in the nucleus then increases the transcription of a number of genes required for T-cell activation, among which IL-2

3. Immunosuppressive Drugs

A. Immunosuppression

- Required for the life of the transplanted kidney to prevent rejection

- Modern protocols combine several agents acting at different sites of the immune response have dropped rates of acute rejection to 10% and increased 1-year graft survival to 90%

- Figure 3 presents the activation of the immune system, together with the proposed site of action of each drug

- Total immunosuppression dose increases the risk of infections and certain malignancies

- Each immunosuppressive drug has its specific non-immune side effects

B. Antibody Agents

- Anti-IL-2 receptor antoginists (non depleting, because the cells are inactivated by not killed)
    * Daclizumab (Zenapax®), basiliximab (Simulect®)
    * Monoclonal antibody that binds to part of the IL-2 receptor surface of T-cell, thus preventing IL-2 from activating T-cells
    * Given at time of transplant and for 1-5 additional doses to prevent (but not treat) rejection
    * These agents have minimal drug specific side effects

- Depleting agents (kill cells)
    * ***OKT3 (Muromonab)***
        - Murine monoclonal antibody against human CD3
        - Prevents the function of the CD3 complex, blocking T-cell activation
        - Used to prevent and treat acute rejection episodes
        - Side effects:
            * Anaphylactic reactions
            * Cytokine release syndrome: fever, chills, malaise, hypotension
            * Infection (cytomegalovirus, CMV)
            * Malignancies (post-transplant lymphoproliferative disorders, PTLD)

Figure 3

Immune system activation and action sites of specific immunosuppressants

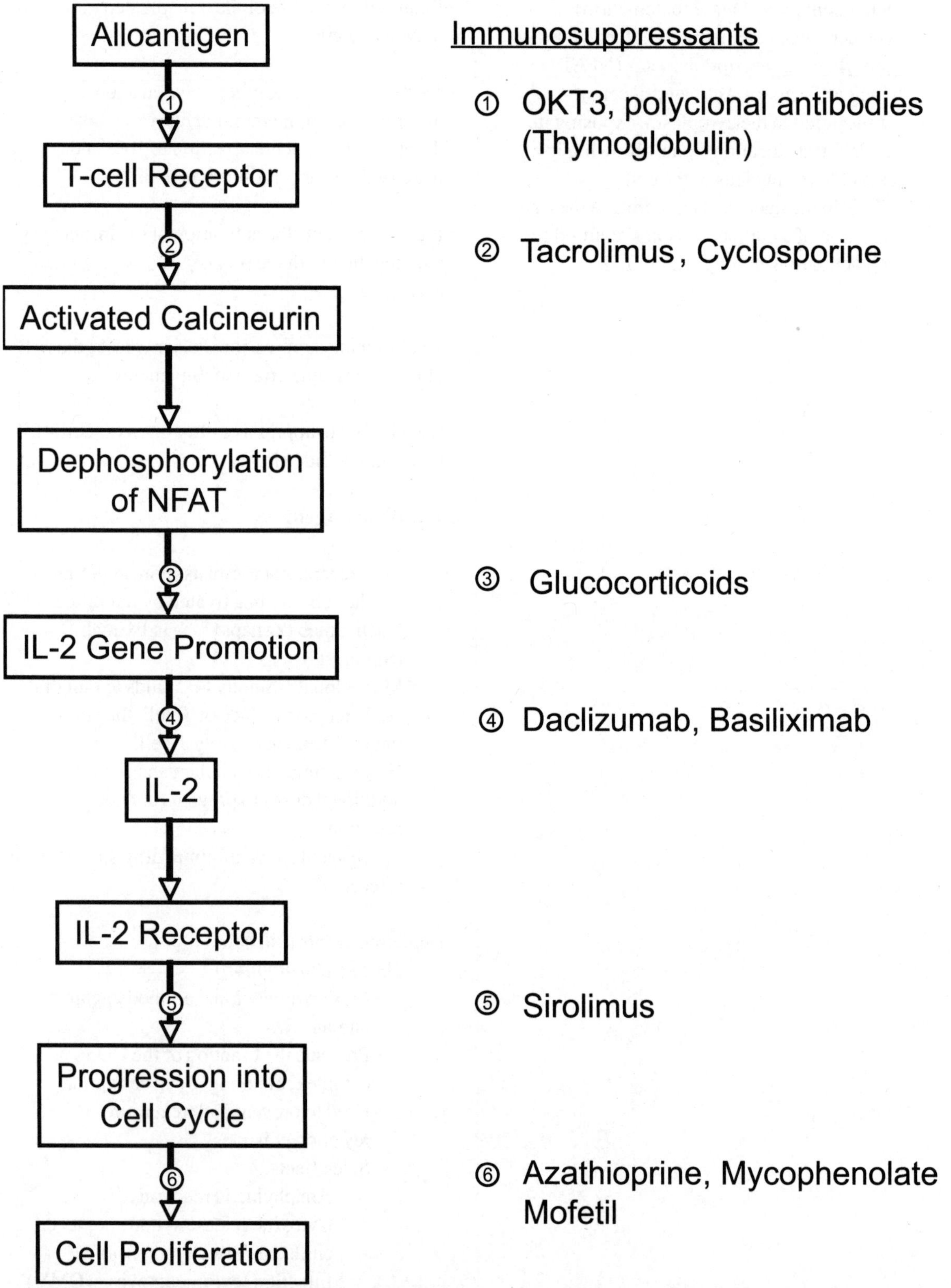

* *Thymoglobulin*
    - Polyclonal antibodies made by immunizing rabbits with human thymocytes
    - Mixture of antibodies against various cell surface antigens
    - Cause profound depletion of T-cells, affecting the functioning of the immune system for weeks
    - Premedication with corticosteroid, acetaminophen and antihistamine is recommended and may reduce the incidence and intensity of side effects
    - Can be used for both induction and to treat acute rejection episodes
    - Side effects:
        * Myelosuppression: leucopenia, thrombocytopenia
        * Cytokine release syndrome: fever, chills, malaise
        * Infection (CMV)
        * Malignancies (post-transplant lymphoproliferative disorders)

C. Calcineurin Inhibitors (CNI)

- Foundation of modern immunosuppression to prevent allograft rejection

- 2 molecules: cyclosporine (Neoral®, Gengraf®) and tacrolimus (Prograf®)

- Interfere with IL-2 gene transcription, by preventing NFAT activation, thus preventing T-cell activation early on

- Side effects
    * Overall relatively similar: both are nephrotoxic, can cause hypertension, reversible neurotoxicity and metabolic abnormalities
    * Cosmetic changes (hirsuitism, gingival hyperplasia and coarsening of facial features) may be more pronounced with cyclosporine
    * Higher incidence of diabetes may be associated with tacrolimus

- Tacrolimus associated with better graft survival in high risk patients

D. Pharmacology and Pharmacokinetic

- Use of these drugs require close monitoring of blood level in order to minimize side effects

- Best correlation between dose and side effect profile is through precise monitoring of the area under the curve (AUC)

- Best approximation of AUC for cyclosporine is through the use of C2 blood level (level found in blood 2h after PO dose)

- Approximation of AUC with trough level (level found in blood just before next dose) is usually used for tacrolimus

- Metabolism is largely hepatic

- Cyclosporine
    * Oral dose: 5-10 mg/kg/day divided BID
    * Target trough 275-350 ng/ml, drop to 175-200 after 6 months

- Prograf
    *Oral dose: 0.1-0.15 mg/kg/day divided BID
    * Target trough 10-15 ng/ml, drop to 6-10 after 6 months

- IV dose is generally one-quarter to one-third of total daily oral dose

- Significant drug interaction, from extensive hepatic metabolism (CYP3A4 enzyme systems)
    * Drugs that may increase blood concentration
    * Calcium channel blockers: diltiazem, verapamil, nifedipine, nicardipine
    * Azole antifungal agents: clotrimazole, fluconazole, itraconazole, ketoconazole, voriconazole
    * Macrolide antibiotics: clarithromycin, erythromycin
    * Other: grapefruit juice, metoclopramide, allopurinol

- Drugs that may decrease blood concentration
    * Anticonvulsivant: carbamazepine, phenobarbital, phenytoin
    * Antibiotics: rifampin, rifabutin, nacfillin

E. Antimetabolites

- These agents interfere with both T- and B-cell proliferation after cellular activation by interfering with nucleotide synthesis required for DNA replication

- Mycophenolate mofetil (CellCept®, Myfortic®) has largely replaced azathioprine (Imuran®) as agent of choice

- Commonly used in combination to prevent acute cellular rejection.

- Side effects
  *Leucopenia and anemia
  *Diarrhea

- Dosage: 1-2 g PO/IV per day

F. Corticosteroids

- Known to prolong allograft survival since 1951

- Mechanism of action is complex and likely involves blockade of multiple inflammatory cytokines at many stages of the activation of the immune system

- Low dose blocks IL-1; high dose blocks IL-2 as well

- Side effects
  * Acne
  * Adrenal cortex suppression
  * Cataracts
  * Dermal atrophy
  * Femoral head aseptic necrosis
  * Glaucoma
  * Glucose intolerance/diabetes mellitus
  * Growth retardation (children)
  * Hirsuitism
  * Hyperlipidemia
  * Hypertension
  * Increased appetite
  * Osteoporosis
  * Peptic ulcers
  * Water and salt retention

- Dosage:
  * High initial dose tapered over weeks or months
  * Solumedrol (250 mg IV every 12 hours for 3 doses) is frequently used perioperatively, then PO prednisone is gradually tapered to 0.1 mg/kd/day over a few months

G. Rapamycin (Sirolimus)

- Most recent immunosuppressive agent introduced

- Distinct mechanism of action from previous immunosuppressive agents: interferes with a cell-cycle specific regulatory kinase (mTOR: mammalian target of rapamycin)

- Dosage: 5-10 mg PO daily

- Blood level
  * Initially 12-15 ng/mL during the first 4 months after transplant
  *4-12 ng/mL thereafter

- Side effects
  * Anemia, leucopenia
  * Hypercholesterolemia
  * Wound complications

H. Acute Rejection

- Suspect rejection after other causes of transplant dysfunction have been ruled out:
  * Dehydration
  * Bacterial or viral infection
  * Drug toxicity
  * Obstruction
  * ATN

- Diagnosis of acute rejection requires a kidney transplant biopsy, usually performed with local anesthesia under ultrasound guidance

- The Banff 97 classification is used to grade the histopathological severity of rejection
  * Grade I: Cellular rejection; interstitial inflammation (>25% of parenchyma) and tubulitis (>4 lymphocytes/tubular cross-section)

* Grade II: Vascular rejection; intimal arteritis
* Grade III: Necrosis; transmural arteritis, arterial fibrinoid necrosis

• Treatment of acute rejection
  * ***Steroidpulse***
    • Will reverse about 75% of first acute rejection, especially if Banff I
    • Typical regimen:
      * 500 mg-1g IV methylprednisolone for 3 days
      * 120-250 mg IV methylprednisolone or PO prednisone for 3-5 days
  * ***Antibody treatment***
    • OKT3 or Thymoglobulin will reverse about 90% of first acute rejection: greater effectiveness at the expense of more side effects
    • Generally reserved for more severe rejection (Banff II or Banff III) or Banff I that does not improve with steroids

• Antibody-mediated acute rejection
  * Immunofluorescence will reveal IgG, sometimes IgM and C3 in the wall of arteries
  * Diffuse peritubular capillary staining for C4d
  * ***Treatment should be aggressive***
    • OKT3/thymoglobulin
    • Intravenous immunoglobulin (IVIg)
    • Plasmapheresis
    • Anti-B cell antibodies

4. Recipient Evaluation

A. Contraindications to Kidney Transplant

• Malignancy
  * Immunosuppressive drugs may unfavorably influence natural history of the malignancy
  * Recommended tumor-free waiting periods for common malignancies
    • Kidney
      * Incidental: no waiting
      * Large, infiltrating lesion: at least 2 years
      * Wilm's tumor: at least 2 years
      * May be wise to remove complex cystic mass before transplant
    • Bladder
      * *In situ*: no waiting
      * Invasive: at least 2 years
      * Beware the need for BCG in immunosuppressed patients
    • Testis, prostate: at least 2 years
    • Breast, skin melanoma, invasive cervical neoplasia: at least 5 years

• Infection
  * Chronic infection precludes transplantation
  * Osteomyelitis and diabetic foot ulcers must be addressed before transplantation
  * Tuberculosis: preferable to wait 1 year after completion of treatment
  * HIV
    • A previous absolute contraindication
    • Now being reconsidered with the success of antiretroviral therapy

• Recurrence of primary disease
  * Diabetes mellitus
    • May recur but low risk (5%-10%) of graft failure
  * Focal glomerulosclerosis
    • May recur rapidly and aggressively in up to 25% of patients after kidney transplant
    • 10%-65% risk of graft failure
  * Polycystic kidney disease
    • Will not recur unless donor also had disease (eg, sibling)
    • Recipients with headaches, other central nervous system symptoms or familial history of aneurysms should be screened for intracranial aneurysms

    • May require native nephrectomy for pain, size, infection or suspicious mass
  * Hyperoxaluria
    • Type 1 hyperoxaluria is an autosomal recessive inborn error of metabolism: missing hepatic alanine glyoxylate aminotransferase
    • Missing enzyme leads to oxalate deposition in the kidneys and eventually ESRD
    • Kidney transplant failure will rapidly occur despite very aggressive management designed to minimize oxalate deposition
    • Require combined liver-kidney transplant
  * Goodpasture's syndrome/disease
    • Autoimmune disorder characterized by glomerulonephritis, circulating anti-glomerular basement membrane (GBM) antibodies (Goodpasture's disease). If diffuse pulmonary hemorrhage is also present, it is referred to as Goodpasture's syndrome
    • Will frequently recur (histopathological evidence deposition of IgG along the glomeruli), but without functional damage to the kidney
  * IgA nephropathy (Berger's disease)
    • IgA deposition in the glomerular mesangium
    • High rate of recurrence in transplanted kidney (40%-60%), but slowly progressive, causing graft failure in 10% of patients

• Noncompliance
  * Past history of noncompliance with medical therapy: at high risk for graft loss
  * Wise to demand period of acceptable compliance before transplant

• Psychiatric illness
  * Any condition (organic mental syndromes, psychosis and mental retardation) that may impair the patient's capacity to understand the transplantation, its demands and complications may be a contraindication to transplant

• Severe extrarenal disease
  * Chronic liver disease and advanced uncorrectable heart disease are contraindications to kidney transplant, but patients may benefit from combined organ transplant
  * Chronic lung disease may prevent safe general anesthesia
  * Severe peripheral vascular disease may preclude arterial anastomosis and endanger limb

B. Urological Evaluation

• Ideally: sterile, continent and compliant urinary tract before transplant

• Obtain voiding cystourethrogram in patients with suspected abnormality

• Even very small bladder may develop normal capacity and compliance after transplantation, unless extensive fibrosis is present

• Transplant is possible with similar outcome in patients with urinary diversion or augments

• Indications for native nephrectomy:
  * Chronic or recurrent acute bacterial pyelonephritis
  * Infected stones
  * Heavy proteiunria
  * Intractable hypertension
  * Polycystic kidney disease: massive kidneys, recurrent infection or bleeding
  * Infected reflux
  * Acquired renal cystic disease with suspicion of adenocarcinoma

• Prostatic enlargement in older men
  * Prostate may be resected before transplant if the patient produces sufficient volume of urine
  * Anuric patients should not be resected: "dry TURP" syndrome (strictures and contractures)
  * Clean intermittent catheterization (CIC) is safe and effective in transplant patients

5. Living Donors

A. Living donors represent more than 50% of kidney transplants performed in the United States

B. HLA-matched cadaveric kidney fares worse than poorly matched living donor kidney

C. Potential advantages of living vs. cadaveric kidney donation

- Better short- and long-term results
- More consistent early function (less delayed graft function) and easier management
- No brain death stress on transplanted kidneys
- Reduced waiting time for recipients
- Ability to time transplant for convenience or medical reasons

D. Potential Disadvantages of Living Kidney Donation

- Immediate risk to the donor
    - * Mortality: 0.02%
    - * Major morbidity: 0.2%
    - * Minor morbidity: 10%
- Long-term morbidity
    - * Possible mild hypertension and proteinuria but rates similar to other family members
    - * Risk of traumatic injury to remaining kidney
    - * Risk of unrecognized renal disease

E. Living Donor Evaluation

- History and physical examination
- Comprehensive laboratory panel plus:
    - *Viral serology
    - *Urine analysis and culture
    - *24-h urine collection for protein and creatinine
- Psychological and social evaluation
- Abdominal/pelvic CT scan with contrast (renal anatomy) or angiogram
- Crossmatch
- Donors >50 years old: chest x-ray, cardiac stress test

F. Exclusion Criteria

- Age less than 18 or greater than 65
- Blood pressure >140/90 (or antihypertensive medication)
- Diabetes or abnormal glucose tolerance test
- Proteinuria >250 mg/day
- Measured glomerular filtration rate <80 mL/min
- Adult polycystic kidney disease families: abnormal CT scan in adult >30 years old
- Hematuria
- Recurrent urolithiasis
- Significant medical history: malignancy, chronic lung or liver disease
- History of thrombosis or thromboembolism
- Abnormal psychological evaluation

G. Donor Nephrectomy

- The best kidney stays with the donor: always transplant the kidney with minor anomaly
- Consider right donor nephrectomy in female of child-bearing age (right-sided hydronephrosis of pregnancy)
- Can be performed open or with laparoscopy
- Institutions with long experience of laparoscopic techniques have excellent outcome, comparable to open technique
- Open donor nephrectomy
    - * Pros
        - Established technique, safe and effective

  - Relatively short operating time
  - Minimal warm ischemia
  - Excellent graft function
* Cons
  - Postoperative pain
  - Longer convalescence
  - Surgical scar, with potential hernia

- Laparoscopic kidney donation
  * Pros
    - Possibly smaller incision
    - Shorter hospital stay
    - Less pain medication
    - Faster return to work
    - Increased donor acceptance
    - Excellent graft function
  * Cons
    - Longer operative time
    - Learning curve may be associated with surgical damage to the kidney
    - Shorter vessels
    - Right kidney laparoscopic nephrectomy may be more challenging
    - Pneumoperitoneum may compromise renal blood flow, with unknown long-term effects

6. Cadaveric Donors

A. Brain Death

- Since 1968, brain death criteria have been used to identify organ donor

B. Expanded Criteria Donors (ECD)

- In an attempt to reduce the discrepancy between available organs and waiting list patients, expanded criteria for cadaveric donation have been used

- An "expanded criteria donor" is:
  * Age >60
  * Age 50-60 and at least 2 of the following:
    - History of hypertension
    - Serum creatinine >1.5
    - Cause of death: cerebrovascular accident

- These organs may not benefit all transplant candidates and are often allocated to older recipients and/or those with urgent need

C. Organ Allocation

- Waiting list
  * National list for "zero mismatch" kidneys (no HLA antigens different between donor and recipient)
  * Regional list for local donors
  * For each donor, a list is generated of patients with the same blood group according to points for:
    - Waiting time
    - High antibody levels
    - Degree of HLA antigen match (esp B-DR)
    - Other local variances (eg, children)

- Tissue typing
  * Panel reactive antibody (PRA): statistical risk of positive crossmatch in a given population
  * Crossmatch
    - Assesses the presence of donor specific antibodies (DSA) in a specific donor-recipient pain
    - Cytotoxic crossmatch is performed by mixing donor cells with serum from the recipient and complement, then assessing viability of donor cells

- Flow cytometry crossmatch also assesses the presence of DSA, using HLA antigens immobilized on very small latex beads
- Flow crossmatch is more sensitive, but less specific because it may identify antibodies that won't destroy donor cells
- Reminder:
    * T-cell crossmatch assesses HLA class I Donor Specific Antibody (DSA)
    * B cell crossmatch assesses HLA class II DSA
- Potential crossmatch results
    * Positive cytotoxic T-cell crossmatch: never transplant
    * Positive T-cell flow crossmatch only: first transplant possible (antibody induction), but do not perform re-do
    * Negative T-cell and positive B-cell cytotoxic crossmatch: first transplant possible (antibody induction), but re-do transplant at very high risk, especially if DSA against HLA-DR are present
    * Positive B-cell flow crossmatch only: second transplant with high titer DSA not recommended
    * Better matching associated with better long-term results when all else equal but donor quality (living donor) trumps HLA matching
    * First 2 healthy recipients with negative cross-match get the kidneys

7. Ischemia-reperfusion Injury and Delayed Graft Function

A. The delayed graft function (DGF) is the failure of the kidney to function immediately, usually defined as need for dialysis in the first week. Ischemia-reperfusion injury (IR) and rejection contribute.

B. IR can promote local inflammation (upregulation of cell adhesion molecules, costimulatory molecules and histocompatibility antigens) that can lead to rejection

C. The resulting DGF is a strong predictor of short-and long-term graft survival, independent of rejection

D. Differential Diagnosis of Delayed Graft Function

- Acute tubular necrosis
- Prerenal renal failure (hemorrhage)
- Vascular stenosis or thrombosis
- Postrenal obstruction (ureteral or Foley obstruction)
- Renal parenchymal injury (nephrotoxic drugs, recurrence of primary renal disease)
- Acute rejection

E. Pulsatile perfusion may improve early function, especially with long cold ischemia times

F. Perioperative maneuvers to reduce the impact of IR

- Adequate hydration
- Mannitol
- Furosemide
- Intra-arterial verapamil
- Low-dose dopamine

8. Surgical Technique and Complications

A. Intraoperative Decisions

- Always attempt to preserve lower pole arteries as they often supply blood to the ureter

- It is acceptable to tie off small upper pole arteries

- Small venous branches can be ligated without consequence

- In cadaveric donors, a short right renal vein can be elongated with the use of the supplied inferior vena cava (almost routinely done for right cadaveric transplant)

- Cadaveric iliac vessels can be used as extenders for both vein or artery

- It is possible to conjoin arterial branches end-side or end-end (Wallace-like) on the bench table, on ice before implantation. Alternatively, 2 separate anastomoses can be performed for arterial branches that are far apart

- Small lower pole arterial branches can be anastomosed end-end with the inferior epigastric artery

- It is possible to use the ipsilateral native ureter end-end without performing a native nephrectomy

- If 2 ureters are present, they can be implanted together (conjoined) or separately

B. Short Ureter

- Sometimes, the transplant ureter will not reach the bladder safely

- How to close a ureteral gap
    * Boari flap
    * Poas hitch
    * Native ureteroureterostomy
    * Native ureteropyelostomy
    * Pyelocystostomy
    * Ileal ureter

9. Surgical Complications

A. Vascular Leak or Thrombosis

- Incidence: 1%-2%

- Re-operation, incurs a high risk to lose kidney

B. Urine Leak or Ureteral Obstruction

- Incidence: 4%-5%

- May require revision of the ureteral anastomosis

- Many endoscopic approaches are available

- Surgery may be preferable for early leaks, necrotic ureter or failure or endoscopic management

C. Lymphocele

- Incidence
    * 5%-10%
    * May be reduced by minimal iliac vessel dissection and ligation of visible lymphatics, as opposed to electrocoagulation

- Presentation
    * Ureteral obstruction: rising serum creatinine
    * Iliac vein compression: ipsilateral leg edema, deep-vein thrombosis

- Small lymphocele may be asymptomatic and does not require treatment

- The larger the lymphocele, the more likely it will be symptomatic and require treatment

- Treatment options
    * Percutaneous drainage
    * Sclerosis
    * Peritoneal window (can be performed open or laparoscopically)

D. Wound Infection

E. Hernia

10. Early and Late Patient Management Issues

A. Early Graft Dysfunction

- Differential diagnosis
  * Acute tubular necrosis (ATN)
  * Acute rejection
  * Drug toxicity
  * Vascular (arterial or venous) compromise
  * Prerenal renal failure (hemorrhage, volume contraction)
  * Postrenal renal failure (ureteral or bladder catheter obstruction)
  * Renal parenchymal injury (nephrotoxic drugs, recurrence of primary renal disease)

- Management
  * Check bladder catheter for patency, irrigate as needed
  * Fluid bolus
  * IV furosemide
  * Check drug levels
  * Renal ultrasound with Doppler or nuclear medicine renal scan to assess patency of vascular anastomosis
  * Transplant biopsy to rule out rejection

B. Long-term Issues

- Chronic allograft nephropathy

- Hypertension

- Diabetes

- Heart disease (it is the most common cause of long term graft loss)

- Infections
  * ***Cytomegalovirus (CMV) infection***
    - Previously referred to as the "42-day fever" from its frequent occurrence around 42 days after transplant
    - May be transmission from donor or reactivation of latent infection
    - Donor and recipient CMV status used to stratify risk: highest risk when donor is positive and recipient is negative
    - Prophylaxis
      * Acyclovir
      * Gancyclovir
      * Valgancyclovir
      * Cytogam (IV Ig from CMV antibody positive blood donors)

    - Target organ affected
      * GI tract (oesophagus, stomach)
      * Liver
      * Glomerulopathy
      * Retinitis
  ****BK virus infection***
    - Named after the initials of the first patients in which it was diagnosed
    - Nonenveloped double-stranded DNA papovavirus
    - Latent in immunocompetent adults, with seroprevalence ranging from 60%-80%
    - Viruria and viremia can be found in 35% and 10% respectively, of transplant patients
    - BK virus nephropathy (BKVN) is found in 5%-10% of transplant patients and can cause renal allograft lost in 50% of those patients
    - Presentation
      * Increased serum creatinine
      * Hemorrhagic cystitis
      * Ureteral stenosis
      * Sterile pyuria
    - Diagnostic
      * Presence of virus in blood and urine (quantified by PCR)
      * DNA hybridization on renal allograft biopsy
    - Management
      * Optimal management has yet to be determined
      * Reduce immunosuppression
      * Stop mycophenolate mofetil and introduce leflunomide (pyrimidine synthesis inhibitor)
      * Antiviral agents: cidofovir (nephrotoxic)

- Erectile dysfunction
  *Possible etiology
    - Drug-induced
    - Widespread atherosclerosis
    - Iatrogenic, if internal iliac artery is used for the arterial anastomosis

* Likely more than 1 etiology present at a given time
* Phosphodiesterase type 5 inhibitors can be used in transplant patients

11. Questions

1. A transplant center is offered a cadaveric kidney from a 53-year-old donor who died from head trauma. Terminal creatinine was 1.6 mg/dL. Patient had a history of hypertension well controlled with 1 drug for 2 years. It is a left kidney with 2 arteries and 2 ureters. Biopsy shows 30% glomerulosclerosis. The most likely reason to turn down this kidney is:

A. High terminal creatinine

B. Donor age

C. 2 ureters

D. 30% glomerusclerosis

E. 2 renal arteries

2. Which of the following is least likely to cause an elevation of serum creatinine in a transplant recipient?

A. High sirolimus level

B. High cyclosporine level

C. Acute rejection

D. BK virus infection

E. Ureteral necrosis

3. A transplant patient has a baseline serum Cr of 1.8 mg/dL and takes tacrolimus, MMF and steroids. Because of persistent hypertension, he is started on an ACE inhibitor. 1 week later the Cr is 3.1 mg/dL. The most likely explanation is:

A. Acute rejection

B. Renal artery stenosis

C. Hypotension and acute tubular necrosis

D. Acute renal vein thrombosis

E. Tacrolimus toxicity since the ACE inhibitor raised the blood levels

Answers

1. D.

2. A.

3. B.

Chapter 10: Urodynamics

Victor W. Nitti, MD

Contents

1. Introduction

The lower urinary tract has two essential functions: **the storage of urine at low pressure** and **the voluntary evacuation of urine.** Low pressures are essential to protect kidneys and assure continence while voluntary evacuation allows for the elimination of urine in social acceptable situations without fear of leakage or overdistension. It is clear that a number of diseases affect the lower urinary tract and disrupt the storage and/or evacuation of urine. This can lead to bothersome symptoms (eg, urinary incontinence or pain from failure to empty) or in some cases potentially harmful sequela. In many cases, a precise assessment of storage and emptying is necessary to optimally treat patients. Urodynamics (UDS) is the dynamic study of the transport, storage and evacuation of urine. It is comprised of a number of tests which individually or collectively can be used to gain information about urine storage and evacuation.

UDS is most useful when history, physical exam and simple tests are not sufficient to make an accurate diagnosis and/or institute treatment. In some cases this may be to obtain an accurate diagnosis for what condition is causing symptoms (eg, lower urinary tract symptoms or incontinence). In others it may be to determine the impact of a disease that has the potential to cause serious and irreversible damage to the upper and lower urinary tract (eg, neurological diseases like spinal cord injury, multiple sclerosis or radiation cystitis). Sometimes profound abnormalities can be found in the relative absence of symptoms.

In order to use UDS in a practical and effective way it is important that the clinician has the proper expertise to know when and why to perform a UDS study. Despite many technical advances in the recording, processing and printing of UDS studies, careful attention to technical details to assure accurate collection of data remains the cornerstone of a good study. Since not all patients undergo UDS for the same reasons, the clinician should "customize" UDS to the patients' symptoms and condition. That means deciding on the questions to be answered before starting each study and designing that study to obtain the answers. It is important to remember that UDS is preformed in an "unnatural setting" and therefore does always duplicate real life. A study that does not duplicate complaints or symptoms when an abnormality is recorded is not necessarily diagnostic. In addition, failure to record an abnormality does not always rule out its existence (eg, failure to demonstrate detrusor overactivity in a patient with urge incontinence).

As mentioned above, one of the most important parts of UDS is its proper performance with careful attention to technical details so that accurate interpretation is possible. It is beyond the scope of this chapter to describe the proper performance of UDS; however, the reader is referred to Schaefer et al for good urodynamic practices and Abrams et al for terminology (see Further Reading).

2. Functional Classification of Voiding Dysfunction

In order to formulate a set of questions to be answered by a urodynamic test, an understanding of the possible causes of symptoms and the possible urodynamic manifestations of a pre-existing condition is necessary. In order to accomplish this, a practical classification of voiding dysfunction is invaluable. The system proposed and popularized by Wein (1982) is simple and allows one to classify voiding dysfunction according to urodynamic findings. In addition, this "functional" classification system helps to clarify treatment options for a given patient.

Functionally abnormalities of the lower urinary tract can be divided into:

1. ***Storage dysfunction*** (failure to properly store urine)

2. ***Emptying dysfunction*** (failure to empty the bladder normally)

3. ***Combined dysfunction*** (failure to store and empty)

Anatomically storage and emptying abnormalities can be caused by:

Bladder dysfunction
a. Overactive (causing failure to store)

b. Underactive (causing failure to empty)

Bladder outlet dysfunction
a. Overactive (causing failure to empty)

b. Underactive (causing failure to store)

Combined bladder and bladder outlet dysfunction

The urodynamic evaluation should help to determine if there is bladder or bladder outlet dysfunction (or both) and whether there is a storage and/or emptying problem. By providing answers to these simple questions the urodynamic test can lead to a correct diagnosis and equally as important, institution of appropriate treatment. Obviously, an understanding of the physiology of urine storage and voiding and the pathophysiology of voiding dysfunction is required to formulate appropriate questions to be answered by a urodynamic study. However, all too often clinicians become caught up in the intricate neurophysiologic aspects of voiding and storage dysfunction and fail to think in practical terms. One should always focus on the possible urodynamic findings in a given case and how each of the findings may ultimately affect treatment. Obviously, these potential findings will be determined by symptoms and/or underlying disease.

3. Simple Tests

There are several simple, noninvasive tests that can be used to evaluate voiding function and perhaps prompt further testing.

Post-void Residual (PVR)

PVR is an excellent assessment of bladder emptying. It can be performed by ultrasound (bladder scan) or catheterization. Elevation of PVR indicates a problem with emptying, but does not tell why.

Uroflowmetry

This is also an assessment of bladder emptying. Normal uroflow is a bell-shaped curve. When the flow rate is reduced or the pattern is altered, this could indicate bladder (underactive) or bladder outlet (obstruction) dysfunction.

4. The Urodynamics Test

The micturition cycle can be divided into 2 phases: the filling (and storage) phase and the emptying phase. Similarly, the UDS can be divided into the same 2 components.

Urodynamics: Filling and Storage

The cystometrogram (CMG) assesses the bladder's response to filling. The CMG can measure filling pressure, sensation, involuntary contractions, compliance, and capacity. Sensation is the part of cystometry that is truly subjective and therefore requires an alert and attentive patient and clinician. There are several subjective parameters that can be recorded during filling that are recognized by the International Continence Society (ICS):

First sensation of bladder filling. First aware of bladder filling.

First desire to void. Feeling that would lead patient to pass urine at next convenient moment, but voiding can be delayed if necessary.

Strong desire to void. Persistent desire to void without fear of leakage.

Urgency. Sudden compelling desire to void.

Normally, the bladder should store urine at low pressure and not contract involuntarily. Once capacity is reached or voluntary voiding is desired, intravesical pressure will increase (voluntary detrusor contraction). In actuality this is preceded by a relaxation of the external sphincter. A normalized adult CMG is depicted on the next page (Figure 1).

Figure 1

A normalized adult CMG

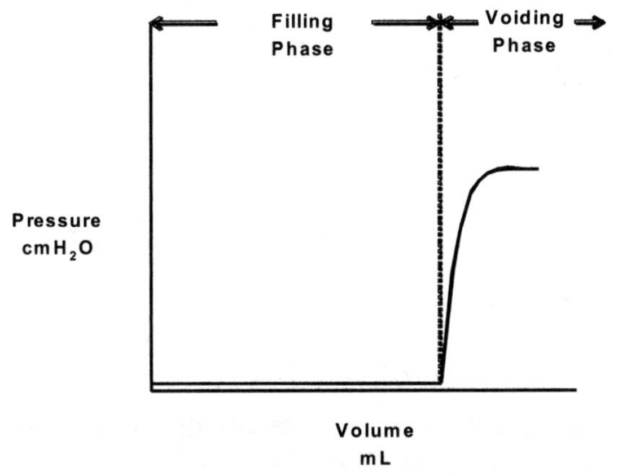

During UDS, bladder pressure is measured by an intravesical catheter (usually transurethral). It is well known that increases in intra abdominal pressure are transmitted to the bladder. Therefore when intravesical pressure is monitored during cystometric studies, it must be realized that this pressure is actually the sum of intra abdominal pressure and the pressure generated by the detrusor itself, either through a contraction or wall tension with bladder filling. The simultaneous measurement of abdominal pressure (Pabd), usually by a rectal or vaginal catheter and vesical pressure (Pves) during urodynamics, provides a means of calculating the true detrusor pressure (Pdet) by subtracting abdominal Pabd from Pves. The ability to calculate subtracted detrusor pressure allows one to distinguish between a true rise in detrusor pressure (either via a contraction or loss of compliance) and the effect of increased abdominal pressure (eg, straining, Valsalva). This is especially important when rises in detrusor pressure are small or when they are accompanied by changes in abdominal pressure (Figure 2).

Adding intra abdominal pressure monitoring gives a better representation of the true detrusor pressure.

In Figure 2A. the total vesical pressure tracing is present (CMG)—note the multiple spikes and rises in pressure. Without having simultaneous monitoring of intra-abdominal pressure, it is impossible if these pressure spikes are due to a rise in detrusor or abdominal pressure.

In Figure 2B. the same tracing is present with intra abdominal pressure monitoring added (multichannel UDS). One can clearly see now that the changes in

Figure 2

Total vesical pressure and intra abdominal pressure

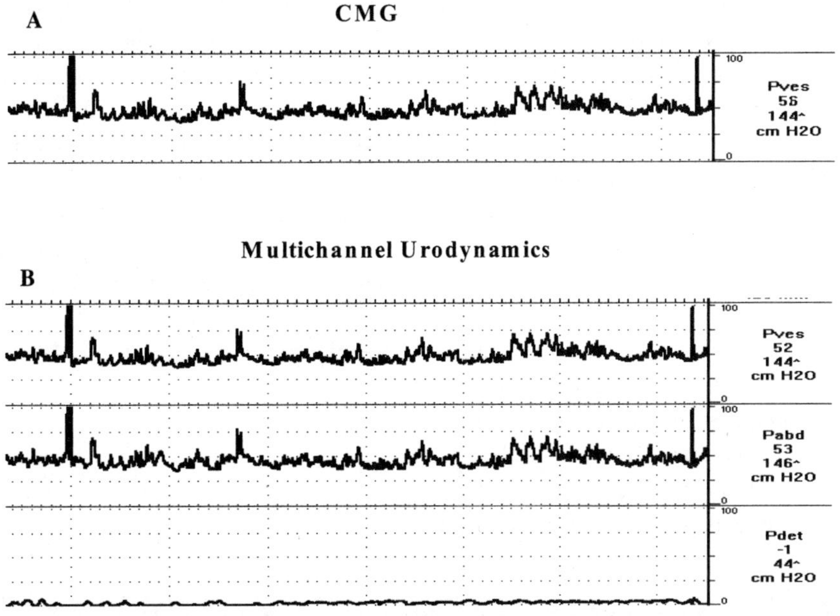

pressure were due to the changes in abdominal pressure. When one looks at the Pdet curve it is noted to be flat and without any rises in pressure.

Abnormalities of Bladder Filling: Detrusor Overactivity and Impaired Compliance

During filling involuntary detrusor contractions (IDC) can occur. These are often associated with urgency and even urge incontinence. Detrusor overactivity (DO) is a urodynamic observation characterized by involuntary IDCs during the filling phase which may be spontaneous or provoked. According to the ICS, DO may be further characterized as neurogenic DO which means it is associated with a relevant neurological condition (eg, spinal cord injury, multiple sclerosis) or ***idiopathic DO*** which means that there is "no defined cause" (non-neurogenic). The term idiopathic is a bit of a misnomer, in that the cause of DO in a non-neurogenic patient may be readily apparent (eg, bladder outlet obstruction, inflammatory process) or may be truly "unknown." Thus, from a practical standpoint, the terms neurogenic and non-neurogenic DO make sense, but do not fit the ICS definitions. (It should be noted that the term neurogenic DO replaced the term detrusor hyperreflexia and the term idiopathic DO replaced the term detrusor instability in the last ICS terminology.)

From a practical standpoint during UDS, DO can further be observed as a single event or multiple IDCs. It can be ***phasic***, or ***terminal*** (occurring at the end of filling). It can also be suppressed or unabortable and may lead to leakage or precipitant micturition. Classifying DO in such a way can be valuable in certain circumstances. For example, overactivity bladder symptoms associated with obstruction have a higher likelihood of resolving with intervention (eg, TURP) when DO is terminal rather than phasic.

The vesicoelastic properties of the bladder, based on its composition of smooth muscle, collagen, and elastin, normally produces a highly compliant structure. Therefore as the bladder fills there is little change in pressure (Figure 3). Compliance relationship between change in bladder volume and change

Figure 3

Detrusor overactivity

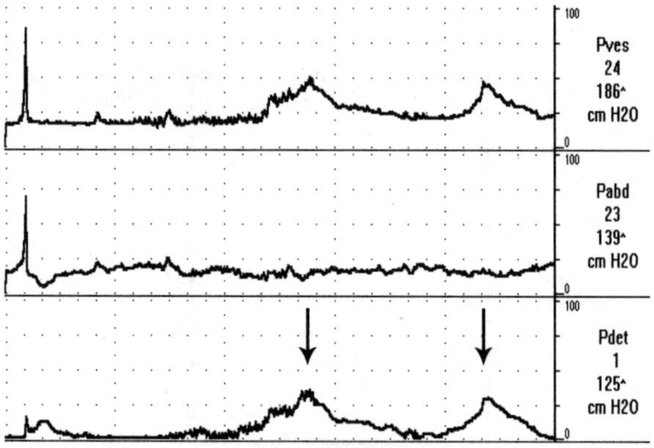

This UDS tracing depicts DO. Note the 2 IDCs (arrows). There is a rise in Pves with no associated rise in Pabd and therefore the subtracted Pdet looks identical to the Pves.

in detrusor pressure (Δvolume / Δpressure) is measured in mL/cm H_2O. The ICS recommends 2 standard points: the Pdet at start of bladder filling (usually zero) and the Pdet at cystometric capacity or before the start of any detrusor contraction that results in significant leakage. Both points are measured excluding any detrusor contractions. Various definitions of impaired compliance have been used (eg, between 10 and 20 mL/cm H_2O); however, there is not a consistent definition based on mL/cm H_2O. In practical terms absolute pressure is probably more useful than a "compliance number" or value. It is well known that storage pressures >40 cm H_2O are known to be harmful to the upper tracts. Impaired compliance is seen in a variety of neurological conditions, especially lower motor neuron lesions such as spina bifida and cauda equina syndrome. It can result from outlet obstruction (anatomical or functional) or structural changes like radiation cystitis or TB. **Impaired compliance with elevated storage pressures is a urodynamic risk factor** and usually needs to be treated to prevent renal damage (Figure 4).

Figure 4

UDS representation of impaired compliance

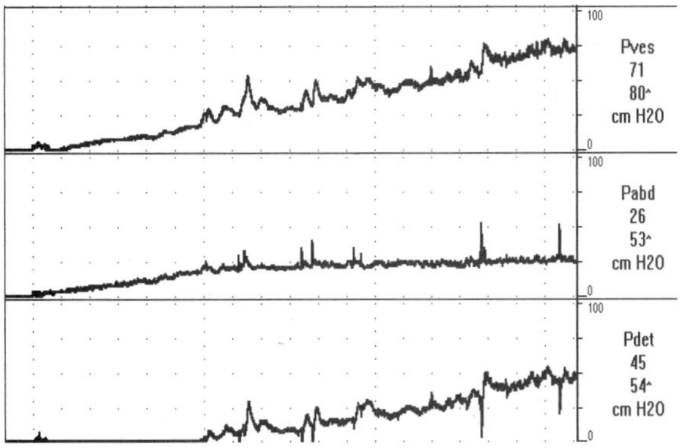

Note the rise in Pves (and Pdet) with bladder filling. The Pdet at the end of filling is approximately 45 cm H_2O, which is a potentially dangerous situation.

Figure 5

Leak point pressure

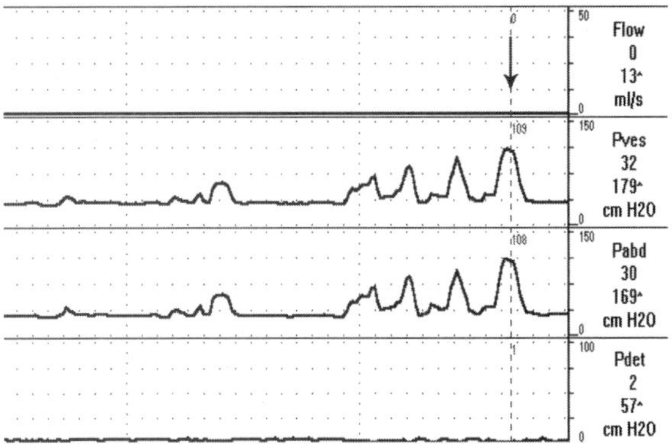

Leak Point Pressures

There are 2 distinct types of leak point pressures that can be measured in the incontinent patient. The two are independent of each other and conceptually measure completely different things. The first is the **abdominal leak point pressure (ALPP)** which is a **measure of sphincter strength** or the ability of the sphincter to resist changes in abdominal pressure. ALPP is defined as the intravesical pressure at which urine leakage occurs due to increased abdominal pressure in the absence of a detrusor contraction. This measure of intrinsic urethral function is applicable to patients with stress incontinence. **An ALPP can only be demonstrated in a patient with stress urinary incontinence.** Conceptually, **the lower the ALPP, the weaker the sphincter.** There is no normal ALPP, as patients without stress incontinence will not leak at any physiologic abdominal pressure (Figure 5).

Attempts have been made to quantify intrinsic sphincter deficiency (ISD) using ALPP. In 1993, McGuire and associates used ALPP to measure 125 women with SUI. When the ALPP <60 cm H_2O, all patients had high grade incontinence with 81% having continuous leakage and 75% having a fixed urethra (no urethral hypermobility). When ALPP was between 61-89 cm H_2O, 80% had pronounced urethral hypermobility and grade moderate to high grade incontinence. When ALPP was >90 cm H_2O, patients had lesser grades of incontinence and minimal to gross urethral hypermobility. The inference is that:

ALPP <60 cm H_2O signifies ISD

ALPP between 60-90 cm H_2O is equivocal (there is a component of ISD)

ALPP >90 cm H_2O indicates little or no ISD

However, from a practical standpoint, **if there is no hypermobility, SUI must be caused by ISD, regardless of the ALPP.** Current technology does not permit a method to distinguish between ISD and hypermobility. Therefore, although these ALPP values are often used, they should be interpreted with caution.

The second type of leak point pressure is **the detrusor leak point pressure (DLPP), which is a measure of detrusor pressure in patients with decreased bladder compliance.** It is defined as the lowest detrusor pressure at which urine leakage occurs in the absence of either a detrusor contraction or increased abdominal pressure.

Figure 6

Pressure in the bladder will continue to increase as the bladder fills

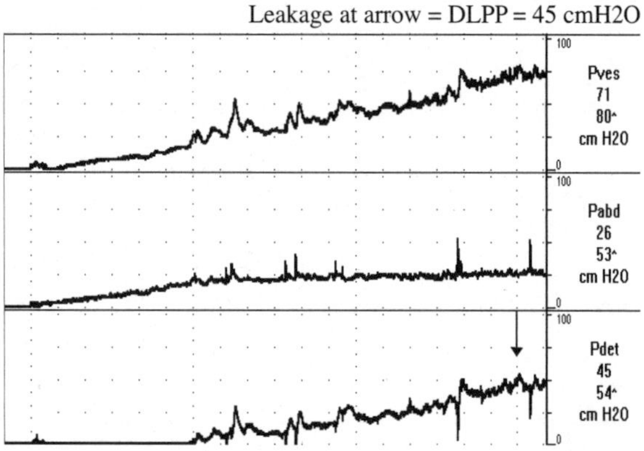

The higher the urethral resistance, the higher the DLPP. One can imagine that in a poorly compliant bladder, if outlet resistance is low, incontinence will occur at a relatively low or "safe pressure. However, if outlet resistance is high, the pressure in the bladder will continue to increase as the bladder fills (Figure 6). There is potentially less incontinence, but eventually the pressure is transmitted to the upper tracts.

From a clinical perspective **DLPP is most useful in patients with lower motor neuron disease affecting the bladder** (spina bifida, spinal cord tumors, after abdominal-perineal resection of the rectum or radical hysterectomy) **and in non-neurogenic patients with low bladder compliance** (after multiple bladder surgeries, radiation and tuberculous cystitis). The higher the DLPP, the more likely is upper tract damage as intravesical pressure is transferred to the kidneys. McGuire documented the deleterious effects that a high leak point pressure has on the upper urinary tracts; leak point pressures greater than 40 cm H_2O result in hydronephrosis or vesicoureteral reflux in 85% of myelodysplastic patients.

In summary, ALPP and DLPP, although **both** called **"leak point pressure"** are completely different. The ALPP measures the sphincter response to increased abdominal pressure. **The lower the ALPP, the "weaker" the sphincter.** The DLPP measures the injured bladder response to increased outlet resistance. **The higher the resistance** (eg, detrusor-external sphincter dyssynergia), **the higher the DLPP,** which is potentially dangerous to the upper tracts.

Urethral Pressure Profilometry

Despite an abundant literature on urethral profilometry, its clinical relevance is controversial. Many urologists do not routinely perform urethral profilmetry. Urethral pressure is defined as the fluid pressure needed to just open a loose urethra. **The urethral pressure profile (UPP)** represents the intraluminal pressure along the length of the urethra in graphic form. Several parameters can be obtained from the UPP:

The urethral closure pressure profile (UCP) is given by the subtraction of intravesical pressure from urethral pressure.

Maximum urethral pressure (MUP) is the highest pressure measured along the UPP.

Maximum urethral closure pressure (MUCP) is the maximum difference between the urethral pressure and the intravesical pressure.

Functional profile length is the length of the urethra along which the urethral pressure exceeds intravesical pressure in women.

In most continent women, the functional urethral length is approximately 3 cm and the MUCP is 40-60 cm H_2O but normal values vary widely.

One caveat of UPP is that its measurement does not diagnose stress incontinence. For example, there is a difference between the urethra of an incontinent patient whose MUCP = 38 cm H_2O and that of a continent women with the same MUCP.

In 2002, the ICS standardization subcommittee concluded that the clinical utility of urethral pressure measurement is unclear. Furthermore, there are no urethral pressure measurements that: 1.) discriminate urethral incompetence from other disorders; 2.) provide a measure of the severity of the condition; 3.) provide a reliable indicator to surgical success, and return to normal after surgical intervention.

Stress-induced Detrusor Overactivity

Sometimes detrusor overactivity can be triggered by a rise in abdominal pressure. Thus the symptom may appear to be stress incontinence, but the condition causing the symptom is actually an involuntary contraction, not sphincteric weakness.

Occult Stress Incontinence

Stress incontinence is demonstrated in a clinically continent woman with pelvic prolapse only when the prolapse is reduced.

Urodynamics: Emptying – The Voiding Phase

Normal voiding accomplished by activation of micturition reflex, which involves:

1. Relaxation of striated urethral sphincter

2. Contraction of detrusor muscle

3. Opening of vesical neck and urethra

4. Onset of urine flow

This occurs as a result of coordination between pontine and sacral micturition centers, with suprapontine input which allows for voluntary control of the micturition reflex.

UDS can evaluate several parameters during the voiding phase including:

1. Detrusor contractility

2. Relaxation of the bladder outlet

3. Coordination of sphincters

According to the ICS, **normal detrusor function** is characterized by a voluntarily initiated continuous contraction that leads to complete bladder emptying within a normal time span, and in the absence of obstruction. **Detrusor underactivity** is when there is a contraction of reduced strength and/or duration, resulting in prolonged bladder emptying and/or a failure to achieve complete bladder emptying within a normal time span. Finally, an **acontractile detrusor** is when there is no demonstrable contraction during UDS. However, when evaluating detrusor function urodynamically, one should correlate UDS with clinical findings. For example, if a patient who normally voids is unable to void during a UDS study, one cannot make a definitive diagnosis of "acontractile detrusor."

The Pressure Flow Relation

Detrusor pressure during voiding is a function of outlet resistance. For a normal detrusor, **the greater the outlet resistance, the higher the detrusor pressure during voiding.** This is accompanied by a reduced flow rate. A healthy bladder is able to overcome obstruction by contracting more forcefully and although flow may be slower, the bladder is able to empty itself. Over time, the detrusor may decompensate and may no longer be able to generate the necessary pressure to overcome obstruction. When this occurs, retention of urine results. **Thus the urodynamic manifestation of bladder outlet obstruction (BOO) is high pressure and low flow** (or more practically speaking, increased pressure and reduced flow). Over time if bladder decompensation results, detrusor underactivity or impaired contractility can result.

In males, obstruction has been defined based on the model of **benign prostatic obstruction (BPO)**. Using clinically obstructed and unobstructed (after TURP) males, several different formulas or nomograms have been created. The ICS nomogram is the one most commonly used today (Figure 7). Using this nomogram and the **bladder outlet obstruction index (BOOI)** derived from it, men can be divided into three groups: obstructed, equivocal and unobstructed.

Based on the slope of the curves, the BOOI is defined as the detrusor pressure at maximum flow rate ($P_{det}Q_{max}$) minus 2 times the maximum flow rate (Q_{max}):

$$\textbf{BOOI} = P_{det}Q_{max} - 2(Q_{max})$$

A BOOI >40 is obstructed; BOOI <20 is unobstructed; and BOOI 20-40 is equivocal for obstruction. This formula and nomogram applies only to males, as female voiding dynamics are different.

Figure 7

ICS nomogram

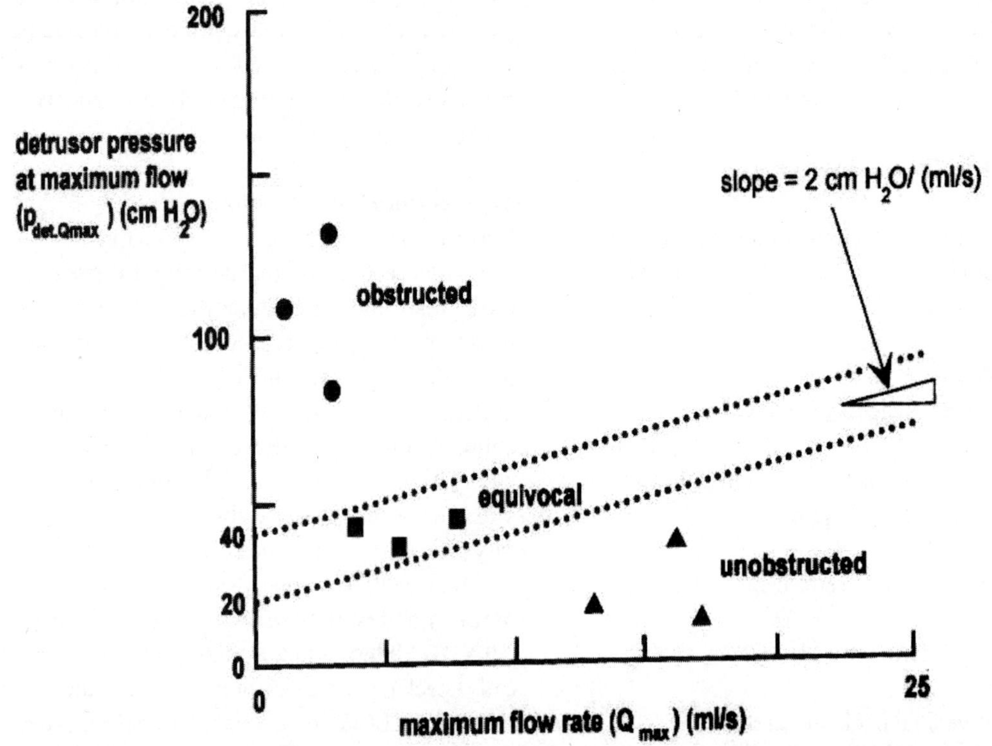

BOO is associated with abnormalities of storage as well. This is presumably due to changes in ultrastructure that occur with obstruction. Detrusor overactivity and impaired compliance occur in conjunction with obstruction. For example, about two-thirds of men with symptomatic BPO have DO and one-half to two-thirds of the time DO resolves with treatment of obstruction. Reduced compliance is also associated with obstruction and has been shown to improve with treatment of obstruction (TURP).

Obstruction in women **cannot** be defined by the ICS nomogram or the BOOI as these **will grossly underestimate female BOO.** This is because normally women void at much lower pressures than men and therefore the obstructed female bladder outlet may not respond as dramatically (or at least with the same pressures) as in the male. Unfortunately there is no condition in women that causes BOO as commonly as BPO in men and therefore creating a consistent standard is difficult. Thus concepts are the same (higher pressure and lower flow), but the values are different and less well defined. Those who are interested are referred to the Further Reading section.

Sphincter Coordination

Normal voiding requires external sphincter relaxation followed by contraction of the detrusor. The external sphincter (and internal sphincter) should remain relaxed until voiding is complete. This is shown below (Figure 8).

Note that the rise in detrusor pressure is ***preceded*** by a fall in urethral pressure and relaxation of the external sphincter as measured by electromyography (EMG). The sphincter and urethral pressure remain low during voiding and then increase when voiding is completed.

The signal source for measurement of the EMG activity of the striated external sphincter is the electrical activity of the external urethral sphincter, the external anal sphincter, or the pelvic floor muscles. Accurate EMG measurement of this relatively low level of electrical activity can be somewhat difficult; however, performance of EMG studies as part of routine urodynamics can be accurate and easily done. **The 2 most commonly used electrodes are surface electrodes and concentric needle electrodes.** Most experts feel that the concentric needle electrode is the superior technique for obtaining a signal source of EMG activity of the striated external sphincter muscles but has the distinct disadvantage of being uncomfortable for the patient, especially if more than one attempt at placement of the electrode is required to obtain an adequate signal. The surface electrodes have a significant advantage compared with the needle electrode regarding patient convenience and comfort. However, the surface electrodes are considered to provide an inferior signal source by some clinicians who routinely perform urodynamic studies, but surface electrodes can provide very good signal source quality if properly used. It is important that the intensity of the EMG signal can determine what the tracing looks like. One should observe relative changes in EMG activity as opposed to raw numbers. (For a more detailed explanation of EMG, see O'Donnell, 1998 in the Further Reading section.)

Normally EMG activity decreases before a voluntary bladder contraction, however it is not abnormal for EMG activity to increase with an involuntary contraction as part of a guarding reflex to inhibit the IDC (Figure 9).

In this case, the patient experienced an IDC which led to increased external sphincter, and an increase in EMG activity. However, shortly after, when the patient voluntarily voids, the sphincter relaxes and EMG activity decreases.

Detrusor-external sphincter dyssynergia (DESD) occurs when there is an involuntary increase external sphincter associated with DO and also with voiding. It is caused by a neurological lesion in the suprasacral spinal cord. DESD can produce profound changes as the detrusor involuntarily contracts against a relatively closed sphincter. This will

Figure 8

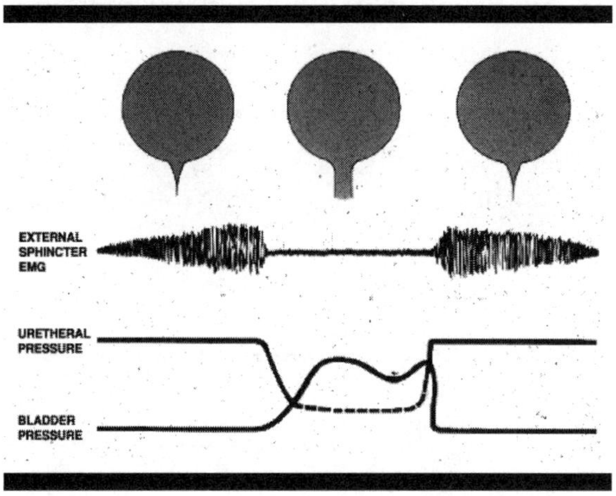

result in high pressures and can even cause impaired bladder compliance over time. DESD is considered a urodynamic risk factor for upper tract deterioration (Figure 10). If there is no neurological lesion, then the dyssynergia is considered a learned behavior (dysfunctional voiding) and can often be "unlearned." True DESD cannot be unlearned and must be treated by bypassing the voiding phase (eg, with intermittent catheterization) or by chemical or surgical ablation of the sphincter. The latter will lead to incontinence.

Figure 9

Not abnormal for EMG activity to increase with involuntary contraction as part of guarding reflex inhibiting IDC

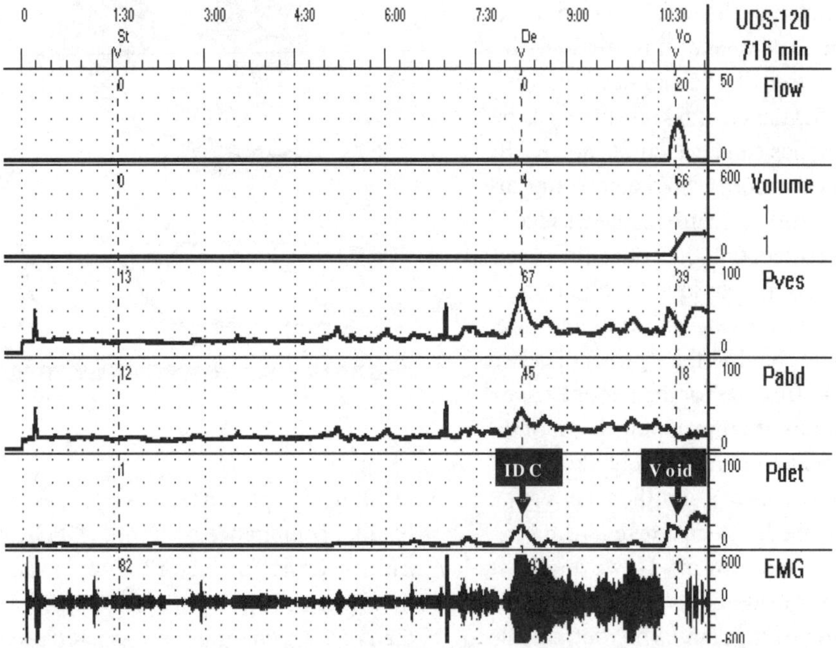

Figure 10

UDS tracing of a patient with myelodysplasia and neurogenic DO and DESD

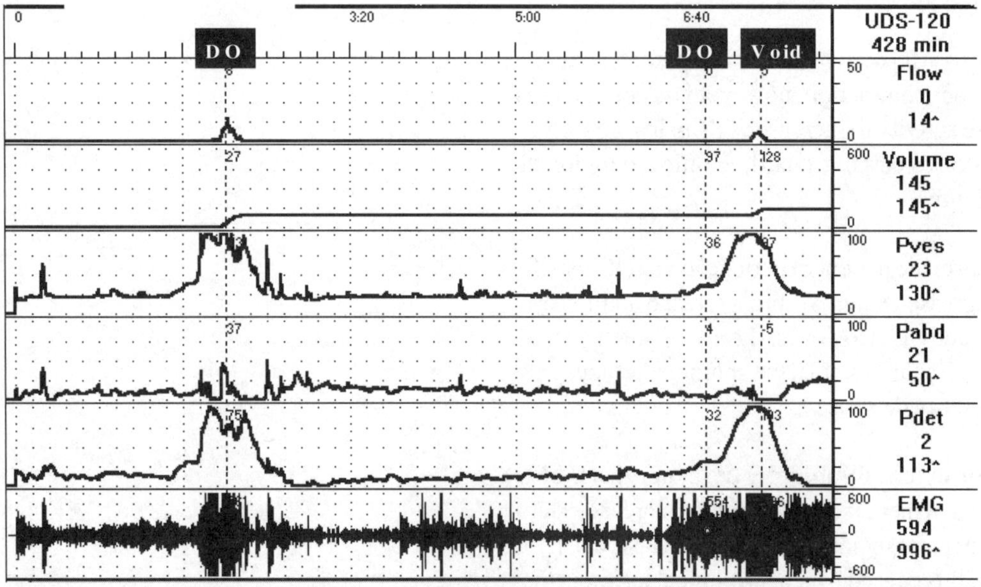

Note the initial IDC associated with DESD and incontinence (measured on the flow channel). With refilling, the UDS is again DO with DESD and then the patient is told to voluntarily void and there is persistent increased EMG activity. As a result there is high pressure, low flow voiding (obstruction from the dyssynergic sphincter).

5. Videourodynamics

Videourodynamics (VUDS) consists of the simultaneous measurement of UDS parameters and imaging of the lower urinary tract. It provides the most precise evaluation of voiding function and dysfunction. VUDS is particularly useful when an anatomic picture is desired, for example:

- In cases of known or suspected anatomical abnormality
- Failure to demonstrate incontinence by conventional methods
- Evaluation of bladder neck (internal sphincter) synergy
- Neurological diseases (or other potentially dangerous causes of voiding dysfunction) where there is associated vesicoureteral reflux. In such cases, reflux volumes and pressures can be measured

VUDS is also useful in the evaluation of suspected female BOO.

VUDS Examples

Figure 11 is a VUDS study of a 45-year-old male with LUTS including frequency, urgency and decreased force of stream. The UDS shows high pressure, low flow consistent with BOO, but in this young man, BPO cannot be assumed. The simultaneous fluoroscopic view of the bladder and outlet taken during voiding shows an incomplete opening

Figure 11

VUDS study of a 45-year-old male with LUTS including frequency, urgency and decreased force of stream

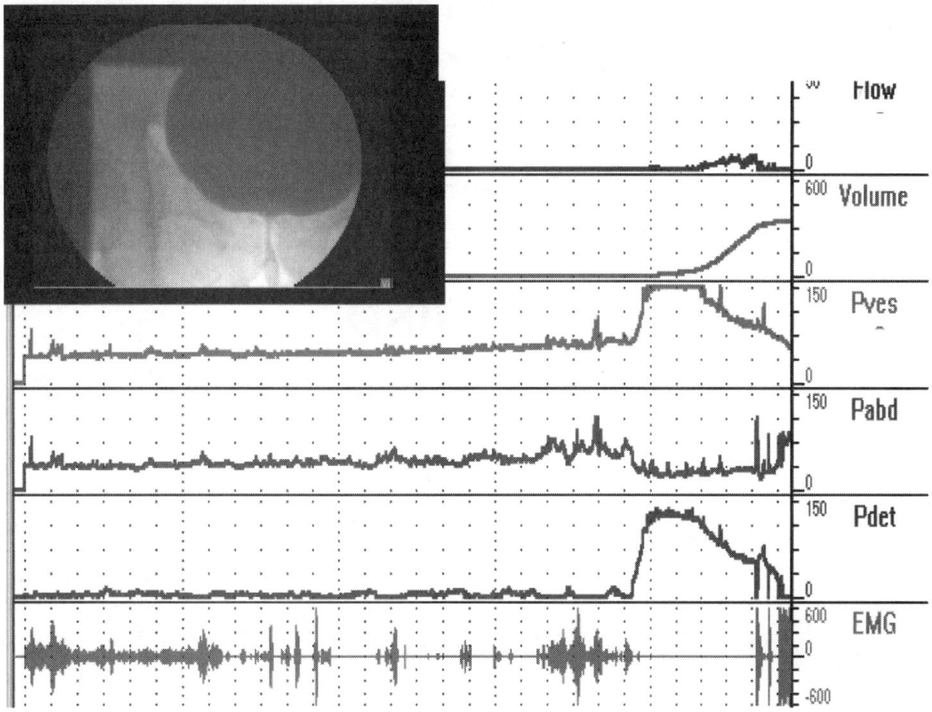

of the bladder neck and the diagnosis of primary bladder neck obstruction can be made.

Figure 12 is a VUDS study of a male with a C1-2 spinal cord injury with suspected DESD and retention of urine, being considered for external sphincterotomy. The UDS shows 2 high pressure IDCs with significant increase in EMG activity, consistent with neurogenic DO with DESD. However, the fluoroscopic picture taken during the second IDC also shows internal sphincter dyssynergia as the bladder neck remains relatively closed. This phenomenon is known to happen in high spinal cord lesions (above the lower thoracic cord). An external sphincterotomy would not be enough to relieve obstruction in this case. An internal sphincterotomy (bladder neck incision) is also needed.

Urodynamic Risk Factors

It cannot be emphasized enough that certain UDS findings are potentially dangerous and usually require intervention. These include:

- **Impaired compliance**
- **DESD**
- **DISD**
- **High pressure DO present throughout filling**
- **Elevated DLPP (>40 cm H_2O)**
- **Poor emptying with high storage pressures**

Figure 12

VUDS study of a male with a C1-2 spinal cord injury with suspected DESD and retention of urine, being considered for external sphincterotomy

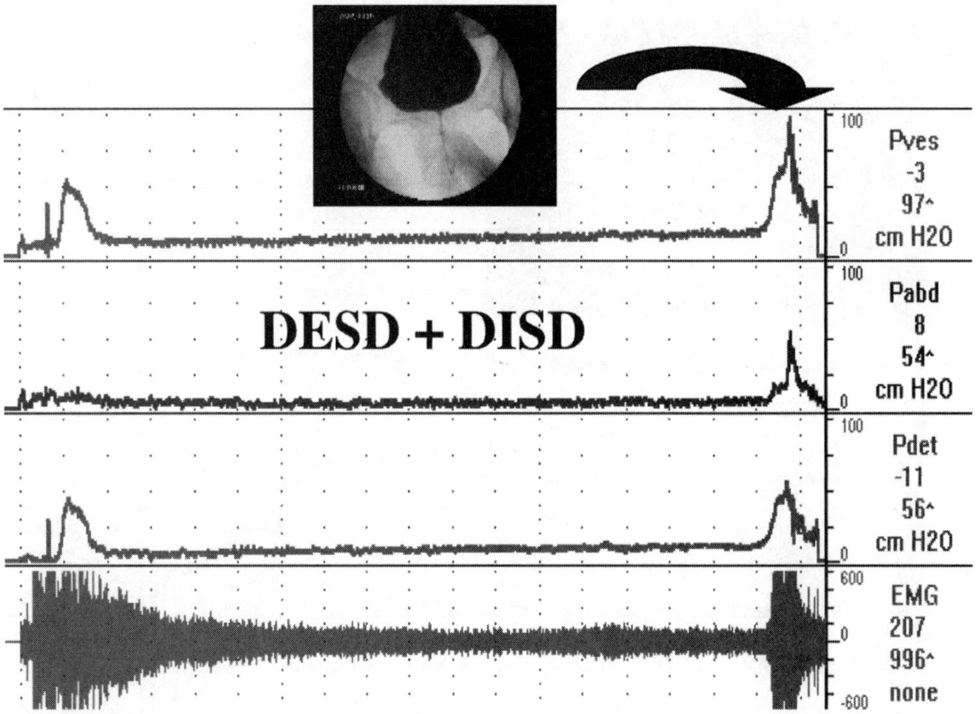

6. Further Reading

1. Abrams P, Griffiths DJ. The assessment of prostatic obstruction from urodynamic measurements and from residual urine. *Br J Urol*. 1979;51:129.

2. Abrams PH, Farrar DJ, Turner-Warwick RT, et al. The results of prostatectomy: a symptomatic and urodynamic analysis of 192 patients. *J Urol*. 1979;121:640.

3. Abrams P. Bladder outlet obstruction index, bladder contractility index and bladder voiding efficiency: three simple indices to define bladder voiding function. *BJU Int*. 1999; 84:14.

4. Abrams P, Cardoza L, Fall M, et al. The standardisation of terminology in lower urinary tract function: report from the standardisation subcommittee of the International Continence Society. *Urology*. 2003;61:37.

5. Akikwala TV, Fleischman N, Nitti VW. Comparison of diagnostic criteria for female bladder outlet obstruction. *J Urol*. 2006; 176:2093-7.

6. Bass JS, Leach GE. Bladder outlet obstruction in women. *Problems in Urology*. 1991;5:141.

7. Blaivas JG, Groutz A. Bladder outlet obstruction nomogram for women with lower urinary tract symptomatology. *Neurourol Urodyn*. 2000;19:553.

8. Blaivas JG. Videourodynamic studies. In: Nitti VW, ed. *Practical Urodynamics*. Philadelphia, PA: WB Saunders; 1998:78-93.

9. Boone TB, Kim YH. Uroflowmetry. In: Nitti VW, ed. *Practical Urodynamics*. Philadelphia, PA: WB Saunders; 1998:27-37.

10. Cespedes RD, McGuire EJ. Leak point pressures. In: Nitti VW, ed. *Practical Urodynamics*. Philadelphia, PA: WB Saunders; 1998:94-107.

11. Chassange S, Bernier PA, Haab F, Roehrborn CG, Reisch JS, Zimmern PE. Proposed cutoff values to define bladder outlet obstruction in women. *Urology*. 1998;51:408.

12. Defreitas GA, Zimmern PE, Lemack GE, Shariat SF. Refining diagnosis of anatomic female bladder outlet obstruction: comparison of pressure-flow study parameters in clinically obstructed women with those of normal controls. *Urology*. 2004;64:675-679.

13. Fleischmann N, Flisser AJ, Blaivas JG, Panagopoulos G. Sphincteric urinary incontinence: relationship of vesical leak point pressure, urethral mobility and severity of incontinence. *J Urol*. 2003;69:999-1002.

14. Griffiths D, Hofner K, van Mastrigt G, et al. Standardization of terminology of lower urinary tract function: pressure-flow studies of voiding, urethral resistance, and urethral obstruction. International Continence Society Subcommittee on standardization of terminology of pressure-flow studies. *Neurourol Urodyn*. 1997;16:1.

15. Griffiths DJ. The mechanics of the urethra and of micturition. *Br J Urol*. 1973;45:497.

16. Huckabay C, Twiss C, Berger A, Nitti VW. A urodynamics protocol to optimally assess men with post-prostatectomy incontinence. *Neurourol Urodyn*. 2005;24:622-626.

17. Lemack GE, Zimmern PE. Pressure flow analysis may aid in identifying women with outflow obstruction. *J Urol*. 2000;163:1823.

18. Leng WW, McGuire EJ. Obstructive uropathy induced bladder dysfunction can be reversible: bladder compliance measures before and after treatment. *J Urol*. 2003; 169:563.

19. Lose G, Griffiths D, Hosker G, et al. Standardisation of urethral pressure measurement: report from the Standardisation Sub-Committee of the International Continence Society. *Neurourol Urodyn*. 2002;21:258-260.

20. Massey JA, Abrams P. Obstructed voiding in the female. *Br J Urol*. 1988;61:36.

21. McGuire EJ. Urodynamic findings in patients after failure of stress incontinence operations. *Prog Clin Biol Res*. 1981;78:351-354.

22. McGuire EJ, Woodside JR, Borden TA. Prognostic value of urodynamic testing in myeloplastic children. *J Urol*. 1981;126:205.

23. McGuire EJ, Fitzpatrick CC, Wan J, et al. Clinical assessment of urethral sphincter function. *J Urol*. 1993;150:1452.

24. Nitti VW, Combs AJ. Urodynamics: when, why and how. In: Nitti VW, ed. *Practical Urodynamics*. Philadelphia, PA: WB Saunders;1998:15-26.

25. Nitti VW, Tu LM, Gitlin J. Diagnosing bladder outlet obstruction in women. *J Urol*. 1999;161:1535.

26. Nitti VW. Cystometry and abdominal pressure monitoring. In: Nitti VW, ed. *Practical Urodynamics*. Philadelphia, PA: WB Saunders; 1998:38-51.

27. O'Donnell PD. Electromyography. In: Nitti VW, ed. *Practical Urodynamics*. Philadelphia, PA: WB Saunders; 1998:65-71.

28. Schafer W. Principles and clinical application of advanced urodynamic analysis of voiding function. *Urol Clin North Am*. 1990;17:553.

29. Schafer W, Sterling AM, Liao L, et al. Good urodynamic practice: report from the standardisation sub-committee of the International Continence Society. *Neurourol Urodynam*. 2002;21:261.

30. Wein AJ, English WE, Whitmore KE. Office urodynamics. *Urol Clin North Am*. 1988; 15:609.

31. Wein AJ. Classification of neurogenic voiding dysfunction. *J Urol*. 1981;125:605.

Chapter 11: Neuropathic Bladder: Voiding Dysfunctions Associated With Neurological Disease

Raymond R. Rackley, MD

Contents

1. Lexicon of Terms and Key Concepts

Bladder Compliance

Bladder compliance (C) is defined as the change in Volume (V) relative to the corresponding change in intravesical or detrusor pressure (Pdet):

C = change V/change Pdet
(expressed as mL/cm H_2O)

- Compliance is generally calculated between two points: the Pdet with the bladder empty at the start of urodynamic filling and the Pdet at either the maximal cystometric capacity or the start of a detrusor contraction
- **Normal bladder compliance should be less than 12.5 mL/cm H_2O**
- Compliance arises from the neuromuscular and biomechanical (collagenous and elastic) components of the bladder wall.
- 3 variables (all of which may be affected by multiple factors) as defined by Laplace's equation come into play:

- **Laplace's equation:**
  T ~ Pdet x R(radius of the bladder)

  1. Wall tension (T)
  2. Detrusor pressure
  3. Bladder volume

- A decrease in bladder compliance (neuromuscular and/or biomechanical properties) can alter bladder wall tension, cause afferent nerve activation, and thereby change bladder sensations and the volume threshold for micturition

Leak Point Pressures

2 pressures obtained during urodynamics measure different aspects of lower urinary tract function:

- Detrusor leak point pressure (DLPP):

  DLLP is defined by the ICS as the lowest detrusor pressure at which urine leakage occurs in the absence of either a detrusor contraction or increased abdominal pressure

- Abdominal leak point pressure (ALPP).

  ALPP is the intravesical pressure at which urine leakage occurs because of increased abdominal pressure in the absence of a detrusor contraction

Smooth vs. Striated Sphincter

The smooth sphincter refers to the smooth musculature of the bladder neck and proximal urethra. This is a physiologic but not an anatomic sphincter and one that is not under voluntary control. The striated sphincter refers to the striated musculature that is a part of the outer wall of the proximal urethra in both the male and the female (this portion is often referred to as the intrinsic or intramural striated sphincter) and the bulky skeletal muscle group that closely surrounds the urethra at the level of the membranous portion in the male and primarily the middle segment in the female (often referred to as the extrinsic or extramural striated sphincter). The extramural portion is the classically described external urethral sphincter and is under voluntary control.

Guarding Reflex

The **guarding reflex** constitutes the efferent limb of a spinal somatic reflex which results in a gradual increase in striated sphincter activity during normal bladder filling and storage. The gradual increase in urethral pressure during bladder filling is due in part to the striated sphincteric element and perhaps in part to the smooth sphincteric element as well. The rise in urethral pressure seen during the filling/storage phase of micturition can be correlated with an increase in efferent pudendal nerve impulse frequency and in EMG activity of the periurethral striated musculature.

Autonomic Hyperreflexia (Dysreflexia)

Autonomic hyperreflexia represents an acute massive disordered autonomic (primarily sympathetic) response to specific stimuli in patients with SCI above the cord level of T6–T8 (the sympathetic outflow).

- It is more common in cervical (60%) than thoracic (20%) injuries
- Onset after injury is variable—usually soon after spinal shock but may be up to years after injury
- Distal cord viability is a prerequisite
- Symptomatically, autonomic hyperreflexia is a syndrome of exaggerated sympathetic activity in response to stimuli below the level of the lesion. The symptoms are pounding headache, hypertesion, and flushing of the face and body above the level of the lesion with sweating. Bradycardia is a usual accompaniment, although tachycardia or arrhythmia may be present. Hypertension may be of varying severity

Detrusor Sphincter Dyssynergia

Sphincter EMG is used to evaluate the striated sphincter complex and the activity of the pelvic floor during bladder filling, storage and voiding. Clinically, the most important information obtained from sphincter EMG is whether there is coordination or discoordination between the external sphincter and the bladder.

- Failure of the sphincter to relax or stay completely relaxed during micturition is abnormal. When it occurs in patients with neurologic disease, it is termed ***detrusor-sphincter dyssynergia***; this typically occurs in patients with suprasacral spinal cord injury in which there is an interruption of the spinobulbar-spinal pathways that normally coordinate the detrusor and the sphincter
- In the absence of neurologic disease, one cannot use the term detrusor-sphincter dyssynergia. Instead, the term ***pelvic floor hyperactivity*** or ***dysfunctional voiding*** is used
- Patients with Parkinson's disease may demonstrate a similar EMG picture that has been termed ***sphincter bradykinesia***. There is a delay in the relaxation of the sphincter at the onset of voiding owing to skeletal muscle hypertonicity

Pseudodyssynergia

Pseudodyssynergia refers to an EMG sphincter "flare" during filling cystometry that is secondary to attempted inhibition of an involuntary bladder contraction by voluntary contraction of the striated sphincter. If a patient has an unstable bladder contraction during filling cystometry, the normal response of the external sphincter is to contract in an attempt to prevent incontinence. This has the same appearance as detrusor-sphincter dyssynergia on an EMG study but is of different significance because it is a voluntary "guarding event."

Spinal Cord vs. Spinal Column in Spinal Cord Injury

Spinal column (bone) segments are numbered by the vertebral level, and these have a different relationship to the **spinal cord segmental level** at different locations. **One must be careful to specify cord versus column level when discussing spinal cord injury.** The sacral spinal cord begins at about spinal column level T12 to L1. The spinal cord terminates in the cauda equina at approximately the spinal column level of L2.

Spinal Cord Shock

Following significant spinal cord injury, a period of decreased excitability of spinal cord segments at and below where the level of injury occurs is known as *spinal cord shock*. It includes a suppression of autonomic activity, as well as somatic activity, and the bladder is acontractile and areflexic.

Cauda Equina Syndrome

Cauda equina syndrome is a term applied to the clinical picture of perineal sensory loss with loss of voluntary control of both anal and urethral sphincter and of sexual responsiveness. This can occur not only secondary to disc disease (severe central posterior disc protrusion) but to other spinal canal pathologic processes as well.

2. Overview of Normal Voiding Function

Innervation of the Lower Urinary Tract

Parasympathetic Nervous System

- Neurotransmitter:

  *Acetylcholine (ganglia and effector sites)

- Receptors:

  *Nicotinic (ganglia and motor endplates)

  *Muscarinic (autonomic effector sites, ie, bladder contractions)

Sympathetic Nervous System

- Neurotransmitter:

  *Acetylcholine (ganglia)

  *Norepinephrine (effector sites)

- Receptors:

  *Alpha (bladder base and neck)—closure of the outlet

  *Betas (bladder body)—detrusor muscle relaxation

Function of the Lower Urinary Tract: 2 Basic Functions

- Bladder filling/urine storage: involves the bladder muscle and bladder outlet

- Bladder/detrusor muscle: there are 3 processes active during bladder filling:

  1. Accommodation of increasing volumes of urine at low pressures with appropriate sensations through 3 activities:

    a. The afferent activity sending sensations to the CNS

    b. The tonic inhibition from the brain inhibits parasympathetic activity c. The inhibition of the parasympathetic system also provided by sympathetic and somatic reflex activity

2. The prevention of involuntary detrusor contractions

3. The prevention of parasympathetic activity

- Bladder outlet: must remain closed by spinal reflex activity that activates sympathetic and somatic nerve pathways **(the guarding reflex)**

- Bladder emptying/urine voiding

- Bladder/detrusor muscle:
  Contraction provided via the process of:

  **Afferent activity: the primary stimulus of micturition reflex is bladder distention that provides afferent activity from stretch receptors*

  **Parasympathetic activity: gives rise to the smooth muscle contraction and inhibits sympathetic reflex*

  **Sympathetic and somatic nerve activity: becomes inactive as voluntary relaxation of the external sphincter initiates the micturition reflex*

  **The Pons/CNS coordinates the bladder and outlet activity*

- Bladder outlet: opens via:

  **Lowering of resistance at the outlet*

  **Absence of anatomic obstruction*

3. General Patterns and Classifications of Neurogenic Voiding Dysfunction

General Comments

- Neurologic disease generally affects lower urinary tract function in a consistent fashion

- Variability of clinical presentation occurs when the following is present:

  **The injury is irritative versus destructive*

  **The injury is partial versus complete*

  **The injury is muticentric versus focal*

  **The injury is specific versus nonspecific*

General Prevalences of Neurogenic Voiding Dysfunction

Central Nervous System Conditions

- *Spinal cord injury: vast majority*
- *Cerebro-vascular accidents: 32%-79%*
- *Dementia: 30%-100%*
- *Parkinson's disease: 40%-70%*
- *Cerebral palsy: 36%*
- *Severe learning disabilities: 12%-65%*
- *Normal pressure hydrocephalus: case reports*
- *Cerebral tumors: case reports*

Central and Peripheral Nervous System Conditions

- *Multiple system atrophy (MSA or Shy-Drager syndrome): 73%*
- *Multiple sclerosis: 52%-97%*
- *Spinal stenosis: 62%*
- *Spine surgery: 38%-60%*
- *Disc disease: 28%-87%*

- *Diabetes mellitus: 25%-87%*

Peripheral Nervous System Conditions

- *Complex pelvic surgery: 20%-79%*
- *Radical hysterectomy: 8%-57%*
- *Guillain-Barré: 25% in case series*
- *HIV: 12% in advanced cases*
- *Herpes: 0.4%*
- *SLE: 0.01%*

Classification Systems of Neurogenic Voiding Dysfunction

General Comments on Classifications Systems

- Due to the diversity of neurological injuries, it has been difficult to have one general system for the entire population of patients with neurogenic voiding dysfunction; ie, no one system is perfect.
- In general, the classification system should do the following:

  * *It should localize the site and type of neurological lesions*

  **It should attempt to outline expected clinical symptoms and presentations*

  * *It should attempt to include conclusions reached from urodynamic testing*

The Functional Classification (Table 1)

Classification of voiding dysfunction can be formulated on a simple functional basis, describing the dysfunction in terms of whether the deficit produced is primarily one of the **filling/storage** or the **emptying/voiding** phase of micturition. There are indeed some types of voiding dysfunction that represent combinations of filling/storage and emptying/voiding abnormalities.

- ***Storage failure** results because of either bladder or outlet abnormalities or a combination.*

  **Bladder abnormalities include involuntary bladder contractions, low compliance, and heightened or altered sensation*

  **Outlet abnormalities include intermittent or continuous decrease in outlet resistance*

- ***Emptying failure** results because of bladder or outlet abnormalities or a combination.*

  **Bladder abnormality includes an inadequate or unsustained bladder contractility.*

  * *Outlet abnormalities include anatomic obstruction and sphincter dyssynergia.*

The ICS Classification System (Table 2)

The storage and voiding phases of micturition are described separately, and within each, various designations are applied to describe bladder and urethral function, as well as bladder sensation.

In general:

- *Detrusor activity: Normal (N), hyperactive (+), or hypoactive/areflexic (-)*
- *Bladder capacity or compliance: Normal (N), high (+), or low (-)*
- *Urethral function: Normal, overactivity (+), or incompetent (-)*
- *Bladder sensation: Normal (N), hypersensitive (+), or hyposensitive/absent (-)*

Table 1

The Functional Classification

I. Failure to Fill/Store

A. Due to Bladder Dysfunction

1. Overactivity
   a. Involuntary contractions
      Neurologic disease or injury
      Bladder outlet obstruction (myogenic)
      Inflammation
      Idiopathic
   b. Decreased compliance
      Neurologic disease or injury
      Fibrosis
      Idiopathic
   c. Combination
2. Hypersensitivity
   a. Inflammatory/infectious
   b. Neurologic
   c. Psychological
   d. Idiopathic
3. Decreased pelvic floor activity (?)
4. Combination

B. Due to Outlet Dysfunction

1. Combination (GSI and ISD)
2. Genuine stress urinary incontinence (GSI)
   a. Lack of suburethral support
   b. Pelvic floor laxity, hypermobility
3. Intrinsic sphincter deficiency (ISD)
   a. Neurologic disease or injury
   b. Fibrosis

C. Due to a Combination of Bladder and Outlet Dysfunctions

II. Failure to Void/Empty

A. Due to Bladder Dysfunction

1. Neurogenic
2. Myogenic
3. Psychogenic
4. Idiopathic

B. Due to Outlet Dysfunction

1. Anatomic
   a. Prostatic obstruction
   b. Bladder neck contracture
   c. Urethral stricture in the male
   d. Urethral compression, fibrosis in the female
2. Functional
   a. Smooth sphincter dyssynergia
   b. Striated sphincter dyssynergia
   c. Dysfunctional voiding

C. Due to a Combination of Bladder and Outlet Dysfunctions

Adapted from: Wein AJ. Pathophysiology and classification of voiding dysfunction. In: Wein, Kavoussi, Novick, Partin, Peters, eds. Campbell-Walsh Urology. *Philadelphia, PA: Saunders/Elsevier; 2007: 1973-1985.*

Table 2

The International Continence Society Classification

Storage Phase	**Voiding Phase**
Bladder Function:	**Bladder Function:**
Detrusor activity: Normal or stable Overactive: Neurogenic Idiopathic	Detrusor activity: Normal Underactive: Acontractile Areflexic
Bladder Sensation:	**Urethral Function:**
Normal Increased or hypersensitive Reduced or hyposensitive Absent	Normal Abnormal: Mechanical obstruction
Bladder Capacity/ Compliance:	Overactivity Dysfunctional voiding, Detrusor sphincter dyssynergia, Nonrelaxing urethral sphincter dysfunction
Normal High Low	
Urethral Function	
Normal closure mechanism Incompetent closure mechanism	

Adapted from Abrams P, Cardozo L, Fall M, et al. The standardization of terminology in lower urinary tract function: Report from the standardization subcommittee of the International Continence Society. Urology. *2003;61:37-49.*

4. Evaluation and Consequences of Neurogenic Voiding Dysfunction Progression

Overview

Evaluation of voiding dysfunction in neurogenic causes should be undertaken to prevent consequences and to determine the goals of treatment:

- Prevent upper urinary tract deterioration
- Restore hygienic and socially acceptable filling and emptying functions of the neurogenic bladder
- Avoidance of infections
- Considerations of bowel and other pelvic organ functions
- Clinical evaluations for neurogenic conditions (other than spinal cord injury) in general:

  1. Tend to correlate poorly with dysfunctions noted on urodynamics
  2. Tend to correlate poorly with clinical symptoms

- Localization of neurogenic injury as a means of predict voiding dysfunction and planning for evaluation:
- ***Lesions above the brainstem*** (CVA, Parkinson's disease, MS, CVA, etc.) between the cortex and the pontine micturition center (PMC) typically result in the following ICS Classification:

  *****Detrusor*** = (+); involuntary bladder contractions (CNS inhibition is lost); rarely is the detrusor acontractile (-)

  *****Sphincter*** = N; Detrusor – sphincter synergy (smooth and striated sphincter synergy)

  *****Sensation*** = N; usually normal

  **Special notes:*

  - *Detrusor areflexia may occur either initially or as a permanent dysfunction*

- *Urinary incontinence may occur due to the detrusor overactivity*

- Spinal cord lesions (myelodysplasia, MS, spinal cord injury, stenosis, or disc disease, etc.) with injuries between the pontine micturition center and S2; ie, above S2 typically result in the following ICS Classification:

  **Detrusor* = (+); involuntary contractions

  **Sphincter* = (+); dyssynergia

  **Sensation* = (-); absent

  **Special notes:*

  - *Those with lesions above T6-8 may develop autonomic dysreflexia*

  - *Incontinence may occur due to detrusor overactivity, but the outlet obstruction can also cause urinary retention*

  - *A careful initial evaluation and periodic follow-up evaluation must be performed to identify and correct the following risk factors and potential complications: bladder overdistention, high-pressure storage, high detrusor leak point pressure, vesicoureteral reflux (VUR), stone formation (lower and upper tracts), and complicating infection, especially in association with reflux.*

  - *Reflux management: The best initial treatment for reflux in a patient with voiding dysfunction secondary to neurologic disease or injury is to normalize lower urinary tract urodynamics as much as possible.*

  - *UTI management: In a consensus reached by the National Institute on Disability and Rehabilitation Research Group (1992), bacteriuria should be treated only when signs or symptoms present.*

Follow-up: In the American Paraplegic Society (APS) Guidelines (1999) for urologic care of SCI, annual follow-up is recommended for the first 5 to 10 years after injury. If the patient is doing well, then follow-up every other year is advised. Upper and lower tract evaluation should be done initially and yearly for 5 to 10 years, then every other year. Urodynamic evaluation was recommended by the APS at the same intervals as upper and lower tract screening. Cystoscopy was recommended annually in those with an indwelling catheter.

- **Disease at S2 and below; and peripheral lesions** (Myelodysplasia, MS, tethered cord, spinal stenosis, polio, etc.) typically result in the following ICS Classification:

  * ***Detrusor*** = (-); acontractile and poor detrusor compliance typically develops

  * ***Sphincter*** = (+); open smooth muscle sphincter, but fixed striated sphincter with loss of voluntary control is the usual finding

  * ***Sensation*** = (-)

  * Special note:
    True peripheral neuropathy can be motor or sensory

- Evaluation of upper and lower urinary tracts

- BMP, serum creatinine, or creatinine clearance in select cases

- Renal ultrasound

- Selective use of renal scans for evaluate renal scarring, function, and obstruction

- Urodynamics (UDS):
  Determining the predominate bladder pressure against which the kidneys drain; while no RCTs had documented beneficial outcomes achieved with UDS information, the overwhelming bulk of evidence supports the use of this testing in neurogenic patients with voiding dysfunction.

  **Determine bladder capacity*

  **Determine bladder/detrusor compliance*

Determine detrusor over/under/normal activity

Determine the detrusor leak point pressure (DLPP):

- The DLPP was first introduced by McGuire and associates for the evaluation of patients with low bladder compliance secondary to myelodysplasia. McGuire found that in myelodysplastic patients with an elevated outlet resistance from a fixed external sphincter, those with a **DLPP greater than 40 cm H_2O were at significantly higher risk for upper tract deterioration (hydronephrosis, reflux) than those with DLPPs less than 40 cm H_2O.** However, while pressures >40 cm H_2O are important, the time over which an elevated pressure is exerted onto the system is also significant.

- Ancillary neurogenic bladder testing: impractical (ice water and bethanecol) or evolving (electro-sensitivity):

*Ice water UDS testing: reveals detrusor overactivity in pathologic conditions; normal bladders or sacral neurogenic lesions have no inducible detrusor contractions, but suprasacral spinal cord lesions will reveal a positive test with inducible involuntary detrusor contractions when using ice-cold water during the filling phase of UDS testing.

*Bethanecol supersensitivity testing with UDS: based on the assumption that denervated/neurogenic bladder will be more sensitive to acetylcholine stimulation than a non-neurogenic acontractile bladder; a positive test reveals a rise in detrusor pressure greater than 15 cm H_2O during the filling after giving sq bethanechol chloride.

* Electrosensitivity testing involves placement of bladder catheter electrode to test for abnormal sensitivities as found in DM, MS, etc.

5. Clinical Presentations of Neurogenic Voiding Dysfunction

Disease at or Above the Brain Stem

- Neurogenic voiding dysfunction secondary to cerebrovascular injury (stroke):

Following the acute CVA event or cerebral shock, acute detrusor areflexia or retention may be present

Common features of chronic impairment include:

Detrusor = (+), Sphincter = N,
Bladder sensation = N

Detrusor overactivity, but normal detrusor compliance

True detrusor dyssynergia does not occur as the lesion is above the pons; pseudodssynergia may occur

Variable sensation; usually intact and often with OAB symptoms

Always consider pre-existing pathology such as BPO and a hypocontractile function

Always consider using urodynamics to document and reveal voiding dysfunction before invasive procedures

- Neurogenic voiding dysfunction secondary to Parkinson 's disease:

Duration and severity of Parkinson's disease does not correlate with urodynamic findings

Voiding dysfunction develops in 35%-70% of cases; detrusor overactivity is the most common finding; Detrusor = (+)

Sphincter bradykinesia and pseudodyssynergia complicate urodynamics;

Impaired contractility may cause hesitancy; Detrusor = (-)

Poorly sustained contractions with obstruction is problematic (DHIC – detrusor hyper-

reflexia and impaired contractility)

**Benign prostatic obstruction with Parkinson's disease is often noted:*

- *Postprostatectomy incontinence (PPI) from TURP – 20% versus 1% in non-neurogenic patients*

- *Risk of PPI is 4% if normal sphincter control exists*

**Sensation is usually intact*

- Neurogenic voiding dysfunction secondary to multiple system atrophy (MSA); also known as Shy-Drager syndrome:

**Voiding dysfunction symptoms precede the diagnosis of MSA (4 years on average) or they present with other symptoms of MSA*

**73% of patients have detrusor overactivity; Detrusor = (+)*

**19% have urinary frequency and urgency without urinary incontinence*

**66% have significant emptying dysfunction with elevated PVRs*

**93% of men have erectile dysfunction*

Disease Primarily Involving the Spinal Cord Above S2

- Neurogenic voiding dysfunction secondary to multiple sclerosis

- 2%-10% of patients with MS present with voiding dysfunction as part of their initial presentation; 80% of MS pts develop voiding dysfunction as part of the condition

**Urodynamic patterns can change in 15%-35% of cases when symptoms change*

**3 basic patterns of voiding dysfunction:*

1. *Detrusor = (+), overactive; Sphincter = N, normal synergy; Sensation = N, normal; this pattern represents 26%-50% of cases*

2. *Detrusor = (+), overactive; Sphincter = (+), dyssynergy; Sensation = N, normal; this pattern represents 24%-46% of cases*

3. *Detrusor = (-), overactive; Sphincter = (?), dyssynergy; Sensation = ?; this pattern represents 19%-40% of cases*

** Pelvic floor and sphincter flaccidity can also occur*

** In most all cases, bladder sensation remains intact*

- Spinal cord injury

* Voiding dysfunction is typically: Detrusor = (+), Sphincter = (+), and Sensation = (-):

* Involuntary detrusor contractions

* Detrusor dyssynergia

* Absent sensation

* ***2 major concepts in treating SCI:***

1. ***Autonomic hyperreflexia (autonomic dysreflexia):***
Treat with terazosin (a selective α_1-adrenergic blocker) for long-term management (3-month study) and prophylaxis. A nightly dose varying between 1-10 mg will reduce severity, whereas erectile function and blood pressure will remain unchanged.

2. ***Detrusor leak point pressure:***
An important concept in urodynamics is the fact that bladder outlet resistance is the main determinant of detrusor pressure and urethral outlet resistance at a moment of flow determines Pdet. If the outlet resistance is high, a higher bladder pressure is needed to overcome this resistance and cause leakage. This high pressure can be

transmitted to the upper tracts, causing reflux and hydronephrosis. However, while pressures >40 cm H_2O are important, the time over which an elevated pressure is exerted onto the system is also significant.

- Myelodysplasia
  - *Voiding dysfunction is more variable than SCI above S2: Detrusor (+,-), Sphincter (+, N, -), Sensation (+, N, -)
  - *At risk for:
    - Upper tract deterioration, reflux
    - Infection
    - Incontinence
    - Carcinoma
    - Sexual dysfunction
    - Bowel dysfunction
- Spinal stenosis
  - *Spinal canal narrowing (congenital or acquired)
  - *Nerve root or cord damage
  - *Ischemia, swelling
  - *Usually presents with low back pain with radiation to the legs, relieved with rest
  - *Variety of bladder and sphincter dysfunctions
  - *Urodynamics and comorbid conditions dictate diagnosis and treatment
- Tethered cord
  - *Primary or secondary (3%-5% of surgical closures for myelodysplasia)
  - *May present in early childhood and up to 80 years of age
  - *Symptoms: urinary incontinence, leg weakness, and backache
  - *Progressive decline without treatment

Disease Distal to the Spinal Cord: Injury Below S2; ie, Sacral Injury

- Radical pelvic surgery: prevalence of voiding dysfunction
  - **Post APR: 20%-60%*
  - **Post-radical hysterectomy:16%-80%*
  - **15%-20% of cases are permanent dysfunctions*
  - **Allow 6 months for apraxia to resolve and/or reinnervation to occur*
  - **Voiding dysfunction: Detrusor = (-), Sphincter = (+), Sensation = N, (-)*
    - *Usually areflexic or hypocontractile detrusor*
    - *Increased risk of detrusor compliance loss*
    - *Bladder neck often open due to sympathetic denervation of compliance loss*
    - *Fixed external sphincter resistance*
  - **Mixed storage and emptying symptoms*
  - **Avoid TURP or outlet surgeries unless carefully studied with UDS*

Miscellaneous Conditions

- Diabetes mellitus
  - *5%-59% of patients with diabetes report symptoms of voiding dysfunction
  - ****Diabetic cystopathy*** is a term used to describe the involvement of the lower urinary tract by this disease.

6. Overview of Treatments for Neurogenic Voiding Dysfunction

* The classic description of voiding dysfunction secondary to diabetes is that of a peripheral and autonomic neuropathy that first affects sensory afferent pathways, causing the insidious onset of impaired bladder sensation. As the classic description continues, a gradual increase in the time interval between voiding results, which may progress to the point at which the patient voids only once or twice a day without ever sensing any real urgency. If this continues, detrusor distention, overdistention, and decompensation ultimately occur. Detrusor contractility, therefore, is classically described as being decreased in the end-stage diabetic bladder.

Voiding Dysfunction: Prioritizing the Medical Goals of Management

- Upper urinary tract preservation or improvement
- Absence or control of infection
- Adequate storage at low intravesical pressure
- Adequate emptying at low intravesical pressure
- Adequate control
- No catheter or stoma
- Social acceptability and adaptability
- Vocational acceptability and adaptability

Reasons to Change or Augment a Given Management Plan

- Upper urinary tract deterioration
- Recurrent sepsis or fever of urinary tract origin
- Lower urinary tract deterioration
- Inadequate storage
- Inadequate emptying
- Inadequate control
- Unacceptable side effects
- Skin changes secondary to incontinence or collecting device

Patient Factors to Consider When Choosing Therapies Outlined in Tables 3 and 4

- Prognosis of underlying disease, especially if progressive or malignant
- General health

Table 3

Therapy to Facilitate Urine Storage/Bladder Filling

Bladder Related (Inhibiting Bladder Contractility, Decreasing Sensory Input and/or Increasing Bladder Capacity)

Behavioral Therapy, Including Any or All of the Following:
Education
Bladder training
Timed bladder emptying or prompted voiding
Fluid restriction
Pelvic floor physiotherapy ± biofeedback

Pharmacologic Therapy
(Oral, Intravesical, Intradetrusor)
- Anticholinergic agents
- Drugs with mixed actions
- Calcium antagonists
- Potassium channel openers
- Prostaglandin inhibitors
- β-Adrenergic agonists
- α-Adrenergic antagonists
- Tricyclic antidepressants; serotonin and norepinephrine reuptake inhibitors
- Dimethyl sulfoxide (DMSO)
- Polysynaptic inhibitors
- Capsaicin, resiniferatoxin, and like agents
- Botulinum toxin

Bladder overdistention
Electrical neuromodulation
Acupuncture and electroacupuncture
Interruption of innervation
- Very central (subarachnoid block)
- Less central (sacral rhizotomy, selective sacral rhizotomy)
- Peripheral motor or/and sensory

Augmentation cystoplasty
(Auto, bowel, tissue engineering)

Outlet Related (Increasing Outlet Resistance)

Behavioral Therapy
- Education
- Bladder training
- Timed bladder emptying or prompted voiding
- Fluid restriction
- Pelvic floor physiotherapy ± biofeedback

Electrical stimulation
Pharmacologic Therapy
- α-Adrenergic agonists
- Tricyclic antidepressants; serotonin and norepinephrine reuptake inhibitors
- β-Adrenergic antagonists, agonists

Vaginal and perineal occlusive and/or supportive devices; urethral plugs
Nonsurgical periurethral bulking
- Collagen, synthetics, cell transfer

Vesicourethral suspension ± prolapse repair (female)
Sling procedures ± prolapse repair (female)
Closure of the bladder outlet
Artificial urinary sphincter
Bladder outlet reconstruction
Myoplasty (muscle transposition)

Circumventing the Problem

Absorbent products
External collecting devices
Antidiuretic hormone-like agents
Short-acting diuretics
Intermittent catheterization
Continuous catheterization
Urinary diversion

Adapted from: Wein AJ. Pathophysiology and classification of voiding dysfunction. In: Wein, Kavoussi, Novick, Partin, Peters, eds. Campbell-Walsh Urology. *Philadelphia, PA: Saunders/Elsevier; 2007:1973-1985.*

Table 4

Therapy to Facilitate Bladder Emptying/Voiding

Bladder Related (Increasing Intravesical Pressure or Facilitating Bladder Contractility)

External compression, Valsalva
Promotion or initiating of reflex contraction
- Trigger zones or maneuvers
- Bladder "training"; tidal drainage

Pharmacologic therapy (oral, intravesical)
- Parasympathomimetic agents
- Prostaglandins
- Blockers of inhibition
  - α-Adrenergic antagonists
  - Opioid antagonists

Electrical stimulation
- Directly to the bladder or spinal cord
- Directly to the nerve roots
- Intravesical (transurethral)
- Neuromodulation

Reduction cystoplasty
Bladder myoplasty (muscle wrap)

Outlet Related (Increasing Outlet Resistance)

At a site of anatomic obstruction
- Pharmacologic Therapy—decrease prostate size or tone
  - α-Adrenergic antagonists
  - 5α-Reductase inhibitors
  - Luteinizing hormone-releasing hormone agonists/antagonists
  - Antiandrogens

Outlet Related (Increasing Outlet Resistance)

- Prostatectomy, prostatotomy (diathermy, heat, laser)
- Bladder neck incision or resection
- Urethral stricture repair or dilation
- Intraurethral stent
- Balloon dilatation of stricture/contracture

At level of smooth sphincter
- Pharmacologic Therapy
  - α-Adrenergic antagonists
  - β-Adrenergic agonists
- Transurethral resection or incision
- Y-V plasty

At level of striated sphincter
- Behavioral therapy ± biofeedback
- Pharmacologic therapy
  - Benzodiazepines
  - Baclofen
  - Dantrolene
  - α-Adrenergic antagonists
- Botulinum toxin (injection)

Urethral overdilation
Surgical sphincterotomy
Urethral stent
Pudendal nerve interruption

Circumventing the Problem

Intermittent catheterization
Continuous catheterization
Urinary diversion (conduit)

Adapted from: Wein AJ. Pathophysiology and classification of voiding dysfunction. In: Wein, Kavoussi, Novick, Partin, Peters, eds. Campbell-Walsh Urology. *Philadelphia, PA: Saunders/Elsevier; 2007:1973-1985.*

Limiting factors: inability to perform certain tasks (eg, hand dexterity, ability to transfer, body habitus)

- Mental status
- Motivation
- Desire to remain catheter or appliance free
- Desire to avoid surgery
- Sexual activity status
- Reliability
- Educability
- Psychosocial environment, interest, reliability, and cooperation of family
- Economic resources

7. Further Reading

1. Abrams P, Cardozo L, Fall M, et al. The standardization of terminology in lower urinary tract function: Report from the standardization subcommittee of the International Continence Society. *Urology*. 2003;61:37-49.

2. Peterson AC, Webster GD. Urodynamic and videourodynamic evaluation of voiding dysfunction. In: Wein, Kavoussi, Novick, Partin, Peters, eds. *Campbell-Walsh Urology*. Philadelphia, PA: Saunders/Elsevier; 2007: 1986-2010.

3. Rackley RR, Appell RA. Evaluation and management of lower urinary tract disorders in women with multiple sclerosis. *Int Urogynecol*. 1999;10(2):139-43.

4. Wein A, Rackley R. Overactive bladder: A better understanding of pathophysiology, diagnosis, and management. *J Urol*. 2006 Mar;175(3 Pt 2):S5-10.

5. Wein AJ. Pathophysiology and classification of voiding dysfunction. In: Wein, Kavoussi, Novick, Partin, Peters, eds. *Campbell-Walsh Urology*. Philadelphia, PA: Saunders/Elsevier; 2007:1973-1985.

6. Wein AJ. Lower urinary tract dysfunction in neurologic injury and disease. In: Wein, Kavoussi, Novick, Partin, Peters, eds. *Campbell-Walsh Urology*. Philadelphia, PA: Saunders/Elsevier; 2007:2011-2045.

8. Questions

1. All of the following statements regarding bladder compliance are true, except:

   A. Bladder compliance is defined as the change in intravesical or detrusor pressure (Pdet) relative to the corresponding change in Volume

   B. Normal bladder compliance is 12.5 mL/cm H_2O

   C. Is calculated between 2 points: the P(det) with the bladder empty at the start of urodynamic filling and the Pdet at either the maximal cystometric capacity or the start of a detrusor contraction (involuntary or voluntary)

   D. Compliance arises from the neuromuscular and biomechanical (collagenous and elastic) components of the bladder wall.

2. The difference between the detrusor leak point pressure (DLPP) and the abdominal leak point pressure (ALPP), 2 pressures obtained during urodynamics that measure different aspects of lower urinary tract function, is the following:

   A. How much fluid is in the bladder when the measurements are obtained

   B. When the Pdet is measured during the filling phase of the urodynamic study in the presence of increased abdominal pressure

   C. When the Pdet is measured during the filling phase of the urodynamic study in the presence a detrusor contraction

   D. The rate of urodynamic filling of the bladder

3. The following statements regarding the smooth and striated sphincter muscle of the bladder outlet and urethra are true, except:

   A. The smooth sphincter refers to the smooth musculature of the bladder neck and proximal urethra.

   B. The smooth muscle is a physiologic and an anatomic sphincter and one that is not under voluntary control.

   C. The striated sphincter refers to the striated musculature that is a part of the outer wall of the proximal urethra in both the male and the female is often referred to as the intrinsic or intramural striated sphincter.

   D. The bulky striated skeletal muscle group that closely surrounds the urethra at the level of the membranous portion in the male and primarily the middle segment in the female is often referred to as the extrinsic or extramural striated sphincter.

   E. The extramural portion is the classically described external urethral sphincter and is under voluntary control.

4. Autonomic hyperreflexia represents which one of the following?

   A. An acute massive disordered autonomic (primarily sympathetic) response to specific stimuli in patients with SCI above the cord level of T6 to T8 (the sympathetic outflow).

   B. Onset after injury is variable—usually soon after spinal shock but may be up to years after injury.

   C. It is more common in cervical (60%) than thoracic (20%) injuries.

   D. Distal cord viability is a prerequisite.

   E. A. and C.

   F. B. and D.

   G. D. only

   H. All the above

5. To differentiate detrusor-sphincter dyssynergia from pelvic floor hyperactivity or dysfunctional voiding, which one of the following statements must be true?:

A. Failure of the sphincter to relax or stay completely relaxed during micturition must be present.

B. Uninhibited contractions on the filling part of the urodynamics must be present.

C. Neurologic disease must be present.

D. Bladder sensation must be absent.

E. Bowel dysfunction must be present.

F. A. and B.

G. C. and D.

H. E. only

I. All of the above

6. Cauda equina syndrome is a term applied to the clinical picture which typically includes which of the following criteria:

A. Loss of voluntary control of anal sphincter

B. Perineal sensory loss

C. Loss of voluntary control of the urethral sphincter

D. Loss of sexual responsiveness.

E. Loss of motor function of the legs

F. A. and C.

G. B. and D.

H. E. only

I. All of the above

7. Spinal cord shock may be characterized by which of the following features:

A. It represents a period of decreased excitability of spinal cord segments at and below where the level of injury occurs

B. It may be short term or chronic

C. It includes suppression of autonomic activity

D. It includes a suppression of somatic activity

E. The bladder is acontractile and areflexic

F. A. and C.

G. B. and D.

H. E. only

I. All of the above

8. Lower urinary tract dysfunction in a classic T10 spinal cord level paraplegic patient after spinal shock has passed would be described as follows:

A. Overactive neurogenic detrusor function

B. Absent bladder sensation

C. Overactive obstructive urethral function

D. Low bladder capacity

E. Normal bladder compliance

F. A. and C.

G. B. and D.

H. E. only

I. All of the above

9. The voiding dysfunction of a stroke patient with urgency incontinence would best be described as follows:

A. Overactive neurogenic detrusor function

B. Normal bladder sensation

C. Normal urethral function

D. Low bladder capacity

E. Normal bladder compliance

F. A. and C.

G. B. and D.

H. E. only

I. All of the above

10. Which of the following comments regarding vesicoureteral reflux in the spinal cord injury (SCI) patients are true:

A. More common in suprasacral injuries

B. Infections are a contributing factor

C. Elevated intravesical pressure during filling and emptying is a contributing factor

D. Persistent reflux can lead to chronic renal damage

E. Risk factor for decreased long term survival in SCI patients

F. A. and C.

G. B. and D.

H. E. only

I. All of the above

Answers

1. A.
Compliance = change Volume / change Pdet (expressed as mL/cm H_2O)

2. B.
DLLP is defined by the ICS as the lowest detrusor pressure at which urine leakage occurs in the absence of either a detrusor contraction or increased abdominal pressure. ALPP is defined as the intravesical pressure at which urine leakage occurs because of increased abdominal pressure in the absence of a detrusor contraction.

3. B.
The smooth sphincter refers to the smooth musculature of the bladder neck and proximal urethra. This is a physiologic but not an anatomic sphincter and one that is not under voluntary control.

4. H. All of the above.
Distal spinal cord viability (incomplete or partial) has to be intact for somatic and sensory stimuli to enter CNS system to trigger the sympathetic outflow.

5. F.
Failure of the sphincter to relax or stay completely relaxed during micturition is abnormal. When it occurs in patients with neurologic disease, it is termed detrusor-sphincter dyssynergia; this typically occurs in patients with suprasacral spinal cord injury in which there is an interruption of the spinobulbar-spinal pathways that normally coordinate the detrusor and the sphincter. In the absence of neurologic disease, one cannot use the term detrusor-sphincter dyssynergia. Instead, the term pelvic floor hyperactivity or dysfunctional voiding is used.

6. I. All of the above.
Loss of leg motor function is not typically seen in Cauda equina syndrome. In addition to all of the above findings, Cauda equina syndrome occurs secondary to disk disease (severe central posterior disc protrusion) and other spinal canal pathologic processes as well.

7. I. All of the above.

8. I. All of the above.
Generally, complete spinal cord lesions above the sacral spinal cord, but below the area of the sympathetic outflow, result in detrusor overactivity, absent bladder sensation, and striated sphincter dyssynergia. While normal bladder compliance may be maintained, reduced bladder capacity is typically noted.

9. I. All of the above.
The most common type of voiding dysfunction after stroke would then be characterized as a failure to store secondary to bladder overactivity, specifically involuntary bladder contractions. The dysfunction would most likely be classified as overactive neurogenic detrusor function, normal sensation, low capacity, normal compliance, and normal urethral closure function during storage; during voiding the description would be normal detrusor activity and normal urethral function assuming that no anatomic obstruction existed. Treatment, in the absence of coexisting significant bladder obstruction or significantly impaired contractility, is directed at decreasing bladder contractility and increasing bladder capacity.

10. I. All of the above.
Surprisingly little is written about vesicoureteral reflux (VUR) in the SCI patient. The reported incidence varies between 17% and 25% of such patients and is more common in those with suprasacral SCI. Contributing factors include: 1) elevated intravesical pressure during filling and emptying; and 2) infection. Persistent reflux can lead to chronic renal damage and may be an important factor in the long-term survival of SCI patients. In the series of SCI patients, persistent reflux was present in 60% of patients of those dying of renal disease. In patients with only transient reflux over a 5- to 15-year period, the urogram was normal in 83%, or calyceal changes were only minimal. It should be noted that high storage and voiding pressures without reflux can be responsible for renal damage.

The best initial treatment for reflux in a patient with voiding dysfunction secondary to neurologic disease or injury is to normalize lower urinary tract urodynamics as much as possible.

Chapter 12: Female Urology and Urinary Incontinence

J. Christian Winters, MD, FACS

Contents

1. Female Urology: Pelvic Organ Prolapse

Anatomy of Pelvic Support

The pelvic floor consists of muscular and fascial tissues acting as a supportive structure which prevents the female pelvic organs from being pushed out by intra abdominal pressure. There are 3 levels of vaginal support. The upper third of the vagina (level I) and uterus are supported by fibers from the uterosacral and cardinal ligaments. This supports the upper vagina above the pelvic diaphragm. These fibers mainly merge into the pericervical ring of connective tissue and into the upper vagina. The middle third of the vagina is attached by the mid-portion of the endopelvic fascia (level II). The anterior wall of the vagina in this location is held in place by the lateral attachments of the pubocervical fascia to the fascia over the obturator internus muscle at the arcus tendineus fascia pelvis (white line) (Figure 1).

The posterior vaginal wall is supported laterally by the lateral attachments of the rectovaginal fascia to the fascia overlying the iliococcygeus muscle. At the lower third of the vagina (level III), the vagina merges with the fascia of the endopelvic fascia and pubourethral ligaments anteriorly to the medial margins of the pubococcygeus. The lower extent of the pubocervical fascia merges into the urogenital diaphragm and the rectovaginal fascia merges into the perineal body. Therefore, in the distal third of the vagina, the endopelvic fascia structures are inserting laterally to the pubourethral ligament and the arcus tendineus, and to the perineal body posteriorly.

Types of Prolapse

Cystocele

There are 4 different areas within the connective tissue support of the bladder that predispose one to cystocele if the connective tissue support fails. There are 4 anatomic defects that can account for the development of cystourethrocele:

a. Paravaginal defect (lateral defect)

b. Transverse defect

c. Midline defect (central defect)

Figure 1

Insertion of lateral vaginal attachments on the arcus tendineus fascia pelvis

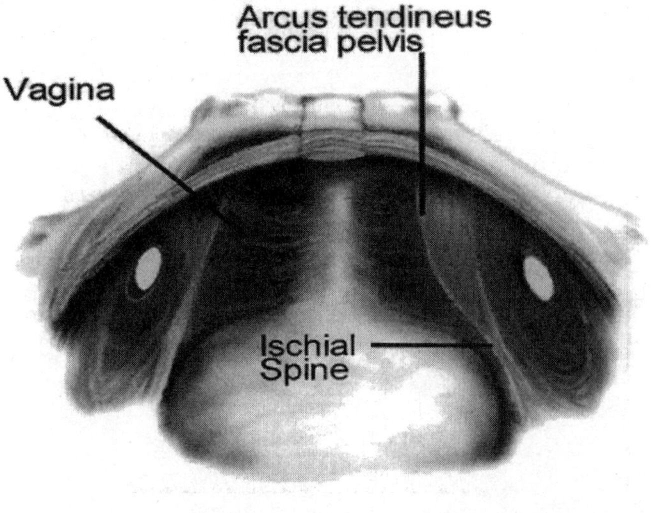

Reprinted with permission: AUA Update Series. Lesson 23, Volume 21; 2002.

d. Distal defect (urethrocele)

The paravaginal defect occurs when a separation of the pubocervical fascia from its lateral attachment to the fascia over the obturator internus muscle occurs at the level of the arcus tendineus fascia pelvis. This represents a break of the pubocervical fascia from the white line. This loss of lateral attachments can occur both unilaterally or bilaterally. Usually, a cystourethrocele is seen when this lateral loss of support occurs, and this defect usually predisposes one to symptoms of stress urinary incontinence.

The transverse defect is a separation of the pubocervical fascia from its attachment to the pericervical ring of tissue at the apex of the vagina (level I). This will allow the base of the bladder to herniate into the anterior vagina. If this occurs in isolation, a proximal cystocele without urethral hypermobility will occur. This usually does not predispose one to stress urinary incontinence as the urethra remains well supported.

The midline defect is any break in the central portion of the hammock like sling of pubocervical fascia upon which the bladder is resting (Figure 2).

Commonly, this condition can create stress incontinence as well because the hammock like break in the pubocervical fascia does involve the area underneath the bladder neck. These occur commonly in patients with paravaginal and lateral defects. However, they are rare in isolation.

The distal defect is an avulsion of the urethral attachment to the urogenital diaphragm as it passes under the pubic symphysis. Essentially, these patients lose the lateral attachment to the urethra, to the arcus tendineus, and pubourethral ligament. In

Figure 2

Break in pubocervical fascia creating central cystocele

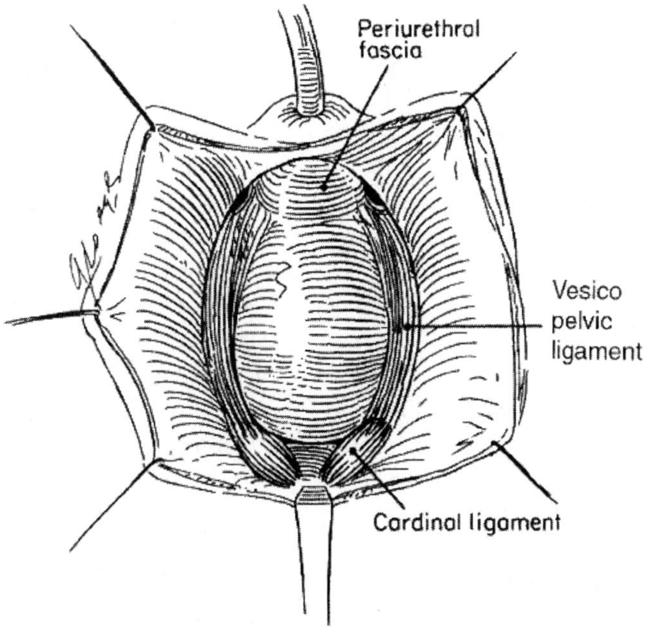

Reprinted with permission: AUA Update Series. Volume 25, Lesson 25; 2006.

addition, these patients lose the anterior attachment of the urethra to the pubic symphysis. This would account for a urethrocele. This condition does predispose one to stress urinary incontinence.

Uterine or Vaginal Vault Prolapse

In patients with a loss of the level I support of the uterosacral ligaments and cardinal ligaments, the apex of the vagina (cervix or vaginal cuff) loses its attachment. Therefore, the apex of the vagina herniates downward as a result of the increased intra-abdominal pressure. This condition will lead to prolapse of the vaginal cuff and/or prolapse of the uterus. Uterine descensus is the result of, and not the cause of, vaginal vault prolapse. It is a result of the loss of level I fascia support that creates uterine or vaginal vault prolapse.

Enterocele

An enterocele is a herniation of the cul-de-sac peritoneum with or without intraperitoneal contents into the fascial layers between the vagina and rectal walls. An enterocele may range from a small bulge posteriorly in the upper part of the vagina to a large defect which protrudes beyond the introitus with visible small bowel internally. The upper aspect of the posterior vaginal wall is where enteroceles occur as a result of a separation of the rectovaginal septum from the level I complex of support. Iatrogenic enteroceles develop after surgical procedures that distort the normal horizontal axis toward the vertical, such as retropubic urethropexy. In approximately 30% of the patients following a Marshall-Marchetti-Krantz bladder neck procedure or a Burch bladder neck suspension, enteroceles have been reported.

Rectocele

The anatomic defect creating a rectocele is similar to the midline defect anteriorly creating a cystocele. As the hammock of rectovaginal fascia overlying the rectum breaks, a bulge of the rectum into the vaginal canal occurs. A transverse defect rectocele occurs simply by a detachment of the perineal body from the rectovaginal fascia. The hammock of recto-vaginal fascia supporting the rectum remains intact but separates from the perineal body. A midline vertical defect is created by a midline separation of the rectovaginal fascia, and a separation of the recto-vaginal fascia can occur from its lateral attachments. Rectoceles are more commonly situated in the mid- to distal aspect of the posterior vaginal wall. These specific anatomic defects are the principles behind site specific reconstruction of posterior defects.

Diagnosis of Pelvic Support Defects

Grading of Prolapse

Many grading systems evaluate the severity of pelvic organ prolapse; however, these systems are fairly subjective, and cross comparison is difficult. Baden and Walker introduced the "half way" system classifying pelvic organ relaxation, allowing one to assess each area of prolapse in relation to the hymen while the patient is straining. The Pelvic Organ Prolapse Quantification examination (POPQ) is a reproducible method to evaluate all quadrants of pelvic floor support. Distinct measurements of various sites are obtained in relation to the hymenal ring in order to define the stage of prolapse. These examination techniques should be emphasized to more adequately standardize pelvic examinations.

Diagnostic Testing

History and physical examination. The evaluation begins with a thorough history. It is important to determine the frequency and characteristics of incontinent episodes. One must determine the type(s) of incontinence present by eliciting information regarding precipitants of the incontinent episode. Did leakage occur with coughing or did it occur with a sensation of needing to void? Are protective pads necessary? If so, what types of pads and how saturated are they? The clinician should understand that it is often very difficult for patients to discuss these symptoms.

A voiding history should be obtained. Day and night time urinary frequency, and any abnormality in urine flow (weak or interrupted) or difficulty initiating the urine stream requiring straining should be assessed. The presence of nocturnal frequency and enuresis is important. A history of recurrent UTI, hematuria or previous bladder suspension may indicate the possibility of an anatomic abnormality.

Other risk factors for bladder dysfunction include: neurologic disease, previous pelvic irradiation, pelvic surgery or pelvic trauma.

Symptoms related to pelvic organ prolapse should be assessed. Vaginal pressure or protrusion is the most common symptom associated with prolapse. Other symptoms include vaginal discharge, back pain, sexual difficulty, dysfunctional voiding or bowel dysfunction. Bowel habits should also assessed. Patients may have difficulty emptying the rectum requiring pressure on the posterior vaginal wall and perineum. Constipation and fecal incontinence are other bowel symptoms that should be elicited.

Medication usage, including over the counter medication, should be documented. Hormonal status and the use of estrogens is important. The obstetrical history including parity, route of deliveries, previous episiotomy and obstetrical complications should be determined.

The use of a questionnaire can facilitate obtaining an accurate history. This ensures that questions concerning the types and severity of incontinence, voiding dysfunction, quality of life impact, and risk factors can be answered by the patient prior to meeting with the clinician. There are incontinence severity scales which are validated instruments to objectively estimate the adverse impact incontinence has on the quality of life. These scales can be compared before and after treatment to assist in outcome assessment. The most commonly used instruments are the Incontinence Impact Questionnaire (IIQ 7) and the Urogenital Distress Inventory Scale (UDI 6).

Physical examination. A thorough physical examination is essential to establish the etiology of urinary incontinence and the presence of concomitant pelvic floor pathology. During the physical examination, every segment of the pelvic floor should be evaluated. The anterior vaginal wall, vaginal apex (or uterus), the upper portion of the posterior vaginal wall, the distal portion of the posterior vaginal wall and the perineum should be separately evaluated. The pelvic examination begins with the patient in the lithotomy position with straining. If all defects of pelvic floor support can be assessed in this position, the exam is then completed. A lower half of a vaginal speculum is utilized to examine for these defects. During examination of the anterior vaginal wall, the urethral support should be established. AQ tip test may be employed with a well-lubricated Q-tip placed at the level of the bladder neck. During straining, a deflection of the Q-tip greater than 30 degrees signifies urethral hypermobility. In many cases, the lack of support and hypermobility of the urethra are obvious with straining, and so therefore, the Q-tip examination is reserved for equivocal examinations only. Additionally, the urethra should be inspected for characteristics of scarring, "kinking," overcorrection or fistula. The characteristic "stove pipe" urethra is still encountered, but usually more subtle findings on examination may indicate postoperative changes that adversely effect urethral function. A stress test is performed in an attempt to elicit stress urinary incontinence. This test should be performed in the lithotomy and standing positions. If loss of urine is seen during the straining maneuver, stress incontinence is likely present. When a cystocele is present, it should be determined if the loss is in the midline (central defect) or if the loss of support is caused by a lateral defect separation of the vagina from its attachments to the pelvic sidewall at the arcus tendineus. With progressive anterior herniation of the vaginal wall, the various anterior defects may be separated utilizing techniques during the physical examination. Most commonly, a surgical sponge stick can be placed into the lateral fornices of the vagina. The lateral fornices of the vagina are elevated anteriorly to try to recreate the attachments of the lateral wall of the vagina to the pelvic sidewall. The patient is then asked to strain once again. If there is no descensus of the vaginal wall maintaining the lateral attachments, the cystocele defect is a predominant lateral defect. A reattachment of the vagina to the pelvic sidewall should correct this patient's problem. However, if elevation of the lateral fornices of the vagina by a sponge stick does not eradicate the prolapse, then there is a central or midline defect cystocele present. This cystocele is created by a loss of the pubocervical fascia hammock below the bladder, causing a central hernia tion of the bladder.

With a speculum then displacing the anterior vaginal wall, the posterior wall of the vagina is assessed.

It is important to distinguish the etiology of prolapse high in the posterior wall as either enterocele or high rectocele. This is accomplished by bimanual recto-vaginal evaluation in the supine and/or standing position to detect enterocele. If a sac or bowel can be palpated during this exam between the rectum and the examiner's finger, this indicates the presence of an enterocele. If no enterocele sac or bowel is palpated between the rectum and the vagina, this defect is most likely a high rectocele. Perhaps the most critical aspect of the exam is to assess the uterine or vaginal apical support. This is usually easier when the cervix is present, as it is a well defined landmark of the vaginal apex. With straining, the descent of a well-supported uterus should not occur and is noted by an absence of cervical descent. The descent of the cervix halfway to the hymenal ring indicates a moderate loss of uterine support. In post-hysterectomy patients, defining the true vaginal apex can be more difficult. The cuff scar and "dimples" at the lateral aspects of the vagina are landmarks that are used to localize the apex. These dimples usually represent the attachments of the uterosacral ligaments. When these landmarks are noted, and the apex of the vagina extends halfway to the hymenal ring with straining, these patients have a significant prolapse of the vaginal vault. This is a difficult aspect of the pelvic examination that warrants attention to detail as apical prolapse can be hidden by large anterior or posterior compartment prolapse or partially reduced by the examining speculum. In most cases, these patients should be evaluated standing with the examiner's fingers placed at the vaginal apex. If the examiner's fingers descend halfway to the hymenal ring or more with straining, vaginal vault prolapse is present.

After the pelvic examination is completed, lower urinary tract function should be assessed. It is known that stress incontinence may develop after the correction of some types of female pelvic organ prolapse. This probably occurs as a result of unmasking occult stress urinary incontinence after the bladder support is restored. Therefore, in all patients with severe prolapse, despite a lack of complaints, lower urinary tract function should be assessed. A urinalysis and residual urine are routinely obtained. A stress test with the reduction of the vaginal prolapse by a pessary or vaginal packing should be performed. Care should be taken not to occlude the urethra during packing as a false negative result may occur. Many of these women may present with concomitant urethral sphincteric deficiency; therefore, the authors prefer urodynamics with vaginal packing to assess abdominal leak point pressures to evaluate urethral function. This is an accurate way to assess abdominal leak point pressures in patients with significant prolapse and allows selection of the most appropriate stress incontinence procedure. All patients should be carefully screened for colorectal dysfunction. Although the vast majority of patients complain of constipation, symptoms of fecal incontinence and/or rectal prolapse should be evaluated.

Urodynamic testing. Urodynamic testing should be considered to rule out occult SUI. Patients with a loss of Level I support generally have greater degrees of prolapse warranting pre operative urodynamic assessment. The urodynamic studies should be performed with a vaginal packing or pessary. In addition to leak point pressure assessment, these studies may provide useful information regarding the voiding characteristics in these women.

Cystoscopy. Although not mandatory in the evaluation of prolapse and incontinence, cystoscopy should be considered in women who have had previous bladder suspension or prolapse repair. Cystoscopy should be performed in women with significant irritative storage symptoms, hematuria or recurrent urinary tract infections. Cystoscopy has been described as an adjunct to help distinguish cystocele from rectocele in select cases.

Fluoroscopic imaging. A voiding cystourethrogram may be helpful to differentiate apical herniation as bladder and/or enterocele. Also, the degree of bladder descensus may be determined. Defecography (defecating proctography) can aid in detection and quantification of rectoceles. Additionally this study can provide functional information regarding the efficiency of rectal emptying. However, correlation of patient symptoms and clinical outcomes has not been correlated to these studies.

Endorectal ultrasound and anorectal manometry. Fecal incontinence is a manifestation of pelvic floor dysfunction such as prolapse and stress urinary incontinence. Manometric systems vary, however testing should follow a defined protocol allowing consistent, reproducible results. Resting pressures are calculated which reflect the resistance provided by the internal anal sphincter. The pressure progressively increases toward the distal end of the sphincter, theoretically acting to maintain continence. Although the normal values are poorly defined, nor mal resting pressures vary between 40 mm Hg and 80 mm Hg. The voluntary squeeze pressure is an assessment of EAS competence. This pressure is actually a cumulative effect of the resting tone and the voluntary squeeze. It is thought that normal squeeze pressures should be approximately twice the resting pressure.

The evaluation of anal incontinence with endoluminal ultrasound provides distinct images of the soft tissues, internal and external anal sphincter complex. The most significant advantage of endoluminal ultrasound is that it provides precise identification of the location and nature of sphincter injury. This is very important when planning surgical repair. Sphincter abnormalities are identified on endoluminal ultrasound in 90% of women with fecal incontinence.

Surgical Correction of Pelvic Organ Prolapse

Anterior Defects (Cystocele)

A central defect cystocele is surgically repaired by the reduction of the prolapsing bladder and reapproximation of the attenuated pubocervical fascia using plicating sutures (Figure 3).

This operation, the anterior colporrhaphy, is the most frequently utilized procedure in the correction of cystocele, and is associated with success rates from 30%-75%. The anterior colporrhaphy only corrects central defects, and the inability to correct other forms of pelvic organ prolapse that commonly present with cystocele is probably a main risk factor in failures of anterior repairs.

A lateral defect cystocele is corrected by the reapproximation of the vagina to the pelvic sidewalls. This operation is completed by placing a row of interrupted sutures from the vagina into the pelvic sidewall at the arcus tendineus, extending all the way to the ischial spine (Figure 4). Multiple sutures are placed to provide support, and this is accomplished abdominally, laparoscopically or transvaginally. When one performs this repair through the vagina, a graft material is usually secured to each pelvic sidewall traversing under the bladder. This provides support to the central cystocele component as well. Graft material commonly used is porcine dermis or polypropylene mesh. Utilizing these techniques, the success rates of these procedures is reported from 80%-95%. There is a higher incidence of complications from the vaginal paravaginal repair when compared to the anterior colporrhaphy.

A transverse cystocele occurs when the pubocervical attachments separate from the level I (cardinal and uterosacral) support which stabilizes the apex of the vagina. In an isolated transverse defect, the cystocele is repaired simply by restoring this support. This is most commonly performed by re establishing cuff support. This explains why many women with cystocele may have correction after an abdominal colpopexy or uterosacral cuff suspension.

Posterior Defects (Rectocele)

A rectocele is repaired by re approximating the rectovaginal fascia together, usually with interrupted sutures in an operation called a posterior colporrhaphy (Figure 5). The operation extends distally toward the perineal body, and involves incorporating levator fascia into the repair distally. In fact, many posterior repairs involve placation and reinforcement of the perineal body. One must take great care not to narrow the vagina excessively, as this may cause sexual dysfunction. Graft materials can be incorporated in this repair, and many have adopted the use of grafts, particularly for repeat repairs. A site specific rectocele repair is accomplished when one re approximates the rectovaginal fascia (which is intact) to the perineal body. This detachment can be responsible for large distal rectoceles that can become symptomatic. This can be accomplished through a small, distal transverse or diamond type incision. Success rates of 66%-75% have been recorded, with the major complications being pain and/or sexual dysfunction.

Enterocele

The most common form of enterocele repair is that

Figure 3

Reapproximation of pubocervical fascia: anterior colporraphy – repair of central cystocele

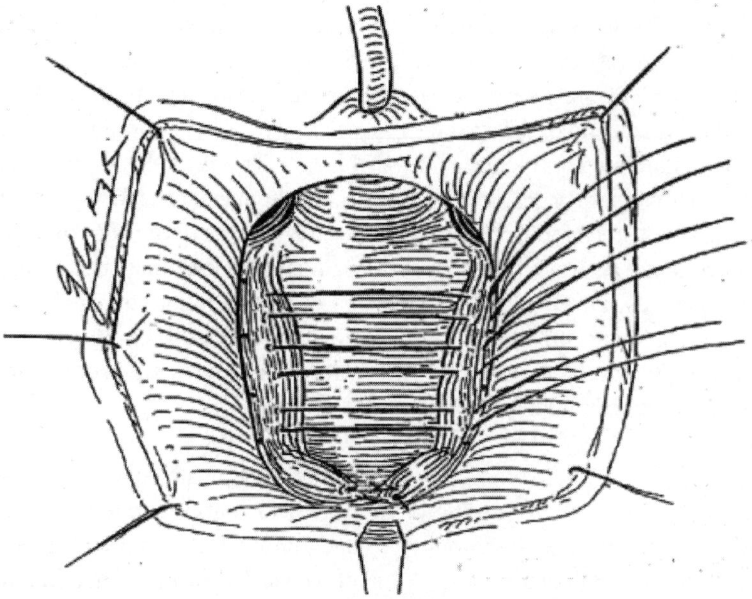

Reprinted with permission: AUA Update Series. Volume 25, Lesson 29; 2006.

Figure 4

Reapproximation of lateral defect: correction of paravaginal defect

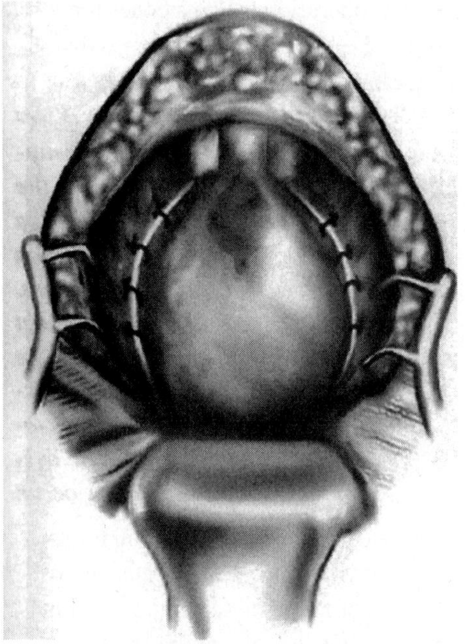

Reprinted with permission: AUA Update Series. Lesson 23, Volume 21; 2002.

of transvaginal sac isolation and closure. The enterocele sac is isolated after making an incision near (or through) the cuff of the vagina. After the sac is dissected out, the bowel contents are reduced, and the sac is closed proximally near the "neck" of the sac. Following this the remaining sac is dissected out and discarded. The enterocele can also be repaired transabdominally. The bowel is manually lifted out of the pelvis, and a cul-de-plasty is performed by closing of the cul-de-sac with permanent, interrupted sutures. The success rates of these procedures is approximately 85%-95%.

Apical Prolapse of the Vaginal Cuff

There are a wide number of procedures to correct apical vaginal prolapse. The importance of recognizing and correcting apical defects is becoming increasingly stressed by vaginal surgeons. This is the means by which the upper vagina is stabilized proximally, and this protects against widening of the genital hiatus. There are a number of abdominal, vaginal and laparoscopic approaches to the correction of apical prolapse, and the surgeon should be well versed to perform several of these procedures. The sacrospinous ligament fixation (SSLF) achieves a functional vagina and vault prolapse cure in 67%-79% of patients. One should place the sutures directly into the body of the sacrospinous

Figure 5

Plication of pararectal fascia, posterior colporraphy

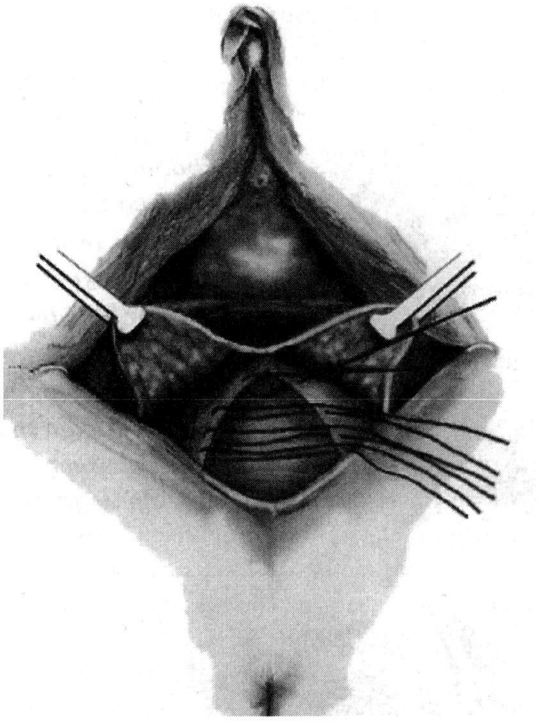

Reprinted with permission: AUA Update Series. Lesson 23, Volume 21; 2002.

ligament as there is a potential for significant vascular or neurologic injury. There is a posterior dis placement and elongation of the vaginal apex after SSLF, which may predispose one to anterior compartment defects. The apex can be sutured directly to the iliococcygeus fascia, or to the uterosacral ligament remnants usually isolated via a transvaginal, intraperitoneal approach. Ureteral patency must be assured after these procedures.

The abdominal sacral colpopexy is one of the most successful ways to correct apical prolapse. This procedure is accomplished via abdominal, laparoscopic or robotic approaches. A graft is utilized to secure the apex of the vaginal to the sacrum. Most authors now fix the graft material to the sacral promontory. A synthetic mesh should be utilized, as there is Level I evidence demonstrating the superiority of permanent mesh materials to biologic graft materials in women undergoing colpopexy. All women should undergo a cul-de-plasty to prevent recurrent enterocele. Success rates as high as 95% have been reported by multiple authors, with an acceptably low graft erosion rate. Complications can include serious bleeding encountered from the presacral venous complex.

2. Urinary Incontinence: Pathophysiology, Evaluation and Treatment

Urinary incontinence is defined as the involuntary loss of urine per urethra. The International Continence Society (ICS) defines incontinence in various domains: The symptom, where a patient or caregivers describe involuntary urine loss; the sign, which is an objective demonstration of urine loss; the urodynamic (UDS) observation, which is incontinence demonstrated during UDS testing; and the condition, which is the lower urinary tract pathophysiology causing incontinence as demonstrated during evaluation.

One must remember that incontinence is a symptom of an underlying disorder, not a disease process. This disorder has significant socioeconomic impact on the quality of life of our patients. More than 20 million Americans are incontinent, and urinary incontinence accounts for at least 30% of nursing home admissions. It is estimated that 650,000 senior citizens restrict activity as a result of incontinence, and as many as 50% of females over the age of 40 experience some episodes of wetting.

Classification of Incontinence

Urinary incontinence is classified in many ways, the most commonly used methods to classify this condition is by way of a symptomatic or functional classification.

A. Symptomatically Defined Classification:

1. Stress Incontinence
2. Urge Incontinence
3. Overflow Incontinence
    a. Retention of large urine volumes precipitates reflex urethral relaxation or unstable bladder contraction.
4. Total Incontinence
5. Transient Incontinence
    a. Extremely important when evaluating incontinence in elderly or patients with significant comorbidity.

B. Functionally Defined Classification:

1. Failure to Empty
    a. Bladder Underactivity
    b. Urethral Obstruction
2. Failure to Store (Urinary Incontinence)
    a. Urethral Incompetence
    b. Bladder Overactivity

Neuroanatomy

Bladder

The bladder consists of smooth muscle which accommodates increasing volumes of urine without increasing its storage pressure. This process of bladder compliance is a unique ability of the urinary bladder facilitating storage of urine. The bladder has a uniform contraction of sufficient magnitude after sphincter relaxation which is responsible for expelling urine. The bladder smooth muscle is innervated by the pelvic nerve arising from the parasympathetic nervous system arising from sacral segments S2-S4. This nerve releases the neurotransmitter acetylcholine. Stimulation of this nerve leads to contraction of bladder via promoting contraction of the smooth muscle. (Thus, anticholinergics medications promote bladder relaxation by inhibiting this process.)

The bladder also contains beta receptors in bladder body, which when stimulated, promotes bladder relaxation. In addition a number of nonadrenergic, noncholinergic receptors (NANC) have been identified within the urothelial lining of the bladder. This implies a potential significance to urothelial (afferent) activity in pathologic conditions of the bladder—OAB, IC, NGB, etc. This is a major emphasis of current research.

Bladder Neck/Proximal Urethra

The bladder neck and proximal urethra consist of smooth muscle abundantly innervated by the sym pathetic nervous system. The hypogastric nerve which arises from the sympathetic nervous system arising from segments T10 L2 releases norepinephrine, causing stimulation of the alpha receptors. This activity promotes contraction of these muscles, causing bladder neck closure and closure of the proximal urethra. This is the major contributor of "passive continence" and is commonly referred to as the "internal sphincter." The pelvic floor striated complex which surrounds the urethra as it exits the pelvic floor comprises the external sphincter complex. This is a voluntary striated muscle, and relaxation of the pelvic floor is essential for efficient bladder emptying. Dysfunction of the striated muscle complex manifests commonly as dysfunctional voiding or detrusor sphincter dyssynergia (in patients with neurogenic bladder). The pudendal nerve, a somatic nerve arising from sacral segments S2-S4 stimulates activity of the pelvic floor striated muscle.

Thus, during urine storage, the sympathetic activity promotes increased resistance of the bladder neck and proximal urethra via the hypogastric nerve, and the external sphincter activity increases via pudendal nerve activity. Increased EMG activity near the end of urinary storage is normal and considered the guarding "reflex."

Micturition

Urine storage is a largely sympathetic function. The voiding cycle is dependent on synergistic outlet reaction and bladder contraction. This activity is regulated via the pontine micturition center located in the pons. Upper cortical centers in the brain controls when voiding will occur, mainly by the inhibitory effect on the pontine micturition center. The pontine micturition center serves as the "on-off" switch to activate the voiding cycle. During storage, sympathetic activity promotes urinary storage by contracting the bladder neck and proximal urethra via the hypogastric nerve. Additionally stimulation of the beta receptors in the bladder body also promote urine storage. When inhibition ceases, the pontine micturition center promotes an inhibition of this sympathetic activity and stimulation of the pelvic nerve (parasympathetic nervous system). This results in bladder contraction in the presence of relaxed sphincter complex.

Etiology of Incontinence

Bladder

The most common bladder cause of urinary incontinence is detrusor overactivity, "overactive bladder." The symptom complex of overactive or bladder may be defined as: urgency, a sudden compelling desire to pass urine that is difficult to defer; urge urinary incontinence, involuntary leakage accompanied by or immediately preceded by urgency; frequency: patient considers that he /she voids too often in the day (>8/ times 24 hours); nocturia, where the patient wakes up >2 times per night to void. The urodynamic observation of overactive bladder is characterized by leakage seen during an involuntary detrusor contraction on cystometry.

There are a number of references to detrusor overactivity with which one must be familiar. Neurogenic detrusor overactivity (formerly detrusor hyperreflexia) is the presence of overactive bladder in patients with known neurologic conditions. Idiopathic detrusor overactivity (formerly detrusor instability) is the presence of overactive bladder activity in a neurologically intact individual without a reversible identifying cause. "Wet" overactive bladder is the presence of urinary incontinence as a result of overactive bladder. "Dry" overactive bladder consists of OAB symptoms (urgency and/or frequency) in absence of incontinence. This represents approximately two-thirds of OAB cases.

There are identifiable, reversible conditions which can cause symptoms of OAB: infection, stones, tumor (CIS), and neurologic disease. Treatment of these conditions is usually met with improvement of symptoms.

During urodynamic studies overactive bladder activity has several different manifestations: involuntary detrusor contractions, abnormal compliance, sensory urgency and a reduction in the cystometric capacity.

Urethral Sphincter

A major cause of urinary incontinence is decreased urethral resistance. In these conditions, the urethra is unable to withstand the forces created by increased intra abdominal pressure and leakage ensues with activity. In these cases the bladder function may be normal, and the leakage occurs because of a lack of urethral closure. This condition is known as stress urinary incontinence. The symptom of SUI has been defined as a complaint of involuntary leakage during exertion or effort, or on coughing/sneezing. The sign of SUI is the observation of involuntary leakage from the urethra at time of exertion or effort ("stress test"). The urodynamic observation of SUI is the occurrence of urinary leakage during filling cystometry associated with increased intra abdominal **pressure in the absence of a detrusor contraction.**

There are evolving theories regarding the etiology of SUI. It appears that women presenting with stress urinary incontinence have a spectrum of varying degrees of intrinsic sphincteric deficiency and a loss of urethral support. The "hammock" hypothesis demonstrates how intact pelvic floor function is necessary to achieve urethral closure during stress activities. The urethra is supported by a hammock of support: the pubocervical fascia extending from each arcus tendineus on the pelvic sidewalls. During increased intraabdominal pressure, the urethra becomes compressed against this structure which closes it. A loss of this supporting network does not achieve urethral closure during times of stress. Patients must have some degree of intrinsic sphincteric deficiency to develop stress incontinence, as it has been observed that there are women with urethral hypermobility who do not leak. The Integral Theory emphasizes that there are 3 very important structures needed to maintain continence during stress: the pubourethral ligament, suburethral vaginal hammock and pubococcygeus muscle. All 3 structures work together by drawing the urethra forward against the pubourethral ligament and closing the urethra. This creates the "dynamic kink" of the urethra that occurs during periods of increased intra abdominal pressure. *The PCM muscle can only contract so much; if there is excessive vaginal laxity, it can't draw the urethra against the PUL to achieve closure.*

Intrinsic sphincteric deficiency (ISD) is a deficiency of the intrinsic urethral closing mechanism. Traditionally the concept of ISD was limited to immobile scarred urethras with little urethral resistance—"stove pipe" urethra. It is now recognized that all women with stress incontinence have some degree of sphincteric deficiency, and that ISD may exist in the presence of urethral hypermobility (in fact, most often does). ISD may be seen in the following situations: neurogenic bladder, autonomic nerve injury, following bladder neck/urethral procedures or after long term urethral catheter. One must understand the degree of ISD in PRIMARY cases. All women with SUI must have some degree of ISD, and those with more significant degrees of ISD should be recognized before selection of therapy.

Other Causes of Incontinence

"Overflow" incontinence, associated with urinary retention and increased PVR. The etiology is variable, either from a reflex urethral relaxation or an unstable contraction of the bladder. This may occur as a result of: outlet obstruction (cystocele/prostate), diabetes and neurogenic retention. There are also anatomic causes of incontinence, which include: fistula, urethral diverticulum, vaginal voiding and ectopic ureters (predominately pediatric). Evaluation of incontinent patients must include methods to rule out these conditions.

The Evaluation of Incontinence

As with all conditions, the evaluation of incontinence begins with a thorough history and physical examination. One should assess the following symptomatology: Does leakage occur with exertion (cough, exercise, etc.)? Does leakage occur with the impending sensation to void? Is there supine leakage or bedwetting (usually in complicated cases)? A very important aspect of the history is: How has incontinence changed the quality of life? How much is the patient bothered by these symptoms? In addition, one should ask if there is pelvic or perineal pain or pressure related to prolapse and/or sexual dysfunction. One should also assess bowel function: constipation, splinting or fecal incontinence. The past history assessment should include the number of pregnancies and vaginal deliveries, and is there were any complications associated with them. Also, was there any history of gynecologic surgery? One should obtain a detailed history of any neurologic disorder, previous bladder suspension or vaginal repair.

On physical examination it is of paramount importance to assess the degree of urethal hypermobility. AQ-tip test can be utilized to quantify the degree of urethral hypermobility. The vaginal examination should assess the presence of: cystocele, enterocele, rectocele, vault or uterine prolapse and perineal body integrity. The quality of the vaginal mucosa should be assessed. A "neurourologic examination" (bulbo cavernosus reflex, cremasteric reflex, perineal sensation) should be considered. A post-void residual (PVR) and stress test are also adjuncts to the physical exam. A urinalysis should be performed on all patients. In patients with any degree of hematuria a work up should be considered as incontinence may be a symptom. A vaginal wet mount should be done if symptomatic discharge is present. x-ray imaging may be obtained (cystogram/defacography) in complex cases of incontinence. Cystograms with straining views is useful in complex cases of incontinence with pelvic organ prolapse.

Urodynamic studies investigate the interaction of detrusor activity and urethral sphincter activity. This is done by measurement of pressure changes within the bladder and urethral sphincter. A cystometrogram measures bladder pressure during filling and voiding. From these measurements one should identify: bladder capacity, bladder sensation, bladder contractility bladder compliance, and the presence (or absence) of involuntary bladder activity. Urethral pressure profilometry or abdominal leak point pressure measurement assesses urethral sphincter function. These studies quantify the intrinsic closing pressures of the urethra. Concomitant EMG activity (patch or needle) is used to assess striated voluntary external sphincter function. However, one must appreciate the tremendous anatomic detail that fluoroscopy provides when assessing sphincter function. Videourodynamics, which is the combination of multichannel urodynamics and fluoroscopy, provides the most comprehensive assessment of anatomy and function of the lower urinary tract.

Treatment of Urinary Incontinence

As with most conditions, an initial conservative approach is desired by most patients. When one selects therapy for urinary incontinence, it is essential to consider the degree of patient bother and also what the patient expectations are. If a patient's major goal is to eliminate nocturia, a sling for coexistent stress urinary incontinence is probably not the best initial approach for her. Whereas, if a woman cannot exercise because of SUI and her expectation is to be able to resume those activities, a sling may be a perfect choice. Conservative therapy really is behavioral modifications, which are effective in stress and urge incontinence. A bladder diary is most helpful, particularly in OAB and nocturnal symptoms. A diary records urinary intake and out put, frequency of voiding, volumes voided and types of urinary accidents. From these data, one can institute measures such as fluid management (monitoring intake) and timed voids. The principle of timed voids is to establish voiding by the clock (by time) as opposed to voiding in response to urge. The bladder volumes remain lower. This facilitates bladder emptying before an involuntary contraction may occur and compensates for the lack of warning time in OAB patients. Expected results include initial improvement in symptoms in up to 90% of women. Drop out rates are high and physicians need to continually remind patients. One should also instruct patients on the avoidance of bladder irritants. This is crucial in patients with urge incontinence. Patients should be taught to avoid: acidic foods, citrus juices and fruits, caffeinated and alcoholic beverages, and spicy foods. Pelvic floor muscle training (PFMT) actually comprises a comprehensive program of pelvic floor physiotherapy and not just Kegel's exercises. The goal is to strengthen the levator support system and enhancing reflex contraction of the pelvic muscles at the time of stress. Many studies report improvement in high proportions of women, although few become dry. Greater improvement is achieved in women who are physically instructed on proper technique and with the addition of biofeedback. This is a most useful modality in women with pelvic pain, dysfunctional voiding and interstitial cystitis.

In combination with the conservative measures above, medications are also efficacious in the management of urinary incontinence. When treating incontinence (failure to store), drugs which promote bladder storage or increase urethral resistance are desirable. The most commonly utilized drugs are antimuscarinic medications which promote urinary storage by blocking the uptake of acetylcholine at the muscarinic receptor level in the bladder. This has been shown to decrease tone and contractility of the bladder. There are a number of widely utilized antimuscarinic (or anticholinergic) medications:

Oxybutynin gel 10% (Gelnique™)
1 packet applied transdermal QD

Oxybutynin IR (gen Ditropan®)
2.5, 5.0 mg BID QID

Oxybutynin ER (Ditropan XL®)
5, 30 mg QD

Oxybutynin TDS (Oxytrol®)
1 patch twice weekly

Tolterodine IR/ER (Detrol® LA)
2, 4 mg QD

Trospium (Sanctura®, Sanctura® XR)
20 mg BID, 60 mg QD

Fesoterodine (Toviaz™)
4 mg BID/, 8 mg QD

Solifenacin (VESIcare®)
5, 10 mg QD

Darifenacin (Enablex®)
7.5, 15 mg QD

There does not appear to be a clear efficacy difference when comparing these medications. One must be aware of the common anticholinergic adverse events (dry mouth and constipation most common) and warn patients of these. There is data to suggest over time many patients stop taking these medications. Whether it is a lack of efficacy, side affects, expense or a combination of all 3 is not known. The concept of muscarinic selectivity improving tolerability is unproven in humans.

The tricyclic antidepressant, imipramine (10, 25 mg TID), has been reported to have a synergistic, additive effect to decrease bladder contractility when combined with anticholinergics. Also, there appears to be some element of bladder smooth muscle relaxation. This drug also has been reported to delay norepinephrine reuptake, thus potentially increasing urethral resistance. One may consider this drug in cases of mixed incontinence. However there are only a small number of case series reporting efficacy. One must be aware of the sedative effects and cardiovascular effects of this medication.

Drugs that increase outflow resistance by increasing sphincteric resistance may also be desirable in the treatment of urinary incontinence. Alpha-agonists which increase the sphincteric tone were previously utilized: ephedrine, pseudoephedrine, phenylephrine or phenylpropanolamine (Entex® LA, Ornade). These agents had limited effect and results were usually transient. One must be aware of the adverse events associated with these medications including hypertension and stroke. In fact, the FDA has eliminated the use of many alpha-agonist medications. It is for these reasons that this treatment modality cannot be recommended at this time in women with stress urinary incontinence. Estrogens have primary usage for menopausal atrophic urethral and vaginal symptoms. Thus, ***topical*** estrogen may be useful in chronic cystitis/UTI or atrophic urethritis. Estrogens have been postulated to stimulate neovascularization of the urethral mucosa with a subsequent increase in alpha receptors, theoretically increasing urethral closing pressure. Several large clinical trials using estrogen and a meta analysis of the literature have demonstrated that estrogen is not effective primary or monotherapy for SUI or urge incontinence. In fact, the Women's Health Initiative Project found that estrogen actually worsened incontinence symptoms. These findings have led many to use estrogen only in cases of urethritis or recurrent UTI in association with vaginal atrophy.

Surgical Management of Incontinence

When conservative therapy fails (or the patient chooses surgery as treatment of choice) there are a number of surgical options that promote bladder storage or increase the urethral resistance. Included is an overview of the many surgical options to promote bladder storage and increase urethral resistance.

Surgical Management of Incontinence:

Overactive Bladder

A. Interstim™ neuromodulation. Stimulation of S3 nerve roots modulates neural activity to bladder

1. Indicated for refractory OAB (urge incontinence or frequency)

2. Indicated for nonobstructed urinary retention.

B. Botulinum toxin: No current FDA approval

1. Prevents release and fusion of acetylcholine

2. Cystoscopic guidance. Multiple injections into detrusor muscle

3. 100-300 units reported

4. Excellent results in randomized controlled trial in neurogenic detrusor overactivity. Trials on going in neurogenic and non neurogenic OAB

5. Temporary response, not known if response will remain sustained after multiple injections

C. Augmentation cystoplasty

1. Bowel augmentation

2. Detrusor myomectomy

D. Denervation: neurectomy, rhizotomy or phenol injections

1. Rarely indicated

E. Future technologies in the treatment of overactive bladder

1. New drugs working on different sites of neurohormonal axis

2. Intravesical delivery systems

3. Bladder instillations

4. Peripheral neuromodulation

Surgical Management of Incontinence: Stress Urinary Incontinence

A. Stress Urinary Incontinence Guidelines Panel (1997)

1. Standard:

a. History: Identify impact on quality of life

b. Physical Exam: positive stress test

c. Urinalysis

d. Other diagnostic tests to evaluate cause of incontinence

2. Retropubic suspensions and sling procedures more efficacious than anterior repairs and pub ovaginal sling procedures for surgical management of SUI

3. Patients must be informed of all options

B. Transabdominal (retropubic) bladder neck suspensions

1. Burch is most common procedure. Question if less obstructing than other retropubic procedures

b. Dry rates of 70%-95% can be expected at 3-5 years follow-up

c. The results are significantly better than transvaginal needle suspensions

d. There is a higher incidence of voiding dysfunction postoperatively

e. Ideal patient: urethral hypermobility and higher leak point pressures

C. Slings. The sling procedure eliminates urethral hypermobility and may provide compression of the urethra, therefore this is the procedure of choice in patients with lower leak point pressures (higher degrees of ISD)

1. Autologous fascial slings—pubovaginal sling

a. Excellent results in all types of SUI

b. Durable results

c. Requires separate fascial harvest, increasing morbidity

2. Allograft and Xenograft slings

a. Encouraging results using graft substitution

b. Intermediate and late failures seen with allograft tissue (fascia and dermis)

c. Variable results reported probably reflects disparity in host acceptance of tissue

d. Encouraging reports using porcine dermis

3. Mid-urethal, tension free synthetic slings; based on integral theory. Placement of mesh to stabilize urethra facilitates pubococcygeus muscle to close urethra during periods of stress

a. TVT: 80% long-term improvement or cure rates (5 years). Significant complications have been reported (8 deaths).

b. "Top down" retropubic variations (TVTTM/SPARC®/LynxTM, etc.) embraced by many urologists.

c. Several studies reveal that SPARC efficacy is comparable to TVT.

d. 2006 Guidelines panel: mid-urethral sling = pubovaginal sling

e. Less incidence of voiding dysfunction post-operatively

f. Transobturator tape—no entry into retropubic space

1. Early data appealing: excellent rates of SUI cure and minimal complications. Less bladder perforation and voiding dysfunction than when compared to TVT

D. Intraurethral injections

1. GAX bovine cross linked collagen injected by either a transurethral or periurethral approach.

a. Improvement or cure rates achieved in 65%-80% of patients utilizing an average of 2.1 injection sessions.

b. Effective in all types of SUI. Although ideal candidate is no hypermobility and ISD

c. 2006 Guidelines panel: 25%-40% cure/improved at 2-4 years.

2. Carbon-coated zirconium beads (Durasphere®)

a. FDA-approved for SUI.

b. Fully biocompatible, no skin test needed.

c. Large size precludes migration, although 1 case report.

d. Efficacy is similar to collagen in multi center trial.

e. Material can be more difficult to inject as beads separate from carrier, and occlude injecting needle. Less since newer formulation released

f. Radiopaque—persistence of material seen on radiographs

3. Calcium hydroxylapatite (Coaptite®):

a. Natural component of bone and teeth

b. Hydroxylapatite spheres suspended in an aqueous gel of sodium carboxylmethylcellulose

c. Migration not reported

d. Biocompatible, no skin test needed

e. Injection technique similar to collagen

f. Efficacy similar to collagen, although less injections required to achieve patient satisfaction

g. Radiopaque—persistence of material seen on radiographs

3. Female Urology: Vesicovaginal Fistulae

Etiology

In underdeveloped countries, birth trauma from prolonged engagement of the fetal head during protracted labor is the most common cause of fistula. In developed countries, fistula formation after hysterectomy is the most common cause, occurring in approximately 1 per 1800 cases. This may occur as a result of suture placement into the bladder with resultant tissue necrosis, or an undetected bladder injury with resultant urine leak through the vaginal cuff establishing a fistulous connection. Less common causes of VVF include: pelvic irradiation, vaginal surgery, foreign body, trauma, and urethral diverticulectomy.

Symptoms

The clinical presentation of VVF may vary depending on the size and location of the fistula. Continuous urine leakage or watery vaginal discharge 7-14 days after a potentially causative surgical procedure is the most common presentation. The amount of leakage can be so severe that all of the bladder contents drain through the fistula, or minimal enough to drain only when the bladder is full or in certain patient positions. In order to make a timely diagnosis, one must be aware of the potential varying presenting symptoms.

Diagnosis

The essential step in diagnosis is suspicion. One must suspect the presence of fistula in order to detect it. A fistula should be suspected in the presence of a watery vaginal discharge in any patient presenting for an incontinence evaluation.

Physical Examination

A physical examination will detect the fistula in most cases. During the physical examination, several associated factors are important to address when planning correction. Fistula size and location are important. Smaller fistula may be approached using more conservative measures. The location of the fistula in the vagina is imperative to identify. Is the fistula located where transvaginal access may be difficult? Fistulas are most commonly in the cuff of the vagina. A small narrowed vaginal canal or fixed cuff may not allow access to the fistula transvaginally. It is also important to assess tissue quality for the presence of inflammation or edema. This is vitally important when timing repair.

Cystogram

A cystogram may be helpful in revealing a unrecognized bladder injury or fistula. A cystogram offers little value in determination of fistula location or size. This study usually does not provide additional information to other methods of diagnosis, therefore it is not usually done unless complex reconstruction is planned.

Cystoscopy

Cystoscopy is essential in the diagnosis of VVF. A fistula should be suspected if mucosal changes, such as a dimple, band of scar tissue, or inflammation are present. Placing a small ureteral catheter into the fistula may assist in determining where the fistula is located in the vagina. The proximity of the fistula to the ureteral orifices, and the presence of other suspected fistula should be assessed cystoscopically. An assessment of the tissue surrounding the fistula should be examined to ensure that it is acceptable to incorporate in a repair. Serial cystoscopic examinations may be needed to assess tissue quality prior to embarking on fistula repair.

Dye Testing

If the diagnosis of VVF remains in doubt after physical examination and cystoscopy, various dye tests can be used to determine if a fistula is present. A "double dye" test can be performed at the bedside. The vagina is packed with four moist gauze pads—one in the right vaginal fornix, and one in the left vaginal fornix. A third pad is placed in the mid-vagina, while the fourth pad is placed at the vaginal opening. The bladder is filled with 1% carmine solution (red), and 10 mL of indigo carmine is injected intravenously. The swabs are removed 15 minutes after injection. A red stain on the mid-vaginal or upper forniceal packs is suspicious for VVF. A blue stain on the pack is suspicious for a ureterovaginal fistula, and a red-stained pad only at the vaginal opening is indicative of urethral leakage. Amore simple diagnosis can be obtained using oral phenazopyridine until the urine is stained orange. The patient then inserts a tampon. The bladder is then filled with a saline/methyline blue solution. After 10 minutes, examination of the tampon is performed. An orange stain at the top of the tampon indicates a ureterovaginal fistula, and a blue stain suggests the presence of a VVF.

Intravenous Pyelogram or Retrograde Pyelography

This is a mandatory test when evaluating VVF. The presence of a ureterovaginal fistula or obstruction may be found in as many as 10%-15% of cases of VVF. Before correction, the ureters must be cleared of any abnormality. In cases where the IVP is indeterminate or the VVF is in close proximity to the ureter, retrograde pyelography should be considered.

Urodynamics

Urodynamic studies are not routinely needed in the evaluation of VVF. Unless the presence of detrusor instability or the competence of the urethral sphincter is in question, urodynamic studies are not needed prior to fistula repair.

CT or MRI

There are only a small number of case reports evaluating the use of these imaging modalities in the diagnosis and management of VVF. The usefulness of these studies appears limited after physical and endoscopic examination. At present, the author has not utilized these imaging modality unless other pelvic pathology is suspected.

Treatment of Vesicovaginal Fistulae

Timing of Repair

Traditionally, repair of fistula was delayed 3-6 months after the offending surgery to allow the edema and inflammation to subside. This can be quite difficult due to the anxiety of the patients. A number of studies have demonstrated that early repair of VVF may be carried out. Early repair of VVF has been reported to have success rates from 90%-100% via abdominal or vaginal approaches.

The timing of the surgical repair should be individualized. Each patient should be examined at frequent intervals to assess tissue integrity. The repair should be performed only when the edema has subsided, necrotic tissue disappeared, and the inflammatory response has resolved. It is important to communicate these principles to the patient. This will restore confidence in the patient that the surgery will be performed at a time that optimizes the chance of a successful outcome. The best chance of success is the first repair—it is much better to do the repair when the tissue quality is best.

Catheter Drainage

Small fistulae or fistulae associated with a foreign body (suture) may respond well to a trial of catheter drainage. If the foreign body can be successfully removed and a small fistulous tract persists, a trial of catheter drainage may result in resolution of the fistula. For catheter drainage to be successful the fistula should be small (few millimeters) and the tissue quality should be excellent. If a fistula will heal with a catheter, there should be no leakage with the catheter in place. If leakage across the fistula stops, the fistulous tract may heal with a 4-week trial of continuous catheter drainage. If continuous drainage is chosen, anticholinergic medication should be given to decrease bladder spasm. If leakage does not stop within one week of the institution of catheter drainage, it is unlikely that the fistula will close with drainage alone.

Fulguration of Fistulous Tract

The theory behind fulguration of the fistulous tract is that the epithelium covering the tract is denuded, promoting closure of the tract. The fistula must be quite small, and a low current is employed which is carried out with a pediatric Bugbee electrode. A low current is utilized, and the fulguration is usually performed through the bladder. There are several small series documenting successful closure of fistula with fulguration. One should not attempt fulguration of larger fistula. A potential adverse effect of fulguration is the destruction of the tissue around the fistula by cautery. This has the potential to actually create a larger fistula defect.

Vaginal Repair

The vaginal approach is preferred as the morbidity of this approach is much less. An abdominal incision is avoided along with opening (bivalving) the bladder. Reduced bladder dissection results in less post operative instability, and potentially shorter catheter time.

Figure 6

Transvaginal VVF fistula repair

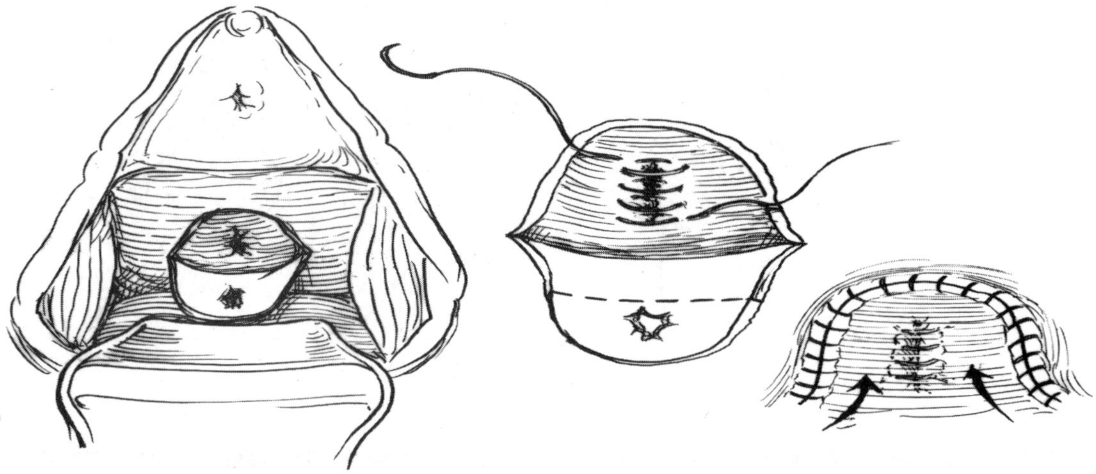

Note: inverting fistula closure covered by vaginal flap.

Figure 7

Abdominal approach

Circumscribing the fistula.

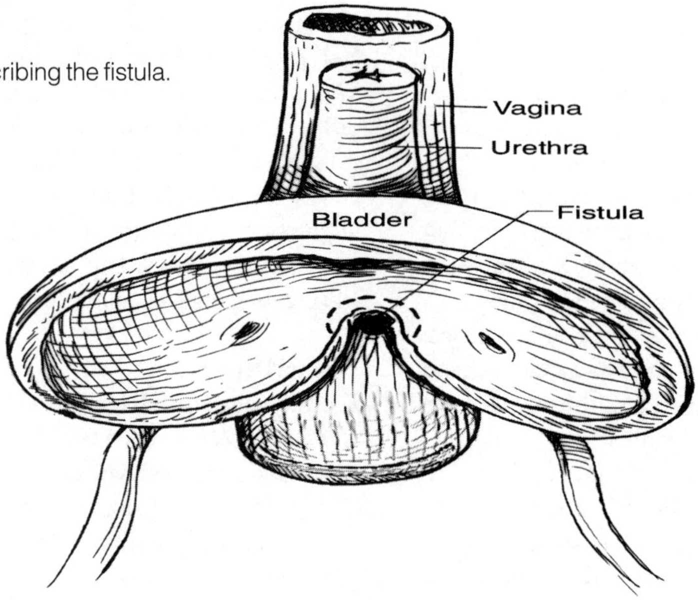

Fistula closure with
omental interposition.

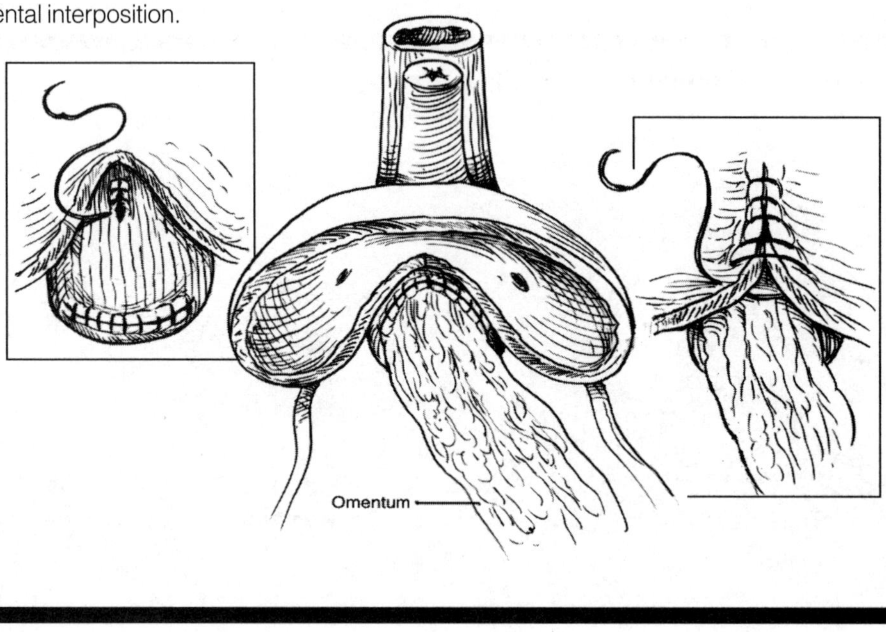

The vaginal repair is usually carried out in the dorsal lithotomy position. Lateral vaginal incisions can provide better exposure if the vaginal capacity is small. An inverted lithotomy position may also be utilized to improve exposure of the vaginal cuff. The principles of transvaginal repair are to isolate the fistula, and close the fistula with multiple-non-overlapping suture lines. Vaginal flaps are created and the fistula is closed without excision of the fistula tract. The sutures utilized to close the fistula should invert the fistula. A second layer, which is placed perpendicular to the fistula, is then used to further invert the closed fistula (Figure 6). The vaginal flap is then advanced over the area of fistula repair and closed with a running suture. A Martius fat pad flap may then be incorporated to add an additional layer to cover the repair. These techniques are associated with 80%-100% success rates.

Abdominal Repair

An abdominal approach should be considered in the following circumstances: high retracted fistula, concomitant ureteral pathology or proximity, multiple fistulae or post-tradiation fistulae. If the surgeon who performs does not repair fistulae frequently, they may favor an abdominal approach. This is important when choosing the route of repair. The surgeon should perform the procedure where he/she is likely to achieve a successful outcome. The principles of the abdominal repair include closure of the fistula with watertight, multiple, non-overlapping suture lines under no tension. Additionally, the abdominal approach affords access to the omentum which is used as interposition tissue. For large (several centimeters) fistulae or hard to reach cuff fistulae the author has had significant success utilizing a transabdominal approach.

The abdominal approach begins with an incision in the midline of the bladder. This incision is carried all the way posteriorly around the fistula, isolating it from the bladder. The bladder flaps are then mobilized in order to minimize tension on the bladder closure. The fistula is closed in 2 layers. After fistula closure, omentum is tacked into position covering the fistula, and the bladder is closed in 2 layers. A suprapubic cystotomy provides large bore catheter drainage for 3-4 weeks (Figure 7). This usually provides more than adequate exposure. Utilizing abdominal approaches, success rates of 90% 100% are routinely achieved.

Partial Colpocleisis (Vaginal Cuff Closure)

In many instances, the fistula is located in the cuff of the vagina. Many times the tissue around the cuff is scarred and friable. Other small fistula may be present or at risk to form after surgery. In some instances the fistula is so small that dye can be seen leaking from a fold of scar in the cuff, but the definite fistula is not identified. It is for these reasons that a partial colpocleisis (Latzko procedure) may be an attractive alternative. The vaginal epithelium is denuded off of the cuff extending 3-4 cm on the anterior and posterior wall of the vagina. Linear sutures are placed 1 cm apart to plicate the soft tissue of the vaginal cuff together, thus closing off the proximal 3-4 cm of the vagina. A second layer is used to reinforce the first suture line. The mucosal margins are re-approximated with a running suture. A catheter is left in for 3 weeks. One potential fear of this procedure is vaginal foreshortening, and patients should be warned of this possibility.

Conclusion

Prompt diagnosis of vesicovaginal fistula is essential. The decision on timing of the surgical repair is individualized, based on the quality of the tissues. Transvaginal approaches are most commonly employed achieving excellent success rates, but similar success rates are achieved using abdominal approaches. The abdominal approach should be considered on all fistulae high in the vagina, which may be difficult to reach via a vaginal approach. The major factor determining the route of repair should be the experience of the surgeon. This will ensure selection of the technique most likely to achieve the best outcome.

4. Female Urology: Urethral and Periurethral Masses

Differential Diagnosis

- Vaginal leiomyoma
- Skene's duct cyst
- Vaginal inclusion cyst
- Ectopic ureter/ureterocele
- Malignancy
- Urethral prolapse
- Urethral caruncle
- Urethral diverticulum
- Vaginal wall cysts

Vaginal Leiomyoma

Vaginal leiomyoma is a benign mesenchymal tumor of the vaginal wall that arises from smooth muscle elements. It presents usually as a smooth, firm mass on the anterior vaginal wall. About 300 cases have been reported—therefore true incidence data is unknown.

These masses may be asymptomatic or cause local symptoms related to the mass effect, such as obstruction, pain and dyspareunia.

These masses are estrogen-dependent and documentation of postmenopausal shrinkage has occurred.

Excision via a transvaginal approach is curative. Local recurrences do not seem to be a problem. Additionally a benign diagnosis can be assured by way of pathologic confirmation.

Skene's Gland Cysts

Skene's gland cysts present as small, cystic masses lateral or inferolateral to the urethral meatus. These lesions do not communicate with the urethral lumen. Adistal, lateral location which displaces the urethral lumen should make one suspicious for a Skene's gland cyst. These are usually quite distal, and displace the urethral meatus, in contrast to urethral diverticuli which are located in the mid- to proximal urethra.

Symptoms can consist of local symptoms due to a mass effect, or commonly as a result of abscess formation, which is a common occurrence with larger Skene's gland masses. These can become exquisitely tender and actually may require marsupialization, aspiration or incision and drainage due to extensive infection. In less complicated cases, excision is the usual treatment. Although these masses don't communicate with the urethra, entry into the distal urethra is not uncommon during excision.

Adenocarcinoma has been reported, but is extremely rare.

Vaginal Wall Cysts

Vaginal wall cysts usually present as small asymptomatic masses on the anterior vaginal wall. These masses can enlarge and cause local symptoms as a result of a mass effect.

Vaginal wall cysts can arise from multiple cell type origins:

- Mesonephric (Gartner's duct cysts)—Found on anterolateral vaginal wall as mesonephric remnants. These patients should have upper tract evaluation. Up to 50% may have Müllerian duct obstruction
- Paramesonephric (Müllerian)
- Endometriotic
- Urothelial
- Epidermoid (inclusion cyst)

Diagnosis is made after excision and pathologic confirmation.

Urethral Mucosal Prolapse

Urethral prolapse presents as a circumferential herniation or eversion of the urethral mucosa through the urethral meatus. This presents a red, engorged, doughnut-shaped lesion that completely surrounds the urethral meatus. The mass may be asymptomatic, or it may present with bleeding, pain or local urinary symptoms.

These occur in 2 populations: postmenopausal women and prepubertal girls. In children it may occur as a result of a deficiency of the muscular attachments of the urethral smooth muscle. This can be aggravated by Valsalva maneuvers or chronic constipation. In postmenopausal women, an estrogen deficiency may aggravate this condition.

Treatment may consist of topical application of estrogen cream and warm baths to reduce inflammation. Removal of urethral prolapse has been accomplished by way of cauterization techniques, ligation around catheters and other means. However, the preferred method is simple excision. Circumferential excision with suture re approximation of the urethral mucosa is usually easily accomplished ,with or without an indwelling catheter.

Urethral Caruncle

Urethral caruncle is an inflammatory condition of the distal urethra, which is most commonly diag nosed in postmenopausal women. The presentation is usually that of a red, engorged, exophytic mass at the urethral meatus, which is covered with mucosa.

These lesions may be etiologically related to urethral prolapse, however this does not represent a true prolapse of the distal urethra. Chronic inflammation can be associated with hemorrhage, swelling, edema, and this inflamed tissue may expand from the urethral meatus due to already weakened muscular and connective tissue.

Pathologic analysis of these lesions is usually consistent with the chronic inflammatory nature. Inflammation, hemorrhage and localized necrosis is commonly seen.

Treatment is usually conservative. Small asymptomatic lesions may be observed, or treated with topical creams, usually estrogen. Larger, symptomatic lesions can be easily excised. Usually traction on the caruncle will expose the base, below which it can be excised. Reapproximation of the mucosa can then follow with a fine, absorbable suture.

Urethral Diverticula

A urethral diverticulum is an epithelial lined, sac-like outpouching that arises from the urethral wall. These diverticuli are usually acquired, but in some instances may be congenital. The reported incidence is between 1.4% and 5%, but the true incidence is not known due to the fact that many small diverticuli are probably not detected. Most cases are thought to be acquired. An infection or obstruction of the periurethral glands can lead to the formation of a periurethral cyst. These cysts gradually enlarge, and then eventually rupture into the urethral wall, allowing urine to enter the cyst, and pool within its confines. Epithelialization then follows completing the transformation into a diverticulum. Stagnation of the urine in the diverticulum can lead to an infectious process which can cause recurrent UTI, stone formation, fistula development and, rarely, malignancy.

The presentation of diverticula is variable. The classic triad of dysuria, dyspareunia and dribbling may occur, but any female with a history of recurrent UTI or dyspareunia should be suspected of having a diverticulum. Other symptoms of a vaginal mass, vaginal pain or even persistent LUTS may be associated with a diverticulum. Many (20%-30%) of these women are asymptomatic.

Most diverticula can be felt on physical examination. This is usually a suburethral mass which may be tender. On compression of this mass, urine or purulent fluid may be seen exiting the urethral meatus. However, this finding is not present on many examinations of diverticuli.

Imaging can assist in the detection of diverticuli. Today it is important also to use imaging to localize and stage diverticuli. As imaging modalities have become more sensitive, one should utilize these images to plan for the surgical repair. For many, the VCUG remains the initial imaging modality. The VCUG done under fluoroscopy is a generally reliable way to diagnose and localize diverticuli. The sensitivity of this modality is reported between 49%-90%. This is an excellent study to screen for coexistent bladder pathology. One should remember to include straining films to assess the bladder neck. An advantage of the VCUG is that it may give a visual confirmation as to the level of urethral origin.

Positive pressure urethrography is another imaging modality with greater sensitivity (85%-100%). The advantages of this study such as excellent detail of the urethra and diverticulum without the need for a patient void seem to be outweighed by the fact that this is a cumbersome procedure for many to perform, and it can be considerably uncomfortable for the patient. Cystoscopy is usually performed in an attempt to localize the ostium of the fistula, and also to look for other causes of LUTS. The ostia are usually seen in about two thirds of cases. Transvaginal ultrasonography has a reported >90% sensitivity in the detection of diverticuli. These images provide anatomic detail regarding the diverticulum and in many cases identification of the ostium. This is a highly operator dependent imaging modality. MRI has taken on a considerable role in the imaging of diverticuli. This permits a noninvasive, high resolution and multiplanar imaging study of diverticuli. Diverticuli appear as areas of decreased signal intensity on T1 images when compared to the surrounding tissues. They have high signal intensity on T2 images. This modality has the best diagnostic accuracy, providing the best anatomic detail regarding the relationship to the urethra, and whether there are any complicating factors: multiple, horseshoe configuration, multiple ostia, etc. This can be a cost-effective option if a limited urethral protocol is followed.

Urodynamics should be strongly considered in women with diverticuli. When doing urodynamics, a fluoroscopic assessment should be considered to assist in localizing the source of leakage. Urodynamics are indicated in women with incontinence, pelvic pain, urinary urgency and incomplete emptying. Ganabathi et al reported that only 37% of women with diverticuli had normal urodynamics, 49% had stress incontinence and 10% had detrusor overactivity. These findings are important, as several authors have documented the safety and efficacy of performing a simultaneous anti incontinence procedure with a diverticulectomy.

The operative approach is a transvaginal urethral diverticulectomy. This is generally done in 4 steps. First, one creates an inverted, U-shaped vaginal incision, creating a broad, based flap. Second, the periurethral fascia is incised transversely. Proximal and distal flaps of periurethal fascia are raised from the diverticulum. The third step is a isolation and excision of the diverticulum. When possible, the diverticulum should be isolated to the ostial urethral attachment to ensure complete excision. Fourth, the urethra is closed longitudinally with 4.0 absorbable suture, followed by a transverse reapproximation of the periurethral fascia in order to avoid overlapping suture lines. The vaginal flap is advanced over the repair and closed. One may safely perform an indicated anti-incontinence procedure in conjunction with a urethral diverticulectomy. In this population, a synthetic sling is contraindicated, and autologous pubovaginal slings are preferred. After the fascia is harvested and a suprapubic tube is placed, the diverticulectomy proceeds in the manner as described above. After dissecting out the diverticular sac, the retropubic space is entered after removing any infectious material. The retropubic space is entered, and the sling sutures are placed into the retropubic space prior to closing the urethral defect. After closing the urethral defect, the periurethral fascia is then closed. The sling is then loosely positioned under the proximal urethra after the periurethral fascia is closed. Placement of a labial fat pad can be done in cases of diverticulectomy where the tissues are thin, and poor healing is of concern.

5. Suggested Reading

1. DeLancey J, Richardson A. Anatomy of genital support. In: *Urogynecologic Surgery.* Gaithersburg, MD: Aspen; 1992,

2. Herbst A, Mishell D, Stenchever M, Droege Mueller W. Disorders of the abdominal wall and pelvic support. In: Stenchever MA, ed. *Comprehensive Gynecology*. 2nd ed. Philadelphia, PA: Mosby Yearbook; 1992:594.

3 Iselin C, Aslan P, Webster G. Transvaginal repair of vesicovaginal fistulas after hysterectomy by vaginal cuff excision. *J Urol.* 1998;160:728.

4. Karram M, Miklos J, Sze E. Pelvic prolapse and lower urinary tract dysfunction in females. In: O'Donnell P, ed. *Urinary Incontinence*. 1st ed. Philadelphia, PA: Mosby Yearbook; 1997:302.

5. Kaser O. The Latzko operation for vesicovaginal fistula. *Acta Obstet Gaenecol Scand.* 1977;56:427.

6. Leach G, Trockman B. Surgery for fistulas and diverticulum. In: Walsh P, Retik A, Vaughn E, Wein A, eds. *Campbell's Urology*. 7th ed. Philadelphia, PA: WB Saunders Co; 1998.

7. Miller E, Webster G. Current management of vesicovaginal fistulae. *Curr Opin Urol.* 2001;11:417.

8. Rashid H, Cos L. Urethral diverticula in the adult female. In: Resnick E, Elder J, Spirnak J, eds. *Critical Decisions in Urology*. 3rd ed. London, England. BC Decker; 2004:302-307.

9. Leach G, Raz S. Vaginal flap technique: A method of transvaginal vesicovaginal fistula repair. In: Raz S, ed. *Female Urology*. Philadelphia, PA: WB Saunders; 1983:372.

10. Rovner E. Bladder and urethral diverticula. In: Wein A, Kavoussi L, Novick A, Partin A, Peters C, eds. Campbell Walsh Urology. 9th ed. Vol 3. Philadelphia, PA: WB Saunders;2007:2361-2391.

11. Winters J, Rackley R, Appell R, Nitti V. Miscellaneous female urologic conditions. In: Nitti V, ed. *Practical Urodynamics*. Philadelphia, PA: WB Saunders; 1998:219 230.

6. Questions

1. A 55-year-old multiparous woman has urge incontinence. Urinalysis is normal and physical exam demonstrates a Grade 3 cystocele. Urodynamics reveal a PVR of 100 cc, involuntary bladder contractions with incontinence, and a detrusor pressure at maximum flow (8 mL/sec) of 50 cm H_2O. When the cystocele is reduced, no stress urinary incontinence can be elicited. The next step is:

   A. Oxybutynin

   B. Doxazosin

   C. Pubovaginal sling

   D. Anterior colporrhaphy

   E. Pubovaginal sling and anterior colporrhaphy

2. A 61-year-old woman becomes incontinent immediately after a transvaginal repair of Grade III cystocele. This is most likely due to:

   A. Detrusor instability

   B. Partial bladder denervation

   C. Underlying urethral deficiency

   D. Surgical damage to the urethral sphincter

   E. Bladder neck and proximal urethral obstruction

3. A 55-year-old woman underwent a midurethral sling for stress incontinence 5 months ago. She now has dysuria, urgency and frequency despite antibiotic treatment for 2 documented UTIs. Urinalysis reveals 2-3 RBC/hpf. Pelvic US reveals a 50 cc PVR. The next step is:

   A. IVP

   B. Uroflowmetry

   C. Filling cystometry

   D. VCUG

   E. Cystoscopy

4. A 60-year-old woman develops vaginal leakage of urine and is found to have a ureterovaginal fistula 5 days after abdominal hysterectomy. Retrograde shows a fistula 2-3 cm above the bladder. Attempts to pass a stent retro and antegrade are unsuccessful. The most appropriate management is:

   A. Observation

   B. Ureteroneocystostomy

   C. Ureteroureterostomy

   D. Perc nephrostomy

5. 3 weeks after an MMK, a 40-year-old woman develops pelvic and suprapubic pain and T 101° F. She experiences difficulty adducting her thighs and has pain to palpation on pubis. The most likely diagnosis is:

   A. Osteitis pubis

   B. Osteomyelitis pubis

   C. Obturator nerve injury

   D. Urinary extravasation

   E. Pelvic abscess

6. A 62-year-old woman complains of UI and difficulty initiating voiding 12 months after a needle suspension for SUI. Her PVR is 120 mL and mid-voiding pressure is 52 cm H_2O during an uninhibited contraction. The best treatment is:

   A. CIC

   B. Ditropan and timed voiding

C. Urethral dilation

D. Removal of suspension suture

E. Transvaginal urethrolysis

7. A 74-year-old female with SUI and DI would like to avoid surgery. The best pharmacologic approach is:

A. Ditropan

B. Detrol

C. Imipramine

D. Terazosin

E. Ephedrine

8. A 75-year-old woman has recurrent cystitis. PE demonstrates Grade I cystocele and atrophic vaginitis. PVR 45 cc. IVP and VCUG are normal. The best management is:

A. Vaginal pessary

B. Oral estrogen

C. Intravaginal estrogen

D. Prophylactic antibiotics

9. A 54-year-old woman S/PXRT for cervical cancer 2 years ago develops micro-hematuria. TUR of a lesion 2 cm above the LUO reveals an inverted papilloma. 3 days post-op she develops a vesicovaginal fistula. The best treatment is:

A. Immediate transvaginal repair

B. Transvaginal repair in 6 months

C. Immediate transabdominal repair

D. Transabdominal repair in 6 months

E. Urinary diversion

10. A 64-year-old female S/PMMK 5 years ago, and transvaginal needle suspension 1 year ago still has severe urinary incontinence. She leaks with and without physical activity. The best diagnostic test is:

A. Urethral pressure profile

B. Video urodynamics

C. Cystometry

D. VCUG

E. CMG EMG

11. A 64-year-old woman has a Grade IV cystocele without urinary incontinence. To determine if she needs a concomitant anti incontinence surgery with the cystocele repair she should undergo:

A. Pelvic MRI

B. Urethral pressure profilometry

C. Urodynamics with a pessary

D. Cysto

E. Uroflow with PVR

Answers

1. D.

This patient suffers from bladder outlet obstruction secondary to a large cystocele as indicated by a high voiding pressure and low flow rate. The obstruction secondarily causes detrusor overactivity and subsequent urge incontinence. Despite reducing the cystocele, no stress incontinence can be elicited indicating good support of the urethrovesical junction. The best treatment is to repair the cystocele with a technique such as anterior colporrhaphy. The absence of stress incontinence precludes the need for a pubovaginal sling and if performed alone is likely to increase the postvoid residual. Although doxazosin can be used for female bladder outlet obstruction, when possible, the best treatment is to correct the underlying abnormality.

2. C.

The most common cause of the onset of urinary incontinence after repair of a large cystocele is underlying urethral dysfunction, which is unmasked by reduction of the cystocele. Cystocele repair should not cause incontinence due to urethral or bladder denervation or obstruction of the proximal urethra. Cystocele repair is typically associated with improvement in both bladder emptying and urge incontinence. Thus, either urethral hypermobility or intrinsic sphincter deficiency is likely to be the cause of incontinence in this setting.

3. E.

Cystoscopy is necessary to exclude the possibility of a foreign body in this setting.

4. B.

In a healthy pt, fistula repair may be undertaken early. Since the attempts to catheterize the ureter failed it is unlikely that this will heal with observation. The more distal portion of the ureter may be injured as well and repair should be done with a ureteroneocystostomy.

5. A.

These are classic signs and symptoms of osteitis pubis. Occurs in up to 2.5% of patients after MMK. Osteomyelitis is possible but far less common than osteitis. Obturator nerve injury (usually secondary to retractors) can occur but typically does not present at 3 weeks (present immediately).

6. E.

This patient is obstructed as evidenced by her elevated voiding pressure and elevated PVR. Ditropan is contraindicated because of the obstruction. CIC will not solve the problem or control the DI. The suspension should be taken down with urethrolysis.

7. C.

Imipramine has both a strong inhibitory action on bladder smooth muscle and a stimulant effect on the bladder outlet. The net result is it promotes urinary storage by preventing DI and increasing urethral resistance.

8. C.

After menopause, diminished levels of glycogen are produced as a result of decreased estrogen production. This alters the vaginal flora resulting in a decrease in the normally dominant lactobacilli. Vaginal pH rises, resulting in an overgrowth of enteric organisms. In a randomized double-blind trial, intravaginal estrogen decreased the incidence of UTIs in postmenopausal women with recurrent UTIs.

9. C.

In a patient with NO evidence of abscess formation or fluid collection, there is little need to wait before fixing the fistula. The abdominal approach provides better access to a radiation induced fistula and allows for an omental pedicle to be interposed between the bladder and vaginal wall.

10. B.

In a patient who has had 2 prior failed surgeries, in-depth testing is required. Only UDS will determine if the pt has involuntary bladder contractions, elevated voiding pressures, low VLLP and urethral hypermobility.

11. C.

Many women develop *de novo* SUI after cystocele repair due to the poor support of the urethra. Pre op UDS should be performed with a pessary or vaginal packing to assess the competence of the bladder neck with proper bladder support. A filling CMG to assess for DI and a VLLP should be performed.

Chapter 13: Medical Management of Urolithiasis

Sean A. Pierre, MD
Glenn M. Preminger, MD

Contents

1. Goals of Medical Management of Urolithiasis

A. Prevent new stone disease

B. Stabilize existing urolithiasis

C. Prevent urologic complications of urolithiasis
- a. Urinary tract obstruction
- b. Urinary tract infection
- c. Renal compromise/end stage renal disease
  - i. Primary hyperoxaluria
  - ii. Hyperuricemia
  - iii. Staghorn renal calculi

D. Prevent nonurologic complications of urolithiasis
- a. Osteodystrophy
  - i. Absorptive hypercalciuria
  - ii. Renal tubular acidosis
  - iii. Primary hyperoxaluria
- b. Cardiomyopathy
  - i. Primary hyperoxaluria
- c. Retinopathy
  - i. Primary hyperoxaluria
- d. Gouty arthritis
  - i. Hyperuricosemia

E. Identify non-urologic conditions predisposing to urolithiasis
- a. Hyperparathyroidism
- b. Gout
- c. Sarcoidosis
- d. GI malabsorptive conditions
- e. Crohn's disease / ulcerative colitis
- f. Biliary disease
- g. Pancreatitis
- h. Bariatric surgery

2. Types of Urolithiasis and Clinical Associations

Table 1

Types of Urolithiasis Based on Stone Composition

Calcium-based	Non-calcium-based
Calcium oxalate monohydrate	Uric acid
Calcium oxalate dihydrate	Ammonium acid urate
	Sodium urate Dihydroadenine Xanthine
Calcium phosphate	Cystine
	Struvite
	Drug-induced (indinavir, ephedrine, triamterene)

3. Diagnoses/Pathophysiology

Table 2

Stone Composition and Possible Clinical Associations

Stone Analysis	Possible Associations
Calcium oxalate	Hypercalciuria Hypercalcemia Hyperoxaluria Hypocitraturia Gouty diathesis Low urine volumes
Ca Phos	Distal renal tubular acidosis Hyperparathyroidism Low urine volumes UTI
Uric acid Ammonium acid urate Sodium urate Dihydroadenine Xanthine	Gouty diathesis Gouty arthritis Gouty nephropathy Gouty tophi Hyperuricosuria Hyperuricosemia Obesity Inborn errors of metabolism (eg, Lesch-Nyhan disease) Myeloproliferative disorder Tumor lysis syndrome EtOH abuse
Cystine	Cystinuria
Struvite	Urinary tract infection

A. Contributors to urolithiasis
- a. Anatomic
  - i. Obstruction (UPJO, stricture, BPH)
  - ii. Renal anatomy (medullary sponge kidney
  - iii. Foreign body (suture, staple, stent)
  - iv. Diverticulum (calyceal, bladder)
  - v. Hydronephrosis
  - vi. Urinary diversion/intestinal substitution
- b. Functional
  - i. Voiding dysfunction (neurogenic)

B. Overall approach to classification of urolithiasis
- a. Type of stones
  - i. Calcium-based
  - ii. Non-calcium-based
- b. Predisposing factors
  - i. Promoter excess
  - ii. Inhibitor deficiency
  - iii. General urine parameters

C. Calcium-based urolithiasis
- a. Promoter excess
  - i. Hypercalciuria
  - ii. Hyperuricosuria
  - iii. Hyperoxaluria
- b. Inhibitor deficiency
  - i. Hypocitraturia
  - ii. Hypomagnesuria
- c. General urine parameters
  - i. Urine acidity ("gouty diathesis")
  - ii. Low urine volumes

D. Non-calcium-based urolithiasis
- a. Promoter excess
  - i. Hyperuricosuria
  - ii. Cystinuria
  - iii. Medications
- b. Inhibitor deficiency
  - i. Hypocitraturia
- c. General urine parameters
  - i. Urine acidity ("gouty diathesis")
  - ii. Low urine volumes
  - iii. Urinary tract infection

4. Calcium-based Urolithiasis

A. Hypercalciuria
- a. Classification
  - i. Hypercalcemic
  - ii. Normocalcemic
- b. Pathophysiology
  - i. Hypercalcemic
    - 1. Increased serum calcium → increased filtered calcium → hypercalciuria
  - ii. Normocalcemic
- c. Most common cause
  - i. Hypercalcemic: primary hyperparathyroidism
  - ii. Normocalcemic: absorptive hypercalciuria
- d. Hypercalcemic hypercalciuria
  - i. Most common causes of 1° hyperparathyroidism
    - 1. Parathyroid adenoma
    - 2. Parathyroid hyperplasia
  - ii. Effects of increased PTH
    - 1. Increase in Ca absorption from GI tract
    - 2. Increase in Ca absorption from kidney
    - 3. Increase in Ca absorption from bone
    - 4. Increase 1,25 OH-Vitamin D production from kidney → increased absorption from GI tract
    - 5. Decreased phosphate resorption from kidney
- e. Normocalcemic hypercalciuria
  - i. Absorptive
    - 1. Increased absorption/reabsorption of Ca from GI tract/bone/kidney → Increased filtered calcium (to keep serum Ca near normal) → hypercalciuria
    - 2. Types I, II, III
  - ii. Renal
    - 1. Distal renal tubule "leaks" calcium into urine → hypercalciuria
  - iii. Resorptive
    - 1. Increased bone demineralization → increased filtered Ca (to keep serum Ca near normal) → hypercalciuria
  - iv. Idiopathic
- f. Absorptive hypercalciuria (AH)
  - i. Classification
    - 1. Type I
      - a. Pathophysiology
        - i. *Increased absorption of Ca from GI tract*
        - ii. **Independent** of dietary Ca content
        - iii. Decreased dietary Ca → negligible effect on urine Ca
        - iv. Increased absorption of Ca → negative feedback → **decreased serum PTH**
    - 2. Type II
      - a. Pathophysiology
        - i. *Increased absorption of Ca from GI tract*
        - ii. **Dependent** on dietary Ca content
        - iii. Decreased dietary Ca → normalization of urine Ca
        - iv. A less severe form of AH Type I
        - v. Because of the increased absorption of Ca → negative feedback → **decreased serum PTH**
  - ii. Renal Hypercalciuria
    - 1. Pathophysiology
      - a. Increased loss of Ca from kidney (distal tubule)
      - b. Loss of Ca → increased serum PTH
      - c. Increased serum PTH → increased GI Ca absorption and increased bone Ca resorption (to keep serum Ca near normal)
    - 2. Net effect
      - a. Normal serum Ca
      - b. Increased urine Ca
    - 3. Most common form of hypercalciuria in pediatric population
  - iii. Resorptive hypercalciuria
    - 1. Pathophysiology
      - a. Increased serum PTH (mild)
        - i. → increased GI Ca absorption
        - ii. → increased bone Ca resorption
      - b. * PTH levels not high enough to cause hypercalcemia
      - c. Most of the increased Ca in the serum is filtered into the urine
        - i. → serum Ca near normal
      - d. Net effect
        - i. Near normal serum Ca
        - ii. Increased urine Ca

B. Hyperuricosuria
(Hyperuricosuric CaOx nephrolithiasis)
- a. How does high urinary uric acid contribute to ***calcium***-based urolithiasis?
  - i. Formation of small uric acid crystals acts as nidus for calcium-based stones—so-called "heterogenous nucleation"

ii. Sodium acid urate may inhibit the effectiveness of naturally occurring inhibitors of stone formation, eg, glycosaminoglycans

b. Classification

i. Hyperuricosemic hyperuricosuria

1. Serum uric acid increased

ii. Normouricosemic hyperuricosuria

1. Serum uric acid normal

c. Uric acid

i. Byproduct of purine metabolism

ii. Precursors: hypoxanthine, xanthine

1. Both more soluble than uric acid

iii. Enzyme involved

1. Xanthine oxidase

2. Hypoxanthine → xanthine → uric acid

3. Same enzyme catalyzes both steps

iv. pKa uric acid = 5.5

1. Thus the insoluble uric acid tends to precipitate out of solution in *acidic urine*

2. **Low urine pH is the primary risk factor for uric acid stones**

3. Urine pH above 5.5 favors formation of CaOx stones, even in the presence of significant hyperuricosuria

d. Risk factors for hyperuricosuria

i. High dietary purine intake (esp. "red meat")

ii. Heritable disorders of purine synthesis

1. Lesch-Nyhan disease

2. Overactivity of PRPP (= PRS =phosphoribosyl pyrophosphate synthetase)

3. Adenosine phospho-ribosyl transferase (APRT) deficiency

iii. Myeloproliferative disorders

1. Secondary to high cellular turnover → increased purine metabolism

iv. Tumor lysis syndrome

1. Significant tumor cell death during therapy, usually chemotherapy

2. 2° to high cellular turnover → increased purine metabolism

v. Medications

1. Probenicid

2. Sulfinpyrazone

C. Hyperoxaluria

a. Classification

i. Primary

ii. Secondary

iii. Enteric

iv. Idiopathic

b. Primary

i. Pathophysiology

1. Increased hepatic *production* → increased serum oxalate → increased filtered oxalate → hyperoxaluria

2. *= 1° Oxalosis*

ii. Subtypes

1. Type I

2. Type II

iii. Type I

Table 3

Comparison of Metabolic Findings in Absorptive Hypercalciuria Types I – III

	Absorptive	**Renal**	**Resorptive**
Serum calcium	Normal	Normal	High Normal/increased
PTH levels	Decreased (secondarily)	Increased (primarily)	Increased
Fasting urinary calcium	Type I: Increased Type II: Normal	Increased	Increased
Intestinal calcium absorption	Increased (primarily)	Increased (secondarily)	Increased (secondarily)

1. More Common
2. Pathophysiology
   a. Excess glyoxylate oxidized to oxalate
   b. Enzyme defect
      i. AGT (alalnine-glyoxylate amino-transferase)
   c. Co-factor for AGT enzyme
      i. Pyridoxine (= Vitamin B_6)
      ii. One of the limiting factors of the reaction
3. Autosomal recessive
   a. Three subtypes
   b. Chromosome 2 (for type I); Chromosome 19 (for types II and III)
4. Present EARLY in life (mean age 5 years old)

iv. Type 2
1. VERY rare
2. Pathophysiology
   a. 2 enzyme deficiencies → increased urine oxalate and glyceric acid
   b. Condition also called L-glyceric aciduria
   c. Enzyme defect
      i. Glyoxylate reductase
      ii. D-glycerate dehydrogenase
   d. Cofactor
      i. NOT pyridoxine

v. Classic findings – 24-hour urine collection
1. Urinary oxalate >100 mg/day

vi. Clinical manifestations: urologic
1. Urolithiasis
   a. Early onset
   b. Recurrent
2. Renal insufficiency
   a. Can be silent in 33%
3. End stage renal disease

vii. Clinical manifestations: non-urologic
1. Pathophysiology
   a. Secondary to oxalate deposition in tissues
2. Heart
   a. Cardiomyopathy
   b. Arrhythmia
3. Bones
   a. Osteodystrophy
   b. Joint pain
4. Eyes
   a. Retinopathy
   b. Maculopathy

c. Secondary (metabolic hyperoxaluria)

i. Pathophysiology
1. Increased hepatic *conversion* of metabolites to oxalate → increased serum oxalate → increased filtered oxalate → hyperoxaluria
2. Hepatic enzymes normal

ii. Risk factors
1. Pyridoxine/vitamin B6 deficiency
   a. Almost like a secondary cause of 1° hyperoxaluria type I
2. Excessive intake of high oxalate-containing food
   a. Spinach
   b. Tea
   c. Chocolate
   d. Nuts
3. Ethylene glycol ingestion
   a. Rare cause of recurrent urolithiasis

d. Enteric

i. Pathophysiology
1. Increased GI Absorption of oxalate → increased filtered oxalate → hyperoxaluria
   a. Small bowel pathology (especially ileum) → decreased bile salt reabsorption → increased chelation of Ca in GI tract → increased free oxalate → increased GI absorption of oxalate
   b. Increased bile salts in colon → increased permeability of colon to oxalate
   c. Diarrhea → loss of Mg → hypomagnesuria
   d. Decrease in oxalobacter formigines
      i. This bacterium metabolizes oxalate in GI tract

ii. Common conditions associated with enteric hyperoxaluria
1. Inflammatory bowel disease (Crohn's/UC)
2. Biliary disease
3. Chronic diarrheal syndromes
4. Pancreatitis/pancreatectomy
5. Small bowel resection
6. Short gut syndrome
7. Small bowel bypass procedures ***(even current bariatric surgery)***
8. Bacterial overgrowth syndromes

iii. Classic findings: 24-hour urine collection
1. Increased urine oxalate
2. Decreased urine Ca
   a. Significant loss in GI tract → Less available for renal excretion

b. Often very low (<100 mg/day)
3. Decreased Urine pH
a. Secondary to HCO_3 loss in GI tract
e. Idiopathic
i. Pathophysiology – theories
1. Abnormal GI tract receptor → increased oxalate absorption
2. Decreased intestinal bacteria which metabolize oxalate

D. Hypocitraturia
a. Pathophysiology
i. Decreased citrate → Decreased chelation of Ca in urine → increased chelation of Ca in urine with other components → calcium urolithiasis
ii. Decreased citrate → decreased chelation of H^+ in urine → Decreased pH → increased risk of urolithiasis (calcium-based and non-calcium based)
b. Pathophysiology
i. **Metabolic Acidosis**
1. Pathophysiology
a. Acidosis → increased chelation of H^+ with citrate in mitochondria → decreased citrate secretion into urine
2. Conditions
a. ***Distal renal tubular acidosis = renal tubular acidosis type I***
b. Chronic diarrheal states
c. Medications: thiazide (causes intracellular acidosis)
d. High dietary protein intake (= Increased acid-ash load)
e. Excessive exercise (lactic acidosis)
f. Idiopathic
ii. Intestinal citrate malabsorption
iii. UTI (formation of enzyme citrate lyase) (Table 4)
c. **Renal tubular acidosis type I = distal renal tubular acidosis**
i. Pathophysiology
1. Inability of Distal Nephron to Secrete H+
ii. Associations
1. Primary
a. Endemic in Thailand
b. Rare hereditary form
c. 80% patients female
2. Secondary
a. Pyelonephritis
b. Urinary tract obstruction
c. Sarcoidosis
d. Renal transplant
e. ATN
f. Analgesic nephropathy
g. Primary hyperparathyroidism
h. Idiopathic hypercalciuria
iii. Findings
1. ***Acidosis*** (systemic)
2. ***Hypocitraturia***
a. Usually severe (<200 mg / day)
b. Pathophysiology
i. Systemic acidosis → increased chelation of H^+ with citrate in mitochondria → decreased citrate secretion into urine
c. Sequelae
i. Urolithiasis (main contributor)
ii. Nephrocalcinosis
iii. bone disease
3. Hypercalciuria
a. Pathophysiology
i. Acidosis → increased dissociation of Ca from serum proteins → increased Ca available for renal filtration
ii. Acidosis → increased demineralization of bone → increased Ca available for renal filtration
b. Sequelae
i. Urolithiasis
ii. Nephrocalcinosis

Table 4

Comparison of Renal Tubular Acidosis Types I, II and IV

	RTA I	RTA II	RTA IV
Nephron segment involved	Distal	Proximal	Depends on disease
Pathophysiology	Inability to secrete H+	Inability to reabsorb HCO_3 (and multiple other species)	Decreased GFR
Association with urolithiasis	Yes	No	No
Acidosis	Non-anion gap Hyperchloremic	Non-anion Gap Hyperchloremic	Early: Non-anion gap. Hyperchloremic Late: (GFR <15-20 mL/min): Anion gap 2° to uremia
Serum K	Low	Low	High
Urine pH	> 5.5	Usu >5.5 but can be <5.5	Usu >5.5 but can be <5.5
Urine citrate	Low	High	Slightly Low
Urine Ca	High	High	Low
Urine HCO_3		Increased	
Special tests	Ammonium chloride loading test	1. FeNa (usu >15%) 2. Bicarbonate loading test	1. Lasix infusion (→ increased urine acidification)
Associations	1. Multiple etiologies 2. Hypophosphatemia	Fanconi syndrome	Causes of end-stage renal disease
Treatment	Treat underlying cause if possible. Urinary alkalinization (K-Citrate, $NaHCO_3$)	1. HCO_3 – supplementation 2. K Citrate	

4. ***Hyperchloremia***
   a. Pathophysiology
      i. Dehydration → increased serum aldosterone → reabsorption of H_2O via Na reabsorption → concomitant Cl reabsorption
   b. Sequelae
      i. Can be an early sign of possible metabolic acidosis
5. ***Hypokalemia***
   a. Pathophysiology
      i. Dehydration → increased serum aldosterone → reabsorption of H_2O via Na^+ reabsorption → concomitant K^+ secretion into urine
      ii. Dehydration → increased serum aldosterone → decreased renal K^+/H^+ antiporter activity → Loss of K+ in urine
   b. Sequelae
      i. Cardiac: arrhythmia
      ii. Musculoskeletal: weakness
      iii. GI: Ileus
6. ***Hyperphosphaturia***
   a. Pathophysiology
      i. Acidosis → increased demineralization of bone → increased Phos available for renal filtration
   b. Sequelae
      i. Osteomalacia
      ii. Growth retardation

iv. Concept of "incomplete" distal renal tubular acidosis
   1. Clinical findings
      a. Mild/absent acidosis
      b. Normal/near-normal serum potassium
      c. Previously known as RTA Type III

E. *Hypomagnesuria*
   a. Pathophysiology
      i. Decreased Mg → decreased chelation of oxalate in urine to form soluble Mg-oxalate complex → Increased free oxalate in urine → increased Ca chelation with oxalate
   b. Etiology
      i. Often associated with hypocitraturia
      ii. GI malabsorptive conditions
         1. Inflammatory bowel disease (Crohn's/UC)
      iii. UTIs

F. *Low urine volume*
   a. Important contributor to all forms of urolithiasis
   b. Can contribute to urine acidity
      i. Dehydration → increased renal Na^+ reabsorption → increased Na^+/H^+ exchanger activity → increased secretion of H^+

G. *Gouty diathesis*
   a. The solubility constants (pKa) for most calcium-based stones are such that they are more likely to form in acidic urine
      i. Exception: calcium phosphate
   b. Patients with gouty diathesis can form either calcium-based or uric acid calculi

5. Noncalcium-based Urolithiasis

A. Gouty diathesis

a. Definition
  i. Urine pH < 5.5
b. Risk factors for gouty diathesis
  i. High dietary purine intake (esp. "red meat")
    1. Increased purines → increased metabolism of purines → increased uric acid production → increased filtered uric acid
  i. High dietary protein intake (esp. "red meat")
    1. amino acid load = "acid-ash" load
  ii. Obesity
    1. Overweight associated with low urine pH
  iii. Heritable disorders of purine synthesis
    1. Lesch-Nyhan disease
    2. Overactivity of PRPP (= PRS = phosphoribosyl pyrophosphate synthetase)
    3. Adenosine phospho-ribosyl transferase (APRT) deficiency
  iv. Myeloproliferative disorders
    1. Secondary to high cellular turnover → increased purine metabolism
  v. Tumor lysis syndrome
    1. Significant tumor cell death during therapy, usually chemotherapy
    2. 2° to high cellular turnover → increased purine metabolism
  vi. Medications
    1. Probenicid
    2. Sulfinpyrazone
  vii. EtOH abuse
    1. Metabolism to organic acids
c. Clinical associations
  i. Gout
    1. Definition
      a. Abnormality of purine metabolism associated with raised but variable serum uric acid levels secondary arthritis
  ii. Gouty arthritis
    1. Often used as a synonym for "gout"
    2. Secondary to deposition of sodium urate crystals in joints
  iii. Gouty nephropathy
    1. Definition
      a. Interstitial nephropathy secondary to uric acid crystal deposition
  iv. Gouty tophi
    1. Definition
      a. Subcutaneous depositions of uric acid in the periarticular tissues giving rise to raised, painless subcutaneous lesions

B. Cystinuria

a. Pathophysiology
  i. Inborn error of metabolism
  ii. Proximal convoluted tubule defect
    1. Defect in transport system for 4 dibasic amino acids ("COLA")
      a. Cystine, ornithine, lysine, arginine
  iii. Why cystine stones rather than other dibasic amino acid stones?
    1. Cystine (pKa 8.3) is relatively insoluble at typical urine pH (5-7)
  iv. Autosomal recessive
  v. Heterogenous nucleation can occur
    1. Can have associated calcium-based urolithiasis (often calcium oxalate)
b. Very few significant nonurinary tract manifestations

C. Infection-based

a. Pathophysiology
  i. UTI → Urinary alkalinization → urolithiasis
  ii. Alkalinizing effect more significant if bacteria contains urease
  iii. E.coli does not produce urease
b. Urease
  i. Metabolizes urea to ammonia and carbon dioxide
  ii. Ammonia → urinary alkalinization → precipitation of urinary calculi with high pKa values
    1. Struvite (magnesium ammonium phosphate)
    2. Calcium phosphate
c. Bacteria reside in the interstities of the calculus
  i. → Difficult (if not impossible) to truly sterilize urine with antibiotic therapy alone
  ii. → Urinary sterilization necessitates removal of all stone material
d. Other possible contributors include factors which increased the risk of UTI
  i. Urinary tract obstruction
  ii. Chronic nonobstructive hydronephrosis
  iii. Neurogenic voiding dysfunction
  iv. Urinary diversion/intestinal substitution

D. Drug-induced calculi

a. Pathophysiology
  i. Drug itself or a metabolite is filtered in the kidney and precipitates out of solution in the urine

ii. Usually requires long-term use of drug
b. Stone types
  i. Indinavir
    1. Protease inhibitor
    2. Used in treatment of HIV infection
  ii. Triamterene
    1. Potassium-sparing diuretic
  iii. Ephedrine
    1. Synthetic alpha-adrenergic agonist

6. Metabolic Evaluation

A. Approaches

a. Abbreviated evaluation
  i. When to perform
    1. Low suspicion of significant metabolic abnormality or contributing pathophysiology
    2. Few/no obvious risk factors for recurrence
  ii. Indications for abbreviated metabolic evaluation
    * All of the following should be true:
    1. First stone episode
    2. Single urinary calculus
    3. Calcium oxalate calculus
    4. Non-staghorn calculus
    5. Uncomplicated clinical course
    6. No anatomic GU anomalies
b. Comprehensive evaluation
  i. When to perform
    1. High suspicion of significant metabolic abnormality or contributing pathophysiology
    2. Risk factors for recurrence present
  ii. Indications for extensive metabolic evaluation
    1. Any of the requirements for abbreviated metabolic evaluation not met
    2. Non-calcium based urolithiasis
      a. Uric acid
      b. Cystine
      c. Struvite
      d. Ca Phos
    3. Medical conditions with increased risk
      a. Gout
      b. Inborn errors of metabolism of purines
        i. Lesch-Nyhan syndrome
        ii. Overactivity of PRS
        iii. APRT deficiency
    4. Myeloproliferative disease
    5. Tumor lysis syndrome
    6. EtOH abuse
    7. GI malabsorptive/diarrheal states
    8. H/O GI surgery
    9. Distal renal tubular acidosis
    10. Hypercalcemia
      a. Hyperparathyroidism
      b. Granulomatous disease
    11. Urinary diversion/intestinal substitution
  iii. High-risk populations
    1. History of recurrent urolithiasis
    2. Family history of stones
    3. Pediatrics
    4. Nephrocalcinosis
    5. Solitary kidney

c. Abbreviated Metabolic Evaluation: Details
  i. History
    1. Dietary Excesses
      a. Purine
      b. Protein
      c. Oxalate
      d. Sodium
    2. Medical conditions which might contribute to urolithiasis
      a. Urologic
      b. Nonurologic
    3. Identification of high-risk populations
      a. History of recurrent urolithiasis
      b. Family history of stones
      c. Pediatrics
      d. Nephrocalcinosis
      e. Solitary kidney
    4. Medications
      a. Indinavir
      b. Triamterene
      c. Ephedrine
      d. Probenicid
      e. Sulfinpyrazole
      f. Chemotherapy
  ii. Physical examination
    1. Head and neck
      a. Palpable mass
        i. Parathyroid adenoma
        ii. Parathyroid hyperplasia
    2. Abdomen
      a. Palpable kidney
        i. Hydronephrosis
      b. Palpable bladder
      c. Voiding dysfunction
    3. Musculoskeletal
      a. Lumbosacral abnormality
        i. Neural tube defect → voiding dysfunction
      b. Painful joint movements
        i. Gouty arthritis
        ii. Primary hyperoxaluria-related
    4. Neurologic
      a. Risk of voiding dysfunction
    5. Cardiovascular
      a. Arrhythmia
        i. Hypokalemia → distal RTA
        ii. Hyperoxaluria
    6. Skin
      a. Gouty tophi
  iii. Urine tests
    1. Urinalysis
      a. pH <5.5
        i. Gouty diathesis
      b. pH >7.5
        i. UTI
    2. Urine culture
    3. Urine microscopy
      a. Crystals
        i. Big one to remember: **benzene-ring appearance = cystine**
  iv. Stone analysis
    1. Calcium-based
      a. CaOx
      b. CaPhos
    2. Non-calcium based
  v. Bloodwork
    1. Electrolytes
      a. Decreased HCO_3
        i. Acidosis, eg, distal RTA
      b. Decreased K
        i. Distal RTA
        ii. Rx
      c. Increased Cl
        i. Metabolic acidosis (eg, distal RTA)
    2. Ca
      a. High
        i. Hyperparathyroidism → check PTH
    3. Phos
      a. Low
        i. Renal hypercalciuria
      b. High
        i. Resorptive hypercalciuria
    4. Uric Acid
      a. High
        i. Gout
  vi. Radiologic imaging
    1. KUB
      a. Low sensitivity (small stones, radiolucent stones, ++ bowel contents)
      b. Tomograms help to increase sensitivity
    2. IVP
      a. Functional component to study
    3. U/S
      a. No radiation
      b. Less sensitive for ureteral calculi
      c. Can assess bladder emptying
    4. CT
      a. High sensitivity and specificity

5. Nuclear renogram
   a. If obstruction in absence of calculus suspected

d. Extensive metabolic evaluation – details
   i. History
      1. Dietary excesses
         a. Purine
         b. Protein
         c. Oxalate
         d. Sodium
      2. Medical conditions which might contribute to urolithiasis:
         a. Urologic
         b. Nonurologic
      3. High-risk groups
         a. History of recurrent urolithiasis
         b. Pediatrics
         c. Nephrocalcinosis
         d. Solitary kidney
      4. Medications
         a. Indinavir
         b. Triamterene
         c. Ephedrine
         d. Chemotherapy
         e. Sulfinpyrazole
         f. Probenecid
   ii. Physical examination
      1. SDA
      2. Head and neck
         a. Palpable mass
            i. Parathyroid adenoma
            ii. Parathyroid hyperplasia
      3. Abdomen
         a. Palpable kidney
            i. Hydronephrosis
         b. Palpable bladder
         c. Voiding dysfunction
      4. Musculoskeletal
         a. Lumbosacral abnormality
            i. Neural tube defect → voiding dysfunction
         b. Painful joint movements
            i. Gouty arthritis
            ii. Primary hyperoxaluria-related
      5. Neurologic
         a. Risk of voiding dysfunction
      6. Cardiovascular
         a. Arrhythmia
            i. Hypokalemia → distal RTA
            ii. Hyperoxaluria
      7. Skin
         a. Gouty tophi
   iii. Urine tests
      1. Urinalysis
         a. pH < 5.5
            i. Gouty diathesis
         b. pH >7.5
            i. UTI
      2. Urine culture
      3. Urine microscopy
         a. Crystals
            i. Big one to remember: **Benzene-ring appearance = Cystine**
      4. 24-hr urine collection
         a. Do 2-3 separate collections initially
            i. Helps to correct for daily variations in diet and fluid intake
         b. Components measured
            i. Volume
            ii. pH
            iii. Ca
            iv. Mg
            v. Phos
            vi. Na
            vii. K
               1. Allows assessment of "compliance" on potassium citrate therapy (value should increase from baseline)
            viii. Creatinine
               1. Value depends on patient characteristics (weight, renal function)
               2. Allows for assessment of "completeness" of collection
               3. If too low (<500 mg/day), consider incomplete collection or dilution with fluid
            ix. Uric Acid
            x. Oxalate
            xi. Citrate
            xii. SO_4
            xiii. Cl
            xiv. Cystine
               1. Have to ask SPECIFICALLY for cystine in some labs
         c. Method of collection
            i. Discard first voided urine on day of collection
            ii. Collect all urine for that day and the first voided urine of the NEXT day

iii. Most containers need to be refrigerated/cooled during the collection process

iv. Stone analysis
1. Calcium-based
a. CaOx
b. CaPhos
2. Non-calcium based

v. Bloodwork
1. Electrolytes
a. Decreased HCO_3
i. Acidosis (eg, distal RTA)
b. Decreased K
i. Distal RTA
ii. Rx
c. Increased Cl
i. Metabolic acidosis (eg, distal RTA)
2. Ca
a. High
i. Hyperparathyroidism → check PTH
3. Phos
a. Low
i. Renal hypercalciuria
b. High
i. Resorptive hypercalciuria
4. Uric acid
a. High
i. Gout

vi. Radiologic imaging
1. KUB
a. Low sensitivity (small stones, radiolucent stones, ++ bowel contents)
b. Tomograms help to increase sensitivity
2. IVP
a. Functional component to study
3. U/S
a. No radiation
b. Less sensitive for ureteral calculi
c. Can assess bladder emptying
4. CT
a. High sensitivity and specificity
5. Nuclear renogram
a. If obstruction in absence of calculus suspected

vii. Special tests
1. "Pak" test (calcium fast and loading test)
a. Allows differentiation of the different types of hypercalciuria
b. Rarely used
i. Mainstays of therapy; absorptive and renal hypercalciuria similar
ii. Other tests can be used to determine presence of resorptive hypercalciuria (serum phos)
c. Uses calcium fasting and loading to exacerbate the differences between the types of hypercalciuria
d. Urine cAMP used as surrogate marker of serum PTH
i. It changes more quickly and reliably with changes in serum Ca
e. Procedure
i. 7 days Low-Ca and Low-Na Diet
ii. Fast from 2100 prior to day of test
iii. Distilled water between 2100 and 0000
iv. At 0700 empty bladder and discard urine
v. Collect urine from 0700-0900 = "Fasting sample"
vi. 1 gm Ca PO
vii. Collect urine from 0900-1300 = "Post-load sample"
viii. Each sample checked for Ca, cAMP and creatinine
f. Results
i. **Absorptive hypercalciuria type I**
1. Fasting urine Ca: High
a. Remember – diet <u>independent</u>
2. Fasting urine cAMP = fasting serum PTH: Low
a. The increased Ca absorption suppresses serum PTH
3. Post-load urine Ca: high
a. GI absorption of Ca still high and independent of diet
4. Post-load urine cAMP = post-load serum PTH: low
a. GI absorption of Ca still high and independent of diet
ii. **Absorptive hypercalciuria Type II**
1. Fasting urine Ca: Low
a. Remember – diet <u>dependent</u>
2. Fasting urine cAMP = fasting serum PTH: normal
a. Because now Ca absorption is normal
3. Post-load urine Ca: high
a. Dietary dependent increase in Ca absorption

4. Post-load urine cAMP = Post-load serum PTH: low
    a. 2° to the increased dietary Ca

iii. **Renal hypercalciuria**
  1. Fasting urine Ca: high
    a. Not related to diet but to distal renal tubule abnormality
  2. Fasting urine cAMP = fasting serum PTH: high
    a. 2° to the Ca loss in urine
  3. Post-load urine Ca: higher
    a. More Ca available for renal filtration
  4. Post-load urine cAMP = Post-load serum PTH: normal
    a. The increased Ca available from GI tract normalizes the serum PTH

iv. **Resorptive hypercalciuria**
  1. Fasting urine Ca: high
    a. Not related to diet
  2. Fasting urine cAMP = fasting serum PTH: high
    a. Primary problem is decreased Phos causing increased serum PTH
  3. Post-load urine Ca: high
    a. Not related to diet
  4. Post-load urine cAMP = post-load serum PTH: high
    a. Again, not related to diet

2. Distal RTA
  a. Blood gases
    i. Acidosis
      1. Consider distal RTA
  b. Ammonium chloride loading test
    i. Allows diagnosis of incomplete distal RTA (mild/absent systemic acidosis, normal/near normal serum K)
    ii. Premise
      1. Primary problem is decreased ability to renally eliminate excess acid → urine pH remains high even when significant acid load delivered
    iii. Procedure
      1. 3 days of an acid load (PO ammonium chloride tabs)
        a. Occasionally done as inpatient because of the risks of symptomatic acidosis and/or hypokalemia
      2. 24-hour urine collection done before and after acid load
    iv. Results
      1. Urine pH >5.5 after acid load: incomplete distal RTA

3. Cystinuria
  a. Sodium nitroprusside colorimetric test
    i. Qualitative rather than quantitative test
    ii. Results
      1. Urine turns magenta color at urine cystine values >75 mg/L

Table 5

Results of Calcium Fast and Loading (Pak) Test for Differentiating Types of Hypercalciuria

Type of Hypercalciuria	Fasting Urine Ca	Fasting Urine cAMP	Post-load Urine Ca	Post-load Urine cAMP
Absorptive Type I	High	Low	High	Low
Absorptive Type II	Normal	Normal	High	Lower
Renal	High	High	Higher	Normal
Resorptive	High	High	High	High

7. Management Strategies

A. Absorptive hypercalciuria

a. Goals – absorptive hypercalciuria type I
  i. Decrease renal filtration of Ca
    1. Decreased dietary sodium
    2. Thiazides (chlorthalidone, indapamide, hydrochlorothiazide)
  ii. Increase urine inhibitors of stone formation
    1. Potassium citrate
  iii. Change general urine parameters
    1. Increased urine output
    2. Urinary alkalization
      a. Potassium citrate
      b. Diet
        i. Moderate calcium intake
        ii. Decreased purine intake
        iii. Decreased animal protein intake
        iv. Increased fiber intake

b. Goals – absorptive hypercalciuria Type II
  i. Decreased renal filtration of Ca
    1. Decreased dietary sodium
    2. Thiazides
  ii. Decreased GI absorption of Ca
    1. Sodium cellulose phosphate (no longer available)
    2. Orthophosphates
  iii. Increased urine inhibitors of stone formation
    1. Potassium citrate
  iv. Change general urine parameters
    1. Increased urine output
    2. Urinary alkalinization
      a. Potassium citrate
      b. Diet
        i. Moderate calcium intake
        ii. Decreased purine intake
        iii. Decreased animal protein intake
        iv. Increased fiber intake

c. Specifics
  i. Decreased dietary sodium
    1. Renal sodium excretion correlates with renal Ca excretion
  ii. Thiazide diuretics (chlorthalidone, indapamide)
    1. Mechanism of action
      a. Inhibits distal tubular Na secretion → concomitant decreased renal Ca excretion
    2. Side effects
      a. Lassitude/sleepiness
      b. Hypokalemia
        i. Often administered with K-citrate or utilize K-sparing diuretic (eg, moduretic – HCTZ + amiloride)
      c. Acidosis (mild)
        i. Secondary to mild hyperuricemia
        ii. Often administered with K-citrate to address this issue
      d. Can unmask subtle hyperparathyroidism
      e. Glucose intolerance
      f. Erectile dysfunction
  iii. Sodium cellulose phosphate (no longer available)
    1. Mechanism of action
      a. Binds Ca in GI tract
    2. Side Effects
      a. GI: nausea, diarrhea
      b. Hypomagnesuria
        i. Binds Mg in GI tract → decreased GI Mg absorption → decreased renal Mg filtration
      c. Hyperoxaluria
        i. Binds Ca and Mg in GI tract → increased free oxalate in GI tract → increased GI oxalate absorption → increased renal oxalate filtration
      d. Negative calcium balance
        i. Secondary increased PTH → bone resorption
  iv. Orthophsophates
    1. Mechanism of action
      a. Bind Ca in GI tract
        i. Side Effects
          1. GI: nausea, diarrhea
          2. Hypomagnesuria
            a. Binds Mg in GI tract → decreased GI Mg absorption → decreased renal Mg filtration
          3. Hyperoxaluria
            a. Binds Ca and Mg in GI tract → increased free oxalate in GI tract → increased GI oxalate absorption → increased renal oxalate filtration
      b. Options
        i. K-Phos neutral
        ii. Neutra-Phos K
        iii. Uro-KP-neutral
  v. Potassium citrate
    1. Mechanism of action
      a. Increases urinary citrate

b. Urinary alkalization
i. Citrate binds to H+
c. Counteracts the K-wasting and Acidotic effects of thiazides
2. Side effects
a. GI intolerance
i. Reduced when taken with food/meals
vi. Diet
1. Decreased purine intake
a. Mechanism of action
i. Decreased purine load → decreased purine metabolism → decreased uric acid production → decreased renal filtration of uric acid → decreased urine acidity → decreased risk of calcium oxalate urolithiasis
b. What to avoid
i. Excessive "red meat," ie, animal protein intake (high purine levels)
2. Decreased animal protein intake
a. Mechanism of action
i. Decreased amino acid load → decreased serum acid load → decreased urine acidity
ii. Decreased amino acid load → decreased serum acid load → decreased consumption of cellular citrate → more citrate available for filtration into urine → decreased hypocitraturia
iii. Decreased amino acid load → decreased metabolism to oxalate → decreased risk of associated calcium oxalate urolithiasis
3. Decreased Sodium Intake
a. Renal sodium excretion correlates with renal Ca excretion
i. Reduction of urinary sodium by 100 mEq / day reduces urinary calcium by 50 mg / day
4. Increased fiber intake
a. Mechanism of action
i. Binds Ca in GI tract
5. Increased urine output
a. Increased fluid intake to keep urine output >2000 mL/day
6. Neutral phosphates
a. Mechanism of action
i. Increased GI absorption of phosphate → increased serum phosphate → negative feedback → decreased vitamin D → decreased GI absorption of Ca
b. Side Effects
i. GI: Nausea, Diarrhea

B. Renal hypercalciuria

a. Goals
i. Decreased Renal Excretion of Ca
1. Thiazides (chlorthalidone, indapamide, hydrochlorothiazide)
2. Decreased dietary sodium
ii. Increased stone inhibitors
1. Potassium citrate
iii. Change general urine parameters
1. Increased urine output
b. Specifics
i. Thiazides
1. Mainstay of therapy of renal hypercalciuria
2. Will correct renal leak of Ca
3. Will maintain positive calcium balance
ii. Decreased sodium intake
1. Renal sodium excretion correlates with renal Ca excretion
iii. Potassium citrate
1. Used in combination with thiazides to prevent hypokalemia with subsequent hypocitraturia
iv. Increased urine output
1. Increased fluid intake to keep urine output >2000 mL/day

C. Resorptive hypercalciuria

a. Goals
i. Decreased Ca resorption from bone
1. Bisphosphonates
2. Surgical removal of parathyroid adenoma or parathyroid hyperplasia
ii. Increased stone inhibitors
1. Potassium citrate
iii. Change general urine parameters
1. Increased urine output
2. Potassium citrate
b. Specifics
i. Surgical removal of parathyroid adenoma or hyperplastic parathyroid tissue best treatment

ii. Orthophosphate
1. Mechanism of action
a. Inhibition of osteoclast activity → counters effect of increased PTH → Decreased bone resorption
b. Possible augmentation of tubular Ca reabsorption → decreased hypercalciuria
c. This may result in negative feedback on PTH production → decreased PTH → decreased bone resorption of Ca
d. Increased urinary citrate excretion
i. Likely secondary to the alkaline nature of orthophosphate (sequesters H^+)
e. Increases urinary pyrophosphate excretion → increased urine stone inhibitor
i. Likely from metabolism of the drug
2. Side effects
a. GI: nausea, diarrhea
iii. Potassium citrate
1. Especially if hypercalciuria not well controlled on orthophosphate therapy
iv. Increased urine output
1. Increased fluid intake to keep urine output >2000 mL/day

D. Hyperuricosuria
a. Goals
i. Decreased stone promoters
1. Diet
a. Decrease dietary purine intake
b. Decrease dietary animal protein intake
c. Decrease dietary sodium intake
2. Allopurinol
ii. Increase stone inhibitors
1. Potassium citrate
iii. Change general urine parameters
1. Increase urine output
2. Urinary alkalization
a. Potassium citrate
b. Specifics
i. Diet
1. Decrease purine intake
a. Mechanism of action
i. Decreased purine load → decreased purine metabolism → decreased uric acid production
ii. Decrease uric acid production → decreased renal filtration of uric acid → decreased urine acidity
b. What to avoid
i. Excessive "red meat" intake (high purine levels)
2. Decrease animal protein intake
a. Mechanism of action
i. Decreased amino acid load → decreased serum acid load → decreased urine acidity
ii. Decreased amino acid load → decreased serum acid load → decreased consumption of cellular citrate → more citrate available for filtration into urine → decreased hypocitraturia
iii. Decreased amino acid load → decreased metabolism to oxalate → decreased risk of associated calcium oxalate urolithiasis
3. Decrease sodium intake
a. Renal sodium excretion correlates with renal Ca excretion
ii. Allopurinol
1. Mechanism of action
a. Inhibitor of xanthine oxidase → decreased uric acid, increased xanthine (more soluble)
2. Side effects
a. Rash
i. Can progress to an exfoliative hemorrhagic dermatitis with systemic vasculitis (rare)
b. Flare of gouty arthritis
c. Xanthine urolthiasis (rare)
iii. Potassium citrate
1. Mechanism of action
a. Urinary alkalinization
i. Increased urinary citrate → increased chelation of urine Ca → decreased chance of associated Ca-oxalate urolithiasis
ii. Increased urinary citrate binds H^+ in urine
iv. Increase urine output
1. Increased fluid intake to keep urine output > 2000 mL/day

E. Primary hyperoxaluria
a. Goals
i. Increased conversion of metabolic intermediates to nonoxalate end products

1. Pyridoxine (= vitamin B6)
ii. Decreased GI oxalate absorption
1. Low oxalate diet
2. Neutral phosphates
iii. Decreased renal oxalate excretion
1. Thiazide
2. Avoid excessive vitamin C
iv. Increased stone inhibitors
1. Potassium citrate
v. Change general urine parameters
1. Increase urine output
2. Urinary alkalization
a. Potassium citrate
vi. **Fix the primary problem**
1. **Liver transplant ± renal transplant**
b. Specifics
i. Pyridoxine (= vitamin B6)
1. Mechanism of action
a. Cofactor for AGT → maximizes the effect of the enzyme
b. Even if the enzyme is not defective (ie, Type 2 primary hyperxolauria), it can help to maximize enzyme activity → minimize oxalate production
ii. Low oxalate diet
1. Avoid foods with high oxalate content
a. Spinach
b. Nuts
c. Chocolate
d. Beets
e. Rhubarb
f. Tea
g. Worcestershire sauce
iii. Neutral phosphates
1. Bind oxalate in GI tract
iv. Thiazide
1. Hypocalciuric effect → decreased Ca available for stone formation
v. Avoid excessive vitamin C
1. Excess ascorbic acid → converted to oxalate
vi. Potassium citrate
1. Mechanism of action
a. Urinary alkalinization
b. Decreased chance of associated calcium oxalate urolithiasis
vii. Increased urine output
1. Increased fluid intake to keep urine output >2000 mL/day

F. Enteric hyperoxlauria
a. Goals
i. Decrease GI oxalate absorption
1. Increased GI chelation of oxalate
a. Low fat diet
b. Bile salt resins
c. Oral calcium supplementation
d. Low oxalate diet
e. Reversal of GI bypass if possible
ii. Increase stone inhibitors
1. Potassium citrate
iii. Change general urine parameters
1. Increase urine output
2. Urinary alkalinization
a. Potassium citrate
b. Sodium bicarbonate
b. Specifics
i. Low fat diet
1. Decreases the chelation of Ca by fats → increased chelation of oxalate by Ca in GI tract
ii. Bile salt resins
1. Decreases the bile salts in GI tract → decreased chelation of Ca with bile salts → increased chelation of oxalate by Ca
iii. Low oxalate diet
1. Avoid foods with high oxalate content
a. Spinach
b. Nuts
c. Chocolate
d. Beets
e. Rhubarb
f. Tea
g. Worcestershire sauce
iv. Oral calcium supplementation
1. Usually as calcium citrate
2. Increased chelation of oxalate in GI tract with extra Ca
3. The extra Ca does not significantly increase the risk of stone formation since these patients have low urine Ca 2° to Ca loss in GI tract
v. Potassium citrate
1. Alkalinizes urine
a. Decreased chance of associated Ca-based urolithiasis
vi. Sodium bicarbonate
1. Many of these conditions associated with increased HCO_3 loss in GI tract
vii. Reversal of GI bypass if possible

G. Hypocitraturia

a. Goals
  i. Increase stone inhibitors
    1. Potassium citrate
  ii. Change general urine parameters
    1. Increase urine output
    2. Urinary alkalinization
      a. Potassium citrate
      b. Sodium bicarbonate
      c. Citrus juice
    1. Lemon juice
    2. Orange juice

H. Hypomagnesuria

a. Goals
  i. Increase stone inhibitors
    1. Magnesium citrate
    2. Magnesium gluconate
    3. Potassium magnesium citrate (not yet FDA-approved)
b. Change general urine parameters
  i. Increased urine output
  ii. Treat concomitant hypocitraturia
    1. Potassium citrate

I. Low urine volume

a. Goals
  i. Change general urine parameters
    1. Increase urine output
b. Specifics
  i. Ideally >3000 mL/day
  ii. Realistically >2000 mL/day
  iii. Usually requires >100 oz fluid/day
  iv. Need to be cognizant of situations where increased fluids required
    1. Exercise
    2. Heat
    3. Illness

J. Gouty Diathesis

a. Goals
  i. Change general urine parameters
    1. Increase urine output
    2. Urinary alkalization
      a. Potassium citrate
      b. Sodium bicarbonate
    3. Citrus juices will not work (no significant change in urine pH)
      a. Decrease acid load
        i. Low purine diet
        ii. Low sodium diet
        iii. Low sugar diet
        iv. High fiber diet
        v. Allopurinol
b. Specifics
  i. Potassium citrate
    1. Urinary alkalization
    2. Decreased acid load
    3. Goal is urine pH 6.5-7.0
  ii. Sodium bicarbonate
    1. Urinary alkalization
    2. Decreased acid load
    3. Goal is urine pH 6.5-7.0
    4. Problem is increase sodium load
  iii. Low purine diet
    1. Decreased acid (especially uric acid)
  iv. Low sodium diet
    1. Decreased urine Ca
  v. Low sugar diet
    1. Decreased ketoacidosis
  vi. High fiber diet
    1. Binds Ca in GI tract → decreased Ca absorption
    2. Decreased intestinal transit time → decreased Ca absorption
  vii. Allopurinol
    1. Indications
      a. Profound hyperuricosuria (urine uric acid >900-1200 g/day)
      b. Hyperuricosemia

K. Cystinuria

a. Goals
  i. Decreased stone promoters
    1. Low methionine diet (rarely effective)
  ii. Increase urinary inhibitors
    1. Urinary cystine-chelating agents
      a. Penicillamine
      b. Thiola (alpha-mercaptopropionylglycine)
      c. Bucillamine (investigational)
      d. Captopril
  iii. Change general urine parameters
    1. Increase urine output
    2. Urinary alkalization
      a. Potassium citrate
      b. Sodium bicarbonate
      c. Acetazolamide
b. Specifics
  i. Low methionine diet

1. Methionine
   a. Essential amino acid metabolized to cystine
   b. Fairly unpalatable → low compliance

ii. Thiola
   1. = alpha-methyl-propionyl-glycine = alpha-MPG
   2. Better side effect profile than penicillamine
   3. Usually first-line treatment for cystinuria

iii. Penicillamine (specifically d-penicillamine)
   1. Forms penicillamine-cystine disulfide: 50x more soluble than cystine
   2. Side effects
      a. Hematologic: agranulocytosis, thrombocytopenia
      b. Dermatologic: pemphigus
      c. Renal: nephrotic syndrome
      d. Rheumatologic: polymyositis
      e. B6 Deficiency → usually add pyridoxine 50 mg PO QD
   3. Cheaper than Thiola

iv. Bucillamine
   1. Better side effect profile than penicillamine
   2. Medication is still investigational

v. Captopril
   1. Captopril-cysteine 200 x more soluble than cystine
   2. Effect not as reliable as other therapies
   3. Rarely used

vi. Potassium citrate
   1. Urinary alkalization
   2. Goal: urine pH approximately 7.0
      a. Greater than this → paradoxical increased risk of CaPhos stone formation

vii. Sodium bicarbonate
   1. Urinary alkalization
   2. Usually added when K-citrate maximized

viii. Increased urine output
   1. Solubility of cystine approximately 250 mg/L of urine
      a. Thus the goal for urinary cystine levels on therapy is <250 mg cystine/L urine

L. Infection-based urolithiasis

a. Goals
   i. Decrease stone promoters
      1. Surgical removal of as much stone material as possible
         a. Ideally, complete stone removal
      2. Correct anatomic/functional abnormalities
         a. UPJO
         b. UVJO
         c. Calyceal diverticulum
         d. Voiding dysfunction
      3. Suppressive antibiotics
         a. Especially where contributing factors difficult to control, eg, neurogenic voiding dysfunction
   ii. Increase stone inhibitors
      1. Urease inhibitors
         a. Acetohydroxamic acid
   iii. Change general urine parameters
      1. Increase urine output
   iv. Treat associated metabolic abnormalities
      1. Metabolic evaluation warranted if stone is "mixed" (ie struvite + calcium)
      2. Metabolic abnormalities rarely found if stone composition is "pure" infection

b. Specifics
   i. Surgical removal of as much stone material as possible
      1. Decreased bacterial load
      2. Decreased urine stasis
   ii. Suppressive antibiotics
      1. Especially where contributing factors difficult to control
         a. Neurogenic voiding dysfunction
         b. Chronic nonobstructive hydronephrosis
   iii. Acetohydroxamic acid
      1. Mechanism of action
         a. Urease inhibitor
      2. Especially where contributing factors difficult to control
         a. Neurogenic voiding dysfunction
         b. Chronic, nonobstructive hydronephrosis
      3. Side effects
         a. Hematologic: anemia, reticulocytosis
         b. Dermatologic: rash
         c. GI: hepatotoxicity, diarrhea, abdominal pain, nausea, vomiting
         d. Teratogenic (avoid use in women of childbearing age)
         e. Other: palpitations, H/A, deep venous thrombosis
   iv. Treat associated metabolic abnormalities
      1. Approximately 50% will have additional metabolic abnormalities

M. Medication-based urolithiasis

a. Goals

i. Decrease stone promoters

1. Stop/change medication

ii. Change general urine parameters

1. Increase urine output

8. Pitfalls of Medical Stone Management

A. Ensure complete 24-hr urine collection

a. 24-hr creatinine as measure of "completeness" of collection

B. New stones/stone growth with 24-hr urine collection volumes → 2000 mL and "normal" parameters

a. Check 24-hr creatinine to ensure patient not adding water/fluid to 24-hr urine collections

C. Increased 24-hr uric acid after initiating K-citrate therapy

a. Decreased urine acidity → increased solubility of uric acid →more uric acid analyzed

D. Citrate level not responding to K-citrate therapy

a. 24-hr urine K should increase with K-citrate therapy

E. Urinary diversions/intestinal substitutions often absorb some urinary components

a. → 24-hr urine collections often unreliable

b. → Often treat presumptively with K-citrate

Table 6

Stone Management Medication Summary

Medication	**Indications**	**Side Effects**	**Dose**	**Other Notes**
Thiazide	Hypercalciuria (absorptive Type I, II; renal) Hyperoxaluria (primary, idiopathic)	Hypokalemia	Chlorthalidone 25-50 mg PO QD Indapamide: 1.25 mg PO QD	High sodium intake will offset effect of thiazide; often administered with K-citrate or amiloride to counter hypokalemic effects; often administered with K-citrate to counter acidotic effects
Orthophosphate	Hypercalciuria (absorptive)	GI intolerance	Each tab has 250 mg Phos 1-2 tabs PO QID	Side-effect profile makes this 2nd line if thiazides ineffective
Bisphosphonate	Hypercalciuria (resorptive)	Hypocalcemia Rash GI intolerance	Alendronate 5-10 mg PO QID Risendronate 5 mg PO qd	Ensure PTH normal before starting medical therapy
Potassium citrate	Hypercalciuria Hyperoxaluria Gouty diathesis Cystinuria	GI intolerance Hyperkalemia	40-90 mEq PO divided BID/TID	Take with meals to avoid GI upset
Sodium bicarbonate	Hyperoxaluria (enteric) Gouty diathesis Distal renal tubular acidosis Cystinuria	GI intolerance Alkalosis	650-1300 mg PO up to QID	

(continued)

Table 6 *(continued)*

Stone Management Medication Summary

Medication	Indications	Side Effects	Dose	Other Notes
Allopurinol	Hyperuricosuria Hyperuricosemia	Rash Xanthine urolithiasis	300-600 mg PO QD	Wait until after acute gouty arthritis attack subsided before starting
d-Penicillamine	Cystinuria	Pyridoxine deficiency, Rash Agranulocytosis Leucopenia Nephrotic syndrome Arthralgia	500-1000 mg PO QID	Side effect profile makes this more of a second-line agent; cheaper than Thiola
Thiola	Cystinuria	Similar to penicillamine but less common and less severe	200-1200 mg PO divided BID-QID	1st line agent
Captopril	Cystinuria	Cough Renal insufficiency	75-150 mg PO QD	Usually 3rd line agent
Acetohydroxamic acid	Infection-based nephrolithiasis	Anemia Rash Hepatotoxicity GI upset DVT	250 mg PO TID/QID	F/U q 3-4 mo required on this medication to monitor for side effects
Pyridoxine	Hyperoxaluria (primary) Cystinuria (if penicillamine being used)		Primary: 200-400 PO QD Adjunct: 50 mg PO QD	
Ca supplementation	Hyperoxaluria (enteric)	Constipation	1-4 gm PO TID with meals	Follow-up urine collections to avoid hypercalcuria Use calcium citrate preparation
Mg gluconate	Hyperoxaluria (primary)	GI intolerance Hyporeflexia Hypotonia/ Muscle paralysis Hypotension Cardiac arrhythmia	Start at 400 or 420 mg PO QD and tailor to response	Side effects usually seen at very high doses
Bile salt resin	Hyperoxaluria (enteric)	GI intolerance	Cholestyramine 1-4 gm PO TID with meals	

9. Questions

Case 1

A 65-year-old African American female with an 8-year history of recurrent stone formation reports having spontaneously passed 35 stones. She has required 3 ureteroscopic laser stone fragmentations and one percutaneous nephrolithotripsy. Current radiographs reveal 3 small stones in the left intrarenal collecting system and 2 in the right. This patient's medical history is significant for inflammatory bowel disease. There is a family history of nephrolithiasis in one sibling.

24-hour Urine Collections

	Normal Range	Initial Visit
Vol	>2000mL/d	1320
pH	5.5-6.7	5.51
Calcium	<200 mg/d	85
Sodium	<200 mg/d	95
Potassium	<60 meq/d	45
Uric Acid	<600 mg/	375
Oxalate	<45 mg/d	78
Citrate	>600 mg/d	<20
Magnesium	>60 mg/d	50
SO_4	<20 mg/d	8
Cystine	0 mg/L	0

Serum Values

	Normal Range	Initial Visit
Sodium	135-145 meq/L	138
Potassium	0.2-4.8 meq/L	3.5
Chloride	98-108 meq/L	107
Bicarbonate	21-30 meq/L	20
Creatinine	0.7-1.4 mg/dL	1.1
Calcium	8.7-10.2 mg/dL	9.2
Phosphorus	2.3-4.3 mg/dL	3.1
Uric Acid	2.5-8.0 mg/dL	4.5
PTH	13-64 ng/mL	48

1. This condition is best described as:

A. Primary hyperoxaluria

B. Gouty diathesis

C. Distal renal tubular acidosis

D. Enteric hyperoxaluria

E. Hyperuricosuria

2. The risk factor most associated with recurrent stone formation secondary to this condition is:

A. Hyperabsorption of oxalate in the jejunum

B. Hyperexcretion of calcium from the distal tubule

C. Diminished citrate absorption in the terminal ileum

D. Hyperabsorption of calcium in the small bowel

E. Increased colonic absorption of free oxalate

3. The optimum treatment for patients with this disorder would include:

A. Calcium supplements, potassium citrate, increased oral fluid intake

B. Dietary restriction of oxalate

C. Thiazides and potassium citrate

D. Allopurinol

E. Pyridoxine

Case 2

A 50-year-old obese Caucasian male is evaluated for a 2-day history of left flank pain without fevers, nausea or emesis. He has a prior history of stone disease for 6 years and has spontaneously passed 4-5 stones. He's had no prior surgeries for calculus disease and family history is negative for nephrolithiasis but positive for gout. No stones are seen on the plain abdominal radiographs. Prior stone composition contains mixed calcium oxalate.

24-hour Urine Collections

	Normal Range	Initial Visit
Vol	>2000mL/d	1300
pH	5.5-6.7	5.12
Calcium	<200 mg/d	140
Sodium	<200 mg/d	170
Potassium	<60 meq/d	35
Uric Acid	<600 mg/d	285
Oxalate	<45 mg/d	35
Citrate	>600 mg/d	220
Magnesium	>60 mg/d	70
SO_4	<20 mg/d	24
Cystine	0 mg/L	0
Serum Values		
Sodium	135-145 meq/L	140
Potassium	3.2-4.8 meq/L	4.2
Chloride	98-108 meq/L	102
Bicarbonate	21-30 meq/L	27
Creatinine	0.7-1.4 mg/dL	0.9
Calcium	8.7-10.2 mg/dL	9.5
Phosphorus	2.3-4.3 mg/dL	2.8
Uric Acid	2.5-8.0 mg/dL	7.7
PTH	13-64 ng/mL	43

4. The most important factor predisposing patients to this metabolic disorder is:

A. Hypercalciuria

B. Low urinary pH

C. Hypocitraturia

D. Low urine volumes

E. Hyperuricosuria

5. The most appropriate medical treatment of this condition is:

A. Allopurinol

B. Thiazides

C. Increased fluids

D. Dietary calcium restriction

E. Potassium citrate

Case 3

A 58-year-old Hispanic female is seen by her family physician with a history of recurrent urinary tract infections treated 3-4 times in the last 18 months. At present she is asymptomatic. She denies a history of nephrolithiasis. Renal ultrasound demonstrates moderate left hydronephrosis and a large density within the renal pelvis with posterior shadowing. KUB with tomography reveals a poorly opacified stone involving the renal pelvis and lower pole calyces. Prior urine cultures have grown *Proteus* and *Klebsiella* species. Following uncomplicated left percutaneous nephrolithotomy, she returns with the following metabolic results:

24-hour Urine Collections

	Normal Range	Initial Visit
Vol	>2000mL/d	1600
pH	5.5-6.7	6.9
Calcium	<200 mg/d	210
Sodium	<200 mg/d	120
Potassium	<60 meq/d	40
Uric Acid	<600 mg/d	360
Oxalate	<45 mg/d	20
Citrate	>600 mg/d	110
Magnesium	>60 mg/d	80
SO_4	<20 mg/d	10
Cystine	0 mg/L	0

Serum Values

	Normal Range	Initial Visit
Sodium	135-145 meq/L	136
Potassium	3.2-4.8 meq/L	3.8
Chloride	98-108 meq/L	98
Bicarbonate	21-30 meq/L	22
Creatinine	0.7-1.4 mg/dL	1.6
Calcium	8.7-10.2 mg/dL	9.5
Phosphorus	2.3-4.3 mg/dL	3.1
Uric Acid	2.5-8.0 mg/dL	6.6
PTH	13-64 ng/mL	28

6. The stone composition of this patient is most likely:

A. Calcium oxalate

B. Uric acid

C. Magnesium ammonium phosphate

D. Cystine

E. Hydroxyapatite

7. The most common cause of recurrent stone disease in a patient having undergone "sand-wich" therapy for a staghorn calculus is:

A. Hypomagnesuria

B. Hyperoxaluria

C. Retained stone fragments

D. Renal tubular acidosis

E. Hypercalciuria

8. Acetohydroxamic acid contributes to reducing infection stone formation by:

   A. Reversing associated metabolic defects

   B. Preventing recurrent urinary tract infections

   C. Alkalinization of the urine

   D. Irreversibly inhibiting urease

   E. All of the above

Case 4

A 12-year-old male is seen for evaluation of recurrent nephrolithiasis. He has spontaneously passed 3 stones over the previous 4 years, and has recently undergone shock wave lithotripsy for 2 without success. He has been treated in the past with an unknown medication, but was discontinued because the parents felt it was of no benefit. Family history is negative for stone disease.

24-hour Urine Collections

	Normal Range	Initial Visit
Vol	>2000mL/d	550
pH	5.5-6.7	5.4
Calcium	<200 mg/d	110
Sodium	<200 mg/d	117
Potassium	<60 meq/d	39
Uric Acid	<600 mg/d	215
Oxalate	<45 mg/d	22
Citrate	>600 mg/d	260
Magnesium	>60 mg/d	80
SO_4	<20 mg/d	7
Cystine	0 mg/L	740

Serum Values

	Normal Range	Initial Visit
Sodium	135-145 meq/L	140
Potassium	3.2-4.8 meq/L	4.1
Chloride	98-108 meq/L	108
Bicarbonate	21-30 meq/L	23
Creatinine	0.7-1.4 mg/dL	0.8
Calcium	8.7-10.2 mg/dL	9.0
Phosphorus	2.3-4.3 mg/dL	4.0
Uric Acid	2.5-8.0 mg/dL	5.9
PTH	13-64 ng/mL	43

9. The likely metabolic diagnosis contributing to this patient's recurrent stone formation is:

   A. Hypocitraturia

   B. Hyperoxaluria

   C. Low urine volumes

   D. Gouty diathesis

   E. Cystinuria

10. Alpha-mercaptopropionylglycine (Thiola®) may be helpful in the management of cystinuria since it:

   A. Acts as a diuretic, further decreasing urinary cystine concentration

   B. Is significantly more effective than d-penicillamine

   C. Can be used as both an oral and intrarenal chemolytic agent

D. Has equivalent efficacy at increasing solubility with reduced toxicity as compared to D-penicillamine

E. Adequately alkalinizes the urine obviating the need for potassium citrate

Case 5

A 19-year-old Caucasian female with a 6-year history of recurrent stone disease is found to have multiple bilateral renal calculi by renal ultrasound during an evaluation for recurrent flank pain. She reports having passed greater than 10 stones in the previous 2 years. Review of the renal ultrasound indicates no evidence of hydronephrosis. KUB and tomograms demonstrate 5 stones on the left and 8 stones on the right, all less than 4 mm in size. She has a strong family history of stones with 3 first-degree relatives and 2 cousins with nephrolithiasis. Stone compositions have been mixed calcium phosphate and calcium oxalate.

24-hour Urine Collections

	Normal Range	Initial Visit
Vol	>2000mL/d	1425
pH	5.5-6.7	6.94
Calcium	<200 mg/d	260
Sodium	<200 mg/d	160
Potassium	60 meq/d	28
Uric Acid	<600 mg/d	410
Oxalate	<45 mg/d	32
Citrate	>600 mg/d	140
Magnesium	>60 mg/d	66
SO_4	<20 mg/d	13
Cystine	0 mg/L	0

Serum Values

	Normal Range	Initial Visit
Sodium	135-145 meq/L	142
Potassium	0.2-4.8 meq/L	3.3
Chloride	98-108 meq/L	107
Bicarbonate	21-30 meq/L	21
Creatinine	0.7-1.4 mg/dL	0.9
Calcium	8.7-10.2 mg/dL	9.2
Phosphorus	2.3-4.3 mg/dL	2.2
Uric Acid	2.5-8.0 mg/dL	4.1
PTH	13-64 ng/mL	58

11. The most definitive test to identify this disorder would demonstrate:

A. Decreased serum parathyroid hormone levels

B. Persistently elevated urine calcium

C. Inability to reduce the urine pH below 5.3

D. Normalization of hypercalciuria

E. Marked increase in urinary uric acid levels with initiation of treatment

Case 6

A 49-year-old Caucasian female with a 4-year history of stone disease has passed 6 stones spontaneously, 3 in the last year. Noncontrast renal CT demonstrates a 2 mm calcification in each kidney without secondary signs of obstruction. Previous stone analysis has revealed a mixed composition of calcium phosphate and calcium oxalate. She had been treated with hydrochlorothiazide in the past but this medication was discontinued after 3 months therapy. Her family history is significant for a brother and grandmother with stones. She is otherwise healthy and has prior surgical history.

24-hour Urine Collections

	Normal Range	Initial Visit
Vol	>2000mL/d	1800
pH	5.5-6.7	5.8
Calcium	<200 mg/d	335
Sodium	<200 mg/d	230
Potassium	<60 meq/d	38
Uric Acid	<600 mg/d	472
Oxalate	<45 mg/d	29
Citrate	>600 mg/d	680
Magnesium	>60 mg/d	70
SO_4	<20 mg/d	15
Cystine	0 mg/L	0

Serum Values

	Normal Range	Initial Visit
Sodium	135-145 meq/L	138
Potassium	0.2-4.8 meq/L	4.3
Chloride	98-108 meq/L	102
Bicarbonate	21-30 meq/L	25
Creatinine	0.7-1.4 mg/dL	1.3
Calcium	8.7-10.2 mg/dL	9.1
Phosphorus	2.3-4.3 mg/dL	2.8
Uric Acid	2.5-8.0 mg/dL	5.1
PTH	13-64 ng/mL	18

12. The primary defect in this condition is considered to be:

A. Primary hyperabsorption of intestinal calcium

B. Hypersecretion of parathyroid hormone

C. Renal leak of calcium

D. Bone disease

E. Excessive dietary intake of calcium-containing foods

Answers

Case 1

1. D.

Enteric hyperoxaluria is a disorder most commonly affecting patients with inflammatory bowel disease, particularly intestinal segments involving the small intestine. Fat malabsorption is the hallmark condition predisposing to saponification and sequestering of calcium to be passed in the stool. Less calcium is available in the GI tract to bind oxalate, thereby allowing more oxalate to be absorbed with a relative increase in urinary oxalate. Primary hyperoxaluria is an autosomal recessive disorder manifest only in the homozygous state. Unless effectively treated early, primary hyperoxaluria typically runs a malignant course with early death from renal failure.

2. E.

Intestinal hyperabsorption of oxalate in patients with enteric hyperoxaluria is the most significant risk factor leading to recurrent calculus formation. Intestinal transport of oxalate is primarily increased because of the effects of bile salts and fatty acids on the permeability of colonic intestinal mucosa to oxalate. The total amount of oxalate absorbed may also be increased because of an enlarged intraluminal pool of oxalate available for absorption. Intestinal fat malabsorption characteristic of ileal disease will exaggerate calcium soap formation, limit the amount of "free" calcium to complex to oxalate, and thereby raise the oxalate pool available for absorption.

3. A.

The initial goals of medical management are to rehydrate and reverse metabolic acidosis. Hydration is at times difficult in some patients as an increase in oral fluids may exacerbate diarrhea. Hydration and potassium citrate will contribute to the reversal of the metabolic acidosis, as well as enhance the excretion of citrate to increase its inhibitory effects on stone formation. Calcium supplements will bind excess oxalate within the intestine thereby reducing intestinal oxalate absorption. Calcium citrate may offer an ideal calcium supplement in this condition as it should reduce urinary oxalate and increase urinary citrate. Thiazides may worsen metabolic acidosis and hypokalemia through its diuretic effects and renal potassium losses. Colon resection may be of benefit in those patients refractory to medical management, as the primary site of intestinal absorption of oxalate is the large bowel.

Case 2

4. B.

Although low urine volumes and hyperuricosuria contribute to the possibility of uric acid stone formation, the most critical determinant of the crystallization of uric acid remains urinary pH. In addition, uric acid stones may be formed in patients with primary gout with associated severe hyperuricosuria and other secondary causes of purine overproduction, such as myeloproliferative states, glycogen storage disease and malignancy.

5. E.

Allopurinol will decrease the production of uric acid by inhibiting xanthine oxidase in the purine metabolic pathway, but is most effective in patients with extremely elevated levels of uric acid (urinary uric acid >1500 mg/day). In addition, increasing total urine volume will decrease the concentration of uric acid to assist in preventing stone formation. However, raising the urinary pH above the dissociation constant of uric acid is the key to prevent recurrent uric acid stone formation and correcting gouty diathesis. The urine pH should be maintained between 6.0 and 6.5. Thiazides and calcium restriction have a limited role in the medical treatment of uric acid stone patients.

Case 3

6. D.

Ascending urinary tract infections with urea-splitting organisms, such as *Proteus* species, will metabolize urea to ammonia. Ammonuria in conjunction with a matrix composed of organic compounds, carbonate apatite, inflammatory cells and bacteria, result in the rapid formation of an "infection" calculus, eventually progressing into a mineralized, dense stone. Bacteria trapped within the stone perpetuate the recurrent urinary tract infections and further stone formation, eventually developing into the classic staghorn calculus.

7. C.

After removal of an infected struvite calculus, the most common cause of recurrent stone formation is failure to completely eradicate the urinary tract infection. Surgical therapy may leave retained fragments of infected stone within calyces, thus allowing infection to persist. Underlying metabolic disorders may also contribute to recurrent stone formation, but persistent infection remains the most important risk factor.

8. D.

Acetohydroxamic acid (AHA), a competitive inhibitor of the bacterial enzyme urease, will reduce the urinary saturation of struvite and retard stone formation. When given at a dose of 250 mg orally three times a day, this medication can prevent the recurrence of new stones and inhibit the growth of existing stones in patients with chronic urea-splitting infections. AHA can also cause dissolution of small stones. However, up to 30% of patients will experience minor side effects, including headache, nausea, vomiting, anemia, rash or alopecia. In addition, 15% of patients have developed deep venous thrombosis while on long-term treatment. Therefore, careful monitoring is required when using this medication.

Case 4

9. E.

Cystinuria is a complex autosomal recessive disorder of amino acid transport involving cystine, ornithine, lysine and arginine. Supersaturation of the urine will occur in patients with the homozygous state. Therefore, it is unusual to see a family history with cystine stones. The age of onset is often in the 1st or 2nd decade of life.

10. D.

d-Penicillamine and alpha-mercaptopropionylglycine are equally effective in their ability to decrease urinary cystine levels. However, studies have demonstrated that alpha-MPG is significantly less toxic than d-penicillamine. Moreover, the side effects that may occur with alpha-MPG are also less severe. However, if a patient has been doing well on d-penicillamine with no significant complications, there is no need to switch medications.

Case 5

11. C.

Renal tubular acidosis is a clinical syndrome of chronic metabolic acidosis resulting from renal tubular abnormalities, while glomerular filtration is relatively well preserved. Although patients may present with many different symptoms and physical findings, renal stone formation is a well-recognized manifestation of distal renal tubular acidosis (dRTA). Patients with the incomplete form of dRTA are not persistently acidemic despite their inability to lower urinary pH with an acid load. These patients are able to compensate for their acidification defect and remain in acid-base balance by increasing ammonia synthesis and ammonium excretion as a buffering mechanism. The initial identification of incomplete dRTA is often a chance finding. Many of these patients will present with recurrent nephrolithiasis or may be referred for evaluation after the discovery of nephrocalcinosis after routine abdominal radiographs. Most patients will have normal serum electrolytes, yet they will have a high-normal urine pH along with significant hypocitraturia. The diagnosis of incomplete dRTA can be confirmed by inadequate urinary acidification after an ammonium chloride loading test.

Case 6

12. A.

The basic abnormality in absorptive hypercalciuria Type I is the intestinal hyperabsorption of calcium. The consequent increase in the circulating concentration of calcium enhances the renal filtered load and suppresses parathyroid function. Hypercalciuria results from the combination of increased filtered load and reduced renal tubular reabsorption of calcium, a function of parathyroid suppression. The excessive renal loss of calcium compensates for the high calcium absorption from the intestinal tract and helps to maintain serum calcium in the normal range.

Chapter 14: Surgical Stone Management

Gary J. Faerber, MD

Contents

1. Shock Wave Lithotripsy (SWL)

Introduction

Shock wave lithotripsy (SWL) by definition is not an endourologic procedure but is certainly the epitome of "minimally invasive surgery." In 1980, Christian Chaussy reported the first successful frag mentation of a urinary calculus using electronically generated shock wave.[1] Since its introduction in 1980, SWL has dramatically revolutionized the management of renal and ureteral stone disease and remains the preferred treatment of renal lithiaisis and proximal ureteral stones (Figure 1).

Physics of Fragmentation

Despite a significant amount of work done in the physics of lithotripsy, the exact mechanism, which results in fragmentation, has not been completely elucidated. Despite the differences in commercially available lithotriptors, the working principles remain similar in that they all produce a characteristic waveform at the focal point, which has a leading edge followed by a tensile wave (Figure 1a). It appears that *cavitation* mechanics plays the major role in fragmentation.

Recent in *vitro* and in *vivo* studies have demonstrated that augmentation of bubble cavitation can also improve stone fragmentation. Methods to

Figure 1

Optimal fragmentation with SWL should result in fragments which should pass easily

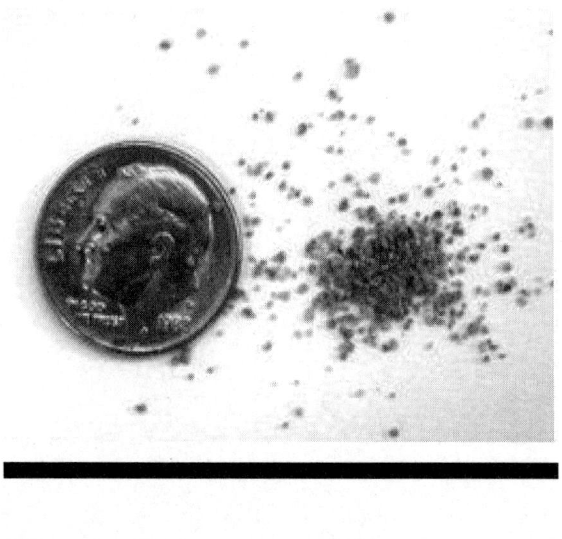

Figure 1a

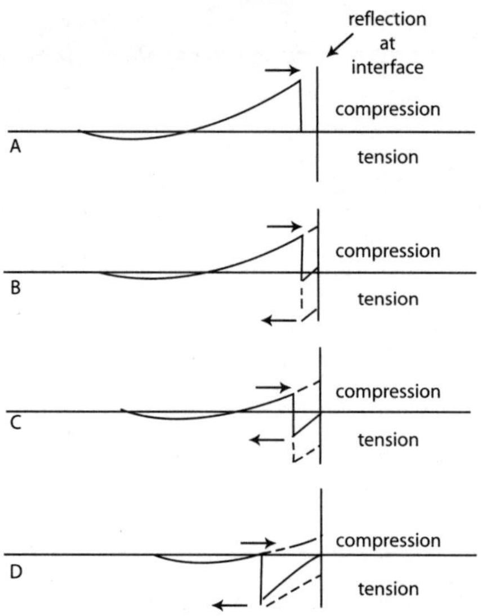

A. Initially, only compressive forces work on the stone reflective surfaces to cause fragmentation.
B., C. After reflection begins, the forces, a short distance from the reflecting surface, create a tensile force pulling in the direction opposite to the compressive forces in the latter part of the shock wave. Together, these opposing forces cause stone fracturing. D. Still later, the tensile (reflected) wave propagates through the stone away from the reflecting free surface.

From Physics and Geometry Pertinent to ESWL. Patrick T. Hunter II, Principles of ESWL eds Robert Reihle Jr. Churchill-Livingstone, New York, NY 1987 pg 26

improve bubble cavitation include optimizing shock wave frequency and the use of an auxiliary shock wave generator.[2,3]

Different Types of Lithotriptors

The Dornier HM3 (Dornier Medical Systems, Inc., Marietta, GA) was the first device designed specifically for extracorporeal fragmentation of urinary lithiasis. Since its introduction over 2 decades ago, design improvements in lithotripsy technology have attempted to maximize stone fragmentation while minimizing renal injury and patient pain during treatment. These modifications have focused mainly on reducing focal point size and increasing aperture (both of which increases peak point pres sure, while decreasing pain at the skin level).

All lithotripsy machines have similar components consisting of: *1) an energy source; 2) a focusing system; 3) an imaging system; and 4) a coupling mechanism*. Unlike the initial HM3 unit, the more contemporary units are multi functional.

The original method of shock wave generation was via a spark gap, or electrohydraulic technique. A high voltage electrical current was generated across an underwater spark gap electrode (F1). This resulted in generation of a high energy pressure wave, which was then focused at a distant point in space (F2) using an ellipsoid reflector. In a piezo electric method, the shockwave is generated by a grid of ceramic or piezoelectric crystals, which are stimulated with a coordinated high energy electrical pulse. Electromagnetically generated shock waves are produced using an electromagnetic coil, which vibrates a metallic membrane.

Focusing in electrohydraulic based lithotriptors is done using a metal ellipsoid. In piezoelectric systems, the ceramic crystals are arranged in a hemi spherical dish. In electromagnetic systems, focusing occurs as a result of either an acoustic lens or a cylindrical reflector.

Localization is accomplished using fluoroscopy, ultrasound, or both modalities with some lithotriptors. Advantages of fluoroscopy include identification of both renal and ureteral calculi and the ability to track migrating fragments during treatment, and the minimal learning curve required to interpret the image. The disadvantage of fluoroscopy is that it employs ionizing radiation and it fails to visualize radiolucent stones or stones which are superim posed over bony structures such as the bony pelvis or the transverse processes. Ultrasound localization provides capability to visualize both radiopaque and radiolucent stones. The learning curve for localizing renal stones is steeper than with fluoroscopy. Small renal stones and proximal ureteral stones in the absence of ureteral dilation may not be visualized. Mid and distal stones are extremely difficult to image solely with ultrasound.

Coupling systems are necessary to effectively transmit the energy created by the shock wave across the skin surface, through the body and finally to the stone. Originally, patients were immersed in water (HM3), but second and third generation devices use small, water filled cushions to provide the air free contact with the skin.

Over 30 shock wave lithotriptors have been marketed by 15 different manufacturers. Earlier systems required dedicated rooms while newer models are portable. All but the HM3 use a water cushion for SW coupling while the HM3 still requires patient immersion (Table 1).

Indications for SWL

The most common indication for a SWL is renal calculous disease. Renal stones <2 cm in diameter, proximal ureteral stones < 1 cm in diameter, and distal stones < 10 mm in diameter can be treated with SWL. Some types of stones are more successfully fragmented with SWL (ie, calcium oxalate dihydrate, uric acid, calcium apatite) compared to more SWL resistant stones (cystine, calcium oxalate monohydrate).

Non urologic indications for SWL include pancreatic and biliary calculi.

Special Considerations

Pediatric Age Group

SWL has been shown to be as efficacious in the pediatric age group as in the adult population (Table 2). Virtually all children require general anesthesia irrespective of whether they are being treated on an older generation, or second or third generation lithotriptor. Modifications may be necessary to accommodate the small child (use of a Stryker frame for HM3), or making the treatment table aperture smaller on the newer generation machines.

Complications resulting from SWL in the pediatric age group have been few. Post treatment skin petecchiae are very common while renal or perirenal hematoma formation is rare. The theoretical concern about how efficiently the smaller diameter pediatric ureter performs has not been realized. Marberger witnessed no hypertension in 22 children

Table 1

Lithotriptors Commercially Available or in Clinical Operation

Company	Machine	Type	Focal Distance (cm)	Focal Zone (W xL)	Peak Pressure at F2 (bar)	Portability
Dornier Medical	HM3	EHL	13	15x90	1300	No
Systems	MFL 5000	EHL	13	10x40	1000	No
	Compact	EMG	13	6.4x70	460*	Yes
	Doli S	EMG				
Medispec	Econolith	EHL	13.5	13x53	726	Yes
Medstone	STS	EHL	15	13x50	350	No
Technomed	Sonolith 4000	EHL	14	12x23	1300	Yes
Medas	Lithoring	EHL	15	12x35	1200	Yes
Direx	Nova	EHL	13.5	5x17	1100	Yes
	Compact	EHL	13.5	5x17	1000	Yes
Seimens	Lithostar	EMG	11.3	11x90	380*	No
	Lithostar Plus	EMG	variable	4x40	650*	No
Karl Storz	Modulith	EMG	16.5	6x30	1000	No
Wolf	Piezolith 2500	PIEZO	10-12	1.5x11	1200	Yes
	Piezolith 3000	PIEZO	10-16.5	4x16.0	1250	Yes

treated with a piezoelectric lithotriptor.[4]There appears to be no significant effect on renal growth or renal function in children treated with SWL.[5] Despite these encouraging findings it is recommended to decrease both the energy delivered and minimize the number of shocks in the pediatric population.

Solitary Kidney

Investigators have demonstrated that SWLcan result in decreased GFR in patients treated for renal lithiasis that have solitary kidneys. Given this find ing, patients with solitary kidneys that are treated with SWLshould have long term monitoring of their renal function.[6,7]

Bilateral Stones

Patients with bilateral stones can be treated either simultaneously or in a staged treatment regimen. Pienckny and Streem demonstrated no difference in renal function in 319 patients who underwent simultaneous bilateral SWL compared to 41 who were treated in a planned, staged fashion.[8] Cass also found no decrease in overall renal function in patients who had bilateral SWL of single stones, but cautioned against bilateral treatment of multiple stones due to a statistically significant decrease in GFR in this cohort.[9]

Anomalous Kidney

Sheir and associates evaluated the safety and efficacy of SWL in a cohort of patients with anomalous kidneys. Their study population consisted of 49 patients with horseshoe kidney, 120 with malrotated kidney, and 29 with duplex kidney who were treated with a second generation lithotripter. Prone positioning was necessary in 38% of the horseshoe kid neys and 31% of the duplex kidneys. Overall stone-free rate for the group was 72%.[10]

UPJ obstruction secondary to a fixed anatomic stricture is a clear contraindication for SWL. In some instances, however, an impacted UPJ stone with stone related edema can mimic the appearance of a UPJ obstruction. Prior radiologic studies may be helpful in determining whether the pelvic dilation is due to a UPJ stricture versus a renal pelvic obstructing stone.

Stones in conduit urinary diversions can be treated with SWL as long as the stone burden is minimal and the stone is located in the kidney where it can be easily localized. Renal stones >1.5 cm in size may be better treated with PCNL and ureteral stones may be better suited for antegrade ureteroscopy.

Spinal Cord Injury

Patients with spinal cord injury (SCI) are susceptible to develop chronic and complicated stone disease over their lifetime. Despite major improvements in the urologic care of the SCI patient, the incidence of stone formation has not changed. Within 10 years of SCI, 7% will develop urinary calculus disease, with the greatest risk occurring in the first 3 months following injury.[11]Risk factors include bone demineralization due to immobility with hypercalciuria, urinary stasis, chronic catheterization, indwelling catheterization, chronic bacteruria, detrusor sphincter dysfunction, and vesicoureteral reflux. 98% of stones in one series were either calcium apatite (calcium phosphate) or struvite (calcium ammonium phosphate) in composition.

Typically, upper tract stones in the SCI population are usually soft and fragment well with SWL. SWL can be considered a first line mode of therapy for upper tract stones <1.5 cm in size. Stone fragment clearance is typically slower in this population, so follow up studies are important in monitoring stone treatment success.

The urinary tracts of SCI patients are typically colonized and patients can develop multi drug resistant organisms. Preoperative urine cultures should be performed so that patients can be placed on proper antibiotic prophylaxis. Patients should be treated with antibiotic prophylaxis for a minimum of 5 7 days in an attempt to sterilize the urine prior to SWL.

Another consideration is the assessment of mobility as it relates to proper positioning at the time of SWL. Various degrees of spinal curvature, limits in extremity due to contracture, and spinal curvature may obviate proper positioning for treatment. Orthopedic hardware may also impede adequate visualization of urinary stones.

Intravenous sedation is usually adequate for the majority of SCI undergoing SWL. Quadriplegics with high level cord injuries can develop autonomic dysreflexia during treatment and standard general anesthesia is recommended.

Overall stone free rates in the SCI population range from 50% 73% at 3 20 months in patients treated with SWL. Those who were not rendered stone free had large stone burdens or had staghorn calculi.[12 14]

Transplant Kidneys

Transplant urinary calculi have been successfully treated with SWL. Patients typically have to be treated in the prone position due to the location of the transplant kidney. In line ultrasound imaging is very helpful in localizing the stone.

Contraindications to SWL

Contraindications to SWL can be categorized into medical and urologic. Absolute medical contraindications are: uncorrected bleeding disorders, uncorrected hypertension, and pregnancy. Relative contraindications are aortic and/or renal artery aneurysm, and cardiac pacemakers.

Urologic contraindications include: Untreated urinary tract infection, urinary obstruction distal to the stone being treated (UPJ, ureteral stricture), severe anatomic or functional alterations in anatomy or physiology which would preclude proper stone elimination (calyceal diverticulum, horseshoe kidney, ectopic kidney, duplicated kidney), and large stone burden. Patient body habitus (morbid obesity, skeletal anomalies) may also preclude treatment with SWL. Finally, there may be technical issues unique to the particular lithotripter being used, which would prevent adequate stone visualization precluding treatment (Table 2).

Preoperative Evaluation

All patients require a thorough history and physical examination. If medically appropriate, patients should have a preoperative CXR and ECG. Cardiology consultation should be requested in patients with cardiac pacemakers and a cardiologist should be on stand by at the time of their procedure to address any concerns or correct any problems with the pacemaker during treatment. Patients should discontinue any drugs (warfarin ((coumadin)), aspirin, clopidogrel ((Plavix®)), etc.), which can interfere with clotting at least one week before treatment.

Table 2

Contraindications to SWL

Medical

Absolute
Uncorrected bleeding diathesis
Uncorrected hypertension
Pregnancy

Relative
Aortic or renal artery aneurysm
Cardiac pacemakers

Urologic

Absolute
Untreated UTI
Urinary obstruction distal to the stone being treated
Inability to visualize stone (skeletal abnormality, body habitus, stone location, radiopacity, stone characteristics, limiting specifications of the lithotripter being used)

Relative
Anatomic or functional alterations (calyceal diverticulum, horseshoe kidney, ectopic kidney, duplicated kidney)
Large stone burden

Urine should be sterile prior to treatment. Patients with infection stones should be on culture appropriate antibiotics prior to treatment.

Preoperative blood studies should include complete blood count, prothrombin and partial thromboplastin time, and in some cases a bleeding time. A type and screen is not necessary but laboratory facilities which can provide a type and screen should be accessible.

Historically, an intravenous pyelography (IVP) was considered obligatory prior to SWL because it provided both a functional and anatomical study of the urinary system. Presently, noncontrast computed tomography has supplanted the IVP as the imaging method of choice in diagnosing renal stone disease. CT usually provides adequate anatomic information of the kidney and collecting system.[15,16] It is important to look at the reconstructed AP image of the CT to see if the stone is radiolucent (especially if the lithotripter being used has only fluoroscopic capability).

Where there is a question of renal function of the kidney being treated, a renal scan may be helpful.

KUB immediately prior to SWL is helpful to confirm the presence of and location of the stone, especially when treating patients on lithotriptors, which rely only on fluoroscopic imaging. In some instances retrograde pyelography at the time of SWL may be necessary to allow for proper visualization of the stone (radiolucent stone or ureteral stone).

Technique of SWL

Technique based on the type of machine one is using: Older model machines such as the HM3 required either general or spinal anesthesia. More contemporary second and third generation machines usually require only intravenous anal gosedation. Patients are placed in a gantry in the HM3 while newer generation machines have a treat ment table in which the patient can lie prone or supine dependent on stone location. For those machines, which require cardiac gating, continuous ECG monitoring is required. Shock waves are delivered either in a gated or ungated fashion. Patients undergoing ungated shock wave lithotripsy with a EHL device should remain continuously monitored as arrythmias may occur which may require the patient to continue treatment "gated." Piezoelectric and electromagnetic generated lithotriptors do not rely on cardiac gated triggering of the shock wave.

Shock wave number and energy levels vary by machine as well as the clinical scenario. A rule of thumb suggests that the lower energy and lower number of shock waves, which provides effective fragmentation, should also result in fewer complications. There is a growing body of evidence suggesting that a slower delivery rate of the shock waves results not only in more successful fragmentation but less renal injury.[17-19]

Postoperative Care

Immediate postoperative care consists of appropriate post anesthesia monitoring. Patients should be adequately recovered from their anesthetic agent(s), should be tolerating oral intake, and should void prior to discharge.

Discharge instructions should include vigorous hydration, return to usual physical activity as tolerated (usually 3 7 days), and straining of urine (for stone collection if stone analysis is unknown). Patients should be given oral pain medications (usually narcotics, nonsteroidal anti inflammatories). Patients who underwent instrumentation at the time of their treatment (cystoscopy with either retrograde catheter placement, or internal ureteral stent placement) should be discharged with antibiotics for 3 5 days. The routine use of preoperative antibiotics prior to SWL is somewhat controversial. Bierkaus and associates and Ilker and associates demonstrated no statistical difference in UTI between those receiving pre operative antibiotics and those that did not. Ameta analysis by Pearle and Roehrborn looked at 8 prospective, randomized, controlled trials and 6 clinical series, with the primary outcome being a diagnosis of a urinary tract infection (UTI) post SWL. A cost analysis was performed comparing a prophylactic strategy (prophylaxis for every patient and treatment for post SWL UTIs) with a treatment only strategy for post SWL. The incidence of post SWLUTIs ranged from 0% to 28% in the control group and from 0% to 7.7% in the patients who underwent prophylaxis. The median probability of a post SWLUTI of 5.7% compared to the drug treatment arms of 2.1%. Relative risk (RR) analysis resulted in an overall RR of post SWLUTIs with prophylaxis versus without prophylaxis of 0.45 (95% CI 0.22 to 0.93) (P = 0.0005).[20-23] Calcium channel blockers and selective alpha 1 blockers can be prescribed to facilitate stone passage.[24-26]

Routine follow up should be arranged in 2 4 weeks with a KUB to assess degree of stone fragmentation and stone passage (Figure 2a, Figure 2b, Figure 2c). Urinalysis and BP should also be checked at this visit. In patients with radiolucent stones, KUB should be substituted with renal ultrasound or renal stone protocol CT. If stone free, then follow up should be tailored based on metabolic findings, patient preference, etc. If patient has residual stone,

Figure 2a

Right renal stone prior to SWL

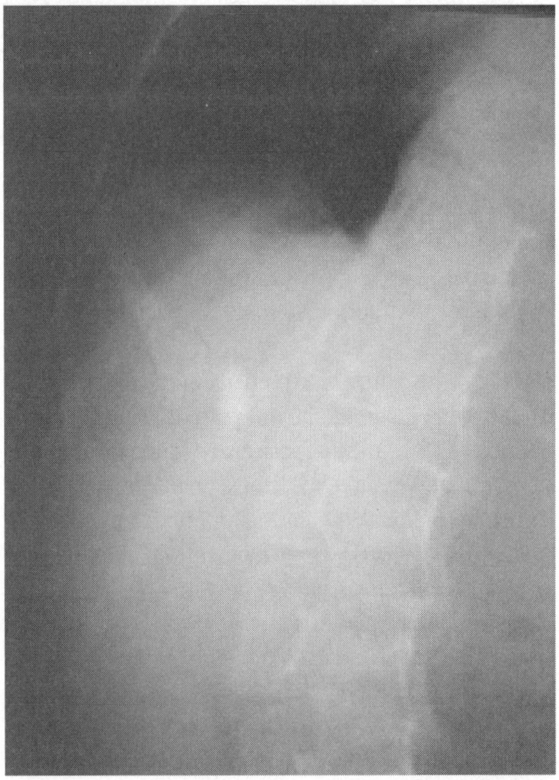

Figure 2b

Follow-up KUB at 4 weeks post-SWL reveals excellent fragmentation and clearance of stone burden

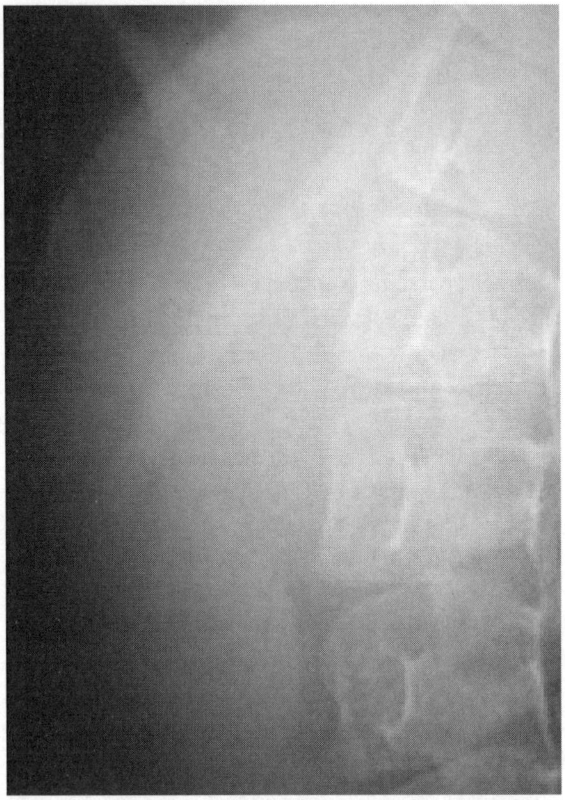

Figure 2c

Subcapsular hematoma of left kidney following left SWL (arrows)

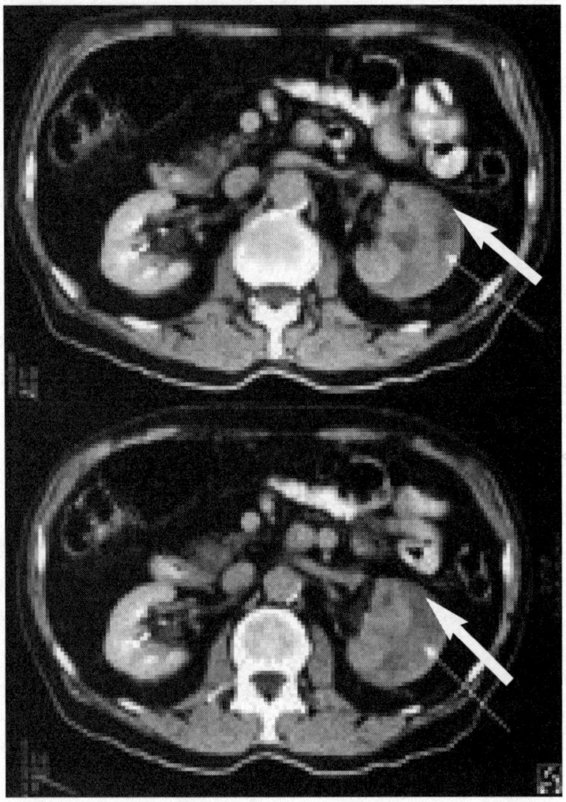

Patient had complete resolution of hematoma on follow-up CT at 6 months.

then follow up at 4 12 week intervals may be warranted based on amount of residual stone, presence of ureteral obstruction, symptoms, etc).

Patients with immediate pain out of the ordinary after treatment should be imaged with either ultra sound or CT to rule out perirenal or subcapsular hematoma. Patients should also be informed to return for medical evaluation for colicky pain that is not responsive to oral pain medication, inability to maintain oral intake, worsening flank or abdominal pain, temperature >38.5°C, or significant hematuria.

Overall Results

Renal

SWL is the most common first line treatment for the majority of renal stones. Despite the HM3 being the original lithotriptor, it is still considered the Cadillac® of lithotriptors based on its superior fragmentation success rate. The modifications made to the second and third generation lithotriptors have allowed for better patient comfort during treatment for poorer stone free rates. Weizer and associates summarized 5 large early series with the unmodified HM3 and demonstrated stone free rates for renal pelvic 76% (48% 85%), upper calyx 69% (46% 82%), middle calyx 68% (52% 76%), and lower calyx 59% (42% 73%). Stone free rates in all these series were dependent on size with stones <10 mm reporting excellent stone free rates. The limited number of comparative studies of the newer generation machines and the continued manufacture and marketing of even more lithotriptors makes it difficult to assess clinical efficacy based on a head to head study. Nonetheless, Weizer and associates provide a comparison of newer generation lithotriptors to the gold standard HM3. These studies confirm the notion that for renal and proximal ureteral stones, the HM3 appears superior.27

Upper Ureteral (in situ, With Stent)

There are two camps of investigators who have argued for better than 20 years over which technology is superior in treating ureteral stones. *Suffice it to say that either SWL or ureteroscopic (URS) treatment are both acceptable treatments for ureteral stones.* Proponents of SWL cite its efficacy, non-invasiveness, and that it can be performed with sedoanalgesia. Proponents of URS cite the high stone free success rate and the expediency over which the procedure can be performed. The AUA Ureteral Stones Guideline Panel meta-analysis showed SWL to have a stone clearance rate of 74% for stones <10 mm and 46% for stones 11 20 mm. More than one session is often required for stone clearance and success rates decrease with successive retreatments. Given these findings the *AUA panel recommended SWL as first line treatment for most patients with stones <10 mm in diameter. Distal stones <10 mm can be either treated with URS or SWL as first line therapy.* Pre stenting does not appear to improve stone free rates but does reduce hospital readmission and emergency room visits.[28-30] Table 3 summarizes several large series in which SWL was used to treat ureteral calculi based on location of stone at the time of treatment.

Table 3

SWL for Ureteral Calculi

Investigator	No. pts	Location	Size	Stone-Free Rates	Retreatment
Pearle	32	Distal	<15 mm	100%	0
Karlsen	33	Prox		58% (3wks) 88% (3 mos)	
Hautmann	45	Distal	<5 mm	78%	14% 2 session 8% 3 session
Hendrikx	69	Distal		51%* (3 mos)	45%
Eden†	404	Distal	8 mm (avg.)	74% (single stone) 50% (mult stone)	
Wu	41	Prox	12.8 mm	61% (1 mos)	
Pardalidis	633	Distal		99%	EQ 92
Lindqvist	24	Prox		95%	1.69
Parker	73	Prox		55%	EQ .51 <10 mm EQ .46 >10 mm

** Stones >11mm, 17% stone-free; stones <11 mm, 75% stone-free*
† 25.9% of patients required URS to render them stone-free

Mid-ureteral Stones

Mid ureteral stones can also be treated with SWL although stone localization can be difficult due to overlying bony structures and body habitus issues.

Lower Ureteral Stones

The case for treatment of lower ureteral stones with URS versus SWL is more controversial. The advantage of SWL over URS is the noninvasiveness of the treatment weighed against the higher retreatment rate, and the higher level of difficulty in localization of the stone. URS has superior stone free rates, is more cost effective and the endoscopic equipment is readily available in most if not all ambulatory surgery centers and hospital operating rooms.

Complications

Complications from SWL can be categorized into immediate and long term. Immediate complications are: tissue injury, bleeding, adjacent organ injury, urinary tract obstruction, post treatment obstruction, and urinary tract infection. Shear stress was originally postulated to be the cause of renal tissue injury. Recent studies however, suggest that SWL induced renal injury may be the result of microvascular injury due to cavitation, which then results in a local inflammatory response resulting in free radical production.[31,32] In most patients, shock waves result in parenchymal edema, which is dependent on number of shock waves and the size of the focal point.[33,34]

Subclinical or subcapsular hematomas can be seen by CT or MRI in up to 25% 30% of patients. Clinically significant subcapsular and perirenal hematomas occur much less frequently with reported rates between 0.24% 4.1%.[35-37] Certain clinical conditions such as hypertension, diabetes mellitus, obesity, and coronary artery disease have been reported to be risk factors.[39,40] The most common and important clinical sign of a hematoma is pain. Patients may also present with tachycardia, hypotension, and significant hematuria. Renal function impairment is uncommon and is seen only in patients with a solitary kidney or in bilateral hematoma following bilateral treatment. Diagnosis is confirmed by CT or ultrasound. Patients should be admitted, placed on bedrest, and serial hematocrits, and imaging should be performed. Reported transfusion rates range from 0% 33%, but typically the vast majority of patients can be managed conservatively. Follow up CT or renal ultrasound every 4 - 8 weeks should be performed to document resolution of the hematoma. Patients should be instructed to avoid strenuous physical exercise until follow up imaging confirms resolution. Patients should also have regular blood pressure checks to ensure that they do not develop renovascular hypertension.

Lung injury (<1%) is the most common nonurologic organ injury and is even more common in children.[41,42] Patients can present with hemoptysis, tachypnea, and decreased oxygen saturation. Pulmonary shielding, with either Styrofoam™ padding or tape provides excellent protection. Intestinal complications are also rare as is pancreatic injury. Proper attention to the blast path is the best preventive measure to avoid these injuries.

Obstruction of the urinary tract by fragments after SWL occur in 5% 10% of cases.[43-45] Predisposing factors include initial stone size, site of stone, renal morphology, shock wave energy. Renal pelvic stones >2 cm, dilated renal pelvis, and ureteric stones between 1 2 cm are all risk factors for steinstrasse formation (Table 4). Patients often present with flank pain and/or colic, fevers, nausea with or without emesis, or they can be completely asymptomatic. Imaging studies should be performed on all patients who are symptomatic or who are in the high risk category. KUB, IVP, CT are useful radiologic studies to diagnose steinstrasse. KUB does not provide any information whether there is any associated hydronephrosis or renal dysfunction. CT is very sensitive in detection of ureteral stone and associated hydronephrosis. CT scan, however, can exaggerate stone fragment size due to volume averaging during image reconstruction. IVP provides both anatomic and physiologic information but may require delayed imaging if there is significant obstruction and delayed function of the affected renal unit. Ureteral stenting appears to decrease the incidence of steinstrasse in patients with stone burdens of 1.5 3.5 cm compared to those with similar stone burdens who were not stented.[46,47] Spontaneous resolution of steinstrasse occurs in 65% 75% of patients.[48,49] Tamsulosin did not appear to improve resolution but did decrease pain symptoms associated with the steinstrasse. Patients who present with fever/UTI/sepsis should undergo percutaneous decompression. Percutaneous decompression, internal stent placement, ureteroscopic stone treatment, or in situ SWL are all treatment options for patients with symptomatic steinstrasse or in patients who have failed medical or nonsurgical treatment.

Urinary tract infection occurs rarely in patients with sterile urine following SWL. Placement on a broad based antibiotic, which is adjusted based on culture and sensitivity, should be implemented whenever a post SWLUTI is suspected. Treatment should be continued for a minimum of 7 10 days in the absence of obstruction and possibly longer if obstruction and/or evidence of acute pyelonephritis are present.

Table 4

Steinstrasse Formation Following SWL

Location	Incidence
Pelvic ureter	74%-84.3%
Iliac ureter	7.8%-4.3%
Lumbar ureter	7%-21%
Overall rate	3.9%-8.7%

Risk factors:	Renal stone	>2 cm 24%
		1-2 cm 16%
		<1 cm 4%
	Ureteral stone	>1 cm 10%
		<1 cm 3%
	Renal pelvis	19%
	Lower calyx	6%
	Middle calyx	10%
	Upper calyx	6%

Fortunately, long term complications of SWL are rare. Long term complications associated with SWL are renal insufficiency, hypertension, and possible metabolic abnormalities. Recently, Krambeck and associates reported on a possible association between prior SWL and the development of diabetes. In their study they identified 600 patients who had undergone SWL at a single institution using a single type lithotriptor (HM3). They then matched this group of patients by age, sex, and year of presentation to a group of stone patients who were treated nonsurgically. Those patients who had been treated with SWL were 1.5 times more likely to develop hypertension and 3.5 times more likely to develop diabetes mellitus than the nonsurgically treated cohort. This appeared to be independent of body mass index, and the size of stone that was treated.[50]

2. Ureteroscopy

Introduction

Advances in fiberoptics, refinements in laser and lithotripsy technology, and miniaturization of the ancillary equipment used in ureteroscopic treatment of upper urinary tract renal calculus disease is one of the more common procedures that practicing urologists perform today.

Rigid Ureteroscopy

Goodman in 1977 described the use of an 11 F pediatric cystoscope to treat ureteral pathology. Richard Wolf Medical Instruments developed an endoscope modeled after the pediatric cystoscope with a 23 cm working length available in 13–16.5 F in diameter, but with the intentional purpose to endoscopically examine and treat ureteral pathology. Working lengths were made longer with lengths up to 39 cm which allowed examination of the renal pelvis. Limitations with these early rigid scopes were the large diameter size, the phenomenon of the "half moon" effect when the scope was bent. The optical systems in today's rigid scopes are fiberoptic, enabling scope manufacturers to significantly decrease the size of the scopes without sacrificing optical clarity. Fiberoptics also allowed the working channels to become larger, and avoided the "half moon" effect. Fiberoptics also led to the development of flexible ureteroscopes which provided acceptable optics, a flexible working tip, and a working channel capable of accepting ancillary instruments. At present rigid and semi rigid ureteroscopes have tip diameters which range from 6.9 to 10 F with single working channels 4.–6.0F and dual working channels from 2.1–5.4 F. ACMI has introduced the DUR-D Digital Flexible ™ which employs a distal CMOS video sensor and built-in LEDs for illumination. Olympus Medical has developed a semi rigid ureteroscope and more recently a flexible ureteroscope where the optical chip is located at the working tip of the scope providing superior optics over the traditional fiberoptic image transmission. Flexible ureteroscopes have tip diameters ranging from 4.9–11.0 F with varying degrees of active primary deflection. The DUR 8E from ACMI has two active deflection points providing even better flexible capabilities. Working channels range from 1.5–4.5 F with most models boasting a 3.6 F channel. Semi rigid ureteroscopes are considerably more durable than their flexible counterparts but undo pressure can result in fracture along the working length of the scope. Improper sterilization, inadvertent laser or other lithotripsy devices too close to the working tip can render these scopes unusable. Flexible scopes, due to the less durable outer and working channel material, the complex working components which allow for active deflection, and the special precautions needed for scope processing, are quite susceptible to scope damage, which may result in progressive decrease in optical performance, decrease in range of active deflection, or the inability to use the working channel. Any and all of these scope malfunctions may render the scope unusable. McDougall and associates reported that the demands placed on the scope by the endoscopists were the usual cause of scope failure, while White and colleague noted a significant number of scope failures caused by personnel charged with maintenance of the ureteroscope.[51,52] In either case, semi rigid, and especially flexible ureteroscopes should be handled with care not only by the operating surgeon but also by the operating room technicians and nursing staff charged with sterilizing or disinfecting the scope between uses. Flexible ureteroscopes have a limited life span and unfortunately should be considered one of the more expensive "disposable" items in the operating room.

Ancillary Equipment in Ureteroscopy

There has been an explosion of both diagnostic and therapeutic endoscopic equipment now available to the endoscopist, including guidewires, catheters, dilators, ureteral sheaths, biopsy forceps, baskets, and lithotripsy devices.

Guidewires

There are numerous guidewires of various sizes and materials. The decision regarding which guidewire to use is based on surgeon preference. Certain guidewires have particular advantages. The 0.035 or 0.038 in Amplatz Super Stiff™ (Microvasive, Boston Scientific, Natick, MA) can be used to straighten a tortuous ureter and place a stent in a ureter with either an intrinsic or extrinsic obstruction. An 0.035 or 0.038 in PTFE nitinol guidewire is invaluable and is the author's preferred wire(s) when performing ureteroscopy. The steerable stiff-angled guidewire can easily be maneuvered beyond

Figure 3

Floppy-tipped guidewire is the wire of choice when trying to place a wire beyond an impacted ureteral stone

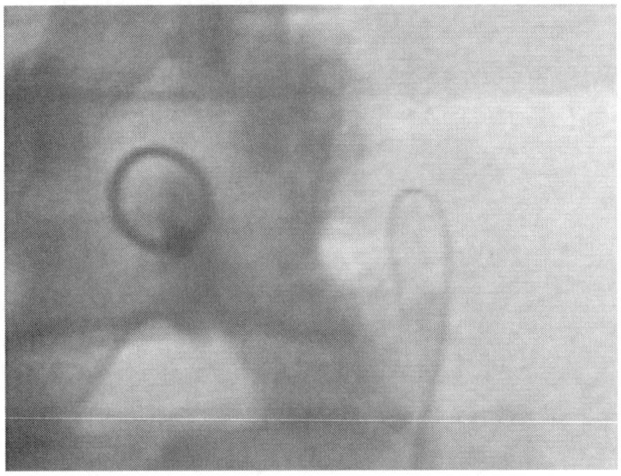

Note how the tip negotiates around the stone not with the tip but with an atraumatic "knuckle."

ureteral stones (even when impacted), as well as negotiate tortuous ureters (Figure 3). Flexible ureteroscopes and post- procedure stents are much more easily placed over this wire because of the guidewire's stiff body and hydrophilic coating. Care is needed when placing a flexible scope over a stiff guidewire to prevent injury to the working channel sheath. In order to reduce injury to the flexible ureteroscope during backloading, a dual floppy tip PTFE nitinol guidewire (Sensor™, Microvasive, Boston Scientific, Natick, MA) was introduced.

A working catheter (5 or 6 F) can be used to perform retrograde imaging studies, facilitate guidewire access to the ureteral orifice, and can be used to assist in manipulating guidewires beyond obstructions (Figure 4). For example, when faced with an impacted stone, the catheter can be placed over the wire up to the level of obstruction to stabilize the wire when can then be successfully negotiated beyond the obstruction. Angled catheters are especially helpful in negotiating tortuous ureters using the aforementioned technique.

Ureteral Dilating Devices

With the development of miniaturized scopes, the need to routinely dilate the ureteral orifice to gain access has decreased dramatically. Despite the decrease in routine dilation of the ureteral orifice, occasionally dilation is necessary and preferred over traumatic injury to the ureteral orifice. Garvin and Clayman demonstrated that dilation of the ureteral orifice with a coaxial balloon dilator was relatively atraumatic and did not lead to long term sequelae such as stricture or reflux.[53] Ureteral dilation can also be achieved with tapered catheters such as the Lieberman catheter (Cook), 8/10 F sheath and obturator (Microvasive, Boston Scientific, Natick, MA) both of which allows secondary placement of a second safety wire. Ureteral access sheaths, (manufactured by Cook, Applied Urolog-

Figure 4

Retrograde pyelogram reveals a mid-ureteral stone

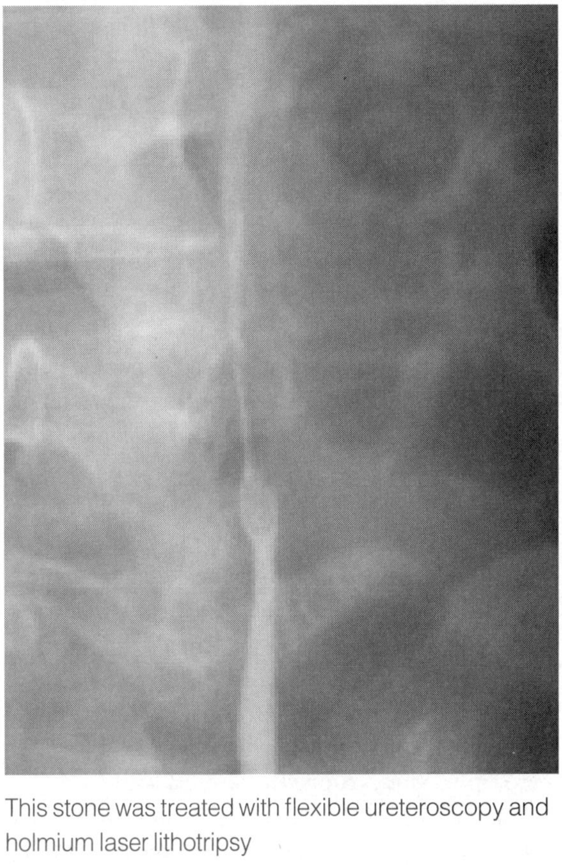

This stone was treated with flexible ureteroscopy and holmium laser lithotripsy ics, Bard and Microvasive) are currently available in inner diameters ranging from 9.5 F to 15 F to lengths ranging from 13-55 cm. The access sheath consists of two components: an inner obturator and an outer cannula, both of which are hydrophilic: allowing for easy placement, withdrawal of the obturator once positioned, and easy maneuvering of the scope within the cannula, and a kink resistent cannula which conforms to the natural curvature of the urethra and ureter. An access sheath can facilitate access to the ureter and allow multiple insertions and withdrawals of the ureteroscope and minimizing the trauma that could accompany repeated passes of the scope. In addition, the access sheath provides continuous drainage of irrigation fluid during ureteroscopy reducing intrapelvic hydraulic pressure while reducing bladder fluid build up obviating the need for periodic bladder drainage during a long ureteroscopic session. The sheaths come in different lengths and diameters, which allow the surgeon to choose the appropriate sheath based on patient size and gender, ureteral width, and stone location. The author typically uses a 11/13 F sheath if using a sheath. Care should be taken during initial placement of an access sheath. An Amplatz Super Stiff wire is usually necessary to place the sheath, especially in ureters, which are not dilated. If the access sheath does not pass easily, then gentle traction, countertraction, may facilitate passage. Kourambas et al reported successful initial placement of an access sheath in over 90% of patients.[54] however that has not been my personal experience. Do not force the sheath because splitting of the ureter can result. In cases where the access sheath cannot be deployed, then placing a temporary stent (5-10 days) will allow passive dilation and result in subsequent successful access sheath placement.

The development of 0-tipped nitinol baskets has been the most important technologic advance in basket technology. They provide atraumatic deployment, excellent irrigation during use, full deflection of the ureteroscope during stone manipulation, excellent memory characteristics with repeated use, and are kink- resistant which also allows multiple deployment and release of stones. The 1.9 F ZeroTip™ Nitinol Stone Retrieval Basket (Microvasive, Boston Scientific, Natick, Mass.) and 1.7 F NCompass™ Nitinol Stone Extractors (Cook Urological, Spencer, Ind.) are both excellent stone retrieval devices. These baskets are the only type of basket the author routinely uses (Figure 5).

Figure 5

Nitinol tipless guidewire allows excellent deflection with superior capture and release of stone

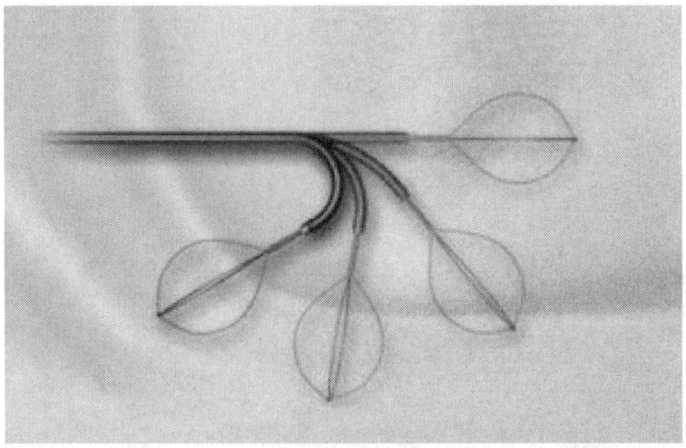

Microvasive, Boston Scientific, Natick, Mass.

Specialty Catheters

Stone Cone™ Nitinol Retrieval Device (Microvasive, Boston Scientific, Natick, Mass.) is designed to sweep multiple stone fragments postintracorpo real lithotripsy, and to prevent proximal migration of fragments during intracorporeal lithotripsy. The sheath is somewhat laser resistant and the coil will release with traction even in a deployed position to allow for device removal.

Lithotripsy Devices

EHL small caliber electrohydraulic probes (1.9F), more flexible than even small quartz fibers used for laser lithotripsy, may be necessary in treating lower pole renal stones. *EHL stone fragmentation occurs as a result of a cavitation bubble*. Concomitant tissue injury and bleeding are more likely to occur with EHL than with holmium laser lithotripsy.

Holmium laser fragments stones through a photothermal mechanism. Holmium laser energy is rapidly absorbed by water so that there is minimal concomitant tissue injury. Fibers in 200 to 100 micron in diameter are available and can tolerate typical energy levels to fragment any and all types of urinary calculi. The smaller diameter fibers by nature are more fragile but allow for more deflection, but also have a tendency to fracture at the tip or along the fiber during laser firing.

Stents

There are multiple stents of varying size, composition, and configuration. There appears to be no real difference in patient stent tolerance despite claims by manufacturers. Stent type is by surgeon preference.

Preoperative Evaluation

As in SWL, patients should undergo a complete history and physical. Urine should be sterile prior to ureteroscopic stone treatment. Patients should be administered preoperative antibiotics.

Bleeding diatheses should be corrected if medically indicated. If normalizing hemostatic parameters are medically contraindicated, ureteroscopy with holmium laser lithotripsy has been safely and successfully performed.[55] Watterson and associates treated 25 patients with uncorrected bleeding diathesis using a holmium laser with an overall stone free success rate of 96% (29/30 procedures). The single patient that suffered from a significant bleeding episode had been treated using EHL.

Operative Technique

C-arm is necessary for ureteroscopy. The urologist should be familiar with the fluoroscopic capabilities and limits if he/she is operating a fixed fluoroscopic unit. All personnel should be properly shielded. Positioning is usually in the lithotomy or modified lithotomy position. Morbidly obese patients may need to be placed in reverse Trendelenburg position so as not to compromise respiratory function. In some cases, flexible URS can be performed with patients in the supine or lateral decubitus position as well.

General anesthesia with endotracheal intubation is preferred. Laryngeal mask anesthesia or spinal anesthesia is also reasonable although kidney movement due to respiratory movement can complicate intracorporeal lithotripsy. *Knowledgeable ancillary assistance is helpful when performing semirigid ureteroscopy but essential in flexible ureteroscopy.*

Irrigation is critical in successful ureteroscopy. Normal saline at body temperature is the irrigant of choice. Simple gravity irrigation is insufficient for adequate flow. There are a number of different systems that vary in complexity and cost. A low cost method employs using a pressure bag, which accommodates a 3 LNS bag inflated to provide flow (Figure 6). Control pump syringes and handheld bulb pump systems can be utilized to augment flow on demand. A more advanced system Level 1 System 1000 (Level 1 Technologies, Rockland, Mass.) provides precision control and warms the system simultaneously.

Postoperative Management

Routine use of stents post-ureteroscopy has not been shown to be necessary. Certain prognostic factors would suggest that stents be used: bilateral ureteroscopy, solitary kidney, ureteral perforation, impacted stone, ureteroscopy >60 minutes, uncorrected bleeding diathesis, ureteroscopy of a struvite or infection stone.[55-59]

Figure 6

Urolock™ adaptor from Microvasive

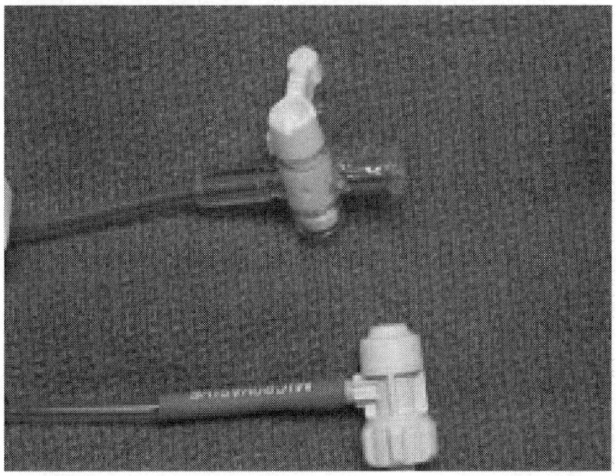

An excellent adaptor which fits on the irrigation port of the ureteroscope. It has a 3-way port for continuous irrigation as well as syringe irrigation when needed. The diaphragm is waterproof but allows repeated placement of lithotripsy and retrieval devices.

Most patients should be discharged on oral antibiotics for 3-5 days. If a stent is left indwelling, consider instructing patients to institute antibiotic pro phylaxis starting 12-24 hours prior to stent removal, continuing for another 24-48 hours.

Counsel patients that mild hematuria and ipsilateral flank discomfort and dysuria is expected following URS. If a stent is left indwelling, also counsel them regarding typical stent related symptoms.

Follow up imaging studies at 2-4 weeks are recommended. KUB or non-contrast CT can be used to assess stone free status. The need for postoperative functional imaging studies is controversial. Weizer and associates recommend a functional imaging study, whereas Bugg and colleagues argue against routine functional imaging.[60,61] Functional studies (IVP, CT with contrast, nuclear renal scan) should be completed in patients with persistent flank pain, persistent or worsening hydronephrosis. Patients with severely impacted stones or patients with traumatic ureteroscopy should also undergo a functional study despite whether they are symptomatic or not (Table 5).

Table 5

Indications for Ureteroscopic Treatment of Renal Stones

SWL failure
Lower pole stone location
Morbid obesity
Musculoskeletal deformities
Bleeding diathesis
Calyceal diverticular stones
Adverse stone characteristic for SWL
Infundibular stenosis
Ectopic or horseshoe kidney

Adapted from Busby JE and Low RK. Ureteroscopic treatment of renal calculi. Urol Clin N Am. *2004;31:90.*

Distal Ureteral Stones

Distal ureteral stones are probably best treated using a semi rigid ureteroscope. A retrograde pyelogram can be performed to confirm the location of the stone(s) and can also delineate the degree of obstruction/impaction of the stone. Through the ureteral catheter, a wire is manipulated beyond the stone into the upper collecting system. Dilation of the ureteral orifice can be accomplished with a balloon dilator or with a tapered catheter. (The author prefers the balloon dilator because of the more uniform dilation which is achieved.) The scope is then placed alongside the wire up to the level of the stone. If the stone is small enough to remove then it is engaged in the basket and removed in toto. Stones which are large or in which the ureteral orifice was not dilated will require fragmentation. Holmium laser is the preferred lithotripsy method. Lithotripsy should be initiated at the leading edge of the stone, which is away from the ureteral wall. As the stone is fragmented, the stone adjacent to the wall will "fall away" from the wall and then can be safely fragmented. During lasering, the aiming beam of the laser can be turned down or off to increase visualization. Periodically, during long laser sessions, the aiming beam should be turned on to assess the integrity of the laser fiber. Care should be taken to adjust the irrigant flow to allow for visualization while preventing proximal migration of fragments. At times stone fragments will impede the view of the main stone. These fragments can either by removed by basketing the stone and placing them in the bladder or by just removing the scope and allowing the fragments to be irrigated out. Stones that are impacted can usually be "manipulated" from the impacted ureteral segment up into the more dilated and "safe" portion of the ureter so that the stone can be fragmented without concern of inadvertent ureteral injury. Impacted stones usually require at least partial laser treatment before they can be safely "manipulated." At the end of treatment a retrograde pyelogram can be performed either via the scope or with catheter after scope removal. This can ensure no injury to the ureter, as well as outlining the upper collecting system configuration, which can allow for proper stent placement (Figure 7a, Figure 7b).

Mid-ureteral Stones

Mid ureteral stones can be treated either with a semi rigid or flexible ureteroscope. *Flexible ureteroscopy is the preferred technique in treating mid ureteral stones*. Semi rigid ureteroscopy of the mid and proximal can be difficult. The author rarely uses a semi rigid scope above the iliac vessels. Relatively easy access to the mid- and proximal ureter with the semi rigid scope can be accomplished in females and in some males (typically ones who have had a stent already indwelling), but the risk of injury to the ureteroscope (shaft bending or fracture) and more importantly ureteral injury appears higher. A guidewire is placed beyond the stone and a safety wire is placed (Figure 8). The safety wire assures that the ureter remains straightened, which significantly improves stone visualization (Figure 9). The flexible scope is placed over the working wire up to the level of the stone either under direct or fluoroscopic (or both) visualization. Alternatively, an access sheath can be placed up to the level of the stone over the working wire. The stone can then be treated as described above. Mid- and ureteral stones are more prone to impaction and care should be taken to avoid injury to the ureter (mid ureteral injuries are more prone to stricture due to its more tenuous blood supply).

Figure 7a

KUB of 36-week gravid woman with severe right flank pain

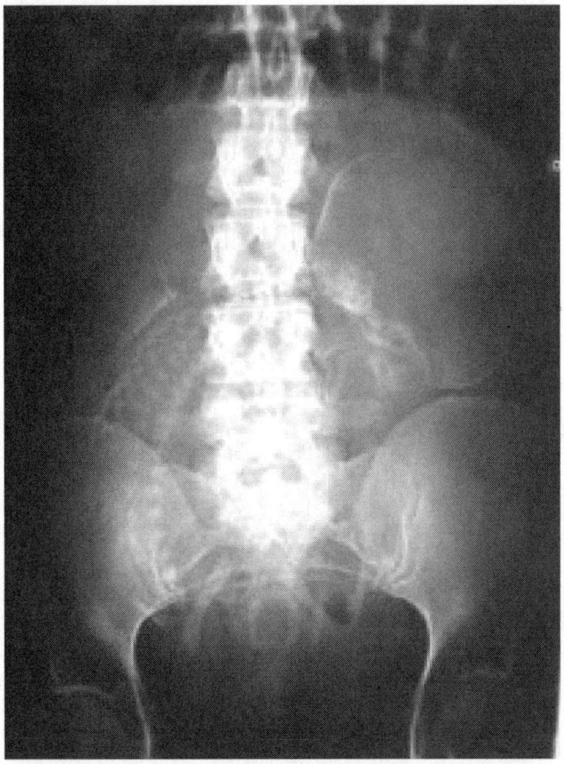

Patient has a distal right ureteral calculus.

Figure 7b

Close-up of KUB reveals this distal ureteral calculus measuring 5x 8 mm

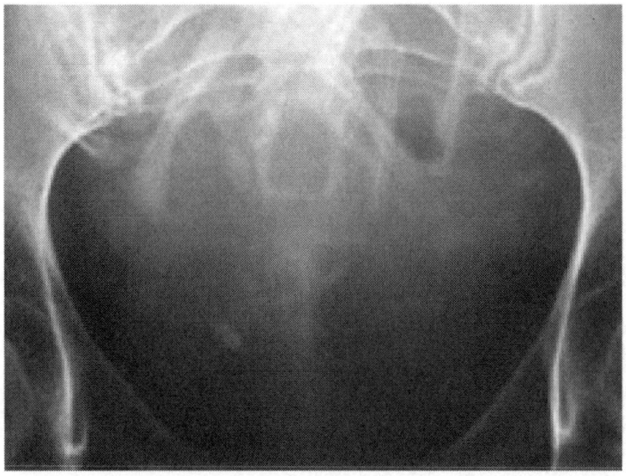

Stone was successfully removed ureteroscopically. Patient had an uneventful postoperative course and had a normal delivery.

Proximal Ureteral Stones

Proximal ureteral stones are best treated using the flexible ureteroscope. Access is similarly achieved as in the technique for mid ureteral stones. Proximal stones and/or partially treated fragments are more prone to proximal migration. Proximal migration can be potentially obviated by using the Stone Cone™ Nitinol Retrieval Device (Microvasive, Boston Scientific, Natick, Mass.). By placing the patient in mild Trendelenburg position the migrating fragments settle either in the renal pelvis or upper pole calyces and are much more readily accessible for further removal or treatment. If using an access sheath, be sure to visually inspect the ureter as you withdraw it to ensure that there has

Figure 8

Endoscopic view of the midureter during passage of the flexible scope up into the collecting system

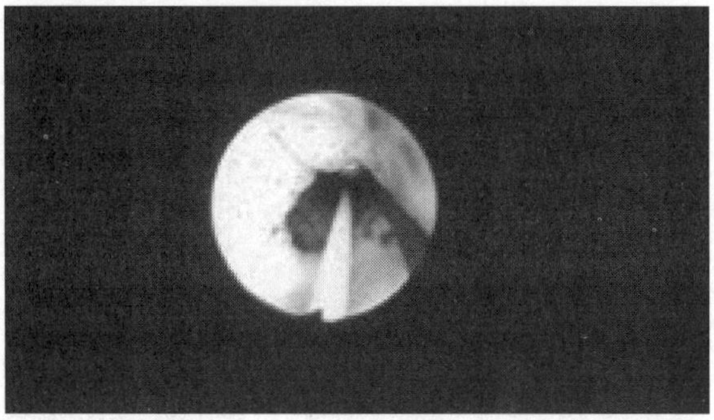

Note the working nitinol guidewire which is being used as the working wire and the Teflon®-coated safety wire.

Figure 9

Endoscopic view of an impacted midureteral stone

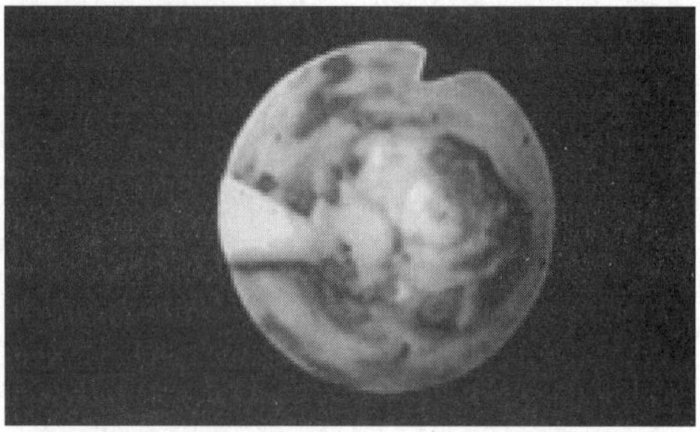

The safety wire keeps the ureter straight and optimizes laser lithotripsy.

been no ureteral injury.

Renal Stones

Renal stones can be successfully treated with retro grade ureteroscopy using a flexible ureteroscope. Access to the kidney is achieved as described above. In some cases in which a renal stone is being treated with lithotripsy and the endoscopist does not plan to remove fragments, a safety wire placement may be obviated. In this case, once successful fragmentation is achieved, a guidewire is placed through the working channel, the scope is withdrawn and a stent can be subsequently placed, if deemed necessary. In most cases, however, a safety wire is recommended (Figure 10). Small stones can be basketed and removed from the kidney and then deposited in the bladder. An access sheath can assist in this type of stone removal. Larger stones can be treated with holmium laser. The author prefers using a 2 F laser catheter (Cook Urological, Spencer, IN) with a 200-micron laser fiber, which provides some level of protection to the ureteroscope working channel during placement of and manipulation of the fiber. The deflection of the scope is not affected by the addition of the fiber but irrigant flow is diminished.[62] The endoscopist should take advantage of the configuration of the collecting system and use it to his advantage when treating renal stones. Renal pelvic stones

Figure 10

Initiation of holmium laser lithotripsy of an upper pole stone

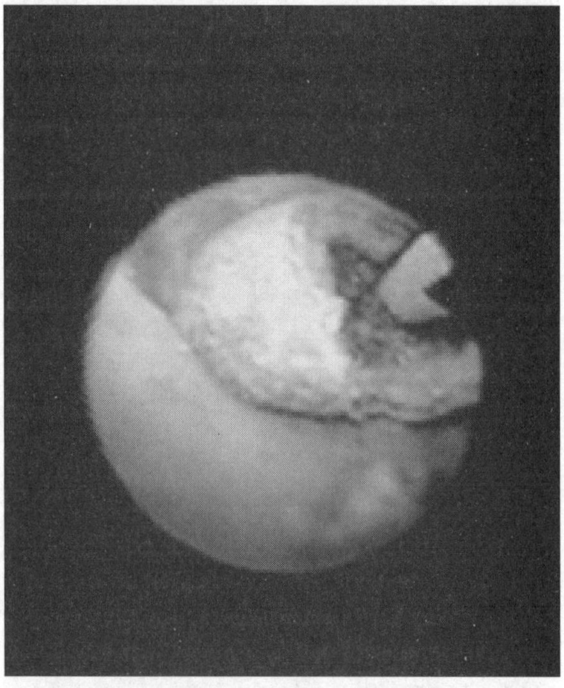

The calyx prevents any migration of the stone during lithotripsy. Note the laser catheter and the laser fiber emanating from the open end.

have a tendency to migrate during lithotripsy. The author recommends actively manipulating renal pelvic stones into an upper pole calyx, which allows a "straight shot" as well as a "backstop" (the upper pole calyx), which prevents any unwanted stone or stone fragment migration. Once in the upper pole, adequate fragmentation can be easily achieved (Figure 11).

Lower pole stones present a challenge. In some cases, patients can be placed in Trendelberg position and the stones can be manually irrigated into a more accessible mid or upper pole calyx (Figure 12). Active repositioning of the stone from the lower pole into an upper pole calyx provides several advantages: easier fragmentation of the stone; decreasing scope fatigue and improving scope life; and reducing working channel injury due to proximal energy dispersal from the laser fiber. In some cases access to some lower pole stones cannot be achieved with a laser fiber in place. Sometimes the stone can be basketed (1.9F baskets provide for more deflection), and then displaced into an upper pole (Figure 13).[63-66] In rare cases in which a large lower pole stone cannot be accessed with a laser and is too large to safely be displaced, EHL using a 1.9 F probe can be employed to fragment the stone, basket and displace the fragment, and then complete the lithotripsy with the holmium laser (Figure 14a, Figure 14b, Figure 14c).

Complications of Ureteroscopy

Complications can be generally classified either by timing (intraoperative vs. early vs. late), or by significance (minor vs. major). Most complications usually occur during or immediately post procedure and major complications are fortunately quite rare.

Intraoperative complications include: mucosal abrasion, ureteral false passage, perforation, extravasation, bleeding, thermal injury, equipment malfunction, ureteral intussusception, and ureteral avulsion.

Figure 11

Flexible ureteroscopy was successful in accessing the lower pole of the left kidney

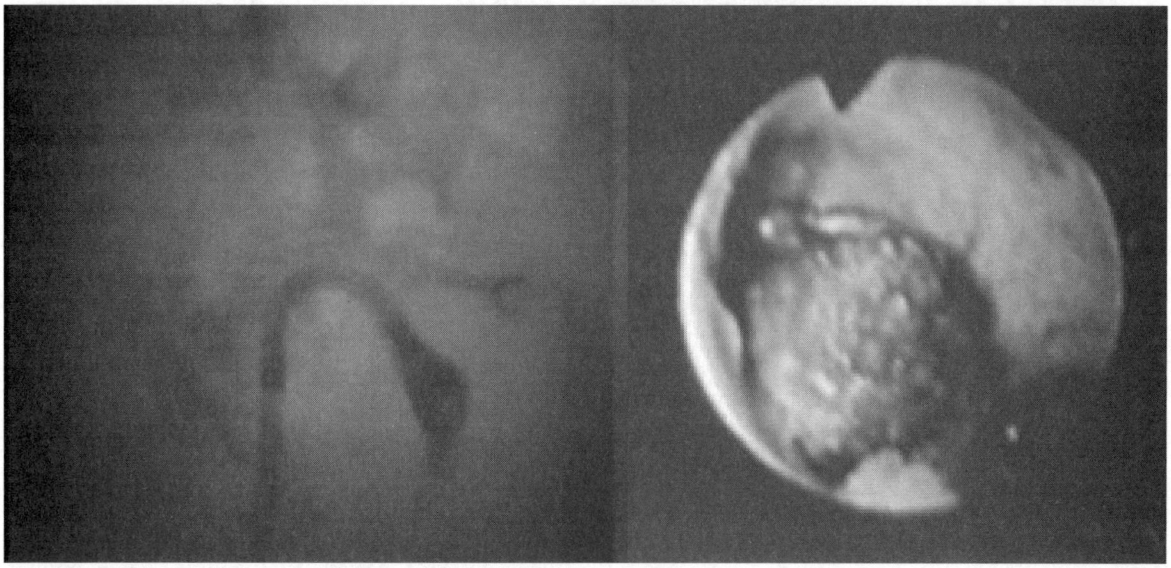

Endoscopy revealed a 6 x 6 mm stone within the lower pole. The stone was displaced into the upper pole where it was successfully fragmented with the holmium laser.

Figure 12

Secondary deflection of ureteroscope into a dependent calyx during diagnostic ureteroscopy for abnormal urine cytologies

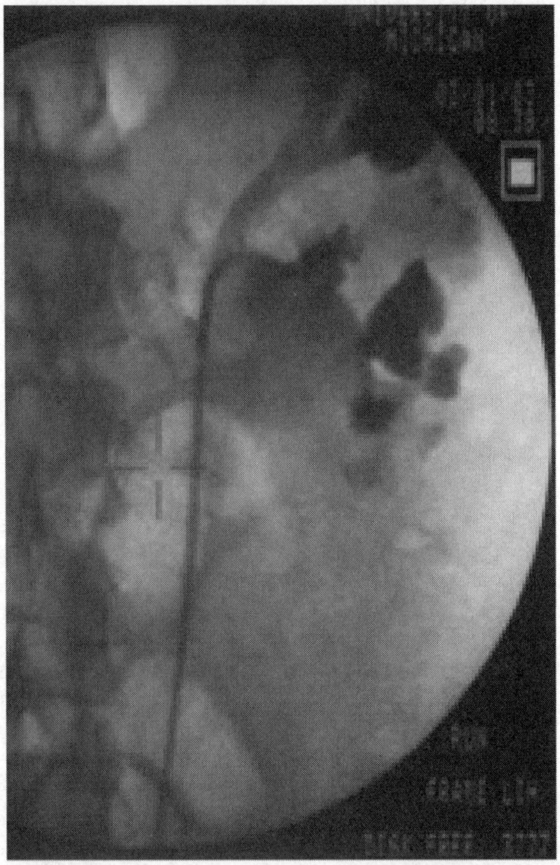

Figure 13

Lower pole stone engaged with nitinol basket and displaced into upper pole for fragmentation

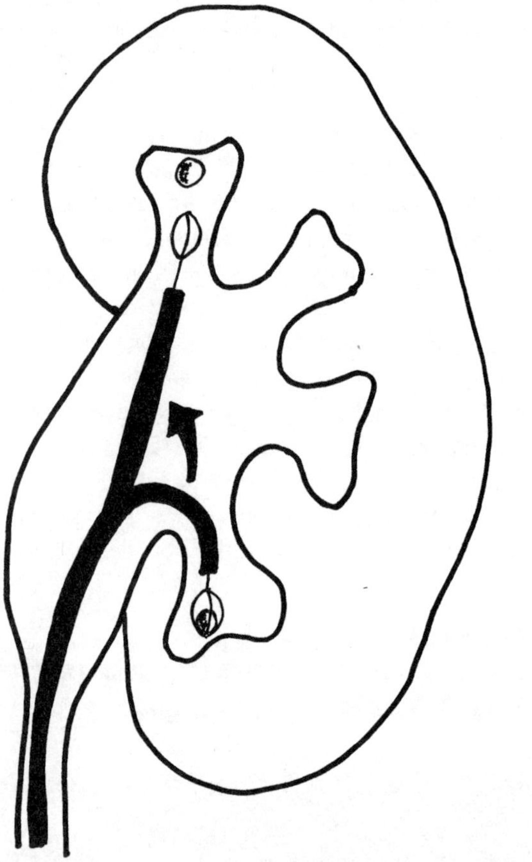

Mucosal abrasion occurs to some extent during all ureteroscopies. Moderate to severe abrasion (especially at the ureteral orifice) can lead to post-operative swelling and edema leading to ureteral obstruction. Careful use of the ureteroscope, atraumatic dilation of the ureteral orifice, and judicious use of ancillary equipment can reduce the risk of significant abrasion injuries. If significant abrasion is apparent, temporary stenting for 7 10 days is the recommended treatment.

Ureteral false passage typically occurs during intubation of the ureteral orifice as well as during negotiation of a guidewire around an impacted stone. Reported false passage rates are between 0.4% 0.9% but is probably an under reported condition.69 False passage at the ureteral orifice often occurs when the catheter does not follow the intramural course of the ureter (ie, males with BPH, gravid females, etc). The guidewire will not advance much beyond the catheter. A retrograde pyelogram may opacify the more proximal ureter and by withdrawing the catheter slightly and using angled guidewire may result in successful negotiation of the false passage. In a severe false passage at the ureteral orifice, placement of the semirigid ureteroscope just within the ureteral orifice can usually allow visualization of the true lumen. The true lumen tends to be inferior and lateral to the false passage, which tends to be medial and superior. A guidewire can be placed up the ureteral lumen and one can continue proceeding with the ureteroscopy. False passage at an

Figure 14a

CT image reveals a large calyceal diverticulum with several calcifications within the large diverticulum

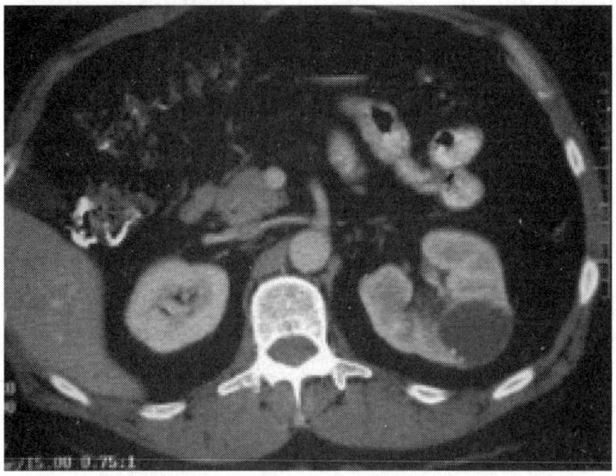

Figure 14c

Endoscopic view of a cluster of small stone within a calyceal diverticulum treated with retrograde ureteroscopy

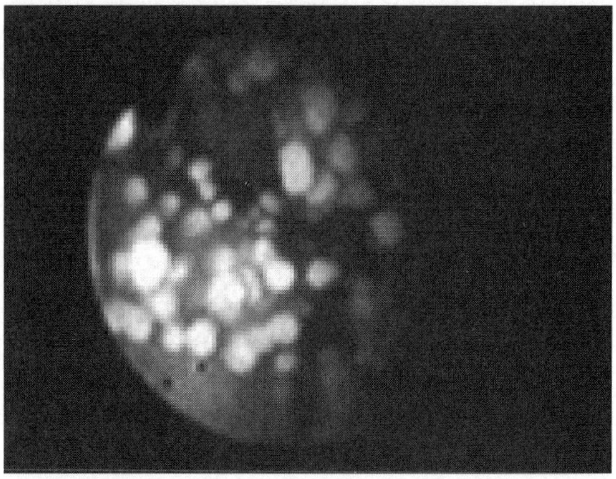

Figure 14b

Flouroscopic image of successful retrograde access into the calyceal diverticulum

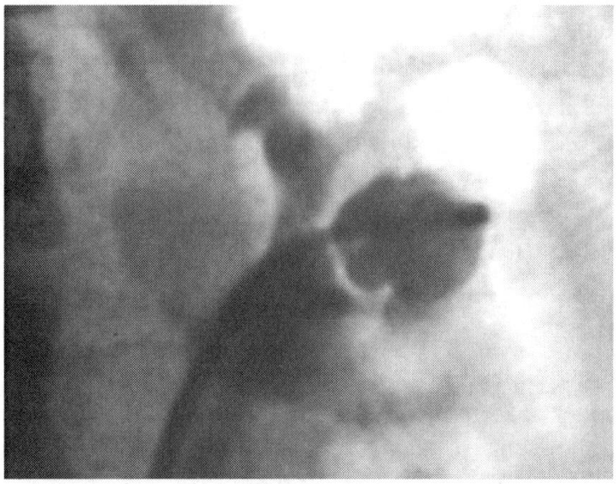

impacted stone is usually apparent when the guidewire does not track up the expected course of the ureter, the floppy tip doesn't "knuckle" or it feels "sticky." In this case the scope can be advanced under direct vision to the level of the stone and a guidewire can be directed beyond the stone under direct vision. The scope can then be withdrawn and a safety wire properly placed using an exchange catheter. Perforations are reported to occur between 1% -15%, with the higher reported incidence rates occurring with larger diameter scopes, complicated stones requiring lengthy procedures, or during treatment of proximal ureteral stones. *Minor perforations can be safely managed with an indwelling ureteral stent for 2-4 weeks.*

Extravasation of small amounts of irrigation fluid is probably common and results in no sequelae. *Saline should be the only irrigant fluid routinely used during ureteroscopic stone treatment.* In over 2,300 ureteroscopies, the author has not had a complication due to fluid overload as a result of significant saline irrigant extravasation. Extravasation of stone material completely outside the ureter has not resulted in any apparent adverse sequelae; however, stone fragments embedded in the ureteral wall appear to be associated with ureteral stricture.[70]

Bleeding is typically minor and self-limiting. Bleeding can impair visualization to the point at which continuing with the procedure may be hazardous. In that case, the procedure should be discontinued, a stent placed, and a plan made on a definitive procedure at a later date.

Thermal injury is due to improper use of a lithotripsy device. EHL energy is much more difficult to control

Table 6

Indications for Percutaneous Stone Removal

Staghorn calculi
Renal pelvis stones >2 cm
Lower pole stones >1.5 cm
SWL-resistant stones
Stones associated with UPJ obstruction
Calyceal diverticular stones
Pts with contraindications for SWL

and extreme care should be used when using this device. *Holmium energy is readily absorbed by water and fortunately has a minimal thermal injury zone of 0.5 to 1 mm.* Significant thermal injury due to holmium laser use is extremely rare.

Equipment malfunction unfortunately does occur and is most likely a combination of exceeding the limited lifespan of the scope, improper use by the endoscopist, or exceeding the physical limits of the scope. Certainly, proper handling, storage, and processing are key to optimizing the lifespan of these delicate instruments. Prior to use the scope should be visually inspected for kinks or bends in the shaft, the integrity of the fiberoptic system, and the deflection mechanism and integrity of the outer and the working sheath of the flexible ureteroscope. The most common intra operative malfunctions occur with the flexible scope and are due to laser fiber damage to the working channel, laser fiber injury to the fiberoptics, or hyper re/de flexion of the scope. Any of these injuries most often render the scope useless and require either major repair or complete scope replacement.

The most-feared intra-operative complications are ureteral avulsion or intussusception, both of which should be completely avoidable. *Avulsion, which is reported to occur around 0.3 % is most commonly due to an attempt to remove a basketed stone from mid or proximal ureter which is too large to safely remove, or incorporating the ureter within the stone basket during stone capture and then attempting to withdraw the basket.*[71] The author strongly advocates the use of nitinol baskets because unlike metal baskets, the tines have superior memory, and stones which are basketed but are too large to be extracted can be disengaged easily. If the stone cannot be disengaged, then cut off the handle of the basket, withdraw the scope leaving the sheathless basket in place. Replace the scope next to the basket and fragment the stone until it can be disengaged from the basket. Be careful not to fracture the tines of the basket as they can be easily lost. Avulsion is recognized when the ureter presents along with the stone. In males it appears as a tubular structure within the bladder, while in females the ureter can be actually be seen emanating from the urethra.

Complete avulsion requires immediate surgical repair. An attempt at laparoscopic repair should only be done by those with exceptional laparoscopic skills; otherwise, it requires an open repair. Distal ureteral avulsions can be repaired with a uretero neocystostomy with or without use of a psoas hitch or boari bladder flap. Mid- and proximal injuries are often more difficult to repair due to the compromised blood supply which occurs at the site of the injury. In mid ureteral injuries, both the proximal and distal ureteral ends should be freshened up, spatulated and anastomosed end to end with fine absorbable sutures over an indwelling ureteral stent.

Blunt dissection around the kidney (especially the upper pole) may be necessary in order to create a tension free anastomosis. A primary UPJ repair can be performed for proximal or UPJ injuries. These can also be difficult because the pelvis may not be dilated like in pyeloplasties done for UPJO. In severe cases, either an immediate auto transplantation or an ileal ureter can be performed. Another option is nonrepairable instances is ligation of the ureter, and percutaneous nephrostomy placement. Finally, in some instances, nephrectomy may be warranted.

Intussusception is a partial thickness mucosal sleeve

injury to the ureter. The mechanism of injury is often similar to avulsion injuries. An attempt at replacement of the ureteral mucosa endoscopically followed by long term internal stent placement may suffice but usually results in long ureteral stricture. Definitive open repair is probably the recommended treatment.

Immediate post operative complications are UTI/sepsis, and obstruction. The risk of infection is 4% 22.5% in several large series. Sepsis occurs less frequently between 0.3% 2.0%.[69] Admission with urine culture, intravenous hydration and intravenous antibiotics are usually necessary to patients with febrile UTIs. Patients with sepsis require aggressive support, which may include ICU admission, blood pressure support, and ventilatory support, in addition to broad spectrum antibiotic cover age. A high index of suspicion for sepsis should accompany any patient who has rigors, has mental status changes, is hypotensive, who is febrile above 102.5°F or is hypothermic < 96°F, who has either a profound leukocytosis or leukopenia.

Ureteral obstruction can occur either as a result of ureteral edema, ureteral spasm, blood clot or residual stone (steinstrasse). Obstruction due to edema, spasm or blood clot is a self-limiting condition and can usually be managed conservatively. In some case of persistent symptoms, stent placement of percutaneous drainage may be necessary. Steinstrasse can occur and can be treated medically with alpha blockers. *In patients with mild steinstrasse who fail medical therapy or are severely symptomatic, stent place ment or definitive URS with stone removal may be necessary. In patients with significant steinstrasse with large stone burden, percutaneous drainage followed by antegrade URS may be necessary.*

Late complications are ureteral stricture disease. Late strictures occur as a result of URS between 0% -4%.[69] Ureteral perforations, impacted stones and use of large diameter ureteroscopes are risk factors in formation of ureteral strictures (Figure 15a, Figure 15b). Roberts and associates reported in one series of 21 patients in which there was a 24% stricture rate in patients who had impacted stones.[72] Early reports with large caliber ureteroscopes cited

Figure 15a

Retrograde pyelogram reveals a severe ureteral stricture at the level of the pelvic vessels

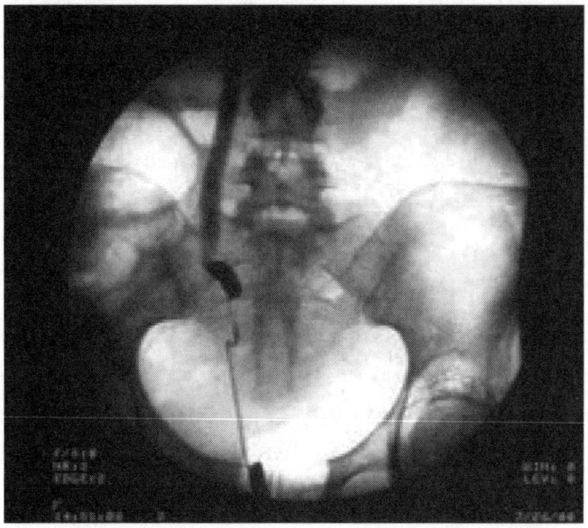

This occurred following attempt at rigid ureteroscopy for a proximal ureteral calculus.

Figure 15b

Patient underwent a boari flap to repair the stricture

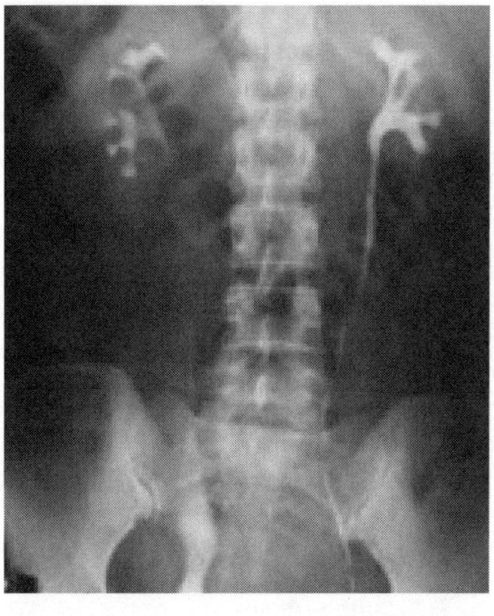

stricture rates of 4% whereas more contemporary series reported stricture rates of <1%.It is unclear whether the more widespread use of access sheaths will result in a higher incidence of stricture formation. An early report by Delvecchio, et al reviewed their experience of 62 patients who underwent URS using a 10/12 access sheath. They reported a 1.4% stricture rate.[73]

Treatment of ureteral strictures is dependent on location and length of stricture, the degree of function remaining in the affected kidney, overall kidney function and patient preference. Short strictures (<1 cm) may be amenable to endoscopic incision. Chronic, long term stenting, or percutaneous drainage may be recommended for patients with significant comorbid conditions. Longer strictures may involve treatment algorithms previously discussed regarding treatment of avulsion injuries.

3. Percutaneous Stone Treatment

Introduction

Goodwin, et al in 1955 described the technique of percutaneous drainage of a kidney for temporary relief of hydronephrosis.[74] 30 years later this technique of kidney access was resurrected to treat stone disease in an endoscopic manner. Percutaneous nephrolithotripsy 30 years later remains an important technique in the urologist's armamentarium in the treatment of upper tract stone disease.

Indications

Indications for percutaneous stone removal are listed in Table 6. CT of the abdomen without contrast is the most common diagnostic survey in patients who present with emergent renal or abdominal complaints. It is the most accurate means of diagnosis for renal stones (Figure 16). The administration of intravenous contrast in conjuction with CT provides an excellent study to define the renal and collecting system anatomy. In addition, CT provides the relationship of the kidneys to other intra abdominal organs, which can facilitate proper per cutaneous approaches to the kidney. A CT urogram provides an excellent radiographic study in this regard. (Figure 17).

Figure 16

Noncontrast CT reveals a right renal stone

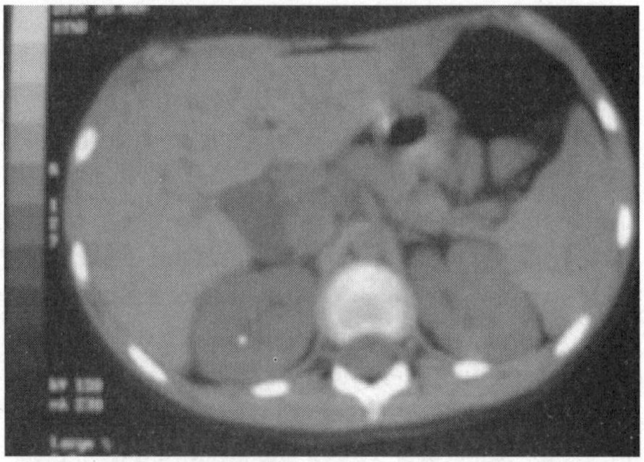

CT is the most accurate radiologic test to detect renal calculi. Calcium-containing stones, cystine, struvite, and uric acid stones are all radiopaque on CT.

Contraindications

Contraindications to percutaneous stone extraction are bleeding diathesis, abdominal anatomy precluding percutaneous access, unusual body habitus (morbid obesity, very long flank kidney length).

Preoperative Evaluation

Standard preoperative evaluation consists of detailed history and physical, correction of a bleeding diathesis, type and screen, and preoperative broad spectrum antibiotic in patients with sterile urine and bacterial specific antibiotic in patients with infection stones. (In patients with struvite stones, consider placing patients on 7-10 day course of bacterial specific antibiotic prior to the planned percutaneous procedure.)

Make a thorough examination of the radiologic imaging in order to plan the proper access(es), approximate the flank kidney length (using CT images), and determine other intra abdominal abnormalities which may call for changes in access (Figure 18, Figure 19a, Figure 19b). The technique of percutaneous stone extraction is specific to the location of the stone, the composition of the stone, other associated renal abnormalities, and body habitus. Percutaneous stone extraction entails the following steps: percutaneous access, tract dilation, stone manipulation, fragmentation, and removal, and drainage post stone extraction (Figure 20).

Figure 17

CT urogram details a complete upper pole staghorn calculus with several smaller lower pole stones

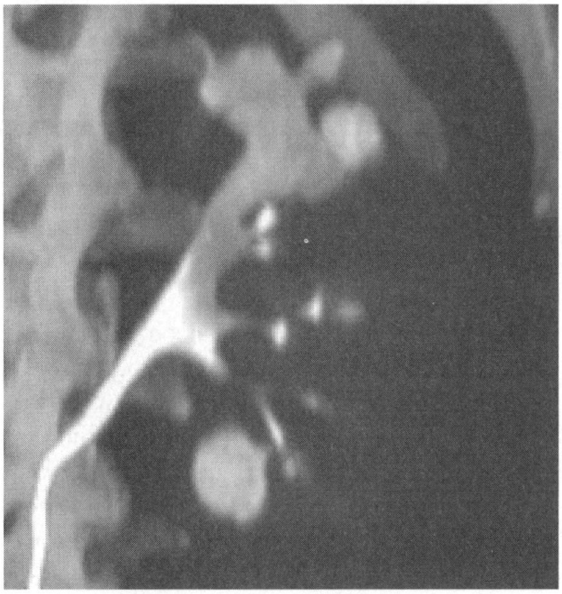

The pelvis and proximal ureter are opacified with contrast and are nondilated.

Technique of PCNL

Percutaneous tract placement can be performed in a staged or as a same session manner. If performed in a staged procedure, it is vital that the urologist com-

Figure 18

KUB of this 8-year-old boy revealed significant left renal stone burden

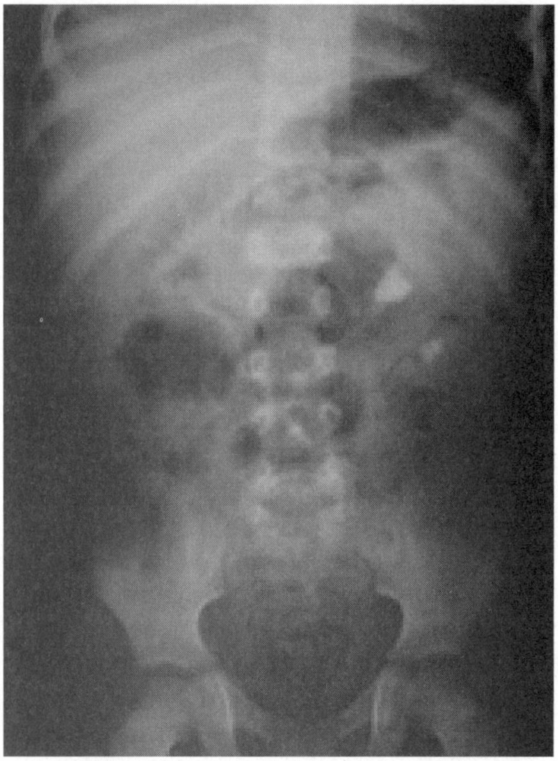

Due to the stone burden patient underwent successful PCNL. Access was obtained via an upper pole puncture. The two lower pole stones were removed using a flexible nephroscope.

Figure 19a

Nephrotomogram reveals a partial lower pole staghorn calculus

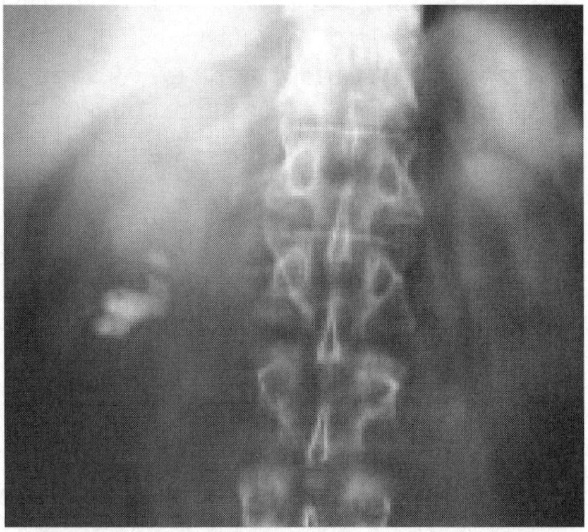

Figure 19b

IVP reveals good function of the right kidney

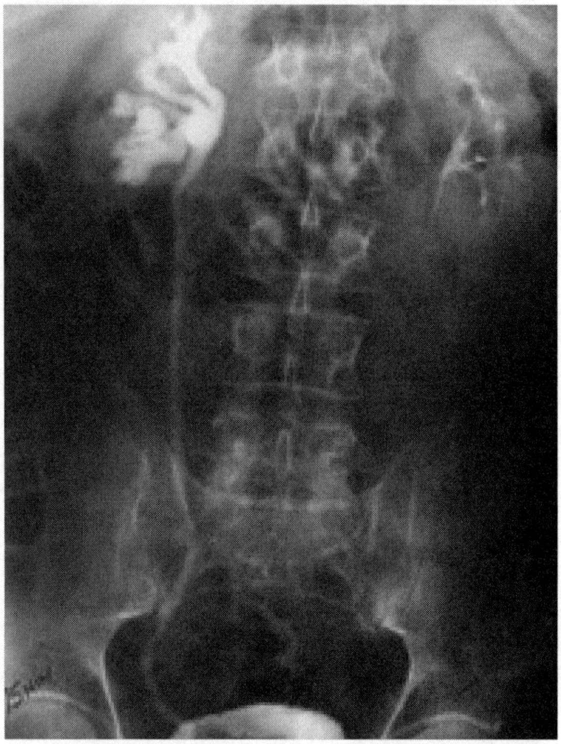

The lower pole also appears to function well despite the large staghorn occupying the entire lower pole moiety. This stone was removed via a posterior lower pole access.

municate to the radiologist which particular access is preferred, which access could be used as an alternate, and finally, which access will not work. Table 7 summarizes the equipment necessary to PCNL. Once access is achieved, drainage is accomplished usually with a small percutaneous catheter (8-14F).

In same session PCNL, patients can be initially placed prone (making sure to properly pad the patient), and flexible cystoscopy with retrograde catheter placement can be performed. An air contrast retrograde pyelogram can be done to outline the collecting system and aid in proper access (air will outline the posterior calyces) (Figure 21a, Figure 21b). This tract is then dilated to 24-30 F with a working sheath and optimally a safety wire securely down the ureter (preferred) or in the collecting system. In the majority of cases, a balloon dilation system is preferred. In cases where there is significant fibrosis of the renal capsule, serial dilation with Amplatz™ renal dilators may be necessary. In patients with horseshoes kidneys or analogous rotational anomalies, the contralateral side is elevated to provide medial rotation of the ipsilateral kidney. In morbidly obese patients who cannot be placed prone (usually due to respiratory issues), percutaneous access can be achieved either in a modified flank or true flank position.[75]

The nephroscope is inserted and blood clots are either removed with suction via the lithotripter probe or with forceps. The urothelium of the calyx should be identified. If the working sheath is too shallow (usually this is indicated by continued tract bleeding, or peri collecting system fat is seen), the scope can be directed into the collecting system and the sheath advanced or the balloon can be replaced more proximally and the sheath advanced over the inflated balloon. Irrigation for stone removal should be with warmed normal saline. Small stones <10 mm in diameter can either be removed whole using

Figure 20

Large right renal cystine stone in a 21-year-old female

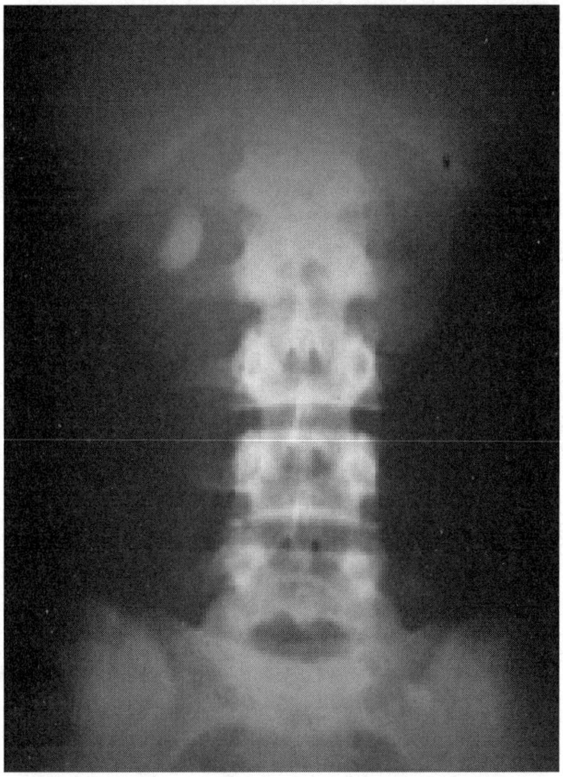

Cystine stones are typically shock-wave resistant. This stone was treated successfully with right PCNL.

graspers, or baskets (Figure 22a, Figure 22b). If when grasping or basketing large stones the stone becomes lodged within the working sheath, the stone can always be removed but counter traction on the sheath may need to be applied to prevent inadvertent sheath displacement. Usually, most stones require fragmentation, which can be accomplished using an ultrasonic suction lithotripter probe. Soft stones (eg, struvite, calcium oxalate dehydrate) can be removed exclusively using the lithotrite. Most stones, however, fragment into various sized fragments which migrate distally. The author prefers to initially fragment stones into relatively larger fragments, which are then removed with graspers. This technique reduces time required to retrieve residual fragments and reduced residual stone incidence. In stones which are ultrasound-resistent (calcium oxalate monohydrate, cystine stones, and some calcium oxalate/uric acid stones), either EHL or holmium laser lithotripsy may be necessary. In the case of using either EHL or holmium laser, the stones are fragmented to sizes which can then be removed with baskets or graspers.

Access to distance stone bearing calyces can usually be accomplished using the flexible nephroscope. Pressure irrigation is usually necessary to provide adequate visualization. Pressurized irrigation also can dilate previously nondilated calyces making their access possible, and can irrigate fragments from these calyces to the renal pelvis for easy suctioning. Inspection of the calyceal system can be facilitated by fluoroscopic injection of contrast via the working channel of the scope. The scope can then be easily directed under both direct and fluoroscopic guidance. Stones which require lithotripsy in calyces accessible only with the flexible scope will require either laser or EHL. 1.9 F EHL probes provide enough irrigation while having no effect on degree of scope deflection and is preferred by the author over holmium laser. If an occlusion catheter is not used or if there is concern regarding ureteral stones, then antegrade flexible ureteroscopy can be performed and stones treated with combination lithotripsy/basketing (Figure 23). In some cases, a second or third percutaneous access may be necessary in cases of significant stone burden. Secondary access may be necessary in cases of staghorn calculi, infundibular stenosis, or duplicated or bifid collecting systems.

Second session nephroscopy can also be performed 1-3 days following initial PCNL in patients with known residual stones or stones seen on follow up radiologic studies (noncontrast CT, renal tomograms, or nephrostrogram). In second stage nephroscopy, working sheaths are usually not necessary in these mature tracts, and therefore, access may be achieved in calyces which had been previously inaccessible.

Post procedural drainage previously was recommended, usually with a large diameter catheter to ensure adequate drainage of the collecting system (oftentimes the urine is bloody and small diameter catheters are prone to clotting off) and tract tampon-

Figure 21a

Gaining percutaneous access of a horseshoe kidney with a large pelvic stone

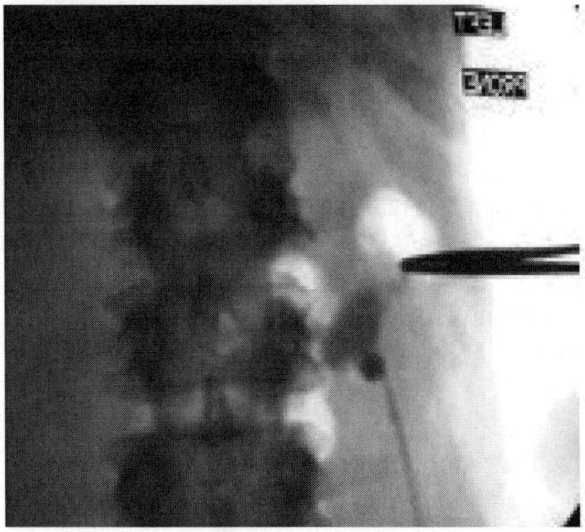

Access is via the upper pole as this portion of the kidney is closest to the skin. The most posterior upper pole calyx is outlined by air which was injected via the catheter. Also the risk of vascular injury is less via an upper pole access. Note the presence of the occlusion balloon catheter which was placed just prior to perc access. This catheter prevents antegrade migration of stone fragments from entering the ureter.

Figure 21b

Nephrostogram after successful PCNL in the horseshoe kidney

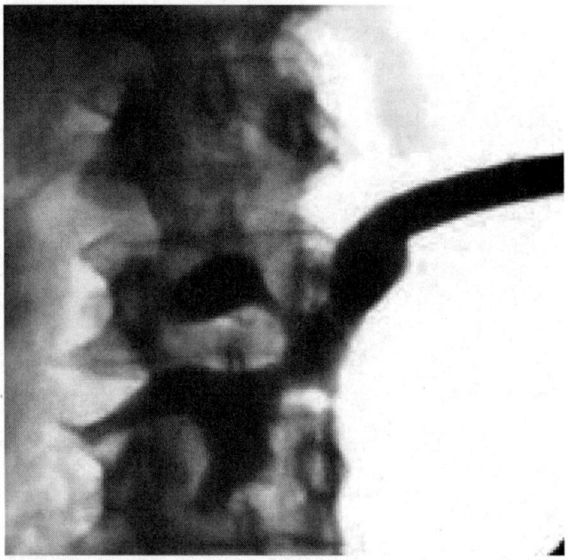

Note the catheter is through the upper pole. Note how medial and anterior the lower pole calyces are.

Figure 22a

Flexible nephroscope was used to access a 1 x 2 cm renal pelvic stone

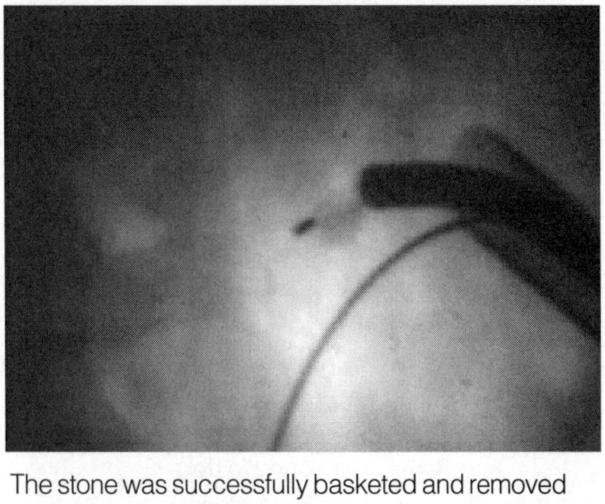

The stone was successfully basketed and removed without the need for lithotripsy.

Figure 22b

Endoscopic view of the stone in the renal pelvis during basket extraction

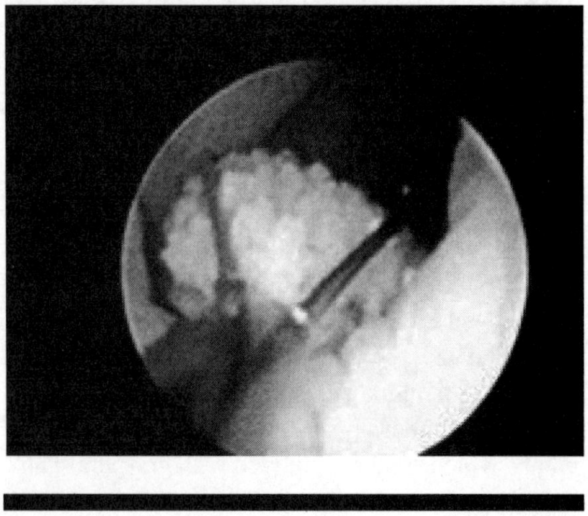

Table 7

Equipment Necessary for PCNL

Access	Retrograde balloon occlusion catheter (allows for RPG during same-session access) Perc access (18-22 G needle) 0.018 in wire, dilator sheath, cumpy catheter, 0.035 in guidewire, 0.035 in Amplatz Super Stiff wire, exchange catheter, balloon dilation catheter, 24-30 F working sheath
Endoscopes	Flexible cystoscope/nephroscope: used to place the retrograde catheter during same-session PCNL, and access to calyceal system not accessible with rigid scope Rigid nephroscope: used for ultrasonic/ laser lithotripsy, removal of large fragments Flexible ureteroscope: used to inspect the ureter if necessary for stones or stone fragments which are located in the ureter.
Ancillary Equipment	Ultrasonic lithotripter with lithotripter probes EHL with EHL probes 1.9-9 F Holmium laser with 200 – 600 micron fibers Stone forceps Stone baskets (0-tipped nitinol preferred)
Drainage	16-24 F Malekot catheters w/without ureteral extenders 10-16 F nephroureteral catheters 8-16 F pig-tail nephrostomy catheters 6-8 F internal ureteral stents

ade. Several authors have reported on successful "tubeless" percutaneous stone removal. Shah and associates reported their experience in 40 patients (45 renal units). The mean stone size in these patients was 33 mm and 23 patients had multiple stones. Three patients had a serum creatinine level of >2 mg/dL (>177 micromol/L). Five patients had successful bilateral simultaneous tubeless PCNL. In all, 51 tracts were required in 45 renal units, 30 of which were supracostal. There was no urine leakage or formation of urinoma after surgery, and no major chest complications in patients requiring a supracostal access tract, except for one with hydrothorax, managed conservatively. Stones were completely cleared in 87% of renal units and 9% had residual fragments of <5 mm.76 Limb and Bellman reported on 112 patients, 86 patients who underwent percutaneous stone extraction and 26 who underwent percutaneous antegrade endopyelotomy. In the group of patients undergoing percutaneous stone extraction, a 93.0% stone free rate was achieved with a mean stone burden of 3.30 cm (2). Patients stayed in the hospital an average of 1.25 days. A total of 5 patients required postoperative transfusions. One patient was found on readmission to have a pseudoaneurysm.[77]

Postoperative Care

Patients are usually admitted post procedure for intravenous antibiotics and pain control. Postoperative imaging can be performed to document stone-free status. Nephrostogram can document the patency of the ureter, and if patent, the nephrostomy can be safely removed. The tract typically seals over within 24 hours. Patients can then be discharged with a light dressing and allowed to return to normal activity in 7-10 days. In cases where the initial nephrostogram reveals persistent extravasation or obstruction, the larger nephrostomy tube can be "down sized" to a 10 F pigtail nephrostomy tube and still discharged. Typically the blood clot or edema causing the obstruction will lyse or resolve within 3 7 days, at which on follow up studies can be removed. Temporary internal ureteral stents can also be placed antegrade at the time of PCNL to ensure patency. These stents can be safely removed as an office procedure at follow up in 2 4 weeks. At this visit, review of the stone analysis, initiation of a metabolic evaluation, and functional studies, if applicable, can be performed.

Figure 23

Antegrade ureteroscopy can be used at the time of PCNL to ensure that there are no retained ureteral stone fragments

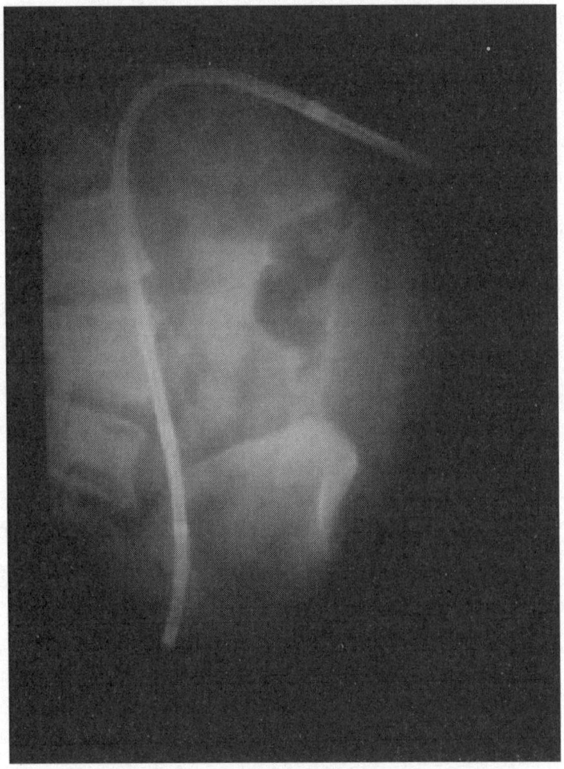

An occlusion balloon catheter can be placed with the balloon inflated at the UPJ or in the proximal ureter which may prevent distal migration of stone fragments during PCNL.

Results

PCNL has been proven to be a safe and efficacious method of removing stones, with success rates from some series ranging from 90% 100% (Figure 24).[73 76] *PCNL is the preferred method recommended by the AUA nephrolithiasis guideline panel for surgically treating staghorn or partial staghorn calculi.* The stone free success rate for PCNL versus

Figure 24

Retrograde pyelogram following most recent SWL demonstrates a large uric acid renal stone without any significant fragmentation

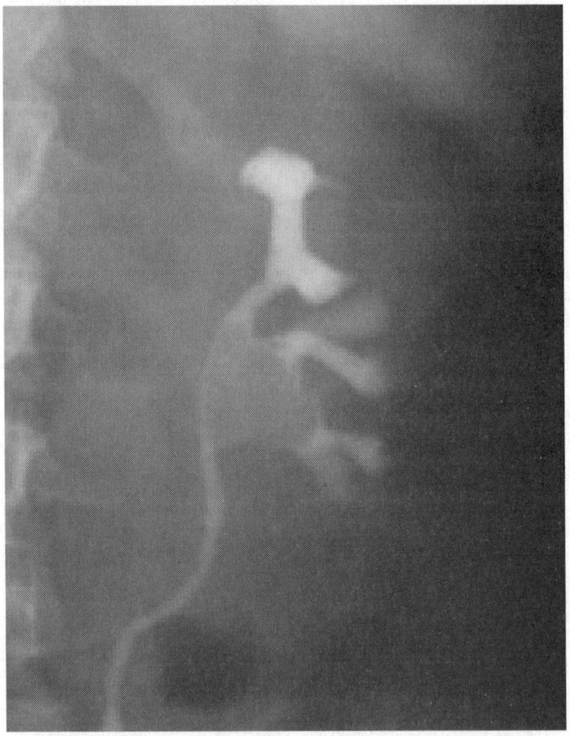

40-year-old woman referred for management of a renal stone. Patient had undergone 4 unsuccessful prior SWLs. Patient underwent successful left PCNL and was rendered stone-free. Patient continues to remain stone-free on an aggressive hydration and alkalinization program.

PCNL+SWL versus SWL alone was 78%, 66%, and 54%, respectively. Open stone surgery was less efficacious than PCNL with a stone free rate of 71%.[77]

Woodside and associates in 1985 described the first successful percutaneous nephrolithotomy in chil dren.[63] They reported on 7 children between the ages of 5 and 18 years of age who underwent PCNL using a technique similar to that described for adult PCNL. They reported a 100% stone free rate with no significant complications. Other investigators have reported their experience in pediatric PCNL with stone free rates of 66% 100% with comparable complication rates similar to adult series.[64]

Complications

Complications in PCNL can be categorized into: access related, endoscopic/stone removal related, immediate postoperative, and late complications and are summarized in Table 8.

The ideal puncture passes through the relatively avascular plane of Brödel into the calyx. The guidewire is then passed through the infundibulum into the renal pelvis. This approach avoids the larger renal vessels, which are anatomically related anteriorly and posteriorly to the major calyceal infundibula. Access can be either via a lower pole or upper pole calyx, depending on the stone, the configuration of the collecting system, and the level of the kidney in relation to adjacent organs. An upper pole access provides excellent access to upper pole stones and to the renal pelvis and proximal ureter but with a higher incidence of pleural injury. Lower pole puncture provides access to the lower pole system and renal pelvis but can limit access to the proximal ureter.

Lacerations or perforations, usually of the renal pelvis, can occur during dilation of the tract or while placing the working sheath and is usually due to over aggressive medial dilation either with the balloon or sequential dilators or inattentive sheath placement. This can be avoided by continuous fluoroscopic imaging during dilation and especially during sheath placement. Counter traction on the balloon is often necessary when placing the sheath. If laceration occurs, a large bore nephrostomy tube should be placed, and the PCN postponed with

Table 8

Complications of PCNL

Access-related
Renal laceration
Bleeding
Perforation
Injury to adjacent organs (pleura, lung, bowel, spleen)
Endoscopic/Stone Removal-related
Bleeding
Extravasation/fluid absorption
Ureteral/pelvic perforation
Immediate
UTI/sepsis
Retained stone fragments
Urinary obstruction
Death
Late Complications
Ureteral stricture
Loss of renal function

external drainage for 24-72 hours to allow healing (Figure 25).

Severe bleeding at the time of access can be arterial (rare) or venous. Venous bleeding is most commonly due to the working sheath being too shallow and not completely within the calyx or collecting system. Repositioning of the sheath is usually successful in decreasing this type of hemorrhage. Arterial bleeding is bright red and is independent of sheath location. Arterial bleeding is usually brisk enough that visualization is completely obscured. If an arterial injury is suspected the procedure should be stopped, and an arteriogram with embolization should be performed.

Figure 25

Right perinephric hematoma following PCN for a large staghorn stone

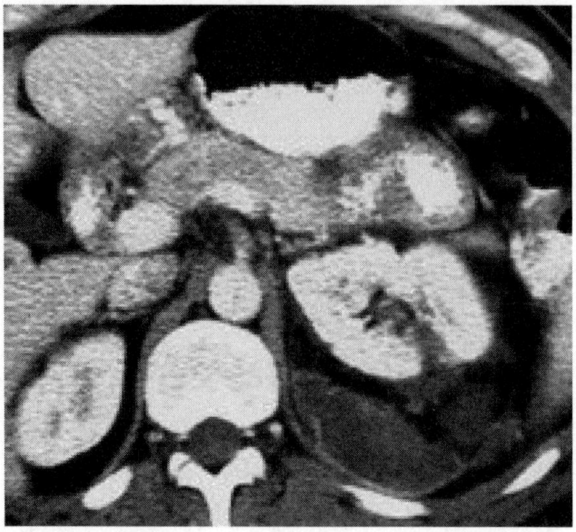

Patient remained asymptomatic and did not require blood transfusion. The hematoma completely resolved within 3 months.

Organs near the kidney are at risk of injury. *Patients undergoing puncture above the 12th rib have an approximate 10% risk of fluid within the pleura.* A supra 11th puncture has a 10% risk of hydrothorax or pneumothorax. A working sheath is highly recommended with upper pole punctures to minimize fluid build up within the pleural space. Fluoroscopic chest examination during and after can often detect a hydrothorax. ACXR in the recovery room is also recommended. Pleural injury should be suspected if there is loss of breath sounds, increase in respiratory pressures, and a decrease in oxygen saturation during the procedure. These symptoms, along with cyanosis, and tachypnea may be present in the immediate postoperative period. If a hydrothorax is diagnosed during the procedure, per cutaneous thoracentesis can be performed to drain the fluid, blood, or urine. Rarely, a chest tube may be necessary.

The incidence of bowel injury is quite rare. Colon injury is approximately 0.2% and is likely to occur in thin patients in which the tract is made too lateral, or in the morbidly obese. Extra peritoneal puncture of the colon can be managed nonoperatively by placement of an internal ureteral stent and withdrawal of the nephrostomy tube into the colon, thereby converting it into a colostomy tube. A follow up injection 7-10 days later of the colostomy tube is performed and if no leak is identified, then the tube can be removed. The internal ureteral stent can be removed in 1-2 weeks. If the puncture is intraperitoneal or if the patient develops fever, chills, or peritoneal signs with an extra peritoneal injury requires open operative repair, usually requiring temporary colostomy. Small bowel injury usu ally requires open or laparoscopic repair.[78 82]

Bleeding during stone extraction is usually due to inadvertent migration of the working sheath. In some cases it may be due to bleeding from the urothelium (most commonly seen in patients with severe inflammatory reaction to the stone with hyperemia of the collecting system). Bleeding can also occur with perforation of the collecting system, usually by placing undue pressure on the stone during ultrasonic lithotripsy or inattentive use of the grasping forceps during stone removal. Bleeding can also occur with avulsion of the infundibulum by placing undue torque with the rigid scope. If bleed ing such as this occurs which prevents adequate visualization, the procedure should be aborted, a drainage tube placed, with plans to repeat the procedure at a later date. Significant venous bleeding can occur at the end of the procedure with removal of the working sheath. If this occurs, a large bore nephrostomy tube (24 F) should be placed, pressure held at the site of the nephrostomy tube for 10 minutes with capping of the tube for 20-30 minutes to allow tamponade within the collecting system. The tube can then be uncapped and the urine will eventually lyse the clot. Gentle clot aspiration of the tube after 30 minutes will assist in providing patency.

Retroperitoneal extravasation of fluid occurs to some degree in all PCNL cases. *It is important to use normal saline to prevent hyposmolar hemolysis and hyponatremia (TURP syndrome).* It is difficult or next to impossible to measure accurately irrigation fluids. Retroperitoneal extravasation is best managed by placement of a nephrostomy tube left indwelling for 24-48 hours. Intraperitoneal extravasation which is manifested by abdominal distention, difficulty with ventilation, abdominal pain can be managed with diuretics in mild cases or peritoneal tap in severe cases.[83, 84]

Ureteral avulsion during percutaneous nephrolithotomy is rare (0.01%) and requires open repair.

Low grade fever (<100.5°F) in the first 12 hours following percutaneous stone is common and may be due to atelectasis or transient bacteremia. Fevers >101.5°F occur less commonly and patients should undergo blood and urine cultures, chest x ray, and continued on a broad spectrum antibiotic. Urosepsis occurs in 0.25 to 1% of patients following PCNL.85Patients with urosepsis should be managed with ICU monitoring, appropriate antibiotic cover age, and blood pressure and ventilatory support.

Deaths associated with percutaneous nephrolithotomy are rare and often related to other comorbid conditions, such as fatal arrhthymias, respiratory failure. Overwhelming sepsis and fatal pulmonary embolus has also been reported.75, 86,87

Hemorrhage due to an arterio venous fistula or pseudoaneurysm typically occurs anywhere from 2 days to 2 weeks following PCNL(Figure 26a, Figure 26b). The most common presentation is an acute bleeding episode 5-7 days postoperatively. *Patients who complain of one episode or intermittent gross hematuria should be suspected of having a fistula or pseudoaneurysm and undergo emergent*

Figure 26a

Patient underwent emergent renal angiogram which revealed a pseudoaneurysm

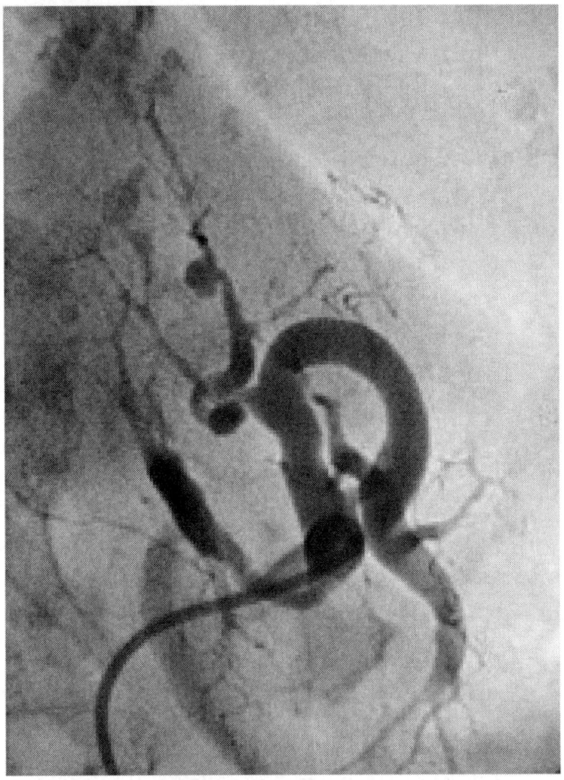

56-year-old male underwent left PCNL. Patient had an episode of gross hematuria 2 weeks following procedure.

Figure 26b

Patient had successful coil embolization with complete resolution of the pseudoaneurysm

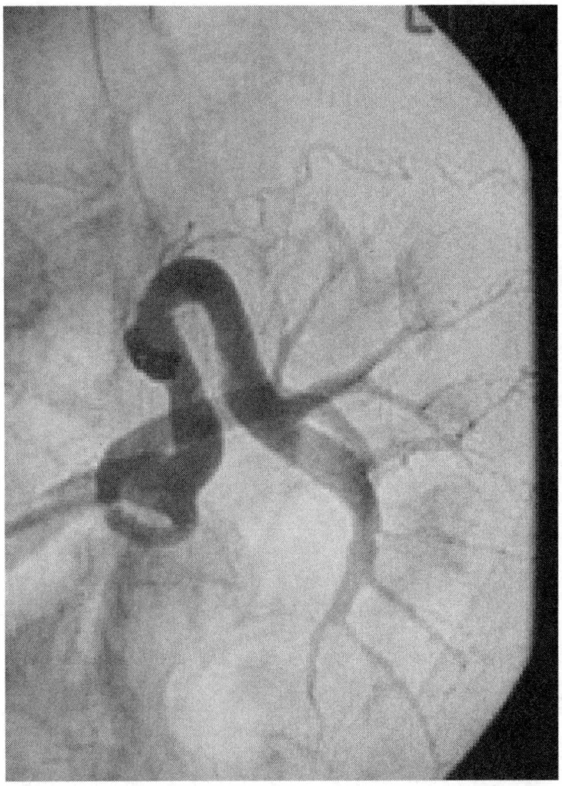

renal arteriography. Treatment for either of these vascular pathologies is selective angio embolization.[88, 89] Long term complications appear to be rare with the most common being ureteral obstruction. Renal dysfunction has been reported but it is unclear whether this was a direct result of PCNL or the natural history of a patient with significant stone disease and chronic UTI.

4. References

1. Chaussy C, et al. First clinical experience with extracorporeally induced destruction of kid ney stones by shock waves. *J Urol.* 1982;127:417.

2. Pace KT, et al. Shock wave lithotripsy at 60 or 120 shocks per minute: Arandomized, dou ble blind study. *J Urol.* 2005;174:595 99.

3. Zhou Y, Cocks FH, Preminger GN, Zhong P. Innovations in shock wave lithotripsy tech nology: updates in experimental studies. *J Urol.* 2004;172:1892 8.

4. Marberger M, Turk C, Steinkogler I. Piezo electric extracorporeal shock wave lithotripsy in children. *J Urol.* 1989;142:349.

5. Thomas R, et al. Effect of extracorporeal shock wave lithotripsy on renal function and body height in pediatric patients. *J Urol.* 1993;149:1082.

6. Cass AS. Renal function after extracorporeal shock wave lithotripsy to a solitary kidney. *J Endourol.* 1994;8:15 19.

7. Chandhoke PS, Albala DM, Clayman RR. Long term comparison of renal function in patients with solitary kidneys and/or moder ate renal insufficiency undergoing extracor poreal shock wave lithotripsy or percutaneous nephrolithotomy. *J Urol.* 1992;147:1226 30.

8. Pienkny AJ, Streem SB. Simultaneous versus staged bilateral extracorporeal shock wave lithotripsy: long term effect on renal function. *J Urol.* 162:151 3, 1999.

9. Cass AS. Renal function after bilateral extra corporeal shockwave lithotripsy. *J Endourol.* 1994;8:395 9.

10. Sheir KZ, Madbouly K, Elsobky E, Abdelkhalek M. Extracorporeal shock wave lithotripsy in anomalous kidneys: 11 year experience with two second generation lithotriptors. *Urology.* 2003;62:10 5.

11. Chen Y, Devivi MJ, Roseman JM. Current trend and risk factors for kidney stones in per sons with spinal cord injury: a longitudinal study.*Spinal Cord*. 2000;38:346 353.

12. Neuwirth H, et al. Use of extracorporeal shock wave lithotripsy in quadriplegic patients. *JAMA*. 1986;256:1295.

13. Lazare JN, Saltzman B, Sotolongo J. Extracorporeal shock wave lithotripsy treatment of spinal cord injury patients. *J Urol*. 1988;140:266 269.

14. Deliveliotis C, et al. Extracorporeal shock wave lithotripsy in paraplegic and quadriplegic patients. *Int Urol Nephrol*. 1994;26:151 154.

15. Colistro R, et al. Unenhanced helical CT in the investigation of acute flank pain. *Clin adiol*. 2002;57:435 41.

16. Mendelson RM, et al. Renal colic: a prospec tive evaluation of non enhanced spiral CT versus intravenous pyelography. *Australas adiol*. 2003;47:22 28.

17. Madbouly K, et al. Slow versus fast shock-wave lithotripsy rate for urolithiasis: a prospective randomized study. *J Urol*. 2005, 173: 127-130.

18. Chacho, J, et al. Does a slower treatment rate impact the efficacy of extracorporeal shock wave lithotripsy for solitary or ureteral stones? *J Urol* 2006, 175: 1370-74.

19. McAteer JA, et al. Treatment protocols to reduce renal injury during shock wave lithotripsy. *Cur Opin Urol*. 2009, 19, 192-95.

20. Bierkaus AF, et al. The value of antibiotic pro phylaxis during extracorporeal shock wave lithotripsy in the prevention of urinary tract infections in patients with urine proven sterile prior to treatment. *Eur Urol*. 1997;31:30 35.

21. Ilker Y, et al. Antimicrobial prophylaxis in management of urinary tract stones by extra corporeal shock wave lithotripsy: is it neces sary? *Urology*. 1995;46:165 7.

22. Deliveliotis C, et al. The necessity of prophy lactic antibiotics during extracorporeal shock wave lithotripsy. *Int Urol Nephrol*. 1997;29:517 21.

23. Pearle MS, Roehrborn CG. Antimicrobial prophylaxis prior to shock wave lithotripsy in patients with sterile urine before treatment: a meta analysis and cost effectiveness analysis. Urology. 1997;49:679 86.

24. Kupeli B, et al. Does tamsulosin enhance lower ureteral stone clearance with or without shock wave lithotripsy?*Urology*. 2004;64:1111 5.

25. Gravina GL, et al. Tamsulosin treatment increases clinical success rate of single extra corporeal shock wave lithotripsy of renal stones.Urology. 2005;66:24 8.

26. Porpiglia F, et al. Role of adjunctive medical therapy with nifedipine and deflazacort after extracorporeal shock wave lithotripsy of ureteral stones.Urology. 2002;59:835 8.

27. Weizer A, Preminger GM. Shock wave lithotripsy: current technology and evolving concepts. AUA Updates. Lesson 36; Vol. 24. 2005;314 323.

28. Bierkins AF, et al. Extracorporeal shock wave lithotripsy for large calculi: the role of ureteral stents. Arandomized trial. J Urol. 1991;145:699 702.

29. Prior JL, Jenkins AD. Use of double pigtail stents in extracorporeal shock wave lithotripsy. J Urol. 1990;143:475 478.

30. Chandkoke PS, et al. Arandomized outcomes trial of ureteral stents for extracorporeal shock wave lithotripsy of solitary kidney or proxi mal ureteral stones. J Urol. 2002;167: 1981 83.

31. Park JK Cui Y, Oh HK Koh GY, Cho KW. Activation of nitric oxide cyclic guanosine monophosphate signaling in kidney by extracorporeal shock wave lithotripsy. *J Urol.* 2003;170:2459 62.

32. Delvecchio F, Auge BK, Munger R, Brown SA, Brizuela R, Zhog P, Preminger GM. Shock wave lithotripsy causes ipsilateral renal injury remote from the focal point: role of regional vasoconstriction. *J Urol.* 2003;169:1526 9.

33. Jocham D. Clinical studies documenting renal change after ESWL. In: *Principles of Extra corporeal Shock Wave Lithotripsy.* New York: Churchill Livingstone; 1978:43.

34. Wilson WT, Miller GL, Morris JS, Fulgham PF, McDougall L, Erdman W, Preminger GM. Morphologic renal changes following piezo electric lithotripsy or spark gap lithotripsy. In: *Shock Wave Lithotripsy II: Urinary and Biliary.* New York: Plenum Press; 1989:19.

35. Knapp PM, et al. Extracorporeal shock wave lithotripsy induced perirenal hematomas. J Urol. 1988;139:700 3.

36. Dhar NB, et al. Amultivariate analysis of risk factors associated with subcapsular hematoma formation following electromagnetic shock wave lithotripsy. J Urol. 2004;172:2271 4.

37. Kostakopoulos A, et al. Subcapsular hematoma due to ESWL: risk factors. Astudy of 4,247 patients.Urol Int. 1995;55: 21 4.

38. Collado Serra A, et al. Renal hematoma as a complication of extracorporeal shock wave lithotripsy.Scand J Urol Nephrol. 1999;33: 171 5.

39. Newman LH, Saltzman B. Identifying risk factors in development of clinically significant post shock wave lithotripsy subcapsular hematomas.Urology. 1991;38:35 8.

40. Kostakopoulos A, et al. Subcapsular hematoma due to ESWL: risk factors. Astudy of 4,247 patients.*Urol Int.* 1995;55:21 4.

41. Malhotra V, et al. Life threatening hypoxemia after lithotripsy in an adult due to shock–wave induced pulmonary contusion. *Anesthesiology.* 1991;75:529 3.

42. Tiede JM, Lumpkin EN, Wass CT, Long TR. Hemoptysis following extracorporeal shock wave lithotripsy: a case of lithotripsy induced pulmonary contusion in a pediatric patient. *J Clin Anesth.* 2001;15:530 3.

43. Coptcoat MJ, et al. The complications of extracorporeal shock wave lithotripsy: management and prevention. *Br J Urol.* 1986;58:578.

44. Soyupek S, et al. Risk factors for the formation of a steinstrasse after shock wave lithotripsy.*Urol Int.* 2005;74:323 5.

45. Madbouly K, et al: Risk factors for the formation of a steinstrasse after extracorporeal shock wave lithotripsy: a statistical model. *J Urol.* 2003;169:292.

46. Al Awadi KA, et al. Steinstrasse: a comparison of incidence with and without J stenting and the effect of J stenting on subsequent management. *BJU Int.* 1999;84:618 21.

47. Sulaiman MN, Buchholz NP, Clark PB. The role of ureteral stent placement in the preven tion of steinstrasse. *J Endurol.* 1999;13:151 5.

48. Fedullo LM et al. The development of stein strassen after ESWL: frequency, natural his tory, and radiologic management. *Am J oentgenol* (AJR) . 1988;151:1145 7.

49. Resim S, Ekerbicer HC, Ciftci A. Role of tamsulosin in treatment of patients with stein strasse developing after extracorporeal shock wave lithotripsy.*Urology.* 2005;66:945 8.

50. Krambeck AE, et al. Diabetes mellitus and hypertension associated with shock wave lithotripsy of renal and proximal ureteral stones at 19 years of followup. *J Urol.* 2006;175:1742 7.

51. McDougall EM, et al. Does the cleaning technique influence the durability of the <9 F flex ible ureteroscope? *J Endourol.* 2001;15: 615 18.

52. White MD, Moran ME. Fatiguability of the latest generation ureteropyeloscopes. Richard Wolf vs. Karl Storz. *J Endourol.* 1998;12:S182.

53. Garvin TJ, Clayman RV. Balloon dilation of the ureter for ureteroscopy. *J Urol.* 1991;146:742 5.

54. Kourambas J, Byrne RR, Preminger GM. Does a ureteral access sheath facilitate ureteroscopy? *J Urol.* 2001;165:780 93.

55. Watterson JD, et al. Safety and efficacy of holmium: YAG laser lithotripsy in patients withbleeding diathesis. *J Urol.* 2002;168:442 45.

56. Hollenbeck BK, et al. Routine placement of ureteral stents is unnecessary after ureteroscopy for urinary calculi.*Urology.* 2001 Apr;57(4):639 43

57. Srivastava A, et al. Routine placement of ureteral stent is unnecessary after ureteroscopy for urinary calculi.*Urology.* 2001;Apr;57(4):639 43.

58. Byrne RR, et al. Routine ureteral stenting is not necessary after ureteroscopy and ureteropyeloscopy: a randomized trial. *J Endourol.* 2002 Feb;16(1):9 13.

59. Borborough PG, et al. Ureteral stenting after ureteroscopy for distal ureteral calculi: a multi institutional prospective randomized controlled study assessing pain, outcomes and complications. *J Urol.* 2001 Nov;166(5):1651 7.

60. Weizer AZ, et al. Routine postoperative imag ing is important after ureteroscopic stone manipulation. J Urol. 2002 Jul;168(1):46 50.

61. Bugg CE, et al. Follow up functional radio graphic studies are not mandatory for all patients after ureteroscopy. *Urology.* 2002 May; 59(5):662 7.

62. Hollenbeck BK, Spencer SL, Faerber GJ. Use of a working channel catheter during flexible ureteroscopic laser lithotripsy. *J Urol.* 2000 Jun; 163(6):1808 9.

63. Auge BK, et al. Ureteroscopic management of lower pole renal calculi: technique of calculus displacement. *J Endourol.* 2001;15;835 38.

64. Kourambas J, et al. Nitinol stone retrieval assisted ureteroscopic management of lower pole renal calculi.*Urology.* 2000;56:935 9.

65. Schuster TG, et al. Ureteroscopic treatment of lower pole calculi: comparison of lithotripsy in situ and after displacement. *J Urol.* 2002;168:34 5.

66. Faerber GJ, Bloom DA. Pediatric endourology. In: Gillenwater JY, Grayhack JT, Howards SS, Duckett JW, eds. Adult and Pediatric *Urology.* St. Louis, Mo: Mosby; 1996:2739 2748.

67. Schuster TG, et al. Ureteroscopy for the treatment of urolithiasis in children. *J Urol.* 2002;167:1813 16

68. Smaldone MC, et al. Endourological management of pediatric stone disease: present status. *J Urol.* 2009, 181: 17-28.

69. Johnson DB, Pearle MS. Complications of ureteroscopy. *Urol Clin N Am.* 2004;31:157 71.

70. Grasso M, et al. Submucosal calculi: endoscopic and intraluminal sonographic diagnostic and treatment options. *J Urol.* 1995;153:1384 89.

71. Stoller ML, Wolf JS. Endoscopic ureteral injuries. In: McAninch JW, ed.*Traumatic and Reconstructive Urology*. Philadelphia, Pa: WB Saunders; 1996:199 211.

72. Roberts WW, et al. Ureteral stricture formation after removal of impacted calculi. *J Urol*. 1998; 159: 723-6

73 Delvecchio FC, et al. Assessment of stricture formation with the access sheath.*Urology*. 2003;61:518 522.

74 Goodwin WE, et al. Percutaneous trocar (needle) nephrostomy in hydronephrosis. *JAMA*. 1955;157:891 94.

75. Faerber GJ, Gow M. Percutaneous nephrolithotripsy in morbidly obese patients. Tech Urol. 1997;3:2 7.

76. Shah HN, et al. Tubeless percutaneous nephrolithotomy: a prospective feasibility study and review of previous reports. *BJU Int*. 2005;96:879 83.

77. Limb J, Bellman GC. Tubeless percutaneous renal surgery: review of first 112 patients. *Urology*. 2002;59:527 31.

78. Reddy PK, et al. Percutaneous removal of renal and ureteral calculi: Experience with 400 cases. *J Urol*. 1985;134:662. Saunders; 1995:179 185.

79. Lee WJ, et al. Percutaneous nephrolithotomy: Analysis of 500 consecutive cases.*Urol adiol*. 1986;8:61.

80. Segura JH, et al. Percutaneous removal of kidney stones: Review of 1000 cases. *J Urol*. 1985;134:1077.

81. Bass RB, et al. Percutaneous ultrasonic lithotripsy in the community hospital. *J Urol*. 1985;33:586.

82. Preminger GM, et al. Chapter 1: AUAGuide line on management of staghorn calculi: Diagnosis and treatment recommendations. J Urol. 173: 2005;1991 2000.

83. LeRoy AJ, et al. Colon perforation following percutaneous nephrostomy and renal calculus removal.*Radiology*. 1985;155:38.

84. Morse RM, et al. Iatrogenic colon and rectal injury injuries associated with urological intervention: report of 14 patients. J Urol. 1988;140:101.

85. Vallencien G, et al. Colonic perforation during percutaneous nephrostomy. *J Urol*. 1985; 134:1185.

86. Kumar A, et al. Isolated duodenal injury during relook percutaneous nephrolithotomy. *Br J Urol*. 1994 Sep;74(3):382 3.

87. Begun FP, et al. Small bowel perforation during percutaneous nephrolithotomy. J *Endourol*. 1989;3:81.

88. Segura JW. Complications of percutaneous lithotripsy. Baltimore, American *Urological Association Stone Update*. February, 1993;355.

89. Carson CC, Nesbitt JA. Peritoneal extravasa tion during percutaneous lithotripsy. *J Urol*. 1985;134:725.

90. Pardalidis NP. Complications of stone treatment. In: Smith AD, ed. *Controversies in Endourology*. Philadelphia, Pa: WB

91. Janetschek G, et al. Morphology of nephrostomy tract after percutaneous stone removal: a case report. *J Endourol*. 1988;2:67.

92. Symons S, et al. Challenge of percutaneous nephrolithotomy in patients with spinal neuropathy. *Int J Urol*. 2006 Jul;13(7):874 9.

93. Cannon GM et al. Renal pseudoaneurysm following percutaneous nephrolithotomy. *Can J Urol.* 2006 Feb;13(1):2984 7.

94. Kessaris DN, et al. Management of hemorrhage after percutaneous renal surgery. *J Urol.* 1995 Mar;153(3 Pt 1):604 8.

Chapter 15: Renal Parenchymal and Upper Urinary Tract Urothelial Neoplasms

Robert G. Uzzo, MD

Contents

1. Renal Parenchymal Neoplasms

A. Epidemiology

- Cancer is the second overall leading cause of death in the United States (following heart disease) and accounts for approximately 1 in 4 deaths. Other leading causes of death include:
  * Cerebrovascular disease (Number 3)
  * Chronic pulmonary diseases (excluding cancer) (Number 4)
  * Unintentional accidents (Number 5)
  * Diabetes (Number 6)
- Over the last 50 years, the death rate due to cancer has changed negligibly while deaths from:
  * Heart disease have dropped more than 2-fold
  * Cerebrovascular disease have dropped more than 3-fold
- In 2003, the number of net deaths from cancer dropped for the first time since 1930
- In 2008, approximately 745,000 men and 692,000 women were diagnosed with cancer. The rates of genitourinary (GU) cancer were as follows:
  * In adult men, GU cancers accounted for nearly 40% of all cancer diagnoses and 16% of all cancer deaths.
    - **Number 1: prostate cancer (33%)**
      * Lifetime probability of diagnosis 1 in 6
      * Accounts for 9% of all cancer deaths in men
    - **Number 4: bladder cancer (6%)**
      * Lifetime probability of diagnosis 1 in 28
      * Accounts for 3% of all cancer deaths in men
    - **Number 6: kidney cancer (3%)**
      * Lifetime probability of diagnosis 1 in 61
      * Accounts for 3% of all cancer deaths in men
  * In **adult women, GU cancers** accounted for approximately 3% of all cancer diagnoses
    - Number 9: kidney cancer (3%)
      * Lifetime probability of diagnosis 1 in 103
    - Number 11: Bladder cancer (2%)
      * Lifetime probability of diagnosis 1 in 85
- **Kidney cancer** is the **most lethal** of all GU neoplasms as a function of percentage of patients diagnosed with the disease who ultimately die of disease
  * **Prostate cancer**
    - Approximately 15% (28,000 deaths/year) of the 186,000 cases diagnosed each year
  * **Bladder cancer**
    - Approximately 201% (14,000 deaths/year) of the 69,000 cases diagnosed each year
  * **Kidney cancer**
    - Approximately 24% (13,000 deaths/year) of the 54,000 cases diagnosed each year
  * **Testicular cancer**
    - Approximately 5% (380 deaths/year) of the 8,090 cases diagnosed each year
- Male-to-female ratio for malignant renal parenchymal lesions is approximately 1.6 to 1
- Primarily a disease of the elderly with peak incidence in the 6th and 7th decades of life
- 10%-20% higher incidence in African Americans for unknown reasons
- 96% of cases are sporadic while 4% are associated with familial syndromes
- The incidence of kidney cancer has increased by a rate of approximately 2% to 4% per year over the last 3 decades. This may be explained by:
  * Increased incidental detection
  * Unidentified environmental influences
- There has been a steady rise in the reported mortality rates attributed to kidney cancer over the last 3 decades

- A slow stage migration has occurred with kidney cancer over the last 3 decades. Current rates of stage at the time the time of presentation are:

  * Localized disease—53%

  * Regionally advanced disease—20%

  * Metastatic disease—22%

- The **only** generally accepted **environmental risk factor** is **tobacco** exposure:

  * Increases relative risk by 1.4 to 2.5

  * All forms of tobacco have been implicated

  * Risk increases with cumulative exposure

B. Molecular Biology

- Relevant kidney cancer genes:

  * **3p25—the *VHL* gene (clear cell RCC)** encodes the VHL protein (pVHL)

  * **A tumor suppressor gene**
    - Tumor suppressor genes **negatively regulate growth**. Their essential function is to prevent uncontrolled proliferative processes including cellular division. Each gene has a corresponding copy of the tumor suppressor gene. **Knudsens's two hit hypothesis** predicts that it only takes one functioning copy to regulate growth, therefore both copies or alleles must be mutated or silenced in order to promote carcinogenesis. In the case of a germline mutation, the offspring inherit a mutated copy of the tumor suppressor from one of their parents. In this scenario, only the second copy of the gene need undergo somatic mutation to induce transformation. This is the case with inherited forms of clear cell kidney cancer associated with the VHL syndrome. In cases of sporadic clear cell carcinoma, the patient is born with two normal copies of the VHL gene, both of which need undergo a somatic mutation to induce transformation

- A small number of established genetic mechanisms are responsible for the majority of known mutations in tumor suppressors

  * **Loss of heterozygosity (LOH)** with or without homozygous deletion
    - Involves the loss of specific chromosomal regions that contain known or presumptive tumor suppressor genes. LOH may be achieved due to a deletion, gene conversion, mitotic recombination, translocation, chromosome breakage and loss, chromosomal fusion or telomeric end-to-end fusions, or whole chromosome loss. This may result in asymmetric loss of a gene or homozygous deletions whereby both copies of the gene are affected
    - LOH is a useful diagnostic marker because of its high level of specificity for transformed cells
    - **Point mutations**
      * Occur at the level of individual nucleotides where substitutions, insertions and deletions may result in frameshift, missense and nonsense mRNA transcripts and ultimately truncated or nonfunctional proteins
    - **Promoter hypermethylation**
      * In most somatic cells, the CpG dinucleotide "islands" in the controlling or promoter region of a gene are normally protected from methylation. Although not a distinct genetic event, promoter hypermethylation is an epigenetic event capable of silencing expression
      * One or more of these events may be responsible for nearly all inherited (germline) and 40%-70% of acquired mutation in VHL responsible for sporadic cases of clear cell RCC

  * **7q31**—the **cMet gene** (papillary RCC) (encodes met protein (**receptor tyrosine kinase family**)

- **An oncogene**

  * Responsible for gain of function molecular events leading to increased cellular growth, differentiation or proliferation through the accumulation of normal sig naling proteins or creation of a mutant activating protein

* Unlike tumor suppressor genes, oncogenes may only require a single mutating event to promote malignant transformation

* **The most common mutating genetic event of the cMet gene is believed to be a point mutation**

* **17p11—The Birt-Hogg-Dubé gene**
    • Tumor suppressor gene
    • Responsible for cases of oncocytoma and chromophobe carcinoma
    • Encodes for the folliculin protein (function unknown)

* **1q42**—The Hereditary Leiomyoma Renal Cell Carcinoma gene (**HLRCC**)
    • A probable tumor suppressor
    • Encodes for the Kreb's cycle protein fumarate hydratase

* **Tuberous Sclerosis Genes**
    • **9q34—TSC 1**
    • **16p13—TSC2**
    • Defects in TSC genes have not been directly linked to cases of RCC

C. Kidney Cancer Syndromes

• There are 4 described hereditary clinical kidney cancer syndromes (Table 1)

* All are **autosomal dominant:**
    • Von Hippel-Lindau (VHL)
    • Hereditary Papillary Renal Carcinoma (HPRC)
    • Birt-Hogg-Dubé (BHD)
    • Hereditary Leiomyoma Renal Cell Carcinoma (HLRCC)

*2 have cutaneous manifestations:
    • **BHD** and **HLRCC**

*No definitive increased ***genetic*** risk of **RCC** with:
    • Acquired renal cystic disease associated with dialysis
    • Autosomal dominant polycystic kidneys
    • Tuberous sclerosis

• **Von Hippel-Lindau**

* Syndrome includes (Table 2):
    • Retinal angiomas (among the earliest finding)
    • Endolymphatic sac tumors
    • Hemangioblastomas of the CNS (benign lesions)
    • Pancreatic cysts and islet tumors
    • Epididymal cystadenomas
    • Renal solid and cystic clear cell carcinoma
    • Pheochromocytomas
        * Most frequently associated with missense mutations of the *VHL* gene that encode for an amino acid substitution

* Relevant molecular pathway
    • A mutated *VHL* gene encodes for a mutated pVHL
    • pVHL regulated by its interactions with elongin and Cul family of proteins
    • The VHL protein complex in the cytoplasm is regulated by the Hypoxia Inducible Factor (HIF)
    • HIF marks the VHL protein complex in the cytoplasm for ubiquitination and degradation
    • If pVHL is mutated, it cannot bind HIF, which then translocates into the nucleus
        * As much as 1%-5% of the human genome may be under some degree of HIF regulation
        * Nuclear accumulation of HIF upregulates VEGF, PDGF, EGF, glucose transport proteins, TGF, erythropoietin, CAIX (important for acid base balance), CXCR4 (a chemokine) and other proteins which regulate cellular growth and development

• **Hereditary Papillary Renal Cell Carcinoma**

* The least common form of hereditary RCC

* All manifestations are confined to the kidney. There are no extrarenal findings

* Characterized by bilateral and multifocal type I papillary RCC

* Histological appearance of all tumors is identical.

Table 1

Familial RCC Syndromes[a]

Syndrome	Gene/Protein	Suppressor/Oncogene	Manifestation
Von Hippel-Lindau (VHL)	3p25/pVHL	Tumor suppressor	Clear cell RCC Cystic RCC Retinal angiomas CNS hemangioblastomas Pheochromocytoma
Hereditary Papillary RCC (HPRCC)	7q34/cMet	Oncogene	Type 1 papillary RCC No extra renal manifestations
Birt-Hogg-Dubé (BHD)	17p11.2/folliculin	Tumor suppressor	Chromophobe RCC Oncocytoma/Oncocytosis Cutaneous fibrofolliculomas Lung cysts pneumothorax
Hereditary leiomyoma RCC (HLRCC)	1q42/fumurate hydratase	Tumor suppressor	Cutaneous leiomyomas Uterine fibroids Type 2 papillary RCC

[a]*All are autosomal dominant*

• **Birt-Hogg-Dubé**

* Manifestations include:
  • Fibrofolliculomas of the head and neck. These lesions are usually painless and develop after the age of 30
  • Pulmonary cysts and spontaneous pneumothorax
  • Multifocal and bilateral renal tumors.
    * Most commonly oncocytoma and chromophobe carcinoma
    * Clear cell and papillary tumors can co-exist

* Other possible associations include nevi, parathyroid adenomas, lipomas, oral mucosal papules, colonic polyps or tumors

• **Hereditary Leiomyoma Renal Cell Carcinoma**

* Manifestations include:
  • Painful cutaneous leoimyomas which can occur anywhere on the body
  • Uterine leiomyomas (fibroids) – early age of onset, multiple and painful
  • Type 2 papillary RCC
    * Typically very aggressive tumors

D. Pathology and Classification (Table 3)

• Renal tumors can be classified by pathological and/or radiographic features

* Pathological classification of renal tumors

* The most common **benign** renal tumors include:

Table 2

Incidence and Age of Manifestations of VHL

Organ	Lesion	% Incidence	Mean Age of Onset (yrs)
Eye	Retinal angioma	25-60	25
CNS	Hemangioblastomas	10-72	33
Adrenal	Pheochromocytoma	10-20	30
Pancreas	Islet cell tumors Cysts	12 20-70	36 36
Epididymis	Cystadenomas	25-60	Unknown
Ear	Endolymphatic sac tumors	10	22

- Angiomyolipomas, oncocytomas, cortical adenomas, cystic nephromas, reninomas (JG apparatus tumors), leimyomas, capsular fibromas, vascular tumors such as arteriovenous malformations and pseudotumors
- Benign inflammatory tumors of the kidney include abscesses and granulomatous diseases such as XGP

* The **most common malignant renal** parenchymal tumors include conventional **(clear cell)**, **papillary**, **chromophobe** and **collecting duct carcinomas**

* Sarcomas of kidney include **leiomyo, lipo, angio, osteogenic, clear cell** and **rhabdomyosarcomas**

* Other tumors of the renal parenchyma include Wilms' tumors, neuroectodermal tumors, carcinoids, lymphoma, or metastases to the kidney

* Most renal cell carcinomas originate from the cells of the proximal collecting tubule with the exception of chromophobes, oncocytomas and papillary carcinomas

- Components of **RCC pathology** include:

  * Histology. The most common histologic types are:
    - **Conventional (clear cell) carcinoma**
      * Accounts for 70%–80% of all RCC
      * Yellow when bivalved, hypervascular with clear or granular cells. **Clear cells contain abundant glycogen and phospholipids**
      * 2%–5% contain sarcomatoid features
      * More aggressive clinical behavior compared with other histologies
      * Appear more likely to respond to immunotherapies and most anti-angiogenic (targeted) therapies
    - **Papillary (chromophilic RCC)**
      * **Second most common** histological type representing 10%–15% of all RCCs
      * More commonly found in subgroups such as those with **end stage renal disease**
      * Contain **basophilic** or **eosinophilic cells** arranged in papillary patterns; however, solid variants are possible
      * **Two subtypes** have been described including **type 1 (more basophilic with scant cytoplasm)** and **type II (more eosinophilic and more aggressive)**

* Tends to be multicentric in as many as 40% of cases
* Grade for grade and stage for stage, prognosis is likely not any different than with conventional RCC

• **Chromophobe RCC**

* Accounts for about 5% of all RCC

* Derived from the cortical portion of the collecting duct or distal tubule

* A perinuclear halo is a typical and a distinctive finding. It is due to microvesicles that stain positive for Hale's colloidal iron, indicating the presence of a mucopolysaccharide unique to RCC

* Studies suggest that the prognosis may be better than for conventional RCC

• **Collecting Duct (Bellini) Carcinomas**

* A rare subtype of RCC accounting for < 1% of RCC

* May occur in a younger population of patients

* Are derived from the medullary collecting system but often extend into the cortex

* Most cases are symptomatic and present at a later stage

* Immunohistochemical and molecular analysis suggest that these tumors resemble urothelial carcinomas

• **Renal Medullary Carcinomas**

* Occurs almost exclusively in association with sickle cell trait and is therefore **most common in African Americans**

* Typically diagnosed in the 3rd decade of life

* Most cases are locally advanced and metastatic at diagnosis

* Highly aggressive. Mean survival is 12 to 15 months

• **Sarcomatoid variants** have been described of almost all histologic types of RCC. It is therefore no longer considered a distinct cell type. They are:
  * Poorly differentiated regions of other histological types
  * Found in 1 to 5% of RCCs, most commonly with conventional or chromophobe RCC
  * Median survival is poor (depending on stage)

• **Grade**

* Nuclear features can be highly variable in RCC

* Grading systems are based on nuclear size, shape and presence or absence of nucleoli
  • Fuhrman's system is the most common classification for conventional RCC
    * Grade 1 and 2 are considered low grade
    * Grade 3 and 4 are considered high grade
  • Papillary (chromophilic) RCC are classified as type 1 (low grade, basophilic) or type II (high grade, eosinophilic)
    * Tumor grade is recognized as an important prognostic variable in RCC

• **Stage**

* Refers to the local, regional and systemic extent of disease

* Historically used the Robson staging system

* Currently uses the 2002 AJCC TNM staging system (Tables 4a and 4b)

* The major improvement of **TNM staging** system over that of Robson is that it **separates tumors with venous involvement**, which can be treated and potentially cured with an aggressive surgical approach, from those with lymphatic invasion. Also, the TNM system **defines the anatomic extent of disease** more explicitly and can be used to facilitate comparisons of data from centers worldwide

* The greatest point of controversy with the 2002 TNM classification of RCC is in the T3a subcategory. Specifically, T3a currently includes patients with extrarenal involvement of the

Table 3

Differential Diagnosis of More Common Adult Renal Tumors

Benign Renal Tumors	Malignant Renal Tumors
Renal Capsular Tumors	**Tumors of the Renal Pelvis and Ureter**
Fibroma	Papilloma
Leoimyoma	Urothelial carcinoma
Lipoma	Squamous carcinoma
	Adenocarcinoma
Renal Parenchymal Tumors	
Oncocytoma	**Renal Parenchymal Tumors**
Adenoma	Conventional carcinoma (clear cell)
Cystic nephroma	Papillary carcinoma
	Chomophobe carcinoma
Vascular Tumors	Collecting duct carcinoma
Hemangiomas	
Hamartoma	**Renal Sarcomas**
Lymphangioma	Leiomyosarcoma
Renal artery aneurysm	Liposarcoma
AV malformation	Angiosarcoma
	Hemangiopericytoma
Pseudotumors	Malignant fibrous histocytoma
Hypertrophic column of Bertin	Rhabdosarcoma
Mesenchymal Tumors	**Other Renal Tumors**
Leiomyoma	Carcinoid
Reninoma (JG tumor)	Lymphoma/leukemia
Metanephric adenoma angiomyolipoma	Metastases
	Wilms' Tumor
	Inflammatory Renal Tumors
	Abscess
	Focal pyelonephritis
	Xanthogranulomatous pyelonephritis
	Tuberculosis

adrenal gland and/or perinephric fat. Adrenal involvement is now well documented as a poor prognostic feature and it has been argued that tumors involving the adrenal should be classified as T4 (contiguous involvement) or M1 (non-contiguous involvement)

E. Evaluation and Imaging

- Clinical staging for RCC begins with a thorough history, physical exam and judicious use of laboratory tests:

Table 4a

AJCC TNM Staging RCC (2002)

Primary Tumor Stage (T)
Tx – Primary tumor cannot be staged
T0 – No evidence of primary tumor
T1 – Tumor confined to kidney and ≤7 cm
T1a – Tumor ≤4 cm
T1b – Tumor 4 cm and ≤7 cm
T2 – Tumor confined to kidney and >7 cm
T3 – Tumor locally advanced within Gerota's fascia
T3a – Involved adrenal and/or perinephric fat
T3b – Involves renal vein or IVC below diaphragm
T3c – Involve IVC above diaphragm
T4 – Tumor invades beyond Gerota's fascia

Regional Lymph Nodes (N)
Nx – Regional nodes cannot be assessed
N0 – No regional nodal involvement
N1 – Metastasis in a single regional lymph node
N2 – Metastases in more than one regional lymph node

Distant Metastases (M)
Mx – Distant metastases cannot be assessed
M0 – No distant metastases
M1 – Distant metastases

Table 4b

TNM Stage Grouping for RCC (2002)

Stage I	T1	N0	M0	
Stage II	T2	N0	N0	
Stage III	T1-T2	N1	M0	
	T3	N0-1	M0	
Stage IV	T4	N0-1	M0	
		Any	N2	M0
		Any	Any	M1

- Symptomatic presentation, significant weight loss (>10% of total body weight), bone pain and poor performance status all suggest advanced disease as do physical exam findings of a palpable mass or lymphadenopathy

- Nonreducing varicocele or lower extremity edema suggests possible venous involvement

- Absence of findings on history and physical exam does not rule out advanced disease

- Abnormal liver function tests, elevated alkaline phosphatase, sedimentation rate or anemia suggest possible advanced disease

- Renal functional assessment should include not only recent serum creatinine, but also a calculation of glomerular filtration rates (GFR) and Chronic Kidney Disease (CKD) stage

  * It has been demonstrated that 20% – 40% of patients presenting with solid renal neoplasms have CKD III or higher at baseline, emphasizing the need for nephron preservation

- Clinical clues will often be helpful in distinguishing a malignant renal mass from other causes (Table 5)

Table 5

Clues for the Differential Diagnosis of the Radiographic Renal Mass

Fever, flank pain, pyuria think inflammatory (pyelonephritis or abscess)
"Problematic stones" — think of XGP
Spontaneous RP bleed — think of underlying RCC
Speckled Ca^{++} — think of possible RCC
Look for fat by MRI, US or CT and consider AML, liposarcoma
For upper pole renal lesions always look for the adrenal
Always assess perirenal soft tissues
For calcified rounded hilar lesion — think about a renal artery aneurysm
Cystic lesions in middle-aged female — think of cystic nephromas

- **Imaging of the renal mass**

  * Radiographic staging of RCC requires a contrast based study demonstrating enhancement (blood flow) of the mass

    - 3 phase CT of the abdomen and pelvis with all 3 phases being done at the same setting is imperative. This is the single best test. Should not rely on a noncontrast CT or a contrast CT performed at different settings, especially on different machines. Enhancement (>15-20 units by CT) of the mass is required
    - MRI pre- and post-gadolinium should be reserved for patients with suspected venous involvement, those with an iodine contrast allergy and those with renal insufficiency
    - Patients with lymphadenopathy >2 cm generally harbor malignancy. Smaller nodes may be inflammatory
    - Venous involvement is best imaged by MRI. The sensitivity of CT for renal vein and IVC involvement is 78%–96%. Venography is reserved for patients with equivocal MRI findings or those with contraindications to MRI
    - Transesophageal echo is an accurate method of determining the cephalad extent of the tumor and may be used intraoperatively. It has no real advantage over MRI in the preoperative setting

  * **Metastatic evaluation** in all cases should include a routine chest x-ray, careful review of the CT findings of the abdomen and pelvis, and liver function tests

    - Bone scan, CNS imaging, and chest CT can all be reserved for symptomatic patients, abnormalities on CXR, abdominal imaging or laboratory studies (ie, elevated alkaline phosphatase), or patients with extensive disease identified by routine studies
    - PET has shown poor sensitivity for routine use in the evaluation of RCC

  * **Renal cysts identified by CT are classified according to the Bosniak system** (Table 6)

    - Bosniak I and II lesions are considered most likely benign and can be followed

- Bosniak IIF lesions require closer follow-up
- Bosniak III and IV lesions should be considered malignant and treated accordingly

* **Ultrasound findings**

- A simple cyst on US should be anechoic, have good through transmission and posterior wall enhancement
  * ***Complex or hyperdense cysts on US may appear to be a solid lesion and read incorrectly as solid renal masses consistent with RCC***
- Fatty lesions such as an angiomyolipoma (AML) appear hyperechoic (white) on US

* **MRI findings**

- A simple cyst on MRI will appear bright on T2 and dark on T1. It will not enhance. A perdense cyst may appear bright on T1 and dark on T2 depending on the age and composition of its contents. It will not enhance
- Fat (ie, from an AML) is generally bright on MRI but depends on technique. Look at subcutaneous fat for an idea as to how the fat looks on that particular MRI sequence

* **Percutaneous biopsy**
- Indications for percutaneous biopsy or aspiration remain limited due to difficulties interpreting limited amount of tissue obtained, sampling errors, and difficulties with differential diagnosis (ie, eosinophilic variants of RCC versus oncocytoma)
- Biopsies should be considered in patient with suspected lymphoma, abscess, or metastatic disease to the kidney. In most cases of patients with a primary malignancy elsewhere, metastases to the kidney are late and are usually accompanied by extensive disease elsewhere. Solitary renal metastases are uncommon

Table 6

Bosniak CT Classification of Renal Cystic Lesions

Bosniak Class	Cancer Risk	Rx	Comments
I (simple cyst)	0%	None unless symptomatic No follow-up needed	No enhancement Smooth, empty
II May be hyperdense (protein/blood)	<10%	None or follow (Bosniak IIF)	Few septa Thin linear calcification No enhancement
III (Indeterminate)	50%	Remove	Thick irregular wall or septa Thick calcifications Moderate septa May enhance Mild to moderate heterogeneity
IV (Cystic RCC)	80%-90+%	Remove	Enhancing nodules

F. Prognosis Factors

- Prognostic factors for RCC can be divided into anatomic, histologic, clinical and molecular categories:

  * Anatomic factors include tumor size, extension, adrenal, venous or lymphatic involvement OR radiographically identifiable metastatic disease
    * Histologic factors include histologic type, nuclear grade, presence of necrosis, sarcomatoid features and invasion of the collecting system

  * Clinical features include performance status, presence of symptoms related to primary or metastases, and weight loss. Also included are possible laboratory factors such as anemia, polycythemia, thrombocytosis, hypercalcemia and/or elevated alkaline phosphatase

  * Numerous molecular prognostic factors have been investigated. Currently none are used routinely in clinical practice

  * The most important prognostic factors remain stage, grade, histology, symptoms at presentation, and performance status

  * Several investigators have combined various prognostic factors into predictive algorithms or nomograms which may help predict recurrence or response to therapy (Table 7)

- 5-year risks of recurrence for local or regional RCC fully excised are approximately:

  * 5%–9% for low-risk disease

  * 20%–25% for intermediate-risk disease

  * 60%–80% for high risk disease

- Metastases from RCC have been reported in nearly every site in the body. Most metastases (50%–75%) are asymptomatic

  * More than 70% of metastases are identified by abdominal imaging and CXR

Table 7

Risk Stratification for RCC

Author	Institution	EOD	Histology	1° endpoint	Presentation
Kattan, et al (2001)	Sloan-Kettering	Local	All	Recurrence	Nomogram
Sorbellini, et al (2005)	Sloan-Kettering	Local	Clear cell	Recurrence	Nomogram
Frank, et al (2002)	Mayo (SSIGN)	Local/ M+	Clear cell	Survival	Algorithm
Zisman, et al (2001)	UCLA (UISS)	Local	All	Survival	Algorithm
Leibovich, et al (2005)	UCLA (SANI)	M+	All	Survival	Algorithm
Motzer, et al (2004)	Sloan-Kettering	M+	All	Survival	Algorithm

* The most common sites of recurrence are lung > bone > liver > adrenal > CNS (Table 8)

* Most recurrences occur within the first 24 months after resection. The risk of recurrence decreases as disease free interval increases

Table 8

Patterns of Recurrent RCC

Site of Recurrence	Median Time to Recur (yrs)
Lung (38%)	1.6
Bone (18%)	1.5
Liver (13%)	1.7
Local 10% (includes adrenal)	1.7
CNS (8%)	2.5

G. Management

- Surgery remains the mainstay of treatment for RCC
- The objective is to resect all tumor with an adequate negative surgical margin
- **Local disease**
  * **Open or laparoscopic/robotic radical nephrectomy**
    - The classic description of the radical nephrectomy includes early ligation of the vessels, removal of the kidney outside Gerota's fascia, excision of the ipsilateral adrenal and complete regional lymphadenectomy
    - The need for complete regional lymphadenectomy in all cases is not well defined and there remains a divergence of clinical practice in this regard, whereas nodal spread of RCC can follow an unpredictable route and there has never been a definitive therapeutic benefit shown with lymphadenectomy
      * Cases of clinically involved lymphadenopathy require resection of all involved nodes where feasible
    - Excision of the ipsilateral adrenal gland has also been controversial. It has been well demonstrated that removal is not routinely necessary in the absence of radiographic involvement unless the primary tumor extensively involves the kidney, is locally advanced or immediately adjacent to the adrenal gland
    - The operative approach to the kidney depends on the size and location of the tumor as well as the body habitus of the patients
      * Open approaches include flank (subcostal, intercostals or with excision of portion of the rib), chevron, or thoracoabdominal (especially useful on the right side with large upper pole tumors, IVC involvement or adjacent organ involvement)
      * Laparoscopic approaches include transabdominal, retroperitoneal or hand assisted
    - **Laparoscopic nephrectomy** has emerged as a **less morbid** and safe option for nearly all cases of localized RCC including large tumors **(<20 cm),** patients with significant prior surgical histories, the morbidly obese and even for cytoreduction or in cases with early venous involvement. Multiple studies have demonstrated the safety and efficacy of laparoscopic nephrectomy in these settings. Robotic approaches may assist in the learning curve but otherwise do not seem to improve pure laparoscopic approaches to nephrectomy or nephroureterectomy
  * **Nephron-sparing surgery (NSS)**
    - Interest in NSS has grown as a result of stage migration due to improved imaging, a greater experience with renovascular surgery, improvements in surgical methods including means to prevent renal ischemic injury, and excellent long-term published outcomes
    - NSS entails complete local excision of the renal tumors leaving the largest possible amount of normal functioning parenchyma. Enucleation of the tumor implies incompleted resection and is not a preferred term for

nephron sparing surgeries for localized kidney tumors. Indications are classified as:

* Absolute—bilateral tumors or a tumor in a anatomically or functional solitary kidney
* Relative—a renal tumor involving kidneys compromised or potentially compromised by systemic disorders which decrease global renal function (diabetes, hypertension, glomerulopathy, etc)
* Elective—an ipsilateral renal tumor in an otherwise healthy individual with two anatomically and functionally normal kidneys
    - The accepted tumor size **cut off** or elective partial nephrectomy is 4 cm; however, lesions up to 7 cm also appear amenable to safe elective partial nephrectomy depending upon the tumor's anatomy

- **Pre-, peri- and postoperative implications of NSS**

* Evaluation for a patient prior to NSS should include all staging considerations as out-lined above. In addition, specific renal imaging such as video three dimensional volume rendered CT may be useful to delineate the relationship of the tumor to the intrarenal vascular supply and collecting system. Additionally, a functional assessment of the contralateral kidney such as a contrast based CT or MRI or a nuclear renal scan is imperative

* Intraoperative considerations should mimic that of a donor nephrectomy with excellent exposure and hemostasis, complete vascular control, and promotion of a brisk intraoperative diuresis. Once these factors are assured, hilar clamping (usually independently with separate arterial and venous clamps), full excision with a negative margin, and detailed reconstruction of the collecting system and renal remnant are essential. Warm ischemic times should be less than 30 minutes and cold ischemic times should be less than 60 minutes whenever possible. Clamping and re-clamping should be avoided and is associated with reperfusion injury

* Patients undergoing NSS for absolute or relative indications, particularly in the case of a solitary kidney, should be told there is a 5%–8% risk of temporary or permanent dialysis associated with NSS depending on the renal tumor anatomy

* Urinary fistula rates are 3%–8% depending on the size of the lesion, the location of the lesion, the ischemic time and the experience of the surgeon. Most fistulae will close after a time with adequate drainage. Some may require a ureteral stent and/or foley catheter to promote healing

* Bilateral synchronous sporadic RCC occurs in 0%–5% of cases and may occur in African American men more commonly. In the case of bilateral RCC, surgeries are usually staged with the less involved size treated first. This provides more options to the surgeon and may reduce the need for perioperative dialysis
    1. Histological concordance rates of bilateral malignant renal masses appear to be as high as 90%

* Cancer specific survival rates depend on the pathological features of the tumor and are reported to be 80%–100% in most series. The risk of local recurrence is 5%–10% and may represent residual disease or de novo tumors secondary to microscopic multifocality

* Patients who undergo NSS, particularly those with a small amount of residual functioning nephrons, may be at **increased risk for hyperfiltration renal injury.** This places patients at increased risk for **proteinuria, focal segmental glomerulosclerosis** and **progressive renal failure.** Efforts to ameliorate the damaging effects of hyperfiltration injury have focused on dietary and pharmacological interventions including dietary restriction of protein (animal studies) and the use of an angiotensin converting enzyme inhibitor

* Nephron-sparing surgery has been associated with significantly lower rates of chronic kidney disease than radical nephrectomy with lower associated rates of comorbidity and mortality

- **Laparoscopic/robotic vs. open NSS:**

  * **The most robust experience exists with open NSS and it should be considered the standard of care for most cases of localized solid renal masses**

  * Laparoscopic NSS presents a considerable technical challenge given the concerns about hemostasis, margin status and reconstruction of the renal remnant. Nevertheless, several series demonstrate good initial results in selected patients, although the reported rates of introperative and postoperative complications (including reoperation rates) are higher than those for open NSS

  * **Laparoscopic NSS** is generally performed via a **transabdominal approach** given the larger working space. Intraoperative ultrasound may facilitate the procedure. Retroperitoneoscopic NSS is feasible in well selected patients

  * Robotics permits a 3D view of the tumor as well as better articulation and may improve perioperative complication rates of minimally invasive partial nephrectomies

    - NSS for patients with VHL represents an absolute indication. Adequate surgical treatment requires excision of all solid and cystic renal lesions. Unfortunately, patients with VHL have multifocal disease which can rarely be excised fully without radical nephrectomy. Several studies demonstrate a 3 cm threshold to intervene in patients with VHL. In these patients, lesions >3cm have been shown to have a greater propensity toward the development of metastases; although there have been reports of smaller lesions associated with metastases. Therefore, NSS may be withheld until the dominant lesion reaches 3 cm. Surgery should then be aimed at "resetting the biological clock" such that all dominant lesions are excised and the renal remnant is watched closely until a dominant lesion reaches 3 cm. Options in this setting include radical nephrectomy with transplantation, attempted NSS or ablative technologies

* **Ablation**

  - Thermal ablative techniques include renal cryosurgery and radiofrequency ablation (RFA)
  - Both can be administered percutaneously or through laparoscopic exposure thus decreasing morbidity and allowing a more rapid recovery
  - Preliminary data suggest that these therapies are effective but the length of follow-up in most studies is quite limited (on average 15–18 months) and long-term efficacy is not established
  - Acceptable candidates for thermal ablations are patients with advanced age, patients with significant comorbidities and those with recurrence after prior NSS
  - Tumors most amenable to ablation are small (< 3.5 cm), peripheral, solid, exophytic lesions remote from major vascular and collecting system structures. These are the same characteristics of the ideal tumor for NSS
  - Heat sinking refers to the dissipation of thermal energy by nearby vascular structures. This is a greater concern with RFA than with cryosurgery. Animal data also suggests there is a greater risk of urinary collecting system injury and fistula formation with RFA than with cryosurgery. Therefore, the type of energy ablation used should be carefully considered for lesions close to the collecting system and larger intrarenal vessels
  - Recurrence and re-treatment rates appear lower with cryosurgery than with RFA. This may be a function of either the application or the technology
  - Lack of enhancement of an ablated mass does not always correspond with histological absence of tumor on biopsy. This troublesome finding is more common with RFA
  - Both ablative techniques cause tumor death by immediate cellular damage and delayed microcirculatory failure
  - The ideal treatment parameters are yet to be fully determined; although most will double, ablate (2 cycles) for a margin of safety

Table 9

Active Surveillance Series in RCC

Study	Institution	N	Mean Lesion Size (cm)	Mean Growth Rate (cm/yr)	Mean F/U Duration (months)
Fujimoto, et al	Sendai Shakaihoken Sendai Hospital, Japan	6	2.47	0.47	29
Bosniak, et al	NYU Medical Center New York	40	1.73	0.36	39
Kassouf, et al	McGill Univ. Health Center Montreal, Canada	26	3.27	0.09	32
Volpe, et al	Princess Margaret Hosp. Toronto, Canada	32	2.48	0.1	35
Wehle, et al	Mayo Clinic Jacksonville, FL US	29	1.83	0.12	32
Kato, et al	Tohoku School of Medicine Sendai, Japan	18	1.98	0.42	27
Sowery, et al	Kingston General Hospital Kingston, Canada	22	4.08	0.86	26
Chawla, et al	Fox Chase Cancer Center Philadelphia, PA	61	2.97	0.20	36
TOTAL		234	2.60	0.28	34

- Imaging concerns remain one of the greatest obstacles to ablative technologies. Real time imaging is best achieved with intraoperative ultrasound; however, most ablations will error overtreatment of the tumor to attain an adequate margin. For this reason, more nephrons may be lost during ablation than excision
- Reported recurrence and/or persistence rates following ablative techniques are between 5%–15%
- Prior tumor ablation makes NSS considerable more difficult and may obviate successful nephron preservation in the future

* **Active surveillance**

- The natural history of untreated small enhancing renal masses presumed to be RCC is becoming better defined whereas previously all tumors were promptly excised
- Elderly patients or those with significant medical risks are offered the opportunity for serial radiographic surveillance to define the growth kinetics of untreated RCC
- Collectively there are approximately more than 500 small renal masses reported in the literature which have undergone a period of

active surveillance for an average of nearly 3 years. In about half of these, pathology is available and in over 80+% RCC was present

- Although the growth kinetics may be some what variable, the rate of radiographic growth in most series is between 0 and 0.86 cm/yr (Table 9)
- As many as 30% of small renal masses show no radiographic growth when followed over a median of 3 years
- The risk of metastatic progression in active surveillance series appears to be quite low at about 1% at a median follow up of 3 years.
- Most series are limited by their retrospective nature and selection biases
- Active surveillance of a small enhancing renal mass requires periodic contrast based cross sectional imaging which is often more frequent initially (every 3–6 months in the first 12 years) and less frequent once stability or slow growth kinetics are established
- Data exist which demonstrate that a judicious period of active surveillance of small localized renal masses in elderly patients or those with co-morbidities followed by delayed intervention as necessary does not place patients at excessive risk for stage or grade progression
- Active surveillance, like any intervention, is a calculated risk

Table 10a

Postoperative Surveillance After Radical Nephrectomy

Stage	History, Exam and Labs	CXR	Mean Age of Onset (yrs)
T1N0M0	Yearly	None (pT1a) Yearly (pT1b)	None (pT1a) Every 2 years (pT1b)
T2N0M0	Yearly	Yearly	Every 2 years
T3N0M0	Every 6 months for 3 years then yearly	Every 6 months for 3 years then yearly	At 1 year then every 2 years

Table 10b

Postoperative Surveillance After Partial Nephrectomy

Stage	History, Exam and Labs	CXR	Mean Age of Onset (yrs)
T1N0M0	Yearly	None (pT1a) Yearly (pT1b)	None (pT1a) Every 2 years (pT1b)
T2N0M0	Yearly	Yearly	Every 2 years
T3N0M0	Every 6 months for 3 years then yearly	Every 6 months for 3 years then yearly	Every 6 months for 3 years then every 2 years

* **Follow-up after definitive treatment for localized RCC:**

  • Surveillance for recurrence is important after surgical excision of RCC
  • Stage-specific surveillance means that follow-up intervals are based upon the likelihood of recurrence as a reflection of the tumor's pathological stage, grade and type
  • All patients should be evaluated periodically with a history, physical examination and selected serum studies (calcium, hemoglobin, liver and renal profiles (including GFR and CKD staging)) yearly or twice yearly
  • Radiographic studies including CXR and CT or MRI are tailored to risk based on stage (Table 10a, Table 10b), grade, and histology.
    * For patients with fully resected T1 RCC, the risk of recurrence is small and many will omit further radiographic studies after the first 2 years
    * For patients with T2 disease, a CXR should be considered yearly and a CT or MRI every 2 years
    * For patients with T3 disease, CXR and body imaging by CT or MRI should be performed every 6 months for 3 years and then yearly
    * Asynchronous renal recurrences in the contralateral kidney occur in 0%–5% of cases and may be higher in African American men. The preferred treatment for a contralateral recurrence is NSS, whereas they are ordinarily identified early and there is often a relative or absolute indication

* **Locally advanced and metastatic disease**

  • Surgery for locally advanced RCC:
  • The principles of surgery for locally advanced RCC remain the same, excision of all localized disease. This ordinarily involves radical nephrectomy, adrenalectomy, regional lymphadenectomy and thrombectomy where appropriate
  • In highly selective cases, NSS may be appropriate and feasible in the setting of node positive disease and/or venous involvement
  • **Principles of surgery for venous involvement include** complete excision with full vascular control

* Involvement of the IVC with RCC occurs in 4%–10% of patients
* In cases of suspected venous involvement, it is imperative to determine the highest level of involvement preoperatively. This is often best staged with an MRV
* Staging includes: level 1 – into the renal vein and ostium, level 2 – extending up the IVC to below the hepatics, level 3 – involving the intrahepatic portion of the IVC, and level 4—extending above the diaphragm
* The prognostic significance of the level of involvement has been controversial
* 5-year survival for fully resected M0 RCC with IVC involvement is reported to be 50% to 70%
* Preoperative angioinfarction may be useful in cases of arterialization of the thrombus or in patients with excessive hilar adenopathy in whom ligating the artery first may be problematic
* For cases of level 1 thrombus, simple milking back of the clot into the renal vein with open or laparoscopic ligation proximally is often sufficient
* For cases of level 2 thrombus, control and sequential clamping of the IVC above and below the clot and the contralateral renal vein after full exposure and ligation of lumbar veins provides a bloodless field
* For cases of radiographic level 3 thrombus, it is may be possible to get above the clot by ligating short hepatics to the caudate lobe of the liver, isolating and selectively clamping the porta hepatis and proceeding as with a level 2 clot. In cases where the hepatic veins are clearly involved, full mobilization of the right lobe of the liver with selective veno-veno bypass has been used successfully
* For cases with level 4 thrombus, cardiopulmonary bypass and hypothermic circulatory arrest is the preferred approach
* Bland thrombus without active RCC may be seen in the IVC below the level of the renal veins. If extensive, it need not be fully resected but consideration should be made for placement of an IVC clip/filter or caval interruption to prevent subsequent embolization.
* Mortality rates associated with radical nephrectomy and IVC thrombus have ranged as high as 5%–10%

* **Cytoreductive Nephrectomy**

  - Removal of the kidney in patients with metastatic RCC is termed cytoreductive
  - In the immunotherapy era, some patients were unable to proceed to systemic therapy, calling into question the benefit of cytoreduction
  - In a randomized prospective trial sponsored by SWOG, the role of cytoreductive nephrectomy was shown to be associated with a statistically significant improved overall survival
  - Selection is key to identifying those most likely to benefit from cytoreductive nephrectomy. Patients should have a good performance status, lower volume metastatic disease, and fewer hepatic or osseous metastases
    * CNS metastases are generally considered contraindications to cytoreduction except in rare circumstances (low volume, low extrarenal disease burden, young healthy patients)
  - Cytoreduction has been successfully performed laparoscopically; however, a laparoscopic approach should not compromise the primary goal which remains excision of all localized disease including involved regional lymph nodes
  - For locally advanced RCC involving adjacent organs such as colon or spleen, cytoreduction is often necessary to control local symptoms. En bloc resection is the primary aim. In selective patients such as those with solitary regional metastases, long term survival is possible with wide excision

* **Metastasectomy**

  - Resection of synchronous or metachronous metastatic RCC (mRCC) is termed metastasectomy
  - Aggressive surgical resection may be associated with favorable long term survival
  - Patients in whom metastasectomy is most often beneficial are those that have "favorable" metastatic biology including **solitary lesions, pulmonary lesions,** and long disease free intervals in the case of metachronous disease
  - Those with multiple, hepatic and/or osseous metastases presenting with synchronous metastatic disease and/or a short disease free interval are poorer candidates for metastasectomy
  - **The Motzer criteria** may be used to stratify the risk of metastasectomy or systemic therapy in patients with mRCC and include performance status, weight loss, serum calcium, LDH, alkaline phosphatase, hemoglobin, platelets and sedimentation rates
  - Local recurrence following radical nephrectomy is uncommon and occurs in about 2%. Only about 40% of local recurrences are isolated meaning the majority of patients with local recurrence also have systemic disease such that an extensive disease evaluation should be pursued
    * Many local recurrences are in adjacent nodes which were not removed at the time of surgery. This emphasizes the importance of adequate preoperative evaluation and surgical resection

* **Systemic Therapies for mRCC:**

  - Multiple adjuvant therapies have been assessed to reduce the risk of recurrence following resection of high risk disease. Of these, only one positive trial has been published using autologous tumor vaccine (Jacham et al). Unfortunately, there were several design and enrollment concerns that limit this study's clinical relevance. Therefore at the current time, the only role for adjuvant treatment of high risk RCC is in the context of a clinical trial
  - There is **no convincing role** for **hormonal or radiation therapies in mRCC** other than for palliation
  - **RCC is a chemoresistant tumor.** Multiple studies have demonstrated a low (2%–6%) response rate to multimodal chemotherapeutic approaches
  - Immunologic therapies have been the preferred treatment for mRCC for the last 2–3 decades. These strategies include cytokines, adoptive immunotherapies and vaccines

* **Cytokines:**
  • **Interferon (IFN) alpha**—a member of a group of pleiotropic proteins with antiviral, immunomodulatory and antiproliferative activities related to modulation of gene expression in selected cell populations. Overall response rates in mRCC to single agent IFN alpha are approximately 12% with only 1.8% complete responses and a median overall survival of 5–15 months
  • **Interleukin 2 (IL 2)**—a T cell growth factor produced by activated T cells which mediates its effect by binding to the IL 2 receptor, which causes expansion of cyto toxic T cells. The overall response rate to IL 2 is approximately 15% with durable complete responses in 6%–8%. IL 2 can be administered in a variety of ways including as a bolus or continuous infusion, or subcutaneously. In the United States, IL 2 was approved on the basis of data from a high dose infusion protocol. The potential side effects includes vascular leak syndrome (hypotension, oliguria, multiorgan failure). Median overall survival for mRCC treated with IL 2 is 12–18 months
  • Cytokine combination therapy with IL 2 and IFN alpha suggest response rates of approximately 19% but with no improve ment in overall survival
* **Adoptive immunotherapy**
  • This strategy involves the transfer of autologous lymphocytes for the treatment of mRCC including lymphokine activated killer (LAK) cells, T cells, and tumor infiltrating lymphocytes (TIL)
  • Randomized trials combining cytokines with adoptive immunotherapy have not shown any improvement in survival. Adoptive immunotherapy remains experimental

* **Vaccines**
  • The use of active specific immunotherapy to indirectly enhance the immune response
  • Vaccines used in RCC include autologous tumor lysate combinations, tumor fused with dendritic cells (an antigen presenting cell), dendritic cell vaccines and heat shock proteins
  • No vaccine trial has demonstrated improvement in survival and therefore these remain investigational
• **Targeted Therapies**
  * With the identification of the VHL gene and subsequent delineation of portions of its pathways, various agents have been investigated which seek to perturb the VEGF pathway for therapeutic benefit
  * Currently specific targeted therapies with activity in RCC carcinoma exist. These have rapidly reached first line status in the treatment of this tumor. The targeted therapies include:
• **Bevacizumab**—an IgG1 monoclonal antibody that binds all isoforms of VEGF thereby inhibiting its signaling by sequestering the circulating ligand. High dose single agent bevacizumab has been shown to increase time to progression compared to placebo although it did not improve overall survival. This was among the first proof of principles that demonstrated that therapies targeting the VEGF pathway could be used for therapeutic benefit. It is currently not being used as a single agent in mRCC. More recent combinations studies (AVOREN) using bevacizumab and interferon alpha as first line therapy in patients with metastatic RCC have demonstrated a statistically significant improvement in progression free survival over either single agent alone. Not yet approved for RCC
• **Sunitinib**—an oral tyrosine kinase receptor inhibitor approved for mRCC that blocks multiple kinases including VEGFR 2, PDGF, cKit and Flt 3. In phase III trials, sunitinib has been shown to have a higher response rate as measured by tumor regression (30%–40%) when compared directly to IFN with a statistically significant improvement in progression free survival. More recent analyses demonstrate that Sunitinib increases overall survival in patients with metastatic RCC. Among the targeted therapies for RCC, radiographic response rates appear to be the most robust with sunitinib. Side effects include fatigue, hypertension, rash, diarrhea, and potentially thyroid and left ventricular dysfunction. Approved for RCC

- **Sorafenib**—an oral tyrosine and Raf kinase receptor inhibitor approved for mRCC. Has demonstrated improvements in progression free survival, tumor regression and stabilization of disease in phase II/III trials. Side effects include nausea, vomiting, diarrhea, fatigue, hypertension, and hand and foot syndrome. Approved for RCC
- **Temsirolimus**—an intravenous inhibitor of mTOR (mammalian target of rapamycin). This agent blocks translation of HIF1. It has been shown in a phase III study of poor risk patients with mRCC to improve overall survival versus IFN. Approved for use in RCC

- **Multimodal therapy**

  * Most cases of advanced RCC are not treated by any one modality alone. The combination of integrated surgery of the primary tumor with selective surgery on metastases and combination or sequential targeted systemic therapies and/or immunotherapies/clinical trials are aimed at prolonging survival in patients with mRCC. Ongoing randomized trials are attempting to validate and refine these strategies

- **Special circumstances**

  * Other malignant neoplasms of the kidney
  * **Sarcomas of the kidney**

    1. Represent **1%–2% of all malignant renal tumors** in adults with a peak incidence in the 5th decade
    2. Renal sarcoma is **less common** but **more lethal** than other genitourinary sarcomas
    3. Differentiation of a renal sarcoma from a sarcomatoid variant of RCC may be difficult. True renal sarcomas are **derived from mesenchymal** elements of the kidney and are typically **surrounded by a pseudocapsule** which is often infiltrated by tumor cells
    4. Often present with metastatic disease **(most often to lung)**
    5. Median survival is months for a high grade renal sarcoma but may be longer for more indolent low grade sarcomas
    6. Most important prognostic variables in renal sarcomas is their **histology, grade** and **margin** status. Leoimyosarcoma (50%–60%) is the **most common type** and may have a female preponderance
    7. **Liposarcoma is the second most common** histology and must be distinguished from angiomyolipoma (AML)
    8. Retroperitoneal sarcomas often involve but do not arise from the kidney
    9. Wide and complete excision are mandatory

- **Renal lymphoma and leukemia**

  1. Renal involvement in patients with hematologic malignancies is commonly found in 34% of patients dying of progressive lymphoma or leukemia at autopsy
  2. Usually a **late manifestation of disease** and represents **hematogenous** spread
  3. Often **asymptomatic**
  4. More common with **non-Hodgkin's** disease than with Hodgkin's variants
  5. Histologically **diffuse forms predominate** over nodular forms
  6. Primary renal lymphoma is very rare given the paucity of lymphoid tissue in the normal kidney
  7. CT characteristics of renal lymphoma include adjacent adenopathy (particularly in uncommon locations for advanced kidney cancer such as in the mesentery), splenomegaly and diffuse enlargement of the kidney which maintains its renoform appearance
  8. If renal lymphoma is suspected, **biopsy** should be performed with **flow cytometry.** Treatment is systemic and the kidney should not be removed
  9. Other clinical clues include **fever, weight loss, fatigue** and **"B" symptoms** of lymphoma

- **Metastatic tumors to the kidney**

  1. Metastatic tumors are the most common kidney tumor. Autopsy studies reveal 12% of patients dying from cancer have metastases to their kidneys
  2. Nearly all represent hematogenous spread
  3. Most common primaries include **lung** (most common solid metastasis to the kidney), **breast, colon and melanoma**
  4. Most often metastatic disease to the kidney is multifocal with small nodules and is associated with metastatic disease elsewhere. Solitary metastases to the kidney are fairly uncommon
  5. If there is uncertainty as to the nature of a renal mass in a patient with a high risk tumor elsewhere, a percutaneous biopsy should be considered

- **Carcinoids of the kidney**

  1. Arise from **neuroendocrine cells** which are not normally present in the kidney
  2. This is therefore an exceptionally **rare renal tumor**
  3. Correlations have been made to **horseshoe kidneys** (increased relative risk **82-fold** over normal kidneys)
  4. Most patients are asymptomatic; a minority will present with carcinoid syndrome (flushing, wheezing, diarrhea)
  5. Should consider evaluation for carcinoid elsewhere such as with colonoscopy or upper GI endoscopy

- **Wilms' Tumor**

  1. Most common abdominal malignancy in children
  2. 3% of Wilms' tumors are seen in adults
  3. Most adult Wilms' in young adults (15–20 years old)
  4. Treatment of adult Wilms' tumor is similar to that in a pediatric population and is multimodal

- Other rare renal malignancies include PNET tumors and small cell carcinomas of the kidney

- **Benign Renal Neoplasms**

  * Oncocytoma

  1. Represents 3%–7% of all solid renal masses
  2. Grossly light brown or mahogany in color, often with a central scar
  3. Microscopically uniform round eosinophilic cells containing a lot of mitochondria
  4. 10%–20% may extend into perinephric fat (pT3a)
  5. Derived from the distal convoluted tubule
  6. May be part of the Birt Hogg Dubé syndrome and be part of the spectrum of chromophobe carcinoma continuum
  7. Cannot be distinguished clinically, radiographically or on percutaneous biopsy from RCC. Like RCC, oncocytoma occurs in middle aged patients with a slight male preponderance
  8. Requires treatment as if it were an RCC (excision, ablation as appropriate)
  9. Death from disease is exceedingly rare. No adjuvant therapy is warranted

- **Angiomyolipoma (AML)**
  1. Benign tumor containing varying amounts of mature adipose tissue, smooth muscle and thick walled vessels
  2. Found in 0.3% of all autopsies
  3. **Female preponderance,** with a potential hormonal dependency (rare before puberty)
  4. Approximately **20%–30%** of AMLs are found in patients with **tuberous sclerosis** (TS) which also has associated mental retardation, epilepsy, and adenoma sebaceum
  5. May present incidentally or after retroperitoneal hemorrhage (Wunderlich's syndrome). (Pregnancy increases the risk of spontaneous hemorrhage.)

6. Diagnosed radiographically with fat on CT, MRI or US. The amount of fat in an AML varies and in 10%+ there may be no fat
7. Occasionally extrarenal occurrences have been reported in lymph nodes or even into the renal vein
8. Uniformly benign clinical course
9. Management depends on size and symptoms. **Most symptomatic AMLs are large and should be resected with NSS approaches.** Even very large AMLs can safely be excised while sparing the kidney
10. A 4 cm cutoff is recognized as one above which as many as 80% of patients develop symptoms including spontaneous bleeding in 10%
11. Selective embolization for bleeding lesions is often effective at stopping the hemorrhage. Primary therapy with embolization has been used but may require repeat treatment

Table 11

Paraneoplastic Syndromes in RCC

Cachexia/fever (cytokines)	20%-33%
Nephropathy (Ig formation)	27%
HTN (renin)	25%
Hypercalcemia metastatic nonmetastatic (PTH-like)	20%
Anemia (cytokine myelosuppression)	20%-40%
Hyperglycemia	10%-20%
Stauffer's[a] (? IL6)	3%-20%
Erythrocytosis (Epo)	1%-8%
Amyloidosism	3%-5%

[a]*Nonmetastatic hepatic dysfunction*

- **Cystic nephroma (Multiloculated cystic nephroma – MLCN)**

1. A benign lesion with a bimodal age distribution. Occurs in young (2–3 year old) boys and middle-aged **(40–50) women**
2. More often symptomatic in adults
3. By definition all are multilocular and therefore appear as Bosniak III or IV cysts
4. No reliable clinical or radiographic means of distinguishing MLCN from cystic RCC
5. Managed surgically with NSS whenever clinically feasible

- **Leiomyoma**

1. Slow-growing benign renal tumor arising from the capsule or peripelvic tissues. Rarely arises from the renal vein
2. No reliable clinical or radiographic means of distinguishing from incidental RCC although clearly capsular location should raise suspicion

- **Juxtaglomerular tumors (reninomas)**

1. A benign hemangiopericytoma derived from the specialized **juxtaglomerular cells**
2. Clinical presentation dominated by **hyper secretion of renin** with **hypertension, hypokalemia, polydipsia, polyuria, myalgias** and **headaches**
3. Female predominance, 3rd to 4th decade of life
4. Often at or near the corticomedullary junction. Often relatively small and amenable to NSS
5. **Cured by excision.** Metastatic disease very rare
6. Should **exclude renal artery stenosis** as cause of hyperreninemia

- **Metanephric adenoma**

1. Benign, occasionally symptomatic, with peak incidence in the 5th decade
2. Small basophilic cells

3. A few reported cases of associated malignant stromal elements
4. No reliable clinical or radiographic means of distinguishing from incidental RCC. Therefore excision, preferably by NSS, is indicated

- **Paraneoplastic syndromes (Table 11)**

1. Found in 20% of patients with RCC.
2. Renal tumors are capable of overproducing 1,25 dihydroxycholecalciferol, renin, erythropoietin, and/or various prostaglandins which may case a myriad of constitutional symptoms.
3. Hypercalcemia may occur in up to 10%+ of patients with RCC and can be due to either bony involvement or the production of parathyroid hormone like peptides. Signs of hypercalcemia include nausea, anorexia, fatigue, and decreased deep tendon reflexes. Management includes hydration, diuretics, and selective use of bisphosphonates and steroids
4. Hypertension can be due to local compression of the renal artery, arteriovenous fistula or overproduction of renin
5. Hypertension can be due to local compression of the renal artery, arteriovenous fistula or overproduction of renin
6. Polycythemia can be due to overproduction of erythropoietin
7. Nonmetastatic hepatic dysfunction (Stauffer's syndrome) has been reported in 3%–20% of RCC cases and is associated with an increase in serum alkaline phosphatase, prothrombin time and/or elevated bilirubin. It may also be due to elevations in interleukin 6
8. In general, paraneoplastic syndromes associated with RCC require nephrectomy

2. Upper Urinary Tract Urothelial Carcinoma

A. Epidemiology and Basic Biology

- Less common than bladder urothelial carcinomas and more often associated with familial syndromes.
- Account for 5%–7% of all renal tumors and 5% of all urothelial tumors.
- Highest incidence in the Balkan states (may account for up to 40% of all renal cancers).
- Peak incidence in 70–79 year age group (mean 65 years old).
- Approximately 60% of upper tract urothelial tumors are in the renal pelvis while 40% are in the ureters.

Table 12

WHO Pathologic Classification of Upper Tract Urothelial Cancers

Papillary Urothelial Lesion
Papillary hyperplasia
Urothelial Papilloma
Papillary urothelial neoplasm of LMP
Low grade urothelial carcinoma
High grade urothelial carcinoma
Flat Urothelial Lesions
Flat urothelial hyperplasia
Flat urothelial atypia
Urothelial atypia of unknown significance
Dysplasia
Carcinoma *in situ*

- Men are affected twice as often, with Caucasians affected twice as often as African Americans

- Risk of developing upper tract urothelial carcinoma in patients with a history of bladder cancer is associated with the stage and grade of the bladder cancer and is highest among patients with CIS in the bladder. This may reflect upward spread of the disease into the distal ureter or simply a "high risk" urothelial phenotype

- Etiology and risk factors

  * **Balkan nephropathy**—a degenerative interstitial nephropathy. Interestingly, bladder cancer rates are not affected

  * **Smoking**—as with bladder cancer, this is the most important modifiable risk factor, increasing the risk 3-fold. Risk appears dose related. Smoking seems to increase the risk of ureteral tumors higher than it does renal pelvic tumors

  * **Coffee** consumption may increase the risk

  * **Analgesic abuse**

  * **Occupational exposure** to coal, asphalt or tar, petroleum, aniline dyes and other amines

  * **Hereditary**—Lynch syndrome II is associated with colon tumors and upper tract urothelial carcinoma. An autosomal dominant defect in the DNA mismatch repair genes hMLH1 and hMSH2

B. Pathology

- Most upper tract urinary cancers are **urothelial**. A small percentage are squamous or adenocarcinomas

- The pathology of upper tract urothelial cancers follows the WHO classification for bladder cancers (Table 12)

- As with bladder tumors, 55%-75% of renal pelvic tumors are low grade and low stage and 85% are papillary

Table 13

Differential Diagnosis of an Upper Tract Filling Defect

1. Radiolucent stone
2. Blood clot
3. Renal papillae
4. Fungus ball
5. Extrinsic vascular compression
6. Renal parenchymal tumor
7. Urothelial cancer
8. Ureteritis/pyelitis cystica
9. Tuberculosis
10. Benign or traumatic ureteral stricture
11. Endometriosis

- In the ureter, invasion is more common than in the bladder

- **Upper tract urothelial carcinomas** are more common in the **lower ureter (70%)** than mid ureter (25%) or upper ureter (5%)

- Patients with **upper tract urothelial cancer** are at risk for developing **bladder cancer**. The magnitude of this risk is likely associated with grade, stage, multifocality, CIS, and other co-risk factors such as smoke exposure

C. Evaluation, Diagnosis, and Imaging

- The most common symptom is hematuria (micro or gross)

- Flank pain may imply obstruction

Table 14

AJCC Staging 2002 for Upper Urinary Tract Urothelial Cancers

Primary Tumor Stage (T)
Tx – Primary tumor cannot be staged
T0 – No evidence of primary tumor
Ta – Noninvasive
Tis – Carcinoma-in-situ
T1 – Invades lamina propria
T2 – Invades muscularis
T3 – Invades sinus/peri-ureteral fat or renal parenchyma
T4 – Invades adjacent organs

Nodal Staging
N1 – Single node ≤ 2 cm
N2 – Nodes 2< x ≤ 5 cm
N3 – Nodes > 5 cm

- **Diagnosis includes:**

  1. Full history and exam

  2. Laboratory evaluation includes liver and renal function tests, urinalysis, and cytologies:
     a. cytology will identify most CIS and high grade tumors but is often falsely negative with low grade tumors
     b. Upper tract washings may be more sensitive than voided urine but likewise may be contaminated from the lower urinary tract
     c. Interpretation of cytologies may be hampered by contrast materials
     d. Baseline serum creatinine, GFR and CKD stage must be obtained and considered during management

  3. Radiographic evaluation
     a. Includes the use of IVP, CT urograms and retrograde pyelograms
     b. The differential diagnosis of a filling defect on these studies is listed in (Table 13)

  4. Endoscopic evaluation
     - **Ureteroscopy** or **nephroscopy**
       a. When combining radiographic evaluations and endoscopy, the diagnostic accuracy of an upper urinary tract defect is approximately 85%–90%
       b. Histologic correlation between ureteroscopic biopsy and final pathology is 78%–90%; however, it is often difficult to get a good specimen given the spatial limitations of small instruments. Therefore, correlation with grade and stage is poor and requires correlation of endoscopic, cytologic and radiographic features

D. Staging and Prognosis

- Staging of upper urinary tract TCC follows TNM Staging guidelines (Table 14).

- Upper tract urothelial carcinomas are generally associated with a poor prognosis with up to 19% of patients presenting with metastatic disease. Prognosis relates to grade and stage and appears better for renal pelvic tumors than for ureteral tumors. In the ureter, invasion is more common than in the bladder. This may be related to a more well-developed muscle layer and the presence of the nearby renal parenchyma in the upper urinary tract

- Upper urinary tract urothelial cancers may spread by direct extension, or by lymphatic or vascular invasion

E. Management

• Laparoscopic/robotic and open approaches

1. As with RCC, treatment for upper tract urothelial cancer can be performed via open or laparoscopic technique. In choosing the approach, clinical and anatomic factors must be considered as well as the comfort level and experience of the surgeon

2. Radical nephroureterectomy <u>and</u> nephron sparing techniques are also available for upper tract urothelial tumors. Nephron sparing approaches should be done for low grade, low stage lesions (open or endoscopic) and for relative or absolute indications as with RCC. NSS options include:

   a. Segmental parenchymal resection
   b. Open pyelotomy with tumor excision and ablation. This is an uncommon means of treatment and generally requires a large extrarenal pelvis and a papillary low grade tumor
   c. Segmental ureteral resection with reconstruction. The type of reconstruction depends on the location and extent of the tumor and includes:
      - Primary end-to-end ureteral anastomosis
      - Direct bladder reimplantation
      - Reimplantation with bladder hitch or flap
      - Ureteral substitution (ie, ileal ureter)

3. Radical nephroureterectomy with excision of a bladder cuff to include the intramural portion of the ureter is considered the gold standard for large, high grade, invasive or multifocal tumors. Ipsilateral adrenalectomy is not considered necessary

   a. Regional lymphadenectomy is usually performed for high-risk tumors as a staging measure. The therapeutic benefit of an extensive lymphadenectomy has not yet been determined but may ultimately be shown to be of similar value as new data demonstrate in bladder cancer

4. Laparoscopic/robotic approaches for upper urinary tract urothelial carcinomas follow the same basic principles as discussed in RCC. Approaches include:

   a. Pure laparoscopic transperitoneal or retroperitoneal surgery
   b. Hand-assisted techniques
   c. Robotic approaches – may assist in the learning curve but otherwise do not seem to improve pure laparoscopic approaches to nephrectomy or nephroureterectomy
   d. Management of the distal and intramural portion of the ureter should not be compromised. Options include:
      - Open excision through the lowest extraction port
      - Aggressive transurethral resection of the ureteral orifice. This should be reserved for proximal, low grade tumors
      - Intussusception (stripping) technique—after laparoscopic nephrectomy, a previously placed ureteral catheter is used to intussuscept the ureter into the bladder where it is excised
      - Transvesical laparoscopic ligation and detachment—performed via two transvesical ports. The ureter is tented up and looped. A Collins knife is then used to circumscribe the orifice
      - Totally laparoscopic excision—requires laparoscopic detrussor incision with dissection of the intramural portion and resection

• Endoscopic

1. Ureteroscopy, pyeloscopy and nephroscopy

   a. Best preserved for low grade, unifocal lesions of the ureter, renal pelvis or upper pole calyx
   b. Steps for retrograde ureteroscopic management include:
      - Endoscopic evaluation and collection of cytologies
      - Biopsy and definitive treatment
        1. Tumor may be debulked with a forceps or basket. The base is then treated with fulguration or laser. Holmium: Yag laser is safer in the ureter because of its shallower penetration (< 0.5 mm). Settings for this laser are energy of 0.6–1 joule with a frequency of 8–10 hertz. Nd:Yag may be better in the pelvis. It

works by coagulative necrosis and has a deeper penetration (5–6 mm). Settings are 5–15 watts for 2 seconds

2. Tumor can be resected with a ureteral resectoscope. Extra care is needed in the mid- to upper ureter

- Antegrade percutaneous management has the advantage of the ability to use larger instruments that can remove a larger volume of tumor. Staging and grading is ordinarily better as well, given the amount of tumor that can be removed. Additionally, lower pole tumors are more easily accessed and topic therapies can more easily be applied. It is best reserved for larger, more extrarenal pelvices

1. Steps include:

    a. Establishment of a nephroscopy tract
    b. Biopsy and definitive therapy
    c. Second look within 2–14 days to allow for adequate healing with rebiopsy and fulguration of the base

2. Results of endoscopic management:

    a. For retrograde management, the overall recurrence rates are approximately 30% and depend on stage, grade, size and focality
    b. Complications of ureteroscopy and their management are similar to endoscopic management of stones
    c. Series for antegrade management are small. Most low grade, smaller, unifocal lesions do well. Higher grade, invasive lesions do worse. Nephroscopy tract seeding appears uncommon

- **Topical and Systemic Therapies:**

1. Instillation therapy
    a. Can be performed antegrade through a nephroscopy tract, retrograde through a ureteral catheter or by reflux up an indwelling ureteral stent
    b. Basic principles include:
        - Rule out infection first
        - Low pressure instillation
    c. Most series are small, retrospective, highly selected and not controlled
    d. The same agents used in bladder cancer have been used in the upper urinary tracts including BCG, mitomycin and thiotepa
    e. The accumulated experience appears encouraging in properly selected patients
    f. Most common complication of upper tract instillation is sepsis

2. Systemic Therapy
    a. Small highly selected series evaluating adjuvant radiation suggest it may decrease local recurrence but not systemic disease
    b. Both induction (neoadjuvant) and adjuvant therapies are reasonable. Neoadjuvant chemotherapy may be a reasonable option for patients with locally advanced disease (into the renal parenchyma or adjacent fat) or bulky regional adenopathy
    c. There are no prospective controlled trials evaluating chemotherapy for upper urinary tract urothelial cancers. Most of the data are extrapolations from bladder cancer series

3. Selected Reading

Cohen HT, McGovern FJ. Renal cell carcinoma. *N Engl J Med*. 2005;353:2477 2490.

Drucker BJ. Renal cell carcinoma: current status and future prospects. *Cancer Treat Rev*. 2005; 31:536 545.

Motzer RJ, Bander NH, Nanus DM. Renal cell carcinoma. *N Engl J Med*. 1996;335:865 875.

Campbell SC, Novick AC, Bukowski RM. Renal tumors. In: Wein AJ, Kavoussi LR, Novick AC, Partin AW, Peters CA, eds. *Campbell-Walsh Urology*. 9th ed. Philadelphia, PA: WB Saunders; 2007:1567.

Epidemiology of RCC

Choyke PL, Glenn GM, Walther MM, et al. The natural history of renal lesions in von Hippel Lindau disease: a serial CT study in 28 patients. *AJR Am J Roentgenol*.1992;159:1229.

Duffey BG, Choyke PL, Glenn G, et al. The relationship between renal tumor size and metastases in patients with von Hippel Lindau disease. *J Urol*. 2004;172:63.

Hock LM, Lynch J, Balaji KC. Increasing incidence of all stages of kidney cancer in the last 2 decades in the United States: an analysis of surveillance, epidemiology and end results program data. *J Urol*. 2002;167:57.

Hollingsworth JM, Miller DC, Daignault S, et al. Rising incidence of small renal masses: a need to reassess treatment effect. *J Natl Cancer Inst*. 2006; 98:1331-1334.

Jemal A, Murray T, Ward E, et al. Cancer statistics, 2005. *CA Cancer J Clin*. 2005;55:10–30.

Molecular Biology and Kidney Cancer Syndromes

Choyke PL, Glenn GM, Walther MM, et al. The natural history of renal lesions in von Hippel Lindau disease: a serial CT study in 28 patients. *AJR* 1992;159:1229.

Duffey BG, Choyke PL, Glenn G, et al. The relationship between renal tumor size and metastases in patients with von Hippel Lindau disease. *J Urol*. 2004;172:63.

Linehan WM, Lerman MI, Zbar B. Identification of the von Hippel Lindau (VHL) gene. Its role in renal cancer. *JAMA*. 1995;273:564–570.

Maher ER, Kaelin WG. von Hippel Lindau disease. *Medicine* (Baltimore).1997;76:381–391.

Seizinger BR, Rouleau GA, Ozelius LJ, et al. von Hippel Lindau disease maps to the region of chromosome 3 associated with renal cell carcinoma. *Nature*. 1988;332:268–269.

Sudarshan S, Linehan WM. Genetic basis of cancer of the kidney. *Semin Oncol*. 2006;33(5):544–551.

Uzzo RG, Novick AC. von Hippel Lindau syndrome: Clinical and molecular considerations for the urologist. *AUA Update Series*. 1999;18: 137–144.

Pathology, Evaluation, Imaging and Prognosis of RCC

Frank I, Blute ML, Cheville JC, et al. Solid renal tumors: an analysis of pathological features related to tumor size. *J Urol*. 2003;170:2217.

Frank I, Blute ML, Leibovich BC, Cheville JC, Lohse CM, Zincke H. Independent validation of the 2002 American Joint Committee on cancer primary tumor classification for renal cell carcinoma using a large, single institution cohort. *J Urol*. 2005;173: 1889.

Frank I, Blute ML, Cheville JC, et al. An outcome prediction model for patients with clear cell renal cell carcinoma treated with radical nephrectomy based on tumor stage, size, grade and necrosis: The SSIGN score. *J Urol*. 2002;168:2395–2400.

Fuhrman SA, Lasky LC, Limas C. Prognostic significance of morphologic parameters in renal cell carcinoma. *Am J Surg Path*. 1982;6:655–663.

Kattan MW, Reuter V, Motzer RJ, et al. A postoperative prognostic nomogram for renal cell carcinoma. *J Urol*. 2001;166:63–67.

Lam JS, Shvarts O, Leppert JT, et al. Renal cell carcinoma 2005: new frontiers in staging, prognostication and targeted molecular therapy. *J Urol*. 2005;173:1853–1862.

Lam JS, Schvarts O, Leppert JT, et al. Postoperative surveillance protocol for patients with localized and locally advanced renal cell carcinoma based on a validated prognostic nomogram and risk group stratification system. *J Urol*. 2005;174:466–472.

Lane BR, Samplaski MK, Herts BR et al: Renal mass biopsy—a renaissance? *J Urol*. 2008; 179(1):20–27.

Lane BR, Kattan MW, Novick AC. Prediction models of renal cell carcinoma. *AUA Update Series*. Vol. 25. Lesson 7. 2006;57–67.

Motzer RJ, Bacik J, Schwartz LH, et al. Prognostic factors for survival in previously treated patients with metastatic renal cell carcinoma. *J Clin Oncol*. 2004;22:454–463.

Zisman A, Pantuck AJ, Dorey F, et al. Improved prognostication of renal cell carcinoma using an integrated staging system. *J Clin Oncol*. 2001;19:1649–1657.

Management of RCC

Chawla SN, Crispen PL, Hanlon AL, Greenberg RE, Chen DY, Uzzo RG. The natural history of untreated renal masses. *BJU Int*. 2007;99(5b):1203–1207.

Clark JI, Atkins MB, Urba WJ, Creech S, Figlin RA, Dutcher JP, et al. Adjuvant high dose bolus interleukin 2 for patients with high risk renal cell carcinoma: a cytokine working group randomized trial. *J Clin Oncol*. 2003;21:31–33.

Coppin C, Porzsolt F, Awa A, Kumpf J, Coldman A, Wilt T. Immunotherapy for advanced renal cell cancer. *Cochrane Database Syst Rev*. 2005 Jan 25;(1).

Crispen PL, Viterbo R, Fox EB, et al. Delayed intervention of sporadic renal masses undergoing active surveillance *Cancer.* 2008; 112(5):1051–1057

Fergany AF, Saad IR, Woo L, et al. Open partial nephrectomy for tumor in a solitary kidney: experience with 400 cases. *J Urol*. 2006;175:1630–1633.

Flanigan RC, Salmon SE, Blumenstein BA, et al. Nephrectomy followed by interferon alfa 2b compared with interferon alfa 2b alone for metastatic renal cell cancer. *N Engl J Med*. 2001; 345:1655–1659.

Gill I, Matin S, Desai M, Kaouk J, et al. Comparative analysis of laparoscopic versus open partial nephrectomy for renal tumors in 200 patients. *J Urol*. 2003;170:64–68.

Gill IS, Remer EM, Hasan WA, et al. Renal cryoablation: outcome at 3 years. *J Urol*. 2005;173:1903–1907.

Hefez KS, Fergany AF, Novick AC. Nephron sparing surgery for localized renal cell carcinoma: impact of tumor size on patient survival, tumor recurrence, and TNM staging. *J Urol*. 1999; 162:1930.

Hegarty NJ, Gill IS, Desai MM, et al. Probe ablative nephron sparing surgery: cryoablation versus radiofrequency ablation. *Urology.* 2006; 68:7–13.

Herr HW. Partial nephrectomy for unilateral renal carcinoma and a normal contralateral kidney: 10 year follow up. *J Urol.* 1999;161:33–35.

Janzen NK, Kim HL, Figlin RA, Belldegrun AS. Surveillance after radical or partial nephrectomy for localized renal cell carcinoma and management of recurrent disease. *Urol Clin N Am.* 2003;30: 843–852.

Jocham D, Richter A, Hoffman L, et al. Adjuvant autologous renal tumour cell vaccine and risk of tumour progression in patients with renal cell carcinoma after radical nephrectomy: phase III, randomized controlled trial. *Lancet.* 2004;363: 594–599.

Kim HL, Belldegrun AS, Freitas DG, et al. Paraneoplastic signs and symptoms of renal cell carcinoma: implications for prognosis. *J Urol.* 2003;170:1742–1746.

Kunkle DA, Haas NB, Uzzo RG. Adjuvant therapy for high risk renal cell carcinoma patients. *Curr Urol Rep.* 2007;8(1):19–30.

Kunkle DA, Egleston BL, Uzzo RG Excise, ablate or observe: the small renal mass dilemma—a meta-analysis and review *J Urol.* 2008 Apr;179(4): 1227–1233

Kunkle DA, Uzzo RG. Cryoablation or radiofrequency ablation of the small renal mass: a meta-analysis *Cancer.* 2008 Nov 15;113(10): 2671–2680.

Matin SF, Ahrar K, Cadeddu JA, et al. Residual and recurrent disease following renal energy ablative therapy: a multi institutional study. *J Urol.* 2006; 176:1973–1977.

Motzer RJ, Rini BI, Bukowski RM, et al. Sunitinib in patients with metastatic renal cell carcinoma. *JAMA.* 2006;295:2516–2524.

Motzer RJ, Bukowski RM. Targeted therapy for metastatic renal cell carcinoma. *J Clin Oncol.* 2006; 10;24(35):5601.

Motzer RJ, Hutson TE, Tomczak P, et al. Phase III randomized trial of sunitinib versus interferon alfa (IFN) in metastatic renal cell carcinoma (mRCC). *N Engl J Med.* 2007 Jan 11;356(2): 115–124.

Neuzillet Y, Lechevallier E, Andre M, et al. Follow up of renal oncocytoma diagnosed by percutaneous tumor biopsy. *Urology.* 2005;66:1181.

Permpongkosol S, Bagga HS, Romero FR, et al. Laparoscopic versus open partial nephrectomy for the treatment of pathological T1N0M0 renal cell carcinoma: a 5 year survival rate. *J Urol.* 2006;176:1984–1989.

Rabbani F, Herr HW, Almahmeed T, Russo P. Temporal change in risk of metachronous contralateral renal cell carcinoma: influence of tumor characteristics and demographic factors. *J Clin Oncol.* 2002;1;20(9):2370–2375.

Rothman J, Crispen PL, Wong YN, et al: Pathologic concordance of sporadic synchronous bilateral renal masses *Urology.* 2008 72(1):138-142.

Sanchez Ortiz RF, Madsen LT, Bermejo CE, et al. A renal mass in the setting of a nonrenal malignancy: when is a renal tumor biopsy appropriate? *Cancer.* 2004;101:2195.

Uzzo RG, Novick AC. Nephron sparing surgery for renal tumors: indications, techniques and outcomes. *J Urol.* 2001;166:6–18.

Varkarakis IM, Allaf ME, Inagaki T, et al. Percutaneous radio frequency ablation of renal masses: results at a 2 year mean follow up. *J Urol.* 2005;174:456–460.

Volpe A, Panzarella T, Rendon RA, et al. The natural history of incidentally detected small renal masses. *Cancer.* 2004;100:738.

Upper Urinary Tract Urothelial Carcinoma

Flanigan RC. Urothelial tumors of the upper urinary tract. In: Wein AJ, Kavoussi LR, Novick AC, Partin AW, Peters CA, eds. *Campbell-Walsh Urology*. 9th ed. Philadelphia, PA: WB Saunders; 2007:163.

Sagalowski AI, Jarrett TM. Management of urothelial tumors of the renal pelvis and ureter. In: Wein AJ, Kavoussi LR, Novick AC, Partin AW, Peters CA, eds. *Campbell-Walsh Urology*. 9th ed. Philadelphia, PA: WB Saunders; 2007:1653.

Chapter 16: Prostate Cancer

Judd W. Moul, MD, FACS
Brent K. Hollenbeck, MD
Kathleen Beekman, MD
Joseph Lattanzi, MD
Maha Hussain, MD

Contents

1. Overview

Prostate cancer is the most common cancer in American men. Despite the fact that this cancer has been diagnosed in an estimated 186,320 American men in the year 2008 and will lead to the death of approximately 28,660 men, there is no universally agreed-upon strategic plan for its diagnosis and management.

Epidemiology

Age

The risk of developing prostate cancer begins to increase at age 50 years in Caucasian men who have no family history of the disease and at age 40 years in African American men and those who have a first-degree relative (father, brother) with prostate cancer. Risk increases with age, but, unlike other cancers, prostate cancer has no "peak" age or modal distribution. There has been a downward "age migration" in the PSA (prostate-specific antigen) era such that the median age at diagnosis is now approximately 60 years old.

Race

The highest incidence of prostate cancer in the world is found in African American men, who have approximately a 9.8% lifetime risk of developing this cancer. This rate is slightly higher than the 8% lifetime risk for Caucasian American men. African American men have an incidence of prostate cancer that is 1.6 times that of Caucasian American men.

The Japanese and mainland Chinese populations have the lowest rates of prostate cancer. Interestingly, although Japanese immigrants to the United States have a higher incidence of prostate cancer than Japanese people living in Japan, their rate is still about half that of Caucasian Americans.

Socioeconomic status appears to be unrelated to the risk of prostate cancer, and the explanation for racial variability is unknown. However, an interplay of diet, hormonal factors and genetics likely accounts for the variability.

Geography

The incidence of prostate cancer is highest in Scandinavian countries (22 cases per 100,000 population) and lowest in Asia (5 per 100,000). Risk may be inversely related to ultraviolet light exposure, as the incidence increases the farther one lives from the equator. However, recent studies show extremely high rates in populations of African heritage, such as Jamaicans.

Etiology and Risk Factors

Family History

Men who have a first-degree relative with prostate cancer have approximately a 2-fold increased risk of developing prostate cancer during their lifetime. An individual who has 2 first-degree relatives with prostate cancer has a 9-fold increase in lifetime risk.

True hereditary prostate cancer occurs in a small number of men and tends to develop at an early age (<55 years old).

Dietary Fat

Studies have suggested that dietary fat may increase the risk of prostate cancer. However, no definitive proof of its role has yet been found.

Vasectomy

Several large epidemiologic studies suggest that vasectomy may increase the relative risk of prostate cancer by as much as 1.85. However, these same studies do not report an increased risk of dying from prostate cancer associated with vasectomy but do indicate a statistically increased risk of dying from lung cancer. These findings argue against an association between vasectomy and prostate cancer. Currently, this association is unproven and does not constitute grounds for fundamental changes in the use of vasectomy.

> An interim report from the European Randomized Study of Screening for Prostate Cancer examined the effect of PSA screening intervals (2 vs. 4 years) on prostate cancer detection rates. The 2-year interval detected more cancers; however, there was no difference in the rates of detection of more aggressive cancers, suggesting that more intensive screening may not always be warranted. (Roobol MJ, Grenabo A, Schroder FH, et al. *J Natl Cancer Inst* 2007;99:1296-1303.)

Sexual Activity/Sexually Transmitted Disease

A large prospective study of more than 29,000 men demonstrated an association between high ejaculatory frequency (more than 21 ejaculations/month) and a decreased risk of prostate cancer, with a lifetime relative risk of 0.67. However, there may be several confounding factors associated with high sexual activity, such as differences in prostate cancer screening or lifestyle. There was no associated increased risk for men in the lowest ejaculatory frequency category. Prevention Active research on chemoprevention of prostate cancer is ongoing. The only prospective randomized trial to demonstrate an effect was the Prostate Cancer Prevention Trial (PCPT), which showed a 24.8% reduction in the risk of prostate cancer among men randomized to receive finasteride (Proscar®) daily vs. those men on the placebo arm. Finasteride as a chemopreventive agent has not been universally accepted, however, because patients in the treatment arm were possibly more likely to exhibit higher-grade prostate cancer. Recent follow-up studies of the PCPT suggest that finasteride probably does not induce high-grade disease, and the observation may be a detection artifact. Other agents under study include vitamin E and selenium, both of which have been associated with a decreased risk of prostate cancer. A large prospective randomized trial to evaluate the effects of these agents in healthy men has recently reported there are no benefits in the prevention of prostate cancer.

Signs and Symptoms

Early-stage Disease

Men with organ-confined prostate cancer often are completely asymptomatic. Men with a large component of benign prostatic hyperplasia often present with bladder outlet obstruction unrelated to prostate cancer.

Locally Advanced Disease

Bladder outlet obstruction is the most common sign of locally advanced prostate cancer. A few men with locally advanced disease present with hematuria, urinary tract infections and irritative voiding symptoms secondary to bladder outlet obstruction.

Advanced Disease

Rarely, men with bulky lymph node metastasis may present with bilateral lower-extremity edema. Men with bony metastasis often present with bone pain and, uncommonly, with lower-extremity weakness or paralysis from spinal cord compression.

Screening and Diagnosis

Prostate cancer screening with PSA and digital rectal examination (DRE) has resulted in not only an increase in prostate cancer detection but also a stage shift. More cancers are now being detected at earlier stages, when they are potentially curable. Prior to screening efforts, most prostate cancers were detected when they produced local symptoms or distant metastases, at which point treatment for cure often was impossible.

Digital Rectal Examination

Prostate biopsy prompted by abnormal findings on DRE, such as nodularity or induration of the prostate, leads to a diagnosis of prostate cancer in only 15%-25% of cases. This rate compares with a prostate cancer prevalence of <5% among men of similar age without an abnormal DRE. Although neither accurate nor sensitive for prostate cancer detection, abnormal DRE is associated with a 5-fold increased risk of cancer present at the time of screening.

PSA

PSA is a serine protease produced by the prostatic epithelium and secreted in the seminal fluid in large quantities. The level of PSA in serum is increased

> Data from the Prostate Cancer Prevention Trial illustrate that there is no "normal" level for PSA. Indeed, there is a continuum of risk that exists, even at low levels of PSA. For example, among men in the placebo arm of the study, 11.1% of men with a serum PSA ≤1 ng/mL had prostate cancer at the end-of-study biopsy. The proportion of men with prostate cancer rose to 30% among those with PSA levels between 3.1 and 4.0 ng/mL, which is still within the "normal" range. (Thompson IM, Ankerst DP, Chi C, et al. *J Natl Cancer Inst* 2006;98:529-534.)

by inflammation of the prostate, urinary retention, prostatic infection, benign prostatic hyperplasia, prostate cancer, and prostatic manipulation. The optimal threshold to recommend prostatic biopsy has come under increasing scrutiny. The overall sensitivity for PSA levels is approximately 70%, but it is not as specific and does not allow for differentiation between indolent and aggressive disease. For example, by using a threshold of 4.1 ng/mL, the majority of cancers in men <60 would potentially be missed. However, a PSA cutoff of 4.1 ng/mL only has a positive predictive value of approximately 30%, meaning 2 out of 3 men would undergo biopsy for benign disease.

A more worthwhile approach for PSA screening may be to use the rate of rise in PSA (PSA velocity) in combination with the absolute PSA value. This approach has been shown to be useful recently in the form of age-adjusted PSA velocity, but accepted guidelines are still controversial.

Another commonly employed test for patients with a PSA level <10 ng/mL is the percent-free PSA level. There is an inverse relationship between the percent-free PSA level and the risk of a cancer diagnosis. Most urologists utilize a cutoff of 10%–25% to prompt a recommendation for biopsy. In men who have never had a prostate biopsy but who have a total PSA level >4.0, a percent-free <25% may suggest a 50%-60% probability of prostate cancer. In men who have had a prior negative biopsy but who have a persistently elevated PSA level >4.0, a percent-free PSA<10% should prompt a repeat biopsy.

Using administrative data, Welch and colleagues found that 32% of Medicare recipients who underwent prostate biopsy were diagnosed with prostate cancer. This is among the first population-based studies to empirically demonstrate detection rates in the PSA era. Further, the incidence rose with age (to 41% among those 80 and older) and with repetitive biopsies. (Welch HG, Fisher ES, Gottlieb DJ, et al. *J Natl Cancer Inst*. 2007;99:1395-1400.)

Current Screening Recommendations

The American Cancer Society and the American Urological Association (AUA) recommend that the PSA test and the DRE should be offered annually beginning at age 50 to men who have a life expectancy of at least 10 years. In high-risk men (African Americans and those with a first-degree relative diagnosed with prostate cancer), screening should be offered at an earlier age (40-45 years-old). Prior to testing, physicians should discuss with their patients the potential benefits of early prostate cancer detection and its implications in the need for subsequent treatment so that patients can make an informed decision about undergoing screening.

There are currently 2 ongoing major prostate cancer screening trials: the Prostate, Lung, Colorectal and Ovarian (PLCO) trial in the United States funded by the National Cancer Institute and the European Organization for Research and Treatment of Cancer (EORTC) trial. The National Comprehensive Cancer Network (NCCN) has recently published aggressive screening guidelines on its website (www.nccn.org). These new controversial guidelines call for baseline PSA levels at a younger age (generally age 40) and suggest that any young man with a PSA level >0.7 ng/mL (median in men aged 40-49) be tested annually. Furthermore, NCCN suggests that biopsy is warranted for a PSA >2.5 ng/mL.

Biopsy

When indicated, prostate biopsy usually is performed as an office procedure by transrectal ultrasonographic guidance using an automated 18-gauge biopsy gun. The procedure is performed with, at most, local anesthesia and carries a risk of significant infection of only 1 in 200 cases. Additional side effects of hematuria and hematochezia are common for 2-3 days following the biopsy. Hematospermia may last for up to 4-6 weeks. Since about the year 2000, prostate biopsy includes laterally directed extended core protocols employing 8-12 biopsy cores per procedure. Multiple studies have demonstrated that the addition of the lateral cores improves the accuracy of biopsy.

If the biopsy result is negative, these men are typically followed conservatively with serial PSA levels and DRE repeated annually. Repeat biopsy is performed only when PSA levels rise at abnormal rates (>0.8 ng/mL/year) or if DRE findings show new nodularity or induration. Men in whom high-grade prostatic intraepithelial neoplasia (PIN) or atypical small acinar proliferation (ASAP) is found on biopsy usually should undergo repeat biopsy, since one-third to one-half will eventually be found to have prostate cancer.

A new test, the UPM-3 urine test, has become more widely available. This test, performed on voided urine after an "attentive" DRE, is based on reverse transcriptase-polymerase chain reaction assay for a PSA product (DD3). It is becoming useful, not as a primary screening test, but to dictate the need for repeat prostate biopsy in men with persistently elevated PSA levels. Recently, the name of this test has been changed to PCA-3.

Pathology

Adenocarcinomas make up the vast majority of prostate carcinomas. A total of 70% of prostate adenocarcinomas occur in the peripheral zone, 20% in the transitional zone and approximately 10% in the central zone.

Other tumor types are relatively rare and include ductal adenocarcinoma, which occurs in the major ducts and often projects into the urethra; and mucinous adenocarcinoma, which secretes abundant mucin and does not arise from the major ducts. Transitional carcinoma of the prostate occurs within the ducts and, to a lesser extent, in the prostatic acini. Typically, primary transitional carcinomas are aggressive cancers that have a poor prognosis. Similarly, neuroendocrine (small-cell) tumors are rare and aggressive, have a poor prognosis, and typically require aggressive surgical and medical management.

> Despite data from the Prostate Cancer Prevention Trial demonstrating the ability of finasteride to reduce the risk of prostate cancer, the adoption of this preventive measure may be hindered by concerns over the induction of high-grade disease in the treatment arm. Recent evidence from 2 different studies suggest that the ascertainment of more high-grade disease in the finasteride arm was due to sampling density bias and the impact of the treatment on prostate volume. (Cohen YC, Liu KS, Heyden NL, et al. *J Natl Cancer Inst*. 2007;99:1366-1374. Lucia MS, Epstein JI, Goodman PJ, et al. *J Natl Cancer Inst* 2007;99:1375-1383.)

Histologic Grade

The grading system developed by Gleason from data accumulated by the Veterans Administration Cooperative Urologic Research Group appears to provide the best prognostic information in addition to clinical stage and is the predominant grading system in widespread use.

Metastatic Spread

Adenocarcinoma of the prostate may spread locally through direct extension into periprostatic fat or via the ejaculatory ducts into seminal vesicles; lymphatically to regional lymph nodes, including the hypogastric and obturator lymph nodes; and hematogenously to bone. The most common sites of bony metastases are the lumbosacral spine (probably related to venous drainage of the prostate through Bastons plexus) and the axial skeleton, but any bone, including the skull and ribs, can be involved. Rare sites of metastatic spread include the liver and lungs.

Prevention

Until 2004, there was no intervention known to prevent prostate cancer. The primary objective of the Prostate Cancer Prevention Trial was to describe the prevalence of histologically proven prostate cancer among men randomized to receive daily finasteride (a 5-alpha-reductase inhibitor that decreases prostate size and serum/prostate dihydrotestosterone levels) or placebo. The authors described a 24.8% reduction in the prevalence of prostate cancer among men taking finasteride, suggesting that it either prevents or delays the appearance of prostate cancer. The caveat of their findings, however, was that these cancers that developed in the treatment arm were of a higher grade. Recent, longer term follow-up studies suggest no increased risk of high-grade disease with finasteride.

Table 1

TNM Staging System of Prostate Cancer

Localized Disease	
T1a	Tumor incidental histologic finding in ≤5% of resected tissue; not palpable
T1b	Tumor incidental histologic finding in >5% of resected tissue
T1c	Tumor identified by needle biopsy (eg, because of elevated PSA level)
T2a	Tumor involves one-half of 1 lobe or less
T2b	Tumor involves more than one-half of 1 lobe but not both lobes
T2c	Tumor involves both lobes
Local Extension	
T3a	Extracapsular extension (unilateral or bilateral)
T3b	Tumor invades seminal vesicle(s)
T4	Bladder invasion, fixed to pelvic side wall, or invasion of adjacent structures
Metastatic Disease	
N1	Positive regional lymph nodes
M1	Distant metastasis

Adapted from Greene FL, Page DL, Fleming ID, et al, eds. AJCC Cancer Staging Manual. *6th ed. New York, NY: Springer-Verlag; 2002.*

Prognosis and Natural History

Staging Systems

The most widely used and universally accepted staging system for prostate cancer is the TNM system (Table 1). In the TNM system, T1 and T2 tumors are confined to the gland, whereas T3 and T4 tumors have local extension.

Risk-adapted Staging

The development of the "Partin Tables" in 1993 ushered in a new era of combining clinical stage, Gleason score, and PSA level to predict pathologic stage after radical prostatectomy. More recently, this has led to the DAmico et al risk groupings for newly diagnosed men with clinically localized disease (Table 2). Patients are divided into 3 risk groups (low, intermediate or high) of occult micrometastases and relapse after initial local therapy. Although not perfect, this system is currently in widespread use and allows a framework for multimodal and multidisciplinary treatment strategies based on risk grouping. Guidelines from both the AUA and NCCN use this system.

Prognosis

The optimal management of patients with prostate cancer varies widely and is highly dependent upon a patient's age, overall health, and tumor risk assessment. The natural history of the disease process can be heterogeneous, ranging from an incidental finding unlikely to result in cancer-specific mortality, to very aggressive, resulting in early widespread metastatic disease and death. Therefore, treating physicians should carefully consider the value of curative therapy with potential toxicity in the context of a patient's comorbidities and life expectancy.

Among patients with clinically localized prostate cancer treated conservatively (observation or hormonal therapy alone), those with a low Gleason score (2-4) have a small risk of dying of their cancer

Table 2

D'Amico et al Risk Stratification for Clinically Localized Prostate Cancer

Low Risk	Diagnostic PSA <10.0 ng/mL and highest biopsy Gleason score ≤6 and clinical stage T1c or T2a
Intermediate Risk	Diagnostic PSA >10 but <20 ng/mL or highest biopsy Gleason score = 7 or clinical stage T2b
High Risk	Diagnostic PSA >20 ng/mL or highest biopsy Gleason score <8 or cinical stage T2c/T3

PSA = prostate-specific antigen

Indicators of the quality of life of prostate cancer care have been developed. However, in a multi-institutional study using the National Cancer Database, Miller and colleagues noted that compliance with the indicators was highly variable and generally more common among those undergoing radiation therapy opposed to those undergoing surgery (Miller DC, Spencer BA, Ritchey J, et al. *Med Care*. 2007; 45:401-409.)

within 15 years (4%-7%). However, those with poorly differentiated tumors (Gleason score 8–10) have a greater risk of dying of prostate cancer than of any other cause, even when the cancer is diagnosed in the eighth decade of life. Indeed, a man diagnosed before the age of 60 with a clinically localized, Gleason score 8–10 prostate cancer has an 87% risk of dying of the disease within 15 years if untreated (Table 3).

D'Amico et al combined a number of national datasets to report 10-year cancer-specific mortality rates for men undergoing radical prostatectomy or external-beam radiotherapy (EBRT) by this risk grouping and age at diagnosis. These 10-year mortality graphs are useful to counsel contemporary-era men contemplating surgery or radiation therapy. Given recent advances in the treatment of metastatic disease, identifying men at high risk for metastatic disease following local therapy is important, as these agents are incorporated earlier in the disease course.

Treatment of Localized Prostate Cancer

There are several treatment options for localized prostate cancer, including radical prostatectomy, EBRT and brachy therapy (interstitial radiation/seeds). Multiple treatment series with each modality have documented the validity of the risk-stratification model based on clinical palpation stage, Gleason score, and serum PSA level. More recently, it has been suggested that biopsy quantification may also be an important factor. Specifically,

Table 3

Risk of Dying of Clinically Localized Prostate Cancer Without Definitive Locoregional Therapy

	Age			
Gleason Score	**55-59**	**60-64**	**65-69**	**70-74**
2-4	4%	5%	6%	7%
5	6%	8%	10%	11%
6	18%	23%	27%	30%
7	70%	62%	53%	42%
8-10	87%	81%	72%	60%

Adapted from Albertsen PC, Hanley JA, Fine J. JAMA. *2005;293:2095-2101.*

counting the number of involved needle biopsy cores or the percentage of each core involved by cancer may be prognostic. Low-risk patients experience a favorable 85%-90% freedom from recurrence, compared with approximately 75% and 35%-50% for the intermediate- and high-risk patients, respectively. Although no randomized studies have been performed, contemporary series, which stratify patients by the risk model, demonstrate remarkably similar outcomes independent of the treatment modality. For this reason, treatment recommendations should be individualized based on patient preference, life expectancy, and discussion of potential toxicities. The AUA's updated clinically localized (T1-T2) prostate cancer guidelines published in 2007 confirm these concepts.

Recent evidence using SEER-Medicare data suggests that older men (those aged 65-80) with low- and intermediate-risk prostate cancer may benefit from aggressive therapy (surgery or irradiation). However, this study did not control for unobserved heterogeneity between patients, which may result in considerable selection bias. (Wong YN, Mitra N, Hudes G, et al. *JAMA* 2006; 296:2683-2693.)

2. Treatment of Clinically Localized Disease (T1, T2)

Radical Prostatectomy

Radical prostatectomy can be performed retropubically through a lower midline incision, an approach that may include pelvic lymph node dissection. Alternatively, some urologists prefer the perineal approach. With the latter approach, a separate incision is required if lymph node removal is desired. Starting in the early 2000s, the robotic-assisted laparoscopic prostatectomy (RALP) began to emerge. By 2008, approximately one-half of radical prostatectomies were performed by this approach. Compared with patients managed with watchful waiting, those treated with radical prostatectomy have a lower risk of distant metastases and improved overall disease-specific survival.

Although the morbidity of radical prostatectomy was a major concern in the past, improvements were made during the 1980s and 1990s. The hazards of anesthesia, risk of blood loss and hospital stay have all been minimized. Nationwide, Medicare data suggest that surgical outcomes are significantly better at those centers performing >40 prostatectomies per year than at other hospitals with a lower surgical volume.

Transfusion is usually unnecessary, and treatment-related mortality is <0.05% at leading prostate cancer centers. The average hospital stay of a man undergoing radical prostatectomy is now approximately 1–3 days at leading referral centers in the United States; several institutions routinely discharge patients within 24 hours. Although urinary incontinence is common in the first few months after prostatectomy, most men recover urinary control; at some leading centers, 90%-98% of men report few or no long-term urinary problems.

Nerve sparing radical prostatectomy is appropriate for men with small-volume disease. It offers those men with good potency prior to surgery the probability of recovering that function following the operation. By permitting better visualization of Santorini's dorsal venous plexus, the apical prostate, the urethra, and the striated urethral sphincter, the nerve-sparing technique also reduces blood loss and improves recovery of urinary continence. In appropriately selected individuals, a nerve-sparing procedure confers no greater risk of prostate cancer recurrence after considering other relevant clinical information (PSA, Gleason score, margin status, seminal vesicle involvement and the presence of extraprostatic spread).

Referral centers have reported that 50%-90% of patients who are fully potent prior to surgery recover erections following a nerve-sparing procedure, but the quality (rigidity and duration) of these recovered erections may be compromised compared with preoperative erections. Erection recovery rates can be higher than 80% in patients <60 years of age and lower in older men. Potency may return anywhere from 2-24 months following surgery. Regardless of potency, sensation of the penis is not changed after this procedure, and men still experience orgasm. Nerve-sparing radical prostatectomy has not compromised cancer control outcomes in well-selected men with early-stage disease. Also, a recent study has suggested that early postoperative use of sildenafil (Viagra®) may facilitate the return of natural erections more quickly. Generally speaking, recovery of erectile function after radical prostatectomy is mediated by age (the younger, the better), pretreatment erectile function (the stronger, the better), and a nerve-sparing approach (bilateral is better than unilateral, which is better than none, which is better than wide dissection).

Laparoscopic Radical Prostatectomy

Laparoscopic prostatectomy was initially described by Schuessler in 1997 but was abandoned because of its technical difficulty and long operative time with little apparent benefit over the conventional technique. A resurgence in the technique was prompted by improved instrumentation and refinements in the procedure itself, although the laparoscopically naive urologist must endure a substantial learning curve (with attendant perioperative morbidity) prior to meeting the outcome standards set by the open technique.

The robotic-assisted laparoscopic prostatectomy (RALP) was developed to overcome some of the difficulties of the standard laparoscopic prostatectomy (eg, intracorporeal suturing). The robotic technique allows for 3D visualization of the operative field and provides for a significantly wider range of movements intracorporeally than do standard laparoscopic instruments. This advance has prompted the assimilation of the technique into the armamentarium of many urologists.

> Volume outcome relationships are evident for a variety of surgeries. Multi-institutional data suggest that the learning curve for radical prostatectomy is steep and does not begin to plateau until at least 250 cases. (Vickers AJ, Ulmert D, Serio AM, et al. *J Natl Cancer Inst* 2007;99:1171-1177.)

Current evidence suggests that in experienced hands, the laparoscopic and robotic techniques have similar oncologic efficacy to that of the open procedure. However, the length of followup (usually <2-3 years) in these studies is limited, suggesting that a measure of caution be taken when interpreting the results. Furthermore, recent studies suggest the learning curve is prolonged, with 200-250 cases necessary before results can be compared with those of experienced surgeons. Long-term effects of these modalities on sexual and urinary health (as measured by a psychometrically valid survey have not been reported, and such data are critical in the context of the prostatectomy patient when evaluating technical results. Though it is a promising advance in the treatment of prostate cancer, published data suggest further research in this area is warranted.

Despite the perception that laparoscopic robotic prostatectomy is "minimally invasive," it actually is an intraperitoneal operation, whereas the open retropubic prostatectomy is a pure retroperitoneal approach. Whether this poses any short- or long-term risk remains unknown. Furthermore, even though the RALP offers excellent visualization, the surgeon does not enjoy the tactile ability associated with the open technique.

Pelvic Lymph Node Dissection

Studies now indicate that regional pelvic lymph node dissection may not be necessary for patients with stage T1c disease if the total Gleason score is <7 and the PSA level is <10.0 ng/mL, (ie, low-risk individuals). Selected intermediate-risk men may also not require this staging procedure, but in high-risk men, it is still considered imperative.

Neoadjuvant Hormonal Therapy

Approximately 15%-35% of men who undergo radical prostatectomy for clinical stage T2 prostate cancer will be found to have pathologic T3 disease following surgery. This finding led some investigators to evaluate the efficacy of neoadjuvant androgen deprivation therapy in prospective clinical trials. Early data from these trials suggested that neoadjuvant hormonal therapy led to a reduction in positive surgical margins. However, these findings need to be considered in a technical context: androgen deprivation therapy causes artifactual changes in prostate morphology that cause difficulties for the pathologic identification of prostate cancer foci.

Indeed, more recent data from prospective studies have shown no proven benefit of neoadjuvant therapy with regard to disease progression-free survival. At present, therefore, it appears that neoadjuvant hormonal therapy does not improve the curative potential of radical prostatectomy but instead is associated with morphologic alterations that complicate the prognostic utility of standard pathology. Consequently, neoadjuvant hormonal therapy with radical prostatectomy is not commonly recommended except as a method to diminish prostate size for technical surgical consideration in selected cases.

Adjuvant Therapy Post-prostatectomy

The potential indications for adjuvant therapy following radical prostatectomy in patients with clinical T1 or T2 malignancy include pathologic evidence of T3 disease, positive nodes, a rising PSA level, and positive surgical margins, among others. Possible adjuvant treatments include radiation therapy and androgen deprivation either alone or in combination. Best available evidence suggests that adjuvant radiation or early salvage radiotherapy (eg, postprostatectomy PSA level <1.0 ng/mL) affords the best results in terms of subsequent biochemical recurrence.

Radiation Therapy

Men with positive margins or pathologic T3 disease following radical prostatectomy are potential candidates for adjuvant EBRT. Some controversy exists as to the efficacy of early postoperative therapy versus intervention once a biochemical failure has been documented.

Valicenti et al demonstrated that the 5-year PSA control rate with immediate postoperative radiation therapy for patients with pathologic T3 disease was 89%, compared with 55% for a matched-pair analysis of surgery alone. Additionally, they demonstrated a favorable dose response in patients receiving EBRT doses above 64.8 Gy.

More recently, Bolla et al reported the results of a randomized, controlled study of observation vs. EBRT in 500 patients with pathologic T3 disease following radical prostatectomy. Although to date there are no data demonstrating an overall survival difference, with a median follow-up of 5 years, the progression-free survival was significantly improved with treatment (74% vs. 53%).

Similarly, a recently published SWOG randomized controlled trial confirms a progression-free survival advantage to adjuvant radiation and even a modest overall survival benefit.

Stephenson et al evaluated a large number of patients with persistent or increasing PSA levels after surgery from five American academic institutions. 45% of patients were free of disease at 4 years after salvage radiation. Patients with no adverse risk features achieved a 4-year progression-free probability of 77%. Patients who experience PSA failure after radical prostatectomy should be restaged with pelvic CT, bone scan and DRE. Patients with no evidence of metastatic disease should be evaluated for adjuvant radiotherapy.

Hormonal Therapy

Significant controversy exists within the academic community as to the timing of initiating androgen deprivation following radical prostatectomy. Clinical trials have documented a benefit only for those patients with nodal involvement.

Treatment Recommendations for Post-prostatectomy Recurrence

Following radical prostatectomy, it is expected that serial PSA levels will become undetectable. Any detectable PSA level (>0.2 ng/mL) following

In a multi-institutional study, 425 men were randomized to receive either external beam radiation or observation following a prostatectomy for pathologic T3 disease. Treatment patients received 60–64 Gy delivered to the prostatic fossa. With a median follow-up of 10 years, the overall survival difference was not statistically significant. However, patients in the treatment group demonstrated a significant improvement in PSA relapse-free survival (10.3 vs. 3.1 years) and in median recurrence-free survival (13.8 vs. 9.9 years); (Thompson IM, Tangen CM, Paradelo J, et al. *JAMA*. 2006;296:2329-2335.)

surgery indicates possible recurrent disease and the need for restaging and possible salvage therapies, including radiation or hormonal therapy, experimental protocols, or observation. However, some patients can develop low levels of detectable PSA after prostatectomy without cancer recurrence, presumably due to small foci of benign prostate tissue in situ. Although there is concern for recurrence when the PSA level is >0.2 ng/mL, most clinicians will wait until a PSA threshold >0.4 ng/mL is reached to assume that the rise in PSA level represents real recurrence.

Definitive Radiation Therapy

EBRT

EBRT utilizes high-energy photons to destroy cancer cells by damaging cellular DNA. Traditional EBRT utilized bony landmarks and standard beam arrangements to deliver dose to the pelvic region. Technologic advances in treatment planning, driven by improved computing power and the incorporation of individualized patient anatomy, have led to dramatic improvements in treatment delivery.

3D conformal EBRT creates 3D representations of target structures (ie, the prostate) and designs highly tailored treatment portals utilizing various angles to create a volume of high radiation dose that conforms to the target shape. The anatomic information used to define the target is generally derived from CT images obtained while the patient is placed in an immobilization device in the precise treatment position. With the selective delivery of dose to the target and avoidance of the surrounding normal tissue, the therapeutic ratio is improved. This approach has permitted the use of doses far higher than tolerable with traditional therapy, with fewer bowel and bladder complications.

Treatment volumes in patients with low-risk disease are designed to encompass the prostate plus a margin for daily variations. Patients with a high risk for periprostatic extension and/or regional lymph node metastasis receive initial pelvic treatment of 45-50 Gy, followed by a coned-down boost to the prostate.

RTOG (Radiation Therapy Oncology Group) 9413 was designed to test the addition of whole pelvic radiation and the timing of androgen deprivation in the treatment of high-risk patients (lymph node-positive potential >15% or locally advanced [Gleason score ≥6 and >cT2c] cancers). At a median follow-up of 59.5 months, Roach, et al noted an improved 4-year disease progression-free survival (60%) among those receiving whole pelvic radiotherapy in conjunction with neoadjuvant androgen deprivation, compared with other treatment arms (44%-50%).

EBRT Dose

The previous standard radiation dose with conventional therapy was 70 Gy given over 7 weeks; however, much recent work has suggested a positive dose response, particularly in the intermediate- and high-risk patient populations. Multiple single-institution experiences have demonstrated that 3D conformal EBRT techniques with doses of 75 Gy and higher can be delivered with minimal toxicities.

A randomized trial from the M. D. Anderson Cancer Center compared 70 Gy given conventionally with 78 Gy delivered with a conformal boost. It showed an advantage in freedom from failure for the higher dose arm in patients with a PSA level >10 ng/mL. Kupelian, et al presented pooled data for nearly 5000 patients from 9 institutions over a narrow time range (1994-1995) to remove treatment technique, stage migration, and lead-time bias. They demonstrated favorable biochemical control outcomes for doses higher than 72 Gy in all risk groups.

The RTOG has completed a dose-escalation trial to assess toxicity with 3D conformal EBRT. In this multi-institutional trial, 78 Gy (prescribed as a minimum to the tumor volume in 2-Gy fractions) was well tolerated, with only 3% of patients experiencing significant (grade 3+) acute gastrointestinal/ genitourinary (GI/GU) morbidity and a 6% rate of significant late toxicity. A comparison trial is being conducted by the RTOG (P0126); it will accrue 1,520 cases and provide information regarding any beneficial effect on mortality with higher radiation doses. Although no standard exists, doses ≥75 Gy with 3D conformal EBRT techniques appear to be well tolerated and improve biochemical response rates.

Intensity modulated radiation therapy (IMRT) is becoming a widely used treatment for prostate cancer. This refinement of conformal therapy employs high nonuniform beam intensity profiles and dynamic multileaf collimation to create even more conformal dose distributions. Further improving the therapeutic index compared with 3D conformal EBRT, IMRT is associated with reduced toxicity, permitting further dose escalations previously unattainable.

IMRT was pioneered in several major centers, and Memorial Sloan-Kettering Cancer Center has reported a series of 772 patients treated with doses between 81 and 86.4 Gy. With a median follow-up of 24 months, the side-effect profile was improved, despite these higher doses, with less than 1% of patients experiencing late grade 3+ GI/GU toxicity. The early PSA relapse-free survival rates for favorable, intermediate and unfavorable risk groups were 92%, 86% and 81%, respectively. Although IMRT is quickly becoming the standard of care at most institutions, some caution should be exercised. The precision of dose delivery and the complexity of treatment planning demand a strong commitment by both physicians and physics personnel to ensure high-quality IMRT.

Androgen Ablation With EBRT

2 potential benefits of the use of transient androgen ablation prior to EBRT have been identified. First, there may be some synergy between the apoptotic response induced by androgen deprivation and radiotherapy that may increase local control. Second, androgen deprivation results in an average 20% decrease in prostate volume. This volume reduction not only may reduce the number of target cells, and thereby improve tumor control, but also may shrink the prostate and, thus, diminish the volume of rectum and bladder irradiated during conformal therapy. Complete androgen blockade can be achieved with luteinizing hormone-releasing hormone (LHRH) agonists plus an oral antiandrogen.

The survival benefits of androgen suppression therapy (AST) for patients with intermediate-risk disease have been uncertain. A recent single-institution prospective trial by D'Amico et al randomized patients with a PSA level >10 ng/ mL, a Gleason score ≥7, or radiographic evidence of extraprostatic disease to receive EBRT (70 Gy) alone or the same EBRT with 6 months of AST. After a median follow-up of 4.5 years, patients treated with combined EBRT and AST were found to have improved disease progression-free, prostate cancer-specific, and overall survival ($P = 0.04$). Although hormone therapy for 3 years has been shown to be beneficial in locally advanced cases, this trial in men with more localized disease showed a benefit to shorter duration of hormone therapy. However, it is not known whether high-dose radiotherapy will obviate the need for AST in this group of patients.

Interstitial Radiotherapy

In the 1970s, the use of permanently placed radioactive iodine implants produced initial results as good as those obtained with other available radiotherapy techniques and posed a small risk of impotence and other morbidity when compared with conventional EBRT and radical prostatectomy. However, ultimate control rates were unacceptable. The technique used (freehand placement of seeds during laparotomy) was found to distribute the radioactive seeds unevenly throughout the gland, and, thus, cold regions may have contributed to the relatively poor outcome.

The advent of improved imaging and seed placement techniques coupled with better patient selection has resulted in vast improvements in cancer control. The perception of fewer side effects in a single outpatient treatment has also contributed to a recent surge in this treatment modality. Transrectal ultrasonography is now utilized to guide seed placement from a transperineal approach, which has corrected the problem of poor seed placement in experienced hands. 2 radioactive seed isotopes have been used: iodine (I-125), with a half-life of 60 days, and palladium (Pd-103), with a shorter half-life (17 days) and subsequent higher dose rate. The advantage of the brachytherapy technique is that substantial dose can be delivered to the prostate with minimal effect on the surrounding tissue.

Although concentrating dose with brachytherapy represents a potential advantage over EBRT, it also highlights the need for appropriate patient selection. Significant dose falloff 2-3 mm beyond placement of the seeds within the gland limits the application of seed monotherapy in patients with potential periprostatic or regional disease extension. Large studies from several leading institutions have now matured and confirm the long-term effectiveness and safety of this approach in low-risk populations. Favorable results have also been reported in selected intermediate-risk patients. Typical monotherapy doses of 145 Gy for I-131 and 125 Gy for Pd-103 are utilized. To date, the data do not support the use of either isotope over the other.

In addition to disease risk factors, certain patient selection factors are important in considering implants. A large prostate size (>60 cc) may make the procedure more challenging, both from the perspective of increased prostate gland swelling due to the increased number of needles and the difficulty of the pubic bone obstructing needle placement. Patients with outlet obstruction symptoms (AUS score >15) have an increased risk of requiring catheterization following implantation. Patients who have undergone prior transurethral resection of prostate (TURP) have been reported to have an increased risk of incontinence; recognizing this risk and placing seeds farther from the defect may help to minimize this risk. Therefore, with proper counseling, patients with small TURP defects may still be considered implant candidates.

For patients with intermediate- or high-risk disease, implants may be combined with EBRT. There is sound logic in combining high-dose therapy to the prostate with an implant and moderate doses of EBRT to the regional tissues to sterilize micrometastatic disease. In this situation, an implant (110 Gy of I-131 or 100 Gy of Pd-104) usually either precedes or follows 20-45 Gy delivered to the pelvis. Some reports have suggested an increase in rectal toxicity with this approach; however, this is likely due to the poor quality of the implant. At least one study from a leading implant center suggested no significant increase in severe early or late GI/GU morbidity with combination therapy. The value of supplemental EBRT needs to be evaluated in comparison to full-dose EBRT in terms of long-term morbidity and cancer control.

High-dose Rate (HDR) Devices
Besides permanent implants, which deliver low dose rate (LDR) radiotherapy, brachytherapy for prostate cancer has been delivered using temporary high-dose rate devices, usually in patients with locally advanced disease. In this technique, a high dose (minimum, approximately 5 Gy) is delivered to the prostate over ≤1 hour by remotely inserting a highly radioactive source into catheters placed into the prostate under ultrasonographic guidance while the patient is under anesthesia. Several treatments are given on separate occasions, and EBRT is used for approximately 5 weeks as well.

More reports are accumulating on the application of HDR brachytherapy to prostate cancer. Various dose-fractionation combinations of HDR with or without combined pelvic EBRT have been employed, with a dose-response relationship apparent in biochemical control. Although the follow-up is short and no prospective randomized trials evaluating this approach have yet been published, it appears that HDR prostate brachytherapy in combination with pelvic EBRT may be effective. The long-term consequences for normal tissue of delivering large doses per fraction using this technique are unclear.

High-Intensity Focused Ultrasound (HIFU) is a relatively new treatment developed and used in Europe. While not currently FDA-approved in the United States, clinical trials are underway. Some patients from the U.S. are also employing "medical tourism" to have the procedure performed in Canada or Mexico.

3. Medications and Devices to Manage Impotence After Prostatectomy EBRT or Brachytherapy

Treatment for postprostatectomy impotence includes the phosphodiesterase inhibitors sildenafil (Viagra), vardenafil (Levitra®), and tadalafil (Cialis®); prostaglandin E1, administered as a urethral suppository (Muse®); intercavernosal injection (Caverject®, Edex®); or vacuum-pump erection aids that are useful for improving erections in men who have poor erectile function after prostatectomy, radiation therapy, or brachytherapy. These therapies are effective in 15%-40% of men with postprostatectomy impotence and in 50%-75% of men with postradiotherapy erectile dysfunction. Insertion of a penile prosthesis is typically offered to patients only after unsuccessful trials with the previously mentioned, less-invasive interventions.

4. Detection and Treatment of Recurrence

Significance and Definition of a Rising PSA Level Post-irradiation

The use of PSA levels following definitive therapy (either radiotherapy or radical prostatectomy) can detect early recurrences that may be amenable to salvage treatment. A rising PSA profile following radiotherapy is unequivocal evidence of the presence of a residual prostatic neoplasm. However, the definition of a rising PSA level after radiation therapy varies in the literature. A1996 consensus conference recommended that PSA failure be considered to have occurred after three consecutive PSA level rises, with the rate of failure defined as halfway between the first rise and the previous PSA level. Moreover, patients with a rising PSA level after irradiation may be a heterogeneous group, including patients with truly localized failure as well as those with metastatic disease. Also, certain patients will have a slowly rising PSA level after irradiation and may not require additional treatment. In patients who do not receive androgen ablation, the 5-year actuarial risk of distant metastasis from the time that the PSA level begins to rise is ~50%. A rapidly emerging key concept in rising PSA levels is PSA velocity, or more specifically PSA doubling time. Multiple recent studies have found that a PSAdoubling time <10-12 months predicts early clinical relapse if biochemical recurrence is untreated.

More recently, a PSA level that has risen 2 ng/mL above the post-radiation nadir PSA is considered a biochemical failure. This is the so-called "Phoenix Definition," based on an ASTRO panel held in that city.

Treatment Recommendations for Recurrence Post-irradiation

In general, men who have clear evidence of a rising PSA level 2 years after definitive radiotherapy for localized prostate cancer should be advised about the options of hormonal therapy (see section 5), salvage surgery, salvage cryotherapy, observation or experimental therapy.

If patients have minimal comorbidity, good life expectancy, and only local evidence of disease recurrence, salvage surgery is an option, but should be preceded by a bone scan, CT scan, cystoscopy and extensive counseling, because urinary difficulties after salvage prostatectomy are substantial and highly prevalent.

5. Treatment of Locally Advanced Disease (T3, T4)

The treatment of patients with locally advanced prostate cancer is centered on a multimodality and multidisciplinary approach, including radiation therapy (EBRT with or without HDR interstitial therapy), androgen ablation plus EBRT, or radical prostatectomy with or without androgen deprivation.

EBRT With and Without HDR Interstitial Therapy

For patients with locally extensive prostate cancer, local failure remains a potential problem after EBRT. This problem has prompted investigations into alternative means to intensify therapy.

One strategy has been to deliver large fractions of radiotherapy using HDR interstitial techniques in combination with EBRT. The large interstitial fractions, which may be on the order of 5 Gy, deliver a high dose to the prostate but spare normal tissues, due to the rapid dose falloff outside the implanted volume. Early experience with this strategy is encouraging, but long-term data on outcome, particularly in patients with locally extensive disease, and on morbidity are awaited.

Patients with locally advanced prostate cancer probably are not good candidates for permanent prostate implants. Patients with stage T3-T4 tumors are at high risk of gross extraprostatic involvement, and this localized therapy may not offer adequate dosimetric coverage of extraprostatic disease.

As mentioned in the previous section, there may be a synergistic effect between hormonal therapy given in conjunction with radiation therapy. In addition to enhancing apoptosis and producing local cytoreduction, the use of early androgen deprivation may possibly delay or even prevent the development of metastatic disease. The current body of evidence from two large randomized trials (RTOG 85-10 and EORTC) suggests that immediate long-term androgen deprivation in conjunction with EBRT improves outcomes among men with locally advanced or high-risk (Gleason score ≥8) prostate cancer compared with radiation therapy alone. An analysis of RTOG 85-31 by Horwitz et al, which employed early indefinite androgen deprivation, demonstrated that patients with locally advanced disease (T3N0) had improved cause-specific failure and distant metastatic failure compared with EBRT alone. Furthermore, a comparison to RTOG 86-10, which studied similar patients treated with only 4 months of hormonal therapy, favored the long-term approach. The EORTC trial randomized 415 patients and demonstrated a 15% overall survival benefit to 3 years of combined therapy versus radiation therapy alone.

Radical Prostatectomy With or Without Adjuvant Therapy

Surgical monotherapy can be considered a reasonable option for patients with locally advanced prostate cancer. Stage T3 disease can be successfully treated with low morbidity and significant reductions in risk of local recurrence, with clinical overstaging (up to 26%) reported by Yamada et al. Well- and moderately-differentiated cancers have cancer-specific survival rates of 76% at 10 years, comparable to those of other treatment modalities.

The Mayo Clinic has one of the largest radical prostatectomy series for T3 disease, consisting of more than 1,000 patients. In this population, of whom 34% received adjuvant therapy, 15-year cancer-specific survival and local recurrence rates were 77% and 21%, respectively. In an Eastern Cooperative Oncology Group (ECOG) trial, referred to as the "Messing Trial", 98 men who were found to have nodal metastases following radical prostatectomy and pelvic lymphadenectomy were randomized to receive immediate androgen deprivation or be followed until clinical disease progression. At a median follow-up of 7 years, 18 of 51 men in the observation group had died, compared with only 4 of 47 in the treatment group ($P = 0.02$).

> Positive margins are not uncommon after radical prostatectomy (37% in this study by Simon et al). Despite these strikingly high rates, approximately only one in five will recur, suggesting that adjuvant therapy is not always necessary (Simon MA, Kim S, Soloway MS. *J Urol*. 2006;175:140-145.)

> Patients with positive lymph nodes at the time of radical prostatectomy who receive immediate androgen deprivation have a survival advantage over those who receive deferred therapy (deferred vs early hazard ratio, 1.84; 95% confidence interval, 1.01-3.35). (Messing EM, Manola J, Yao J, et al. *Lancet Oncol*. 2006;7:472-479.)

Treatment of Node-positive Disease

Whether any local treatment adds to the overall survival duration in patients with known nodal involvement is debatable. Until recently, the standard of care had been to perform frozen-section pathologic analysis on pelvic lymph nodes at the time of radical prostatectomy, prior to removal of the prostate. If this analysis revealed micrometastases, radical prostatectomy was thought to be contraindicated. Although retrospective in nature, recent data from several American centers, including one large study from the Mayo Clinic, have reported a survival benefit in men who undergo radical prostatectomy despite the presence of micrometastases to regional pelvic lymph nodes. These men tend to do better and survive longer when started on early hormonal therapy, either with orchiectomy or an LHRH agonist.

Radiation Therapy

There are also compelling data that long-term survival is achievable in these patients with combination radiation and hormonal therapy. Data from the M. D. Anderson Cancer Center indicate a benefit to pelvic/prostate radiation therapy plus immediate hormonal manipulation compared with hormones alone. A subset analysis of patients with node-positive disease from RTOG 85-31 revealed immediate hormonal therapy plus radiation therapy resulted in 5- and 9-year cause-specific survival rates of 84% and 76%, respectively. Therefore, aggressive locoregional therapy appears to be effective in this cohort of unfavorable patients.

6. Treatment of Advanced Systemic Disease

Defining Advanced Disease

Metastatic Prostate Cancer

The most common sites of metastatic disease are the bone and pelvic and abdominal lymph nodes. Other, less common sites include the liver and lungs. Complications of metastatic prostate cancer include pain, fatigue, skeletal fractures, spinal cord compression, urinary outlet obstruction and failure to thrive. First-line hormonal therapy for men with metastatic prostate cancer delays these complications.

Rising PSA Level

A large series of more than 2000 patients treated with radical prostatectomy at Johns Hopkins University demonstrated that approximately 17% of cases recurred, with only 5.8% being local disease. In the remaining patients, disease recurred initially with either a rise in PSA level alone (9.7%) or evidence of clinical metastases (1.7%).

Outcomes for men with only a rising PSA level can vary greatly. Time to PSA recurrence (< vs. >2 years), PSAdoubling time (< vs. >9 months), and Gleason score (8-10 vs. 5-7) are among the important factors for predicting the development of metastatic disease and survival. The major developments for hormonal therapy in advanced prostate cancer were achieved prior to routine PSA testing and were often complicated by problematic study design. There are no prospective data that confirm a benefit to early hormonal therapy for men with a rising PSA alone. However, for patients with a rising PSA level who are at high risk for the development of metastases, some physicians agree that early hormonal therapy is likely to benefit this group of patients as well as those with radiologic evidence of metastatic disease.

First-line Therapies for Advanced Disease

The standard first-line treatment of advanced prostate cancer, regardless of whether local treatment has been applied, is to ablate the action of androgens by medical or surgical means. For the majority of patients, androgen ablation can result in a decline in PSA level, palliation of disease-related symptoms and regression of metastatic disease on imaging.

Bilateral Orchiectomy

The advantages of orchiectomy over other means of castration include an immediate decline in testosterone levels and ease of compliance for patients. Given these advantages, however, many men still opt for medical castration, with the potential advantage of intermittent hormonal therapy. In addition, the psychological impact of orchiectomy can be significant. Nonetheless, bilateral orchiectomy may be appropriate for a select group of patients.

LHRH Analogs

LHRH agonists, such as leuprolide (Lupron®, Eligard®, Viadur®), goserelin (Zoladex®), and triptorelin (Trelstar®) interfere with the normal pulsatile secretion of LH from the pituitary gland, resulting in an eventual decline in serum testosterone levels. The effect is reversible with cessation of therapy. Because LH is initially increased with LHRH agonists, testosterone levels may actually increase initially as well. This finding can result in a transient rise in PSA levels and potential growth of metastatic sites. Because of this initial "flare response" with LHRH agonists, consideration should be given to the administration of an antiandrogen prior to the LHRH, especially in patients who are at risk for complications from the disease (such as spinal cord compression, worsening pain or urinary outlet obstruction; Table 4).

Pure LHRH antagonists (abarelix [Plenaxis®]) and degarelix have been approved by the FDA. Their main advantage is the lack of an LHRH surge or flare, and are indicated in men with impending spinal cord compression or other now uncommon clinical scenarios where a flare could be harmful. Abarelix was rarely associated with an anaphylactic reaction and was withdrawn from the market. Degarelix, a second compound in the class, was FDA-approved in December 2008 and is not associated with any anaphylactic reactions.

Antiandrogens

Antiandrogens function to block the binding of dihydrotestosterone (DHT) to the androgen receptor, blocking the translocation of the DHT-androgen receptor complex into the nuclei of cells. There are 2 general classes: steroidal and nonsteroidal. Steroidal antiandrogens include cyproterone and megestrol. The most commonly used antiandrogens include the nonsteroidal agents flutamide, bicalutamide (Casodex®), and nilutamide (Nilandron®). These agents differ slightly in their affinity for the androgen receptor and their side-effect profiles.

Typically, antiandrogens are used in combination with surgical or medical castration. Some trials comparing antiandrogens alone with LHRH analogs have shown similar efficacy, but more recent trials suggest that monotherapy with antiandrogens may be inferior in terms of time to disease progression and possibly survival. For example, a randomized trial of monotherapy with high-dose bicalutamide (150 mg daily) compared with flutamide plus goserelin demonstrated that patients treated with bicalutamide monotherapy had fewer side effects, such as loss of libido or erectile dysfunction, and trended toward improved quality of life. However, in patients with radiographic evidence of metastases, bicalutamide monotherapy was associated with a small 6-week decrease in survival (hazard ratio, 1.3). Despite this finding, for men who are intolerant to the side effects of LHRH analogs or for those without metastatic disease, monotherapy with antiandrogens can be considered after careful discussion with patients.

Antiandrogen monotherapy with flutamide or bicalutamide is also sometimes used to treat PSA recurrence. Used alone or in combination with a 5-alpha reductase inhibitor (finasteride or dutasteride), this approach is associated with fewer side effects than traditional androgen suppression therapy, but the approaches have not been approved by the US FDA. A significant downside is nipple tenderness or gynecomastia, but this "peripheral blockade" approach may preserve potency and libido.

Combined Androgen Blockade

Combined androgen blockade (CAB) refers to the elimination of testicular androgens in combination with blockade of adrenal androgens, generally with an LHRH analog and an antiandrogen agent.

The use of CAB is somewhat controversial. Several randomized trials comparing LHRH antagonists alone vs. CAB have demonstrated a survival benefit

Table 4

Hormonal Approaches to the Treatment of Advanced Prostate Cancer

Method	Mechanism of Action	Side Effect
Surgical castration	Removal of testicular androgens	Hot flashes (50%), psychological effects
Diethylstilbestrol (DES)	Inhibition of gonadotropin secretion	Gynecomastia, cardiovascular risks at high doses
LHRH analogs (goserelin, leuprolide, triptorelin)	Inhibition of gonadotropin secretion	Hot flashes (50%), less gynecomastia than with DES, fatigue
Antiandrogens (bicalutamide, flutamide, nilutamide)	Blockade of binding of dihydrotestosterone to its receptor	Abnormal liver function studies, diarrhea (10%)

LHRH = luteinizing hormone-releasing hormone

The American Society of Clinical Oncology recently published guidelines for the initial management of androgen-sensitive (recurrent, metastatic) prostate cancer. Based on the literature, immediate androgen deprivation was associated with a moderate decrease in prostate cancer mortality and a moderate increase in other causes of mortality. Currently, there is no definitive evidence favoring the early initiation of androgen deprivation in this population. (Loblaw DA, Virgo KS, Nam R, et al. *J Clin Oncol*. 2007; 25:1596-1605.)

with CAB. However, in one of the largest trials conducted by the United States Intergroup, more than 1300 men were randomized to undergo orchiectomy vs. orchiectomy plus flutamide. There was no significant advantage to CAB in terms of time to disease progression or overall survival. Some investigators believe that bicalutamide, a more potent agent, may be associated with greater survival when used as part of CAB.

The American Society of Clinical Oncology recommends the routine use of CAB over monotherapy with an LHRH antagonist or orchiectomy (2007 updated guidelines).

Diethylstilbestrol (DES)

Estrogen administration, in the form of DES, also produces chemical castration. DES inhibits prostate growth, primarily through the inhibition of the hypothalamic-pituitary-gonadal axis, which blocks testicular synthesis of testosterone and thus lowers plasma testosterone levels. Since doses higher than 3 mg/d cause significant cardiovascular mortality, DES has fallen out of favor as a first-line therapy to induce castration.

Ketoconazole (Nizoral®)

Ketoconazole is an antifungal agent that can inhibit adrenal and testicular steroid synthesis at higher doses, leading to a decline in adrenal and testicular androgens. It has the benefit of a rapid decline in testosterone, which can be useful for patients who present emergently with a complication of newly diagnosed advanced disease. Ketoconazole is started at a dose of 200 mg TID and increased to a total dose of 400 mg TID. Ketoconazole is associated with significant side effects (such as fatigue, nausea and vomiting), however, and must be given with supplemental hydrocortisone to avoid symptoms of adrenal insufficiency. Because of the side effects, its use is more common in the second-line setting, where responses can be expected in 20%-40% of patients following progression with CAB.

Early vs. Late Treatment

Whether to treat patients early with hormonal therapy or wait until patients become symptomatic has been tested in a large European trial conducted by the Medical Research Council. Men were randomized to receive immediate hormonal therapy (orchiectomy or an LHRH analog) vs. delayed therapy which was initiated with symptomatic progression. Men who were treated with early therapy were less likely to experience urinary obstructive symptoms requiring intervention, pathologic fractures, and cord compression than those treated in the delayed arm (Table 5). The survival benefit was less clear, however, because many of the men in the delayed arm died before they received any hormonal therapy. This study was also complicated by the initiation of PSA monitoring during the study period. Many patients and physicians currently are not comfortable delaying therapy until the onset of symptoms while the PSA level is rising; this fact limits the applicability of its findings in the modern era.

Other smaller trials have examined this issue as well. A Cochrane Database review was conducted in 2002; it demonstrated an increase in progression-free survival and a small, but significant, improvement in survival with early hormonal therapy.

Treatment Recommendations

Just as for localized disease, initial treatment for advanced prostate cancer must be individualized. A patient who presents with a rising PSA level only after local treatment and a slow PSAdoubling time, a prolonged time to PSA recurrence, and a low initial Gleason score may not require immediate therapy, especially if there are other more significant comorbidities. However, a patient with multiple metastatic sites will need immediate treatment, generally with orchiectomy or CAB initially followed

Table 5

The Incidence of Complications From Advanced Prostate Cancer With Immediate vs Deferred Androgen Deprivation

Complication	Immediate	Deferred
Pathologic fracture	2.3%	4.5%
Spinal cord compression	2.0%	5.0%
Ureteric obstruction	7.0%	11.8%
Extraskeletal metastases	7.9%	11.8%

by monotherapy with an LHRH analog, to prevent the sequelae of metastatic disease, such as fracture, spinal cord compression, and ureteral obstruction. Ketoconazole may be considered as the initial systemic therapy for patients presenting with cord compression as the first presentation of prostate cancer. Given the overall limitations of hormone therapy, all appropriate patients should be offered access to clinical trials.

For patients with a rising PSA level who are at high risk for the development of metastases, a discussion regarding the potential advantages to early treatment and an explanation of the lack of randomized prospective data are warranted. Some investigators favor early treatment for these patients based on the data from the Medical Research Council trial and the Cochrane Database review, understanding that this information is extrapolated from data obtained prior to PSA testing and from patients with clinical and radiographic metastases.

Second-line Hormonal Therapies

Outcomes with initial androgen ablation can vary from responses that last from months to years; they also vary as a function of the Gleason grade, pretreatment PSA velocity, and extent of disease at the time of initiating treatment. Once PSA levels begin to rise with androgen ablation, the disease is often referred to as "hormone refractory" or "castrate resistent." This term is actually a misnomer, because preclinical data suggest that tumors may become hypersensitive to androgens, resulting in worsened disease if androgen ablation is removed entirely. Moreover, many patients have disease that remains sensitive to further hormonal manipulations, such as second-line antiandrogens, steroids or ketoconazole.

An example of this sensitivity to hormonal manipulation is exemplified in the antiandrogen withdrawal response. Up to one-third of patients with a rising PSA level while receiving treatment with an antiandrogen will have a decline in PSAlevel and or clinical regression with antiandrogen withdrawal. The mechanism of this response has not been fully elucidated but supports the hypothesis that the androgen receptor remains important in progressive disease.

Although second-line hormonal therapy has demonstrated benefit in terms of PSA levels and response, there are no data to demonstrate a survival advantage with second-line hormonal therapy. Its role has further come into question, with data that support the use of docetaxel (Taxotere®) chemotherapy for men with metastatic androgen-independent prostate cancer to improve survival. It is unknown whether the survival benefit with docetaxel is limited after multiple hormonal therapies.

For patients with a rising PSA level only, timing of chemotherapy is even less clear. The Eastern Cooperative Oncology Group attempted a trial comparing ketoconazole/hydrocortisone with docetaxel in patients with a rising PSA level but no evidence of metastatic disease after hormonal therapy, but the trial was closed early due to lack of accrual. Until prospective data are available, physicians will need to counsel patients carefully on the different options and timing of those options available at the time of progression, including second-line hormonal manipulation, chemotherapy and, especially, clinical trials.

Chemotherapy for Androgen-independent Disease

Docetaxel

The role of chemotherapy has changed significantly over the past several years with the results of two

Table 6

Chemotherapy Regimens for Prostate Cancer

Drug/Combination	Dose and Schedule
Mitoxantrone/Prednisone	
Mitoxantrone	12 mg/m^2 IV on day 1
Prednisone	5 mg PO BID
Repeat cycle every 21 days.	
Tannock IF, Osoba D, Stockler MR, et al. *J Clin Oncol.* 1996;14:1756-1764.	
Docetaxel/Estramustine	
Docetaxel	60 mg/m^2 on day 2 every 21 days
Estramustine	280 mg orally on days 1 to 5 every 21 days
Dexamethasone	60 mg orally given as a premedication before docetaxel
Petrylak DP, Tangen CM, Hussain MHA, et al. *N Engl J Med.* 2004;351:1513-1520.	
Docetaxel/Prednisone	
Docetaxel	75 mg/m^2 IV every 3 weeks
Prednisone	5 mg orally BID started on day 1
Note: Standard docetaxel premedication should be given prior to the administration of docetaxel	
Tannock IF, de Wit R, Berry WR, et al. *N Engl J Med.* 2004;351:1502-1512.	

Table prepared by Ishmael Jaiyesimi, DO.

large randomized trials demonstrating a survival benefit for men with androgen-independent metastatic prostate cancer treated with docetaxel based chemotherapy (Table 6). Investigators from the Southwest Oncology Group randomized patients to receive mitoxantrone (Novantrone) plus prednisone versus docetaxel (60 mg/m^2) plus estramustine and dexamethasone every 3 weeks. Patients in the docetaxel arm had a significant improvement in survival by 2 months.

A second trial by Tannock et al showed a similar survival benefit of 2 months with docetaxel (75 mg/m^2) plus prednisone given every 3 weeks compared with mitoxantrone and prednisone. These trials were the first to demonstrate a survival benefit with chemotherapy in advanced prostate cancer and have sparked numerous studies involving docetaxel in combination with newer agents. Toxicities of docetaxel include myelosuppression and neuropathy, both of which can be dose-limiting.

Mitoxantrone Plus Prednisone

Mitoxantrone (12 mg/m^2) plus prednisone has been approved for use in advanced prostate cancer based on improvement in palliation of pain and quality of life over prednisone alone despite no improvement in overall survival.

Bisphosphonates

Bone metastases from prostate cancer are associated with increased bone formation around tumor deposits, resulting in characteristic osteoblastic metastases. However, concomitant with the osteoblastic activity is a marked increase in bone resorption and osteolysis, which can be inhibited by bisphosphonates.

Studies of bisphosphonates in prostate cancer have demonstrated mixed results. A combined analysis of 2 multicentered, randomized, controlled trials comparing pamidronate with placebo in men with androgen-independent progressive prostate cancer demonstrated no benefit in terms of skeleton-related events or palliation of symptoms. A phase III trial with an oral bisphosphonate, clodronate, demonstrated no difference in either symptomatic bone metastases or prostate cancerrelated deaths when compared with placebo.

A phase III trial demonstrated a reduction in skeleton-related events for men with androgen-independent metastatic prostate cancer with a more potent bisphosphonate, zoledronic acid (Zometa®). However, it is important to note that this trial did not show an improvement in quality of life with zoledronic acid, nor did it demonstrate a reduction in the development of new metastases.

At this time, the recommendation for zoledronic acid in prostate cancer is limited to men with androgen-independent prostate cancer. It is important to recognize the limitations of this therapy and to understand that there is no defined role for its use in men with androgen-dependent prostate cancer. Although these men are at higher risk for osteoporosis, less potent oral bisphosphonates may be a more reasonable approach, given the longterm side effects associated with zoledronic acid (renal insufficiency and osteonecrosis of the mandible).

Newer Therapies

Several new therapies for men with prostate cancer (some as single agents and some with chemotherapy) are under investigation, with promising early results. They include the endothelin receptor antagonist 204054, the VEGF inhibitor bevacizumab (Avastin®), and a new class of antimicrotubule agents (the epothilones). There are ample preclinical and early clinical data to suggest that all of these agents may have activity against prostate cancer, but no definitive trials to establish their role have yet been performed. These agents are still considered investigational. Several trials are evaluating the combinations of docetaxel and bevacizumab, docetaxel and 204054, and docetaxel and a vaccine.

More recently, a better understanding of the androgen synthesis and metabolic pathways related to hormone-refractory prostate cancer is emerging. Newer, more potent antiandrogens are under intense study.

Radiation Therapy for Palliating Bone Metastasis

Radiotherapy is effective in controlling local pain associated with skeletal prostate metastasis. In general, a treatment regimen of 30 Gy over 10 treatments results in rapid and durable local symptom control and a reduced dependence on analgesics.

For patients with more extensive bone involvement causing pain that may be difficult to address with localized EBRT, alternatives include wide-field irradiation (ie, hemibody irradiation) or systemic administration of radioactive, bone-seeking isotopes that can deliver therapeutic doses to skeletal metastatic disease. Radioactive isotopes used in this fashion include strontium-89 chloride (Metastron®) and samarium SM 153 lexidronam (Quadramet®).

7. Suggested Reading

Albertsen PC, Hanley JA, Fine J, et al. 20-year outcomes following conservative management of clinically localized prostate cancer. *JAMA*. 2005;293: 2095-2101.

Bill-Axelson A, Holmberg L, Ruutu M, et al. Radical prostatectomy versus watchful waiting in early prostate cancer. *N Engl J Med*. 2005;352:1977-1984.

D'Amico AV, Chen MH, Roehl KA, et al. Preoperative PSA velocity and the risk of death from prostate cancer after radical prostatectomy. *N Engl J Med*. 2004;351:125-135.

D'Amico AV, Moul JW, Carroll PR, et al. Cancer-specific mortality after surgery or radiation for patients with clinically localized prostate cancer managed during the prostate-specific antigen era. *J Clin Oncol*. 2003;21:2163-2172.

D'Amico AV, Moul JW, Carroll PR, et al. Surrogate end point for prostate cancer-specific mortality after radical prostatectomy or radiation therapy. *J Natl Cancer Inst*. 2003;95:1376-1383.

D'Amico AV, Renshaw AA, Sussman B, et al. Pretreatment PSA velocity and risk of death from prostate cancer following external beam radiation therapy. *JAMA*. 2005;294:440-447.

Freedland SJ, Humphreys EB, Mangold LA, et al. Risk of prostate cancer-specific mortality following biochemical recurrence after radical prostatectomy. *JAMA*. 2005;294:433-439.

Lawton CA, Winter K, Grignon D, et al. Androgen suppression plus radiation versus radiation alone for patients with stage D1/pathologic node-positive adenocarcinoma of the prostate: Updated results based on national prospective randomized trial Radiation Therapy Oncology Group 85-31. *J Clin Oncol*. 2005;23:800-807.

Moul JW, Wu H, Sun L, et al. Early versus delayed hormonal therapy for prostate-specific antigen only recurrence of prostate cancer after radical prostatectomy. *J Urol*. 2004;171:1141-1147.

Sharifi N, Gulley JL, Dahut WL. Androgen deprivation therapy for prostate cancer. *JAMA*. 2005;294: 238-244.

Smith MR, Kabbinavar F, Saad F, et al. Natural history of rising serum prostate-specific antigen in men with castrate nonmetastatic prostate cancer. *J Clin Oncol*. 2005;23:2918-2925.

Stephenson AJ, Shariat SF, Zelefsky MJ, et al. Salvage radiotherapy for recurrent prostate cancer after radical prostatectomy. *JAMA*. 2004;291:1325-1332.

Thompson IM, Ankerst DP, Chi C, et al. Operating characteristics of prostate-specific antigen in men with an initial PSA level of 3.0 ng/mL or lower. *JAMA*. 2005;294:66-70.

Thompson IM, Pauler DK, Goodman PJ, et al. Prevalence of prostate cancer among men with a prostate-specific antigen level < or = 4.0 ng per milliliter. *N Engl J Med*. 2004;350:2239-2246.

Sanda MG, Dunn RL, Michalski J, et al. Quality of life and satisfaction with outcome among prostate-cancer survivors. *N Engl J Med*. 2008;358(12):1250-1261.

Thompson IM Jr, Tangen CM, Paradelo J, et al. Adjuvant radiotherapy for pathologically advanced prostate cancer: a randomized clinical trial. *JAMA*. 2006;296(19):2329-2335.

Lippman SM, Klein EA, Goodman PJ, et al.HYPERLINK "http://www.ncbi.nlm.nih.gov/pubmed/19066370?ordinalpos=3&itool=EntrezSystem2.PEntrez.Pubmed.Pubmed_ResultsPanel.Pubmed_RVDocSum" Effect of selenium and vitamin E on risk of prostate cancer and other cancers: the Selenium and Vitamin E Cancer Prevention Trial (SELECT). *JAMA*. 2009;301(1):39-51.

Gaziano JM, Glynn RJ, Christen WG, et al. HYPERLINK "http://www.ncbi.nlm.nih.gov/pubmed/19066368?ordinalpos=4&itool=EntrezSystem2.PEntrez.Pubmed.Pubmed_ResultsPanel.Pubmed_RVDocSum" Vitamins E and C in the prevention of prostate and total cancer in men: the Physicians' Health Study II randomized controlled trial. *JAMA*. 2009;301(1):52-62.

Lu-Yao GL, Albertsen PC, Moore DF, et al. Survival following primary androgen deprivation therapy among men with localized prostate cancer. *JAMA*. 2008;300(2):173-181.

Trock BJ, Han M, Freedland SJ, et al. HYPERLINK "http://www.ncbi.nlm.nih.gov/pubmed/18560003?ordinalpos=6&itool=EntrezSystem2.PEntrez.Pubmed.Pubmed_ResultsPanel.Pubmed_RVDocSum" Prostate cancer-specific survival following salvage radiotherapy vs. observation in men with biochemical recurrence after radical prostatectomy. *JAMA*. 2008;299(23):2760-2769.

Zheng SL, Sun J, Wiklund F, et al. Cumulative association of five genetic variants with prostate cancer. *N Engl J Med*. 2008;358(9):910-919.

Walsh PC, DeWeese TL, Eisenberger MA. Clinical practice. Localized prostate cancer. *N Engl J Med*. 2007;357(26):2696-2705.

Bañez LL, Hamilton RJ, Partin AW, et al. Obesity-related plasma hemodilution and PSA concentration among men with prostate cancer. *JAMA*. 2007;298(19):2275-2280.

Thompson I, Thrasher JB, Aus G, et al for the AUA Prostate Cancer Clinical Guideline Update Panel. Guideline for the management of clinically localized prostate cancer: 2007 update. *J Urol*. 2007;177(6):2106-2131.

Chapter 17: Non-Muscle Invasive Bladder Cancer

Michael A. O'Donnell, MD

Contents

1. Epidemiology

Basic Statistics

- Median age 70 years old but rare in women < 40 years old
- Male:female ratio 3:1
- 68,000 new cases (incidence) in 2008; prevalence ~ 9X incidence
- 4th most common cancer in men; 9th most common in women
- Ethnic predominance Caucasians > African Americans > Hispanics > Asians BUT higher death rate in women and in African Americans
- Presentation: 75% non-muscle invasive; 20% muscle-invasive; 5% metastatic

Risk Factors

- Cigarette smoking
  - Smoke is potent source of urothelial carcinogens especially biphenyl amines
  - Dose response relationship to development of bladder cancer (especially > 40 pack years)
  - Increases hazard ratio to develop bladder cancer by 2-4 fold
  - Responsible for ~ 50% males cases; ~ 30% female but women are catching up
  - 15-20 year latency time
  - Quitting reduces risks but never down to non-smoker
  - New evidence that second-hand smoke is contributor
- Environmental/Occupational Exposure
  - Responsible for ~20 % of cases
  - First occupationally-identified cancer (Rehn 1895 in aniline dye industry)
  - Exposure to chemicals in following industries: aluminum, dye, paint, petroleum, rubber, textile, printing
  - Higher risk professions: truck drivers, hairdressers, dry cleaners, paper manufacturers, rope/twine makers, dental technicians, apparel manufacturers, plumbers
- Analgesic abuse: phenacetin (removed in 1987)
- Pelvic radiation: eg, cervical/anal/prostate cancer
- Cyclophosphamide: 4 to 9-fold increased risk
- Chronic cystitis: indwelling catheters, bilharziasis (for squamous cell carcinoma)
- Miscellaneous: arsenic, bracken fern, Balkan nephropathy, *Aristolochia fangchi* (Chinese weight loss herb); associated with bilateral upper tract cancers

Genetics

- Positive family history in 8% cases
- Relative risk increases ~2-fold with family history but non-hereditary
- Rare familial syndrome: (Lynch syndrome II) with defect in DNA mismatch repair
- No specific gene locus yet identified
- Polymorphisms in detoxification mechanisms contribute to higher susceptibility to environmental carcinogens
  - Smokers: Slow acetylators have 40% higher risk than fast acetylators
  - Glutathione S-transferase M1 null (~2-fold increased risk; tobacco independent)

2. Histology

- 90%-95% transitional cell carcinoma (TCC) in United States and Europe
- ~5% squamous cell carcinoma (SCC) EXCEPT
  * Increased incidence in spinal cord injury patients or those with chronic infection or foreign bodies
  * Up to 80% of bladder tumors are SCC in endemic regions of *Schistosoma hematobium* infection (Egypt, Sudan, Saudi Arabia, Africa)
- 0.5%-2% adenocarcinoma
  * Usually arise from urachus or trigonal region
  * Especially prevalent in cases of prior bladder extrophy
  * Majority have associated history of long-term inflammation or infection
  * Nonurachal adenocarcinomas of the bladder must be distinguished from extension of colorectal primary, usually by colonoscopy
  * Most common type associated with ureterosigmoidostomy
  * Signet cell variant associated with very aggressive behavior
- Transitional cell carcinoma with mixed features such as squamous or glandular differentiation
  * Treatment same as for TCC
- Other variant cancer histology of clinical significance (<1% incidence). Usually invasive at time of presentation.
  * Small cell or neuroendocrine cancer
    - May be pure or mixed with high-grade TCC
    - Stains positive with neuroendocrine markers, such as neuron specific enolase, synaptophysin or chromogranin
    - Unlike other forms of bladder cancer, primary treatment is systemic chemotherapy (VP-16 plus cisplatinum)
  * Micropapillary cancer
    - Thought to be a highly aggressive variant of TCC
    - Aggressive surgery indicated for non-metastatic disease
    - Superficial forms relatively resistant to BCG therapy (primary cystectomy advocated)
    - Muscle-invasive and advanced forms relatively resistant to systemic chemotherapy
  * Carcinosarcoma
    - Very aggressive cancer with mixed epithelial and mesenchymal malignant elements
  * Sarcomatoid carcinoma
    - Sometimes mistaken for carcinosarcoma because of sarcoma-like appearance but proven by immunostaining to contain only epithelial elements
  * Metastatic cancers—may include renal cell, ovarian, melanoma, etc.
- Potential premalignant lesions
  * Leukoplakia—squamous metaplasia with keratin; precursor for squamous cell carcinoma ~ 20%
  * Cystitis glandularis—glandular metaplasia of von Brunn's nests from chronic inflammation; possible precursor to adenocarcinoma.
  * Inverted papilloma—not malignant but associated with TCC elsewhere
  * NOTE: mild-moderate dysplasia is most often reactive in nature and not associated with malignancy while severe dysplasia is synonymous with carcinoma in situ (CIS)
- Benign tumors
  * Squamous metaplasia—common in 50% females, 10% males
  * Nephrogenic adenoma
    - Metaplastic urothelial response to trauma, infection, radiation, or chronic immunosuppression

- Associated with hematuria, dysuria and frequency
- Treated by TURBT and conservative cystoscopic follow-up

* Cystitis cystica and follicularis—inflammatory lesions of bladder

* Pseudosarcoma—spindle cell tumor associated with prior surgery

* Malacoplakia—chronic reaction to ongoing urinary tract infection

3. Molecular Characterization

Transitional Cell Carcinoma

- Most common chromosomal abnormality is loss of large segments of chromosome 9, especially 9q in low-grade TCC

- 2 proposed pathways: proliferative (loss of 9q) for low-grade cancers vs. dysplastic (p53 mutation) for high-grade cancers

- Frequent aneuploidy of chr 3, 5, 7, 17; (*Note:* tetraploidy is not considered abnormal—found in umbrella cells)

- Locus defects in p53, retinoblastoma (Rb), H-ras, p16 (CDKN2), p21 (WAF1) and p27 (Kip1)

- Markers of aggressivity include:

  * HIGH p53, Ki-67 (MIB-1), matrix metalloproteinase (MMP) immunostaining (Note: mutant p53 shows up as increased staining due to reduced degradation)

  * HIGH Urokinase-type plasminogen activator (uPA) serum level

  * LOW Rb, E-cadherin, and p27 immunostaining

Squamous Cell Carcinoma

- Frequent chromosomal alterations of 9p

- Mutation of CDKN2 (p16) 3X more frequent than in TCC

Adenocarcinoma

- Poorly defined at present

4. Clinical Presentation and Initial Work-up

Signs and Symptoms

Hematuria

- Found in 80%-90% of cases; (70%-80% gross hematuria)
- Typically visible, intermittent, painless and present throughout urination
- Bladder cancer is the most common cause of gross hematuria in patients > 50 yr old
- Often initially ignored by patients and physicians alike (especially female patients)
- Differential diagnosis: UTI, calculi, renal cancer, glomerulonephritis, trauma, BPH, others
  - * Consider clinical context (age, gender, risk factors) and details of hematuria
  - * All noninfectious gross hematuria of unknown etiology requires urologic work-up (upper tract study, cytology and cystoscopy)
- Irritative voiding symptoms (dysuria, urgency)
  - * Found in 20%-30% of cases, ~ half without hematuria
  - * May be misattributed to (interstitial) cystitis and prostatitis
  - * More common with high-grade aggressive disease, especially CIS and SCC
- Special signs and symptoms
  - * Mucosuria—passage of mucus sometimes seen with adenocarcinoma

Physical Exam

- Rarely abnormal in early disease states
- Conditions associated with advanced disease
  - * Palpable pelvic mass and/or flank pain
  - * Abnormal digital rectal exam may reveal extension into prostate
  - * Bloody urethral discharge or mass may indicate urethral or prostatic involvement
  - * Inguinal and distant lymphadenopathy
  - * Weight loss and cachexia
- Exam under anesthesia (EUA) important clinical staging step
  - * Fixed mass after transurethral resection (TUR) = clinical (c) T4
  - * Palpable mass after TUR = cT3

Laboratory Evaluation

- Urinalysis with microscopic exam
- Urine culture with sensitivity
- Urine cytology—especially helpful if indicative of high-grade disease
  - * A positive cytology showing high-grade dysplastic cells should be considered cancer until proven otherwise
  - * A positive cytology showing clusters of low-grade papillary clumps may be inaccurate, due to instrumentation or stones
- Electrolytes, BUN and creatinine
- Newer FDA-approved urine-based test support diagnosis but do not stand alone to make diagnosis
  - * These include BTA-Trak, BTA-Stat, nmp-22, BladderChek, UroVysion FISH, and ImmunoCyt

Imaging Studies

- Intravenous pyelogram (IVP) or CT urogram should be performed prior to cystoscopy and biopsy (TUR) to evaluate for obstruction and possibility of upper tract TCC (2% in early disease; up to 20% in advanced disease)
- Retrograde pyelograms sometimes necessary if upper tract studies are inconclusive
- Chest x-ray to rule out metastatic disease
- Bone scan not routinely performed unless high clinical suspicion of bone metastasis
- Renal and/or bladder ultrasound not required in majority of cases
- MRI may substitute for CT scan for clinical staging

5. Cystoscopic Evaluation and Initial Resection

- Cystoscopy is currently the gold standard for bladder cancer diagnosis
  - * No substitutes are adequate including urine marker tests or radiologic studies
  - * Office flexible cystoscopy initially for most cases of hematuria after upper tract studies
  - * If imaging or cytology highly suggestive of bladder cancer then office cystoscopy can be deferred in lieu of cystoscopy with biopsy or TUR under anesthesia
- Visual features of aggressive vs. nonaggressive lesions
  - * Small papillary lesions on a stalk are accurately classified visually >90% of time as low-grade, noninvasive bladder tumors
  - * Large tumors with a broad base or nodular configuration and areas of necrosis are more likely to be high-grade and invasive (at least stage T1)
  - * Red velvety flat lesions are typical of CIS especially in the setting of a highly suspicious or positive urine cytology
- TUR for complete removal of all suspicious lesions
  - * Avoid excess cautery for accurate histological assessment
  - * Cold cup resection alone with fulguration of base and periphery is appropriate for small papillary tumors
  - * Laser treatment (Holmium, YAG, KTP) is not appropriate at first tumor setting
  - * Detrusor muscle is required for all stage T1 lesions for accurate staging to rule out muscle-invasive disease
    - Understaging rate is up to 50% for high-grade stage T1 disease if detrusor muscle (muscularis propria) is absent. ***CAUTION***: wisps of muscle within the submucosa (muscularis

mucosa) can be mistaken for true detrusor muscle

- Even with true detrusor muscle present and not involved by cancer there is a 10%-20% understaging rate along with a 30%-50% chance of leaving residual tumor behind in T1 lesions
- Strongly recommended that all high-grade T1 lesions undergo a repeat TUR within 2-6 weeks of initial resection
  * Reduces understaging rate to <10% if confirms no muscle invasion
  * Improves response to intravesical immunotherapy with BCG and intravesical chemotherapy with mitomycin if done routinely
  * Provides prognostic information for later decision making
    - If no disease or only stage Ta residual then progression rare
    - If residual CIS only then progression ~25%
    - If residual T1 then progression ~75% by 2 years
- Special circumstance—tumor in diverticulum
  * Ta disease may be safely removed with caution if technically feasible
  * T1 disease, especially if high-grade, may be under-staged and easy to perforate; consider partial cystectomy/diverticulectomy if isolated and technically feasible
- Complications of TUR
  * Bleeding (early or delayed)
  * Bladder perforation
    - Often associated with obturator reflex (can be mitigated by neuromuscular blocking agents or local anesthetic block)
  * Need to distinguish intraperitoneal (often dome) from extraperitoneal – consider intraoperative cystogram
    - Most extraperitoneal perforations can be managed conservatively
    - Some intraperitoneal perforations can be managed conservatively
      * Small, not associated with infected urine—conservative
      * Large, associated with potential peritonitis, or bowel injury – repair (can be done laparoscopically)
  * Important points in acute management
    - If small and late in TUR can finish resection (switch from water to glycine, reduce pressure). Check for TUR syndrome.
    - If large, associated with bleeding or early in TUR back out, return at another time
    - If associated with bowel injury, repair immediately

- Directed biopsies of suspicious lesions is always appropriate

- Random biopsies

  * Not appropriate if mucosa is normal and tumor appears papillary and noninvasive with negative cytology

  * Appropriate when cytology is positive yet tumor appears papillary and noninvasive

  * Appropriate when visually aggressive tumors are present

  * Appropriate when contemplating partial cystectomy or other bladder-sparing approaches to rule out coincident CIS

Table 1

Comparative Aspects of FDA-approved Urinary Markers

Marker	PoC	Description	Sn 1°	Sn 2°	Sp 1°	Sp 2°	Comment
Hg-dipstick	X	Urine hemoglobin dipstick	52	40	82	87	Often first screen; nonspecific
Cytology		Lab reference standard	48	35	94	94	Sensitive up to 70% with grade 3
Cytometry		Flow DNA histogram for ploidy	60	60	80	82	Equaled to cytology in direct comparison
BTA Stat®	X	Human complement factor-H related protein	70	58	75	73	False positive with inflammation or blood
BTA Trak		Same-quantitative ELISA	69	71	65	66	False positive with inflammation or blood
BladderChek	X	Nuclear matrix protein in mitotic spindle	56	50	86	87	False positive with inflammation
NMP22		Same-quantitative ELISA	73	71	80	73	False positive with inflammation
ImmunoCyt		Panel of 3 monoclonal Abs applied to same cytology sample	83	67	80	75	Interobserver variability
FISH		4 probes for polysomy of Chr 3, 7, 17 or loss of 9p21	84	79	95	70	Not affected by BCG or inflammation; anticipatory positives

6. Role of Urinary Marker Tests in Initial Diagnosis

- Available FDA-approved markers (Table 1)
  - * Fluid-based
    - BTA Trak (quantitative) and BTA Stat® (qualitative—point of care)
    - NMP22 (quantitative) and BladderChek® (qualitative—point of care)
  - * Cell-based
    - ImmunoCyt™ —immune assisted cytolog
    - FISH—fluorescent *in situ* hybridization (aneuploidy of chromosomes 3, 7, 17; loss of 9p21 ((CDKN2)) locus)
    - Cytology—current standard
  - * All new marker tests suffer from reduced specificity
    - Cytology has a specificity of ~95% meaning that a frankly positive cytology for high-grade dysplastic cells should be assumed to indicate cancer until proven otherwise
    - False-positive tests are common wi h new markers
      - * Urine based assays less accurate with hematuria, infection or inflammation present (eg, from stones)
      - * Some tests (FISH) pick up positives months before they are cystoscopically visible (so-called anticipatory positive)
  - * All new marker tests have improved sensitivity over cytology
    - BUT still miss 20%-40% of cases (more sensitive for higher grade cancers)
    - NONE completely rule out cancer nor obviate need for cystoscopy as initial evaluation
    - CAN help stratify patients for higher or lower risk of cancer and help direct intensity of efforts for cancer work-up
    - BEST when used in conjunction with cystoscopy
  - * Utility of new urine markers in non-TCC cases is not established

Table 2

TNM Staging System for Bladder Cancer

Mucosa	Stage 0a Stage 0is	Ta Tis	N0	M0
Submucosa	Stage I	T1	N0	M0
Muscularis	Stage II	T2a T2b	N0	M0
Adventicia	Stage III	T3a T3b	N0	M0
Prostatic invasion	Stage IV	T4a		
Outside bladder		T4b (pelvic sidewall)	N0	M0
		Any T	N1-N3	M0
		Any T	Any N	M1

Figure 1

Relationship of 1973 WHO to 1998 WHO/ISUP

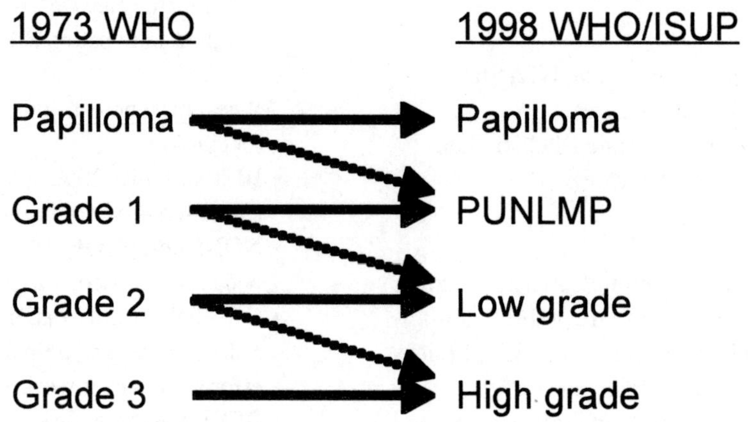

From Lerner SP, Konety BR, Skinner EC.
AUA 2006 Annual Meeting Course 60PG syllabus, Non-muscle invasive bladder cancer: risk-adapted treatment.

Table 3

Relationship of 1973 WHO and 1998 WHO/ISUP Grade to Progression

		Progression	
WHO 1973	**Cases %**	**45 mo**	**90 mo**
Papilloma	5.2	0	0
G1	31.3	11	11
G2	59	11	24
G3	4.5	60	60

		Progression	
WHO ISUP-1998	**Cases %**	**45 mo**	**90 mo**
Papilloma	2.2	0	0
LMP	21.6	8	8
Low grade	54.5	10	13
High grade	21.6	23	51

From Samaratunga H, Epstein JL. Urology. *2002;60(2):315-319.*

7. Pathological Staging and Grading

- TMN system for staging (Table 2)

  * Non-muscle-invasive groups include:
    - Stage Ta—mucosally confined
    - Stage Tis (CIS)—carcinoma *in situ*
      * Flat lesion confined to the mucosa
      * Always high-grade
      * Thought to be precursor for invasive disease
      * Nonamenable to surgical resection due to multifocal nature and tendency to spread widely along surface, sometimes invisibly
    - Stage T1—invasive into lamina propria (submucosa)
      * Usefulness of further substaging to early or deep invasion (T1a, T1b) is still controversial due to lack of consistent landmarks and inconsistent prognostic utility. Does not predict response to intravesical therapy.
      * Associated lymphovascular invasion (LVI) is a poor prognostic sign
        - Increased chance of under-staging (up to 88% in one series)
        - Increased chance of occult lymph node metastasis
        - Decreased survival
        - Advocated by some to justify
      * Early cystectomy
      * Neoadjuvant (upfront) chemotherapy prior to cystectomy

- Grading system of urothelial neoplasms

  * Concordance rates for grade between different pathologists only about 50%-60% using the three-tier grade 1, 2, 3 system in effect since 1973

  * As a result, a new classification system with more rigorous standards was proposed in 1998 by the World Health Organization (WHO)/ International Society of Urologic Pathology (ISUP) (Figure 1)

  * Urologic community is currently in a state of flux between acceptance of 1998 vs. 1973 systems, in part due to long historical familiarity and prognostic utility of older 1973 system

  * New classification system results in greater number of high-grade lesions but retains prognostic utility for progression (Table 3)

8. Risk Factors Associated with Recurrence and Progression

- Grade

  * Recurrence at 2 years: papilloma (~20%) < PUNLMP (~40%) < LG TCC (60%-70%) < HG TCC (~80%)

  * Progression at 4/8 years: papilloma (~0%/0%) < PUNLMP (~8%/8%) < LG TCC (10%/13%) < HG TCC (23%/51%)

- Stage

  * Recurrence—minor influence Ta versus T1

  * Progression—significantly higher for T1 or CIS (5%-7% per year)

- Prior recurrence rate (primary, recurring ≤1 per year, recurring >1 per year)

  * Primarily affects recurrence

- Multifocality (single, 2-7 tumors, >8 tumors)

  * Primarily affects recurrence

- Tumor size (<3 cm, >3 cm)

  * Primarily affects recurrence

  * Some affect on progression in multifocal high-grade cases

- Concomitant CIS

  * Primarily affects progression especially for T1 disease

- Tumor presence at initial 3-month cystoscopy

  * Primarily affects recurrence (strong predictor)

- Risk Classification Scheme

  * Low risk (~50%)
    - Low-grade (grade 1-2) solitary, primary Ta papillary tumors
    - Progression rate <5% at 5 years)

  * Intermediate risk (~35%)
    - Recurrent Ta/T1 low-grade
    - Multifocal Ta/T1 low-grade
    - Progression rate <10% at 5 years

  * High-risk (~15%)
    - Any high-grade Ta or T1
    - Any CIS
    - Progression rate 25%-50% at 5 years (highest for multifocal T1G3 + CIS)

9. Intravesical Therapy

Treatment Options

- Single dose immediate postoperative (post-TUR) intravesical chemotherapy

  * Appropriate agents:
    - Mitomycin: bioreductive alkylating agent
    - Doxorubicin (adriamycin) or epirubicin (not used in US): topoisomerase inhibitor and DNA intercalator
    - Thiotepa: alkylating agent (low molecular weight 189 permits absorption)

  * Inappropriate agents: BCG (DANGER: sepsis!), interferon (ineffective)

  * Appropriate setting: after resection of any suspected non-muscle-invasive papillary tumor, single or multiple

  * Contraindications: suspected bladder perforation, excessive bleeding, known allergy

  * Technique: instillation of drug for 30-60 minutes dwell time; administered within 6 hours of TUR for maximum benefit (ineffective after 24 hours)

  * Toxicity:
    - <5% incidence of moderate-severe cystitis with appropriate use
    - With perforation: potential severe local tissue reaction or peritonitis (not thiotepa) or transient myelosuppression (especially thiotepa)

  * Expected benefit (Class I medical evidence of effectiveness)
    - 12%-15% absolute reduction in recurrence rate out to 3+ years
    - 25%-50% relative reduction in recurrence
    - Sufficient as sole therapy for low risk solitary tumors
    - Insufficient as sole therapy for intermediate or high risk or multifocal tumors (supplement with additional chemotherapy or immunotherapy)

- Multidose delayed intravesical chemotherapy

  * Appropriate agents: mitomycin, doxorubicin (adriamycin), epirubicin, thiotepa. (Gemcitabine and docetaxel under investigation.)

  * Appropriate setting: started 1-4 weeks after TUR for intermediate risk patients

  * Contraindications: known allergy or intolerance, concurrent infection

  * Technique: instill drug for 1-2 hours weekly for 6-8 weeks

  * Optimization techniques for maximum benefit of mitomycin ~ doubles disease free rate
    - Reduce urine output by relative dehydration
    - Completely empty bladder prior to instillation
    - Increase concentration (40 mg in 20 cc water)
    - Alkalinize urine with oral bicarbonate to reduce acid degradation (for mitomycin)

  * Maintenance therapy (usually monthly) of unclear benefit but recently supported by 2007 AUA meta-analysis

  * Toxicity:
    - Chemical cystitis (frequency, urgency, hematuria) in 10%-40% of patients
      * Mitomycin > adriamycin > epirubicin > thiotepa
      * 5%-10% delay or dropout due to intolerance
    - Drug-specific
      * Mitomycin: genital/palmar skin rash (~10%), bladder contracture (~2%)
      * Adriamycin: allergic reaction (~1%)
      * Thiotepa: myelosuppression (~13%), dose and frequency dependent; requires weekly complete blood count monitoring

  * Expected benefit
    - 12%-15% absolute reduction in recurrence rate out to 3+ years
    - Soft evidence that mitomycin is superior to adriamycin and thiotepa
    - Appropriate treatment for intermediate risk papillary tumors with or without prior immediate postoperative dose (especially multifocal cases)

  * Limitations

- Failure of one chemo agent increases failure likelihood of another chemo agent
- Limited activity (not first line) for CIS
- Ineffective against BCG failures as single agent therapy
- No evidence of effect on tumor progression

- Multidose immunotherapy with BCG

  * Appropriate setting: started 2-6 weeks after TUR for intermediate or high-risk patients

  * Contraindications:
    - Traumatic catheterization (bleeding/pain/instrumentation) – ABORT!
    - Recent gross hematuria (within 24 hours)
    - Unresolved urinary tract infection
    - Significant immunosuppression/ HIV (mild immunosuppression with inhaled or low-dose steroids or methotrexate allowed with close monitoring)
    - Active autoimmune disease (rheumatoid arthritis, lupus, scleroderma, etc.) especially if on Remicade® (TNF receptor antagonist)
    - Known allergy
    - NOT reflux, remote history of treated TB, positive PPD, prosthetic devices (small increased risk)

  * Technique: instill drug for 1-2 hours weekly for 6 weeks

  * Maintenance therapy
    - Usually 3-week miniseries at 3 months then every 6 months for up to 3 years
    - At least 1 year of maintenance is necessary to achieve full benefit (superiority over chemotherapy and reduction in risk of early progression)

  * Expected benefit
    - Average absolute 30% reduction in recurrence rate
    - Superior to chemotherapy (except perhaps in low-risk group)
    - Favored in higher risk groups by risk/benefit ratio
    - Treatment of choice for CIS, stage T1 high-grade disease
    - Shown to reduce progression risk by ~ 30%
    - Recent study showed survival benefit versus epirubicin

  * Mechanism of action:
    - Associated with T-helper type 1 immune response (increased IL-2 and interferon-gamma)
    - Opposed by T-helper type 2 response (increase IL-4 and IL-10)
    - Likely involvement of neutrophils, T-cells and NK cells

  * Toxicity:
    - Cystitis (frequency, urgency, hematuria)
      * Common (>50% of patients) >> chemotherapy
      * ~10% delay or dropout due to intolerance
      * Techniques to improve tolerance include:
        - Traditional symptom relieving drugs (anticholinergics, pyridium—try FIRST)
        - BCG dose reduction
        - Spacing treatments out 2 weeks apart
        - Decreasing dwell time
        - Adding ofloxacin 8 and 20 hours after BCG
        - Isoniazid X 3 days will NOT reduce side effects or incidence of serious BCG infection
    - Flu-like symptoms
      * Fever, chills, myalgias, arthralgias (up to 25%)
      * High fever >39.5 C° or recurring after 24 hours may be sign of serious BCG infection
    - Infection/inflammation related
      * Severe in ~ 5% total
      * Usually require 3-6 months of anti-TB medication (BCG is resistant to most conventional antibiotics including cephalosporins)
      * Single agent isoniazid—INH (300 mg daily) for moderate severity cases
      * Double or triple therapy with INH, rifampin (600 mg daily), and ethambutol (1200 mg daily) for severe cases
      * Vitamin B6 (pyridoxine) supplementation recommended
      * Cycloserine now recognized as INEFFECTIVE
      * Pyrazidimine (para-aminosalicylic acid) ineffective

    * Fluoroquinolones have activity as 3rd line agents
  - Oral or systemic steroids useful adjunctive to diminish inflammatory side effects (fever, sweats) and/or hypersensitivity side effects (arthralgias, myalgias) in severe cases

* Organ-specific manifestations
  - Prostatitis (~40% asymptomatic, <5% symptomatic)
    * May result in rise in PSA or abnormal DRE (resolves on own)
    * Treat only if symptomatic (with anti-TB meds)
  - Epididymitis (<2%)
  - Distant organs (<1%)
    * Lung, liver, kidney, bone
    * Sometimes miliary pattern (lung)
  - Sepsis (<0.5%)
    * Can be fatal
    * Usually result of traumatic catheterization
    * Rapid onset with hypotension and cardiovascular collapse
    * Early use of steroids (in addition to antibiotics) can be life-saving by blocking inflammatory cascade

* Hypersensitivity/allergy related (rare <5%)
  - Rash (2%-5%)
  - Reiter's syndrome (arthritis, uveitis, conjunctivitis)
  - Polyarthritis

- Intravesical treatment by risk group classification (supported by both 2007 AUA and 2008 EAU Guidelines Commissions)

  * Low-risk group
    - Single dose immediate (within 6 hours) chemotherapy after TUR
    - TUR alone and wait for 3 month cystoscopy result (less optimal)

  * Intermediate-risk group
    - Single dose immediate chemotherapy after TUR
    - Additional 6-week course of chemotherapy especially if multifocal
    - 6-week course of BCG with maintenance in place of chemotherapy or if prior failure of 6-week course of chemotherapy

  * High-risk group
    - Single dose immediate chemotherapy after TUR (for papillary tumor)
    - Additional 6-week course of BCG plus maintenance for minimum of 1 year if achieve disease-free status

10. Indications for Immediate Cystectomy for Apparent Non-Muscle Invasive Disease

- Strong indications
  - * Unfavorable variant histology
    - Micropapillary TCC
    - Small cell carcinoma (upfront systemic chemotherapy indicated before cystectomy)
    - Squamous cell carcinoma (potential for partial cystectomy if limited to diverticulum)
    - Adenocarcinoma (often under-staged)
  - * Lymphovascular invasion in stage T1 (associated with high risk of clinical under-staging; consider systemic neoadjuvant chemotherapy)
  - * Bulky incompletely resectable multifocal stage T1 high-grade
  - * Recurrence of stage T1 high-grade or CIS after BCG failure X 2
  - * Prostatic stromal invasion with TCC
  - * High-grade T1 disease in a bladder diverticulum (often under-staged)
  - * Dysfunctional bladder (bladder cripple) with recurrent disease
- Relative indications
  - * Stage T1 high-grade still present after repeat TUR
  - * Recurrence of stage T1 high-grade after BCG failure X 1
  - * Multifocal stage T1 high-grade with CIS at primary presentation
  - * Recurrent nonstromal prostatic involvement with TCC
- Impact of delay
  - * Patients developing muscle invasion while on surveillance do no better and perhaps worse than those presenting with de novo muscle invasion
  - * High-risk disease present 6 months after BCG has higher risk for progression
  - * Delay of more than 2 years after initial presentation for high-risk disease associated with reduced cancer-specific survival

11. Surveillance Plan Based on Risk Classification

- Upper tract studies
  * None required for low risk if initial work-up is negative
  * Every 2 years for multifocal or frequent recurrences in bladder
  * Every 1-2 years for high-risk groups
  * Whenever cytology becomes positive without visible lesion in bladder
- Cystoscopy
  * Low-risk:
    - If initial 3 month cystoscopy negative, safe to wait until 12 months for next cystoscopy then 1-2 X per year
    - If no recurrence by 5 years then chance of future recurrence <5%
  * Intermediate- and high-risk:
    - Every 3 months X 2 years, then every 6 months X 2 years, then annually
- Cytology
  * Low-risk: not necessary if initial cytology is negative
  * Intermediate- and high-risk: recommended quarterly
- Biopsies
  * Directed biopsies for any suspicious lesions on cystoscopy
  * Random biopsies optional initially to evaluate treatment response for high-grade disease, especially CIS
  * Random biopsies if cytology becomes suspicious or positive (required)
- Ancillary urine markers (NMP22, FISH, BTA)
  * In general, reduced sensitivity vs. initial diagnosis. May miss up to 50%.
  * Not a substitute for cystoscopy
  * False (and anticipatory) positive rate is a problem
  * Positive ancillary test by itself is NOT an indication for treatment
  * Positive ancillary test does increase risk of future recurrence and may be useful in increasing rigor of surveillance
- Office-based treatment of recurrent tumors
  * Laser or electrofulguration appropriate for papillary non-invasive appearing tumors in patients with prior documented low-intermediate risk disease (non-high-grade, noninvasive)
  * Delay in treatment of small papillary noninvasive appearing tumors until larger in those with prior low-intermediate (non-high-grade non-invasive) disease is safe (average growth rate ~ 2 mm per month)
  * Office biopsy if uncertain

12. Work-up for Positive Cytology

- Reliability

  * 95% accurate if unequivocally positive for high-grade dysplastic cells

  * False positives more common for "papillary clusters" especially in presence of stones or instrumentation

  * Ileal loop or neobladder cystology accurate if positive but must inform cytopathologist that specimen from bowel segment to avoid false positive

- Localizing source of positive cytology

  * Check bladder first
    - Biopsy any suspicious lesions
    - Random biopsies even if no visible lesions

  * Check upper tracts
    - Upper tract studies (IVP, CT urogram, MRI urogram, retrograde pyelogram)
    - Ureteral wash specimens with barbotaged saline (done before retrograde)
    - Ureteroscopy for radiographically suspicious lesions or localizing cytology (not useful for routine evaluation)
    - Incidence of upper tract disease > 20% in setting of prior bladder CIS previously treated with BCG even with complete response (median time 5 years)
    - *Note:* positive upper tract cytology unreliable in presence of visible bladder tumors or biopsy positive CIS due to contamination
    - May treat with topical BCG via stents or antegrade instillation

  * Check prostatic urethra
    - Cold cup or TUR urethral strip biopsy (between 5:00 - 7:00 most useful)
    - Incidence > 20% in setting of prior bladder CIS previously treated with BCG even with complete response (median time 1 year)
    - Deeper tissue TURP helpful to rule out prostatic stromal invasion (submit superficial and deep resections as separate specimens).
    - Transrectal ultrasound biopsy most useful if palpable nodule on DRE
    - Lesser forms of prostatic TCC – CIS, ductal or acinar TCC may respond to BCG with or without formal TURP (not required)

  * GYN source should be checked in women with negative workup

  * Rare prostate cancer source (~3%) usually with Gleason score ≥7

  * Failure to identify source of positive cytology despite above work-up will eventually yield bladder source in ~ 80% of cases

  * Positive cytology should generally be treated once localized with BCG if otherwise appropriate

13. Treatment of Intravesical Therapy Failures

- Intravesical chemotherapy failures will respond to BCG similarly to previously untreated patients
- BCG failures will seldom respond to single agent conventional intravesical chemotherapy
- BCG failures X1 will often respond to a 2nd course of BCG (30%-50% response)
- BCG failures X 2 respond very poorly to another course of BCG (<20% response)
- In general, patients with high-risk disease should be offered cystectomy after BCG failure X 2
- Patients refusing cystectomy or with medical contraindications to cystectomy or those with lower risk disease may be offered alternative therapy
  * Low-dose BCG plus interferon (40%-50% 2-year disease free status; best for BCG failures X 1)
  * Interferon alone (<15% 2-year disease free status)
  * Investigational chemotherapy (gemcitabine, docetaxel, combination/sequential therapy)
  * Photodynamic therapy (rarely available, bladder contractures common)
  * Radiation therapy (not appropriate for CIS, low-grade, or papillary disease; possibly useful for select cases of stage T1 high-grade disease)
  * Other investigational agents ideally under auspices of clinical trials

14. Methods of Chemoprevention

- Scant evidence that high-dose antioxidant vitamins (A, B1, 2, 3, 5, 6, 12; C, D, E, folate, zinc) can reduce recurrence of low grade noninvasive papillary cancers after BCG treatment
  * Potential harm of high vitamin A
    - Hepatotoxicity for doses approaching 40,000 IU
    - Higher rates of lung cancer in current smokers receiving vitamin A supplementation
- No convincing evidence for DFMO or vitamin A analogues, such as finretinide
- Smoking cessation recommended—higher recurrence and progression rate for continued smokers
- Higher intake of fruit and vegetables associated with decreased risk
- Higher intake of fat and cholesterol associated with increased risk
- Higher intake of nonchlorinated water >6 cups/day associated with decreased risk
- Oral lactobacilli has been linked to improved response rates to intravesical chemotherapy

15. Recommended Reading

1. Kirkali Z, Chan T, Manoharan M, et al. Bladder cancer: epidemiology, staging and grading, and diagnosis. *Urology*. 2005;66 (suppl 1):4-34.

2. Garcia-Closas M, Malats N, Silverman D, et al. NAT2 slow acetylation, GSTM1 null genotype, and risk of bladder cancer: results from the Spanish Bladder Cancer Study and meta-analyses. *Lancet*. 2005;366:649-659.

3. Sorensen FB, Sasaki M, Fukuzawa S, Yamabe H, Olsen S, Yoshida O. Qualitative and quantitative histopathology in transitional cell carcinomas of the urinary bladder. An international investigation of intra- and interobserver reproducibility. *Lab Invest*. 1994;70:242-254.

4. Eble JN, Young RH. Carcinoma of the urinary bladder: a review of its diverse morphology. *Semin Diagn Pathol*. 1997;14:98-108.

5. Mitra AP, Datar RH, Cote RJ. Molecular pathways in invasive bladder cancer: new insights into mechanisms, progression, and target identification. *J Clin Oncol*. 2006;24:5552-5564

6. Lee R, Droller MJ. The natural history of bladder cancer. Implications for therapy. *Urol Clin North Am*. 2000;27:1-13.

7. Zhang J, Gerst S, Lefkowitz RA, Bach A. Imaging of bladder cancer. *Radiol Clin North Am*. 2007;45:183-205.

8. Jakse G, Algaba F, Malmstrom PU, Oosterlinck W. A second-look TUR in T1 transitional cell carcinoma: why? *Eur Urol*. 2004;45: 539-546.

9. Golijanin D, Yossepowitch O, Beck SD, Sogani P, Dalbagni G. Carcinoma in a bladder diverticulum: presentation and treatment outcome. *J Urol*. 2003;170:1761-1764.

10. Collado A, Chechile GE, Salvador J, Vicente J. Early complications of endoscopic treatment for superficial bladder tumors. *J Urol*. 2000;164:1529-1532.

11. Oosterlinck W. Guidelines on diagnosis and treatment of superficial bladder cancer. *Minerva Urol Nefrol*. 2004;56:65-72.

12. Bassi P, De Marco V, De Lisa A, Mancini M, Pinto F, Bertoloni R, Longo F. Noninvasive diagnostic tests for bladder cancer: a review of the literature. *Urol Int*. 2005;75:193-200.

13. van Rhijn BW, van der Poel HG, van der Kwast TH. Urine markers for bladder cancer surveillance: a systematic review. *Eur Urol*. 2005. 47:736-748.

14. Platz CE, Cohen MB, Jones MP, Olson DB, Lynch CF. Is microstaging of early invasive cancer of the urinary bladder possible or useful? *Mod Pathol*. 1996;9:1035-1039.

15. Smits G, Schaafsma E, Kiemeney L, Caris C, Debruyne F, Witjes JA. Microstaging of pT1 transitional cell carcinoma of the bladder: identification of subgroups with distinct risks of progression. *Urology*. 1998;52:1009-1013.

16. Lopez JI, Angulo JC. The prognostic significance of vascular invasion in stage T1 bladder cancer. *Histopathology*. 1995;27:27-33.

17. Lee CT, Montie JE, Zhang YX, Dunn RL, Wood DP. Lymphovascular invasion is an independent predictor of survival in cT1 bladder cancer. *J Urol*. 2005;173 (suppl):911A.

18. Samaratunga H, Makarov DV, Epstein JI. Comparison of WHO/ISUP and WHO classification of noninvasive papillary urothelial neoplasms for risk of progression. *Urology*. 2002;60:315-319.

19. Millan-Rodriguez F, Chechile-Toniolo G, Salvador-Bayarri J, Palou J, Vicente-Rodriguez J. Multivariate analysis of the prognostic factors of primary superficial bladder cancer. *J Urol*. 2000;163:73-78.

20. Sylvester RJ, van der Meijden AP, Oosterlinck W, et al. Predicting recurrence and progression in individual patients with Stage Ta T1 bladder cancer using EORTC risk tables: a combined analysis of 2596 Patients from Seven EORTC Trials. *Eur Urol*. 2006;49(3):466-465.

21. Holmang S, Hedelin H, Anderstrom C, Johansson SL. The relationship among multiple recurrences, progression and prognosis in patients with stage Ta and T1 transitional cell carcinoma of the bladder followed for at least 20 years. *J Urol*. 1995;153:1823-1827.

22. Fitzpatrick JM, West AB, Butler MR. Superficial bladder tumors: the importance of recurrence pattern following initial resection. *J Urol*. 1986;135:920-924.

23. O'Donnell MA. Practical applications of intravesical chemotherapy and immunotherapy in high-risk patients with superficial bladder cancer. *Urol Clin North Am*. 2005; 32:121-131.

24. Lamm DL, Riggs DR, Taynelis CL, Nseyo UO. Apparent failure of current intravesical chemotherapy prophylaxis to influence the long-term course of superficial transitional cell carcinoma of the bladder. *J Urol*. 1995; 153:1444-1450.

25. Sylvester RJ, Oosterlinck W, van der Meijden AP. A single immediate postoperative instillation of chemotherapy decreases the risk of recurrence in patients with stage Ta T1 bladder cancer: a meta-analysis of published results of randomized clinical trials. *J Urol*. 2004 Jun;171(6: 1):2186-2190.

26. Au JL, Badalament RA, Wientjes MG, et al. International Mitomycin C Consortium. Methods to improve efficacy of intravesical mitomycin C: results of a randomized phase III trial. *J Natl Cancer Inst*. 2001;93:597-604.

27. Thrasher JB, Crawford ED. Complications of intravesical chemotherapy. *Urol Clin North Am* 1992;19:529-539.

28. Sylvester RJ, van der Meidjen AP, Lamm DL. Intravesical bacillus Calmette-Guérin reduces the risk of progression in patients with superficial bladder cancer: a meta-analysis of the published results of randomized clinical trials. *J Urol*. 2002; 168:1964-1970.

29. Bohle A, Jocham D, Bock PR. Intravesical bacillus Calmette-Guérin versus mitomycin C for superficial bladder cancer: a formal meta-analysis of comparative studies on recurrence and toxicity. *J Urol*. 2003;169:90-95.

30. Sylvester RJ, van der Meijden AP, Witjes JA, Kurth K. Bacillus Calmette-Guérin versus chemotherapy for the intravesical treatment of patients with carcinoma in situ of the bladder: a meta-analysis of the published results of randomized clinical trials. *J Urol*. 2005;174:86-91.

31. Lamm DL, Blumenstein BA, Crissman JD, et al. Maintenance BCG immunotherapy for recurrent Ta, T1 and carcinoma in situ transitional cell carcinoma of the bladder: a randomized Southwest Oncology Group study. *J Urol*. 2000;163:1124-1129.

32. Saint F, Patard JJ, Maille P, et al. Prognostic value of a T helper 1 urinary cytokine response after intravesical bacillus Calmette-Guérin treatment for superficial bladder cancer. *J Urol*. 2002;167:364-367.

33. Martinez-Pineiro JA, Martinez-Pineiro L, Solsona E, et al for the Club Urologico Espanol de Tratamiento Oncologico (CUETO). Has a 3-fold decreased dose of bacillus Calmette-Guérin the same efficacy against recurrences and progression of T1G3 and Tis bladder tumors than the standard dose? Results of a prospective randomized trial. *J Urol*. 2005;174:1242-1247.

34. Andius P, Fehrling M, Holmang S. Intravesical bacillus Calmette-Guerin therapy: experience with a reduced dwell-time in patients with pronounced side-effects. *BJU Int*. 2005;96:1290-1293.

35. Bassi P, Spinadin R, Carando R, Balta G, Pagano F. Modified induction course: a solution to side-effects? *Eur Urol.* 2000;37 suppl 1:313-2.

36. Colombel M, Saint F, Chopin D, Malavaud B, Nicolas L, Rischmann P. The effect of ofloxacin on bacillus Calmette-Guérin induced toxicity in patients with superficial bladder cancer: results of a randomized, prospective, double-blind, placebo controlled, multicenter study. *J Urol.* 2006;176:935-939.

37. Lamm DL, Steg A, Boccon-Gibad L, et al. Complications of bacillus Calmette-Guerin immunotherapy:review of 2,602 patients and comparison of chemotherapy complications. *Prog Clin Biol Res.* 1989;310:335.

38. Babjuk M, Oosterlinck W, Sylvester R, Kaasinen E, Böhle A, Palou-Redorta J. EAU guidelines on non-muscle-invasive urothelial carcinoma of the bladder. J; European Association of Urology (EAU). *Eur Urol.* 2008;54:303-314.

39. Hall MC, Chang SS, Dalbagni G, Pruthi RS, Seigne JD, Skinner EC, Wolf JS Jr, Schellhammer PF. Guideline for the management of nonmuscle invasive bladder cancer (stages Ta, T1, and Tis): 2007 update. *J Urol.* 2007; 178:2314-2330.

40. Stein JP. Indications for early cystectomy. Urology. 2003;62:591-595.

41. Nieder AM, Brausi M, Lamm D, et al. Management of stage T1 tumors of the bladder: International Consensus Panel. *Urology.* 2005;66 (suppl 1):108-125.

42. Herr HW, Badalament RA, Amato DA, Laudone VP, Fair WR, Whitmore WF Jr. Superficial bladder cancer treated with bacillus Calmette-Guérin: a multivariate analysis of factors affecting tumor progression. *J Urol.* 1989;141:22-29.

43. Kamat AM, Gee JR, Dinney CP, et al. The case for early cystectomy in the treatment of nonmuscle invasive micropapillary bladder carcinoma. *J Urol.* 2006;175:881-885.

44. Siefker-Radtke AO, Dinney CP, Abrahams NA, Moran C, Shen Y, Pisters LL, Grossman HB, Swanson DA, Millikan RE. Evidence supporting preoperative chemotherapy for small cell carcinoma of the bladder: a retrospective review of the M. D. Anderson cancer experience. *J Urol.* 2004;172:481-484.

45. Morgan JD, Bowsher W, Griffiths DF, Matthews PN. Rationalization of follow-up in patients with noninvasive bladder tumors. *Br J Urol.* 1993;72:135-142.

46. Bradford TJ, Montie JE, Hafez KS. The role of imaging in the surveillance of urologic malignancies. *Urol Clin North Am.* 2006;33:377-396.

47. Donat SM, North A, Dalbagni G, HerrHW. Efficacy of office fulguration for recurrent low grade papillary bladder tumors less than 0.5 cm. *J Urol.* 2004;171:636-639.

48. Soloway MS, Bruck DS, Kim SS. Expectant management of small, recurrent, noninvasive papillary bladder tumors. *J Urol.* 2003,170:438-441.

49. Schwalb MD, HerrHW, Sogani PC, Russo P, Sheinfeld J, Fair WR. Positive urinary cytology following a complete response to intravesical bacillus Calmette-Guerin therapy: pattern of recurrence. *J Urol.* 1994;152:382-387.

50. O'Donnell MA, Boehle A. Treatment options for BCG failures.*World J Urol.* 2006;24: 481-;487.

51. Catalona WJ, Hudson MA, Gillen DP, Andriole GL, Ratliff TL. Risks and benefits of repeated courses of intravesical bacillus Calmette- Gu駻in therapy for superficial bladder cancer. *J Urol.* 1987;137:220-224.

52. Steinberg G, Bahnson R, Brosman S, Middleton R, Wajsman Z, Wehle M. Efficacy and safety of valrubicin for the treatment of Bacillus Calmette-Guérin in refractory carcinoma in situ of the bladder. The Valrubicin Study Group. *J Urol*. 2000;163:761-767.

53. Joudi FN, Smith BJ, O'Donnell MA; , et al for the National BCG-Interferon Phase 2 Investigator Group. Final results from a national multicenter phase II trial of combination bacillus Calmette- Guérin in plus interferon alpha-2B for reducing recurrence of superficial bladder cancer. *Urol Oncol*. 2006;24:344-348.

54. Akcetin Z, Todorov J, Tuzel E, et al. Radiochemotherapy after transurethral resection is an effective treatment method in T1G3 bladder cancer. *Anticancer Res*. 2005; 25:1623-1628.

55. Fleshner N, Garland J, Moadel A, et al. Influence of smoking status on the disease-related outcomes of patients with tobacco associated superficial transitional cell carcinoma of the bladder. *Cancer*. 1999;86: 2337-2345.

56. Lamm DL, Riggs DR, Shriver JS, vanGilder PF, Rach JF, DeHaven JI. Megadose vitamins in bladder cancer: a double-blind clinical trial. *J Urol*. 1994;151:21-26.

57. Moyad MA. Bladder cancer prevention. Part I: what do I tell my patients about lifestyle changes and dietary supplements? *Curr Opin Urol*. 2003;13:363-378.

58. Moyad MA. Bladder cancer recurrence: Part II. What do I tell my patients about lifestyle changes and dietary supplements? *Curr Opin Urol*. 2003;13:379-383.

59. Naito S, Koga H, Yamaguchi A, et al, Kyushu University Urological Oncology Group. Prevention of recurrence with epirubicin and lactobacillus casei after transurethral resection of bladder cancer. *J Urol* 2008; 179:485-490.

16. Questions

1. A 43-year-old woman whose 55-year-old brother was recently diagnosed with bladder cancer seeks advice from you regarding her own risk. Her history is notable for pelvic radiation 9 years earlier for cervical cancer. She smokes 1-1/2 packs per day since age 20, drinks 4-5 cups of artificially sweetened coffee per day, and works as a hair stylist specializing in colorization. She had frequent UTIs as a child. Which of the following would constitute legitimate risk factors for the development of bladder cancer in her case?

A. Female gender, pelvic radiation, smoking

B. Pelvic irradiation, smoking, coffee consumption, prior UTIs

C. Family history, pelvic radiation, smoking, artificial sweetener use

D. Pelvic radiation, smoking, occupation

E. Female gender, family history, prior cervical cancer

2. 2 years after resection of a stage T1 high-grade lesion with glandular differentiation from the right lateral wall and BCG therapy with maintenance X 1 year, a suspicious lesion is found in a similar location and resected. Histology reveals a nephrogenic adenoma. Which of the following statements best reflects the clinical significance and implication of this result?

A. This is a premalignant lesion that is strongly associated with the subsequent development of adenocarcinoma. The lesion should be re-resected then closely followed cystoscopically with periodic biopsies.

B. This is a variant form of transitional cell carcinoma associated with a high probability of muscle invasion, lymph node involvement or distant metastasis. Radical cystectomy is indicated with possible adjuvant chemotherapy depending on the findings.

C. This is a variant form of bladder carcinoma with a strong predisposition to metastasize and should be treated with cisplatinum.

D. While not malignant, this lesion is strongly associated with recurrence. A repeat BCG induction course with further maintenance therapy should be started.

E. This is a benign inflammatory lesion. Only routine periodic cystoscopy is required.

3. Which of the following immunohistochemistry profiles for a bladder tumor would be associated with the most aggressive tendencies?

A. High p53 and Rb staining, low Ki67 and E-cadherin

B. High p53 and Ki67 staining, absent Rb and E-cadherin

C. High Rb and E-cadherin, low p53 and Ki67

D. High Ki67 and Rb, low p53 and E-cadherin

E. Low p53, Rb, E-cadherin and Ki-67

4. A 65-year-old otherwise healthy man with gross hematuria and negative CT urogram has a 1.5 cm lesion found on cystoscopy that is subsequently resected to reveal stage T1, high-grade TCC with deep invasion of the submucosa but no involvement of the scant muscle present. The most appropriate next step would be:

A. Bring patient back for circumferential biopsies around the tumor resection bed as well as random bladder biopsies to determine suitability for a partial cystectomy.

B. Begin a course of BCG therapy 3 weeks later with plans to cystoscope and possibly biopsy 6 weeks after completing the BCG therapy.

C. Strongly advise the patient to consider radical cystectomy at this point given the aggressive nature of the disease

D. Re-resect the patient within the next 4 weeks to determine whether there is residual disease or deeper disease present

E. No further treatment at present. Use the results of the 3-month cystoscopy to determine whether further treatment is indicated

5. A 69-year-old otherwise healthy woman has a 2.5 cm tumor identified on cystoscopy for work-up of recurrent painless gross hematuria. An IVP is negative and voided cytology is negative for tumor cells. The appropriate management plan would be:

A. Transurethral resection under anesthesia with random bladder biopsies

B. Transurethral resection with administration of mitomycin within the first few hours of surgery provided there is no significant bleeding or perforation recognized

C. Transurethral resection with bilateral ureteral wash cytologies

D. Transurethral resection with administration of BCG within the first few hours of surgery provided there is no significant bleeding or perforation recognized

E. Office biopsy of the lesion under local anesthesia to determine grade as a guide for future management

6. Which of the following is false regarding papillary neoplasms of low malignant potential (PUNLMP)?

A. They encompass some formerly described papillomas and grade 1 transitional cell carcinomas

B. Because they are essentially benign entities they do not require periodic cystoscopic follow-up

C. They recur with a cumulative frequency approaching 40% but progress in less than 10% of cases with long-term follow-up

D. They tend to be rather small and are always low-grade

E. They represent an entity distinct from papilloma in the new 1998 WHO/ISUP grading system

7. Which of the following intravesical agents is unlikely to cause local tissue inflammation or necrosis if administered in the presence of an unsuspected bladder perforation?

A. Thiotepa

B. BCG

C. Mitomycin

D. Doxorubicin

E. Epirubicin

8. A 64-year-old man is diagnosed with primary stage Ta low-grade bladder cancer in 3 separate locations, the largest one of which (3.5 cm) is suggestive of early lamina propria invasion. Detrusor muscle present and not involved. He currently requires Remicade for severe rheumatoid arthritis. Because a small bladder perforation was noted at the time of his initial TUR he did not receive any immediate postoperative intravesical chemotherapy. What would be the best treatment now based on risk/benefit considerations?

A. Observation only with cystoscopic surveillance at 3 months

B. Re-resection with deep biopsies of tumor base and immediate instillation of mitomycin

C. Begin a full course of BCG therapy 3 weeks later with plans for subsequent maintenance therapy to reduce progression risk

D. Begin a 6-week course of mitomycin with no definitive plans for maintenance at this time

E. Return to operating room for more complete staging evaluation including random bladder biopsies, upper tract washes, and prostatic urethral biopsies

9. A patient calls 6 hours after receiving his fourth scheduled treatment with BCG complaining of frequency, urgency, light red urine without clots and a temperature of 38.8° C with some chills. The most appropriate response to this situation would involve:

A. Reassurance that these symptoms are common with BCG treatment and that they will most likely clear up on their own

B. Inform the patient that he should immediately report to the emergency room for evaluation and potential admission for 24-hour observation

C. Call in prescriptions for an anticholinergic medication and 7-day course of ciprofloxin to start immediately with instructions to call back if temperature exceeds 39.5 C, relapses within next 48 hours or is associated with worsening symptoms

D. Call in a prescription for isoniazid to take for next 7 days and then for three days preceding each subsequent BCG treatment

E. Admit to hospital for possible BCG sepsis with treatment including triple anti-tuberculosis therapy (isoniazid, rifampin, ethambutol) and steroid therapy

10. A 72-year-old woman undergoes TUR of a 4 cm bladder tumor with immediate instillation of mitomycin C. Pathology report returns 5 days later revealing poorly differentiated transitional cell carcinoma invasive into the lamina propria with focal areas of micropapillary disease. Detrusor muscle is present and not involved. Pre operative CT urogram was negative for any apparent disease outside the bladder. Treatment at this point should involve:

A. Re-resection of the tumor site which, if negative, should be followed expectantly with quarterly cystoscopy and cytology

B. Re-resection of tumor site which, if negative, should be followed by a full 6-week course of BCG therapy with full cystoscopic restaging at 3 months

C. Re-resection of the tumor site which, if positive for residual T1 disease, should prompt an immediate cystectomy

D. Immediate cystectomy presuming remainder of metastatic workup is negative

E. Neoadjuvant systemic chemotherapy X 3-4 cycles, then planned cystectomy

Answers

1. D.

Female gender is associated with a lower risk. Coffee consumption, artificial sweetener use, occasional UTIs and prior cervical cancer are unrelated to risk. Besides pelvic radiation, smoking and occupational exposure to permanent hair dyes, family history is the only other legitimate risk factor in this case.

2. E.

Nephrogenic adenomas are benign lesions associated with prior trauma, surgery, chronic inflammation or infection. They do not predispose to further cancers. Answer A. would be appropriate for cystitis glandularis, answer B. would be appropriate for the micropapillary variant and answer C. would be appropriate for the small cell variant of bladder cancer.

3. B.

High p53 staining is associated with p53 mutation, a process that inhibits self-destructive apoptosis of cancer. Ki67 is a marker of proliferation. High values indicate a faster growth rate. Rb functions as a cell cycle brake. Loss of Rb promotes cancer cell proliferation. E-cadherin is a cell surface molecule that keeps cells fixed in place. Loss of E-cadherin is associated with increased invasive and metastatic potential. The least aggressive profile for comparison would be answer C.

4. D.

Essentially all stage T1 high-grade cancers should be re-resected because of the high chance of both residual disease or unsuspected muscle invasion. While BCG therapy is appropriate for completely resected and accurately staged T1 high-grade cancer, if the tumor is under-staged and actually T2 this 3 month delay (also found in answer E.) will be potentially harmful. Radical cystectomy or partial cystectomy is premature unless there are extenuating circumstances (multifocal or bulky T1, associated lymphovascular invasion for radical; tumor in diverticulum for partial).

5. B.

A single dose of intravesical chemotherapy delivered with 6 hours of TUR will significantly decrease the risk of recurrence for low-risk bladder cancer at minimal risk to the patient. Choice D., giving BCG, is contraindicated for high chance of inducing BCG sepsis. Neither random biopsies (A.) nor ureteral cytologies (C.) are indicated in the setting of low-grade disease with negative voided cytology. An office bladder biopsy (E.) in this new bladder cancer patient adds nothing to the management since TUR remains the most definitive initial diagnostic and therapeutic maneuver.

6. B.

PUNLMPs do recur with moderate frequency and occasionally progress, thus they are not strictly benign and deserve periodic follow-up.

7. A.

Although it will cause transient myelosuppression, as a non-vesicant agent it will not lead to a severe local tissue reaction if extravasated. Mitomycin and the anthracyclines, doxorubicin (adriamycin) and epirubicin, are all vesicant drugs with a high potential for local tissue damage. BCG can also cause a localized or systemic infection in such a circumstance.

8. D.

A 6-week course of mitomycin will reduce the relative chance of recurrence by over 30%. Although perhaps even more efficacious, BCG (C.) is contraindicated in patients taking the TNF receptor blocker Remicade because of the elevated risk of BCG infection. Observation alone is unsatisfactory in this intermediate risk patient whose recurrence risk with multifocal disease exceeds 60% and with a modest progression rate of 5%-15%. Re-resection (B.) is not unreasonable but not required in the setting of low-grade disease, equivocal early lamina propria invasion and clearly negative detrusor involvement. Likewise, answer E. is overly aggressive in the setting of low-grade disease.

9. C.

It is unclear at this point whether the patient is having a normal but exaggerated transient immune reaction to BCG, iatrogenic standard bacterial UTI or early signs of serious BCG infection. Treatment of irritative voiding symptoms is appropriate but fever >38.5 but <39.5 should prompt treatment. Since fluoroquinolone antibiotics are active against most standard bacterial UTIs and BCG they are a reasonable first choice until the patient declares himself through either higher fever (≥39.5), relapsing fever after 48 hours or worsening constitutional symptoms. At that point the patient should report for medical evaluation, possible in-hospital evaluation, and institution of more specific antituberculosis drug therapy (B.). Extended outpatient isoniazid monotherapy is appropriate for milder forms of BCG infection although it will not prevent the onset of fever and sepsis if administered for 3 days around the time of BCG instillation (D.). Triple drug antibiotic therapy and steroids would be appropriate for BCG sepsis with hemodynamic compromise (E.).

10. D.

Micropapillary disease is poorly responsive to conservative measures (A.) or to BCG therapy (B.) resulting in reduced survival. Any delay in therapy (including re-resection) is potentially dangerous (C.). Neoadjuvant chemotherapy (E.) has not been shown to be of any benefit in clinically localized disease for this variant form of bladder cancer.

Chapter 18: Bladder Cancer

Seth P. Lerner, MD, FACS

Contents

1. Natural History and Staging

Bladder cancer is the 4th most common cancer in men and the 10th in women. Significant progress has been made in the management of invasive cancer and we have learned much about multimodal therapy. The urologist plays a central role in integrating surgery, chemotherapy and radiation therapy in order to achieve the goal of long-term cancer control. This chapter will focus on the evaluation and treatment of patients with muscle invasive and metastatic bladder cancer. Since transitional cell is the most common histology much of the talk is focused on this entity. I will mention certain aspects of the treatment of other histologies. I will also cover the most pertinent aspects of urinary diversion. Specific references are provided with some of the material in order to provide more in depth review and a bibliography is provided at the end as well.

Natural History

The majority (80%) of patients with muscle invasive cancer present de novo as their first manifestation of bladder cancer. The remaining 15%-20% progress from non-muscle invasive cancer after treatment with intravesical therapy. **Deaths due to bladder cancer invariably occur as a result of distant metastases present at the time of loco-regional therapy.** Progression of cancer after definitive loco-regional therapy commonly occurs within the first 2 years after treatment. Late recurrences are more common after perioperative systemic chemotherapy and often occur in unusual sites including the central nervous system, bowel serosa and peritoneum. One must consider muscle invasive bladder cancer as a systemic disease and design treatment strategies around the integration of treatment targeting the loco-regional disease (bladder and pelvic lymph nodes) and occult visceral metastatic disease according to pathologic risk factors.

Histology

Primary cancers of the bladder arise from the urothelium and transitional cell is by far the most common cell type. Squamous cell predominates in Middle Eastern countries where bilharziasis is endemic and occurs more frequently in women in Western countries and in the setting of chronic indwelling catheters and recurrent infection. Adenocarcinomas of the bladder are uncommon but occur in the bladder base/trigone area and patients with exstrophy are at higher risk. Surgical treatment of urachal adenocarcinoma is partial cystectomy and the biology is similar to colorectal adenocarcinoma. **Small cell neuroendocrine cancer is also a rare variant and may be the predominant histology or mixed with TCC. This phenotype is easily distinguished by immunohistochemistry expressing synaptophysin and chromogrannin. Treatment requires neoadjuvant chemotherapy (cisplatin and etoposide) followed by radical cystectomy or radiation therapy. Small cell may also be associated with paraneoplastic syndromes including ectopic ACTH production, hypercalcemia and hypophosphatemia.**

There have been other unusual variants reported including ***lymphoepithelioma-like cancers*** which have a better prognosis than high grade invasive TCCs, though treatment is similar stage for stage. **The micropapillary variant resembles ovarian papillary serous cancer and is very aggressive.** It tends toward high grade, high stage and is frequently associated with lymphatic and vascular invasion.[1] Radical cystectomy is the treatment of choice as this phenotype typically does not respond to chemotherapy directed at TCC. Rhabdomyosarcoma is seen both in children and adults and leiomyosarcoma is seen in adults. Primary lymphoma of the bladder is rare but the bladder may be involved in up to 10% of cases of systemic lymphoma.

Clinical and Pathologic Staging (Table 1)

The T stage denotes the clinical stage which is determined prior to definitive therapy. The depth of invasion determined on the TURBT specimen and the bimanual exam under anesthesia determine the clinical stage. Pathologic stage is derived from the cystectomy specimen. Clinical understaging is more common that overstaging (which does occur, however).

The 1997 TNM staging schema introduced a modification from prior staging schemes. Prior to 1997, T2 was inner half of muscle and T3a was outer half. T3b represented all levels of perivesical fat invasion. In the current system **T2a and T2b represent inner and outer half of muscle, respectively, and T3 is split into T3a (microscopic) and T3b (macroscopic, or visible on gross inspection of the cystectomy specimen). T4a prostate requires established stromal invasion,** which can occur via the urethra or as direct extension via the bladder neck or posteriorly into the seminal vesicles or periprostatic tissue. **CIS of prostatic urethra or ducts does not upstage, as outcome is determined by the primary bladder cancer stage.**[2] Node and metastases staging is similar to other GU malignancies. Positive nodes above the common iliac bifurcation are classified as N+M1 disease. The UICC and AJCC staging systems are uniform in the 6th edition of American Joint Committee On Cancer (AJCC) staging manual

Table 1

TNM Staging Bladder Cancer

Primary Tumor	
T1	— Lamina propria invasion
T2a	— Inner half muscularis propria
T2b	— Outer half muscularis propria
T3a	— Perivesical fat; microscopic
T3b	— Perivesical fat; macroscopic
T4a	— Invades prostate, seminal vesicles, vagina, uterus, or rectum; mobile, no fixation
T4b	— Pelvic sidewall, abdominal wall; fixed
Nodes	
N1	— Single node ≤ 2 cm diameter
N2	— Single node >2 ≤ 5 cm, or multiple nodes none > 5cm
N3	— lymph node >5 cm diameter
Metastases	
M1	— visceral metastases or lymph nodes above the common iliac bifurcation

AJCC/UICC 1997; 2002.

Staging Pitfalls

European Association of urology (EAU) Guidelines require muscularis propria in the TURBT specimen for accurate staging. Without this understaging of T1 disease is common and outcomes for T1 cancer are worse with no muscularis propria in the specimen.

T1 vs. T2
There are fine muscle bundles called muscularis mucosa present within the lamina propria (Figure 1a and Figure 1b). There are blood vessels in this area as well. These muscle bundles may be

Figure 1a

Muscularis mucosa of the lamina propria

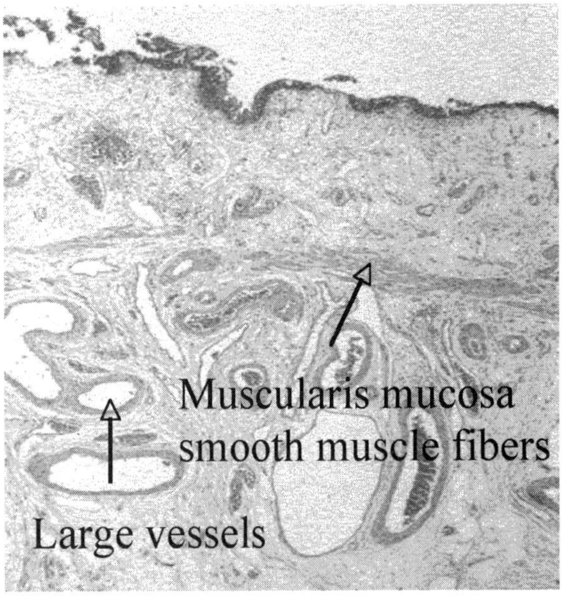

The muscularis mucosa of the lamina propria can be identified in up to 80% of bladder specimens and is recognized by fine muscle bundles and large vessels.

Figure 1b

Lamina propria and deep portions of the muscularis propria

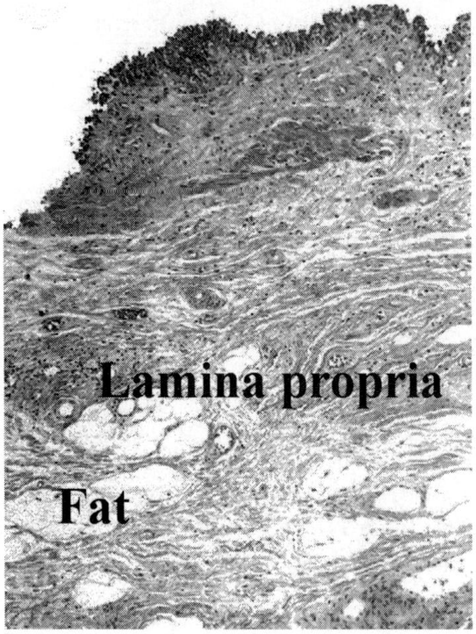

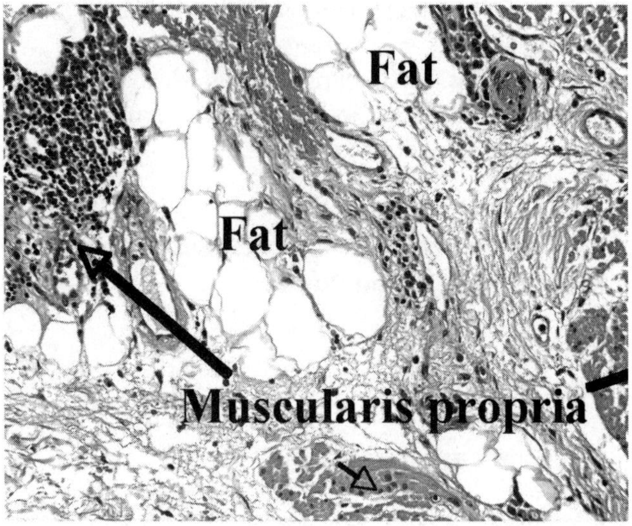

Fat can be observed in lamina propria and deep portions of the muscularis propria.

confused with the muscularis propria leading to overstaging of a T1 tumor as T2. In addition, recent data suggests that **up to 40% of patients initially diagnosed as T1 who undergo cystectomy are pathologic T2.** The management of patients with high grade T1 tumors is challenging. It is imperative to accurately stage these patients prior to embarking on intravesical therapy. We therefore routinely re-resect patients with T1G3 tumors before determining appropriate therapy.

Indications for initial cystectomy for T1 disease include:

- Size >3cm
- Micropapillary histology
- Lymphovascular invasion
- Recurrent high grade T1 cancer

T2 vs. T3
Fat can be observed in the lamina propria and deep portions of the muscularis propria and should not be confused with perivesical fat invasion. Stage T3 requires cancer in fat in the absence of muscle bundles.

Staging the Bladder and Urethra

There are 4 pieces of critical information to obtain in order to plan appropriate therapy:

1. Does the local tumor cause upper tract obstruction and is there a concomitant upper tract tumor which also needs treatment?
2. What is the T-stage of the tumor assessed by bimanual exam under anesthesia?

T2a — nonpalpable

T2b — induration; no mass

T3 — 3D mass, mobile

T4a — invades adjacent structures

T4b — fixed; not mobile

3. Determine stage and depth of invasion with TURBT and status of the remaining bladder urothelium with directed biopsies.

4. Determine the status of the bladder neck (female) and prostatic urethra (male).

TURBT—Goals in Staging the Primary Tumor

- Establish histology
- Assess for lymphatic/vascular invasion—a risk factor for metastases
- Depth of penetration
- Complete resection not necessary when cystectomy anticipated
- Directed biopsies to establish status of mucosa regarding CIS
- Stage bladder neck/urethra

  * In men, a negative prostatic urethra biopsy is associated with a negative apical urethra margin, obviating the need for intraoperative frozen section

    - Biopsies of the prostatic urethra should be done in all patients prior to radical cystectomy. Using a resectoscope, take a full loop from the mid-prostate to the mid- to the distal verumontanum and 5 and 7 o'clock adjacent to the verumontanum. This is where there is the highest concentration of prostatic ducts where CIS is most likely to be found. The full thickness chip allows the pathologist to see the interface between the urethra mucosa, the prostatic ducts and stroma. This method is the most accurate means of staging the prostatic urethra

  * Bladder neck biopsies are a surrogate for urethra involvement in women when considering orthotopic diversion

Goals of Additional Staging

- Further assess primary bladder tumor

  * Local extent

  * Involvement of adjacent organs

- Assess regional and distant lymph nodes – computed tomography
- Determine presence of visceral metastases directed to the most common sites: lung, liver and bone – computed tomography, MRI, bone scintigraphy.

Incidence of Pelvic Node Metastases

The incidence of pelvic node metastases (%) is directly related to the depth of invasion of the primary tumor and the presence of lymphovascular invasion.

	P0-P1	P2	P3	P4
8 series	0–6	6–30	27–59	43–59

The most common sites of visceral metastases are the lung, liver and bone. Following chemotherapy, unusual sites including CNS and the peritoneum may occur but are generally not a focus of staging at initial presentation.

Staging Evaluation— Regional and Metastatic Disease

Routine

- Chest x-ray
- Laboratory

* Electrolytes, BUN, creatinine, CBC

* Liver function tests, alkaline phosphatase

- Computed tomography (CT) abdomen and pelvis

  * T3 and T4 primary tumors

  * Elevated liver function studies

  * Rationale: preoperative histologic confirmation of pelvic nodal or liver metastases alters treatment

Optional

- Computed tomography chest (obtain with the following)

  * Abnormal chest x-ray or history suggests lung metastases

  * T4 or N+ disease by clinical staging

- Bone scintigraphy

  * Elevated alkaline phosphatase; bone pain

  * T4 or N+ disease by clinical staging

- MRI

  * Contrast allergy or to resolve equivocal bone scan

- PET/CT—no defined role to date for routine staging for nodal or visceral metastases. Can be helpful in resolving nodal or visceral metastatic disease when these findings will determine the use of chemotherapy or surgery

Several commercially available serum biomarkers (CA-125, CA-19.9) have been reported to be elevated in patients with advanced disease and may provide a marker that correlates with disease and response to therapy but this is not standard.

2. Treatment

Goals

The treatment strategy for invasive bladder cancer should achieve complete eradication of the locoregional disease including the primary tumor and regional lymph nodes. Treatment should also include occult regional node and visceral metastases when the risk of this occurring is high enough using neo-adjuvant or adjuvant chemotherapy. Patients should have volitional control of urination via the retained urethra or by a continent catheterizable stoma in properly selected patients. Treatment related morbidity should be minimized wherever possible.

Extent of Surgery

Radical cystectomy provides excellent local control of the primary tumor and should include in men the bladder, prostate and seminal vesicles and in women the bladder, ovaries, uterus/cervix and anterior vagina. In sexually active women, vaginal preservation and or reconstruction must be discussed preoperatively. The rate of involvement of the uterus, cervix and ovaries is uncommon.[3] Preservation of the vagina and uterus provides better support for a neobladder and the pelvic floor.[4] Aposterior-based invasive cancer in women is a relative contraindication to urethral preservation in women and mandates careful attention to the margin on the vagina and including at least a small strip of anterior vaginal wall in order to maintain a negative surgical margin.

Pelvic and Iliac Lymphadenectomy

A bilateral pelvic lymphadenectomy including the external and internal iliac and obturator lymph nodes is required for radical or partial cystectomy. The true perivesical nodes are embedded in the perivesical fat and can harbor metastatic disease.

An extended node dissection that starts at the origin of the inferior mesenteric artery or the aortic bifurcation including the common iliac and presacral lymph nodes provides accurate staging, and may increase the total lymph node count and improve survival. In patients with T3 or T4 tumors the nodes proximal to the common iliac bifurcation are involved in up to one half of patients with node metastases.[5]

Grossly Positive Node Metastases

The management of patients with grossly involved lymph nodes must include treatment of systemic micrometastatic and loco-regional disease. If recognized on pre-operative imaging and outside the true pelvis, CT-guided biopsy should be done to establish histology. If positive, then chemotherapy should be initiated followed by cystectomy. When adenopathy is encountered at time of cystectomy, frozen section should be performed to confirm the presence of metastasis and extended lymph node dissection and radical cystectomy should be performed. Cystectomy should not be performed when:

1. Lymph node metastases are unresectable due to bulk or proximal extent above the common iliac vessels

2. There is evidence of extensive peri-ureteral disease

3. The bladder is fixed to the pelvic sidewall

4. Tumor is invading the rectum

Morbidity and Mortality

The major complication rate is 15%-25%, with gastrointestinal and genitourinary tract the most common problems. Prolonged ileums, bowel obstruction, urine leaks and urinary tract infection are common problems encountered. Metabolic problems and dehydration occur more frequently in the elderly and are a common reason for readmission in the early postoperative period. Most of these complications can be managed conservatively. Mortality rates dropped dramatically with improved antibiotics, better pulmonary and cardiac care and modern anesthesia. I quote my patients a 0%-3% mortality risk based predominantly on the risk of postoperative pulmonary embolus, myocardial infarction and sepsis.

Management of the Urethra

The risk of urethral TCC following cystectomy is influenced by the presence and extent of involvement of the prostatic urethra and prostatic stroma, with stromal invasion carrying a risk of approximately 30% (none < focal CIS < diffuse CIS < ductal/acinar involvement < stromal invasion). Men should undergo urethrectomy if CIS is diffuse within the prostatic urethra or ducts or if there is prostatic stroma invasion. (Figure 2) Some feel that the only indication is cancer at the apical urethra margin. Small low-grade papillary tumors of the urethra can be resected prior to cystectomy and the urethra retained if there is no other indication for urethrectomy. **The probability of developing a second primary TCC of the retained urethra is lower with orthotopic diversion compared to cutaneous diversion.**[6]

Cystectomy in women historically included the urethra. New data indicate that the distal two-thirds of the urethra serves as an adequate sphincter mechanism innervated by the pudendal nerve and is infrequently involved with transitional cell cancer.[7,8] Limiting dissection to above the endopelvic fascia will preserve the innervation. **Cancer at the bladder neck or urethra or a T4 tumor involving the anterior vagina are contraindications to urethra preservation and orthotopic neobladder.** Urethra cancer is always associated with bladder neck cancer, so biopsy findings of the bladder neck are an excellent surrogate for preoperative staging of the female urethra (Figure 3).

Nerve-sparing Cystectomy

Nerve-sparing cystectomy is appropriate in patients who are potent and sexually active and have clinically organ-confined cancer and no evidence of local extension intraoperatively. There is no negative impact on local recurrence and approximately 40% can achieve erections satisfactory for intercourse. The results are age-dependent, similar to that observed for nerve-sparing radical prostatectomy. Nerve-sparing may improve continence in patients with a neobladder but this may also simply reflect better dissection at the apex of the prostate and preservation of the urethra sphincter complex.[9]

Carcinoma *In Situ* (CIS) of the Ureter

- Atypia, dysplasia does not require any action

- Attempt should be made to achieve a negative margin on the ureter, but do not compromise on ureteral length

Figure 2

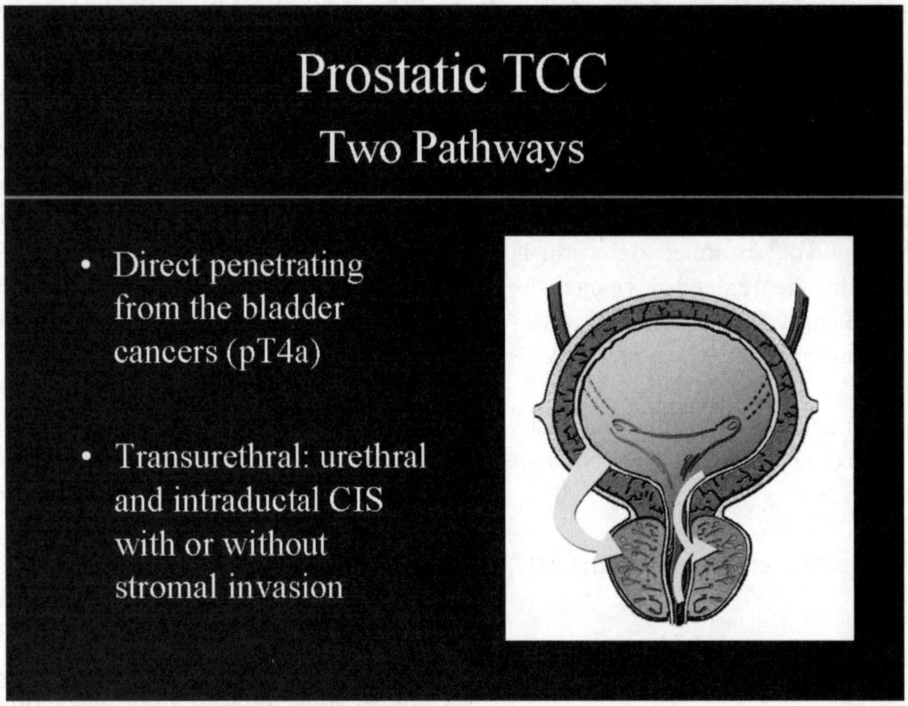

Mapping study of location of transitional cell carcinoma in the female bladder (n = 36). All patients with cancer in the urethra also had cancer at the bladder neck.

- Cancer recurrence at the anastamosis is rare even with a positive margin
- Nephrectomy is not indicated for CIS of the ureter
- CIS of the ureter is not independently associated with a worse outcome
- Incidence of upper tract tumors after orthotopic neobladder is 2.4%-17%[10]
- Monitor with IVP or CT and voided cytology if CIS of lower tract or ureter

Outcome

Survival following radical cystectomy is driven by pathologic tumor stage and the status of the pelvic lymph nodes (Table 2).[11] Within each stage category, positive nodes have a negative impact on survival. The combination of P3 or P4 and positive lymph nodes is associated with a particularly bad prognosis and is an indication for adjuvant chemotherapy.

Prostatic Involvement

CIS involving the prostatic urethra, ducts or acini (no stromal invasion) does not adversely affect prognosis following cystectomy as the outcome is driven by the primary stage of the bladder tumor.[2] As mentioned, prostatic CIS does not change the stage, which is determined by the stage of the bladder tumor.

Prostatic stromal invasion occurs via prostatic urethra (noncontiguous) or as direct invasion (contiguous) from the primary bladder tumor via the bladder neck or posteriorly via penetration of the periprostatic tissues and/or seminal vesicles. This is true T4 disease and carries an adverse prognosis. Some

Table 2

Survival Following Radical Cystectomy According to Pathologic Tumor Stage and Node Status

Stage	% with Positive Nodes	5-year Survival: Node Negative	5-year Survival: Node Positive
pT2	6%-31%	64%-83%	34%-66%
pT3	27%-64%	17%-46%	11%-27%
pT4	45%-59%	0%-33%	11%-27%

Lerner SP, Skinner DG. Radical cystectomy for bladder cancer. In: Comprehensive Textbook of Genitourinary Oncology. *2nd ed. Philadelphia, PA: Lippincott Williams & Wilkins; 2000:425-447.*

Table 3

Survival and Recurrence-Free Probability According to Number of Positive Lymph Nodes (LN)

No. of Pos.	N	Recurrence-Free Probability	Survival
LN		5y ± SE	5y ± SE
0	127	76 ± 4.8%	68 ± 5%
>1	14	43 ± 11%	51 ± 11%
>5	10	40 ± 10%	42 ± 17%
>6	8	13 ± 12%	33 ± 18%
>10	5	20 ± 18%	20 ± 18%

Baylor College of Medicine, 2003.

Figure 3

Map of severe dysplasia, CIS and cancer

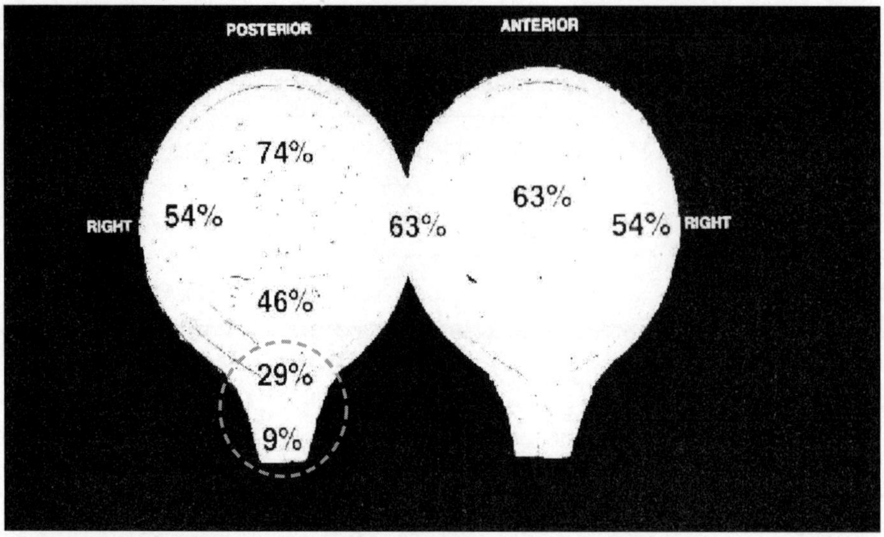

studies suggest that direct invasion from the primary bladder tumor is associated with a worse prognosis compared to invasion via noncontiguous involvement of the prostatic urethra.[12] There is a category of lamina propria invasion of the prostate that is contiguous with prostatic CIS that is included in T4 stage but carries a prognosis similar to prostatic CIS only.[13] When these patients are excluded from T4 the difference in outcome between invasive phenotypes disappears.

All of the following may impact survival:

- Number of lymph nodes removed

  * Important in both node-negative and node-positive patients

- Number of positive lymph nodes
- Percent of nodes involved with cancer
- Pathologic stage of the primary tumor
- Extranodal extension

In node-negative patients, an inadequate node dissection will likely miss node metastases leading to understaging of the cancer. In node positive patients the number of positive nodes has a direct impact on prognosis. A recent term of "lymph node density" has been introduced that reflects the number of positive nodes divided by the total number of nodes removed.[14] The pathologic stage also influences the outcome in node positive patients. Extranodal extension of cancer is a poor prognostic feature.

Impact of Age

- Advance age (≥80) is associated with higher incidence of stage pT3/T4 [15]
- Higher recurrence rates may be due to lower use of peri-operative chemotherapy in elderly patients

Monitoring for Recurrence

Monitoring is focused on early detection of asymptomatic recurrence and imaging directed at abnormalities suggested in the history and physical exam. **Most recurrences occur within the first three years after cystectomy in patients who have not been treated with systemic chemotherapy.** Local pelvic recurrence may be detectable by an abnormal DRE or bimanual. Patient with an orthotopic diversion may present with urinary retention as the first indication of local pelvic recurrence. Sciatic pain suggests local recurrence or pelvic bone metastases. Gross hematuria may occur as a result of pelvic recurrence invading a neobladder. The most common distant sites are lung, liver and bone, and a chest x-ray, lab work directed to bone marrow, liver function and bone metastases (alkaline phosphatase) should be performed at each visit. There are no data to support or refute a rationale for CT or MRI though many perform these at annual followup for the first few years. **Central nervous system metastases may occur late (after 3 years) in patients who have received chemotherapy.** Bowel obstruction may also occur late as a manifestation of intraperitoneal metastases.

Urethra recurrences are new tumors—so-called second primary tumors. Urethral wash cytology is sensitive for identifying urethra TCC and should be performed at least annually in patients with any CIS in the cystectomy specimen (or pre-cystectomy biopsies). Upper tract tumors are uncommon following cystectomy though the risk can be as high as 25% at 10 years in patients with CIS.[16] In these patients, an IVP or CT with intravenous contrast and urine cytology should be performed annually. Predictors in cystectomy patients also include urethra TCC and patients with a positive ureter margin should be monitored as well.

Indications for Secondary Urethrectomy

- Positive urethral wash cytology and biopsy confirmation of urethral cancer
- Bloody urethral discharge mandates urethroscopy and biopsy
  - If cancer confirmed usually invasive and difficult to cure
- Urethrectomy should include urethral meatus
  - Local therapies including 5FU are generally ineffective

3. Alternatives to Radical Cystectomy

Radical TURBT

- Initial occurrence of bladder cancer
- No CIS
- Size ≤3 cm
- T2 (no palpable mass)—T3 tumors are not amenable to complete TUR and T4 tumors are not eligible as by definition they are invading surrounding structures
- Not in dome or high posterior wall due to risk of bowel injury
- **Re-resect at 3 months to assure complete removal of the tumor.** If tumor persists at this time, then radical cystectomy or radiation should be considered
- Disadvantages
  - No pathologic node staging
  - Lifelong surveillance—up to 25% require cystectomy

When these criteria are followed, the long-term survival is comparable to radical cystectomy.[17,18]

Partial Cystectomy

The indications for partial cystectomy are similar to radical TURBT with one exception – the location. **Tumors should be in a location suitable to bladder preservation – usually on the dome and away from the ureteral orifices.** Bilateral pelvic lymphadenectomy should be performed at the time of surgery for pathologic staging of the nodes. Long-term relapse rates are high despite these strict criteria. This option has a definite role in patients who have had an objective response to neo-adjuvant chemotherapy. The tumor site can be resected in patients with a complete response (CR) in order to pathologically assure complete tumor removal, and in patients with a partial response and the tumor location is amenable to partial cystectomy (the gold standard, however, is radical cystectomy in patients who experience a PR).

In the unique situation of urachal adenocarci noma, partial cystectomy is the preferred surgi cal method for local control. This should be done using a closed technique in order to avoid tumor spill of this highly implantable tumor, with en bloc resection of posterior rectus sheath, urachus and dome of bladder.

External Beam Radiotherapy
External beam irradiation has a very long track record in the treatment of patients with invasive TCC of the bladder. In the United States, it has generally been used for patients who are not surgical candidates. In Europe it has enjoyed a strong role for decades as a primary treatment option. As monotherapy it is best used for patients with significant pulmonary or coronary artery disease for whom the risks of surgery are prohibitive and for whom multi-agent cytotoxic chemotherapy is not an option. The doses range from 55-65Gy delivered in daily fractionation. **Poor prognostic features include the presence of hydronephrosis, locally advanced tumors (stages T3b and T4) and patients who are anemic.**

The 5-year survival probabilities are influenced by the clinical stage of the tumor (5-year survival: T2- 26 = 59%; T3-10 = 52%). Patients with bulkier tumors do not fare as well and maximal debulking of the primary tumor with TURBT should be performed when feasible. CIS is resistant to radiation. This may be present at the time of initial diagnosis or develop subsequent to radiation, and so the bladder must be monitored lifelong. Patients may require additional intravesical therapy to control CIS. Today, radiation is rarely given as monotherapy. At a minimum, a radiosensitizing chemotherapy drug should be administered along with the radiation. **The most commonly used drugs are cisplatin, 5-FU and docetaxel**, and it is estimated that response rates to radiation are increased by 10%-15%.

4. Integrated Treatment Strategies

Radical Cystectomy and Preoperative Radiation
- 6 randomized trials: TCC (4); Bilharzial SCCa (2)

- Meta-analysis

    * Odds ratio 0.94 (95% CI 0.57 - 1.55)

    * Potential survival benefit and better local control with bilharzial cancer

    * No role in contemporary radical cystectomy for TCC

- **No role for postoperative radiation— toxicity too high**

- In the case of documented local recurrence, pelvic irradiation can be performed safely

Neoadjuvant Chemotherapy
Rationale. Neoadjuvant chemotherapy is utilized to treat micrometastic disease present at the time of cystectomy in order to reduce the risk of, or delay the emergence of, measurable metastatic disease and improve long-term survival. The benefit is the primary tumor is in place and response to chemotherapy can be objectively assessed. It is possible that an otherwise unresectable tumor (T4b or M1 nodes—proximal to the common iliac bifurcation) can be downstaged and become resectable. The disadvantages are related to errors in clinical staging; the potential for overtreating patients who would otherwise be cured with surgery alone and the potential that ineffective chemotherapy may delay definitive local therapy.

There have been several randomized trials of neoadjuvant chemotherapy where chemotherapy followed by cystectomy or radiation have been compared to surgery or radiation alone (Table 4). The eligibility criteria for these trials included patients with T2-T4 tumors and N+ disease. Both the MRC/EORTC and the SWOG studies showed improved survival for the patients who received neo-adjuvant chemotherapy.[19,20] In the SWOG neoadjuvant chemotherapy trial, patients received three cycles of M-VAC followed by cystectomy or cystectomy alone. **There was an approximate 2.5 year improvement in median survival and the 5 year survival probability was improved by 15%.**

Figure 4

Neo-adjuvant Chmotherapy Meta Analysis 5% Survival Advantage

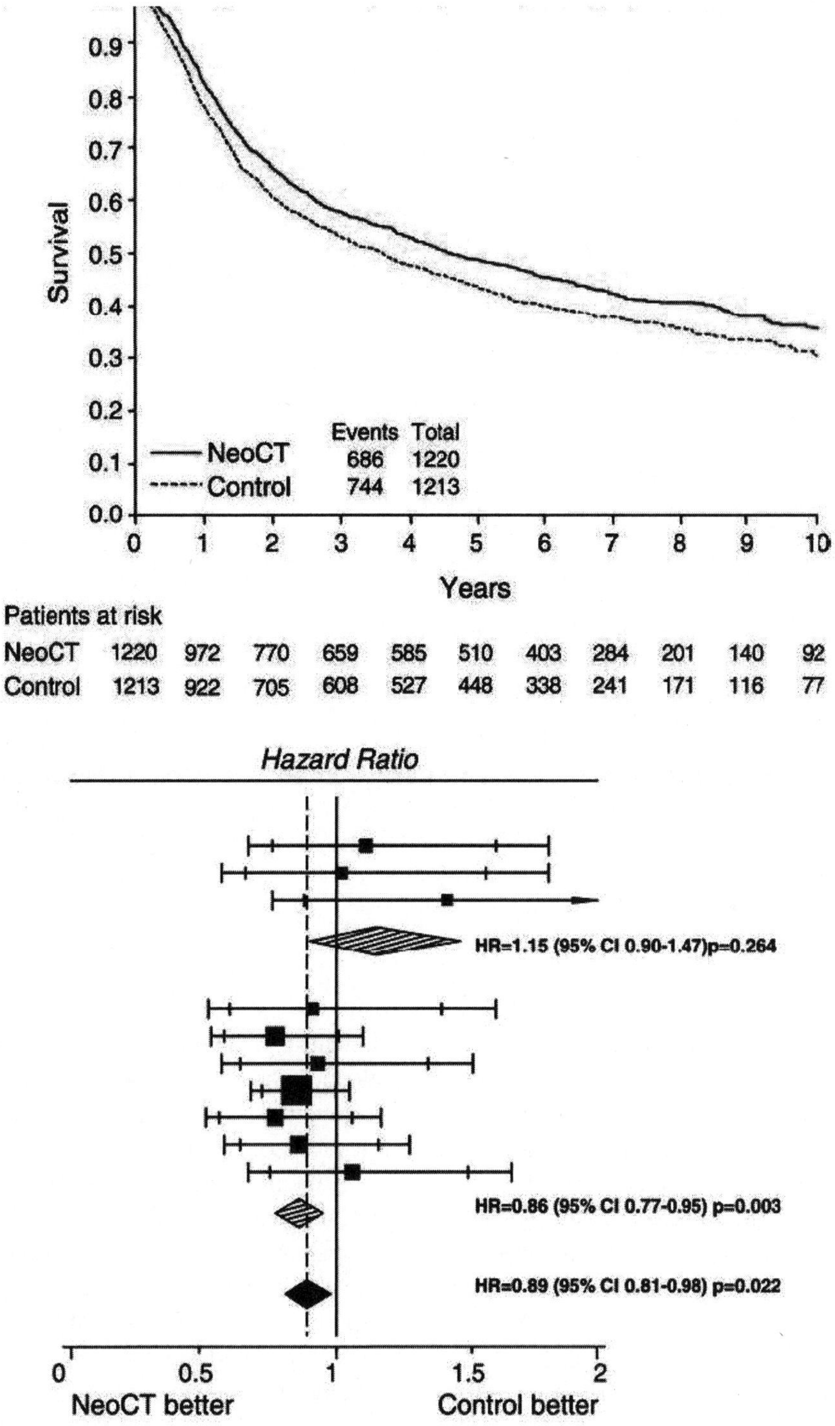

- Individual patient data from 11 randomized trials
- 9% survival benefit with platinum based combination chemotherapy

Reprinted from Vale, CL. Neoadjuvant Chemotherapy in Invasive Bladder Cancer: Update of a Systematic Review and Meta-Analysis of Individual Patient Data. Eur Urol. *48, 202-206. 2005. With permission from Elsevier.*

Table 4

Neoadjuvant Chemotherapy Randomized Trials

	Regimen	Benefit? Progression	Survival
CUETO	Cisplatin	No	No
NORDIC	Cisplatin/Dox +	NS	Yes (T3,T4a)
	XRT		
MRC/EORTC	CMV	No	Yes
SWOG	M-VAC	Yes	Yes
GUONE	M-VAC	?	No
Egypt	Carbo/MTX/Vbl	?	Yes
Nordic II	Cisplatin/Mtx	No	No

Dox = Doxorubicin; XRT = external beam irradiation; NS = not significant; CMV = cisplatin, methotrexate, vinblastine; M-VAC = methotrexate, vinblastine, adriamycin, cisplatin; Carbo = carboplatin; MTX = methotrexate

The only chemotherapy regimens that have shown this benefit are M-VAC and CMV (see discussion of metastatic disease later for more details on these regimens). **A recent meta-analysis using individual patient data found a 5% overall survival advantage for neoadjuvant chemotherapy and a 9% advantage for multi agent platinum based regimens but none for single agent chemotherapy (Figure 4).**

In summary, the benefit of neoadjuvant chemotherapy for patients with non-organ confined tumors is generally accepted. The complication rate of cystectomy is not materially affected by neo-adjuvant chemotherapy.[21]

There are still unresolved issues, however. Better staging modalities that provide more accurate clinical staging will provide more precise patient selection. As new agents are introduced into the treatment of patients with metastatic disease, their role in a neoadjuvant setting has yet to be evaluated. Many medical oncologists are using Gemcitabine/cisplatin, but randomized clinical trials testing this regimen in the peri-operative setting have not been reported. The molecular determinants that predict response to treatment are a subject of intense research and will provide more precise targeted therapy options in the future. Since the randomized trials to date have not been powered for subset analysis, there remains a question as to the relative benefit for patients with or without nodal metastases.

Table 5

Adjuvant Chemotherapy Randomized Trials

	Regimen	Progression	Survival
Skinner, et al (1988)	CISCA	Yes	No
Stockle, et al (1992)	M-VA(E)C	Yes	Not eval.
Studer, et al (1994)	Cisplatin	Not eval.	No
Freiha, et al (1996)	CMV	Yes	No
Bono, et al (1989)	Cisplatin + MTX	No	No

CISCA = cisplatin, cyclophosphamide, adriamycin; M-VA(E)C = methotrexate, vinblastine, adriamycin (epirubicin), cisplatin; CMV = cisplatin, methotrexate, vinblastine; MTX = methotrexate

Figure 5

Strategy for integrating radical TURBT, radiation and chemotherapy

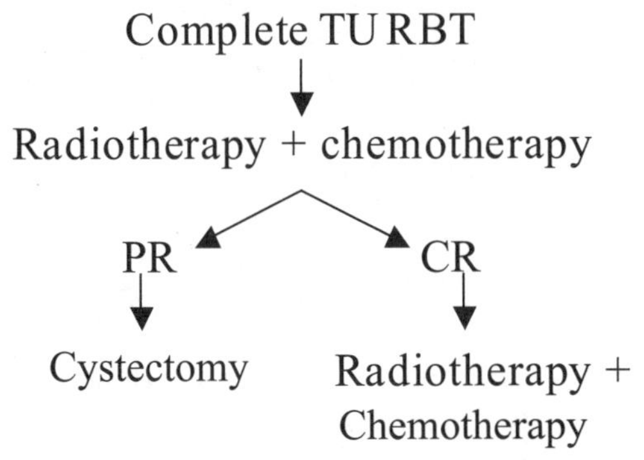

Adjuvant Chemotherapy

Rationale. The rationale for adjuvant chemotherapy (treatment given to treat a risk of recurrence following definitive local therapy) is based on pathologic staging of the primary tumor and lymph nodes. Chemotherapy is therefore given to the patients most at risk for having residual micrometastatic disease and local therapy is given up front when the patient is in the best physical condition. Chemotherapy is given when there is minimal (micrometastatic) disease burden. The disadvantage is there is no measurable disease which allows objective measurement of response and there is the potential that the patient may not recover fully from surgery in a timely fashion to receive chemotherapy.

5 randomized trials have been published to date (Table 5). There is clear evidence that adjuvant chemotherapy had a positive impact on time to progression but this did not translate to a long-term survival benefit. Adjuvant chemotherapy can be administered safely following cystectomy.
Most trials allow treatment up to 12 weeks following surgery which should provide more than adequate time for recovery. **None of the studies, however, was performed in such a way as to be definitive, primarily due to the fact that the three studies using multi agent chemotherapy did not have the statistical power to detect such improvement.**

Many feel it is appropriate based on the trials showing a benefit to neoadjuvant chemotherapy and surgery to offer adjuvant chemotherapy in the case of patients with nonorgan-confined cancers after complete pathologic staging of the cystectomy specimen and pelvic lymph nodes. A trial at M.D. Anderson demonstrated similar results when chemotherapy was administered as all neoadjuvant vs. split between neo and adjuvant.[22] Unfortunately, several new randomized adjuvant chemotherapy trials were closed early due to slow accrual, so we may not have level I evidence to support this approach and therefore use our knowledge of the natural history of invasive bladder cancer to guide decision-making for now.

Trimodal Therapy

Trimodal therapy starts with as thorough a TURBT as possible (Figure 5). Patients respond to radiotherapy best with minimal bulk of tumor. Chemotherapy is then integrated with definitive radiation (for doses see description of external beam radiation earlier in this chapter). Patients who have a partial response (PR) go on to cystectomy and patients who have a complete response (CR) receive additional radiation and chemotherapy. The chemotherapy serves to enhance the response to the radiation and to treat micrometastatic disease. 5-year survival probabilities are 40%-50% and approximately one-fourth to one-third of patients require cystectomy.

5. Molecular Biology

Transitional cell carcinoma is a multitude of diseases with variable biologic manifestations. Molecular alterations facilitate a fuller understanding of the biology of the disease, identify potential targets for therapy and correlates of response to treatments. P53 plays a significant role in the development of CIS and high grade invasive cancer. The retinoblastoma tumor suppressor gene (RB) is also important. The effects of these 2 genes are modified by p21 and p14/16, respectively. **Fibroblast growth factor receptor 3 (FGFR3) has recently been implicated in the development of Ta papillary disease.**

P53 is a tumor suppressor gene and a key cell cycle regulator. Its normal function is control of the G1/S transition. It mediates its activity through the induction of p21. **p53 is induced in response to DNA damage induced by chemotherapy or radiation, leading to cell cycle arrest and induction of apoptosis.**

Figure 6

Positive p53 immunohistochemistry

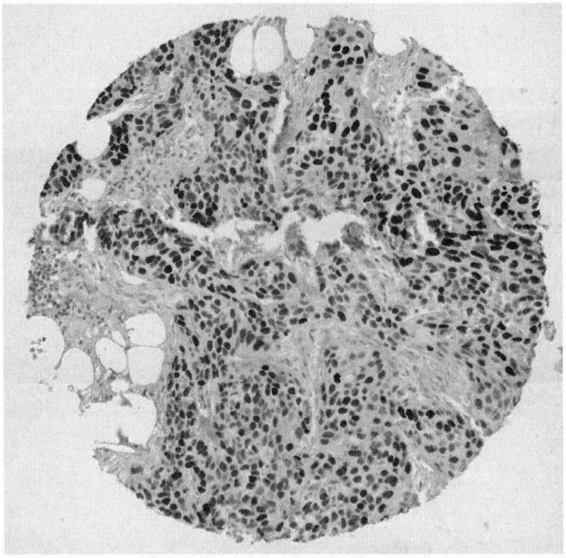

Positive p53 immunohistochemistry on a high-grade invasive TCC with intense nuclear immunoreactivity indicating altered p53 protein.

- Located on short arm of chromosome 17 (17p)

- Gene product is a key protein involved in cell-cycle regulation

- Inhibits phase-specific cell-cycle progression (G1-S)

- Mediates its control through transcriptional activation of p21 WAF1/CIP1

- DNA damage ↑ → p53 wild type ↑ → p21→ cell cycle arrest and induction of apoptosis

Role in Bladder Cancer

- **P53 altered in half of invasive bladder cancers**

- P53 immunohistochemistry a good surrogate for p53 gene mutation

Recent studies suggest that it adds prognostic value to mutation analysis.

- Mutated p53 protein has a prolonged half-life compared to wild type (Figure 6)

  * A positive nuclear stain indicates mutant protein

  * ≥10% of cells positive correlates with p53 gene mutation

The original study from USC[23] demonstrated the effect p53 alterations have on prognosis was confined to patients with organ-confined node negative cancer and served as the basis for a clinical trial that attempts to validate this observation prospectively and determine whether M-VAC adjuvant chemotherapy can improve the survival in p53 positive patients. This trial closed early and p53 did not predict outcome nor did chemotherapy clatter prognosis in patients with altered p53 status.

Retinoblastoma (Rb) tumor suppressor gene

- Located on long arm of chromosome 13 (13q)

- **Rb is altered in up to 50% of invasive bladder cancers**

- Inactivation of the RB gene is more frequent in high grade and advanced stage TCC

- Alteration of RB expression has been associated with disease progression and decreased survival

Immunohistochemical analysis is the most reliable means of determining RB status. A negative or a strong intense staining of more than 50% of the cells is evidence of the altered state. A heterogeneous stain is the normal phenotype. P16 is a cyclin-dependent kinase inhibitor, and it competes for the binding of D-cyclins by CDK 4 and 6, which ultimately have an impact on RB function. When it is bound to the CDKs, P16 inhibits the phosphory lation of RB, which thereby inactivates RB, preventing progression through the cell cycle.[24]

When both p53 and RB pathways are normal, the risk of progression and death after cystectomy is minimal. When one or the other is altered the risk is higher and when both are altered the risk is highest. These biomarker alterations add additional independent prognostic in addition to pathologic tumor stage and lymph node status.

- Less than 5% of patients initially present with metastatic bladder cancer beyond the pelvic lymph nodes

- 50% of patients with muscle invasive bladder cancer will progress to metastatic disease despite curative local therapy

- The median duration of survival following the diagnosis of metastatic bladder cancer is 2 years

Liver, lung and bone are the most common sites after pelvic node metastasis. CNS metastases are more common after chemotherapy as this appears to be a privileged site.

- Autopsy study of 367 patients; pT2-pT4[25]

- Sites

Regional nodes (90%)	Pleura (16%)
Liver (47%)	Kidney (14%)
Lung (45%)	Adrenal gland (14%)
Bone (32%)	Intestine (13%)
Peritoneum (19%)	

The best results with chemotherapy are achieved in patients who are asymptomatic and lymph node only metastases, with approximately one-third of patients surviving 3 years. Patients with symptoms and/or visceral sites of metastases fare much worse. These data are for transitional cell cancer or TCC with mixed histology. **Chemotherapy for patients with primary squamous cell or adeno-carcinoma is not standardized and generally felt to not be as effective.**

M VAC is the gold standard combination chemotherapy regimen. Patients with a neobladder or continent cutaneous diversion should have a catheter placed during hydration with cisplatin in order to avoid overdistension of the reservoir and with the methotrexate in order to avoid absorption of methotrexate across the bowel and subsequent high serum methotrexate levels. M-VAC is administered according to the following schedule and cycles every 28 days. Chemotherapy for measurable metastatic disease is usually given for 6 cycles (neoadjuvant or adjuvant therapy is given for 3-4 cycles).

Methotrexate	(30 mg/m^2)	Days 1, 15, 22
Vinblastine	(3 mg/m^2)	Days 2, 15, 22
Adriamycin	(30 mg/m^2)	Day 2
Cisplatin	(70 mg/m^2)	Day 2

The original long-term, follow-up study from Memorial Sloan-Kettering demonstrated the requirement for a complete response to chemotherapy with or without surgery in order to achieve a survival benefit.[26] One-half of the complete responses (CR) achieved in 39% of patients were durable, resulting in an estimated 20% cure rate. **Failure to achieve a CR is not compatible with long term survival.** Consideration should be given to resection of solitary metastatic sites that persist after chemotherapy.

CMV is another regimen commonly used. The difference between M-VAC and CMV is that CMV uses a higher dose of cisplatin (100 mg/m^2) and adriamycin is not used. Though no clinical trials have ever compared the two regimens they are generally felt to be equivalent in efficacy. Comparisons of multi-agent therapy to single agent cisplatin clearly show the inferiority of single agent cisplatin (Figure 7).

Several randomized trials have led to the following conclusions in metastatic or unresectable locally advanced disease (Table 6):

1.) **Combination chemotherapy (with M VAC) is superior to single agent cisplatin;** 2.) M-VAC is superior to CISCA(cisplatin, cyclophosphamide, adriamycin); 3.) Dose intensification (HD = high dose) and use of growth factors has not resulted in improved survival; 4.) The recent industry sponsored trial of gemcitabine and cisplatin **(GC) suggested that GC is equivalent to M VAC for the treatment of metastatic disease with less toxicity** (Figure 7). GC had higher

Figure 7

Metastatic bladder cancer: M-VAC vs. gemcitabine/cisplatin – overall survival

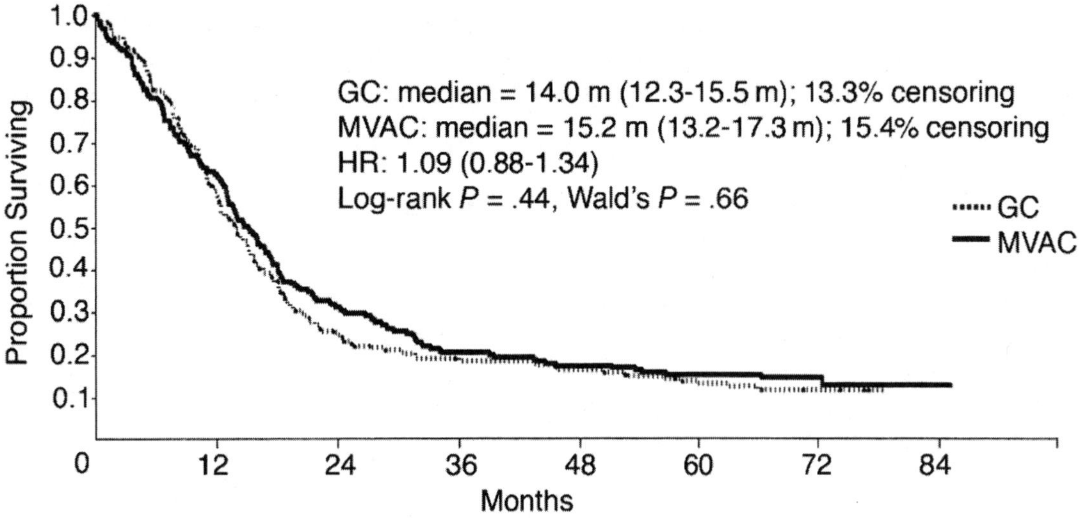

No. of patients at risk:

203	118	50	36	30	23	7	0	GC
202	125	62	40	34	29	9	1	MVAC

With permission. von der Maase H, et al. Metastatic bladder cancer: M-VAC vs. gemcitabine/cisplatin – overall survival. J Clin Oncol. *2005;23:4602-4608.*

Table 6

Randomized Clinical Trials in Metastatic or Unresectable Locally Advanced Urothelial Cancer

		n	**RR**	**MDS**	**Results**
Intergroup	M-VAC	126	39%	12.5	M-VAC> DDP
	DDP (cisplatin)	120	12%	8.2	
MDACC	M-VAC	65	65%	11.1	M-VAC > CISCA
	CISCA	55	46%	8.3	
EORTC	HD-MVAC	134	62%	14.5	HD-MVAC
	M-VAC	129	50%	14.1	± > M-VAC
Lilly	GC	164	49%	13.8	M-VAC ± = GC
	M-VAC	151	46%	14.8	

HD = high dose RR = recurrence rate MDS = median disease-free survival incidence of grade 3 and 4 anemia and thrombocytopenia whereas M-VAC had a higher incidence of grade 3 and 4 neutropenia.

M-VAC is still a standard of care for metastatic bladder cancer. GC is used increasingly as it is easier to administer and there is a perception of equivalency and less toxicity. The median survival is 12-15 months and performance status and visceral metastases influence response to chemotherapy.

Taxanes

- The taxanes paclitaxel (Taxol®_) and docetaxol (Taxotere®_) are active in this disease

    * **Work by disrupting microtubule assemble during S phase**

- Taxol/carboplatin has been studied extensively

    * Complete response rates vary from 0%-40%

    * **This is widely felt to be is an inferior regimen as front-line treatment**

    * May have a role as salvage therapy

- Taxanes are being added to other regimens including a 3-drug regimen of gemcitabine, cisplatin and paclitaxel which is being compared to gemcitabine and cisplatin in a Phase III EORTC trial

7. Urinary Diversion

The urologist planning cystectomy should review the options of a conduit, continent cutaneous diversion requiring intermittent catheterization, and orthotopic neobladder. Particular techniques utilized reflect training experience and bowel segment preferences. Patient factors and underlying health influence this choice as well. Options and considerations include:

- *Incontinent*

    * Conduit

- Ileum, transverse colon

- *Continent*

    * Ureterosigmoidostomy

    * Orthotopic

    * Catheterizable stoma

- **Considerations**

    * Choice of bowel segment

    * Patient selection

    * Surgical technique

    * Functional outcomes

    * Metabolic consequences

Neils Kock, a Swedish general surgeon, described principles of urinary diversion that have withstood the test of time.[27] **Capacity is assured by detubularization, which disrupts the circular smooth muscle, thereby decreasing wall tension and folding, which decreases the intraluminal pressure according to LaPlace's law (pressure = wall tension/radius). Separation of the urinary and fecal streams virtually eliminates the risk of cancer in the intestinal segment.** The patient should achieve social continence. The need to prevent reflux is frequently debated. It is highly unlikely that reflux of colonized urine in a low pressure system is harmful. Antireflux mechanisms may however promote "stretching" of the reservoir, thereby increasing capacity and decreasing intraluminal pressures. Minimizing the risk of electrolyte absorption reduces the risk of chronic acidosis and bone resorption.

Continent Cutaneous Diversion

Right colon reservoirs rely on a detubularized segment that includes the cecum, ascending colon and hepatic flexure and proximal transverse colon based on the ileocolic and right colic arteries with collaterals from the marginal artery of Drummond. The segment is usually 30 cm long and is opened between the 2 anterior tinea to the base of the appendix which is excised or utilized as the catheterizable channel, if it has an adequate lumen, by laying it in a trough created in the bed of an anterior tinea. **The continence mechanism of these reservoirs relies on the ileocecal valve, which is plicated in the case of the Indiana[28] and Florida[29] pouches, or intessucepted and stapled in the case of the Mainz Pouch (which can also be utilized for an orthotopic neobladder).[30] The Kock pouch utilizes ileum and an intessucepted and stapled nipple valve is created for both the afferent (ureter) and efferent limbs (catheterizable channel).[31]** The continence and anti-reflux mechanisms of the T- pouch are created with a serosal-lined extraluminal valve.[32]

Other Options for a Continent Catheterizable Stoma

The Mitrofanoff principle was originally described for the appendix which is tunneled in an antireflux fashion into the native bladder or laid in a trough created along a colon tinea. Today the principle is applied in a variety of tapered intestinal segments that can be utilized for a catheterizable stoma. Monti (from Brazil) has described a technique of utilizing short segments of ileum that are detubularized and rolled into a tube for construction of an efferent catheterizable channel using the Mitrofanoff principle.[33] The Benchekroun valve is a 14 cm segment of ileum that is folded inward along its entire length and can be used with a variety of reservoirs.[34] The long-term durability has been questioned recently, with a high rate of stenosis observed.

Patient Selection

- Life expectancy >1 year
- Strong self-image and desire to be "bag free"
- Manual dexterity
    - * Lifelong requirement for intermittent catheterization
- **Normal or nearly normal renal function**
    - * ClCr ≥50 mL/min
    - * Cr ≤2.0 mg/dL
- Normal or nearly normal bowel function
    - * Some recommend colonoscopy prior to surgery if a colon reservoir will be used. Patients with signs or symptoms suggesting colon disease or patients at increased risk for colon cancer should definitely have this done

While I personally feel that patients should be offered the choice of continent diversion in all settings, it may not be appropriate for patients who are having cystectomy as palliation.

The right lower quadrant is the most common stoma site and should be selected in consultation with the enterostomal therapist. **The umbilicus has the advantage of concealability and it is simple to perform. The umbilicus is the shortest distance to traverse which makes it advantageous in obese patients.** Quality of life studies indicate that the continence rates are higher than for orthotopic diversion.

Orthotopic Urinary Diversion

Lilien and Camey were perhaps the first to popularize orthotopic bladder replacement demonstrating that continence could be achieved first with non detubularized ileum (Camey I) then detubularized ileum (Camey II).[35] The "hemi Kock" pouch adapts the Goodwin cup patch technique for a low pressure reservoir and an intessucepted ileal nipple valve to prevent reflux. The Studer pouch relies on the same Goodwin cup patch technique, then a long (15-20 cm) afferent limb which is refluxing. The ileal neobladder creates a low pressure reservoir by detubularizing a long segment of ileum and reconfiguring to a W or M configuration. The ureters are reimplanted in an end-to side fashion or in a serosal-lined extraluminal trough. The T-pouch, developed at USC, adapts this concept of a serosal-lined trough to create a non-refluxing afferent limb that does not require use of staples.

The ileocolic neobladder utilizes detubularized cecum, ascending colon and terminal ileum, and the ureters are implanted end-to-side in the colon segment. Investigators at Johns Hopkins reported a 12 year experience in 96 patients. Bladder neck contracture was the most common complication. Olsson has popularized the use of absorbable staples to construct a detubularized right colon reservoir.[36] The sigmoid colon is an excellent option especially when the sigmoid is redundant as it easily reaches into the pelvis. The ureters can be implanted in an end-to-side or non-refluxing tinea reimplant fashion.

Advantages of Small Bowel

- **Lower pressures than colon**
- Reliably reaches the urethra
- Facilitates taking ureters high (eg, XRT, CIS)
- Low incidence ureteral stricture (4%)
- Urine is frequently sterile

(NB: Very low incidence of late complications)

Ureteral Implantation

The end to side ureterointestinal anastamosis is reliable with a low stricture rate of approximately 4%. It was described by Wayland Leadbetter for use with an ileal conduit and with the original description of the conduit by Bricker. It can be used in virtually any setting where a ureter is implanted into bowel. **LeDuc described a nonrefluxing ureter reimplant that is associated with a higher stricture rate.** When implanting a ureter into colon, the end-to-side works quite well as reflux is not a major

Table 7

Sites of Absorption of Various Substances Thoughout the GI Tract

	Stomach	Duodenum	Jejunum	Ileum	Terminal Ileum	Colon
Carbohydrates	X	X	X	X		
Protein		X	X	X	(X)	
Calcium		(X)	(X)			
Iron		(X)	(X)			
Water-soluble vitamins			X	X		
Vitamin B_{12}				((X))	X	
Bile acids				(X)	X	
Sodium, chloride, ware				X	X	X

X-absorption, (X)-limited absorption and ((X))-very limited absorption occurs. Only absorption of bile acids and vitamin B_{12} are restricted to a single area, namely the ileum, and other absorptive tasks may when needed be taken over by different parts of the bowel.

concern. Many surgeons prefer a tinea reimplant that is non-refluxing. The major advantage is that it can be performed without opening the bowel. **The Wallace technique brings the spatulated ends of both ureters together in a single implant.** The major disadvantage is that both ureters are at risk if a stricture occurs, or any other type of distal obstruction. More recently, Ghoneim described a method of reimplantation into an ileal neobladder where the ureter is laid into an extraluminal serosal lined trough that is non-refluxing. Along discussion at the AUA in 2005 concluded that there was no role for an anti-reflux anastamosis with an orthotopic neobladder.

Patient Selection for Orthotopic Diversion

The patient must have **normal sphincter** function and this can be assessed by a careful history and physical exam. **The retained urethra should not be at significant risk for developing cancer** (see earlier in invasive bladder cancer section). The patient should understand the rehabilitation period during which they will require pads and be highly motivated to work through this period in order to achieve social continence. Elderly patients or patients with locally advanced tumors (P3b, P4 or N+) or those who have had prior pelvic irradiation are not routinely excluded. The complication rate is not materially affected by neo-adjuvant chemotherapy. **Orthotopic Diversion in Women**

Women with normal sphincter function are excellent candidates for orthotopic reconstruction. Patients who may require urethra or bladder neck suspension can also be considered but may be at higher risk for requiring intermittent catheterization. **Any evidence of cancer at the bladder neck or urethra is an absolute contraindication. T3 or T4 tumors of the posterior bladder are relative contraindications as it may not be possible to get an adequate margin distally. The distal two-thirds of the urethra is critical to normal sphincter function and must be preserved. Dissection below the endopelvic fascia must be avoided in order to avoid damage to the pudendal nerve which innervates this portion of the urethra.** Approximately 20% of patients will require intermittent catheterization (some refer to this as "hypercontinence"). This phenomenon is much more common in women than in men.

Daytime continence is achieved in a high percentage of patients regardless of age or gender. During sleep, older patients have a higher rate of incontinence. As the bladder fills and intraluminal pressures rise, resting urethra pressure does not increase to compensate for the rise in neobladder pressure, resulting in incontinence. Most patients need to void once or twice at night in order to reduce the risk of incontinence. **Urinary retention in men is uncommon and must raise the possibility of local pelvic recurrence.** Urethral anastamotic strictures are also uncommon in both men and women. The following data are from the author's experience in a consecutive group of patients:

Daytime	59/69 (86%)
<65	37/42 (88%)
>65	22/27 (81%)
Night	37/68 (54%)
<65	26/41 (63%)
>65	11/27 (41%)

Conduit Urinary Diversion

- Advantages
  * Simple to perform
  * Easy to manage—high satisfaction rate
- Disadvantages
  * Fear of odor and leakage
  * External appliance
  * Restricted social and sexual activities
- Bowel segment
  * Terminal ileum – no prior irradiation
  * Transverse colon – prior pelvic irradiation
  * Avoid a long loop which leads to stasis of urine

Ileal Conduit

- Patient selection

  * No motivation to be free of an appliance

  * Manual dexterity

  * Elderly patient who needs something simple

  * Palliative surgery

- Stoma—usually placed in the right lower quadrant in consultation with an enterostomal therapist after examining the patient in the lying, sitting and standing positions.

  * Turnbull loop ileostomy—Eliminates risk of stomal stenosis

  * Rosebud end stoma—creates a nipple that minimizes urine contact with skin

- Enterostomal therapist

  * Consult preoperatively for counseling and marking stoma site for best results

Physiology

Stomach

The stomach is used more in the pediatric population especially in children with renal insufficiency. **The stomach absorbs carbohydrates and makes intrinsic factor which is important for absorption of B12 by the terminal ileum.** The metabolic consequences include B12 malabsorption and alkalosis which is associated with hypokalemia and hypochloremia. Reduced hydrochloric acid secretion results in loss of feedback on gastrin secretion which may produce peptic ulcers and hematuria, the so-called **hematuria dysuria syndrome**.

Jejunum

Jejunum should not be used except as a last resort. The jejunum secretes sodium and chloride and absorbs hydrogen ions and potassium. **The primary pathophysiology is dehydration that is related to large water shifts and the subsequent stimulation of aldsoterone.** This facilitates sodium reabsorption in the distal tubule and collecting duct in exchange for potassium and protons. What follows is potassium diuresis with low urine sodium concentration perpetuating the problem. Exchange of urinary potassium for hydrogen results in acidosis. (Mills, RD, Studer, UE. *J Urol*. 1999:1057) The **metabolic abnormality consists of metabolic acidosis accompanied by hyperkalemia, hyponatremia and loss of chloride.** The patient may complain of nausea, emesis and fatigue. The treatment is hydration and sodium chloride.

Ileum and Colon

- Secretes sodium and bicarbonate

- Absorbs ammonium, hydrogen chloride

  * Ammonium is principle mechanism of acidosis

- **Hyperchloremic metabolic acidosis**

  * Total body potassium deficit

  * Hypocalcemia, hypomagnesemia, hyperamonemia

- Symptoms

  * Fatigue, anorexia, diarrhea

- Treatment

  * IV hydration plus bicarbonate

  * Potassium supplementation

Table 7 describes sites of absorption throughout the GI tract. The reference is a comprehensive review of GI physiology pertinent to interposition in the urinary tract.

Complications

An inevitable consequence of orthotopic or continent cutaneous diversion is a reduction in the absorptive capacity of the bowel. Most patients will ultimately adapt to this but some do experience a change in bowel function. The loss of the ileocecal valve in the case of right colon reservoirs may contribute to loose stools or diarrhea. **Diarrhea is usually due to fat malabsorption and bile salts irrita-**

tion of the colon. Metamucil works by adding bulk to the stool and this is what I try first. Subsequent management is anti-motility drugs which are usually successful. **Cholestyramine** will absorb excess bile salts and is usually effective in patients that do not respond to antimotility agents. **B12 deficiency is a consequence of malabsorption related to the loss of the distal terminal ileum or use of a large segment of distal ileum.** Other risk factors include radiation exposure to the terminal ileum. Loss of B12 is insidious and takes several years, though it has been reported earlier.[38] I recommend annual monitoring of B12 levels and replacement if deficiency is identified. Treatment should be initiated prior to symptoms. Parenteral B12 shots are reliable and there are now oral formulations that can be administered as well.[39] **Osteoporosis can occur as a result of acidosis causing depletion of bone phosphate stores.** Patients with renal insufficiency are at higher risk.

Other Complications

- Cholelithiasis
  - * Decreased bile acids causes lithogenic oversaturation of bile
  - * Incidence: 9% with resection 30-50 cm ileum; 35% with resection 100 cm
  - * No documented increased risk in urinary diversion
- Renal calculi
  - * ***Decreased bile acids; fat malabsorption and binding of intestinal calcium; increased oxalate***
  - * Chronic bacteriuria and struvite stones
  - * Dehydration
- Reservoir calculi—usually form on foreign body

Small stones can be treated with standard endoscopic techniques. **Repeated manipulation of a continent cutaneous stoma should be avoided, and so large stones are best treated with a percutaneous or open technique.**

Secondary Cancer

- Rare
- 0% in over 2000 patients
  - * 1 patient recurrent lymphoma (Kock Pouch)
- Colonoscopy pre-op for at risk patients prior to colon reservoir procedures
- Recommend pouch endoscopy annually starting at 3 years post-op
- There area case reports of typical adenocarcinoma of the colon forming in an Indiana Pouch and I have treated two patients for this recently–9 and 10 years following cystectomy.
- **Highest risk in ureterosigmoidostomy**
  - * Contact of feces and urine[40]
  - * **After 10 years: annual colonoscopy—risk increases dramatically to up to 25-50 times the normal population**

8. References

1. Kamat AM, Gee JR, Dinney CP, et al. The case for early cystectomy in the treatment of non-muscle invasive micropapillary bladder carcinoma. *J Urol*. 2006;175(3 Pt 1):881-885.

2. Esrig D, Freeman JA, Elmajian DA, et al. Transitional cell carcinoma involving the prostate with a proposed staging classification for stromal invasion. *J Urol*. 1996;156(3):1071-1076.

3. Chang SS, Cole E, Smith JA Jr, Cookson MS. Pathological findings of gynecologic organs obtained at female radical cystectomy. *J Urol*. 2002;168(1):147-149.

4. Ali-El-Dein B, Gomha M, Ghoneim MA. Critical evaluation of the problem of chronic urinary retention after orthotopic bladder substitution in women. *J Urol*. 2002;168(2):587-592.

5. Vazina A, Dugi D, Shariat SF, Evans J, Link R, Lerner SP. Stage specific lymph node metastasis mapping in radical cystectomy specimens. *J Urol*. 2004;171(5):1830-1834.

6. Stein JP, Clark P, Miranda G, Cai J, Groshen S, Skinner DG. Urethral tumor recurrence following cystectomy and urinary diversion: clinical and pathological characteristics in 768 male patients. *J Urol*. 2005;173(4):1163-1168.

7. Stein JP, Esrig D, Freeman JA, et al. Prospective pathologic analysis of female cystectomy specimens: risk factors for orthotopic diversion in women. *Urology*. 1998;51(6):951-5.

8. Stenzl A, Draxl H, Posch B, Colleselli K, Falk M, Bartsch G. The risk of urethral tumors in female bladder cancer: can the urethra be used for orthotopic reconstruction of the lower urinary tract? *J Urol*. 1995;153(3 Pt 2):950-955.

9. Kessler TM, Burkhard FC, Perimenis P, et al. Attempted nerve sparing surgery and age have a significant effect on urinary continence and erectile function after radical cystoprostatectomy and ileal orthotopic bladder substitution. *J Urol*. 2004;172(4 Pt 1):1323-1327.

10. Stenzl A, Bartsch G, Rogatsch H. The remnant urothelium after reconstructive bladder surgery. *Eur Urol*. 2002;41(2):124-131.

11. Stein JP, Lieskovsky G, Cote R, et al. Radical cystectomy in the treatment of invasive bladder cancer: longterm results in 1,054 patients. *J Clin Oncol*. 2001;19(3):666-675.

12. Njinou Ngninkeu B, Lorge F, Moulin P, Jamart J, Van Cangh PJ. Transitional cell carcinoma involving the prostate: a clinicopathological retrospective study of 76 cases. *J Urol*. 2003; 169(1):149-152.

13. Shen SS, Lerner SP, Muezzinoglu B, Truong LD, Amiel G, Wheeler TM. Prostatic involvement by transitional cell carcinoma in patients with bladder cancer and its prognostic significance. *Hum Pathol*. 2006;37(6):726-734.

14. Stein JP, Cai J, Groshen S, Skinner DG. Risk factors for patients with pelvic lymph node metastases following radical cystectomy with en bloc pelvic lymphadenectomy: concept of lymph node density. *J Urol*. 2003;170(1): 35-41.

15. Clark PE, Stein JP, Groshen SG, et al. Radical cystectomy in the elderly: Comparison of survival between younger and older patients. *Cancer*. 2005;103(3):546-552.

16. Herr HW, Cookson MS, Soloway SM. Upper tract tumors in patients with primary bladder cancer followed for 15 years. *J Urol*. 1996; 156(4):1286-1287.

17. Herr HW. Transurethral resection of muscleinvasive bladder cancer: 10-year outcome. *J Clin Oncol*. 2001;19(1):89-93.

18. Solsona E, Iborra I, Ricos JV, Monros JL, Casanova J, Calabuig C. Feasibility of transurethral resection for muscle infiltrating carcinoma of the bladder: long-term follow-up of a prospective study. *J Urol*. 1998;159(1): 95-98; discussion 98-99.

19. Neoadjuvant cisplatin, methotrexate, and vinblastine chemotherapy for muscle-invasive bladder cancer: a randomised controlled trial. International collaboration of trialists. *Lancet*. 1999;354(9178):533-540.

20. Grossman HB, Natale RB, Tangen CM, et al. Neoadjuvant chemotherapy plus cystectomy compared with cystectomy alone for locally advanced bladder cancer. *N Engl J Med*. 2003; 349(9):859-866.

21. Hall MC, Swanson DA, Dinney CP. Complications of radical cystectomy: impact of the timing of perioperative chemotherapy. *Urology*. 1996;47(6):826-830.

22. Millikan R, Dinney C, Swanson D, Sweeney, et al. Integrated therapy for locally advanced bladder cancer: final report of a randomized trial of cystectomy plus adjuvant M-VAC versus cystectomy with both preoperative and postoperative M-VAC. *J Clin Oncol*. 2001;19(20):4005-4013.

23. Esrig D, Spruck CH 3rd, Nichols PW, Chaiwun B, Steven K, Groshen S, et al. p53 nuclear protein accumulation correlates with mutations in the p53 gene, tumor grade, and stage in bladder cancer. *Am J Pathol*. 1993; 143(5):1389-1397.

24. Xu HJ, Cairns P, Hu SX, Knowles MA, Benedict WF. Loss of RB protein expression in primary bladder cancer correlates with loss of heterozygosity at the RB locus and tumor progression. *Int J Cancer*. 1993;53(5):781-784.

25. Wallmeroth A, Wagner U, Moch H, Gasser TC, Sauter G, Mihatsch MJ. Patterns of metastasis in muscle-invasive bladder cancer (pT24): An autopsy study on 367 patients. *Urol Int*. 1999;62(2):69-75.

26. Sternberg CN, Yagoda A, Scher HI, Watson RC, Geller N, Herr HW, et al. Methotrexate, vinblastine, doxorubicin, and cisplatin for advanced transitional cell carcinoma of the urothelium. Efficacy and patterns of response and relapse. *Cancer*. 1989;64(12):2448-2458.

27. Faxen A, Kock NG, Sundin T. Long-term functional results after ileocystoplasty. *Scand J Urol Nephrol*. 1973;7(2):127-130.

28. Rowland RG. Present experience with the Indiana pouch. *World J Urol*. 1996;14(2):92-98.

29. Webster C, Bukkapatnam R, Seigne JD, et al. Continent colonic urinary reservoir (Florida pouch): long-term surgical complications (greater than 11 years). *J Urol*. 2003;169(1):174-176.

30. Lampel A, Fisch M, Stein R, Schultz-Lampel D, et al. Continent diversion with the Mainz pouch. *World J Urol*. 1996;14(2):85-91.

31. Skinner DG, Lieskovsky G, Boyd S. Continent urinary diversion. *J Urol*. 1989;141(6):1323-1327.

32. Stein JP, Skinner DG. The craft of urologic surgery: the T-pouch. *Urol Clin North Am*, 2003;30(3):647-661xi.

33. Monti PR, Lara RC, Dutra MA, de Carvalho JR. New techniques for construction of efferent conduits based on the Mitrofanoff principle. *Urology*. 1997;49(1):112-115.

34. Benchekroun A, Essakalli N, Faik M, Marzouk M, Hachimi M, Abakka T. Continent urostomy with hydraulic ileal valve in 136 patients: 13 years of experience. *J Urol*. 1989;142(1): 46-51.

35. Lilien OM, Camey M. 25-year experience with replacement of the human bladder (Camey procedure). 1984. *J Urol*. 2002;167(2 Pt 2):1161-1167; discussion 1168.

36. Kirsch AJ, Hensle TW, CAOlsson. Rapid construction of right colon pouch: initial clinical experience. *Urology*. 1994;43(2):228-231.

37. Mills RD, Studer UE. Metabolic consequences of continent urinary diversion. *J Urol*. 1999;161(4):1057-1066.

38. Steiner MS, Morton RA, Marshall FF. Vitamin B12 deficiency in patients with ileocolic neobladders. *J Urol*. 1993;149(2):255-257.

39. Lane LA, Rojas-Fernandez C. Treatment of vitamin b(12)-deficiency anemia: oral versus parenteral therapy. *Ann Pharmacother*. 2002; 36(7-8):1268-1272.

40. Crissey MM, Steele GD, Gittes RF. Rat model for carcinogenesis in ureterosigmoidostomy. *Science*. 1980;207(4435):1079-1080.

Chapter 19: Penile and Urethral Cancer

Kenneth W. Angermeier, MD

Contents

1. Premalignant Penile Lesions

Cutaneous Horn

- Solid protuberance resulting from cornification of the epithelium over a preexisting skin lesion
- Associated with human papillomavirus (HPV) type 16
- Should be excised for accurate histologic evaluation

Lichen Sclerosis (LS)

- Also known as balanitis xerotica obliterans (BXO) (Figure 1)
- Symptoms: pain; pruritis; bleeding; decreased urinary stream
- White patch on the prepuce or glans that often involves the urethral meatus
- May be associated with glanular or coronal fissures, advancement of foreskin onto the glans, meatal stenosis and/or urethral stricture
- Biopsy recommended to confirm diagnosis
- Previous reports have documented an association with squamous cell carcinoma
- Treatment: topical steroid cream (betamethasone); circumcision; possible need for meatotomy or urethral reconstruction

Leukoplakia

- Whitish plaques often involving the urethral meatus
- Biopsy necessary to confirm diagnosis and rule out malignant change
- Associated with squamous cell carcinoma in situ and verrucous carcinoma
- Treatment: surgical excision; circumcision to eliminate chronic inflammation

Figure 1

Chronic lichen sclerosis with deformity of the urethral meatus

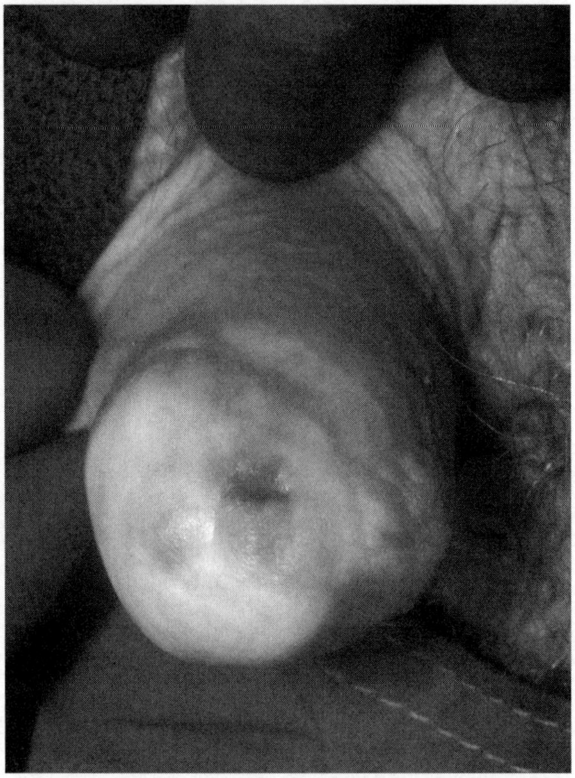

Reprinted with permission of the Cleveland Clinic

2. HPV-Related Lesions

Bowenoid Papulosis

- Pigmented papules of the penile shaft in younger men
- Associated with HPV-16
- Biopsy histologically consistent with squamous cell carcinoma (SCC) in situ, but clinical course is invariably benign
- Treatment: electrodessication; 5-fluorouracil (FU) cream; laser; surgical excision

Condyloma Acuminatum

- Papillomatous genital lesions generally considered to be benign (Figure 2)
- Associated with HPV-6 and -11 most typically
- Histologically characterized by the koilocyte—a cell with an atypical nucleus surrounded by an empty cavity
- Subclinical flat "acetowhite" lesions may be detected by applying 5% acetic acid to the genitalia
- Treatment: 5% imiquimod cream; topical podophyllin; intralesional interferon; laser; electrocautery; surgical excision
- Associated in some cases with development of SCC of the penis

Verrucous Carcinoma (Buschke-Lowenstein tumor)

- Large condyloma that displaces and invades adjacent tissues
- Associated with HPV-6 and 11
- Histologically no evidence of malignant change and does not metastasize
- Treatment: cryosurgery; surgical excision with close follow-up for recurrence

Figure 2

Condyloma accuminata

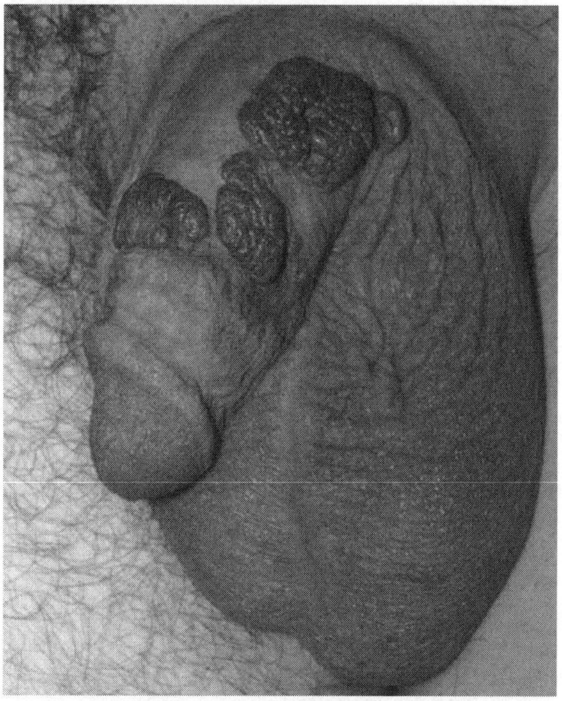

Reprinted with permission of the Cleveland Clinic

3. Penile Squamous Cell Carcinoma

Carcinoma *in Situ*

- Erythroplasia of Queyrat: SCC in situ on the glans or prepuce; red, velvety, well-marginated lesion (Figure 3)

Figure 3

SCC *in situ* of the glans penis extending into the distal urethra

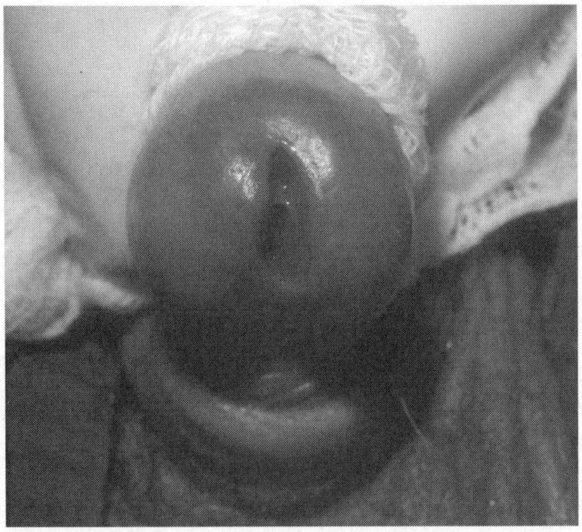

Reprinted with permission of the Cleveland Clinic

- Bowen's disease: SCC in situ located on penile shaft
- May progress to invasive carcinoma in 10% of cases
- Treatment: 5-FU cream; laser; surgical excision including circumcision

Invasive SCC

- Accounts for 0.4%-0.6% of cancers among men in the United States and Europe
- Primarily occurs in the preputial cavity of uncircumcised older men
- Neonatal circumcision virtually eliminates risk of developing invasive SCC (not so for circumcision performed later in life)
- Associated most commonly with HPV-16, but also with HPV-18, -31, -33
- Additional risk factors: poor hygiene, smoking, phimosis, number of sexual partners, LS
- If untreated, most patients will die of their disease within 2 years

Presentation

- Primary tumor may be a nonhealing ulcer, papule, indurated mass or exophytic growth

Figure 4

Large invasive penile SCC

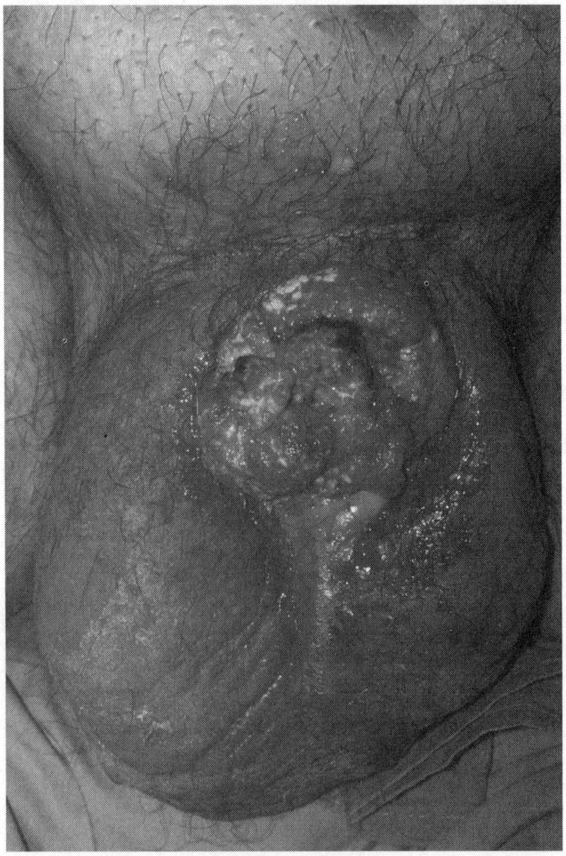

Reprinted with permission of the Cleveland Clinic

- Most common location is on the glans penis (46%), followed by the prepuce (21%)
- May be associated with penile bleeding or purulent discharge
- Rarely may present as an inguinal mass or draining abscess due to nodal metastases if the primary tumor is obscured by phimosis

Diagnosis

- Delay in diagnosis is common
- Biopsy is necessary to confirm the diagnosis and assess depth of invasion, tumor grade and presence of vascular invasion
- Basaloid and sarcomatoid histological variants are more aggressive
- At diagnosis, thorough palpation of inguinal regions for lymphadenopathy is essential
- Computed tomography (CT) may be helpful in the assessment of inguinal nodes in an obese patient or those with a history of inguinal surgery, and of the pelvic nodes when the inguinal nodes are palpable
- Magnetic resonance imaging (MRI) is the best study to obtain additional information about the extent of the primary tumor in some cases when considering organ-sparing surgery

Staging and Prognosis

AJCC Staging for Penile Cancer

Primary Tumor (T)

TX	Primary tumor cannot be assessed
T0	No evidence of primary tumor
Tis	Carcinoma in situ
Ta	Noninvasive verrucous carcinoma
T1	Tumor invades subepithelial connective tissue
T2	Tumor invades corpus spongiosum or cavernosum
T3	Tumor invades urethra or prostate
T4	Tumor invades other adjacent structures

Lymph Nodes (N)

NX	Regional nodes cannot be assessed
N0	No regional lymph node metastases
N1	Metastasis in a single regional lymph node
N2	Metastases in multiple or bilateral superficial inguinal nodes
N3	Metastases in deep inguinal or pelvic nodes

Distant Metastasis (M)

MX	Distant metastasis cannot be assessed
M0	No distant metastasis
M1	Distant metastasis

- The most important factor determining survival is the extent of lymph node metastases
- Factors associated with ultimate cure following surgical treatment of lymphadenopathy include unilateral nodal involvement, ≤2 positive nodes, no extranodal tumor extension and no pelvic metastases

Surgical Treatment—Primary Tumor

Laser Therapy

- Advantage of eliminating tumor with preservation of surrounding tissues and penile function
- Best suited for Tis, small Ta, T1 tumors and for patients with manageable T2 tumors who refuse more aggressive surgical treatment
- CO_2 laser primarily suitable for Tis
- Most commonly used laser overall: Nd:YAG

- Try to achieve a 3-5 mm margin around the tumor

- Local recurrence rate approximately 20%

Mohs Micrographic Surgery

- Excision of tissue in thin layers with immediate microscopic examination and tumor mapping to eliminate malignancy with maximal preservation of local tissues

- Requires significant technical support and surgeon experience

- Useful for Tis or small superficially invasive tumors

- Local recurrence rates 6%

Conservative Surgical Excision

- Recent studies have indicated that a 2 cm surgical margin may not always be required for effective local control of SCC penis

- Excisional biopsy with primary closure

- Circumcision

- Glans tumor excision with defect closure using a outer preputial flap or a split thickness skin graft (STSG)

Figures 5a-d through 6: Surgical glans defect covered with outer preputial flap

Figure 5a

Superficial glans tumor

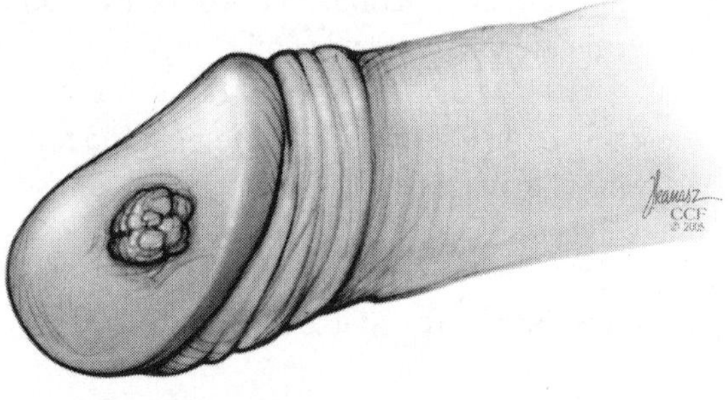

Reprinted with permission of the Cleveland Clinic

Figure 5b

Outer preputial flap outlined

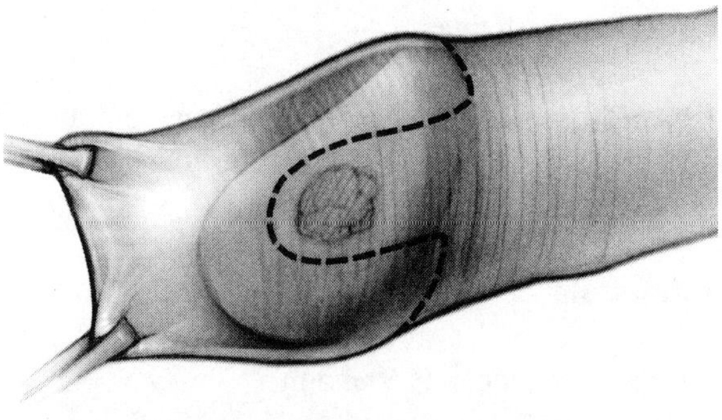

Reprinted with permission of the Cleveland Clinic

Figure 5c

Tumor excised and circumcision performed

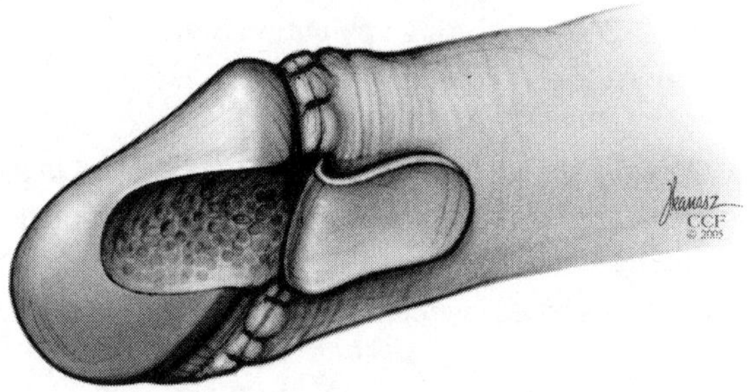

Reprinted with permission of the Cleveland Clinic

Figure 5d

Glans defect filled with outer preputial flap

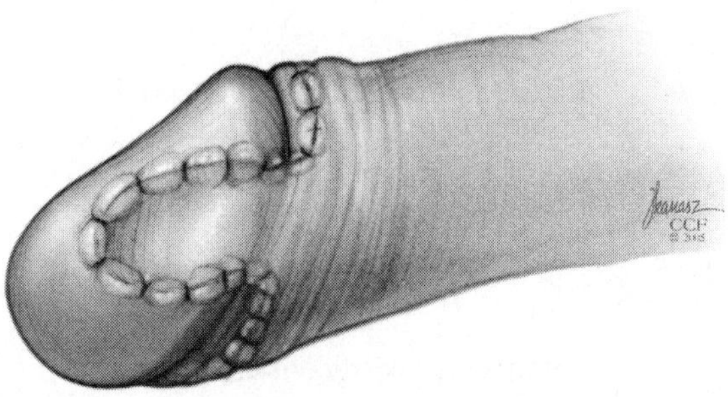

Reprinted with permission of the Cleveland Clinic

Figure 6

STSG to glans penis following excision of extensive SCC *in situ*

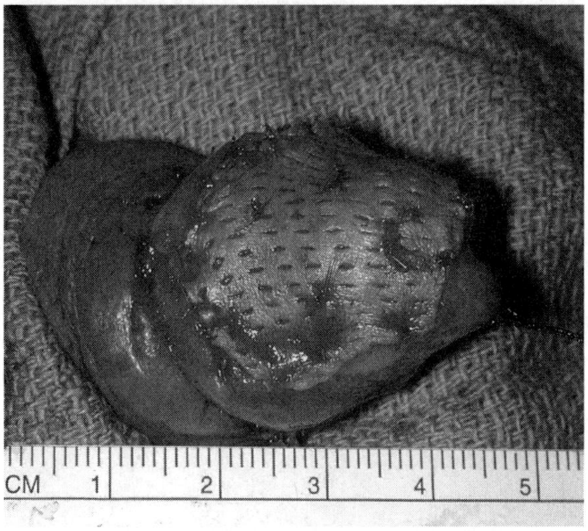

Reprinted with permission of the Cleveland Clinic

Figures 7a-7d: Partial penectomy

Figure 7a

Incision with ligation and division of dorsal penile vessels

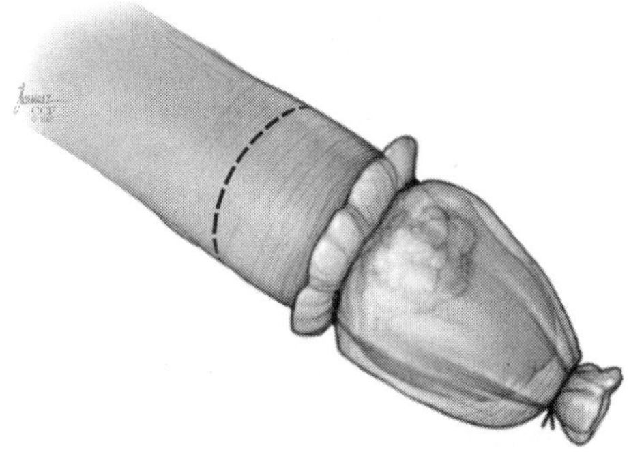

Reprinted with permission of the Cleveland Clinic

Figure 7b

Corpora transected and urethra spatulated

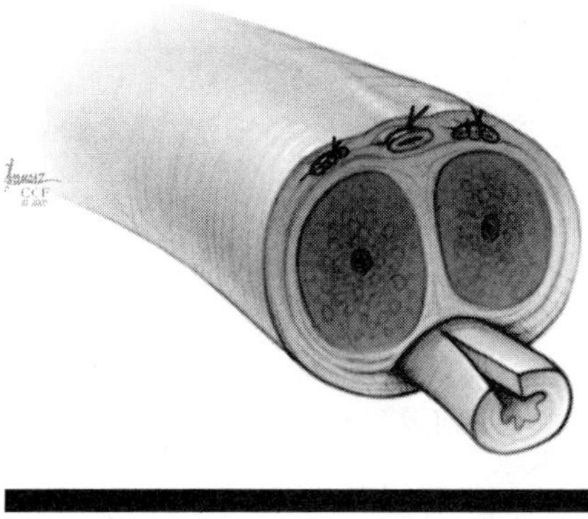

Reprinted with permission of the Cleveland Clinic

Figure 7c

Glans defect filled with outer preputial flap

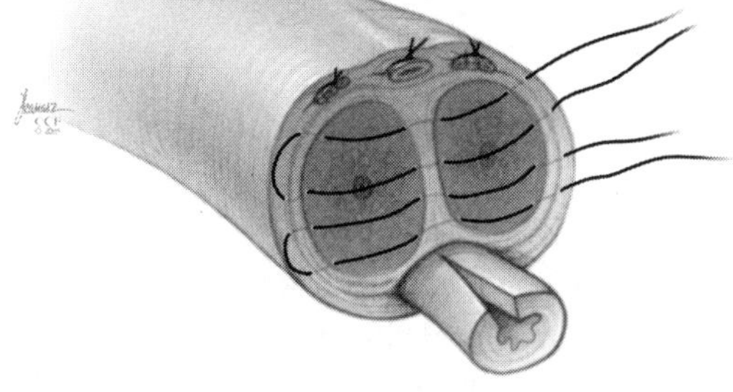

Reprinted with permission of the Cleveland Clinic

Figure 7d

Final closure with creation of urethrostomy

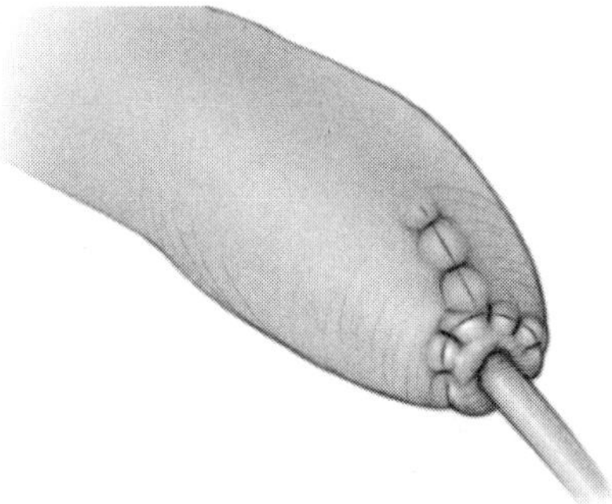

Reprinted with permission of the Cleveland Clinic

- Glansectomy: complete removal of the glans penis with preservation of the corporal bodies

- Intraoperative frozen sections are critical to help confirm complete tumor excision

- Recently reported local recurrence rates 8%-11%

- Requires careful long term follow-up

Partial Penectomy
- Most commonly performed surgical procedure for the treatment of the primary tumor in patients with invasive SCC

- Amputation of the penis at least 2 cm proximal to the tumor (Figures 7a-7c)

- Additional goal is to preserve the ability to void in a standing position

- Provides excellent local control with a recurrence rate of 0%-8%

- Adequate sexual function postoperatively: 20%

Total Penectomy
- Indicated for penile tumors whose size or location would not allow an adequate surgical margin and preservation of upright voiding (Figures, 8a-8e)

- Amputation of the penis at the base at the level of the suspensory ligament

- Creation of perineal urethrostomy

- Excellent local control rates have been reported

Figures 8a-8e: Total penectomy

Figure 8a

Incision

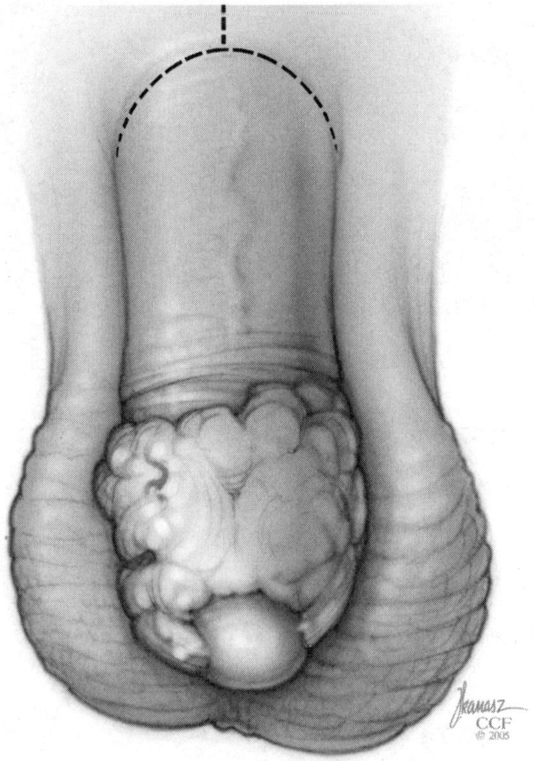

Reprinted with permission of the Cleveland Clinic

Figure 8b

Transection of the corpora near the level of the pubis

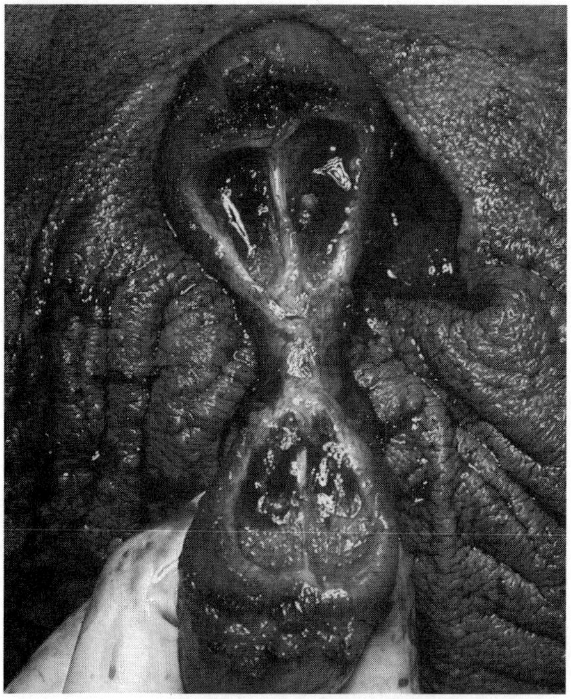

Reprinted with permission of the Cleveland Clinic

Figure 8c

Mobilization of the remaining urethra off of the proximal corporal bodies

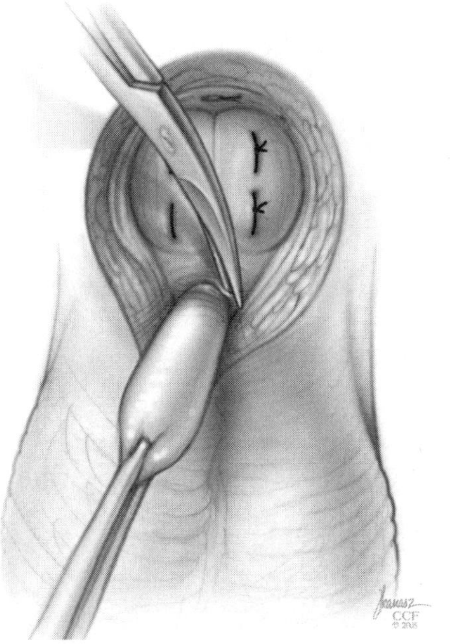

Reprinted with permission of the Cleveland Clinic

Figure 8d

Transposition of the urethra through a perineal incision

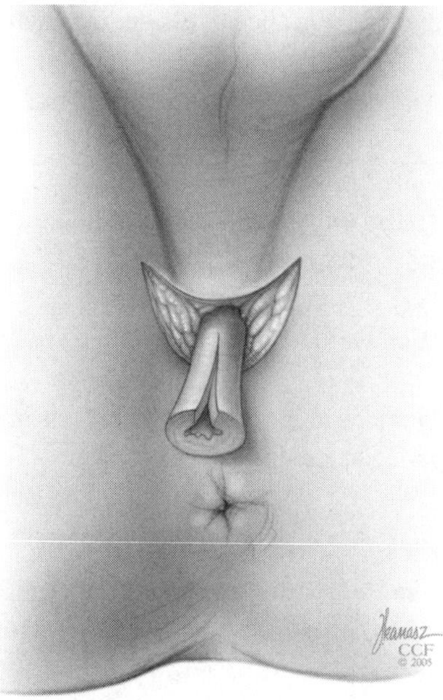

Reprinted with permission of the Cleveland Clinic

Figure 8e

Completion of perineal urethrostomy

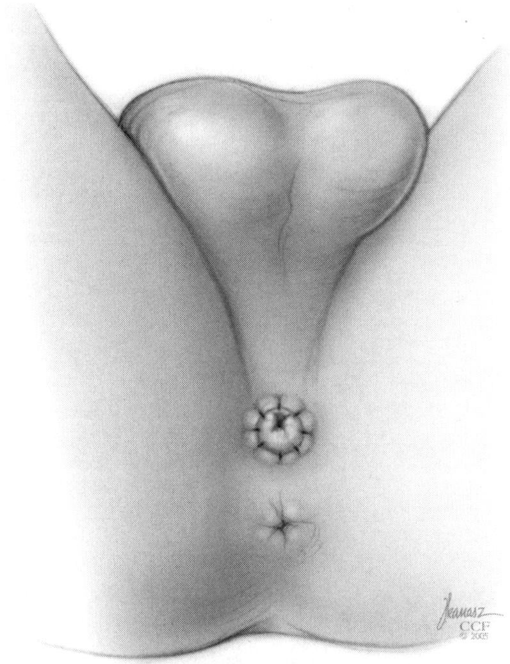

Reprinted with permission of the Cleveland Clinic

Management of Regional Lymph Nodes

Anatomy

- SCC spreads initially to the regional lymph nodes before the occurrence of distant metastases
- First echelon drainage is to the inguinal lymph nodes
- Metastatis from the primary tumor to the superficial nodes may occur bilaterally
- Superficial nodes:

  * 4-25 nodes in the deep membranous layer of the superficial fascia of the thigh

Figure 9

Superficial inguinal lymph nodes and branches of the saphenous vein

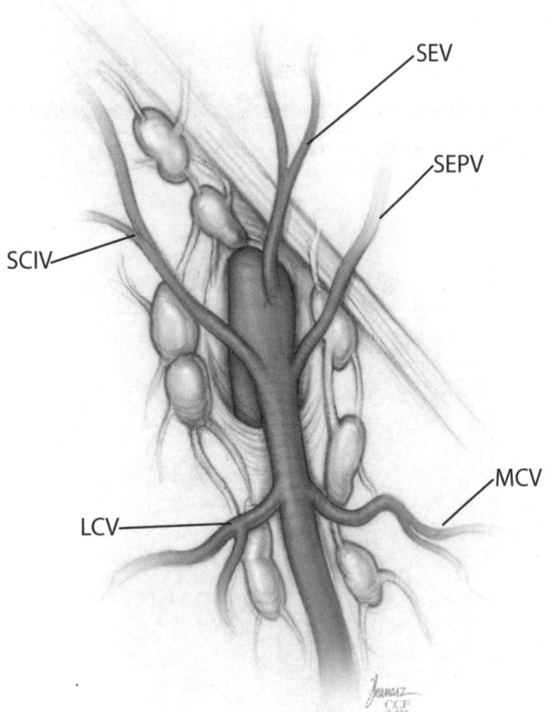

SEV, superficial epigastric; SEPV, superficial external pudendal; MCV, medical cutaneous; LCV, lateral cutaneous; SCIV, superficial circumflex iliac

Reprinted with permission of the Cleveland Clinic

- Deep nodes
  * Within the femoral canal medial to the femoral vein, and between it and the lacunar ligament
  * Most cephalad node in this group is the lymph node of Cloquet
- Second echelon drainage is from the deep inguinal nodes to the ipsilateral external iliac nodes

Figure 10

Deep inguinal lymph nodes

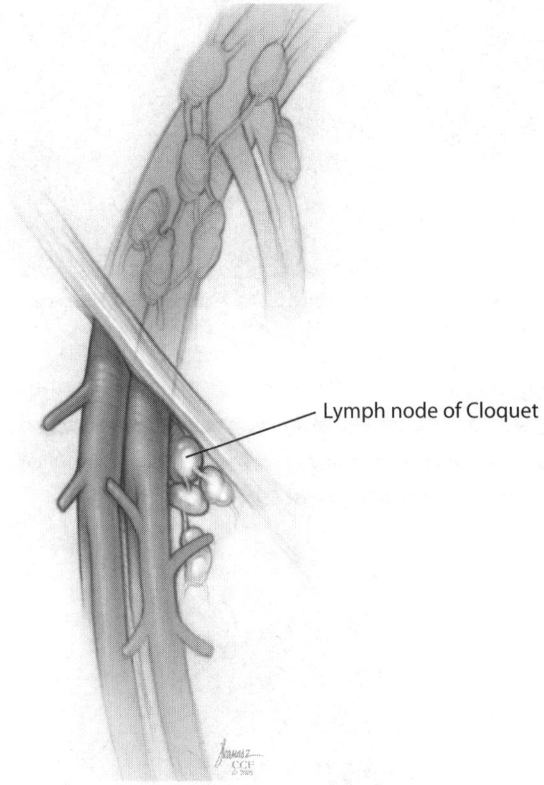

Reprinted with permission of the Cleveland Clinic

Observation

- In the setting of palpably negative groins, observation of the inguinal regions is reasonable for the following tumors due to the low risk of metastatic disease:

  * Tis, Ta

  * T1, grade I or II and no vascular invasion

Antibiotics

- Traditional teaching has been administration of antibiotics for 4-6 weeks in the setting of palpable inguinal lymph nodes as they may be inflammatory and resolve sparing the patient an operation

- This approach is reasonable in patients who are at low risk of having metastatic disease

- However, when lymphadenopathy is marked and metastatic disease is strongly suspected, antibiotics will help decrease the inflammatory component but surgical treatment should not be unduly delayed

Sentinel Node Biopsy (SNB)

- Proposed by Cabanas in 1977

- Impetus for a conservative approach to the inguinal nodes was the significant morbidity associated with inguinofemoral lymphadenectomy

- A finger is inserted through a small incision parallel to the inguinal crease and toward the pubic tubercle, where the lymph node is palpated and excised.

- This technique was ultimately found to result in a significant number of false negative exams and has been abandoned.

- However, recent improvement of the false negative rate of SNB to 18% has been noted with technical modifications including: lymphoscintographic imaging of the sentinel node, lymphatic tracking using injection of blue dye around the primary tumor, inguinal ultrasonography with fine needle aspiration of abnormal nodes, intraoperative palpation of the wound and extended pathologic analysis of the excised specimen

Modified Inguinal Lymphadenectomy

- Key aspects:

  * Shorter skin incision

  * Exclusion of the area lateral to the femoral artery and caudal to the fossa ovalis

  * Preservation of the saphenous vein

  * Elimination of sartorius transposition

- Removal of the superficial nodes within the described area and the deep nodes medial to the femoral vein to the level of the inguinal ligament

Figure 11

Modified inguinal lymphadenectomy

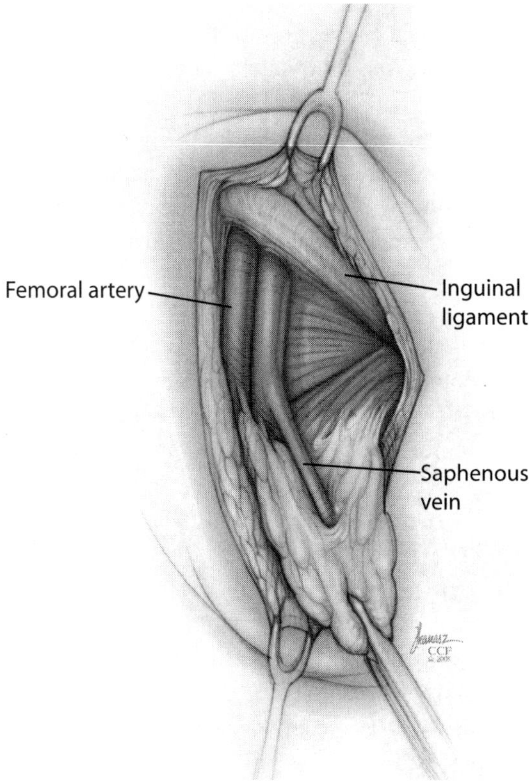

Lymph node packet is medial to the femoral artery and includes superficial and deep inguinal nodes

Reprinted with permission of the Cleveland Clinic

- Indications:

  * Patients with a primary tumor that places them at increased risk for inguinal metastases and clinically negative groins on examination should undergo bilateral modified inguinal lymphadenectomy

    - Stage T2 or greater

    - Stage T1—grade III SCC

    - Vascular invasion

  * Palpably negative groin with metastatic disease involving the contralateral side

- However, if metastatic disease develops in an inguinal region unilaterally at a later date after initial treatment of the primary tumor, contralateral inguinal lymphadenectomy in the absence of palpable disease is not necessary

- During the procedure, if frozen section examination demonstrates metastatic disease, the procedure is converted to a standard extended inguinofemoral lymphadenectomy

- Ipsilateral pelvic nodes are virtually never positive in the lymphadenectomy when the inguinal nodes are negative

- Complications (usually self-limited): seroma (25%), lymphorrhea (10%), wound infection or necrosis (0%-9%), temporary lower extremity edema (20%)

Radical Ilioinguinal Lymphadenectomy

- Indicated in patients with resectable metastatic adenopathy and may be curative when the disease is limited to the inguinal nodes.

- Aggressive lymphadenectomy is associated with potential cure in 30%-60% of cases

- Removal of superficial and deep inguinal lymph nodes within an area outlined:

  * Superiorly by a line drawn from the superior margin of the external inguinal ring to the anterior superior iliac spine (ASIS)

  * Laterally by a line drawn from the ASIS inferiorly for 20 cm

  * Medially by a line drawn from the pubic tubercle for 15 cm

  * Inferiorly by the inferior boundary of the femoral triangle (Figure 12)

Figure 12

Areas for removal of superficial and deep inguinal lymph nodes

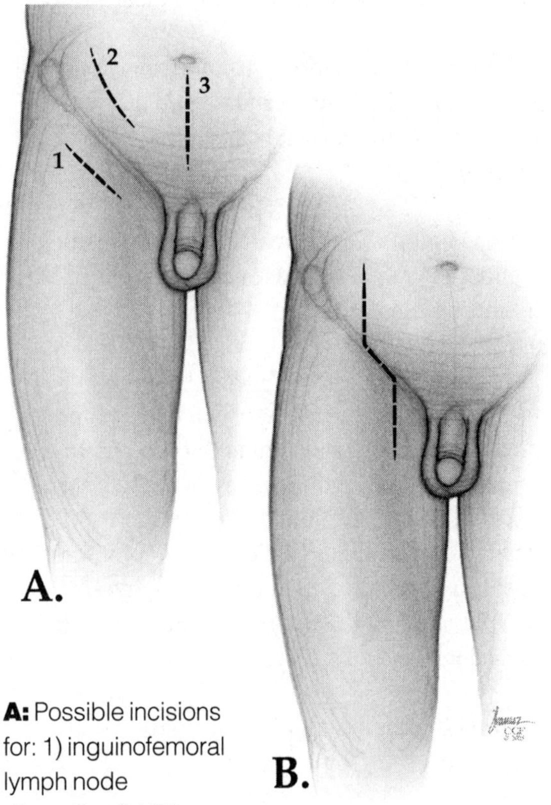

A: Possible incisions for: 1) inguinofemoral lymph node dissection (LND); 2) Unilateral pelvic LND; 3) Bilateral pelvic LND
B: Single incision approach for ilioinguinal LND

Reprinted with permission of the Cleveland Clinic

- Possible incisions (Figures13a-13b)
- Fascia lata is opened longitudinally over the sartorius muscle at the lateral boundary of the dissection
- Care is taken to avoid the femoral nerve located lateral to the femoral artery and below the iliacus fascia
- Saphenous vein is usually ligated and resected with the specimen, but may be preserved in selected cases of low volume metastatic disease
- Detach sartorius muscle from ASIS and rotate to cover exposed femoral vessels (Figures 14a-14b)
- Pelvic lymphadenectomy is generally indicated in the setting of positive ipsilateral inguinal nodes, and should include the distal common iliac, external iliac and obturator nodes
- Contemporary complication rates: Minor 40%-50%; Major (marked lymphedema, flap necrosis, symptomatic lymphocele) 5%-21%

Figures 13a-13b: Dissections for radical inguinofemoral LND

Figure 13a

Initial dissection for radical inguinofemoral LND with exposure of superior border defined by the external oblique fascia

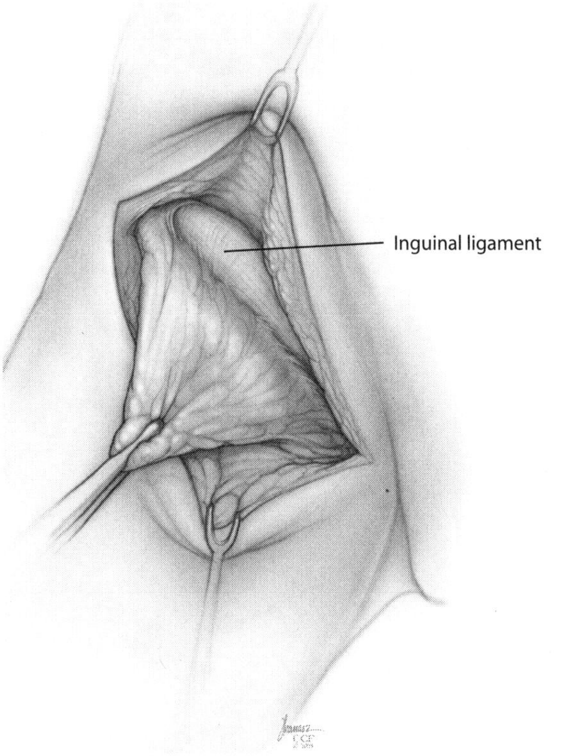

Reprinted with permission of the Cleveland Clinic

Figure 13b

Inferior dissection during radical inguinofemoral LND with removal of lymph node packet from the inferior border of the femoral triangle

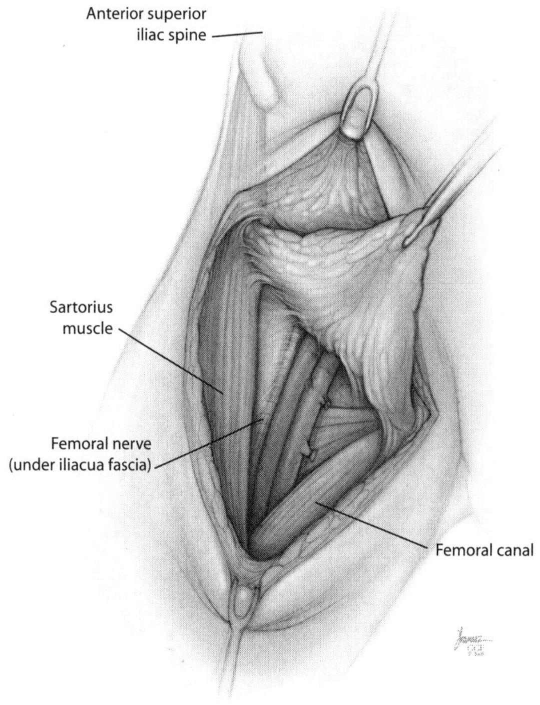

Reprinted with permission of the Cleveland Clinic

- Palliative ilioinguinal lymphadenectomy is reasonable in selected patients with surgically incurable disease to prevent complications of infection, chronic abscess with foul-smelling drainage or life-threatening femoral hemorrhage

Radiation Therapy

- Very little role in treatment of penile SCC
- May be considered for treatment of selected primary tumors:
    * Small, superficial, noninvasive lesions on the glans penis
    * Patients who refuse surgery
- External beam radiotherapy or brachytherapy have been used
- Local control rates are inferior to surgical therapy, and a significant number of patients will require subsequent penectomy
- Complications: urethral fistula, urethral stricture, necrosis, pain, edema
- Radiation therapy to the inguinal areas is not as effective as surgical therapy, and may result in significant complications of skin ulceration or breakdown and lymphedema

Chemotherapy

- Indicated for unresectable locoregional tumor or distant metastatic disease
- Sites of distant metastases: lung, bone, liver
- Most commonly used agents: cisplatin, bleomycin, methotrexate
- Responses to multi-drug regimens are partial and generally of short duration
- In patients with unresectable locoregional disease, chemotherapy may allow subsequent tumor resection in some cases.

Figures 14a-14b: Left saphenous-sparing inguinofemoral LND

Figure 14a

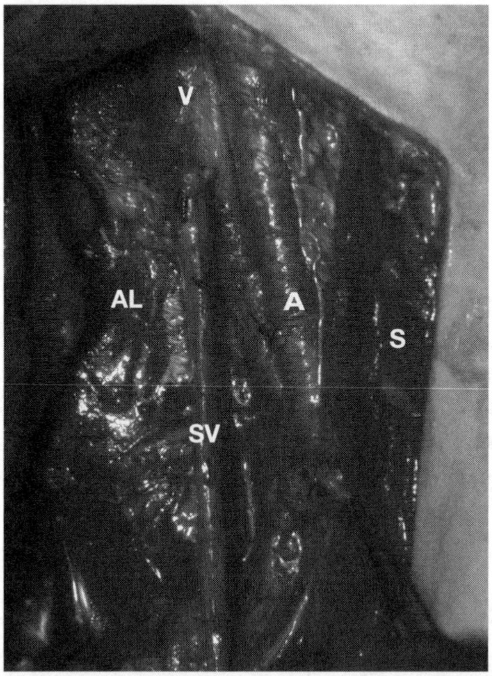

Adductor longus = AL; Femoral vein = V
Femoral artery = A; Sartorius = S; Saphenous vein = SV
Reprinted with permission of the Cleveland Clinic

Figure 14b

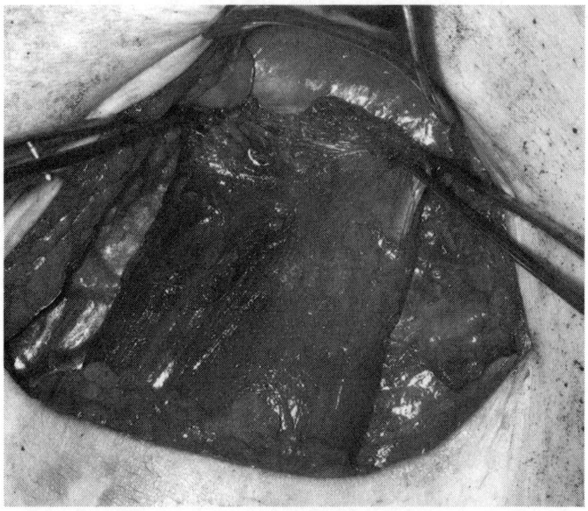

Reprinted with permission of the Cleveland Clinic

4. Uncommon Penile Cancers

Melanoma

- Brown or bluish black papule or ulceration, most typically on the glans penis
- Surgery is treatment of choice

  * Foreskin lesion—circumcision

  * Glans penis—partial penectomy

  * Penile shaft—partial or total penectomy

- Prognosis depends on tumor stage and extent of lymph node metastasis

Sarcomas

- Very rare

Epithelioid Sarcoma
- May mimic Peyronie's disease clinically with corresponding delay in diagnosis

Kaposi's Sarcoma
- Tumor of the reticuloendothelial system
- Raised, painful bluish papule or ulcer
- Often associated with human herpesvirus 8 and AIDS

Others
- Angiosarcoma, leiomyosarcoma, malignant fibrous histiocytoma, osteosarcoma,

Treatment
- Aggressive local tumor excision with partial or total penectomy if needed
- Wide surgical margins are necessary as local recurrences are typical of sarcomas
- Withdrawal of immunosuppression or radiotherapy may be effective in some cases of Kaposi's sarcoma

Metastatic Disease

- Most commonly from cancer of the bladder, prostate or rectum
- Most frequently presents as priapism (Figures 15a-15b)
- Tumor usually infiltrates one or both corpora cavernosa; mass lesions may occur but are less common
- Associated with advanced disease, and subsequent survival is often limited

Figure 15a

Priapism related to corporal infiltration by hormone refractory prostate cancer

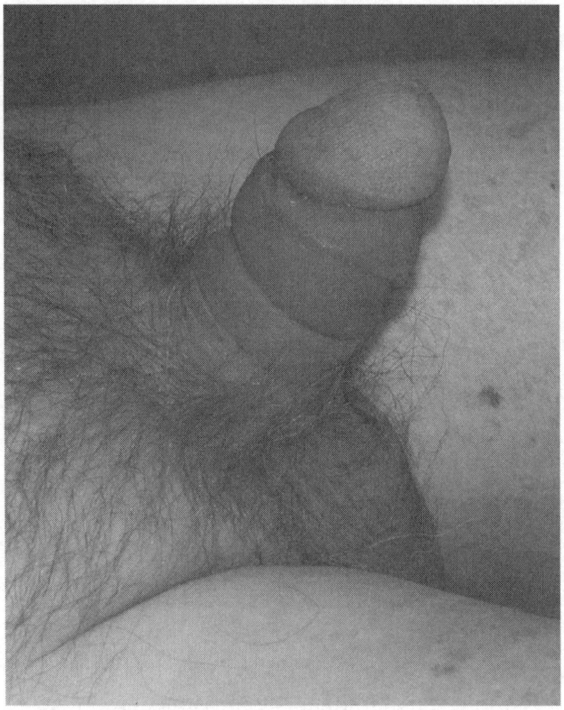

Reprinted with permission of the Cleveland Clinic

Figure 15b

Resolution of priapism following external beam radiotherapy

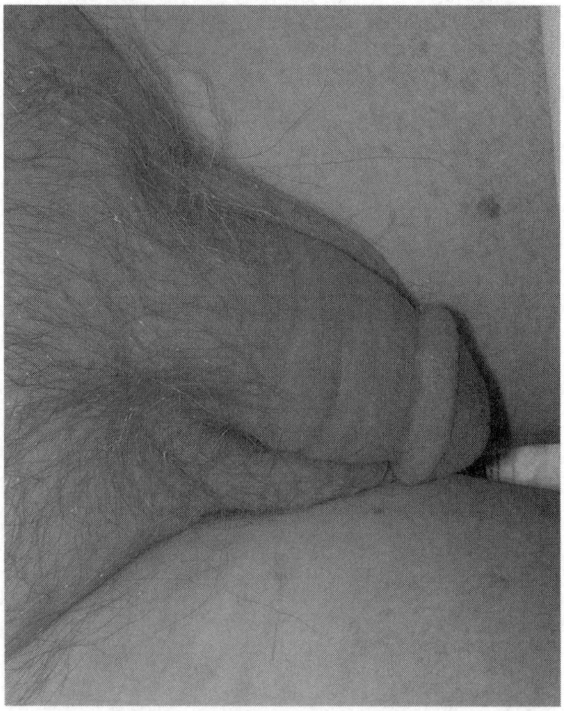

Reprinted with permission of the Cleveland Clinic

5. Male Urethral Cancer

General

- Rare and usually presents in the 5th decade of life
- Etiologic factors:
  * Chronic inflammation due to urethral stricture, urethritis, sexually transmitted disease
  * Probably HPV-16
- Onset is usually insidious and a high index of suspicion is needed
- Presenting symptoms:
  * Urethral bleeding
  * Palpable mass
  * Obstructive voiding symptoms (Figure 16)

Figure 16

Cystoscopic view of SCC of the bulbous urethra

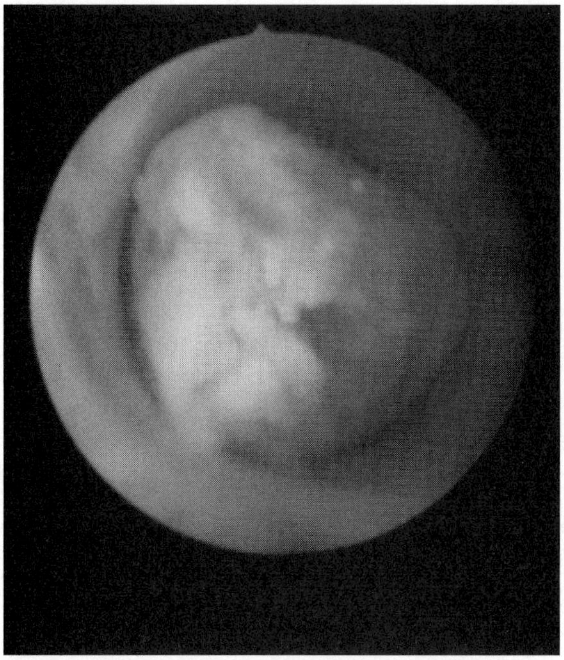

Reprinted with permission of the Cleveland Clinic

Anatomy and Pathology

- Tumor location:
  * Bulbomembranous urethra (posterior urethra): 60%
  * Penile urethra (anterior urethra): 30%
  * Prostatic urethra: 10%
- Tumor pathology:
  * Bulbomembranous urethra:
SCC—80%;
transitional cell carcinoma (TCC)—10%;
adenocarcinoma —10%
  * Penile urethra—SCC 90%; TCC 10%
  * Prostatic urethra—TCC 90%; SCC 10%
- Spread is by direct extension to adjacent structures including corpus spongiosum and periurethral tissues
- Lymphatic spread:
  * Anterior urethra—superficial and deep inguinal nodes
  * Posterior urethra—pelvic nodes
- Palpable inguinal nodes occur in 20% of patients and always represent metastatic disease

Evaluation and Staging

- Cystoscopy with biopsy
- Bimanual examination under anesthesia
- Urine cytology is not very reliable for diagnosis of primary urethral carcinoma, with sensitivity being greatest in men with TCC
- CT scan to evaluate for metastatic disease
- MRI is helpful in detecting invasion of the corpora cavernosa (Figure 17)

Figure 17

MRI of patient with a locally extensive SCC of the bulbous urethra

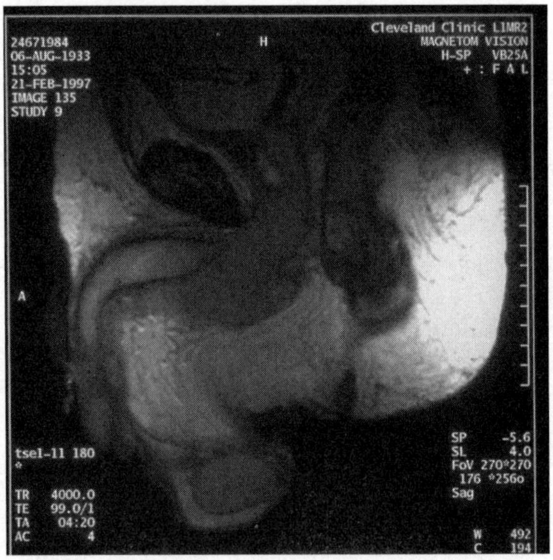

Reprinted with permission of the Cleveland Clinic

TNM Staging System for Urethral Cancer

Primary Tumor (T)

Tx	Primary tumor cannot be assessed
T0	No evidence of primary tumor
Ta	Noninvasive papillary, polypoid or verrucous carcinoma
Tis	Carcinoma *in situ*
T1	Tumor invades subepithelial connective tissue
T2	Tumor invades corpus spongiosum, prostate, or periurethral muscle
T3	Tumor invades corpus cavernosum, beyond prostate capsule, anterior vagina, bladder neck
T4	Tumor invades other adjacent organs

Regional Lymph Nodes (N)

Nx	Regional lymph nodes cannot be assessed
N0	No regional lymph node metastasis
N1	Metastasis in a single lymph node, 2 cm or less in size
N2	Metastasis in a single lymph node 2-5 cm in size or multiple nodes with none > 5 cm
N3	Metastasis in a lymph node > 5 cm

Distant Metastasis (M)

MX	Presence of distant metastasis cannot be assessed
M0	No distant metastasis
M1	Distant metastasis

Surgical Treatment

- Anterior urethral cancer is more amenable to surgical control and the prognosis is better when compared to posterior urethral cancer

Penile Urethra

- Superficial, low grade tumors: transurethral resection, local excision, distal urethrectomy

- Infiltrating tumors (Figure 18)

  * Distal half of the penis: partial penectomy

- Ilioinguinal lymphadenectomy is indicated in the presence of palpable inguinal adenopathy in the absence of pelvic or distant metastatic disease

- As opposed to penile cancer, prophylactic or early inguinal lymphadenectomy in the absence of palpable adenopathy has not been shown to be of benefit

Bulbomembranous Urethra

- Poor survival figures have been reported for all forms of treatment, but it appears that radical excision offers the best chance for local and long-term disease control

- Early, small lesions have been successfully treated with transurethral resection or segmental urethral excision, but tumors appropriate for this are very rare.

- Standard surgical treatment for invasive posterior urethral cancer is total penectomy with cystoprostatectomy, and may include resection of the inferior aspect of the pubic rami (Figure 19)

- Proximal penile shaft: total penectomy

- Large pelvic floor defects may require a rectus abdominis muscle flap or myocutaneous flap for closure

Radiotherapy and Chemotherapy

- Radiation as monotherapy is generally reserved for patients with early-stage lesions of the anterior urethra who refuse surgery

- Combination of radiation and chemotherapy has shown some success in a small number of patients with localized and metastatic urethral cancer

- Patients with advanced stage or metastatic disease are most commonly treated with a multimodal approach

Urethral Cancer Recurrence After Cystoprostatectomy

- Approximately 40% of urethral recurrences are diagnosed within 1 year after cystoprostatectomy with a median time to diagnosis of 18 months

- Cutaneous diversion

  * Incidence of urethral recurrence: 2.1%-11.1%

  * Prostatic stromal invasion by TCC increases risk of urethral recurrence

  * Post-cystectomy monitoring: Urethral wash cytology

  * Symptoms: urethral bleeding, discharge or mass

  * CT and/or MRI may be needed to assess for metastatic disease or local tumor extension

  * Treatment: Total urethrectomy including the urethral meatus (Figures 20a-20d)

- Orthotopic diversion

  * Incidence of urethral recurrence: 0.5%-4%

  * Negative frozen section of distal prostatic urethral margin at the time of cystoprostatectomy results in low incidence of recurrence

Figure 18

Penile mass due to TCC of the penile urethra following previous cystoprostatectomy for TCC of the bladder

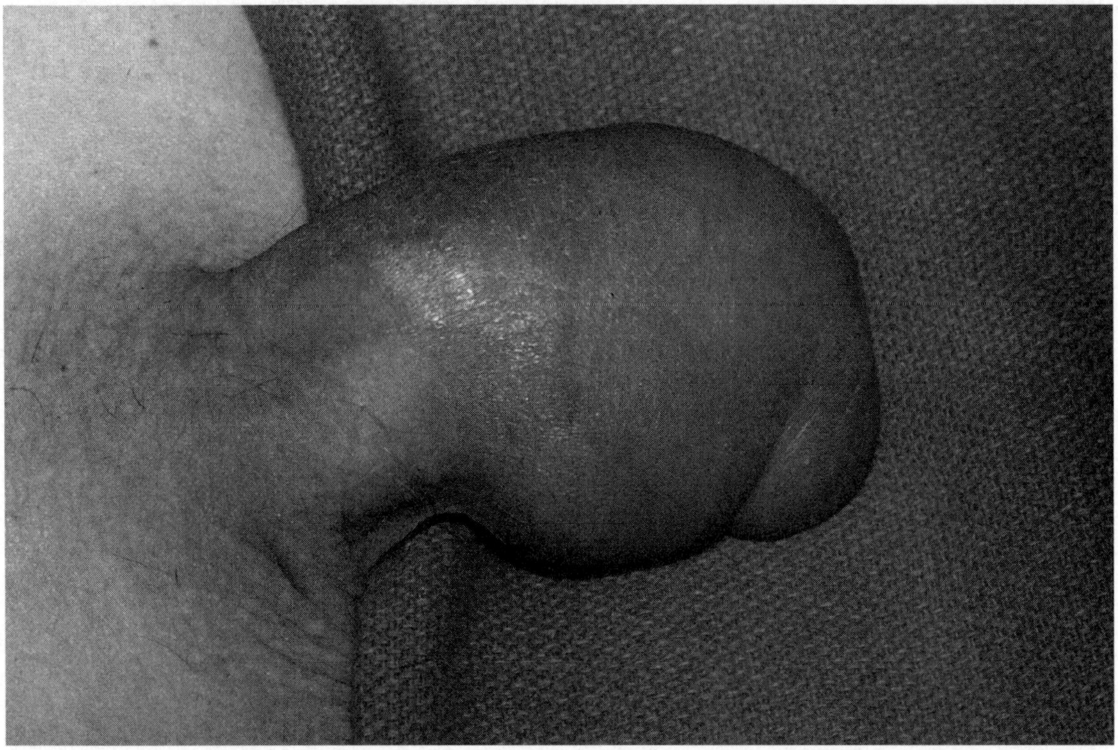

Reprinted with permission of the Cleveland Clinic

Figure 19

Surgical specimen from total penectomy, urethrectomy, cystoprostatectomy and inferior pubectomy for a large bulbous urethral SCC

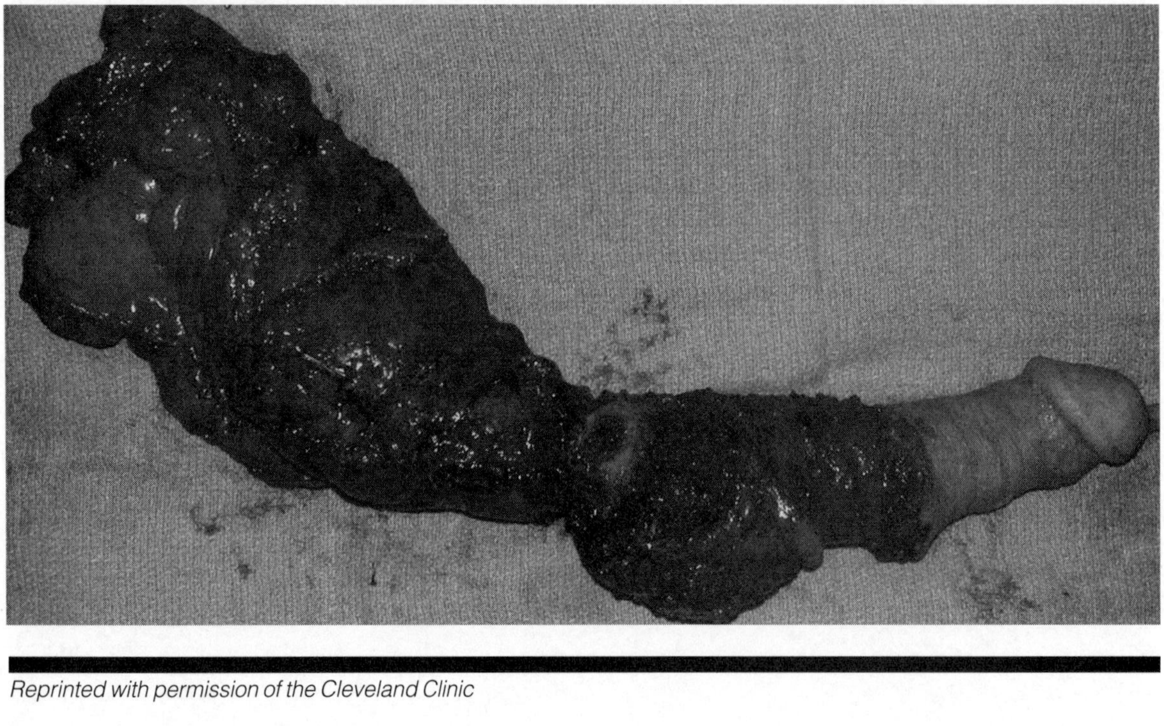

Reprinted with permission of the Cleveland Clinic

Figures 20a-20d: Secondary urethrectomy following previous cystoprostatectomy

Figure 20a

Perineal incision

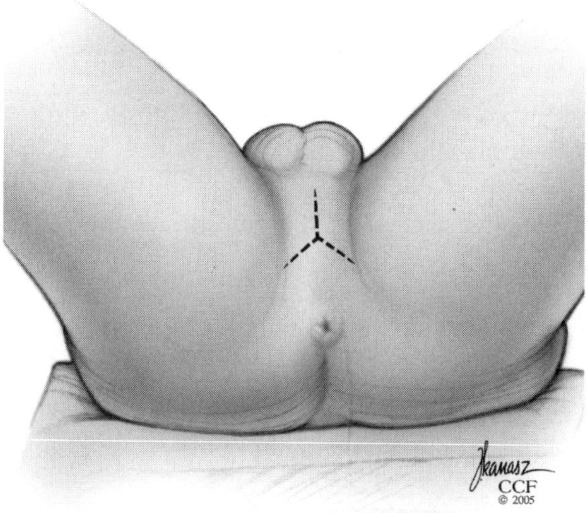

Reprinted with permission of the Cleveland Clinic

Figure 20b

Division of bulbospongiosus muscle to expose the bulb of the corpus spongiosum, and initial dissection of the urethra off the corporal bodies

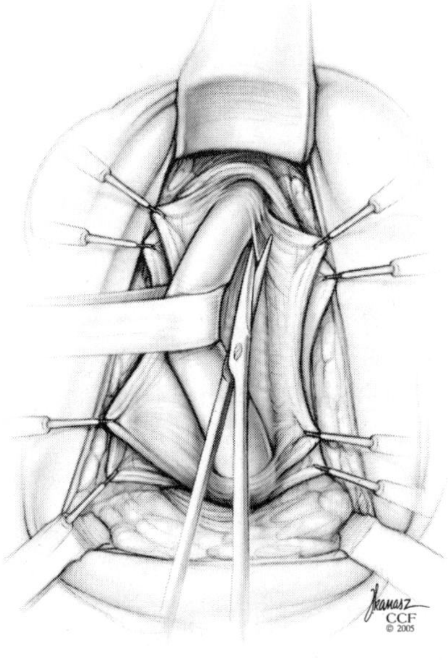

Reprinted with permission of the Cleveland Clinic

Figure 20c

Distal urethral dissection which then connects to the proximal dissection at the level of the distal shaft

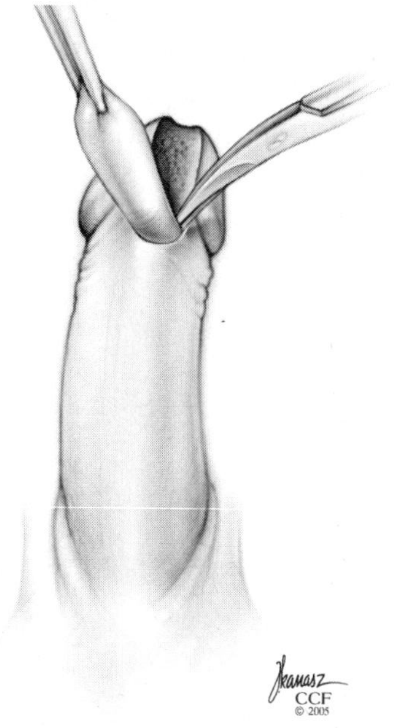

Reprinted with permission of the Cleveland Clinic

Figure 20d

Sagittal view demonstrating posterior bulb dissection and location of the bulbar arteries

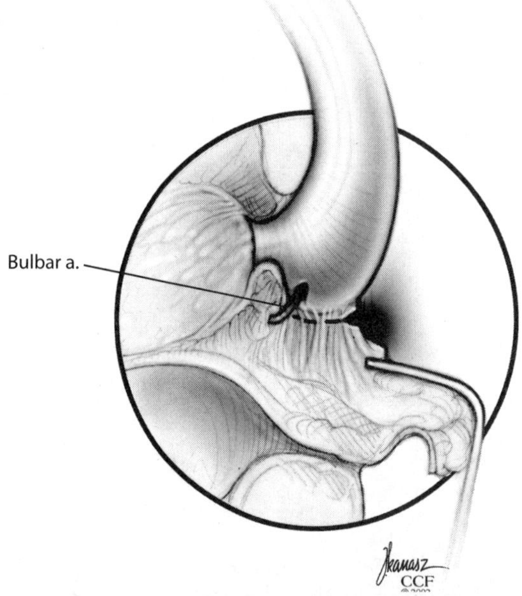

Reprinted with permission of the Cleveland Clinic

* Post-cystectomy monitoring: Voided urine cytology

* Symptoms: hematuria, urethral discharge or mass

* Treatment: Total urethrectomy with excision of a cuff of pouch adjacent to the anastomosis and cutaneous diversion often using a portion of the existing neobladder

6. Female Urethral Cancer

General

- Urethral cancer is the only urologic malignant neoplasm that is more common in women than men

- Rare: 0.02% of all female cancers

- Most commonly diagnosed in the fifth and sixth decades of life

- Etiology: leukoplakia, chronic irritation, caruncles, polyps, HPV

- 5% arise within a diverticulum

- Symptoms: obstructive voiding, dysuria, urinary frequency, urethral bleeding or mass

Anatomy and Pathology

- Divisions of female urethra

    * Anterior—Distal third

    * Posterior—Proximal two-thirds

- The distal third of the urethra may be excised without compromising continence

- Lymphatic drainage

    * Anterior urethra—superficial and deep inguinal nodes

    * Posterior urethra—iliac and obturator nodes

- Pathology

    * SCC 50%-70%

    * Adenocarcinoma 25% (increased incidence within urethral diverticula)

    * TCC 10%

- Evaluation
  * Cystoscopy with biopsy
  * Bimanual examination under anesthesia
  * CT to evaluate for metastatic disease
  * MRI is best test for imaging local urethral anatomy and tumor extent

Treatment

- Most studies have not detected any significant differences in survival based on histologic tumor subtype

- Distal urethral carcinoma tends to be low stage and is associated with improved survival compared to proximal tumors

- Most significant prognostic factor for local control and survival is the anatomic location and extent of the primary tumor

Distal Tumors

Surgery

- Circumferential distal urethrectomy (70%-90% cure rate)

- Complications: meatal stenosis, incontinence

* Ilioinguinal lymphadenectomy only when palpable disease and no distant metastases

Radiotherapy

- May use external beam, brachytherapy or combination of both

- 5-year survival rates equivalent to surgery in some series

- Complications: incontinence, stricture, fistula, infection

Proximal Tumors

More likely to be high stage and invade the bladder and vagina

Surgery

- Anterior exenteration with wide vaginal excision and pelvic lymphadenectomy

- Suboptimal cure rates with surgery alone have led to recommendations for multimodality therapy in most cases

Multimodality Therapy

- Radiotherapy + chemotherapy (5-FU and mitomycin C for SCC; MVAC for TCC)

- Radiotherapy + anterior exenteration

7. Further Reading

1. Agrawal A, Pai D, Ananthakrishnan N, et al. The histological extent of the local spread of carcinoma of the penis and its therapeutic implications. *BJU Int*. 2000;85:299-301.

2. Bandieramonte G, Lepera P, Marchesini R, et al. Laser microsurgery for superficial lesions of the penis. *J Urol*. 1987;138:315-319.

3. Bevan-Thomas R, Slaton JW, Pettaway CA. Contemporary morbidity from lymphadenectomy for penile squamous cell carcinoma: The M.D. Anderson cancer center experience. *J Urol*. 2002;167:1638-1642.

4. Bissada NK, Yakout HH, Fahmy WE, et al. Multi-institutional long-term experience with conservative surgery for invasive penile carcinoma. *J Urol*. 2003;169:500-502.

5. Clark PE, Stein JP, Groshen SG, et al. The management of urethral transitional cell carcinoma after radical cystectomy for invasive bladder cancer. *J Urol*. 2004;172:1342-1347.

6. Coblentz TR, Theodorescu D. Morbidity of modified prophylactic inguinal lymphadenectomy for squamous cell carcinoma of the penis. *J Urol*. 2002;168:1386-1389.

7. Colberg JW, Andriole GL, Catalona WJ. Long-term follow-up of men undergoing modified inguinal lymphadenectomy for carcinoma of the penis. *Br J Urol*. 1997;79:54-57.

8. Culkin DJ, Beer TM. Advanced penile carcinoma. *J Urol*. 2003; 170:359-365.

9. Dalbagni G, Zhang ZF, Lacombe L, et al. Male urethral carcinoma: Analysis of treatment outcome. *Urology*. 1999;53:1126-1132.

10. Dalbagni G, Donat SM, Eschwege P, et al. Results of high dose rate brachytherapy, anterior pelvic exenteration and external beam radiotherapy for carcinoma of the female urethra. *J Urol*. 2001;166:1759-1761.

11. Dimarco DS, Dimarco CS, Zincke H, et al. Surgical treatment for local control of female urethral carcinoma. *Urol Oncol*. 2004;22: 404-409.

12. Fleming ID, Cooper JS, Henson, DE, et al. Penis. *AJCC Cancer Staging Manual*. American Joint Committee on Cancer. 5th ed. Philadelphia, PA: Lippincott-Raven, 1997: 215-217.

13. Forman JD, Lichter AS. The role of radiation therapy in the management of carcinoma of the male and female urethra. *Urol Clin North Am*. 1992;19:383-389.

14. Haas, GP, Blumenstein, BA, Gagliano RG, et al. Cisplatin, methotrexate, and bleomycin for the treatment of carcinoma of the penis: A Southwest Oncology Group Study. *J Urol*. 1999;161:1823-1825.

15. Hardeman S, Soloway MS. Urethral recurrence following radical cystectomy. *J Urol*. 1990;144:666-669.

16. Hoffman MA, Renshaw AA, Loughlin KR. Squamous cell carcinoma of the penis and microscopic pathologic margins. How much margin is needed for local cure? *Cancer*. 1999;85:1565-1568.

17. Horenblas S, van Tinteren H, Delemarre JFM, et al. Squamous cell carcinoma of the penis. II. Treatment of the primary tumor. *J Urol*. 1992;147:1533-1538.

18. Horenblas S, Jansen L, Meinhardt W, et al. Detection of occult metastasis in squamous cell carcinoma of the penis using a dynamic sentinel node procedure. *J Urol*. 2000;163:100-104.

19. Licht MR, Klein EA, Bukowski R, et al. Combination radiation and chemotherapy for the treatment of squamous cell carcinoma of the male and female urethra. *J Urol*. 1995;153:1918-1920.

20. Malloy TR, Wein AJ, Carpiniello VL. Carcinoma of penis treated with neodymium YAG laser. *Urology*. 1988;31:26-29.

21. McDougal WS, Kirchner FK, Edwards RH, et al. Treatment of carcinoma of the penis: The case for primary lymphadenectomy. *J Urol*. 1986;136:38-41.

22. McDougal WS. Carcinoma of the penis: Improved survival by early regional lymphadenectomy based on the histological grade and depth of invasion of the primary lesion. *J Urol*. 1995; 154:1364-1366.

23. Mohs FE, Snow SN, Larson PO. Mohs micrographic surgery for penile tumors. *Urol Clin N Amer*. 1992;19:291-304.

24. Oberfield RA, Zinman LN, Leibenhaut M, et al. Management of invasive squamous cell carcinoma of the bulbomembranous male urethra with co-ordinated chemo-radiotherapy and genital preservation. *Br J Urol*. 1996;78:573-578.

25. Parra RO. Accurate staging of carcinoma of the penis in men with nonpalpable inguinal lymph nodes by modified inguinal lymphadenectomy. *J Urol*. 1996;155:560-563.

26. Pietrzak P, Corbishley C, Watkin N. Organ-sparing surgery for invasive penile cancer: Early follow-up data. *BJU Int*. 2004;94: 1253-1257.

27. Slaton JW, Morgenstern, N, Levy DA, et al. Tumor stage, vascular invasion and the percentage of poorly differentiated cancer: Independent prognosticators for inguinal lymph node metastasis in penile squamous cancer. *J Urol*. 2001;165:1138-1142.

28. Ubrig B, Waldner M, Fallahi M, et al. Preputial flap for primary closure after excision of tumors on the glans penis. *Urology*. 2001;58:274-276.

29. Zeidman EJ, Desmond P, Thompson I. Surgical treatment of carcinoma of the male urethra. *Urol Clin N Amer*. 1992;19:359-372.

8. Questions

Penile Urethral Cancer

1. Where do penile cancers most commonly arise?

   A. Shaft

   B. Prepuce

   C. Frenulum

   D. Glans

   E. None of the above

2. Which of the following is not a risk factor for invasive SCC?

   A. Phimosis

   B. Number of sexual partners

   C. Smoking

   D. Poor hygiene

   E. Alcohol intake

3. What is the most important prognostic factor for survival in patients with penile cancer?

   A. Primary tumor stage

   B. Extent of lymph node metastasis

   C. Presence of vascular invasion

   D. Primary tumor grade

   E. Medical comorbidities

4. The following statements pertaining to conservative surgical excision for penile carcinoma are true, except for which one?

   A. Glansectomy and circumcision remove the entire contents of the preputial cavity

   B. Large defects after glans tumor excision may be covered with a flap of outer preputial skin

   C. Frozen section biopsies are usually not needed during these procedures

   D. Careful postoperative long-term surveillance is necessary

   E. Circumcision alone may be sufficient to treat certain preputial tumors

5. Which of the following statements about partial penectomy is most accurate?

   A. It provides for normal sexual function in over 70% of men

   B. It is performed less often than total penectomy

   C. Postoperative voiding is through a perineal urethrostomy

   D. It results in local recurrence rates of less than 10%

   E. It requires division of the penis at least 3 cm proximal to the tumor

6. Which of the following statements regarding the progression of penile cancer is true?

A. Metastasis initially involves the superficial inguinal nodes

B. Metastatic spread from the primary tumor is usually unilateral

C. Metastasis initially is hematogenous to the lung, liver or bone

D. Metastasis initially involves the deep inguinal nodes

E. Crossover from the inguinal nodes to the contralateral pelvic nodes is common

7. Observation of the inguinal regions is reasonable when there is no palpable adenopathy and the primary tumor demonstrates all of the following, except?

A. Tis

B. T1, grade II

C. Vascular invasion

D. Ta

E. T1, grade I

8. All of the following statements pertaining to modified inguinal lymphadenectomy are true, except for:

A. The saphenous vein is preserved

B. It is indicated for management of palpable inguinal lymphadenopathy

C. The dissection excludes regions lateral to the femoral artery

D. The thigh incision is shorter than that used for standard ilioinguinal lymphadenectomy

E. Both superficial and deep inguinal nodes are included in the surgical specimen

9. Which of the following statements regarding ilioinguinal lymphadenectomy is true?

A. Rotation of the gracilis muscle is performed to cover the femoral vessels

B. It is done only for palliation

C. Complications are few and minor in nature

D. The saphenous vein may be preserved in the setting of low volume metastatic disease

E. Pelvic node dissection is necessary even if the unilateral inguinal nodes are negative

10. What is the most frequent site of urethral cancer in the male?

A. Fossa navicularis

B. Prostatic urethra

C. Pendulous urethra

D. Penoscrotal urethra

E. Bulbomembranous urethra

11. Which of the following statements concerning distal urethral cancer in the male is true?

A. Most common histologic type is transitional cell carcinoma

B. Penectomy is usually indicated for tumors infiltrating the corpus spongiosum

C. Prognosis is worse than for bulbomembranous urethral cancer

D. In the absence of palpable inguinal nodes, early inguinal lymphadenectomy is indicated

E. Conservative surgical therapy is never effective

12. What is the most common histologic type of proximal urethral cancer in women?

A. Squamous cell carcinoma

B. Transitional cell carcinoma

C. Adenocarcinoma

D. Melanoma

E. Sarcoma

13. What is the most significant prognostic factor for local control and survival in female urethral cancer?

A. Age at presentation

B. Histologic type

C. Anatomic location and extent of primary tumor

D. Hematuria

E. Presence of urethral diverticulum

Answers

1. D.
Penile cancers occur most commonly on the glans penis (48%) followed by the prepuce (21%).

2. E.
There is no evidence linking penile cancer to alcohol intake.

3. B.
The presence and extent of inguinal lymph node metastasis are the most important prognostic factors for survival in patients with SCC penis.

4. C.
Frozen section biopsies are often a critical component of conservative surgery for penile cancer to help ensure complete tumor excision.

5. D.
Partial penectomy results in a local recurrence rate of 0%-8%. It provides for adequate sexual function in a low percentage of men, is performed more commonly than total penectomy, does not result in a perineal urethrostomy and traditionally is done with a 2 cm tumor margin.

6. A.
Metastasis initially occurs to the superficial inguinal nodes, and this may be unilateral or bilateral. Progression is subsequently to the deep inguinal nodes and then the pelvic nodes. Distant metastasis occurs late. Pelvic nodes will not be positive if the ipsilateral inguinal nodes are negative.

7. C.
Vascular invasion in the primary tumor is an indication for modified inguinal lymphadenectomy in the setting of clinically negative groins.

8. B.
In the setting of palpable adenopathy, more extensive complete ilioinguinal lymphadenectomy is indicated.

9. D.
In the setting of low volume metastatic disease, the saphenous vein may be preserved in order to try to decrease the risk of postoperative complications. The sartorius muscle is used to cover the femoral vessels, and the procedure may carry a chance of cure in 30%-60% of cases when pelvic nodes are not involved.

10. E.
In males, urethral cancer occurs most commonly in the bulbomembranous urethra (60%), followed by the penile urethra (30%) and prostatic urethra (10%).

11. B.

Penectomy is indicated for tumors infiltrating the corpus spongiosum. The most common histologic type is SCC and the prognosis is better than that for bulbomembranous cancers. Early or prophylactic has not been shown to be advantageous in urethral cancer. Some cases of early or superficial distal urethral cancer may be managed effectively with conservative surgical therapy.

12. A.

SCC is the most common histologic type of proximal urethral cancer in women.

13. C.

The most significant prognostic factor for local control and survival in women with urethral cancer is the location and extent of the primary tumor.

Chapter 20: Testicular Cancer

Jose J. Correa, MD
Wade J. Sexton, MD

Contents

1. Histologic Classification

Management recommendations for the patient with a newly diagnosed testicular cancer are principally dependent upon an accurate histologic description of the primary tumor. Radiographic staging studies and serum tumor markers further define the options available to the patient and provide an initial glimpse of a patient's long-term prognosis.

Table 1 demonstrates the classification of germ cell and non-germ cell tumors. Germ cell tumors account for 90% - 95% of all testicular tumors and are composed of five basic cell types: **seminoma, embryonal cell carcinoma, yolk sac tumor, choriocarcinoma and teratoma.** A broad classification is recognized between seminomas and nonseminomas and is important for determining the management of locoregional disease and distant metastases. Over half of all primary tumors consist of more than one cell-type and are known as mixed germ cell tumors. Germ cells tumors arise from plurpotential cells, which explain the different germ cell elements in the primary tumor or its metastatic sites. Adequate tissue sampling and appropriate use of tumor markers establishes the diagnosis with near certainty.

Non-germ cell tumors account for 5%-10% of testicular tumors and broadly include the sex cord-gonadal stromal tumors (ie, leydig cell and sertoli cell tumors), lymphoid and hematopoietic tumors, and metastatic tumors from other primary neoplasms.

Seminoma

Classic Seminoma

Seminomas comprise the **most common type of germ cell tumor (approximately 45%)** and the most common histology found in men over the age of 35. The classic seminoma accounts for 80%-85% of seminomatous germ cell tumors. The **testicle is usually enlarged** and when cut has a bulging homogeneous gray-white appearance. Microscopically, there are relatively large cells with clear cytoplasm arranged in uniform sheets, lobules, or columns. The supporting stroma shows varying amounts of lymphocytic infiltrate or granulomatous reaction, which is thought to represent a host response to the tumor. There are occasional mitoses and little variation in the nuclear arrangement. Syncytiotrophoblastic elements occur in 20%-25% of seminomas and account for the bHCG (beta-human chorionic gonadotropin) production by some of the tumors.

Seminoma With High Mitotic Index

Originally classified as an anaplastic seminoma, now this seminoma variant is referred to as a seminoma with a high mitotic index. Stage for stage, this tumor has the same prognosis as a classic seminoma, although there are several features that suggest a more aggressive and more lethal behavior. These variants show increased mitotic activity averaging 3 mitoses per high power fields, more cellular atypia and more nuclear pleomorphism. The tumors have a higher rate of local invasion, an increased rate of metastatic spread, and a higher rate of bHCG production. Morphologically, these tumors closely resemble embryonal cell carcinoma and account for 5%-10% of all seminomas.

Spermatocytic Seminoma

Spermatocytic seminomas account for less than 5% of all seminomas. They occur most commonly in men over the age of 40 years and approximately 5% of patients have bilateral disease. Unlike other germ cell tumors that can involve the ovary, retroperitoneum, or mediastinum, spermatocytic seminomas only involve the testicle. Grossly, the tumors are large with a yellowish, soft, mucoid appearance to the cut surface. The cells vary in size and have deeply pigmented cytoplasm and closely resemble different phases of maturing spermatogonia. The nuclei of most cells have a characteristic filamentous chromatin distribution. Once the diagnosis is confirmed following radical orchiectomy, no further treatment is warranted as these tumors behave in a benign manner. Only rarely are spermatocytic seminomas associated with sarcomas. The sarcomas are typically undifferentiated, although on occasion there may be differentiated forms such as rhabdomyosarcoma. The sarcoma elements metastasize extensively.

Table 1

Testicular Tumors

Germ Cell Tumors

- **Precursor Lesion: Intratubular germ cell neoplasia (carcinoma *in situ*)**
- **Tumors of one histologic type**

Seminoma

- Seminoma
  - o Variant: seminoma with syncytiotrophoblastic cells
- Spermatocytic seminoma
  - o Variant spermatocytic

Nonseminoma

- Embryonal Carcinoma
- Yolk Sac Tumor
- Trophoblastic tumors
  - o Choriocarcinoma
  - o Trophoblastic neoplasms other than carcinoma
  - o Monophasic choriocarcinoma
  - o Placental site trophoblastic tumor
- Teratoma
  - o Dermoid Cyst
  - o Monodermal teratoma
  - o Teratoma with somatic type malignancies

- **Tumors of more than one histologic type (mixed forms)**
- Mixed embryonal carcinoma and teratoma (Teratocarcinoma)
- Mixed teratoma and seminoma
- Choriocarcinoma and teratoma/embryonal carcinoma
- Others

Miscellaneous tumors of the testis

- Carcinoid tumor
- Tumors of ovarian epithelial type
- Nephroblastoma
- Paraganglioma

Lymphoid and hematopoietic tumors

- Lymphoma
- Plasmacytoma
- Leukemia

continued

Table 1 (continued)

Sex Cord/ Gonadal-Stromal Tumors

- **Pure forms**
  - Leydig cell tumor
  - Malignant Leydig cell tumor
  - Sertoli cell tumor
    - o Sertoli cell tumor lipid rich variant
    - o Sclerosing sertoli cell tumor
    - o Large cell-calcifying sertoli cell tumor
  - Malignant Sertoli cell tumor
  - Granulosa cell tumor
    - o Adult type granulosa cell tumor
    - o Juvenile type granulosa cell tumor

- **Tumors of the thecoma/fibroma group**
  - Thecoma
  - Fibroma

- **Sex cord/gonadal-stromal tumor incompletely differentiated**
- **Sex cord/gonadal-stromal tumor, mixed forms**
- **Malignant sex cord/gonadal-stromal tumor**
- **Tumors containg both germ cell and sex cord/gonadal- stromal elements**
  - Gonadoblastoma
- **Germ cell sex cord/gonadal-stromal tumor, unclassified**

Tumor of the collecting duct and rafe
- Adenoma
- Carcinoma

Secondary tumor
(Metastases)

Adapted from: Eble J.N., *Sauter G, Epstein* J.I., *Sesterhenn* I.A, eds. World Health Organization classification of tumors. Pathology and genetics of tumors of the urinary system and male genital organs. Lyon, MA: *IARC Press; 2004.*

Nonseminomas

Embryonal Carcinoma

Pure embryonal cell carcinoma comprises only 3%- 4% of germ cell tumors but embryonal cells are present in variable amounts in up to 40% of tumors with mixed histologic types. Embryonal histologies are most common during the third decade of life and are less common in adolescent males between 15-20 years. These germ cell elements have not been described in pre-pubertal testes. **Pure embryonal cell carcinomas** may be associated with **elevated levels of serum AFP. Syncytiotrophoblastic cells** are scattered throughout the tumor and are responsible for **bHCG elevation** in patients with embryonal histologies. Grossly, the tumors are typically smaller with a poorly defined capsule. The cut surface appears grayish-white with areas of hemorrhage and necrosis. Microscopically, there are malignant appearing epithelioid cells arranged in glands or tubules. Cell borders are indistinct and there is frequent nuclear overlap. The cytoplasm is pale, eosinophilic, or vacuolated, and the nuclei have a see-through appearance with prominent nucleoli and numerous mitoses. Lymphovascular invasion and involvement of epididymal and paratesticular structures are common. These findings are of prognostic importance.

Yolk Sac Tumor

The yolk sac tumor is the **predominant tumor in infants and children.** In adults, pure yolk sac tumors account for a very small percentage of testicular neoplasms (2%). Yolk sac elements are present in up to 40% of mixed germ cell testicular neoplasms and are responsible for the **production of AFP.** Grossly, the tumor appears soft, homogeneous, grey-yellow and greasy. It is poorly encapsulated. Microscopically, there are at least 10 different patterns of yolk sac elements, which can make it difficult to distinguish particularly in mixed patterns. Epithelioid cells form glandular or ductal structures and are arranged in columns, papillary projections or solid islands. The individual cells are small and range from cuboidal and columnar to flat. The cells have poorly defined borders and a vacuolated cytoplasm containing glycogen and fat. The nuclei are of variable sizes and there are frequent mitoses. The endodermal sinus pattern is characterized by **Schiller-Duval bodies**—papillary structures with a central fibrovascualr core covered by a layer of cuboidal tumor cells.

Choriocarcinoma

Pure choriocarcinomas account for less than 1% of germ cell neoplasms. Clinically, the primary tumors are often very small and may not be palpable. The actual size of the tumor depends on the extent of local hemorrhage. Patients typically present with symptoms due to extensive metastatic disease. Traditionally, there are two distinct cell types that must be present to satisfy the definition of a choriocarcinoma—**syncytiotrophoblasts** and **cytotrophoblasts**. However, monophasic choriocarcinomas consisting of only cytotrophoblastic or intermediate trophoblastic cells have been reported. The syncytiotrophoblasts produce bHCG and the cells may be large, multinucleated or mononuclear. There is abundant and often vacuolated, eosinophilic cytoplasm, and the nuclei are large and hyperchromatic. The cytotrophoblasts have pale staining cytoplasm and distinct cell borders. Cytotrophoblast nuclei have 1 or 2 nucleoli.

Teratoma

Teratomas constitute approximately 35% of germ cell tumors in infants and children. In adults, teratomas are found in only 2%-7% of testis tumors in pure form, but 45%-50% of mixed germ cell tumors contain teratoma. Most always, these tumors contain more than one germ cell layer in different stages of maturation. Mature elements look like benign tissues derived from normal endoderm, ectoderm, and mesoderm. Immature elements consist of undifferentiated primitive tissues from the three germ cell layers. Teratomas in children are benign as they are diploid, lack chromosomal imbalances and do not show gains of isochromosome (12p). In postpubertal patients, teratomas are **hypotriploid**, demonstrate chromosomal imbalances including a gain of i(12p), and have the potential for metastatic spread. Since mature and immature teratomas have the same genetic changes and biologic potential specific for prepubertal and postpubertal patients, they are no longer subclassified into mature and immature categories.

Grossly, teratomas are often large and inhomogeneous. The cut surface reveals cystic regions containing lakes of mucinous or gelatinous material interspersed among areas of solid tissue. There is a haphazard arrangement of enteric or salivary glands, respiratory epithelium, fat, smooth or striated muscle, cartilage, bone, glial or neuroectodermal tissues. Although the tumor appears benign, lymphovascular invasion may be present which supports its metastatic potential. Pure teratoma or teratoma found in mixed germ cell tumors is resistant to both radiation and chemotherapy. Rarely, teratomas will harbor somatic-type malignancies such as adenocarcinoma and rhabdomyosarcoma, identical to cancers found at other organ sites. Some patients with metastatic teratomas that undergo malignant degeneration of a single cell type respond to chemotherapy regimens directed towards the specific malignant cell observed. Unfortunately, the prognosis for patients with malignant transformation (particularly at distant sites) is poor.

Mixed Germ Cell Tumors

Approximately 60% of germ cell tumors contain more than one histologic pattern. Of these, 59% contain seminoma, 41% contain yolk sac tumor, and 47% contain embryonal carcinoma and teratoma. Syncytiotrophoblast cells are found in 42% of mixed germ cell tumors, although pure choriocarcinoma typically spreads to distant sites unaltered. The most frequent combination is embryonal carcinoma, yolk sac tumor, teratoma, and syncytiotrophoblasts with or without seminoma. A **polyembryoma** consists of a mixture of yolk sac tumor and embryonal cell carcinoma forming **embryoid bodies** which are ovoid structures consisting of a cavity surrounded by loose mesenchyma associated with syncytiotrophoblasts and occasionally teratoma. Each cell type has invasive and metastatic capabilities.

Burned-out Germ Cell Tumors

Few patients with metastatic cancer lack clinical evidence of a primary testicular tumor. The pathologic examination of the orchiectomy specimen occasionally reveals an area of scar or hemorrhage. This finding is most common in patients with pure choriocarcinoma and has been proposed in patients with pure teratoma and discordant pathology at metastatic sites. Less than 10% of patients with "pure seminoma" have clinical evidence of nonseminomatous metastases at distant sites. However, 30%-45% of patients who die from apparent metastatic pure seminoma actually have nonseminomatous elements. These findings support the fact that some germ cell elements regress or burn out in the primary specimen. Mixed tumors that contain seminoma are managed as nonseminomas.

Intratubular Germ Cell Neoplasia: Carcinoma *in Situ*

Testicular carcinoma *in situ* (CIS) is thought to be the precursor of all invasive germ **cell tumors except spermatocytic seminoma** in adults and the **pediatric testicular tumors (yolk-sac and mature teratoma).** This supposition is supported by the presence of CIS in nearly 100% of testicular parenchyma adjacent to the primary invasive tumor. Histologically, the malignant germ cells are large with abundant pale cytoplasm, irregularly outlined nuclei with one or two prominent nucleoli, and located at the periphery of the seminiferous tubules between normal appearing sertoli cells. Testicular CIS has been studied carefully in Scandinavian countries where the reported incidence of CIS is approximately 1%. This correlates well with the lifetime risk for the development of invasive testis cancer in this at risk population of men. Reports indicate that 50% of patients with CIS found on testicular biopsy developed invasive tumors within five years of diagnosis if left untreated. The overall incidence of testicular CIS in the general population is low. However, there are groups of patients at risk for the development of CIS, including: patients with a history of contralateral testicular cancer (5%-6%), cryptorchidism (3%-5%), an atrophic contralateral testis with unilateral testis cancer (30%), an extragonadal germ cell tumor (40!) and intersex or sexual ambiguity (25%-100%). The data are controversial regarding the presence of infertility and any increased risk for testicular CIS. In patients with known invasive germ cell tumors, the finding of contralateral testicular microlithiasis on ultrasound increases the risk of harboring carcinoma in situ in that testicle. However, testicular microlithiasis was not felt to be associated with invasive testicular germ cell tumors in asymptomatic populations with no risk factors for CIS or testicular cancer. Patients at risk for testicular CIS and potentially for invasive germ cell tumors should be offered either careful surveillance, or testicular biopsy following a discussion of the potential risks and benefits of diagnosis and therapy.

2. Epidemiology, Risk Factors, Presentation and Diagnosis

Incidence

In 2008, there was a projected incidence of 8090 new testicular cancer cases and 370 deaths related to testicular cancer within the United States. Testicu lar cancer is the most common solid tumor among American men aged 20-34 and the second most common solid tumor in men 35-40 years. The lifetime probability of developing testicular cancer is approximately 1 in 300, and the risk of dying from the disease is about 1 in 5000. The age-adjusted incidence of testis cancer varies worldwide and is highest in Scandinavian countries (Norway and Denmark—9.3 cases per 100,000 men), intermediate in the United States (5.4 cases per 100,000 men) and lowest in Africa and Asia. American black males have a rate of 0.9 per 100,000 men, which is believed to be 10 times higher than the incidence rate in Africa.

Age and Histology

Seminoma is the most common histologic type of germ cell tumor with a peak incidence between 35 and 39 years. Most spermatocytic seminomas and malignant testicular lymphomas occur in men over the age of 50 years. Generally, nonseminomatous tumors occur in younger patients in the 20-30 year age group. **Pure yolk sac tumor and pure teratoma are the predominant histologic subtypes in pediatric groups.** Both yolk sac tumor and teratoma are present in older patients, typically as germ cell elements in mixed nonseminomatous tumors. Teratoma is a benign tumor in prepubertal patients but has metastatic potential in adolescents and older men.

Bilateral Testicular Cancers

Bilateral testicular germ cell tumors occur in 1%-4% of patients. The synchronous presentation of bilateral tumors is less common (17%-30% of patients) than the metachronous development of a second contralateral tumor (70%-83%). Most metachronous tumors occur at a median of 5 years from diagnosis of the incident tumor. Seminoma is the predominant histology in synchronous and metachronous tumors. Although patients with a primary testicular tumor have an elevated risk for contralateral CIS or the development of a second contralateral invasive germ cell tumor, contralateral testis biopsies are not recommended routinely as the prognosis for patients with a second germ cell tumor is excellent. Fortunately, the long-term disease free survival in patients with bilateral germ cell tumors approaches 90%. Careful surveillance of the contralateral testicle including monthly self-testicular examinations is mandatory.

Risk Factors

Table 2 lists factors reported to increase one's risk for the development of a testicular cancer. Several reasons are postulated to explain why tumorigenesis might occur in cryptorchid patients. These reasons include: abnormal germ cell morphology, increased temperature exposure, interference with the testicular blood supply, endocrine dysfunction and gonadal dysgenesis. Interestingly, in cryptorchid patients who develop testicular malignancies, 5%-10% of the germ cell tumors actually develop in the normal descended contralateral testicle. This finding is consistent with testicular biopsy data indicating an elevated risk for CIS in the contralateral testicle of patients with testicular maldescent. Orchiopexy facilitates appropriate clinical surveillance of the involved gonad. Until recently, no data indicated that orchiopexy prevented the development of CIS and invasive germ cell tumors. A systematic literature review and meta-analysis by Walsh and colleagues, suggests that a prepubertal orchiopexy may decrease the risk of testicular cancer. This study showed an average 3-fold increased risk of tumorigenesis in men when orchiopexy was delayed (10-11 years or later) or was not performed, compared to patients who underwent surgery earlier. A separate meta-analysis which included another large cohort study confirmed Walsh's findings. There were potential confounding factors as the early orchiopexy group may have included patients who might have experienced spontaneous testicular descent making them a sub-group of low risk patients that may have influenced the results of the meta-analyses.

Table 2

Possible Risk Factors for Testicular Cancer

Risk Factor	Risk Increase [a]
Cryptorchidism	3 - 14X
Metachronous testis cancer	2 - 4X
Positive family history	5X
Diethylstilbestrol exposure	2.5 - 5X
Gonadal dysgenesis	50X
Androgen insensitivity syndrome	15X

[a] = Increase in relative risk compared to

Testicular trauma does not cause testicular cancer. The traumatic event likely leads to an increased awareness of testicular pathology and indirectly facilitates tumor detection. Hormonal fluctuations and estrogen exposure are postulated to cause changes in germ cells leading to the development of testicular cancer. Hormonal imbalances may play a causative role in cancer development particularly in patients with testicular atrophy. Patients might experience decreased feedback inhibition for gonadotropin secretion, which could be the driving force for malignant transformation of an already damaged germinal epithelium.

In a recent case-control study of 369 men with testicular germ cell tumors between 18-44 years of age, compared to 979 age matched controls, Daling and colleagues found a correlation between marijuana use and testicular germ cell tumors, particularly nonseminomas. The frequency of use (daily or weekly) vs. marijuana use less than once per week also increased the risk of developing a testicular tumor.

Presentation and Diagnosis

On average, there is a mean delay of 5 months from the onset of initial symptoms to the diagnosis of testicular cancer. The responsibility for this diagnostic delay is both patient and physician related. Patients are reluctant to seek medical attention for testicular pathology due to ignorance, embarrassment, fear, denial or inadequate access to medical care. Physicians misdiagnose testicular tumors as hernias, hydroceles, spermatoceles, epididymo-orchitis and trauma-related pathology. These diagnoses as well as others such as testicular torsion are part of the differential diagnosis in patients with a testicular mass. However, a mass should be considered a testicular cancer until proven otherwise. A scrotal ultrasound is an important adjunctive study available in equivocal cases. If local signs and symptoms are attributed to an infectious process such as epididymitis, a normal physical exam must be documented during immediate follow-up. Unfortunately, patients with symptoms due to metastatic disease on occasion are subjected to unnecessary procedures, biopsies or abdominal explorations, prior to the recognition of a clinically obvious testicular mass. Occasionally, patients may be found to have abdominal metastases suggestive of an extragonadal germ cell tumor. A scrotal ultrasound should be performed to rule out the testicle as the source of a primary germ cell tumor. Impalpable tumors or evidence for small burned out tumors may be visible with ultrasonography.

The most common presenting signs and symptoms in patients diagnosed with testis cancer are listed in Table 3.

Seminomas tend to expand within the testis as a **painless, rubbery mass,** whereas **nonseminomatous** tumors often have more **discrete and irregular characteristics.** However, these distinctions are not always evident. Patients with nonseminomas are more likely to complain of **testicular pain.** The presenting complaint in patients with metastatic disease might include: **back pain due to bulky lymphadenopathy; dyspnea, cough or hemoptysis** from numerous pulmonary lesions; gastrointestinal disturbances such as anorexia, nausea, emesis and possibly even hemorrhage due to bowel involvement; neck mass secondary to supraclavicular lymph node involvement; bone pain due to skeletal metastases (seminoma patients); and even lower extremity edema from occlusion of the inferior vena cava.

Table 3

Most Common Presenting Signs and Symptoms and Their Frequency

Painless mass or swelling	40%- 55%
Pain ± mass or swelling	25%- 50%
Sign or symptom related to mets	5%- 20%
History of trauma	3%- 13%
Gynecomastia or breast tenderness	1%- 5%
Incidental finding	<5%

The impact of the delay in the diagnosis has being addressed by a recent European population based study that included 542 patients. The study confirmed a delay in diagnosing seminoma of 4.9 ± 6.1 months compared to 2.8 ± 4.0 months for nonseminomas. The delay in diagnosis led to a statistically significant impact on the 5 year survival rate only in the patients with nonseminoma. This study stresses the importance of early detection and management.

Patterns and Mechanisms of Spread

Testicular germ cell tumors have highly predictable patterns of spread. The tunica albuginea of the testis acts as a natural boundary for most testicular tumors preventing involvement of the epididymis and the testicular cord. Tumors confined to the testicle and the tunica albuginea most always spread directly to the retroperitoneal lymph nodes through lymphatic channels that course with the testicular cord and gonadal veins before fanning out medially into the retroperitoneum after crossing over the ureter. The primary landing zone for left-sided tumors is the left para-aortic region bounded by the left renal vein, ureter and the aorta above the inferior mesenteric artery. Less common locations of primary spread from left-sided tumors include the pre-aortic and the interaortocaval regions. **The primary landing zone** for **right-sided** testicular tumors is the **interaortocaval region beneath the left renal vein**, followed by the paracaval and the preaortic regions. In many cases, lymphatic drainage crosses over from right to left, therefore **left para-aortic lymph node involvement** occurs more commonly in patients with **right testicular primaries.**

Primary testicular tumors with epididymal or cord involvement may spread to pelvic or inguinal lymph node basins. Iliac or inguinal node involvement must be considered for cryptorchid patients, patients with scrotal wall involvement and patients who have had prior inguinal surgery or procedures that would disrupt the normal lymphatic flow from the primary tumor. Patients with advanced retroperitoneal lymph node metastases may have pelvic or inguinal metastases from retrograde lymphatic spread. **Suprahilar or retrocrural lymph node involvement is less common for low volume retroperitoneal disease.** In patients with advanced retroperitoneal lymphatic metastases, both of these locations are more common sites of nodal involvement and require careful scrutiny on preoperative radiographic imaging studies and during retroperitoneal lymph node dissection (RPLND).

Lymphatic drainage above the retroperitoneum is to the **cisterna chyli, thoracic duct**, and usually to the **left supraclavicular lymph nodes.** Extranodal visceral and distant metastases result from either direct hematogenous dissemination (common with choriocarcinoma) or through lymphaticovenous communications. The most direct communication is the junction of the thoracic duct and the subclavian vein, although in the setting of bulky retroperitoneal lymph node metastases, small lymphaticovascular communications develop in the retroperitoneum allowing for subsequent vascular tumor emboli and distant progression or visceral involvement of testicular cancer. Rarely, distant progression occurs in the absence of retroperitoneal lymph node involvement. Lymphatic channels may bypass the retroperitoneum altogether and communicate directly with the cisterna chili or the thoracic duct. This pattern of lymphatic drainage and the possibility of direct hematogenous spread accounts for the small percentage of patients who relapse (most commonly in the lungs) following a negative RPLND for clinical stage I disease.

3. Clinical Staging

Accurate staging of testicular germ cell tumors is critical to the process of treatment decision making. Staging requires a combination of serum tumor markers, radiographic studies, and precise interpretation of the histologic findings and tumor type(s) following radical orchiectomy. In 1997 (updated in 2002), the American Joint Committee on Cancer (AJCC) adopted a staging system applicable to patients with seminomas and nonseminomas (Tables 4 and 5). The system is unique in that tumor marker levels have been incorporated into the staging criteria emphasizing the importance of serum tumor markers in determining prognosis.

Tumor Markers

Tumor markers are important for testicular cancer diagnosis, staging, determining prognosis, monitoring treatment response, and for detecting relapse. There are two main classes of tumor markers: **oncofetoproteins (AFP and bHCG)**, which are associated with embryologic development, and **cellular enzymes lactate dehydrogenase (LDH)** and **placental alkaline phosphatase (PLAP)**. PLAP is a marker of advanced disease (particularly for seminoma) and is utilized rarely for clinical purposes.

Alpha-fetoprotein (AFP)
AFP is a 70 kilodalton single-chain glycoprotein and it is the predominant serum-binding protein in the fetus. AFP is synthesized in the **fetal yolk sac, liver and intestine**. Peak gestational levels occur during weeks 12–4, and then begin to fall after 16 weeks until the AFP level is minimally detectable after the first year of life. Beyond 1 year, the AFP level should be less than 10 ng/ml. The serum half-life of AFP is 5-7 days. After the first 6 weeks of post-natal life, AFP elevations can be detected in several benign and malignant conditions other than germ cell tumors including: **normal pregnancy; ataxia telangiectasia; hereditary tyrosinemia; liver toxicity** related to chemotherapy, **anesthetics, antiepileptics, hepatitis and alcoholism; and cancer of the lung, stomach, pancreas and liver** (seen in 70% of patients with hepatocellular carcinomas). AFP may be elevated in patients with pure **embryonal cell carcinoma, teratocarcinoma, yolk sac tumors** and in patients with other mixed germ cell tumors. **AFP levels are normal in patients with pure choriocarcinoma and pure seminoma**. If the

Table 4

2002 AJCC TNMS Staging System for Testicular Cancer

Primary Tumor (T)

pTx	Primary tumor cannot be assessed (radical orchiectomy has not been performed)
pT0	No evidence of primary tumor (eg, scar)
pTis	Intratubular germ cell neoplasia / carcinoma *in situ*
pT1	Tumor limited to testis and epididymis; no lymphovascualr invasion; may invade tunica albuginea but not tunica vaginalis
pT2	Tumor limited to testis and epididymis; lymphovascualr invasion present or there is invasion of tunica vaginalis
pT3	Direct cord invasion ± lymphovascular invasion
pT4	Direct scrotal invasion ± lymphovascular invasion

Regional Lymph Nodes (N) – Clinical

Nx	Regional lymph nodes cannot be assessed
N0	No regional lymph node mets
N1	Lymph node mass, single or multiple nodes, ≤2 cm in greatest dimension
N2	Lymph node mass, single or multiple nodes, 2-5 cm in greatest dimension
N3	Lymph node mass >5 cm

Regional Lymph Nodes (N) – Pathologic

pNx	Regional lymph nodes cannot be assessed
pN0	No regional lymph node mets
pN1	Lymph node mass ≤2 cm; or ≤5 positive nodes, none >2 cm in dimension
pN2	Lymph node mass 2-5 cm; or >5 nodes positive, none >5 cm; or (+) extranodal extension
pN3	Lymph node mass >5 cm

(continued)

Table 4 *(continued)*

2002 AJCC TNMS Staging System for Testicular Cancer

Distant Metastasis (M)

Mx	Distant mets cannot be assessed	
M0	No distant mets	
M1	Distant mets	
M1a	*Nonregional nodal or pulmonary mets*	
M1b	*Distant mets other than nonregional nodal or pulmonary*	

Serum Tumor Markers (S)

Sx	Markers not available or performed	
S0	Markers within normal limits	
S1	LDH hCG (mIU/mL) AFP (ng/mL)	<1.5 x normal and <5000 and <1,000
S2	LDH hCG (mIU/mL) AFP (ng/mL)	1.5 - 10 x normal or 5,000 - 50,000 or 1,000 - 10,000
S3	LDH hCG (mIU/mL) AFP (ng/mL)	>10 x normal or >50,000 or >10,000

Data according to 2002 American Joint Committee on Cancer (AJCC). AJCC Cancer Staging Manual. *6th ed. New York, , NY: Springer-Verlag; 2002.*

Table 5

TNMS Stage Grouping for Testis Cancer

Stage				
0	pTis	N0	M0	S0
IA	pT1	N0	M0	S0
IB	pT2-4	N0	M0	S0
IS	pT1-4	N0	M0	S1-3
IIA	any T	N1	M0	S0/1
IIB	any T	N2	M0	S0/1
IIC	any T	N3	M0	S0/1
IIIA	any T	any N	M1a	S0/1
IIIB	any T	N1-3	M0	S2
	any T	any N	M1a	S2
IIIC	any T	N1-3	M0	S3
	any T	any N	M1a	S3
	any T	any N	M1b	any S

Data according to 2002 American Joint Committee on Cancer (AJCC). AJCC Cancer Staging Manual. *6th ed. New York, NY: Springer-Verlag; 2002.*

AFP is elevated in patients with histologically pure seminoma, the primary specimens should be re-evaluated to exclude the presence of other germ cell elements, or areas of scar that could be representative of burned-out germ cell elements other than seminoma. Patients with a histologically pure seminoma and an elevated AFP are managed like other patients broadly classified as having nonseminomas.

Human Chorionic Gonadotropin (HCG)
HCG is a 38 kilodalton protein secreted by placental syncytiotrophoblasts to maintain the viability of the corpus luteum. In healthy men, only minute amounts of bHCG are detected (<5mIU/mL). There are two subunits of HCG. The **alpha subunit** is homologous with the pituitary glycoprotein hormones (leutinizing hormone, follicle stimulating hormone, thyroid stimulating hormone). The **beta subunit** of HCG (bHCG) is 70% homologous with the leutinizing hormone (LH) beta chain but it has a unique amino acid c-terminal extension that allows the production of specific antibodies used to target the purified bHCG subunit in radioimmunoassay techniques. The serum-half life of bHCG is 24-36 hours. Like AFP, bHCG can be elevated in both benign and malignant conditions. Given the cross reactivity with LH, it is important to remember that conditions resulting in an elevated LH (ie, hypogonadism) can falsely elevate bHCG levels. An intramuscular injection with 200 mg testosterone can help to distinguish cancer related elevations of bHCG from cross-reaction with LH. Other conditions leading to elevated levels of bHCG include marijuana use and cancers of the liver, pancreas, stomach, lung, breast, kidney or bladder. **bHCG levels** are **elevated** in every patient with **choriocarcinoma**, 40%-60% of patients with embryonal cell carcinoma, and 10%-25% of patients with pure seminoma due to syncytiotrophoblastic elements.

Lactate Dehydrogenase (LDH)
LDH is a 134 kilodalton cellular enzyme produced by muscle, liver, and numerous other organs and may be falsely elevated with hemolysis. Elevation of LDH is nonspecific and must be taken into consideration with other tumor markers and staging studies. However, evidence points to the utility of LDH as a marker of tumor volume or a marker of advanced disease—particularly for bulky seminoma. LDH elevation has a direct relationship with

disease burden and with the stage of a patient's malignancy. Along with AFP and bHCG, LDH is a component of the TNMS staging system and the degree of elevation carries prognostic significance.

Tumor Marker Elevation

A significant percentage of patients with nonseminomatous germ cell tumors have an elevation of either bHCG or AFP (or both markers) prior to undergoing radical orchiectomy (Table 6). The degree of marker elevation in these patients with nonseminomas helps to stratify patients into good, intermediate and poor risk groups according to the International Germ Cell Consensus Classification. Smaller numbers of patients with pure seminomas have elevated bHCG or LDH (Table 6). Typically, if bHCG levels in seminoma patients are abnormal, the serum levels will be less than 100 mIU/mL to 200 mIU/mL. Rarely does a patient with a pure seminoma have an elevated bHCG beyond 500 mIU/mL. Contrary to the prognostic significance of diagnostic marker levels in patients with nonseminomas, the degree of HCG elevation in patients with seminomas prior to orchiectomy has no apparent affect on patient outcome or prognosis. Low level marker elevation following radical orchiectomy for clinical stage I patients can be due to any of the aforementioned benign or malignant conditions associated with elevated bHCG, AFP or LDH. In general, however, persistent marker elevation indicates the presence of systemic disease and patients should be considered to have occult metastases.

Monitoring Treatment Response

Serum tumor markers are very useful for monitoring treatment response and disease relapse. Markers often provide the first evidence of relapse (including patients with normal markers at presentation) while on surveillance for clinical stage I disease, or following therapy for known or suspected metastatic disease. As demonstrated in Table 6, not every patient with a germ cell malignancy will present with elevated markers. However, the initial value of a marker provides an early indication of prognosis, and generally, the degree of marker elevation correlates with tumor burden. **Markers should decline** according to their known kinetics following radical orchiectomy (in the absence of occult metastases), and following radiation or chemotherapy when patients are treated for systemic disease. A rate of marker normalization that is less than the expected rate of decline, or persistent marker elevation despite therapy, indicates that there is continued marker production from viable germ cell elements due to incomplete resection, tumor persistence, drug resistance or relapse.

Two-thirds of patients with bulky metastatic disease will have a marker surge after initiating chemotherapy, which causes an early prolongation of the marker half-life. After the marker surge, the rate of normalization is proportional to the amount of viable germ cell tumor. However, normal tumor markers do not signify disease absence. Approximately 10% of patients with normal markers after chemotherapy have viable nonteratoma germ cell tumor confirmed histologically following post-chemotherapy retroperitoneal lymph node dissection (RPLND). Based on risk factors for micrometastases, 20%-50% of patients with normal markers and clinical stage I diseases are proven to have metastatic germ cell tumor at the time of their primary RPLND. Persistent marker elevation is indicative of systemic disease. A patient, whose **markers remain elevated** following **radical orchiectomy** or induction chemotherapy, should be treated with **primary chemotherapy or second line/salvage chemotherapy** respectively. Patients with persistently elevated markers prior to primary RPLND or postchemotherapy RPLND most always relapse.

Radiographic Studies

Scrotal Ultrasound

Ultrasonography is an extension of the physical examination and can confirm the presence of a testicular tumor which usually has the appearance of a hypoecohic parenchymal mass. While a scrotal ultrasound is not required for the diagnosis of a testicular cancer, the study has several important applications. A scrotal ultrasound is useful to exclude testicular tumors in patients with hydroceles or testicular inflammatory conditions (epididymitis, orchitis) where an adequate physical examination is often significantly limited or the diagnosis of a testicular mass is in question. An ultrasound is a requirement for any patient suspected to have an extragonadal germ cell tumor (EGCT). The scrotal ultrasound might reveal a small impalpable tumor or a suspicious area potentially representative of a

Table 6

Frequency of Raised Markers at Testis Cancer Diagnosis

	Marker	Number	Percentage (%)	Range (%)
Stage I seminoma				
	bHCG	31/298	10	5 - 40
	LDH	5/18	27	0 - 33
Metastatic seminoma				
	bHCG	38/146	26	13 - 61
	LDH	41/75	55	33 - 70
Stage I nonseminoma				
	AFP	103/196	53	48 - 75
	bHCG	55/196	28	24 - 46
	AFP or bHCG	115/196	57	24 - 75
Metastatic nonseminoma	AFP	439/716	61	59 - 74
	bHCG	421/760	55	40 - 68
	AFP or bHCG	414/515	80	70 - 92

bHCG = beta human chorionic gonadotropin; AFP = alpha-fetoprotein
Adapted from Rustin GJ, et al. Consensus statement on circulating tumour markers and staging patients with germ cell tumours. Prog Clin Biol Res. *1990;357:277-284.*

burned out germ cell tumor. It is extremely important to establish the testicle as the site of origin as the prognosis is significantly worse for patients with primary mediastinal EGCTs compared to patients with testicular primaries or primary retroperitoneal EGCTs.

Scrotal ultrasonography is utilized increasingly during the workup of infertility, orchalgia, scrotal swelling, varicoceles, and patient or physician detected scrotal pathology. An ultrasound performed for these indications occasionally reveals an incidentally detected scrotal mass. Some tumors are small and palpable on physical examination, but not large enough to have been noticed by the patient. Other incidentally detected testicular lesions are impalpable. In patients with no retroperitoneal pathology and normal tumor markers, many incidentally detected, impalpable lesions have benign histologies. Germ cell tumors are confirmed pathologically in smaller numbers of patients. Patients with small testicular tumors are candidates for testis sparing surgery. If organ preservation is considered, the lesions must be approached through a standard inguinal incision, the vascular pedicle (testicular cord) should be controlled, and intraoperative ultrasound utilized to confirm tumor location. Intraoperative frozen sections of the tumor and the surrounding testicular parenchyma are required to determine if testis sparing surgery is feasible or if radical orchiectomy is indicated. Infrequently, false negative intraoperative frozen sections occur. Patients should be informed of this risk and the possibility that a subsequent radical orchiectomy may be required.

Abdominal Imaging

Abdominal computed tomography (CT). CT is the modality of choice for staging the retroperitoneum (including the para-aortic, interaortocaval, paracaval, retrocrural, suprahilar, presacral and pelvic lymph node regions) and evaluating the abdominal viscera. Arterial and venous phases of the CT permit the precise definition of aberrant and accessory vascular structures (ie, accessory renal arteries). A detailed understanding of a patient's vascular anatomy is important for patients who are candidates for an RPLND. However, the CT does not distinguish benign lesions (fibrosis) from teratoma and viable non-teratomatous germ cell elements such as embryonal cell carcinoma. For clinical stage I disease, the CT scan is unable to detect micrometastases, which is the reason treatment decisions following radical orchiectomy are based upon tumor histology (tissue types and relative percentage of germ cell elements) and other risk factors (tumor markers and pathologic characteristics) that help to predict the presence or absence of occult metastatic disease.

Magnetic resonance imaging (MRI). MRI has no distinct advantage over CT for abdominal imaging. Like the CT scan, the MRI does not distinguish benign from malignant lesions. The MRI is useful for evaluating patients suspected to have obstructed vessels, particularly the inferior vena cava (IVC). Complete IVC obstruction due to tumor infiltration or venous thrombosis infrequently occurs in patients with bulky retroperitoneal lymphadonepathy. Preoperative knowledge of this scenario and whether the patient has established collateral venous return helps the surgeon to determine if IVC resection is an option and whether an interposition graft would be required.

Positron emission tomography (PET). PET has a limited role in the staging and evaluation of patients with metastatic testicular cancer. PET studies detect viable malignant germ cells, but the study does not distinguish teratoma from fibrosis. Therefore, in patients with nonseminomatous germ cell tumors, the recommendation for surveillance, RPLND or adjuvant chemotherapy is based on clinical staging and risk factors for metastases in patients with clinical stage I disease and low volume clinical stage II disease. Likewise, nonseminomatous patients with postchemotherapy residual masses and normal tumor markers require surgical consolidation regardless of the PET scan results. On the contrary, the PET scan is highly predictive for residual tumor following chemotherapy in patients with clinical stage II or III seminomas. Traditionally, surgery is recommended for patients based on the size of the residual mass and the probability of finding viable germ cells. Following chemotherapy, 13%-27% of residual tumors ≥3 cm harbor viable seminoma compared to 0 to 3! of residual tumors <3 cm. The PET scan helps to clarify which patients would benefit from an RPLND. In one series, PET had a positive predictive value and a negative predictive value of 100% and 96%, respectively, for predicting the presence or absence of viable tumor in patients with residual masses following chemotherapy. In the setting of a residual mass, the results of a PET scan can significantly influence disease management and spare some patients a technically challenging and sometimes incomplete surgical resection. In a recent prospective multicenter trial of 20 patients that underwent RPLND for residual masses following chemotherapy for metastatic seminoma, the results of PET were correlated with histological findings from the retroperitoneal specimens. The negative predictive value of PET was 100% whereas the positive predictive value was only 25%. The negative predictive value was independent of the tumor size (1-13 cm). It is plausible that the false positive PET scans identified the desmoplastic reaction and inflammation associated with treated, non-viable seminoma as the studies were performed at a median of 28 days following the completion of chemotherapy. Additional evaluation regarding the utility of PET will be necessary. However, in the setting of a residual mass following chemotherapy for metastatic seminoma, a negative PET scan might potentially spare some patients a technically challenging and sometimes incomplete surgical resection.

Chest Imaging

In clinical stage I disease, the risk of chest involvement is less than 5%. Many urologists believe that a posterioanterior and lateral chest x-ray is adequate to image the chest in patients with no evidence of abdominal metastases. Practically, many patients undergo simultaneous CT of the chest and abdomen. The disadvantage with this approach is the common finding of indeterminate subcentimeter pulmonary lesions. Over time many of these lesions do not change in size and are interpreted to be benign. Rarely does a chest CT alter management for patients with clinical stage I disease although when an abnormality is demonstrated, dual therapy might be avoided by the administration of induction chemotherapy. However, the risk of chest involvement is approximately 40% in the setting of an abnormal abdominal CT, under which circumstances more sensitive chest imaging with CT is required.

4. Management of the Primary Tumor

Radical Orchiectomy

A radical orchiectomy is most always the initial step in the management of a patient with a testicular tumor that is suspicious for a germ cell neoplasm. A precise histological interpretation of the germ cell type(s) and amount(s) as well as a description of the primary T stage is critical to determining subsequent options for disease management.

Some patients with advanced disease are very symptomatic at presentation. A radical orchiectomy can be temporarily delayed when tumor markers and clinical staging are diagnostic of a germ cell malignancy. It is important to initiate induction chemotherapy to ensure that the patient experiences no delay in receiving systemic treatment. Following chemotherapy, a radical orchiectomy is performed as a single procedure or concurrent with an RPLND. Removing the primary tumor is always recommended as viable germ cell tumor and teratoma are found in 8%-25% and 32%-42% of patients, respectively.

A radical orchiectomy provides excellent local control for most every patient managed according to sound oncologic principals and cures many patients with clinical stage I testis cancer. The procedure involves the complete excision of the testicle, its surrounding tunics, and the entire spermatic cord just proximal to the level of the internal inguinal ring. A 5-7 cm incision is made parallel to the inguinal ligament approximately 2 cm above the pubic tubercle and carried down to the external oblique aponeurosis. The incision can be extended over the upper scrotum for patients with very large tumors. The fascia is incised along the direction of its fibers down through the external ring. The ileoinguinal nerve is identified and preserved. The cord is completely mobilized and elevated with a penrose drain. Dissection proceeds towards the pubic tubercle careful to incorporate all of the cremasteric fibers and perforating cremasteric vessels, which must be secured. The cord is wrapped with a penrose drain and clamped as a tourniquet just below the internal ring. With manual pressure and eversion of the ipsilateral hemiscrotum, the testicle and the tumor are delivered into the operating field. The gubernacular attachments are released and the radical orchiectomy is completed by dissecting the cord 1-2 cm into the internal inguinal ring and separately ligating and dividing the vas deferens and the cord vessels. Silk ties or suture ligatures should be utilized in order to identify the gonadal vein stump if the patient undergoes an RPLND. Scrotal or retroperitoneal hemorrhage is the most common complication following a radical orchiectomy. Close attention to hemostasis and careful ligation and division of the cord structures must be ensured. Following irrigation, the wound is closed by approximating the external oblique fascia, Scarpa's fascia, and the skin.

Partial Orchiectomy

Patients with a tumor in a solitary testicle and patients with bilateral testicular tumors are considered for testis-sparing surgery. Advantages of organ preservation include the prevention of androgen deprivation and the subsequent need for lifelong hormonal supplementation, and the preservation of fertility in smaller numbers of patients. Several guidelines must be respected when treating patients with an organ-sparing approach: patients should have normal preoperative serum levels of leutinizing hormone and testosterone; a partial orchiectomy should be approached through an inguinal incision and oncologic principals of dissection for a radical orchiectomy must be followed; the operative field must be draped to prevent tumor contamination; the tumor is localized with intraoperative ultrasonography; cold ischemia should be utilized during tumor excision; and tumors should be small (ie, <20 to 25 mm diameter). Frozen section for margins and biopsies of the surrounding tumor bed should be accomplished to ensure complete excision of the tumor and to determine the presence of intratesticular germ cell neoplasia or carcinoma in situ (CIS); adjuvant local irradiation should be considered for patients with CIS in the parenchymal bed; patients must be highly motivated and compliant with strict follow-up guidelines. Local recurrences are very rare for patients with CIS managed with postoperative radiation. However, local recurrences are possible in patients followed without adjuvant radiation and thus some patients require a delayed orchiectomy.

There is a role for testis-sparing surgery in patients with incidentally detected, impalpable, small intraparenchymal tumors and a normal contralateral testicle. Most of these patients have normal markers and no other clinical or radiographic evidence of disease. Several reports indicate that 50%-80% of small lesions (particularly <10 mm greatest diameter) have benign histologies (Leydig cell, Sertoli cell and other benign forms). **Seminoma is the most common germ cell histology.** The principals of management are identical to those described for testis-sparing procedures in patients with solitary testicles or bilateral tumors.

Scrotal Violation

The traditional surgical approach to a radical orchiectomy involves an inguinal incision and high ligation of the spermatic cord. However, scrotal violations (scrotal orchiectomy, incisional biopsy, fine needle aspiration) occur in 4%-17% of patients with testicular malignancies. Scrotal violation is associated with an increased risk of local recurrence particularly when tumor is found in a scrotal wall specimen. The traditional recommendation for managing patients with scrotal violation includes a hemiscrotecotmy, which is a disfiguring procedure for some patients. Although debatable, many urologists believe that scrotal violation excludes otherwise acceptable patients from surveillance protocols.

Recent reports question the need for a formal hemiscrotectomy in the patient with a scrotal violation. Scrotal violation, increases the risk of a local recurrence from <1%, up to 3%-6%. In a smaller series of patients, there were no local recurrences with scrotal violation, provided that surgical margins were negative and the spermatic cord was uninvolved by tumor. Furthermore, no significant differences in distant recurrence rates or survival have been demonstrated in patients with scrotal violation.

Sheinfeld, et al summarized the following management principals for patients with scrotal violation:

1. In patients with low-stage seminoma, the radiation portals should extend to the ipsilateral groin and scrotum. Side effects include an increased risk of infertility.

2. Low-stage nonseminoma patients undergoing RPLND should have simultaneous wide excision of the scrotal scar and the remaining testicular cord.

3. Patients who received at least induction chemotherapy should have the scrotal scar and the remaining cord structures excised at the time of postchemotherapy RPLND, although local relapse is rare following systemic chemotherapy.

4. Formal hemiscrotectomy and extensive groin dissection are no longer recommended.

Intratular Germ Cell Neoplasia: Carcinoma *In Situ*

Several factors must be taken into consideration when deciding upon treatment for patients with testicular carcinoma in situ including age, fertility concerns, status of the contralateral testicle, the presence of unilateral vs. bilateral testicular CIS, the presence of testicular atrophy, and patient compliance. Certainly, the major concern with carcinoma in situ is the possibility of developing an invasive germ cell tumor. It has been reported that 50% of patients with intratesticular germ cell neoplasia (CIS) will develop an invasive neoplasm within 5 years if left untreated. Tumor markers are not elevated in patients with CIS unless an invasive neoplasm is present.

Testicular biopsy remains the gold standard for the diagnosis of testicular CIS. In the United States, contralateral testicular biopsies are not performed routinely for patients with invasive germ cell tumors. Biopsies are more often considered or recommended if patients have contralateral testicular atrophy, intersex disorders, extragonadal germ cell tumors, cryptorchidism, and as part of an infertility evaluation. In the presence of a normal contralateral testicle, most would agree that a radical orchiectomy is the treatment of choice for patients with CIS. Hypogonadal patients who require hormonal supplementation and patients with compromised fertility also should be considered for a radical orchiectomy. It is important to remember that many patients with invasive germ cell tumors or CIS are subfertile at the time of diagnosis.

There are other management options besides radical orchiectomy for patients with solitary testicles and CIS, or the uncommon patient diagnosed with CIS and a normal contralateral testicle. Options include observation, radiation, and chemotherapy. Short-term observation may be a reasonable approach for the patient seeking to father children in light of the protracted natural history of CIS. However, he must be counseled regarding the risks and benefits of this approach including the development of an invasive germ cell tumor that could result in the need for a radical orchiectomy, or lead to anorchia. The benefits of radiation include cancer cure as well as the preservation of endocrine function. However, all men who receive testicular radiation become infertile. Testicular radiation causes a Sertoli cell only pattern on subsequent testicular biopsies. Lower dosages of radiation (14 Gy) have been compared to higher dosages (up to 20 Gy standard) to determine the effects on carcinoma *in situ* and Leydig cell function. Regardless of the radiation dose, some patients still require testosterone supplementation over time and testosterone replacement does not appear to be radiation dose dependent. Furthermore, relapse of CIS has been reported following irradiation with 14 Gy. The 20 Gy dose remains the standard dose for testicular CIS although 16-18 Gy dosages are likely as efficacious as higher dosages. Chemotherapy is not recommended as primary treatment for testicular CIS unless it is planned as adjuvant therapy for high-risk patients or for patients with metastatic disease. In patients with known CIS prior to chemotherapy, the estimated cumulative risk of CIS 5 and 10 years after treatment is 21% and 42%. These patients must be followed closely with biopsies. Radiation therapy is offered for recurrence.

5. Retroperitoneal Lymph Node Dissection (RPLND)

There are many rationales for performing an RPLND for testis cancer: 1.) The retroperitoneal lymph nodes are usually the first site and often the only site of metastatic spread from testicular cancers; 2.) RPLND alone cures 50%-90% of patients with node positive low-volume nonseminomas (pN1 or pN2 disease); 3.) Up to 25% of patients with pN1 or pN2 disease harbor teratoma in their nodal specimens following primary RPLND which is resistant to both chemotherapy and radiation; 4.) Relapse rates following a negative RPLND are less than 5%-10%, are rarely in the field of surgical dissection, and usually are due to pulmonary metastases or elevated markers; 5.) Current radiographic modalities understage roughly 15%-50% of clinical stage I patients depending on risk factors for micrometastases; 6.) Albeit uncommon, late relapses following primary chemotherapy usually occur in the retroperitoneum, have a poorer prognosis and are usually chemorefractory; and 7) Untreated retroperitoneal metastases are most always fatal. Based on these and other observations, RPLND is a critical component in the management of patients with testicular germ cell tumors.

Technique and Exposure

Prior to the surgical procedure, patients should be counseled regarding options for sperm banking even if nerve-sparing procedures are planned. A mechanical bowel preparation is self-administered the day prior to surgery. The surgeon should have an intimate knowledge of the patient's clinical stage to include tumor distribution, overall tumor burden, and his vascular anatomy. Vascular anomalies are not uncommon. Up to 20% of patients have accessory renal arteries. Occasionally, a patient will have a retroaortic renal vein that could be mistaken for a lumbar vein. Up to date tumor markers should be obtained as most (80%) patients with elevated markers fail a primary RPLND. Induction chemotherapy is recommended for patients with new or persistent marker elevation following orchiectomy. Very few patients with elevated markers following second line and salvage chemotherapy regimens undergo an attempted desperation RPLND. Unfortunately, the outcome for this subset of patients is poor.

Open RPLND

An open RPLND is usually performed through a midline abdominal incision (although thoraco-abdominal approaches have been utilized as well with the advantage of easier access to the ipsilateral suprahilar region). An incision extends from the xiphicostal junction to just below the midpoint between the umbilicus and the pubic symphysis. The falciform ligament is divided to prevent injury to the hepatic capsule during elevation of the chest wall. Self-retaining retractors are positioned. The degree of bowel mobilization depends on the extent of surgical dissection. A peritoneal incision is made medial to the inferior mesenteric vein along the root of the small bowel mesentery, and carried from the cecum to the ligament of Treitz up towards the splenic flexure of the colon. The fourth portion of the duodenum is mobilized superiorly. For bulky adenopathy, or for added exposure, the inferior mesenteric vein can be suture ligated and divided. The posterior peritoneal incision is carried around the cecum and the ascending colon is mobilized along the paracolic gutter to the foramen of Winslow. The duodenum is kocherized off of the underlying vena cava and the large and small bowel is detached from the underlying retroperitoneum and great vessels to the level of the right and left renal hilum. The superior mesenteric artery is identified above the left renal vein and care taken to avoid unnecessary direct compression of the vessel during bowel retraction. Likewise, the pancreas is carefully padded and retracted to avoid injury. The omentum, transverse colon, right colon and small bowel are placed on the anterior chest wall surrounded by moistened, warmed, laparotomy pads. The bowel should be inspected frequently throughout the case to ensure adequate vascular perfusion. The descending colon and the splenic flexure are mobilized such that the medial aspect of the underlying left kidney, the left renal hilum, and the gonadal vein are completely visualized. The inferior mesenteric artery is usually left intact although division is required sometimes based on the volume of tumor. The common iliac arteries are visualized and dissected just beyond their bifurcation.

Anatomical boundaries and landmarks are carefully identified prior to proceeding with the surgical dissection. The superior boundary of dissection includes the right and left renal artery and renal vein. In low stage disease, retrocrural or suprahilar involvement is uncommon. With advanced disease, these regions should be carefully scrutinized prior to surgery with abdominal imaging, and then palpated intraoperatively. Lateral boundaries of dissection include the ureters and the ipsilateral gonadal veins. The inferior boundary courses along the common iliac vessels to their bifurcation distally. The posterior boundaries are the anterior spinous ligament and the psoas muscle fascia, which are identified during the course of the lymphadenectomy. The lymphatic tissue is dissected away from the medial aspect of the ureters. The gonadal vein is divided at the level of the renal vein (left side primary) or the inferior vena cava (right side primary) and dissected into the ipsilateral internal inguinal ring for complete excision. If nerve sparing is planned, a prospective nerve dissection is initiated once the surgical boundaries are established (although care should be taken inferiorly along the common iliacs to avoid injury to nerve trunks beyond the hypogastric plexus). The hypogastric plexus and the postganglionic sympathetic fibers are prospectively identified, meticulously dissected and gently elevated with vessel loops. As the dissection proceeds and as aorta and IVC are mobilized, the sympathetic ganglia and the sympathetic chains are more easily identified and the sympathetic structures are preserved to maintain emission and antegrade ejaculation. The left side postganglionic fibers course over top of the aorta and should be dissected prior to initiating the split and roll maneuver. The lymphatic tissue is split along the anterior surfaces of the inferior vena cava and the aorta, the renal veins and the iliac arteries. The IVC and the aorta are rolled laterally and medially identifying lumbar arteries and veins, which are ligated and divided to disengage the great vessels from the posterior abdominal wall. During the lymphadenectomy, great care is taken to carefully dissect and expose the renal arteries, which are at the superior extent of the dissection. Accessory renal arteries should be considered. Lymphatics require precise control with surgical clips or ties, particularly at the peripheral limits of dissection. Particular attention to lymphostasis is required inside the right crus of the diaphragm under the right renal artery where lymphatics course to join the cisternae chyli. Failure to achieve good control of the lymphatic vessels results in postoperative chylous leaks in a small percentage of patients—more common following postchemotherapy RPLNDs.

Laparoscopic RPLND

Compared to an open RPLND, a laparoscopic RPLND offers patients several potential advantages including: decreased blood loss, **decreased perioperative morbidity, decreased length of hospitalization, quicker convalescence and favorable cosmetic results.** In a recent review of laparoscopic RPLND series, including studies comparing open and laparoscopic approaches, the operating time was longer for laparoscopic procedures (204 vs. 186 min), but the complication rate (15.6% vs. 33%), reintervention rate (1.4% vs. 6.6%) and hospital stay (3.3 vs. 6.6 days) favored the laparoscopic technique ($P<0.05$). In experienced hands, the principals of dissection during the lymphadenectomy should be identical to open techniques (ie, templates of dissection, disengagement of the IVC and aorta form the posterior abdominal wall, nerve sparing) although some investigators report limiting the dissection anterior to the lumbar vessels. Median local and distant cancer control rates are comparable between laparoscopic RPLND and open RPLND with few in-field relapses and few distant recurrences. The number of lymph nodes resected is reportedly higher with open techniques compared to laparoscopic procedures and these findings need to be carefully considered when addressing the therapeutic nature of a lap RPLND. Presently, however, most patients with positive retroperitoneal nodes are treated with adjuvant chemotherapy regardless of their risk for disease relapse. Thus, it is difficult to determine the therapeutic potential of laparoscopic RPLND as a sole treatment option for patients with pathologic node-positive disease.

Primary Landing Zones and Template Dissections

Carefully documented anatomic studies and detailed mapping studies of RPLND pathology specimens clarify the patterns of spread from the primary testicular tumor and help to define the most common sites of lymph node involvement. For left sided tumors, the first echelon of lymph node drainage is the infrahilar left para-aortic and preaortic regions followed by the inter-aortocaval lymph nodes. Left to right crossover to the paracaval region is uncommon for low stage or low volume disease. Practically, there is very little nodal tissue in the precaval and the paracaval location during a primary RPLND. If the patient has positive nodes during a left modified template dissection, the paracaval tissue can easily be resected during mobilization of the inferior vena cava, which is required for prospective nerve sparing, and complete excision of the interaortocaval nodes. Lymphatics from right-sided testicular tumors drain primarily to the interaortocaval lymph nodes followed by the precaval and the preaortic regions. Intraoperative node mapping studies in patients undergoing primary RPLND reveal that right to left crossover to the para-aortic nodes occurs in roughly 20% of patients with pathologic node positive disease. Thus, the preaortic and para-aortic nodes should be removed for right modified template dissections. Table 7 demonstrates the retroperitoneal regions that must be dissected at a minimum to maximize the oncologic efficacy of a primary RPLND. Consideration should be given towards performing a full bilateral RPLND for patients with multiple microscopic positive nodes and certainly for gross lymphadenopathy identified during primary RPLND to maximaize the oncologic efficacy of the lymph node dissection.

Emission, Ejaculation, and Nerve Preservation

Normal antegrade ejaculation involves the precise coordination of 3 events. During orgasm, the bladder neck closes and there is seminal emission, followed by ejaculation. Sympathetic nerves originate from the T12 to L4 spinal cord levels. The nerves enter the paravertebral sympathetic ganglia, then post-ganglionic nerves course medially to form a plexus of nerves (hypogastric plexus) overlying the aorta concentrated between the inferior mesenteric artery takeoff and the aortic bifurcation (Figure 1). The sympathetic fibers travel from the hypogastric plexus via the pelvic plexus to innervate the vas deferens, seminal vesicles, bladder neck, and prostate. Ejaculation occurs via neural input from sacral and lumbar spinal cord levels.

Pudendal somatic innervations from S2 to S4 facilitates relaxation of the external urethral sphincter and contraction of the bulbourethral and perineal muscles. Injury to the sympathetic ganglia, the postganglionic nerves, and the hypogastric plexus

Table 7

Primary Landing Zones and Templates for Modified Primary RPLND

	Predominant Landing Zones	Minimum Dissection in Modified Template
Left side template	Para-aortic[a] Preaortic Interaortocaval	Para-aortic Preaortic Inter-aortocaval Ipsilateral common iliac Precaval
Right side template	Inter-aortocaval[a] Precaval Preaortic	Interaortocaval Precaval Preaortic (above IMA) Paracaval Para-aortic (above IMA) Ipsilateral common iliac

RPLND = retroperitoneal lymph node dissection; IMA = inferior mesenteric artery; [a]= primary landing zone

Figure 1

Sympathetic nerves originating from the T12 to L4 spinal cord levels

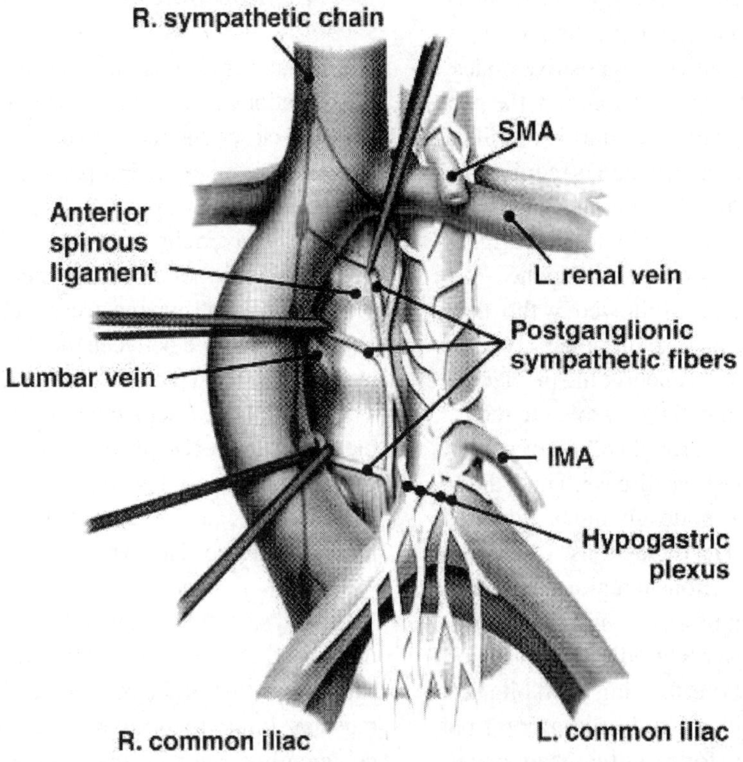

during the course of an RPLND, causes failure of emission and retrograde ejaculation. Traditionally, bilateral infrahilar RPLNDs were performed for low stage disease. Rates of ejaculatory dysfunction were prohibitively high with bilateral non-nerve sparing techniques. Prospective nerve sparing techniques and modified template dissections were described and performed which decreased the rates of ejaculatory dysfunction to less than 5% while maintaining oncologic efficacy. Postganglionic nerves and the hypogastric plexus are prospectively identified and meticulously dissected coursing over the common iliac arteries and above the distal aorta. Dissection proceeds proximally towards the ganglia and the sympathetic trunks. Prospective nerve dissections are possible with primary or postchemotherapy RPLNDs. However, nerve preservation should not compromise the therapeutic aspects of the surgical procedure.

Complications of RPLND

A primary RPLND is generally very well tolerated. Minor complications (5%-15% of patients) and major complications (5%-7% of patients) are uncommon and occur more predominantly in patients undergoing bilateral RPLND compared to template dissections (Table 8). The development of a small bowel obstruction requiring exploration and lysis of adhesions occurs in 1% or less of patients. Emission and antegrade ejaculation is preserved in 93%- 99% of patients undergoing nerve-sparing procedures. Most minor complications are related to wound infections and atelectasis, and usually do not prolong hospitalization.

The rate of complications related to postchemotherapy surgery is 20%-25%. Pulmonary complications account for the majority of minor and major problems

Table 8

Complications of Retroperitoneal Lymph Node Dissection

Primary RPLND

Minor	**Major**	**Delayed**
Wound infection	DVT/PE	Death (rarely reported)[a]
Pneumonia/atelectasis	Bowel injury	DVT/PE
Prolonged ileus	Pancreatitis	Hydronephrosis
UTI	Unplanned nephrectomy	Ventral hernia
Lymphocele	Chylous ascites	
Bleeding requiring transfusion	Bowel obstruction (1%)	Ejaculatory dysfunction (0%-7%) in nerve-sparing cases
	Vascular injury	

Postchemotherapy RPLND

Wound infection	Pulmonary (prolonged ventilation, bleomycin toxicity, pneumonia, PE)	Death (1%)[a]
Pneumonia / atelectasis	DVT/PE	DVT/PE
Prolonged ileus	Bowel obstruction (2%)	Gastric ulcer
UTI	Chylous ascites (2%)	Hydronephrosis
Lymphocele	Ureteral injury	Ventral hernia
Bleeding requiring transfusion	Pancreatitis	Ejaculatory dysfunction
	Renal infarction	
	Unplanned nephrectomy or organ resection	
	Bowel injury	
	Gastrointestinal bleeding	
	Hemorrhage	

UTI= urinary tract infection; DVT= deep vein thrombosis, PE= pulmonary embolus
[a]= immediate or delayed

in the postoperative setting and are experienced by 8%-10% of patients overall (Table 8). Bleomycin is used routinely as part of a standard chemotherapy protocol. A side effect of bleomycin is pulmonary interstitial fibrosis, which causes a restrictive pattern lung disease and a probable oxygen diffusion deficiency. Both during surgery and in the perioperative setting, it is important to judiciously manage intravenous fluids and balance crystalloid and colloid administration to prevent pulmonary edema and increasing inspired oxygen demands. Aggressive pulmonary physiotherapy is mandatory.

Renovascular injuries and gastrointestinal complications account for the majority of the remaining complications in postchemotherapy patients. Injury to the renal vessels may result in the development of hypertension, renal atrophy, or result in the need for an unplanned nephrectomy. Small bowel obstructions often are successfully managed with nasogastric tube decompression. Exploration is reserved for patients who exhibit signs or symptoms of toxicity or who fail to respond to conservative measures. Causes of a prolonged ileus include: mechanical obstruction, pancreatitis, urinomas, retroperitoneal or mesenteric hematomas, bowel ischemia and bowel infarction.

Chylous ascites occurs in 2%-7% of patients overall, and can be associated with IVC resection, suprahilar dissections, and hepatic resections. Careful lymphatic stasis must be ensured throughout the course of dissection, particularly inside the right diaphragmatic crus where lymphatics course to the cisternae chyli. Most patients with chylous leaks experience abdominal distention, prolonged ileus or pleural effusions (more common with retrocrural dissections). The physical exam reveals a fluid wave. A paracentesis is both diagnostic and therapeutic and may be required on multiple occasions. The fluid is typically milky, demonstrating high fat and high-protein content. Up to 80% of patients are managed successfully with combinations of conservative measures including repeated paracentesis, diuretics, total parenteral nutrition and low fat diets with medium chain triglycerides. Smaller numbers of patients require peritoneovenous shunts, which unfortunately are associated with high surgical revision rates.

6. Management of Nonseminoma

The management of nonseminomatous germ cell tumors (NSGCT) is approached very systematically (**Figures 2 and 3**). With careful risk stratification based on the precise interpretation of the orchiectomy specimen and the clinical staging studies, as well as the careful integration of surgery and chemotherapy, most patients with NSGCT have very favorable outcomes.

Clinical Stage 1 and Low-Volume Clinical Stage 2 NSGCT

There are three management options available to patients with clinical stage I disease and normal markers (cT1-4, N0, M0, S0; normal markers prior to orchiectomy, or normalization of markers following radical orchiectomy). These options include surveillance, or primary treatment with either chemotherapy or RPLND. A risk adapted management approach is based on the accurate interpretation of the patient's primary pathology, as well as his staging studies. Each management option should be discussed with the patient as part of his counseling following radical orchiectomy. Patients should be counseled regarding sperm banking prior to therapy.

Stage IS NSGCT

Patients with clinical stage IS disease have persistent serum tumor marker elevation or new marker elevation following orchiectomy and require full induction chemotherapy (BEP x 3 or EP x 4). Elevated markers imply that the patient has systemic disease and he is unlikely to be cured by primary RPLND alone. Up to 80% of patients with elevated markers prior to RPLND will relapse.

Risk Factors for Occult Metastases in Clinical Stage I NSGCT

Risk factors for the presence of occult micrometastases for clinical stage I seminoma and clinical stage I NSGCT are listed in Table 9. The most important and the most consistent risk factors for relapse in patients with NSGCTs include elevated serum tumor markers, the presence of lymphovascular invasion (LVI), and the presence of majority embryonal cell carcinoma (EC). MIB-1 staining has been evaluated as a risk factor for occult metastases as well. MIB-1 is a monoclonal antibody developed for application in paraffin-embedded tissues, and it is used to measure the immunohistochemical

Table 9

Reported Risk Factors for Micrometastases and Relapse in Clinical Stage I Seminoma and NSGCT

Seminoma
Elevated serum tumor markers
Lymphatic or vascular invasion
Primary tumor size >4-6 cm
Rete testis invasion
NSGCT
Elevated serum tumor marker
Majority embryonal cell carcinoma (>50%)
Lymphatic or vascular invasion
MIB-1 staining
Absence of yolk sac elements
Higher T stage (T2-T4)
Large tumor size (>4-6 cm)

expression of Ki-67 (a nuclear antigen found in all cycling human cells and a marker for cellular proliferation). The results of MIB-1 staining are mixed. MIB-1 staining was found to be a promising marker for predicting the presence of occult metastases in some studies whereas MIB-1 staining in other reports did not correlate with the pathological stage in patients with clinical stage I NSGCT. Patients with normal markers, LVI, and high percentage EC, have at least a 40%-50% risk of relapse due to micrometastases. The presence of one risk factor (either LVI or majority EC) decreases the risk of relapse to 20%-40%, whereas the absence of both risk factors decreases the risk of relapse to less than 20%. Over 70% of patients with clinical stage I pure EC have occult metastases detected at RPLND.

Surveillance

Surveillance following radical orchiectomy is an option available to many patients who would otherwise be over-treated and subjected to an unnecessary RPLND or to unnecessary chemotherapy. The rationale for considering surveillance is based on the following observations: current radiographic imaging studies have improved diagnostic accuracy, radical orchiectomy alone cures the majority of patients with clinical stage I tumors, and early relapses can be cured with cisplatin-based chemotherapy. Surveillance studies consistently show that 25%-35% of patients (regardless of risk factors) will relapse while on observation. The majority of relapses occur within one year (median time to relapse approximately 5-6 months). Relapses beyond the 2nd year are rare, although late relapses have been reported and long-term follow-up is mandatory. Generally, 60% of relapses involve the retroperitoneal lymph nodes (± other sites), 30-45% of patients have normal markers at relapse, and 20% of patients will have a marker-only or a lung-only relapse. The type of relapse directs subsequent therapy (Figure 2). Patients detected to have a low-volume retroperitoneal relapse with normal markers (stage IIA) should be considered for a primary RPLND. Patients with stage IIB disease or other patterns of relapse should be considered for standard induction chemotherapy. The overall survival for patients entered onto surveillance protocols ranges from 96%-100%. The optimal candidate for surveillance has cT1, N0, M0, S0 disease (normal markers, normal radiographic studies), a low % EC, and no LVI. The patient should be highly motivated, compliant, and have consistent access to surveillance protocols.

Primary Chemotherapy

In order to avoid the side effects and the potential morbidity of an RPLND, several studies have examined the role of primary chemotherapy in high-risk patients (clinical stage IB). Relapse rates following 2 cycles of cisplatin-based chemotherapy range from 2%-4%. Patients with clinical stage IS disease and patients with clinical stage IIA and IIB disease who elect primary chemotherapy require standard induction dosages (3 courses BEP or 4 courses EP). Primary chemotherapy is utilized more frequently in Europe compared to the United States. The disadvantages of primary chemotherapy include both short and long-term chemo-related toxicity: **renal insufficiency, neuropathy, ototoxicity, myelosuppression, alopecia, mucositis, infertility, pulmonary fibrosis and Raynaud's phenomenon.** Toxicity is less with 2 cycles BEP compared to standard induction regimens.

Figure 2

Low-stage NSGCT

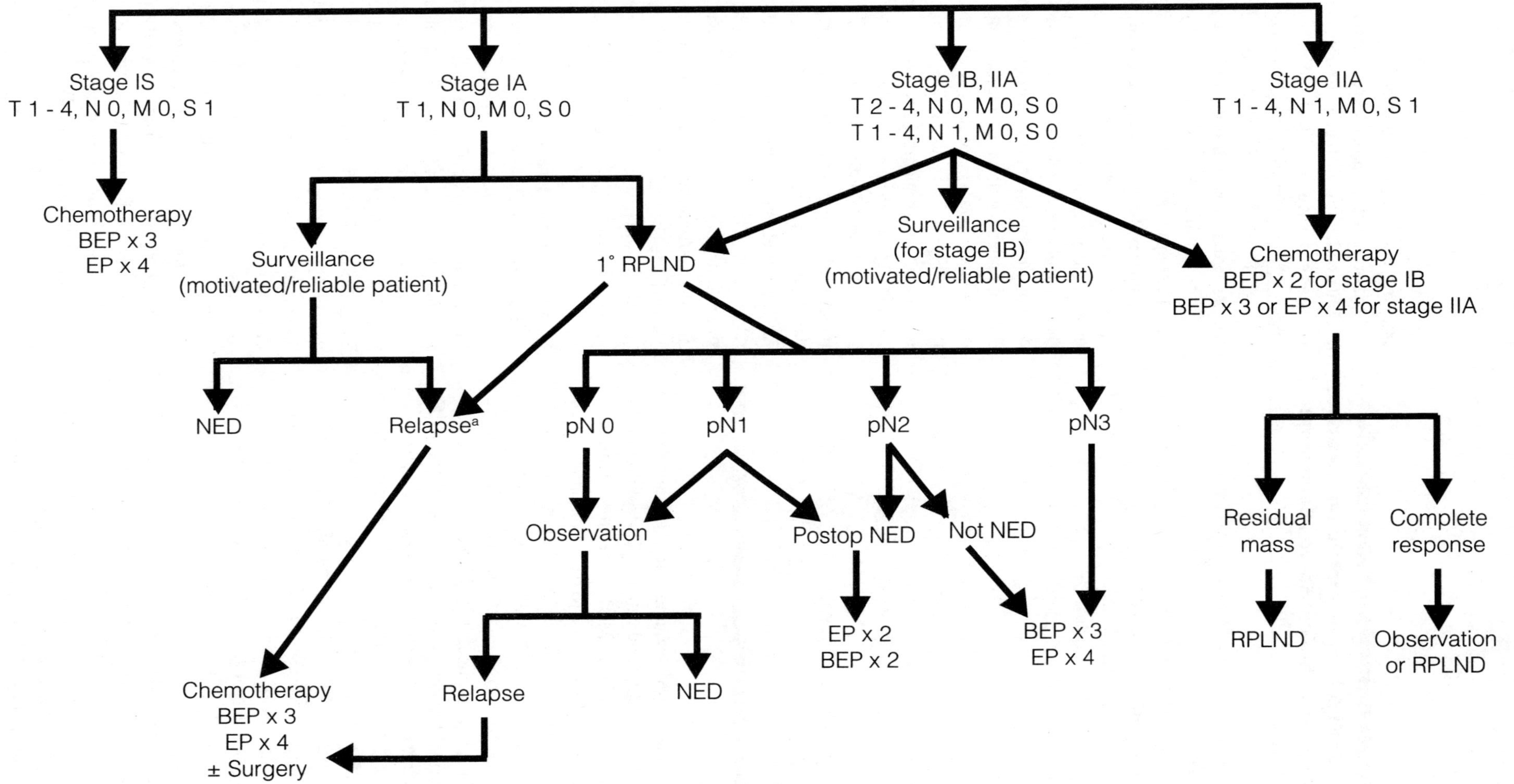

[a] Depending on type of relapse (Marker positive or extraretroperitoneal mets – induction chemotherapy) (Marker negative and retroperitoneal mass – primary RPLND); BEP = bleomycin, etoposide, cisplatin; EP = etoposide, cisplatin

Modified from Sheinfeld J. 2005 AUA Review Course: Testis Cancer (lecture).

Figure 3

High-stage NSGCT

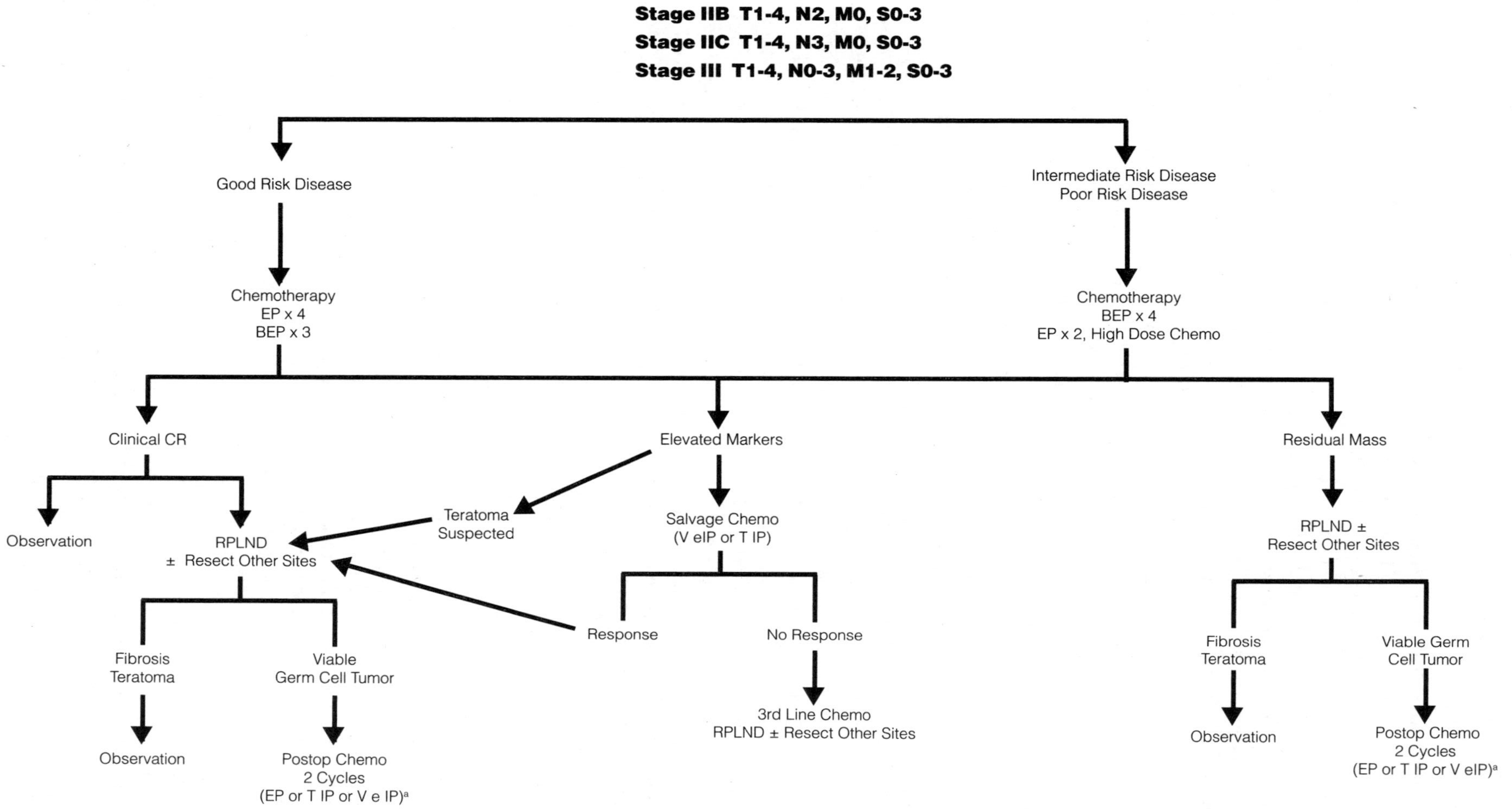

[a] Postop chemo given if patient received induction chemotherapy only; BEP = bleomycin, etoposide, cisplatin. Modified from 2005 AUA

Retroperitoneal Lymph Node Dissection (RPLND)

In the United States, a primary RPLND remains the favored management option for many patients with clinical stage I disease or low volume clinical stage II disease (stage IIA and some stage IIB) and normal serum markers. In patients with clinical stage I disease, candidates for a primary RPLND include intermediate to high-risk patients (based on risk factors for occult micrometastases) with normal serum tumor markers, and poorly compliant patients. An RPLND is diagnostic; it is therapeutic as a sole treatment modality in 50% to 90% of patients with pathologic N1 and N2 metastatic cancer; and it "secures" the retroperitoneum from disease recurrence, as in-field relapses are rare when the RPLND is performed by experienced surgeons. Pathologic stage I patients have a relapse rate of 5% to 10% following a negative RPLND. Most always, the relapse occurs out of the field of dissection (lung, marker, or combination). Nerve-sparing dissections are accomplished with tremendous success in most every patient undergoing a primary modified template or bilateral RPLND. A bilateral RPLND should be considered for patients determined to have multiple microscopically positive nodes during surgery, and for patients who are found to have previously undiagnosed gross lymphadenopathy. The morbidity of a primary RPLND is very low, and associated mortality is negligible.

A primary RPLND is an option for clinical stage IIA and stage IIB patients with normal markers. The surgeon should have a low threshold to perform a bilateral nerve sparing dissection in this setting. Stage IIB patients are candidates for a primary RPLND if only lymph node metastases are present and located within the primary landing zone. If there are multifocal metastases, lymph node metastases outside the primary landing zones, or if the patient is symptomatic, primary induction chemotherapy is recommended.

A recent randomized phase III trial conducted by The German Testicular Cancer Study Group compared primary RPLND with one course of primary chemotherapy (BEP) following orchiectomy for clinical stage I testis cancer. A total of 382 patients were randomized into each treatment arm and the mean follow up after surgery or chemotherapy was 4.7 years. There was a 7.59% difference in the 2-year recurrence free survival rate favoring chemotherapy (2 recurrences with chemo, 13 recurrences with RPLND). 7 of the surgical patients recurred solely within the retroperitoneum or within the inguinoscrotal region. Study sites included both specialized centers with experience in the surgical management of testicular cancer as well as community hospitals with low volume RPLND experience. In addition, longer patient follow up is required to determine if there will be more recurrences in the chemotherapy arm as the mean time to delayed relapse following primary chemotherapy is approximately 6 years.

Adjuvant Chemotherapy Following Primary RPLND

The decision to recommend chemotherapy following an RPLND is based upon the pathologic stage, the completeness of resection, the status of the tumor markers, and patient compliance. The randomized, prospective Testicular Cancer Intergroup Study revealed that 2 courses of cisplatin-based adjuvant chemotherapy most always prevents relapse in patients with pathological Stage II testicular cancer treated with orchiectomy and retroperitoneal-lymph-node dissection. Survival was similar in patients with pathologic stage II disease randomized to observation and treated with standard induction chemotherapy at the time of relapse. Relapse is uncommon for patients with pathologic N1 testis cancer (5 or fewer positive lymph nodes, all nodes ≤2 cm in size, and no extranodal extension) and studies reveal that up to 90% of patients with N1 disease are cured following RPLND alone. Thus, observation is the standard of care for completely resected, compliant patients with normal markers following RPLND. However, patients with pathologic N2 disease (more than 5 positive nodes, any node greater than 2 cm, extranodal extension) have a higher risk of relapse with observation (~ 50%). 2 cycles of adjuvant chemotherapy (BEP x 2 or EP x 2) are recommended for this group of patients following RPLND. Patients with elevated markers post-op, remaining unresected retroperitoneal tumor, or distant disease, as well as patients with pathologic N3 disease following RPLND, require induction chemotherapy (BEP x 3 or EP x 4).

Advanced NSGCT (Clinical Stage IIB-IIC, Clinical Stage III)

Primary Chemotherapy

The prognosis of patients with advanced NSGCT has been classified according to a validated model published by the International Germ Cell Cancer Collaborative Group (1997). The classification stratifies patients into good, intermediate and poor risk groups based on the levels of tumor markers (AFB, β-HCG, LDH) and the poor risk prognostic factors of metastases to organs other than the lungs (Table 10, Figure 3). Patients with advanced stage NSGCT are initially treated with platinum-based chemotherapy. Induction chemotherapy in good risk patients consists of 3 courses BEP (bleomycin, etoposide, cisplatin) or 4 courses EP (etoposide, cisplatin) based on the results of randomized clinical trials showing equivalent response rates and survival. Intermediate risk and poor risk patients require 4 courses of BEP as induction therapy. Poor risk patients often present with bulky lymphadenopathy, severe symptoms and malnourishment, making treatment delivery even more challenging.

However, chemotherapy should be started as soon as possible. While response and remission rates approach 60%-70% with front-line therapy, many poor risk patients relapse or die from disease. Second line therapy consists of conventional chemotherapy (TIP-paclitaxel, ifosfamide, cisplatin; or VeIP-vinblastin, ifosfamide, cisplatin) or high-dose chemotherapy (with or without autologous bone marrow transplantation or stem cell support). In patients who receive ifosfamide, mesna should be used before and after each dose of ifosfamide to prevent hemorrhagic cystitis.

Postchemotherapy Residual Mass

Surgery plays a critical role in the management of patients with advanced NSGCT. Following induction chemotherapy, 10%-15% of patients are found to have viable tumor in their retroperitoneum and up to 40% of patients will have residual teratoma. There is some controversy regarding patient selection for a postchemotherapy RPLND. Generally, patients with a residual mass and normal tumor markers following chemotherapy should undergo a post-chemotherapy RPLND. However, the definition of a normal CT scan and a residual mass varies among many centers of excellence. Definitions of a normal CT include no residual mass, residual lymph nodes < 1 cm, or residual lymph nodes <1.5 to 2 cm. Currently, there are no widely accepted clinical parameters or radiographic studies that differentiate residual viable germ cell elements (embryonal cell, yolk sac, choriocarcinoma, seminoma) from teratoma or fibrosis in the residual mass. In addition, the absence of teratoma in the primary tumor does not preclude its presence in the retroperitoneum. PET scans may suggest the presence of viable non-teratomatous germ cell tumor, but its utility in NSGCT patients is limited by its inability to differentiate teratoma from fibrosis. Most centers recommend observation for patients who experience a complete response to chemotherapy and reserve surgery for a detectable residual mass regardless of dimension, although there are advocates of performing postchemotherapy RPLNDs for all patients who had clinical node positive disease before chemotherapy, regardless of the postchemotherapy CT findings. The later approach is based on the reported incidence of residual teratoma in up to 15% of patients with "normal" CT scans prior to postchemotherapy RPLND. Although the biological potential of teratoma in this setting is debatable, the presence of unresected teratoma could account for some of the few late relapses in patients who experience complete responses with induction chemotherapy. The overall relapse rate in patients undergoing a complete RPLND and who were found to have teratoma or fibrosis in the resected specimen is 5%-10%. A recent report finds that in patients with only teratoma in the resected specimen following initial postchemotherapy RPLND, the 10-year probability of freedom from recurrence was 80%. The size of the residual mass and IGCCCG risk classification were significant predictors of disease recurrence. In the patients that recurred, one-half recurred with viable germ cell tumor and one-half recurred with teratoma (including some with malignant transformation). Nevertheless, observation is standard for patients with completely resected teratoma or fibrosis, whereas patients with completely resected viable germ cell tumor in the surgical specimen following induction chemotherapy derive a survival benefit from two additional courses of chemotherapy.

Table 10

International Germ Cell Consensus Classification

		Seminoma	
Risk Level	**Good**	**Intermediate**	**No Patients Classified as Poor Prognosis**
Primary site **Extent of mets** **Marker status**	Any primary site AND No nonpulmonary visceral mets AND Normal AFP Any hCG Any LDH	Any primary site AND Nonpulmonary visceral mets AND Normal AFP Any hCG Any LDH	
Patient (%)	90%	10%	
5 year PFS	82%	67%	
5 year OS	86%	72%	
		Nonseminoma	
Primary site **Extent of mets** **Marker status**	Testis/RP primary AND No nonpulmonary visceral mets AND Good Markers LDH <1.5 x nl; hCG <5000; AFP <1000	Testis/RP primary AND No nonpulmonary visceral mets AND Intermediate markers LDH >1.5 – 10x nl or hCG >5000 – 50,000 or AFP >1000 – 10,000	Mediastinal primary OR Non-pulmonary visceral mets OR Poor markers LDH >10x nl or hCG >50,000 or AFP >10,000
Patient (%)	56%	28%	16%
5 year PFS	89%	75%	41%
5 year OS	92%	80%	48%

PFS = progression free survival; OS = overall survival

Data from International Germ Cell Cancer Collaborative Group. International Germ Cell Consensus Classification: a prognostic factor-based staging system for metastatic germ cell cancers. J Clin Oncol. *1997;15(2):594-603.*

There are several rationales for resecting residual teratoma. **First**, teratoma may grow, invade or obstruct vital organs and become unresectable (growing teratoma syndrome). **Second**, teratoma is radioresistant and chemoresistant. **Finally**, 2%-8% of teratomas undergo malignant transformation to non-germ cell elements such as sarcoma and adenocarcinoma. These tumors do not respond to standard cisplatin-based chemotherapy regimens. Chemotherapy tailored to the malignant histology is recommended although surgical resection remains the mainstay of therapy. The prognosis for patients with teratoma and malignant degeneration is significantly compromised.

Most patients that relapse with testicular cancer do so within the first 2 years. However, long-term follow-up is necessary for all patients with testicular cancer secondary to the possibility of late relapses. A late relapse is defined as a tumor recurrence beyond 2 years after primary therapy and occurs in 2%-3% of patients following a complete response. Patients at all stages of disease are at risk. The median time to a late relapse is 7 years (range 2-32 years) and the most common site of recurrence is in the retroperitoneum or in the chest. Patients are managed best with surgical resection, as chemotherapy alone is rarely effective. Viable germ cell tumor and teratoma are found in 80% and 20% of surgical specimens respectively. Unfortunately, the long-term disease-free survival in patients who suffer a late relapse is poor (reported to be approximately 25%).

Patients with persistently elevated markers following induction chemotherapy require second-line or salvage chemotherapy with very few exceptions (ie, mild false elevations of markers due to liver toxicity, hypogonadism, etc.). In patients who respond to second line and other salvage chemotherapy regimens, the importance of a complete resection cannot be understated. The histologic characteristics of resected metastatic sites after salvage chemotherapy are significantly different from patients undergoing RPLND after induction chemotherapy. Viable nonteratomatous germ cell tumor, teratoma and fibrosis are found in 50%, 40%, and 10% of patients respectively. Postoperative chemotherapy does not improve disease specific survival for patients with viable germ cell elements following salvage chemotherapies (an important distinction from patients with viable germ cell elements in the completely resected specimen following standard induction chemotherapy). Furthermore, only select patients benefit from an RPLND in the setting of marker elevation or disease progression after aggressive systemic chemotherapy (desperation RPLND). Generally, a desperation RPLND is discouraged when markers remain elevated after salvage regimens as resection is often incomplete due to associated bulky retroperitoneal and visceral disease. However, 20%-30% of patients who are completely resected in a desperation attempt may experience long-term disease free survival.

The oncologic principles and the techniques of a postchemotherapy RPLND are similar to those discussed previously with the following caveats:

1. A full bilateral retroperitoneal node dissection is the standard of care. There is a variable distribution of metastases outside the boundary of a modified dissection following chemotherapy, and it is difficult to differentiate tumor from fibrosis intraoperatively.

2. There is no defined role for only excision or biopsy of the residual nonseminomatous mass.

3. Chemotherapy results in tremendous fibrosis making vascular dissection significantly more difficult.

4. Retrocrural and suprahilar dissections are required more often.

5. Complete surgical resection often involves adjacent organ resections (kidney, adrenal, bowel, liver, etc.) and vascular resections, particularly for bulky disease.

6. Prospective nerve-sparing procedures are feasible depending on the bulk of tumor, but not at the expense of cancer control and complete tumor excision. Every effort should be made to completely resect all retroperitoneal disease during the initial RPLND as a complete resection significantly influences relapse and survival. Overall, relapse rates following an initial RPLND (regard-

less of risk group) approach 20%. However, following repeat RPLNDs, relapse rates range from 35%-50% and disease-free survival is negatively impacted.

Resection of Nonretroperitoneal Sites

Small numbers of patients require resection of abdominal viscera or distant metastatic sites. Consistent with findings in the postchemotherapy retroperitoneal mass, the size of the mass at distant sites does not correlate with the pathological findings (ie, the presence or absence of viable tumor or teratoma). Likewise, the potential for histologic discordance between the resected retroperitoneal residual mass, and the tumor excised from distant sites is well established and reported to be approximately 35%. Simultaneous excision of retroperitoneal and pulmonary or mediastinal disease is an option, particularly if all disease can be excised through a single incision.

7. Management of Seminoma

Approximately 70% of patients with pure seminoma present with Stage I disease. Metastases to the retroperitoneum or to pulmonary and visceral sites are less common and occur in 20% and 10 % of patients respectively. The disease characteristics of seminoma differ significantly from patients with NSGCTs (70% of whom have metastatic disease at presentation). According to the Internation Germ Cell Consensus Classification, 90% of patients with seminoma are classified as having a good prognosis. Contrary to patients with NSGCTs, no patient with a pure seminoma is classified as having a poor prognosis (Table 10). Nevertheless, metastatic seminoma can be fatal. At the time of death, most patients have liver and lung involvement. Additionally, 50% of patients have bone metastases and 25% of patients have brain metastases. Many of those dying of disease actually have nonseminomatous germ cell elements in metastatic sites.

Stage I Seminoma

There are 3 management options for patients with stage I seminoma; surveillance, chemotherapy; and radiation (Figure 4).

Surveillance

Surveillance has emerged as an acceptable option for many patients with clinical stage I testicular seminoma. This option is based on the results of several prospective trials that reveal cancer specific survival rates ranging from 98%-100% in patients entered onto surveillance protocols following radical orchiectomy. In addition, while the short-term side effects of low-dose radiation therapy are minimal, there are still concerns regarding infertility, bowel toxicity, and the possible association of radiation therapy with secondary malignancies. Regardless of risk factors, approximately 15%-20% of patients relapse on surveillance indicating the presence of occult micrometastases at the time of diagnosis. Similar to patients with NSGCT, there are several pathologic variables that predict which patients have the greatest risk for harboring occult disease (Table 9). 2 risk factors (rete testis invasion and tumor size >4 cm) were examined for their prognostic capabilities in a pooled multivariate analysis of 3 separate surveillance trials of patients with clinical stage I seminoma. If both risk factors were present, the 5-year relapse rate was 31%, com-

Figure 4

Seminoma

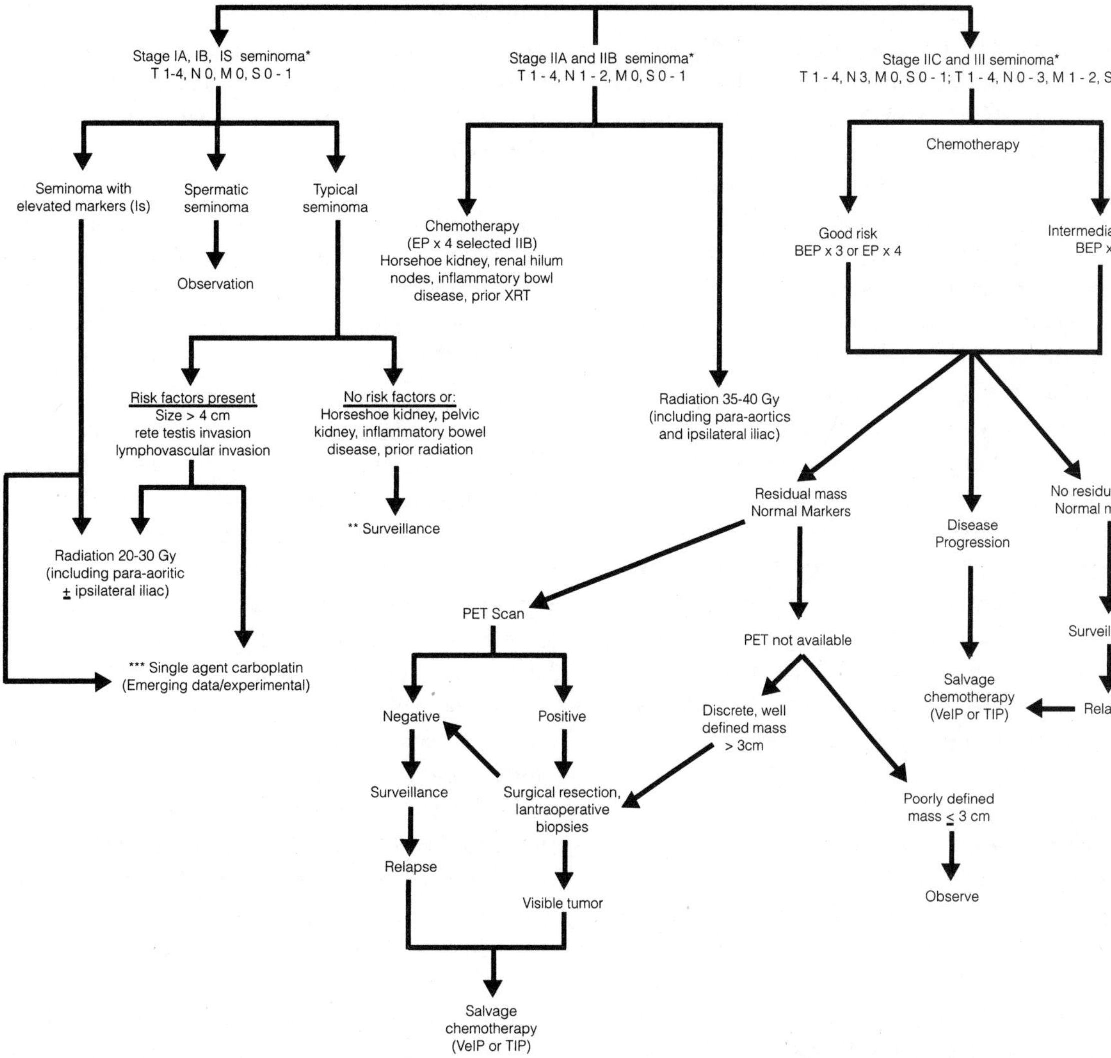

* elevated b-HCG < 100-200ng/m1 usually require no change in management for State I, IS, IIA, IIB seminoma

** Relapse on surveillance - restage and treat accordingly

*** Radiation therapy currently remains standard of care

BEP = Bleomycin, etoposide, cisplatin
EP = Etoposide, cisplatin
VeIP = Vinblastin, ifosfamide, cisplatin
TIP = Paclitaxel, ifosfamide, cisplatin

pared to 16% with 1 risk factor, and 12 % with no risk factors. In other studies, the presence or absence of LVI was identified as an important prognostic factor for relapse.

The majority of relapses in patients with clinical stage I seminoma occur in the para-aortic and in the interaortocaval lymph nodes (80%-90%), with a median time to relapse between 12 and 18 months following radical orchiectomy. Long-term follow-up is critical, as late relapses beyond 5 years have been reported. Most patients that relapse are treated with radiation therapy and of the 10%-20% of patients who experience a second relapse almost all are salvaged with systemic chemotherapy. The overall survival of patients who elect surveillance is approximately 98% which is similar to that reported for patients treated with primary adjuvant radiation. The major disadvantage with surveillance for stage I seminoma is the fact that a reliable serum tumor marker does not exist for the disease. Thus, surveillance protocols depend heavily on radiographic imaging studies. The optimal candidate for surveillance is the reliable patient with a pure seminoma, normal markers, a tumor size <4 cm, no rete testis invasion, and no evidence for lymphovascular invasion.

Primary Chemotherapy

Single agent carboplatin has been investigated as adjuvant therapy in patients with clinical stage I seminoma. Prospective nonrandomized trials show that two courses of carboplatin in high-risk patients are effective in preventing relapse while systemic toxicity appears acceptable. Furthermore, recent interim results from the prospective, randomized Medical Research Council trial of radiation compared to single dose carboplatin shows similar relapse rates for each treatment option. Longer follow-up will be required to confirm the preliminary therapautic equivalence between carboplatin and radiotherapy in the treatment of stage I seminoma, and whether side effects will favor one treatment over the other. Similar to radiotherapy, there are concerns regarding the overtreatment of patients with clinical stage I seminoma and the unnecessary exposure to potentially harmful long-term side effects of adjuvant chemotherapy. Thus, at the present time, single agent chemotherapy for clinical stage I seminoma remains experimental.

Radiation

Radiation has been the treatment of choice for most patients with clinical stage I seminoma following radical orchiectomy. Traditionally, 35 Gy was administered to the para-aortics and the ipsilateral iliacs in a hockey-stick fashion. Prophylactic mediastinal and left supraclavicular radiation was offered to many patients as well. However, supradiaphragmatic (mediastinal and supraclavicular) radiation is no longer recommended as it compromises a patient's ability to receive subsequent therapy and it potentially increases the patient's risk of developing delayed radiation-related complications and secondary malignancies. Currently, most centers recommend 25 Gy only to the para-aortic nodes, which has equivalent recurrence rates and overall survival rates compared to radiation directed towards both the para-aortics and the ipsilateral iliacs. Additionally, gastrointestinal and hematologic side effects, and adverse effects on spermatogenesis, are less with para-aortic radiation only. The only caveat is that patients require pelvic CTs as part of their follow-up protocol. In a randomized controlled trial Jones and colleagues compared radiation therapy for 625 patients with stage I seminoma using 20 Gy vs. 30 Gy. Patients treated with 30 Gy had significantly more side effects and work related limitations one month following the completion of therapy. However, by three months post-therapy, there was no difference between the groups. The median follow-up was 61 months and 10 and 11 relapses occurred in the 30 Gy and 20 Gy groups respectively. In summary no significant difference was found in terms of recurrence but patients in the 20 Gy group experienced less morbidity with an earlier return to work.

The effectiveness of radiation therapy for clinical stage I seminoma is well documented. Relapse rates range between 0%-7% following adjuvant radiation, and overall 5 to 10 year survival rates are 96%-100%. Contraindications to radiation therapy include prior abdominal radiation, a history of inflammatory bowel disease, and the presence of a horseshoe or pelvic kidney. Under these circumstances, patients can be treated with adjuvant chemotherapy or enter a surveillance program.

Stage IIA and IIB Seminoma

Patients with stage IIA and IIB seminoma are traditionally treated with adjuvant radiation. The dose of radiation is 35 to 40 Gy and the radiation treatment fields include the ipsilateral external iliac, the bilateral common iliacs, the paracaval and the para-aortic nodes (high enough to cover the cisterna chyli). The radiation portal extends from the T10 to T11 region superiorly, to L4 inferiorly. Radiation to the kidney is avoided due to sensitivity of the renal parenchyma to the radiation. Thus, chemotherapy (Epx4) is preferred in clinical stage IIB patients that have lymphadenopathy particulary close to the renal hilum. In patients that have a retained spermatic cord or scrotal contamination, the treatment fields can be widened to incorporate the operative site. The contralateral testicle should be shielded.

The 5-year survival rate for clinical stage IIA and IIB patients combined approaches 90%. Many patients who relapse can be salvaged with cisplatin-based chemotherapy. Patients with clinical IIC seminoma (N3, node >5 cm) are best managed with systemic chemotherapy as relapse rates with radiation monotherapy exceed 50%. Patients with prior abdominal radiation, a history of inflammatory bowel disease, renal hilum nodes, or with a horseshoe or pelvic kidney, should be treated with systemic chemotherapy as well.

Stage IIC and Stage III Seminoma

Cisplatin-based regimens are highly effective for patients with bulky disseminated testicular seminoma. Response rates exceed 90% and up to 90% of responders remain disease free for prolonged periods of time. Many patients who progress or who relapse following induction chemotherapy can be salvaged with standard second line chemotherapy regimens. Adifficult aspect of management involves the seminoma patient with the postchemotherapy residual mass (Figure 4). Most would agree that observation is warranted for residual masses <3 cm in size as viable tumor is rarely present in the pathological specimen (0%-3%). In addition, data indicate that 50% of residual masses resolve or disappear during surveillance (median 12.5 months). However, in patients with a residual mass ≥3 cm in size, identifiable tumor is found in 13%-27% of patients undergoing post-chemotherapy biopsies or an attempted RPLND. The challenging aspect of care in a patient with a residual mass who would otherwise be recommended to undergo surgical excision is influenced by the extreme difficulty encountered during surgical dissection. Patients with bulky seminoma exposed to chemotherapy have an intense post-chemotherapy desmoplastic reaction that involves the retroperitoneal lymph nodes occupied by seminoma. An RPLND or an excision of the mass is often incomplete due to the peritumoral fibrosis (which is much denser than the fibrosis encountered in NSGT postchemotherapy masses). In addition, patients with bulky seminoma only rarely have teratoma in the post-chemotherapy residual mass (likely representative of unrecognized NSGCT components in the primary testicular tumor). In order to avoid unnecessary surgery and higher rates of surgical morbidity in this patient population, PET/CT has been studied to determine its predictive capabilities in defining the presence or absence of viable tumor. Recent studies examining the utility of PET for advanced seminoma demonstrate negative predictive values of 100% in patients with residual masses following chemotherapy. The positive predictive value of PET varies and may be influenced by the timing of the study following chemotherapy and the possibility of detecting activity related to the tumor associated desmoplastic reaction in response to chemotherapy. However, in the setting of a residual mass, the results of a PET scan significantly influences disease management (Figure 4). The patient with a residual mass ≥3 cm and a negative PET can be spared a technically challenging and sometimes incomplete surgical resection. Careful follow-up is mandated to detect disease relapse in the absence of surgical resection or biopsies.

8. Sex Cord/ Gonadal Stromal Tumors

Sex cord stromal tumors compromise approximately 5% of testicular neoplasms in adults, with a higher prevalence in the pediatric population (10 - 30% of all testicular neoplasms). These tumors originate from cells in the sex cords (Sertoli cell and granulosa cell tumors) or from the testis stroma (Leydig cell tumors). In general, patients with sex cord /stromal tumors present with a testicular mass or with signs and symptoms related to the secretion of testosterone or estrogen. Most tumors are benign although 10%-15% of Leydig cell tumors and 10%-20% of Sertoli cell tumors are considered malignant.

Leydig cell tumors

Leydig cell tumors account for 1 to 3% of all testicular tumors and they are the most common of the non-germ cell tumors. Patient presentation occurs at any age, but most commonly between 20 and 60 years. The 20% of Leydig cell tumors that occur in prepubertal patients are considered benign. While most patients present with a palpable mass, 30% present with signs and symptoms such as virilization, gynaecomastia or decreased libido related to androgen or estrogen secretion. Because some patients present with endocrine related symptoms before a palpable mass is recognized, it is important to have a high index of suspicion for a testicular tumor (ie. gynaecomastia of unknown origin) and include an ultrasound examination of the scrotum and testicles during the work-up of endocrine-associated complaints.

Characteristically, these tumors are small, yellow-brown and well circumscribed. Microscopy reveals polyhedral cells with round eccentric nuclei, eosinophilic cytoplasm and occasional characteristic inclusions (Reinke's crystals). The histopathological features that predict malignant behavior include large tumor size (>5 cm), lymphatic or vascular invasion, increased mitotic activity and involvement of the spermatic cord. The tumors can metastasize to the retroperitoneum, lung, liver and bone.

Radical inguinal orchiectomy is the treatment of choice. CT of the abdomen and pelvis should be performed to rule out metastases if histopathological features suggest malignant potential. The role of RPLND in the management of malignant Leydig cell tumors or in the setting of metastatic disease is unclear, yet has been offered to some patients either primarily or following chemotherapy for retroperitoneal metastases. Response to chemotherapy and radiotherapy in the metastatic setting has been limited. Surveillance (including CT) is recommended every 6 months for 2 years for patients without malignant features and more frequently for those with potential malignant tumor.

Sertoli cell tumors

Sertoli cell tumors account for less than 1% of testicular tumors. While patients present at any age, the presentation and diagnosis usually occurs before age 20 and up to third of patients present with gynaecomastia. Most tumors are benign although 10% have malignant features and can metastasize (retroperitoneal nodes, lung and bone). Tumors usually are well circumscribed, white or yellow and firm, with focal cystic areas. Histologically, the tumors have tubular formations lined by elongated Sertoli cells with moderate to abundant cytoplasm, pale to intense eosinophilic quality and large cytoplasmic vacuoles in half of the cases. In some areas the tumor is solid and can be confused with seminoma. Features suggestive of malignancy include: mitotic figures, cellular and nuclear pleomorphism, large tumor size and necrosis.

Radical orchiectomy is the treatment of choice. Successful management with RPLND has been reported in patients with retroperitoneal involvement. The value of chemotherapy and radiation therapy for malignant disease is uncertain.

The large-cell calcifying Sertoli cell tumor subtype that occurs most commonly in pediatric patients can be associated with Peutz-Jeghers syndrome (gastrointestinal polyposis and mucocutaneous pigmentation) and with Carney syndrome (pituitary adenomas, mucocutaneous pigmentation and cardiac myxomas).

Gonadoblastoma

Gonadoblastomas occur almost exclusively in patients with intersex disorders (complete androgen insensitivity, male pseudohermaphroditism and

Turner syndorme) and gonadal dysgenesis (45,X/46,XY). These rare tumors account for lass than 0.5% of all testis neoplasms. 80% of the patients are phenotypically female and 20% are phenotypically male.

Radical orchiectomy is the treatment of choice and a contralateral prophylactic orchiectomy Is recommended when gonadal dysgenesis is present because of the high incidence of contralateral disease (50%). Rarely, the gonadoblastoma develops into a malignant germinoma (seminoma) that most often is successfully managed with systemic chemotherapy.

9. Lymphoid, Hematopoietic and Metastatic Tumors

Lymphoma

In the testicle, lymphoma can occur as a primary tumor, as the initial manifestation of clinically occult systemic disease or as the site of recurrent disease. Lymphoma is the most common testicular neoplasm in patients over 60 years. Either metachronous or synchronous bilateral testicular involvement occurs in 38% of patients. Most patients experience diffuse, painless enlargement of the testicle, and 30% of patients have systemic constitutional symptoms including weight loss, anorexia, and fever. Radical orchiectomy is diagnostic although the prognosis is poor for most affected patients with less than 50% 5-year disease-free survival. Patients with lymphoma confined to the testis have a more favorable outcome.

Leukemia of the testis

The testis is a common site of recurrence of leukemia mainly in children (acute lymphocytic leukemia). Primary leukemia of the testis is rare. Bilateral testicular Involvement occurs in half of the cases. Biopsy is diagnostic, and the treatment of choice is testicular irradiation combined with chemotherapy.

Metastatic tumors

Metastatic tumors to the testis are rare aside from hematopoeic conditions such as lymphoma or leukemia. The most common primary tumor types reported to metastasize to the testis include: prostate, lung, gastrointestinal tract, melanoma and kidney. Most cases are found incidentally at the time of autopsy.

10. Further Reading

Book Chapters and Websites

Eble eds. Sauter G, Epstein JI, Sesterhenn IA eds. World Health Organization Classification of tumors. Pathology and Genetics of tumors of the Urinary System and Male Genital Organs. Lyon, MA: IARC Press;2004.

National Comprehensive Cancer Network (NCCN) *Clinical Practice Guidelines in Oncology: Testicular Cancer.* v1. 2007. www.nccn.org

Richie JP, Steele G. Neoplasms of the testis. In: Walsh PC, Retik AB, Vaughan ED, Wein AJ, eds. *Campbell's Urology.* Philadelphia, PA: Saunders; 2002:2876-2919.

Ries LAG, Melbert D, Krapcho M, et al, eds. SEER Cancer Statistics Review, 1975-2005, National Cancer Institute. Bethesda, MD, http://seer.cancer.gov/csr/1975_2005/, based on November 2007 SEER data submission, posted to the SEER web site, 2008.

Sheinfeld J, McKiernan J, Bosl GJ. Surgery of testicular tumors. In: Walsh PC, Retik AB, Vaughan ED, Wein AJ, eds. *Campbell's Urology.* Philadelphia, PA: Saunders; 2002:2920-2944.

Histologic Classification

Berthelsen JG, Skakkebaek NE, Sorensen BC, Morgensen P. Screening for carcinoma in situ of the contralateral testis in patients with germinal testicular cancer. *Br Med J.* 1982;285(6536):1683-1686.

Burke AP, Mostofi FK. Spermatocytic seminoma: a clinicopathologic study of 79 cases. *J Urol Pathol.* 1993;1:21-32.

Donadio AC, Motzer RJ, Bajorin DF, et al. Chemotherapy for teratoma with malignant transformation. *J Clin Oncol.* 2003;21(23):4285-4291.

Floyd C, Ayala AG, Logothetis CJ, Silva EG. Spermatocytic seminoma with associated sarcoma of the testis. *Cancer.* 1988;61(2):409-414.

Giwercman A, Thomsen JK, Hertz J, et al. Prevalence of carcinoma in situ of the testis in 207 oligospermic men from infertile couples: prospective study of testicular biopsies. *BMJ.* 1997;315(7114):989-991.

Hoei-Hansen CE, Rajpert-De Meyts E, Daugaard G, Skakkebaek NE. Carcinoma in situ testis, the progenitor of testicular germ cell tumours: a clinical review. *Ann Oncol.* 2005;16(6):863-868.

Holm M, Hoei-Hansen CE, Raipert-De Meyts E, Skakkebaek NE. Increased risk of carcinoma in situ in patients with testicular germ cell cancer with ultrasonic microlithiasis in the contralateral testicle. *J Urol.* 2003;170(4 Pt 1):1163-1167.

Mostofi, FK. Proceedings: Testicular tumors. Epidemiologic, etiologic, and pathologic features. *Cancer.* 1973;32(5):1186-1201.

Motzer RJ, Amsterdam A, Prieto V, et al. Teratoma with malignant degeneration: diverse malignant histologies arising in men with germ cell tumors. *J Urol.* 1998;159(1):133-138.

Peterson AC, Bauman JM, Light DE, McMann LP, Costabile RA. The prevalence of testicular microlithiasis in an asymptomatic population of men 18 to 35 years old. *J Urol.* 2001;166(6): 2061-2064.

Sesterhenn IA, Davis CJ. Pathology of germ cell tumors of the testis. *Cancer Control.* 2004;11(6):374-387.

Skakkebaek NE, Berthelsen JG, Muller J. Carcinoma-in-situ of the undescended testis. *Urol Clin North Am.* 1982;9(3):377-385.

Tickoo SK, Hutchinson B, Bacik J, Mazumdar M, Motzer RJ, Bajorin DF, Bosl GJ, Reuter VE. Testicular seminoma: a clinicopathologic and immunohistochemical study of 105 cases with special reference to seminomas with atypical features. *Int J Surg Pathol.* 2002;10(1):23-32.

Epidemiology, Risk Factors, Presentation and Diagnosis

Che M, Tamboli P, Ro JY, et al. Bilateral testicular germ cell tumors: twenty-year experience at M. D. Anderson Cancer Center. *Cancer*. 2002;95(6):1228-1233.

Daling JR, Doody DR, Sun X, et al. Association of marijuana use and the incidence of testicular germ cell tumors. *Cancer.* 2009 Feb 9. [Epub ahead of print]

Hentrich M, Weber N, Bergsdorf T, Leidl B, Hartenstein R, Gerl A. Management and outcome of bilateral testicular germ cell tumors: Twenty-five year experience in Munich. *Acta Oncol*. 2005;44(6): 529-536.

Holzbeierlein JM, Sogani PC, Sheinfeld J. Histology and clinical outcomes in patients with bilateral testicular germ cell tumors: the Memorial Sloan Kettering Cancer Center experience 1950 to 2001. *J Urol*. 2003;169(6):2122-2125.

Huyghe E, Muller A, Mieusset R, Bujan L, et al. Impact of diagnostic delay in testis cancer: results of a large population-based study. *Eur Urol*. 2007;52(6):1710-1716.

Jemal A, Siegel R, Ward E, et al. Cancer statistics, 2008. *CA Cancer J Clin*. 2008;58(2):71-96.

Pettersson A, Richiardi L, Nordenskjold A, Kaijser M, Akre O. Age at surgery for undescended testis and risk of testicular cancer. *N Engl J Med*. 2007. 3;356(18):1835-1841.

Richie JP, Steele G. Neoplasms of the testis. In: Walsh PC, Retik AB, Vaughan ED, Wein AJ, eds. *Campbell's Urology*. Philadelphia, PA: Saunders; 2002:2876-2919.

Sheinfeld J, McKiernan J, Bosl GJ. Surgery of testicular tumors. In: Walsh PC, Retik AB, Vaughan ED, Wein AJ, eds. *Campbell's Urology*. Philadelphia, PA: Saunders; 2002:2920-2944.

Tuazon E, Banks K, Koh CJ, et al. Re: Prepubertal orchiopexy for cryptorchidism may be associated with lower risk of testicular cancer. *J Urol*. 2008;180(2):783-784; author reply 784-5.

Walsh TJ, Dall'Era MA, Croughan MS, Carroll PR, Turek PJ. Prepubertal orchiopexy for cryptorchidism may be associated with lower risk of testicular cancer. *J Urol*. 2007;178(4 Pt 1):1440-1446.

Clinical Staging

Becherer A, De Santis M, Karanikas G, et al. FDG PET is superior to CT in the prediction of viable tumour in postchemotherapy seminoma residuals. *Eur J Radiol*. 2005;54(2):284-288.

Bruns F, Raub M, Schaefer U, Micke O. No predictive value of beta-hCG in patients with stage I seminoma—results of a long-term follow-up study after adjuvant radiotherapy. *Anticancer Res*. 2005;25(3A): 1543-1546.

Carmignani L, Gadda F, Gazzano G, et al. High incidence of benign testicular neoplasms diagnosed by ultrasound. *J Urol*. 2003;170(5):1783-1786.

Connolly SS, D'Arcy FT, Gough N, McCarthy P, Bredin HC, Corcoran MO. Carefully selected intratesticular lesions can be safely managed with serial ultrasonography. *BJU Int*. 2006;98(5):1005-1007.

De Santis M, Becherer A, Bokemeyer C, et al. 2-18fluoro-deoxy-D-glucose positron emission tomography is a reliable predictor for viable tumor in postchemotherapy seminoma: an update of the prospective multicentric SEMPET trial. *J Clin Oncol*. 2004;22(6):1034-1039.

Flechon A, Bompas E, Biron P, Droz JP. Management of postchemotherapy residual masses in advanced seminoma. *J Urol*. 2002;168(5): 1975-1979.

International Germ Cell Cancer Collaborative Group. International Germ Cell Consensus Classification: a prognostic factor-based staging system for metastatic germ cell cancers. *J Clin Oncol*. 1997;15(2): 594-603.

Johns PL, Lawrentschuk N, Ballok Z, et al. 18F-fluorodeoxyglucose positron emission tomography in evaluation of germ cell tumor after chemotherapy. *Urology*. 2004;64(6):1202-1207.

Muller T, Gozzi C, Akkad T, Pallwein L, Bartsch G, Steiner H. Management of incidental impalpable intratesticular masses of ≤5 mm in diameter. *BJU Int*. 2006;98(5):1001-1004.

Powell TM, Tarter TH. Management of nonpalpable incidental testicular masses. *J Urol*. 2006;176(1):96-98.

Puc HS, Heelan R, Mazumdar M, et al. Management of residual mass in advanced seminoma: results and recommendations from the Memorial Sloan-Kettering Cancer Center. *J Clin Oncol*. 1996;14(2):454-460.

Richie JP, Steele G. Neoplasms of the testis. In: Walsh PC, Retik AB, Vaughan ED, Wein AJ, eds. *Campbell's Urology*. Philadelphia, PA: Saunders; 2002:2876-2919.

Schwartz BF, Auman R, Peretsman SJ, et al. Prognostic value of BHCG and local tumor invasion in stage I seminoma of the testis. *J Surg Oncol*. 1996;61(2):131-133.

Sheynkin YR, Sukkarieh T, Lipke M, Cohen HL, Schulsinger DA. Management of nonpalpable testicular tumors. *Urology*. 2004;63(6):1163-1167.

Sturgeon CM, Duffy MJ, Stenman UH, et al. National Academy of Clinical Biochemestry laboratory medicine practice guidelines for use of tumor markers in testicular, prostate, colorectal, breast, and ovarian cancers. *Clin Chem*. 2008;54(12):e11-e79

Management of the Primary Tumor

Aki FT, Bilen CY, Tekin MI, Ozen H. Is scrotal violation per se a risk factor for local relapse and metastases in stage I nonseminomatous testicular cancer? *Urology*. 2000;56(3):459-462.

Berthelsen JG, Skakkebaek NE, Sorensen BC, Morgensen P: Screening for carcinoma in situ of the contralateral testis in patients with germinal testicular cancer. *Br Med J*. 1982;285(6536):1683-1686.

Capelouto CC, Clark PE, Ransil BJ, Loughlin KR. A review of scrotal violation in testicular cancer: is adjuvant local therapy necessary? *J Urol*. 1995;153(3 Pt 2):981-985.

Carmignani L, Gadda F, Gazzano G, Nerva F, et al. High incidence of benign testicular neoplasms diagnosed by ultrasound. *J Urol*. 2003;170(5):1783-1786.

Christensen TB, Daugaard G, Geertsen PF, von der Masse H. Effect of chemotherapy on carcinoma in situ of the testis. *Ann Oncol*. 1998;9(6):657-660.

Connolly SS, D'Arcy FT, Gough N, McCarthy P, Bredin HC, Corcoran MO. Carefully selected intratesticular lesions can be safely managed with serial ultrasonography. *BJU Int*. 2006;98(5):1005-1007.

Heidenreich A, Weissbach L, Holtl W, Albers P, Kliesch S, Kohrmann KU, Dieckmann KP; German Testicular Cancer Study Group. Organ sparing surgery for malignant germ cell tumor of the testis. *J Urol*. 2001;166(6):2161-2165.

Hinz S, Schrader M, Kempkensteffen C, et al. The role of positron emission tomography in the evaluation of residual masses after chemotherapy for advanced stage seminoma. *J Urol*. 2008 Mar;179(3):936-940; discussion 940. Epub 2008 Jan 22.

Leibovitch I, Baniel J, Foster RS, Donohue JP. The clinical implications of procedural deviations during orchiectomy for nonseminomatous testis cancer. *J Urol*. 1995;154(3):935-939.

Leibovitch I, Little JS Jr, Foster RS, Rowland RG, Bihrle R, Donohue JP. Delayed orchiectomy after chemotherapy for metastatic nonseminomatous germ cell tumors. *J Urol*. 1996;155(3):952-954.

Muller T, Gozzi C, Akkad T, Pallwein L, Bartsch G, Steiner H. Management of incidental impalpable intratesticular masses of ≤5 mm in diameter. *BJU Int*. 2006;98(5):1001-1004.

Ondrus D, Hornak M, Breza J, et al. Delayed orchiectomy after chemotherapy in patients with advanced testicular cancer. *Int Urol Nephrol*. 2001;32(4):665-667.

Petersen PM, Giwercman A, Daugaard G, et al. Effect of graded testicular doses of radiotherapy in patients treated for carcinoma-in-situ in the testis. *J Clin Oncol*. 2002;20(6):1537-1543.

Powell TM, Tarter TH. Management of nonpalpable incidental testicular masses. *J Urol*. 2006;176(1): 96-98.

Sheinfeld J, McKiernan J, Bosl GJ. Surgery of testicular tumors. In: Walsh PC, Retik AB, Vaughan ED, Wein AJ, eds. *Campbell's Urology*. Philadelphia, PA: Saunders; 2002:2920-2944.

Skakkebaek NE, Berthelsen JG, Muller J. Carcinoma-in-situ of the undescended testis. *Urol Clin North Am*. 1982;9(3):377-385.

Steiner H, Holtl L, Maneschg C, Berger AP, Rogatsch H, Bartsch G, Hobisch A. Frozen section analysis-guided organ-sparing approach in testicular tumors: technique, feasibility, and long-term results. *Urology*. 2003;62(3):508-513.

Retroperitoneal Lymph Node Dissection (RPLND)

Abdel-Aziz KF, Anderson JK, Svatek R, Margulis V, Sagalowski AI, Cadeddu JA. Laparoscopic and open retroperitoneal lymph-node dissection for clinical stage I nonseminomatous germ-cell testis tumors. *J Endourol*. 2006;20(9):627-631.

Albers P, Seiner R, Krege S, et al. Randomized phase III trial comparing retroperitoneal lymph node dissection with one course of bleomycin and etoposide plus cisplatin chemotherapy in the adjuvant treatment of clinical stage I Nonseminomatous testicular germ cell tumors: AUO trial AH 01/94 by the German Testicular Cancer Study Group. J Clin Oncol. 2008;26(18):2966-2972.

Albqami N, Janetschek G. Laparoscopic retroperitoneal lymph-node dissection in the management of clinical stage I and II testicular cancer. *J Endourol*. 2005;19(6):683-692.

Donohue JP, Zachary JM, Maynard BR. Distribution of nodal metastases in nonseminomatous testis cancer. *J Urol*. 1982;128(2):315-320.

Donohue JP, Foster RS, Rowland RG, Bihrle R, Jones J, Geier G. Nerve-sparing retroperitoneal lymphadenectomy with preservation of ejaculation. *J Urol*. 1990;144(2 Pt 1):287-291.

Eggener SE, Carver BS, Sharp DS, Motzer RJ, Bosl GJ, Sheinfeld J. Incidence of disease outside modified retroperitoneal lymph node dissection templates in clinical Stage I or IIA nonseminomatous germ cell testicular cancer. *J Urol*. 2007;177(3): 937-943.

Evans JG, Speiss PE, Kamat AM, et al. Chylous ascites after postchemotherapy retroperitoneal lymph node dissection: review of the M.D. Anderson experience. *J Urol*. 2006;176(4 Pt 1):1463-1467.

Janetschek G, Hobisch A, Peschel R, Hittmair A, Bartsch G. Laparoscopic retroperitoneal lymph node dissection for clinical stage I nonseminomatous testicular carcinoma: long-term outcome. *J Urol*. 2000;163(6):1793-1796.

Poulakis V, Skriapas K, de Vries R, et al. Laparoscopic retroperitoneal lymph node dissection: does it still have a role in the management of clinical stage I nonseminomatous testis cancer? A European perspective. *Eur Urol*. 2008;54(5):1004-1015.

Rassweiler JJ, Scheitlin W, Heidenreich A, Laguna MP, Janetschek G. Laparoscopic retroperitoneal lymph node dissection: does it still have a role in the management of clinical stage I nonseminomatous testis cancer? A European perspective. Eur Urol. 2008;54(5):1004-1015.

Ray B, Hajdu SI, Whitmore WF Jr. Proceedings: Distribution of retroperitoneal lymph node metastases in testicular germinal tumors. *Cancer.* 1974;33(2):340-348.

Sheinfeld J, McKiernan J, Bosl GJ. Surgery of testicular tumors. In: Walsh PC, Retik AB, Vaughan ED, Wein AJ, eds. *Campbell's Urology.* Philadelphia, PA: Saunders; 2002:2920-2944.

Steiner H, Peschel R, Janetschek G, et al. Long-term results of laparoscopic retroperitoneal lymph node dissection: a single-center 10-year experience. *Urology.* 2004;63(3):550-555.

Stephenson AJ, Bosl GJ, Motzer RJ, et al. Retroperitoneal lymph node dissection for nonseminomatous germ cell testicular cancer: impact of patient selection factors on outcome. *J Clin Oncol.* 2005;23(12):
2781-2788.

Weinstein M. Lymphatic drainage of the testes. *Atlas Urol Clin North Am.* 1999;7:1-7.

Weissbach L, Boedefeld EA. Localization of solitary and multiple metastases in stage II nonseminomatous testis tumor as basis for a modified staging lymph node dissection in stage I. *J Urol.* 1987;138(1):77-82.

Management of Nonseminoma

Amato RJ, Ro JY, Ayala AG, Swanson DA. Risk-adapted treatment for patients with clinical stage I nonseminomatous germ cell tumor of the testis. *Urology.* 2004;63(1):144-148.

Baniel J, Foster RS, Gonin R, Messemer JE, Donohue JP, Einhorn LH. Late relapse of testicular cancer. *J Clin Oncol.* 1995;13(5):1170-1176.

Brenner PC, Herr HW, Morse MJ, et al. Simultaneous retroperitoneal, thoracic, and cervical resection of postchemotherapy residual masses in patients with metastatic nonseminomatous germ cell tumors of the testis. *J Clin Oncol.* 1996;14:1765-1769.

Carver BS, Shayegan B, Serio A, Motzer RJ, Bosl GJ, Sheinfeld J. Long-term clinical outcome after postchemotherapy retroperitoneal lymph node dissection in men with residual teratoma. *J Clin Oncol.* 2007 Jan 29; [Epub ahead of print].

Cullen MH, Stenning SP, Parkinson MC, et al. Short-course adjuvant chemotherapy in high-risk stage I nonseminomatous germ cell tumors of the testis: a Medical Research Council report. *J Clin Oncol.* 1996;14(4):1106-1113.

Donohue JP, Leibovitch I, Foster RS, Baniel J, Tognoni P. Integration of surgery and systemic therapy: results and principles of integration. *Semin Urol Oncol.* 1998;16(2):65-71.

Fox EP, Weathers TD, Williams SD, et al. Outcome analysis for patients with persistent nonteratomatous germ cell tumor in postchemotherapy retroperitoneal lymph node dissections. *J Clin Oncol.* 1993;11:1294-1299.

Gels ME, Hoekstra HJ, Sleijfer DT, et al. Thoracotomy for postchemotherapy resection of pulmonary residual tumor mass in patients with nonseminomatous testicular germ cell tumors: aggressive surgical resection is justified. *Chest.* 1997;112:967-973.

Heidenreich A, Schenkmann NS, Sesterhenn IA, et al. Immunohistochemical expression of Ki-67 to predict lymph node involvement in clinical stage I nonseminomatous germ cell tumors. *J Urol.* 1997;158(2):620-625.

Heidenreich A, Sesterhenn IA, Mostofi FK, Moul JW. Prognostic risk factors that identify patients with clinical stage I nonseminomatous germ cell tumors at low risk and high risk for metastasis. *Cancer.* 1998;83(5):1002-1011.

Logothetis CJ, Samuels ML, Trindade A, Johnson DE. The growing teratoma syndrome. *Cancer.* 1982;50(8):1629-1635.

Motzer RJ, Amsterdam A, Prieto V,et al. Teratoma with malignant degeneration: diverse malignant histologies arising in men with germ cell tumors. *J Urol*. 1998;159(1):133-138.

Pohar KS, Rabbani F, Bosl GJ, Motzer RJ, Bajorin D, Sheinfeld J. Results of retroperitoneal lymph node dissection for clinical stage I and II pure embryonal carcinoma of the testis. *J Urol*. 2003;170(4 Pt 1):1155-1158.

Sexton WJ, Wood CG, Kim R, Pisters LL. Repeat retroperitoneal lymph node dissection for metastatic testis cancer. *J Urol*. 2003 Apr;169(4):1353-1356.

Sogani PC, Perrotti M, Herr HW, Fair WR, Thaler HT, Bosl G. Clinical stage I testis cancer: long-term outcome of patients on surveillance. *J Urol*. 1998;159(3):855-858.

Stephenson AJ, Bosl GJ, Motzer RJ, et al. Retroperitoneal lymph node dissection for nonseminomatous germ cell testicular cancer: impact of patient selection factors on outcome. *J Clin Oncol*. 2005;23(12):
2781-2788.

Vergouwe Y, Steyerberg EW, Eijkemans MJ, Albers P, Habbema JD. Predictors of occult metastasis in clinical stage I nonseminoma: a systematic review. *J Clin Oncol*. 2003;21(22):4092-4099.

Williams SD, Stablein DM, Einhorn LH, et al. Immediate adjuvant chemotherapy versus observation with treatment at relapse in pathological stage II testicular cancer. *N Engl J Med*. 1987;317(23):1433-1438.

Management of Seminoma

Aparicio J, Germa JR, Garcia del Muro X, Maroto P, Arranz JA, Saenz A. Risk-adapted management for patients with clinical stage I seminoma: the Second Spanish Germ Cell Cancer Cooperative Group study. *J Clin Oncol*. 2005;23(34):8717-8723.

Dossmann M, Zagars G. Postorchiectomy radiotherapy for stages I and II testicular seminoma. *Int J Radiat Oncol Biol Phys*. 1993;26:382-390.

Flechon A, Bompas E, Biron P, Droz JP. Management of postchemotherapy residual masses in advanced seminoma. *J Urol*. 2002;168(5):
1975-1979.

Fossa SD, Horwich A, Russell JM, et al. Optimal planning target volume for stage I testicular seminoma: A Medical Research Council randomized trial. Medical Research Council Testicular Tumor Working Group. *J Clin Oncol*. 1999;17(4):1146.

Jones WG, Fossa SD, Mead GM, et al. Randomized trial of 30 versus 20 Gy in the adjuvant treatment of stage I Testicular Seminoma: a report on Medical Research Council Trial TE18, European Organization for the Research and Treatment of Cancer Trial 30942. *J Clin Oncol* 2005;23:1200-1208.

International Germ Cell Cancer Collaborative Group. International Germ Cell Consensus Classification: a prognostic factor-based staging system for metastatic germ cell cancers. *J Clin Oncol*. 1997;15(2):594-603.

Oliver RT, Mason MD, Mead GM, et al. Radiotherapy versus single-dose carboplatin in adjuvant treatment of stage I seminoma: a randomised trial. *Lancet*. 2005;366(9482):293-300.

Puc HS, Heelan R, Mazumdar M, Herr H, et al. Management of residual mass in advanced seminoma: results and recommendations from the Memorial Sloan-Kettering Cancer Center. *J Clin Oncol*. 1996;14(2):454-460.

Travis LB, Fossa SD, Schonfeld SJ, et al. Second cancers among 40,576 testicular cancer patients: focus on long-term survivors. *J Natl Cancer Inst*. 2005;97(18):1354-1365.

von der Masse H, Specht L, et al. Surveillance following orchidectomy for stage I seminoma of the testis. *Eur J Cancer*. 1993;29A(14):1931-1934.

Warde P, Gospodarowicz MK, Panzarella T, et al. Stage I testicular seminoma:results of adjuvant radiation and surveillance. *J Clin Oncol*. 1995;13:
2255-2262.

Warde P, Jewett MA. Surveillance for stage I testicular seminoma. Is it a good option? *Urol Clin North Am*. 1998;25(3):425-433.

Warde P, Specht L, Horwich A, et al. Prognostic factors for relapse in stage I seminoma managed by surveillance: a pooled analysis. *J Clin Oncol*. 2002;20(22):4448-4452.

Sex Cord / Gonadal Stromal Tumors

Dilworth J, Farrow G, Oesterlin J. Non-germ cell tumors of the testis. *Urology* 1991; 37:399-412.

Conkey DS, Howard GC, Grigor KM, et al. Testicular sex cord-stromal tumours: the Edinburgh experiencee 1988-2002, and review of the literature. *Clin Oncol*. 2005;17:322-327.

Grem JL, Robins HI, Wilson KS, et al. Metastatic Leydig cell tumor of the testis: report of three cases and review of the literature. *Cancer*. 1986;58:2116-2119.

Ulbright TM, Amin MB, Young RH. Tumors of the testis, andexa, spermatic cord and scrotum. *Atlas of tumor pathology, farc 25, ser 3*. Washington, DC: Armed Forces Institute of Pathology. 1999: 1-290.

Chapter 21: Benign Prostatic Hyperplasia and Bladder Calculi

James C. Ulchaker, MD, FACS
Alexis E. Te, MD

Contents

1. Epidemiology, Pathophysiology and Natural History of BPH

Benign prostatic hyperplasia (BPH) is one of the most common diseases of elderly men. It often is associated with lower urinary tract symptoms (LUTS) that interfere with normal daily activities and sleep patterns. The prevalence of BPH is dependent upon age, with initial development usually after age 40. By age 60, the prevalence of BPH is greater than 50% and by age 85 it is as high as 90%. The prevalence of bothersome symptoms also increases with age. About half of all men who have a histologic diagnosis have moderate to severe LUTS.[1]

Long-term data from population based studies have recently become available, yet the risks of complications and morbidities from untreated BPH remain uncertain. It is unclear whether a patient with a specific symptom complex will develop complete urinary retention over a certain period of time. Many patients are bothered by LUTS with varying degrees of bother even with the same frequency and severity of symptoms. Generally, patient perception of BPH severity, as well as the degree of interference with the patient's lifestyle, should be the primary consideration in choosing appropriate therapy.

BPH is defined by histologic evidence of stromoglandular hyperplasia. BPH is not mutually inclusive with LUTS, which is defined by the presence of irritative and/or obstructive symptoms, or with bladder outlet obstruction (BOO), which is defined by the presence of urodynamic obstruction.

The natural history of BPH shows that symptoms worsen in 55% of patients, remain stable in 30% of patients and improve in 15% of patients.[2] Prostate size increases with age at a rate of 0.6 mL/year.[3] Men with prostate volume >40 cc are 3 times as likely to have elevated symptoms, twice as likely to be bothered by symptoms and twice as likely to experience interference with normal daily activities.[4] Men with prostate size >30 cc have a 3-fold risk for acute urinary retention (AUR).[5] The estimated prostate growth rates increase by 1.6% per year across all ages.[6] Higher baseline prostate volume is associated with higher rates of prostate growth.

The risk factors for prostatectomy are a change in size and force of stream, a sensation of incomplete voiding and enlarged prostate on digital rectal exam.[7] The risk of AUR/prostate surgery increases with the number of risk factors—1 risk factor (9%), 2 risk factors (16%) and 3 risk factors (37%). Men over age 70 years with 3 risk factors have 11 times higher risk than men aged 40 years.[5] Complications of BPH progression include worsening of symptoms, such as increase in bother and decrease in quality of life. Clinical progression can also result in retention, hematuria, urinary tract infection (UTI), bladder stones and renal failure, which may require surgical intervention.[8] Treatment of BPH is based on relieving bladder outlet resistance to increase urinary flow rate.

The pathophysiology of BPH and resulting lower urinary tract symptoms of BPH are intertwined. The basic pathophysiology of benign prostatic hyperplasia at the cellular level that leads to overall gland enlargement has not been well elucidated but is clearly dependent on hormonal factors and other related growth factors. The growth and maintenance of the prostate gland is dependent on dihydrotestosterone and is affected by changes in hormonal environment from aging. Such changes occur in testosterone, estrogen and other growth factors which influence apoptosis and prostate growth. These changes may also affect prostate tissue composition of stromoglandular epithelial hyperplasia as well as alpha adrenergic tone and innervation. The over all impact of these factors results in overall gland enlargement. However, the prostate gland can be anatomically divided into several zones: the peripheral zone, the central zone and the transition zone. The changes in prostate size and muscle tone, mainly in the central and transition zone which surround the urethra, affect urinary flow through the prostatic urethra, narrowing the flow and creating bladder outflow obstruction. This functional urodynamic obstruction produces compensative changes in bladder that increase bladder pressure to overcome the outlet resistance. This results in a progressive detrusor hypertrophy with resulting decrease in compliance and capacity over time. Detrusor overactivity can also occur from this process. Overall, these changes produce symptoms of frequency, urgency, nocturia, slow urinary stream and incomplete emptying that potentially can progress to urinary retention.[9]

2. Evaluation of BPH and LUTS

Current medical therapies for BPH include alpha adrenergic blockers, which reduce sympathetic tone, and 5-alpha reductase (5AR) inhibitors, which reduce volume. Thermotherapies, which include needle ablation, microwave therapy, water induced thermotherapy, and laser treatments, reduce volume and open channels. Surgery, such as transurethral resection of the prostate (TURP) and open prostatectomy, remove volume and open channels. All of these treatments seek to improve urinary flow and symptoms by reducing bladder outlet obstruction.

Brief Summary of the AUA BPH Guidelines

In 2006, the American Urological Association updated the BPH recommendations of the 1994 clinical practice guidelines. The new guidelines make minimal modifications to the recommended diagnostic methods for detecting and assessing the severity of BPH, based on expert clinical judgment. The guidelines update existing statements on patient management. Extensive literature searches were conducted, and critical reviews and syntheses were used to evaluate empirical evidence and significant outcomes of all currently available treatment approaches.

The new AUA guidelines provide an algorithm (Figure 1) as a framework for diagnosis and treatment of BPH. Individual patients may present differently, so clinicians should exercise clinical judgment and act in the patient's best interest.[10]

Noninvasive Evaluation

The treatment of bladder outflow obstruction can be improved by using urodynamic parameters. However, all rationally designed studies for BPH should incorporate a relevant medical history focusing on the nature and duration of symptoms, previous surgical procedures, sexual function and current medications. A focused physical examination should be performed of the suprapubic area, including a digital rectal exam. An AUA symptom score and bother score, urinalysis, free urinary flow rate, postvoid residual (PVR), PSA, when appropriate, and voiding diary should also be performed.

Free uroflowometry is an objective efficacy parameter consistently utilized in evaluation of BPH therapies. It may predict response to therapy, especially surgery, using a maximum flow rate (Q_{max}) of <10 mL/sec, which is consistent with obstruction, vs. a Q_{max}>15 mL/sec and LUTS, which is consistent with a non-BPH diagnosis. There are test-retest variability issues, and there is no established flow rate cut off value, and no predictive value for medical therapeutic response.

PVR is an excellent indication of bladder emptying. It may prompt additional testing, including renal ultrasound and creatinine levels. There is

Figure 1

American Urological Association BPH treatment guidelines

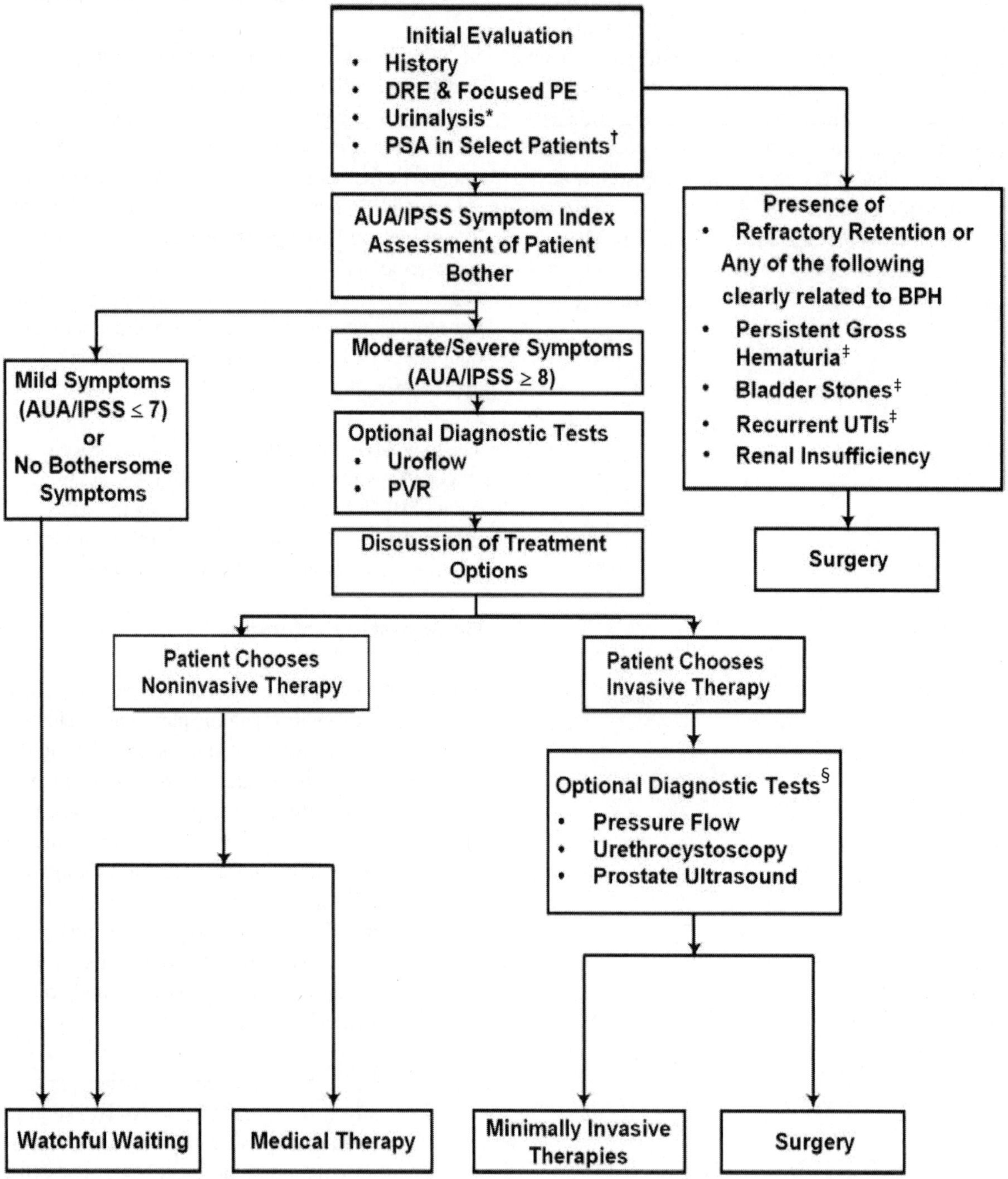

** In patients with clinically significant prostatic bleeding, a course of a 5 alpha-reductase inhibitor may be used. If bleeding persists, tissue ablative surgery is indicated.*

† Patients with at least a 10-year life expectancy for whom knowledge of the presence of prostate cancer would change management or patients for whom the PSA measurement may change the management of voiding symptoms

‡ After exhausting other therapeutic options as discussed in detail in the text.

§ Some diagnostic tests are used in predicting response to therapy. Pressure-flow studies are most useful in men prior to surgery.

AUA, American Urological Association; DRE, digital rectal exam; IPSS, International Prostate Symptom Score; PE, physical exam; PSA, prostate specific antigen; PVR, postvoid residual urine; UTI, urinary tract infection considerable within patient variability, which limits the predictive value of PVR. There is no proven correlation between PVR and the development of UTIs in patients with obstruction.

No definitive volume guidelines exist. Clinicians may monitor patients with watchful waiting or use medical therapy for patients with high PVR. There is an increased risk of overall progression, symptom progression, and AUR in higher PVR groups.[11]

The pivotal Medical Therapy of Prostatic Symptoms (MTOPS) study concluded that high baseline PVR predicts progression in placebo treated, but not actively treated, patients. Patients experiencing AUR had higher PVR at baseline and on treatment, and at their last visit before an event in all treatment groups. However, compared to age, prostate specific antigen (PSA) and prostate volume, PVR is a weak predictor of progression.[11]

Role of Pressure Flow Studies

Urodynamics have a utility in assessing bladder function and confirming bladder outlet obstruction in men with LUTS. BPH associated with BOO may cause LUTS. Patients with BPH have a greater risk to develop urinary retention. More than 10% of men in their 70s will experience AUR. While it makes sense that those with severe BOO are at highest risk for retention, clinical utility of pressure flow studies in the management of LUTS and BPH is controversial and currently not recommended for routine use.

However, pressure flow studies are the best modality available to diagnose obstruction. They provide an understanding between BPH, LUTS and BOO, are useful in monitoring therapy and assessing morbidity, and are good for counseling patients about postoperative expectations. Basic pressure flow studies are performed by measuring simultaneously bladder pressure with a catheter placed transurethrally, abdominal pressure with a catheter placed transrectally, and a urinary flow meter. Generally, bladder outlet obstruction is defined by simultaneous high bladder pressure and low urinary flow rate. Several nomograms are utilized to grade obstruction such as the Abram-Griffith nomogram. More invasive procedures, such as transrectal ultrasound (TRUS) and prostate biopsy, can confirm prostate size, confirm prostate anatomy for invasive therapy, assess the presence of intravesical component, assess the presence and size of the middle lobe, assess the risk of progression and assess the presence of prostate cancer.

Endoscopic evaluation of the lower urinary tract is not recommended in an otherwise healthy male with an initial evaluation consistent with BOO, unless the treatment alternatives being contemplated depend on the anatomical configuration of the prostate, or hematuria is present.

Are flow rates, PVRs, TRUS, prostate biopsy and urodynamics necessary? Some points clinicians need to consider when making a decision about BPH evaluations include: reproducibility; correlation with symptoms severity and improvement; studies to refine technique and usefulness; the need for surgical intervention or diagnosis; and monitoring for efficacy and morbidity risk. Are these evaluations necessary? They definitely are useful and integral to BPH management.[12]

BPH treatment is symptom driven. The goals of treatment are to relieve LUTS, treat BOO, and to treat and prevent morbidities, including retention, UTIs, obstructive uropathy and stones. The basis for treatment is decreasing bladder outlet resistance/obstruction. While symptom severity does not correlate well with urodynamic obstruction severity, removing the obstruction often results in symptom relief. Urodynamic obstruction severity correlates well with morbidities, such as retention, obstructive uropathy, hematuria, infection and stones.

Factors to consider in the treatment of BPH include the symptom severity based on AUA guidelines, risk reduction in morbidity and progression, the patients overall health and age/life expectancy, expected durability of symptom relief, treatment side effects, whether the treatment is reversible (medications) or permanent (surgery), and the patient's needs and expectations.

Before initiating any threapy, one must first discuss behavioral modifications that may contribute to voiding dysfunction, such as concomitant drugs, regulation of fluid intake (especially in the evening), lifesyle changes and dietary advice (especially the avoidance of excess alcohol, caffeine and highly seasoned or irritative foods).

Medical Therapy Mechanism of Action

Medical therapy is designed to either relax the prostate gland with alpha blockers or to shrink the gland with 5AR inhibitors. Alpha blockers have a dynamic component by relaxing the prostate smooth muscle and bladder neck, decreasing overall prostatic tone, and improving urinary flow rate and therefore symptoms. 5AR inhibitors affect the static component by decreasing prostate size, improving urinary flow rate, and improving symptoms. Although more gradual than alpha blockers, 5AR inhibitors not only shrink the prostate but also stunt prostate growth, and therefore affect the natural history of BPH and delay progression of disease. Both types of drugs can decrease detrussor pressure by 10 cm H_2O and cause a mild decrease in BOO. Symptom relief is provided via increased Q_{max} and decreased PVR, as well as influencing receptor factors (eg, innervation, such as alpha 1D and antimuscarinic). A little bit goes a long way to relieving symptoms, but may be too late or not enough to relieve symptoms or impact morbidity risk leading to more invasive therapeutic options.

The Old vs. New Alpha-Adrenergic Blockers

The original alpha-adrenergic blockers, such as prazosin, terazosin and doxazosin, were initially FDA-approved for the indication of hypertension. The original formulations required dose titration for BPH indications due to the risk of orthostatic hypotension, dizziness and fatigue. Advancements in uroselectivity via receptor selectivity (alpha 1A and D) and sustained release formulations influencing the pharmacokinetic release profile have progressed the concept of uroselectivity. At least 3 discrete alpha 1 adrenergic subtypes have been identified.[13,14] In general, alpha 1A receptor blockers affect the prostate, alpha 1B blockers affect vascular tone, and alpha 1D blockers affect the bladder. This concept led to the development of uroselective drugs with minimal vascular side effect profiles and effective once a day formulations that do not require titration, such as tamsulosin and alfuzosin. In the current AUA BPH guidelines, at the FDA-approved dosage, efficacy is presumed to be equivalent among all FDA-approved BPH alpha-adrenergic blockers: terazosin, doxazosin, tamsulosin and alfuzosin. The differences between the various alpha-adrenergic blockers appear to lie in their tolerability and side effect profiles (Table 1).

Prevention and Treatment Role of 5-Alpha Reductase Inhibitors

Prostate growth and maintenance is dependent on male androgens. Dihydrotestosterone is the main active male hormone affecting prostate growth and development. Testosterone is converted to dihydrotestosterone by 5-alpha reductase (5AR). Two 5AR isoenzymes have been identified that convert testosterone to dihydrotestosterone (Table 2). The first 5-alpha reductase blocker is finasteride, which is only a type 2 5AR inhibitor. Type 2 actions are mainly in the prostate gland and account for about 70% of dihydrotestosterone production. The other and more recently marketed 5AR inhibitor is dutasteride. This drug is a dual inhibitor, blocking both type 1 and type 2 5-alpha reductase. With this drug's current formulation and long half-life,

Table 1

Alpha-Adrenergic Blockers for BPH

Agent	Receptor Selectivity	Plasma t 1/2	Extended Release Formulation	Duration of Action	Inhibitor Mechanism
Phenoxybenzamine	$\alpha 1$, $\alpha 2$	24 hr		72-96 hr	Irreversible
Prazosin	$\alpha 1$	2-3 hr		4-6 hr	Reversible
Terazosin	$\alpha 1$	2-4 hr		Up to 18 hr	Reversible
Doxazosin	$\alpha 1$	22 hr	yes	Up to 24 hr	Reversible
Tamsulosin	$\alpha 1$	14-5 hr	yes	Up to 24 hr	Reversible
Alfuzosin	$\alpha 1$	3-10 hr	yes	Up to 24 hr	Reversible

dihydrotestosterone is lowered by greater than 90%. Both drugs have demonstrated efficacy and durability in long term responders and, more importantly, have been demonstrated to decrease progression not only of symptoms, but also towards retention and surgery. Both drugs will lower the serum PSA by approximately 50%, and may have the side effects of diminished ejacualation and libido, and erectile dysfunction. They are primarily indicated in symptomatic patients with prostate size greater than 30 mL or PSA greater than 1.4 ng/mL.[15,16]

MTOPS: The Role of Combination Therapy

The large MTOPS clinical trial found that a combination of the 2 drugs finasteride and doxazosin was significantly more effective than either drug alone for preventing progression of BPH, especially in men at high risk for disease progression.[17,18] Finasteride, a 5AR inhibitor, and doxazosin, an alpha-1 receptor blocker, together reduced the overall risk of BPH progression by 66% compared to placebo. The combined drugs also provided the greatest symptom relief and improvement in urinary flow rate. Doxazosin alone reduced overall risk of progression by 39% and finasteride alone by 34% compared to placebo. The combination treatment and finasteride alone also significantly reduced the risk of invasive therapy by 67% and 64%, respectively. (Doxazosin did not reduce the long term risk of invasive therapy.) Most invasive treatments in MTOPS were transurethral or open surgeries to remove prostate tissue. Other invasive therapies included transurethral incision, microwave or laser therapy, and prostatic stents.

MTOPS found that combination therapy was especially effective in men with prostates larger than 40 cc or serum PSAs above 4 ng/mL.[18] The study shows that combination therapy offers dramatically greater and longer lasting relief from symptoms and, over time, that 5 AR inhibitors shrink the prostate and actually prevent growth so that fewer men are at higher risk for progression of symptoms, developing retention, and proceeding to surgery. This study is a benchmark for identifying men at risk for BPH progression, and who may benefit most from combination therapy. The study helps alleviate the concern that medical treatment might initially relieve symptoms but mask problems related to continuing prostate growth (Table 3).

Table 2

5-Alpha Reductase Inhibitors

Finasteride	
Inhibits type 2 5AR	
Reduces Serum DHT levels by about 70%	
Reduces intraprostatic DHT levels by about 80%	
Reduces serum PSA by about 50%	
6-8 hour half-life	
Dutasteride	
Inhibits both type 1 and type 2 5AR	
Reduces serum DHT levels by more than 90%	
Reduces intraprostatic DHT levels by more than 90%	
Reduces serum PSA by about 50%	
5 week serum half-life	

Ekman P. Drug Safety. *1998;18:161-170. Ekman P.* Scand J Urol Nephrol. *1999;(suppl 203):15-20. Bartsch G, et al.* Eur Urol. *2000;37:367-380. Bartsch G, et al.* World J Urol. *2002;19:413-425.*

The large CombAT study is an ongoing, multicenter, randomized, double-blind, parallel group study, evaluating whether the combination of dutasteride and tamsulosin is more effective than either monotherapy alone for improving symptoms and longterm outcomes in men with moderate to severe LUTS and BPO. To date, 2-year analysis is available. It also confirms that combination therapy provides a significantly greater degree of benefit than either drug alone.[19]

Complementary Therapies: Phytotherapies or Nutriceuticals?

More and more men with symptoms of BPH are treating themselves with phytotherapies or nutriceuticals sold over the counter. Two of the most commonly used phytotherapies are *Serenoa repens* (saw palmetto) and *Pygeum africanum*. Little is known about the long term effects of these agents, and most American physicians are reluctant to discuss or recommend them to patients because only a modest number of published reports have appeared in the peer reviewed medical literature. The available literature supports the hypothesis that these compounds may have some beneficial effects on BPH symptoms, but there are no statistically significant reports of rigorously conducted clinical trials on the long term effects (both beneficial and adverse) and on patient-reported outcomes.

To fill the gap in this information, the National Institutes of Health organized a randomized, double blind clinical trial called Complementary and Alternative Medicine for Urological Symptoms (CAMUS). The objective of the study is to analyze whether *Serenoa repens* (saw palmetto) impacts clinically on clinical BPH.[20]

Role of Anticholinergic Therapy with LUTS

There is a high prevalence of overactive bladder (OAB) in men, and the symptoms are often bothersome. OAB and BPH often coexist. Irritative symptoms can persist after BPH treatment. Men with LUTS/BPH are generally treated with alpha blockers, but may also have OAB. Men treated for BOO and BPH with alpha blockers and surgical therapy can continue to have persistent OAB symptoms.

Antimuscarinic therapy has shown statistically significant effectiveness on OAB symptoms in men. Men with LUTS and confirmed BOO are generally initially treated first for BPH/ LUTS. An antimuscarinic can be added as appropriate if OAB symptoms persist. Several published studies demonstrate antimuscarinic agents such as tolterodine can be utilized effectively for symptom treatment of men with no increased risk for AUR.[21-24] Although tolterodine has been the single agent recently evaluated in studies specifically for the symptomatic treatment of men, many agents have historically been utilized in the symptomatic treatment of men, including agents such as oxybutynin. Many OAB trials have also included men in their treatment population and many studies are under way that are evaluating the symptomatic treatment of men with many other available antimuscarinic agents approved for the indication of OAB. However, monitoring of PVRs is probably a wise precaution when utilizing antimuscarinic agents in men at risk for retention.[21, 25, 26–27]

4. Interventional Therapies

The rationale for interventional therapies for the treatment of BPH to improve lower urinary tract symptoms or treat urinary retention is based on relieving bladder outlet obstruction due to the prostate growth impingement on the prostatic urethra. Traditionally, for decades, the standard of care was to offer either transurethral resection of the prostate (TURP) or open prostatectomy to reduce prostatic bladder outlet obstruction. These procedures are associated with well-known quality of life complications, such as impotence and incontinence, as well as life-threatening complications, such as bleeding with a well-defined but low mortality rate. As a result, a plethora of alternative options have developed, from medical therapy to minimally invasive therapy to traditional surgical therapy. The options and alternatives are many (Table 4).

Table 3

Summary of Large North American Studies that Evaluated 5-Alpha Reductase Monotherapy

	Finsteride Study Group[1]	VA Cooperative[2]	PLESS[3]	MTOPS[4]	Dutasteride Multicenter[5]
Year published	1992	1996	1998	2002	2002
Follow-up (years)	1	1	4	5	2
Number of patients	895	1229	3040	3047	4325
Mean Prostate Volume	59	36.2	54	31.2	55
Change in AUASS	1.7	NS	2	1	2.2
Change in Qmax	1.8	NS	1.7	0.8	1.6
RR in AUR	NR	NR	57	66	57
RR in BPH surgery	NR	NR	55	62	48

NS = not significant; NR = not reported

1. *Gromley GJ, et al.* N Engl J Med. *1992;327:1185-1191.*
2. *Lepor H, et al.* N Engl J Med . *1996;335:533-539.*
3. *McConnell JD, et al.* N Engl J Med. *1998;338:557-563.*
4. *McConnell J, et al.* N Engl J Med. *2003;349:2387-98.*
5. *Roehrborn, et al.* Urology. *2002;60:434-441.*

Office Analgesia

Physicians use their own discretion in choosing an analgesic. Risks increase as the physician moves from 2% intraurethral Xylocaine® jelly (transurethral instillation) to non-steroidal anti-inflammatory drugs (NSAIDs) and analgesics in combination with sedative/hypnotics (IM/PO); perineal or transrectal pro-static block; IV sedation (for example with morphine and/or versed); and spinal or epidural anesthesia. Light general anesthesia and general anesthesia are the most risky in the office setting.

Many office-based analgesia therapies are available:

- Preop medications—Ativan®, Vicoprofen®, Celebrex®, Ditropan XL®
- Periop medications—Intravesical chilled lidocaine/marcaine solution, Ultracet®, hyoscyamine, intraurethral lidocaine
- Postop medications—Alpha blockers, such as Flomax®, Uroxatral®, Vioxx®, ibuprofen or other NSAIDs
- Also available are local anesthetic blocks, prostate blocks and pudendal nerve blocks

Office-based analgesia generally does not include intravenous sedation, but if applied should include monitored anesthesia support. A variety of oral anxiolytic agents and analgesics are available, as well as local infiltrating anesthesia agents. Awareness of toxicity dosage is important as well as monitoring of patients after the procedure is completed. Cardiopulmonary arrest support equipment is necessary, and one should be aware of vasovagal events. Vital signs monitoring is also important as well as proper consideration of anesthesia surgical assessment risk when treating patients in the outpatient setting.

Thermotherapies

Invasive management of BPH has changed over the past 15 years, with the number of cases of transurethral resection of the prostate (TURP) decreasing from more than 250,000 per year to about 100,000 per year. Minimally invasive thermotherapy has become an option to surgical, as well as, medical therapy. It offers acceptable efficacy with tolerability and a low threat of adverse events, and expands the treatment population.

Table 4

Invasive Treatment Options for BPH

Minimally Invasive Thermotherapy
Nonsite specific therapies TUMT® (transurethral microwave thermotherapy) 4 commercial variations
WIT™ (Water-Induced Thermotherapy)
Debulking Minimally Invasive Surgery
TVP® (transurethral electrovaporization)
PVP (photoselective laser vaporization)
HoLEP (holmium laser enucleation)
HoLAP™ (holmium laser ablation)
Saline bipolar TURP
TUIP (transurethral incision of prostate)
Site-specific Therapies
Electrical radiofrequency ablation TUNA™ (transurethral needle ablation)
Laser ILC (interstitial laser coagulation)
Major Surgery
TURP
Open prostatectomy

Treatment Principles of Thermotherapies

Dependent on the temperature that is reached in the tissue, a clinician can either coagulate or vaporize tissue. A photothermal effect is induced when the tissue temperature stays below 100° C, and tissue gets coagulated. Photoablative (vaporization) effects occur when the tissue temperature reaches past the boiling point of 100° C, and tissue is vaporized. The total energy delivered during lesion formation (measured in joules) is determined by the relationship between the power delivered (watts) and time exposure (seconds). **Minimally invasive thermotherapy generally has a therapeutic effect** using a coagulative necrotic approach. The process of targeted heating above 50° C but below 100° C allows a gradual process of edema, inflammation followed by coagulation necrosis, and gradual atrophy. Conceptually, alpha-adrenergic receptor destruction is also thought to influence symptom relief.

Current Technologies and Their Differences

TUNA. In 1996, the FDA approved the minimally invasive transurethral needle ablation (TUNA) system for the treatment of BPH. Needle electrodes deliver low level radiofrequency energy precisely into the target tissue. Shields help to protect the urethra from thermal damage. The radiofrequency energy thermally devascularizes and denervates the target tissue, creating necrotic lesions. The radiofrequency energy decreases prostate size by 10%–15% by heat and dehydration. The heat energy produced and the result ing thermal effect is determined by the amount of tissue contact, length of the needle and wattage.

TUMT. The use of microwaves in the prostate was introduced in the 1990s with transurethral microwave thermotherapy (TUMT). TUMT uses microwave heating to create temperatures greater than 45° C, which is the minimum cytotoxic level of tissue. In order to create the high intraprostatic temperature, water-cooling is often used at the urethra to maintain patient comfort levels. It is this combination that creates an effective, yet minimally invasive treatment.

A handful of TUMT systems are available, each with different technical characteristics based on microwave antenna design, cooling design, duration of treatment, and bladder balloon design. The goal of treatment is to denervate and reduce the prostate volume. This is accomplished by tissue coagulation via heat.

The temperature in the prostate depends on 3 parameters: the microwave power (watts), which heats the tissue; the blood flow, which cools down the heated tissue; and heat conduction, which redistributes the heat. Of these, the microwave power and the blood flow are the most important factors to obtain therapeutic temperatures.

Both cooled and non-cooled systems are in use. Next generation microwave systems provide significantly more benefit to the patient, without the limitations of early microwave systems and interstitial therapies. Cooling allows generation of greater intraprostatic tissue temperatures (50° C–80° C), preserves urethral mucosal tissue and decreases morbidity. High tissue temperatures produce a large volume of necrosis in a short time. The coolant makes the procedure more comfortable for the patient and protects adjacent healthy tissue. With low temperature, non-cooled treatment, the hottest point is at the urethra and diminishes rapidly.

The Targis Cooled Thermo Therapy™ (Urologix) was one of the first anesthesia-free, minimally invasive BPH treatments designed for in-office use. It uses proprietary microwave technology to precisely deliver targeted high energy deep to the diseased tissue while leaving other nontargeted areas intact. The low temperature coolant protects the urethra during energy delivery, enhancing patient comfort and minimizing recovery times.

This system has been reported to have high durability in cases 5 years after treatment. It can be performed in an office or outpatient setting in about 1 hour. The urologist places the microwave delivery system, which is on the tip of the flexible catheter, into the bladder and inflates a standard urological balloon for positioning. The system's patented dipole antenna is then positioned in the prostatic urethra. The coolant emitted from the catheter simultaneously protects the urethra.

The Prolieve® System (Boston Scientific) provides water cooled balloon dilation TUMT. The treatment begins with intraurethral lidocaine 10 minutes prior to catheter placement, then proceeds to inflation of a 46F dilatation/prostatic compression balloon of the transurethral catheter. This system features a quick power ramp up to thermotherapy temperatures. Thermotherapy is delivered for about 45 minutes at a maximum of 50 watts as heated fluid is circulated in the prostate balloon. During a 5-minute cool down period, the prostate balloon remains inflated and the bladder is filled with 180 cc. The catheter is removed, and a voiding trial is begun.

The CoreTherm® (ProstaLund) provides feedback treatment with a temperature monitoring probe that is inserted into the prostate from the catheter. The temperature probe contains multiple temperature transducers to map the temperature distribution in the prostate along the probe. The microwave power and the treatment time are varied according to these readings. Intraprostatic temperature monitoring allows control by the treating physician, who can estimate the prostate volume treated.

The TMX 2000™ (Thermatrx) provides the lowest energy but is not a cooled system. The antenna directs heat and energy to the appropriate target (periurethral tissue) but does not direct heat to sensitive tissues (bladder neck and external sphincter). Low energy and low power are required to achieve tissue necrosis without cooling, on average 6–7 watts. A known and reproducible dose of heat is applied. Actual periurethral tissue temperature is continuously measured. Multiple treatment coil lengths ensure the optimal dose of heat is applied to the appropriate tissue of every prostate. The TMX 2000 can treat prostatic lengths (bladder neck to veru) of 2.5 cm and longer.

Analysis and Review of Thermotherapy Efficacy and Safety

Microwave technologies are not created equal. The paradigms for treatment vary. There are differences in power (maximum power: Thermatrx 23 watts, Prolieve 50 watts, Cooled ThermoTherapy 75 watts, CoreTherm 80 watts), delivery, urethral cooling, the efficacy and safety profile, and in the published peer-review literature. Thermatrx has low power and no urethral cooling. CoreTherm has high power and intraprostatic temperature monitoring. Targis has high power and urethral cooling. At low blood flow rates, the CoreTherm adds safety by reducing the microwave power and avoiding a possible overtreatment. At high blood flow, the CoreTherm adds efficacy by increasing the microwave power. Finally, the available efficacy data of themotherapies have been criticized for a number of issues, including a concern over the quality of comparative controls, plethora of positive data from single center studies rather than multicenter studies, issues of sham versus true effects within the efficacy parameters, appropriate direct comparator issues, technology changes occurring faster then clinical experience accumulated, no significant effect on PSA or prostate volume, high or unreported retreatment rates, and inability to predict which patients would benefit.[28–32]

Electrosurgical Techniques

The standard TURP. Successful treatment of BPH is measured by a decrease of symptom score, increase in peak flow rate and Qmax, and decrease of bother score. Absolute indications for surgery include refractory urinary retention, recurrent UTI, recurrent gross hematuria, renal insufficiency, bladder stones due to BPH, and large bladder diverticulum due to BPH.

The gold standard surgical treatment for BPH since the 1930s has been TURP, which has an 80%–85% success rate. This surgical procedure may lead to bleeding, dilutional hyponatremia (TUR) syndrome, and anesthetic risk. About 10%–15% of patients need retreatment at 10 years.

During the TURP procedure, the surgeon uses a resectoscope's wire loop to remove the obstructing tissue one piece at a time. The pieces of tissue are carried by the fluid into the bladder and then flushed out at the end of the operation. The standard TURP is an electrosurgical procedure that is performed in an aqueous environment. Basically, electrical current is carried through an insulated sheath to a wire loop that on contact with tissues creates electrosurgical heat that enables the wire to cut the tissue. It is important that the liquid medium be nonionic to maintain high current density in the wire loop for efficient electrosurgical cutting of target tissue. Historically, the irrigating solution first utilized was sterile distilled water. However, a well-known complication related to water irrigation fluid absorption via open venous channels during resection (dilutional hyponatremia) can occur in addition to bleeding related to the open venous channels. The absortion of sterile water into the bloodstream produces not only hemodynamic shifts, but also osmotic and electrolyte shifts between tissue and cellular compartments resulting in seizures. With sterile water, hemolysis also occurred resulting in renal failure due to myoglobinemia. Eventually, nonionic normo-osmotic irrigation fluids were developed, such as glycine irrigation, which are utilized today. However, these fluids were still nonionic (hyponatremic), and dilutional hyponatremia is still a risk. Management of this "TUR syndrome" generally consists of diuresis of free water with a diuretic and careful management of fluid electrolyte status with IV electrolyte solutions replacement with frequent serum electrolyte monitoring. A regional anesthetic such as a spinal is generally preferred for a TURP because impairment of congnitive function is an early and key diagnostic finding of significant dilutional hyponatremia.

Of interest, TURP is not recommended for large prostates since prolonged resections have a significant increased risk for dilutional hyponatremia as well as bleeding requiring transfusion. In fact, modern-day TURP has a higher mortality rate in the United States than open prostatectomy. As such, TURP is considered invasive along with open prostatectomy. This well known complication is generally avoided with the advent of bipolar TURP as well as other energy modialities, such as laser therapy, which does not require a nonionic irrigation solution.

In the United States, 97% of all surgical procedures for BPH are TURP. TURP leads to large changes in Q_{max} (+125%) and PVR (+74%). The probability of surgical complications or UTI is about 15% and probability of bleeding is 2%. There is no definitive evidence that TURP causes delayed mortality.

If surgery is indicated, TURP or a TURP-like procedure is still the best option. Morbidities are technique-and technology-related, which are getting better every year. If obstruction is the issue, this is the best pathway to treatment.[33]

Open prostatectomy. Standard TURP has its limitations that make it less than ideal for large prostate glands. A TURP for a large gland requiring a long resection time is a higher risk for bleeding requiring transfusion and for TUR syndrome. Additionally, transurethral resection in a large prostate is technically challenging since instrumentation length may be inadequate, and concurrent large bladder stones removal or diverticula repair may warrant an open procedure. Therefore, open prostatectomy continues to have a role in the management of bladder outlet obstruction in large prostates.[34]

Advancements in minimally invasive techniques have allowed these procedures to be performed both laparoscopically, robotically, and most recently through single port technology. However, its limitations include an intense learning and significant expertise in the field of advanced laparoscopic techniques.[35–37]

Electrovaporization and bipolar saline TUR. An electrosurgical modification of TURP combines 2 electrosurgical effects into 1 action. Vaporization is utilized in cutting, and desiccation is utilized in coagulation. The clinician uses a spiked, fluted or grooved roller bar to direct current through the resectoscope.

Five reported series of 240 patients have compared electrovaporization to standard TURP. Both procedures led to 55% improvement in AUA Symptom Score, more than 100% peak urinary flow, no incontinence, more than 75% retrograde ejaculation and no mortalities. Electrovaporization led to fewer transfusions and catheterizations and shorter hospital stays.

The advantages of electrovaporization include an efficacy that approaches TURP, similar improvement in IPSS, Qmax about 1 mL/sec less, decreased morbidity, less catheterization time, less hospital time and earlier return to work. Disadvantages include limitation on gland size and operative time. Modern design modifications of monopolar electrovaporization include various new optimal probe designs as well as various electrovaporative thick loops. Equally important are microprocessor controlled generators that optimize current delivered against variable electrical tissue resistance to optimize electrosurgical effects.

Finally, there are new designs that incorporate bipolar technology that eliminate the use of glycine and allow the advantageous use of normal saline irrigation, which reduces the risk of dilutional hyponatremia. Several competing technologies have variations in the optimal electrode design, optimal generator characteristics and competing bipolar technology designs. Available randomized peer review data suggest that the technique of surgical debulking is similar to that of standard TURP, and short term efficacy data by several authors suggest outcomes similar to TURP. However, the bipolar technology has an overall superior safety profile due to the increased hemostatic qualities of the electrovaporization technique, and the utilization of normal saline irrigation with the decreased risk of dilutional hyponatremia.[38–42]

Laser Therapies in BPH

Principles of laser tissue interactions. In the late 1980s, lasers became a novel way to open a wider channel and improve voiding dynamics for BPH. This cutting edge technology has been demonstrated to be minimally invasive and safe. Efficacy, both short-term and long-term, varies by the type of laser utilized, expertise of the surgeon, effective debulking of tissue and general technique applied. Individual techniques may vary greatly, but the 2 main tissue effects are coagulation and vaporization. Coagulation results in necrosis, gradual atrophy and sloughing of necrotic tissue, (ie, a debulking of the prostate). The laser also causes tissue and water to vaporize and results in an instantaneous debulking of prostatic tissue.

Interstitial laser coagulation (ILC). Interstitial laser coagulation of the prostate is a minimally invasive coagulative technique using an 830 nm diode laser system. It is technically a thermotherapy utilizing a site specific approach and a laser energy source. The only available commercial system was the Indigo Dye Laser System by Ethicon Endosurgery. It is no longer being commercially produced. It was a readily transportable, low-power, diode laser device that used a 15–20 watt variable power source.

ILC was an office-based technique that used local anesthesia. The fiber was introduced via a transurethral approach directly into the prostate. The laser transmitted energy through the fiber to a 2-cm long, light-diffusing tip that was passed via a cystoscope. The laser application time was 90 seconds. An ellipsoid lesion of tissue coagulated around the axis of the fiber. The affected area had a diameter of 1.5–2 cm and a length of 2 cm corresponding to the length of the energy diffusing fiber tip.

The advantages of the ILC were that it was a minimally invasive, office-based procedure, which required minimal anesthesia, had modest clinical outcomes, with no significant sexual side effects and minimal morbidity. Its disadvantages included a long catheterization, no immediate symptomatic relief, high incidence of UTI and an unsatisfactory re-treatment rate.

Limited randomized, controlled trials are available, but several published series suggest moderate improvement in AUA Symptom Score and peak flow rates with minimal long-term side effects compared to TURP.[43–45]

The high-power, 532 nm wavelength KTP photoselective laser vaporization prostatectomy (PVP). Photoselective laser vaporization prostatectomy with the KTP laser is the newest advance in laser technology and has gained fast popularity due to ease of use and powerful vaporization efficiency to its remove prostate tissue. The 532 nm wavelength is fully transmitted through water so that there is no energy absorption in the irrigant and the laser is selectively absorbed by hemoglobin, producing efficient prostate tissue removal with hemostasis. The coagulation zone depth is 1-2 mm with a side firing optical fiber in non-contact mode. The end point is a TURP-like cavity. Prospective, multicenter studies and single center studies report efficacy and durability to 3 years with high-risk patients and patients with large glands being effectively treated. Recent advancements have produced a more powerful 532 nm wavelength laser (120W) utilizing a diode laser source.[46–49]

Holmium enucleation and ablation techniques. The holmium YAG laser delivers energy in a pulsatile manner using a thermo mechanical mechanism of action. The laser emits a beam of 2150 nm, which has high absorption in water as well as hemoglobin. This creates a high temperature vapor bubble that explodes and has a thermo mechanical vaporization impact that is hemostatic on its target.

HoLEP. Holmium laser enucleation of the prostate (HoLEP) produces results that are similar to TURP with fewer complications (less intraoperative bleeding). In this procedure, a holmium laser is used to incise the prostate tissue and the end of the endoscope is then utilized to push and enucleate prostatic tissue into the bladder. The enucleated tissue is then removed with a morcellator. The benefits of HoLEP over traditional surgery include a shorter hospital stay, shorter catheterization time, and shorter recovery time. However, this procedure is technically difficult.

HoLAP. Holmium laser ablation of the prostate (HoLAP) uses a laser to vaporize obstructive prostatic tissue in a side fire approach like the 532 mm wavelength laser but is limited to small glands. The decision whether to use HoLAP or HoLEP is based primarily on the size of the prostate. Ablation usually is performed when the prostate is smaller than 40 cc. HoLA P offers the same advantages as PVP when compared to TURP. Patients who undergo HoLAP usually do not require overnight hospitalization and in most cases, the catheter is removed the same day or the morning following the procedure. There is only 1 published single series with long-term follow-up. More data is needed before any significant conclusions are made.[50–54]

Miscellaneous Devices: other technologies at wavelengths such as 980 (Evolve) and 2150 (Thullium) exist, however, little to no peer-reviewed data exists for these technologies.

Urethral Stents. This is an area which has been investigated for many years. The early stents had significant discomfort and perineal pain, and thus, fell out of favor. Newer stents have optimistic early results.

5. LUTS, Sexual Function, and Dysfunction with Medical and Surgical Treatment

The impact of medical therapies on sexual function is less than surgical treatments because it is reversible. Surgical therapies may cause retrograde ejaculation. Retrograde ejaculation may occur with minimally invasive thermotherapy (about 5%-10%), PVP (30%-40%), transurethral incision of the prostate (20%-30%), TURP (about 80%-90%) and open prostatectomy (about 80%-90%).

6. Metabolic Syndrome, Lower Urinary Tract Symptoms and BPH

Recent studies have suggested a link between hypertension, symptomatic BPH and sexual dysfunction.[51] This relationship has directed researchers and clinicians to study a relationship between lower urinary tract symptoms (LUTS) and the presence of a metabolic syndrome.[56] In fact, recent epidemiologic findings support a relationship by linking obesity, hypertension, cardiovascular disease with BPH, lower urinary tract symptoms and sexual dysunction.[57,58] These findings have been supported by a hypothesis demonstrated in animal studies that a link exists between autonomic nervous system overactivity and the pathophysiological development of urinary symptoms from progressive bladder dysfunction, due to prostatic hyperplasia and prostatic bladder outlet obstruction.[59–61] Sympathetic overactivity appears to be part of the metabolic syndrome and development of LUTS secondary to BPH. Metabolic syndrome has been described as a collection of abnormalities, including obesity, dyslipidemia, hypertension, impaired glucose metabolism, elevated C reactive protein (chronic inflammation) and autonomic sympathetic overactivity with insulin resistance, such as correlated, hypothesized, underlying pathogenic mechanisms.[62–65]

7. Etiology, Pathogenesis and Presentation of Bladder Calculi

Bladder calculi account for 5% of urinary calculi and usually occur because of bladder outlet obstruction, neurogenic voiding dysfunction, infection, or foreign bodies. Supernaturation of the urine in the bladder may subsequently develop and heterogeneous nucleation around a nidus may occur. In addition, aggregation results in crystal growth and stone formation.[66] Nutritional deficiencies combined with a low protein and high carbohydrate diet have been implicated in the pathogenesis of pediatric bladder lithiasis, in Africa and the Middle East.[67] Furthermore, dehydration, diarrhea, fever and infection decrease urine production and enhance crystallization. The composition of bladder calculi are influenced by both the pH and the degree of saturation of the urine.[68] Most calculi are of mixed composition and consist of calcium oxalate, uric acid, or struvite if infection is present.[69]

Diet, voiding dysfunction and uncorrected anatomic abnormalities, such as posterior urethral valves and veicoureteral reflux, predispose children to bladder stones. In men, several factors, such as urethral stricture, BPH, bladder diverticulum and neurogenic bladder, are all associated with bladder calculus formation. In women, the majority of vesical calculi are secondary to prolapse, female pelvic surgery, neurogenic bladder or foreign bodies. There are numerous reports concerning bladder migration of intrauterine devices and intravaginal accessories, including pessaries, diaphragms and cerclages. In both genders, spinal cord injury and indwelling Foley catheters can predispose one to bladder stone formation.

The typical symptoms of a bladder stone are intermittent and painful voiding with terminal hematuria. The pain may be referred to the tip of the penis, along the course of the second and third sacral nerve, or to the scrotum. In children, the pain may be referred to the perineum through the third and fourth sacral nerves. Lastly, more than 50% of bladder calculi are not discernable on plain X-rays. The most accurate mean of diagnosis remains cystoscopy.[70]

Treatment of Bladder Calculi

If conservative treatment is desired in a child, their diet can be altered by the addition of phosphorous, protein, vitamins and magnesium, which can significantly decrease the incidence of vesical lithiasis, especially in endemic areas. In adults, irrigation of the bladder with an alkaline solution or Renacidin has been reported to be beneficial for some stones.

Open surgery remains the main treatment of bladder calculi in children. In adults, the classical treatment for bladder calculi is endoscopic transurethral disintegration with mechanical cystolithotripsy, lithalopaxy ultrasound, electrohydraulic lithotripsy (EHL), Swiss Lithoclast and holmium: (YAG laser lithotripsy). Traditionally, treatment of large (>4 cm) vesical calculi has been via open surgery. Extracorporeal shock wave lithotripsy should not be considered as a first-line therapy for the vast majority of adults with bladder lithiasis. Percutaneous procedures are rarely performed, but numerous modalities are currently in development. Elimination of all stone material is essential during any of these procedures, or the remaining stone material will serve as a nidus for future recurrent stone formation

8. Recommended Reading and References

Recommended Reading

1. *Guideline on the Management of Benign Prostatic Hyperplasia*. American Urological Association; 2003. Updated 2006. http://www.auanet.org/guidelines/bph.cfm

2. Wein, Kavoussi, Novick, Partin and Peters, eds. The prostate. In: *Campbell Walsh Urology*. 9th ed. Vol. 3, section XVI. Philadelphia, PA: Saunders Elsevier; 2007:2677–2895.

3. Kirby, McConnell, Fitzpatrick, Rhoerborn and Bolye, eds. *Textbook of Benign Prostatic Hyperplasia*. 2nd ed. London, England: Taylor and Francis; 2005.

4. Smith, Badlani, Bagley, et al, eds. *Smith's Textbook of Endourology*. 2nd ed. London, England: BD Decker; 2007:603-740.

5. Kaplan SA, Partin AW, Atala AJ, eds. *Minimally Invasive Procedures in Urology*. Boca Raton, FL: Taylor and Francis;2005.

References

1. Guideline on the Management of Benign Prostatic Hyperplasia. Diagnosis and Treatment Recommendations. Chapter 1; p1. American Urological Association; 2003 (updated 2006). http://www.auanet.org/guidelines/bph.cfm

2. Kirby RS, Fitzpatrick P. *Benign Prostatic Hyperplasia*. Health Press; 1995.

3. Girman CJ, Jacobsen SJ, Rhodes T, Guess HA, Roberts RO, Lieber MM. Association of health related quality of life and benign pro static enlargement. *Eur Urol*. 1999;35(4): 277-284.

4. Jacobsen SJ, Jacobson DJ, Girman CJ, et al. Natural history of prostatism: risk factors for acute urinary retention. *J Urol*. 1997;158(2): 481-487.

5. Kirby RS. The natural history of benign pro static hyperplasia: what have we learned in the last decade? *Urology*. 2000;56(5 suppl 1):3-6.

6. Rhodes T, Girman CJ, Jacobsen SJ, Roberts RO, Guess HA, Lieber MM. Longitudinal prostate growth rates during 5 years in ran domly selected community men 40 to 79 years old. *J Urol*. 1999;161(4):1174-1179.

7. Arrighi HM, Guess HA, Metter EJ, Fozard JL. Symptoms and signs of prostatism as risk fac tors for prostatectomy. *Prostate*. 1990;16(3): 253-261.

8. Roehrborn CG, McConnell JD. In: Walsh PC, et al. *Campbells' Urology*. 8th ed. Philadelphia, PA: WB Saunders Co; 2002:1297-1330.

9. Veltri R, Rodriguez R. Molecular biology, endocrinology, and physiology of the prostate and seminal vesical. In: Wein, Kavoussi, Novick, Partin, Peters, eds. *Campbell-Walsh Urology*. 9th ed. Philadelphia, PA: Elsevier; 2007:2677-2726.

10. *Guideline on the Management of Benign Prostatic Hyperplasia*. Diagnosis and Treatment Recommendations; Chapter 1: p7. American Urological Association; 2003 (updated 2006). http://www.auanet.org/guidelines/bph.cfm.

11. Roehrborn CG. Definition of at risk patients: baseline variables. *BJU Int*. 2006;97 (suppl 2):7-11; discussion 21-22.

12. Te AE, Ikeguchi EF, Choi J, Kaplan SA. Urodynamics and benign prostatic hyperplasia. In: Kirby RS, McConnell JD, Fitzpatrick JM, Roehrborn CG, Boyle P, eds. *Textbook of Benign Prostatic Hyperplasia*. 2nd ed. Oxford, England: Isis Medical Media; 2002.

13. Foglar R, Shibata K, Horie K, Hirasawa A, Tsujimoto G. Use of recombinant alpha 1 adrenoceptors to characterize subtype selectiv ity of drugs for the treatment of prostatic hypertrophy. *Eur J Pharmacol*. 1995;288(2):201-207.

14. Hatano A, Takahashi H, Tamaki M, Komeyama T, Koizumi T, Takeda M. Pharma cological evidence of distinct alpha 1 adreno ceptor subtypes mediating the contraction of human prostatic urethra and peripheral artery. *Br J Pharmacol*. 1994;113(3):723-728.

15. Roehrborn CG, Bruskewitz R, Nickel JC, et al. Proscar Long Term Efficacy and Safety Study Group.Sustained decrease in incidence of acute uri nary retention and surgery with finasteride for 6 years in men with benign prostatic hyperplasia. *J Urol*. 2004;171(3):1194-1198.

16. Roehrborn CG, Marks LS, Fenter T, et al. Efficacy and safety of dutasteride in the four year treatment of men with benign prostatic hyperplasia. *Urology*. 2004;63(4):709-715.

17. Wysowski DK, Farinas E. Finasteride in benign prostatic hyperplasia. *N Engl J Med*. 2004;350(13):1359-1361; author reply 1359-1361.

18. McConnell JD. Medical Therapy of Prostatic Symptoms (MTOPS) Research Group. The long term effects of doxazosin, finas teride, and the combination on the clinical progression of BPH. *N Engl J Med*. 2003; 349: 2387-2398.

19. Roehrborn CG. The Effects of Dutasteride, Tamsulosin, and Combination Therapy on Lower Urinary Tract Symptoms in Menwith Benign Prostatic Hyperplasia and Prostatic Enlargement: 2-Year Results from the CombAT Study. *J Urol*. 2008:179(2):616-621.

20. Complementary and Alternative Medicine for Urological Symptoms (CAMUS) Clinical Trial. http://www.niddk.nih.gov/patient/camus/CAMUS.htm.

21. Jaffe WI, Te AE. Overactive bladder in the male patient: epidemiology, etiology, evaluation, and treatment. *Curr Urol Rep*. 2005;6(6):410-418.

22. Kaplan SA, Walmsley K, Te AE. Tolterodine extended release attenuates lower urinary tract symptoms in men with benign prostatic hyper plasia. *J Urol*. 2005 Dec;174(6):2273-2275; discussion 2275-2276.

23. Jumadilova Z, Zyczynski T, Paul B, Narayanan S. Urinary incontinence in the nursing home: resident characteristics and prevalence of drug treatment. *Am J Manag Care*. 2005 Jul;11(4 suppl):S112-S120.

24. Lee JY, Kim HW, Lee SJ, Koh JS, Suh HJ, Chancellor MB. Comparison of doxazosin with or without tolterodine in men with symp tomatic bladder outlet obstruction and an over active bladder. *BJU Int*. 2004;94(6): 817-820.

25. Corcos J, Casey R, Patrick A, et al for the Uromax Study Group. Adouble blind ran domized dose response study comparing daily doses of 5, 10 and 15 mg controlled release oxybutynin: balancing efficacy with severity of dry mouth. *BJU Int*. 2006;97(3):520-527.

26. Dmochowski RR, Nitti V, Staskin D, Luber K, Appell R, Davila GW. Transdermal oxybu tynin in the treatment of adults with overactive bladder:combined results of two randomized clinical trials. *World J Urol*. 2005;23(4): 263-270.

27. Gonzalez RR, Te AE. Overactive bladder and men: indications for anticholinergics. *Curr Urol Rep*. 2003;4(6):429-435.

28. Gonzalez RR, Te AE. How do transurethral needle ablation of the prostate and transurethral microwave thermotherapy compare with transurethral prostatectomy? *Curr Urol Rep*. 2003;4(4):297-306.

29. Shabbir M, Kirby RS. Fact or fiction: what do the benign prostatic hyperplasia data tell us? *Curr Urol Rep*. 2005;6(4):243-250.

30. Mattiasson A, Wagrell L, Schelin S, et al. Five year follow up of feed back microwave thermotherapy versus TURP for clinical BPH: a prospective randomized multicenter study. *Urology*. 2007;69(1):91-96.

31. Te AE. Editorial comment on five year follow up of feedback microwave thermotherapy ver sus TURP for clinical BPH: a prospective ran domized multicenter study. *Urology*. 2007;69(1):96-97.

32. Walmsley K, Kaplan SA. Transurethral microwave thermotherapy for benign prostate hyperplasia: separating truth from marketing hype. *J Urol*. 2004;172(4 Pt 1):1249-1255.

33. Santarosa RP, Te AE, Kaplan SA. Transurethral resection, incision and ablation of the prostate. In: Graham SD, ed. *Glenn's Urologic Surgery*. 5th ed. Philadelphia, PA: Lippincott, Williams & Wilkins; 1998: 921-931.

34. Sandhu JS, Te AE. Open prostatectomy. In: Kaplan SA, Cabelin M, eds. *Atlas of Urologic Clinics of North America*. Philadelphia, PA: WB Saunders; 2002.

35. Sotelo R, Spaliviero A, Garcia-Segui A, et al. Laparoscopic Retropubic Simple Prostatectomy. *J Urol*. 2005 Mar:173(3):757-760.

36. Sotelo R, Clavijo R, Carmona O, Garcia O, et al. Robotic Simple Prostatectomy. *J Urol*. 2008:179(2):513-515.

37. Desai MM, Aron M, Canes D, et al. Single-Port Transvesical Simple Prostatectomy: Initial Clinical Report. *Urology*. 2008: 72(5):960-965.

38. Cabelin MA, Te AE, Kaplan SA. Transurethral vaporization of the prostate: current techniques. *Curr Urol Rep*. 2000;1(2):116-123.

39. Hon NH, Brathwaite D, Hussain Z, et al. A prospective, randomized trial comparing conventional transurethral prostate resection with PlasmaKinetic® vaporization of the prostate: physiological changes, early complications and long term follow up. *J Urol*. 2006; 176(1):205-209.

40. Seckiner I, Yesilli C, Akduman B, Altan K, Mungan NA. Aprospective randomized study for comparing bipolar PlasmaKinetic® resection of the prostate with standard *TURP. Urol Int*. 2006;76(2):139-143.

41. de Sio M, Autorino R, Quarto G, et al. Gyrus bipolar versus standard monopolar transurethral resection of the prostate: a randomized prospective trial. *Urology*. 2006; 67(1):69-72.

42. Tefekli A, Muslumanoglu AY, Baykal M, Bin bay M, Tas A, Altunrende F. Ahybrid tech nique using bipolar energy in transurethral prostate surgery: a prospective, randomized comparison. *J Urol*. 2005;174(4 Pt 1): 1339-1343.

43. Terada N, Arai Y, Okubo K, et al. Interstitial laser coagulation for management of benign prostatic hyperplasia: long term follow up. *Int J Urol*. 2004;11(11):978-982.

44. Kursh ED, Concepcion R, Chan S, Hudson P, Ratner M, Eyre R. Interstitial laser coagulation versus transurethral prostate resection for treating benign prostatic obstruction: a randomized trial with 2 year follow up. *Urology*. 2003;61(3):573-578.

45. Norby B, Nielsen HV, Frimodt Moller PC. Transurethral interstitial laser coagulation of the prostate and transurethral microwave ther motherapy vs. transurethral resection or inci sion of the prostate: results of a randomized, controlled study in patients with symptomatic benign prostatic hyperplasia. *BJU Int*. 2002; 90(9):853-862.

46. Lee R, Gonzalez RR, Te AE. The evolution of photoselective vaporization prostatectomy (PVP): advancing the surgical treatment of benign prostatic hyperplasia. *World J Urol*. 2006;24(4):405-409.

47. Te AE, Malloy TR, Stein BS, Ulchaker JC, Nseyo UO, Hai MA. Impact of prostate specific antigen level and prostate volume as pre dictors of efficacy in photoselective vaporization prostatectomy: analysis and results of an ongoing prospective multicentre study at 3 years. *BJU Int*. 2006;97(6):1229-1233.

48. Te AE, Malloy TR, Stein BS, et al. Photoselective vaporization of the prostate for the treat ment of benign prostatic hyperplasia: 12 month results from the first United States multicenter prospective trial. *J Urol*. 2004; 172(4 Pt 1):1404-1408.

49. Te AE. The next generation in laser treatments and the role of the green light high performance system laser. *Rev Urol*. 2006;8 (suppl 3):S24-S30.

50. Gupta N, Sivaramakrishna, Kumar R, Dogra PN, Seth A. Comparison of standard transurethral resection, transurethral vapour resection and holmium laser enucleation of the prostate for managing benign prostatic hyper plasia of >40 g. *BJU Int*. 2006;97(1):85-89.

51. Elzayat EA, Elhilali MM. Holmium laser enucleation of the prostate (HoLEP): the endourologic alternative to open prostatectomy. *Eur Urol*. 2006;49(1):87-91.

52. Tan AH, Gilling PJ. Lasers in the treatment of benign prostatic hyperplasia: an update. *Curr Opin Urol*. 2005;15(1):55-58.

53. Tan AH, Gilling PJ, Kennett KM, Fletcher H, Fraundorfer MR. Long term results of high power holmium laser vaporization (ablation) of the prostate. *BJU Int*. 2003;92(7): 707-709.

54. Tooher R, Sutherland P, Costello A, Gilling P, Rees G, Maddern G. Asystematic review of holmium laser prostatectomy for benign prostatic hyperplasia. *J Urol*. 2004;171(5): 1773-1781.

55. McVary KT. Autonomic nervous system over activity in men with lower urinary tract symptoms secondary to benign prostatic hyperplasia. *J Urol*. 2005;174:1327-1433.

56. Kasturi S, Russell S, McVary KT. Metabolic syndrome and lower urinary tract symptoms secondary to benign prostatic hyperplasia. *Curr Urol Rep*. 2006;7(4):288-292.

57. Hammarsten J. Clinical, anthropometric, metabolic and insulin profile of men with fast annual growth rates of benign prostatic hyper plasia. *Blood Press*. 1999;8:29-36.

58. Meigs JB. Risk factors for clinical benign prostatic hyperplasia in a community based population of healthy aging men. *J Clin Epidemiol*. 2001;54:935-944.

59. McVary KT. Growth of the rat prostate gland is facilitated by the autonomic nervous system. *Biol Reprod*. 1994;51:99-107.

60. Golomb E. Spontaneous hyperplasia of the ventral lobe of the prostate in aging, genetically hypertensive rats. *J Androl*. 2000;21: 58- 64.

61. Steers WD. The spontaneously hypertensive rat: insight into the pathogenesis of irritative symptoms in benign prostatic hyperplasia and young anxious males. *Exp Physiol*. 1999; 84:137-147.

62. Haffner SM. The metabolic syndrome: inflammation, diabetes mellitus, and cardiovascular disease. *Am J Cardiol*. 2006;97:3A-11A.

63. Hammarsten J. Components of the metabolic syndrome risk factors for the development of benign prostatic hyperplasia. *Prostate Cancer Prostatic Dis*. 1998;1:157-162.

64. Rohrmann S. Serum C reactive protein concentration and lower urinary tract symptoms in older men in the Third National Health and Nutrition Examination Survey (NHANES III). *Prostate*. 2005;62:27-33.

65. Reaven GM. Hypertension and associated metabolic abnormalities: the role of insulin resistance and the sympathoadrenal system. *N Engl J Med*. 1996;334:374-381.

66. Papatsoris AG, Varkarakis I, Dellis A, Deliveliotis C. Bladder lithiasis: frpm open surgery to lithotripsy. *Urol Res*. 2006:34:163-167.

67. Ali SH, Rifat UN. Etiological and clinical patterns of childhood urolithiasis in Iraq. *Pediatr Nephrol* 20:1453-1457.

68. Schwartz BF, Stoller ML. The vesical lithiasis. *Urol Clin North Am*. 2006;27:333-346.

69. Menon M, Resnick MI. Urinary lithiasis: etiology, diagnosis, and medical management. In: Walsh PC, Retik AB, Vaughan ED, Wein AJ, eds. *Campbell's Urology*. 8th ed. WB Saunders, eds. pp:3229.

70. Drach GW. Urinary lithiasis: etiology, diagnosis, and medical management. In: Walsh PC, Retik AB, Stamey TA, Vaughan ED, eds. *Campbells Urology*. 6th ed. Philadelphia, PA: WB Saunders:2140.

Chapter 22: Surgical Disease of the Adrenal Gland

Jay T. Bishoff, MD

Contents

1. Objectives

- The objective of this chapter is to help urologists pass board and recertification examinations.
- Given the complexity of surgical adrenal disease, a review of this topic can be overwhelming.
- Recognizing this fact, I have provided a chapter in outline form, to be a concise and rapid overview of adrenal disorders.
- On any given examination, there will only be a few questions covering the topic of the adrenal gland.
- The questions at the end of the chapter are provided to cover commonly tested adrenal topics.

2. Embryology

- The adrenal cortex derives from mesoderm.
- The medulla develops from neuroectoderm.
- Heterotopic adrenal tissue is usually associated with the kidney and its development, but in the case of renal agenesis or solitary kidney the adrenal gland, on the affected side, is found in the normal position.

3. Anatomy

Size

- The average size of the adrenal gland is:
  * Length: 5 cm
  * Width: 3 cm
  * Depth: 1 cm
  * Weight: 5 gm

- The fetal adrenal gland weighs as much as 10 grams, almost twice the size of the adult gland.

- The reason is that the fetal cortex is much larger and is believed to have a role in embryogenesis and homeostasis.

- After birth, the fetal cortex regresses during the first 6 weeks of life.

- Ratio of adrenal to kidney weight is:
  * Neonate 1:3
  * Adult 1:30

Location

- The adrenal gland is located in the retroperitoneum. It is triangular in shape and is contained in its own sub-compartment within Gerota's fascia.

Blood Supply

- Arterial supply
  * Receives 7 cc/gram minute
  * There are 3 commonly described arterial sources of flow:
    1. ***Inferior phrenic artery is the main arterial supply***
    2. Aorta
    3. Renal artery

- The adrenal may have gonadal branches which are seen in 60% of fetal dissections

- Arterial vessels are rarely seen during surgery, but the surgeon must know of their location and use hemostatic instrumentation to prevent bleeding.

Venous Drainage

- Single main adrenal vein is the most important surgical structure

- ***Right adrenal gland*** drains directly into the posterior aspect of the inferior vena cava. The right sided adrenal vein is usually very short and easily torn during dissection.

- ***Left adrenal gland*** drains directly into the renal vein. The insertion is usually overlying the aorta and is usually medial to the insertion of the left gonadal vein on the renal vein. The left side can have a significant sized Phrenic Branch as well.

Nerve Supply

- The ***adrenal medulla is innervated by sympathetic branches*** which trigger the release of the medullary hormones:
  * ***Epinephrine***
  * ***Norepinephrine***

- The adrenal cortex has no known innervations

Lymphatic Drainage

- The adrenal gland drains to:
  * Lateral aortic nodes
  * Nodal chains running from the renal artery to diaphragm

- Adrenal carcinoma requires an extensive lymphadenectomy at the time of adrenalectomy

Hormone Production

- The adrenal cortical steroids have a *common precursor with the conversion of cholesterol to pregnenolone.*

Hormone Release

- Corticotrophin-releasing hormone (CRH) is synthesized in the hypothalamus and arrives at the pituitary through the portal blood system.

- CRH results in the release of ACTH from the pituitary gland and *ACTH stimulates cortisol release from the adrenal gland.*

- Adrenal androgen production is also influenced by ACTH as well as other factors (DHES, DHEAS).

- *However, the primary control of Aldosterone secretion from the zona glomerulosa is angiotinsen II, not ACTH.*

Adrenal Cortex

- Developed from mesoderm.

- Contains three distinct zones easily remembered from the pneumonic "GFR."

- Each zone secretes adrenal steroids derived from the basic structure of cholesterol changed to pregnenolone.

Figure 1

Adrenal cortex hormone production: steroid production chart

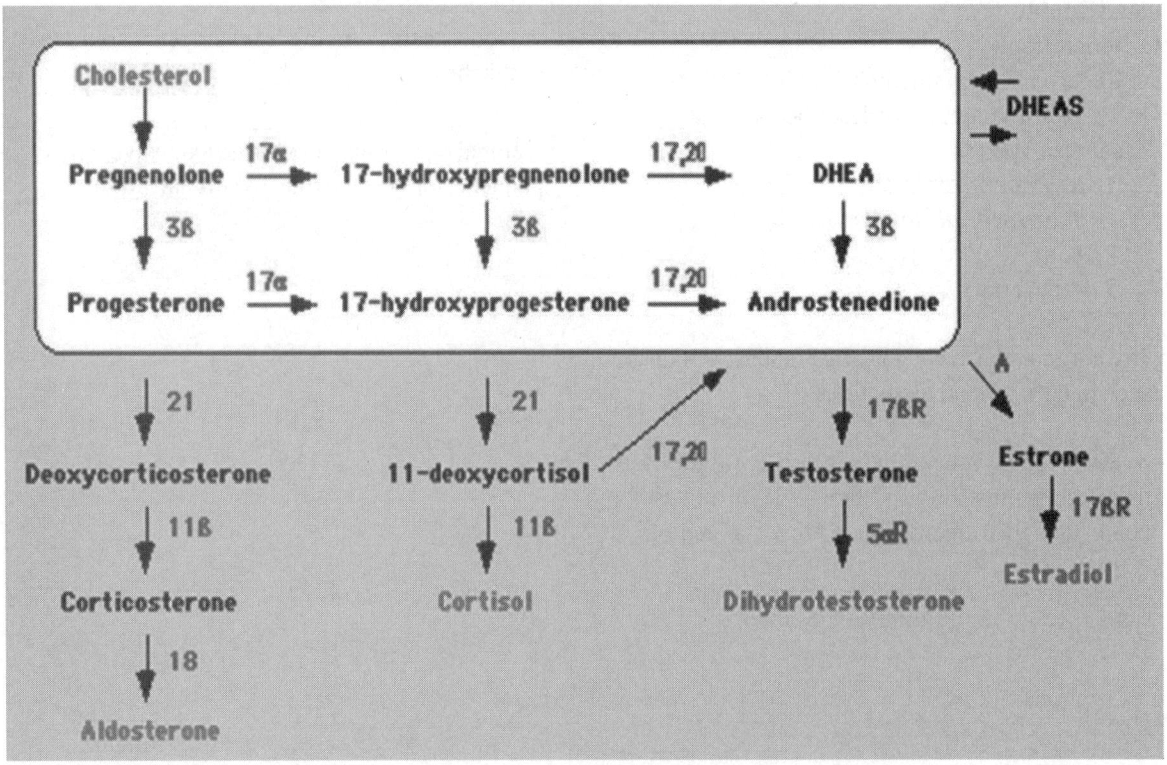

- Zona glomerulosa (outer) production of aldosterone
- Zona fasciculata (middle) production of cortisol
- Zona reticularis (inner) production of sex steroids

Figure 2

Hypothalamic – pituitary – adrenal axis

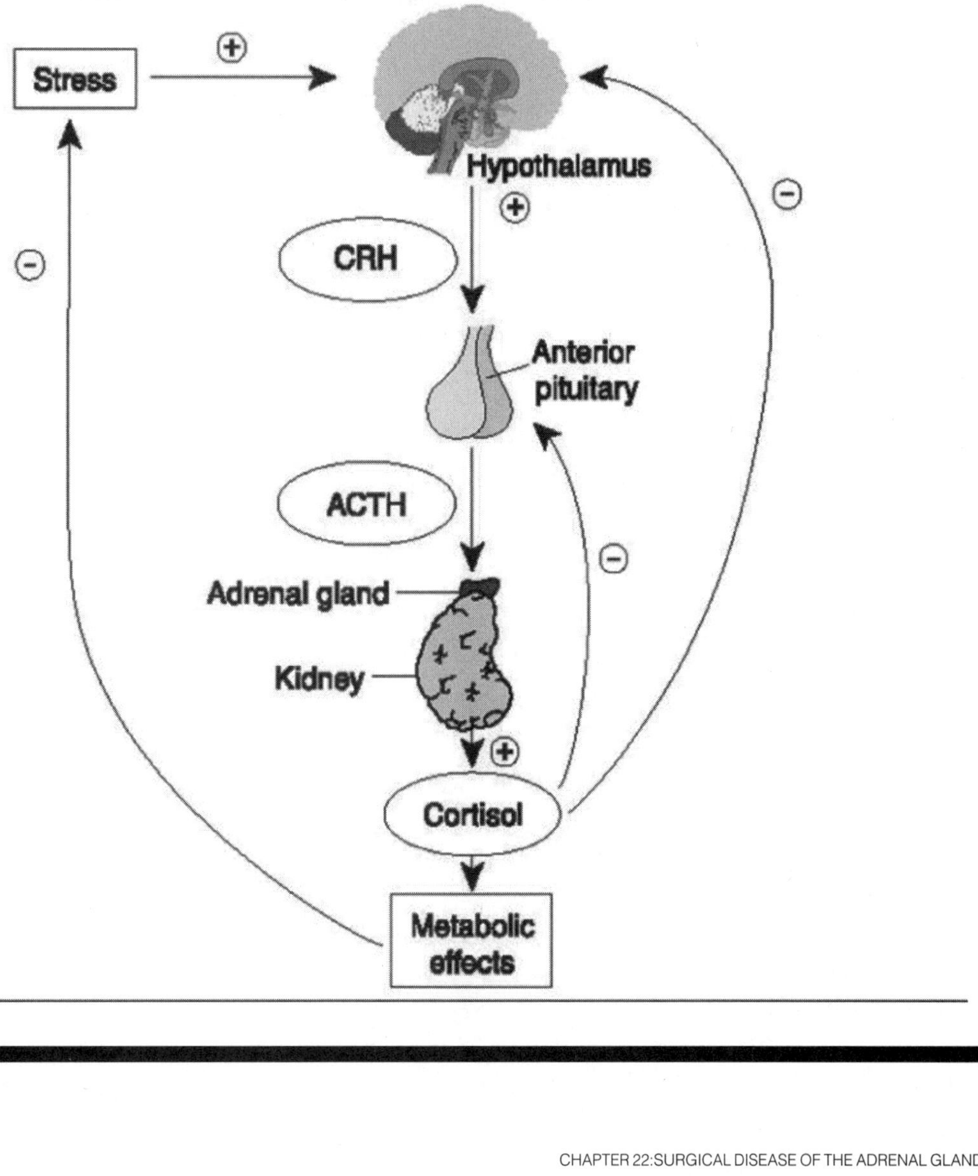

5. Specific Adrenal Cortex Steroid Description

Aldosterone

- Produced in the zona glomerulosa

- ***Primary stimulus for aldosterone release is angiotensin II***

- Other stimuli for release of aldosterone include:
  - * ACTH
  - * Decreased serum sodium
  - * Elevated serum potassium
  - * The juxtaglomerular apparatus located in the afferent arterioles of the kidney senses decreased renal perfusion and as a result releases renin.

- Renin from the kidney cleaves a single bond on angiotensinogen releasing angiotensin I.

- ACE (angiotensin converting enzyme) splits two amino acids off of angiotensin I to make angiotensin II.
  - * *Note:* In the past it was believed that ACE from the lungs was the major site of conversion of AI to AII. More recently it has been discovered that ACE is also found in kidney, duodenum, ileum and the uterus. Current thoughts are that the peripheral sites play an equal role to the lung in conversion of AI to AII

- ***Angiotensin II directly stimulates the adrenal glomerulosa cells to release aldosterone.***

- Aldosterone activates Na-K pump in nephron: which results in the retention of Na and water (water follows Na)

Glucocorticoids

- Glucocorticoids are responsible for a vast array of different physiologic functions in the body:
  - * Salt retention
  - * Skeletal and cardiac contractions
  - * Protein catabolism
  - * Inhibit bone formation
  - * Inhibits collagen synthesis
  - * Increases vascular contractility
  - * Anti-inflammation
  - * Anti-immune activity
  - *Maintains normal GFR

Cortisol

- ACTH and cortisol have diurnal variation; they are normally: high in the AM, low PM

- Both ACTH and cortisol inhibit CRH release by feedback

Androgens

- Sex steroid secretion by the adrenal gland is stimulated by ACTH not gonadotropins.

- Sex steroid secretion by the adrenal gland is of minor physiologic importance, except in disease states.
  - * ie, elevated concentrations in women with hirsuitism from adrenal tumors

- The exact control mechanisms for adrenal androgens have not been determined.

6. Adrenal Medulla

- Distinct from cortex embryologically derived from neuroectoderm

- Secretes cathecolamines sympathetic stimulation

- Stored in secretory cells

- Preganglionic neurons trigger release

Catecholamines

- ***Large chromaffin cells secrete mainly epinephrine, but also secrete norepinephrine and dopamine.***

- ***Precursors to catecholamines are dietary tyrosine and phenylalanine***
  * Site of production of catecholamines: adrenal, CNS, adrenergic nerve terminals.

- Healthy humans circulating catecholamines
  * ***Norepinehprine*** 73%
  * Epinephrine 14%
  * Dopamine 13%

- Phenylethanolamine-N-methyltransferase (PNMT) enzyme from the medulla converts through methylation of norepinephrine which gives you epinephrine.

- PNMT is located in the adrenal medulla. Therefore, if a patient has an excess of ***both*** epinephrine and norepinephrine, the tumor is in the adrenal gland and not in other sites of chromaffin tissue.

- Excess ***norepinephrine and epinephrine source is adrenal pathology***

Epinephrine/Norepinephrine

- Catecholamine secretion from neural sympathetic nerves

- Half-life is only 20 seconds

- Metabolism:
  * Catechol-*O*-methyltransferase and monoamine oxidase break down the catecholamines to produce the break-down products:
    - Primary ***Urine vanillylmandelic acid (VMA)***
    - Secondary Metanephrine and normetanephrine

7. The Incidental Adrenal Tumors

- CT, MRI, US are more commonly performed than in the past

- Body imaging has become a new addition to the physical examination

- 0.5%-5% of abdominal CTs show abnormal adrenal glands

- Incidental adrenal finding
  * Found at autopsy in 2%-8%

- Carcinoma almost never seen at autopsy
  * 85% of adrenal tumors are nonfunctional and benign
  * Significant cost of evaluation unless streamlined
  * Balance of costs and benefits

- Definition of an incidental mass
  * Mass >1 cm
  * Discovered on examination for nonadrenal purpose
  * Absence of signs or symptoms of adrenal disorder

- Questions to be asked:
  * Is the mass functional?
  * Are there any physical signs or symptoms?
  * Is there biochemical evidence of activity?
    1. Pheo screen
    2. Potassium level
    3. Glucocorticoid screen
  * Is the mass malignant?
  * Is there any history of another malignancy?
  * Is imaging suggestive of malignancy?

Nature of Incidentially Found Adrenal Mass N = 2005

- (Young WF, et al. *Endocrinol Clin N Am.* 2000)

- In a review of 2005 incidentally-discovered adrenal masses, the percentages of different findings were:

- ***Nonfunctioning adenoma*** 82%

- Functioning adenoma
  * Cushing's syndrome 5%
  * Pheochromocytoma 5%
  * Aldosteronoma 1%

• Malignancy
  * Adrenal metastasis 3%
  * Adrenal cortical ca. 4%

Nature of Mass
• Medical history and size are important characteristics

• Adrenal metastasis
  * 6% have no history of cancer
  * 50% have a positive history of cancer

• Adrenal cortical carcinoma
  * Only 2% of all masses are cortical carcinoma
  * However, 65% of masses >6 cm are cortical carcinoma

Other (Rarer) Possibilities to be Included in Your Differential Diagnosis
• Myelolipoma/lipoma has CT findings that are similar to that of renal angiomyelolipoma (fat) (Figure 3).

Figure 3

Bilateral myelolipomas

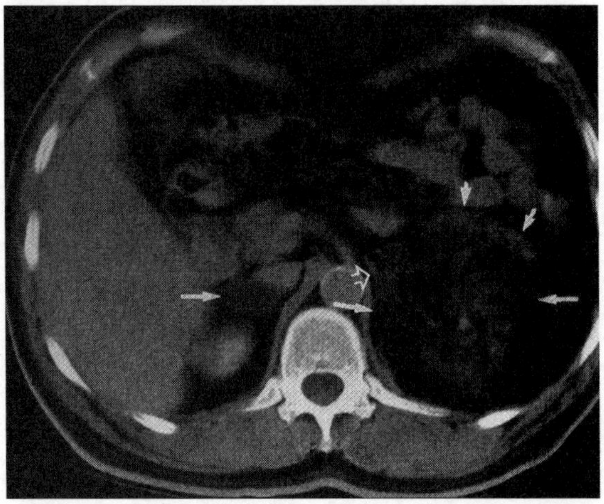

Bilateral myelolipomas seen in a 64 y/o male with large left-sided and smaller right-sided masses, demonstrating fat content on CT imagining consistent with myelolipoma

• If the adrenal gland has fat density material, it is by definition a benign myelolipoma

• Adrenal cyst/hematoma benign cysts can be followed and may be true cysts or pseudo-cysts
  • Ganglioneuroma
  • Neuroblastoma

• Findings after-work up:
  * If the patient has no overt signs or symptoms endocrine activity or positive findings discovered during a metabolic after work-up are rare:
    • Cushing's 5%
    • Pheochromocytoma 2%
    • Aldosteronoma <1%

This point is very important! If the patient has a known primary cancer, the adrenal mass will be metastatic from the primary site 50% of the time. Therefore, consideration of and work-up for other cancers is warranted in the patient with an incidentally found adrenal mass.

Subclinical Cushing's Syndrome
• This is a real entity and often misunderstood by urologists as not clinically significant

• Total 24° cortisol production is often normal in these patients, but they still have significant pathology

• Subtle changes often occur such as the loss of diurnal variation of cortisol secretion

• Prognosis is variable with 3 different possibilities

  * Normalization
  * Persistence
  * Progression to full clinical Cushing's

• Subclinical Cushing's is an indication for adrenalectomy and should be considered in the differential diagnosis of the incidental adrenal mass.

Incidental Adrenal Mass Initial Evaluation
• History and physical exam

• Look for signs of hormonal syndromes

• Search for occult malignancy

- CXR

- Stool for occult blood

- Mammogram (in women)

The Limited Endocrine Evaluation is Very Useful to Determine the Presence of:
- Pheochromocytoma

- Aldosterone-producing adenoma

- Cortisol-producing adenoma

Extent of Endocrine Evaluation Remains Controversial
- Most limited evaluation consists of three simple tests:

- Serum potassium if hypertensive R/O aldosteronoma

- (Unlikely if not hypertensive, but can be difficult to diagnosis if on diuretics, K replacement and other antihypertensive medications)

- Plasma metanephrines: most sensitive test for pheochromocytoma

- 24-hour urine cortisol

- The low-dose dexamethasone suppression test is most sensitive for "subclinical" Cushing's syndrome, but 24-hour urine cortisol is a good start

Diagnosis: Endocrine Evaluation
- The indications for a complete endocrine evaluation include:
  1. Findings on examination and H&P suggestive of an excess of specific hormone
  2. Positive findings on limited evaluation screening tests

Hypertension Caused by an Adrenal Source is Rare
- 15% of adult population is hypertensive

- Only 1% is adrenal in origin
  1. 0.5% primary hyperaldosteronism
  2. 0.2% pheochromocytoma
  3. 0.2% Cushing's syndrome

8. Imaging of the Incidental Adrenal Tumor

- *Most incidental adrenomas are nonfunctional.*

- If not a metastasis then usually a nonfunctioning adenoma.

- Rarely adrenal cortical carcinoma.

- Uncertain progression of nonfunctional adenoma complicates issue.

- Strategies and criteria for radiographic imaging continue to evolve, but some general guidelines are available to help in the decision for imagining.

Diagnosis: Imaging
- It is rare for a nonfunctional adenoma to become functional.

- Most series report no progression of small adenomas to cancer.

- Three series do report the occurrence of adrenal cortical carcinoma in small tumors.

- Kloos, et al, 1997: Found 3 cancers in patients with initial adrenal tumors ranging in size from 3-5 cm who did not have follow-up.

- Linos, et al, 1997: Reported on 3 patients with tumors measuring 2.6-2.9 cm that were found to be carcinoma.

- Zaluaka, et al,1998: Reported on a series of 311 incidental adrenal tumors and found 22 adrenal carcinomas (7%) ranging in size from 3.2-20 cm.

- The small adrenal carcinoma is rare but reported. For examination purposes it is probably safe to use 5 cm as the cut-off to be carcinoma. For functional tumors the surgeon should always be concerned about the presence of carcinoma and treat it accordingly during surgery.

Diagnosis: MRI
- *BOTH carcinoma and pheochromocytomas are hyper-intense on T2 images (ie, they "light up" as they go from T1 to T2)*

- Intensity of the adrenal gland on T2 relative to liver < 0.8 suggests cortical adenoma

Figure 4a

Benign adenoma hypo-intense on T1 MRI

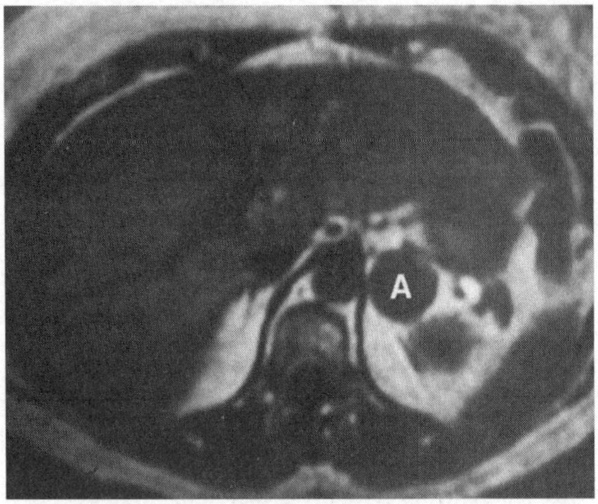

Figure 4b

Hypo-intense on T2 MRI

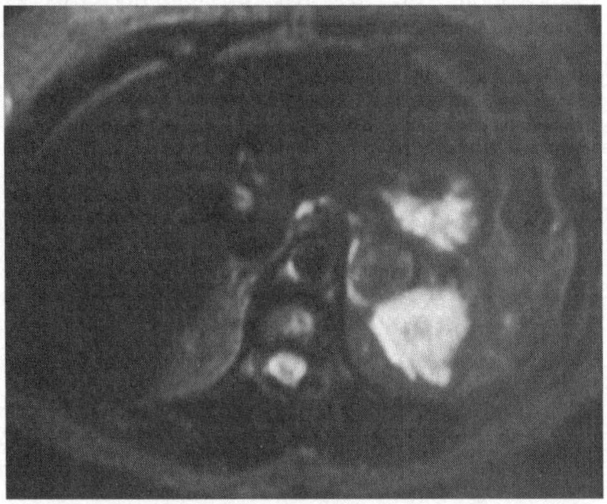

- Chemical-shift MRI

  * Signal from cortical adenomas drops out in opposed phase

Diagnosis: CT Adenoma Characteristics

- Sharp margins
- Smooth and homogenous
- Lipid-rich
- Most have density <10 HU on noncontrast images
- Values for cancer and pheochromocytoma are much higher.
- Density reduces at least 60% on initial contrast density at scan delayed 15 min.

Diagnosis: Imaging Criteria

Study Indicating Adenoma

	Sens	Spec
* CT density < 10 HU	71%	98%
† CT washout > 60%	100%	100%
* MRI T2 intensity < 0.8 compared to liver	80%	80%
* Loss of signal on chemical shift MRI	95%	100%
NP-59 scintigraphy	93%	100%

* All evaluating for fat content
† Becoming more widely accepted

Diagnosis: Nuclear Scintigraphy

- NP-59 (131I-6b-iodomethyl-norcholesterol) taken up by adrenal cortex (ie, adenoma) not space occupying lesion (cancer, pheochromocytoma)
- MIBG taken up preferentially by pheochromocytoma

Figure 5a

Adrenal metastasis often appear heterogeneous on T1 images

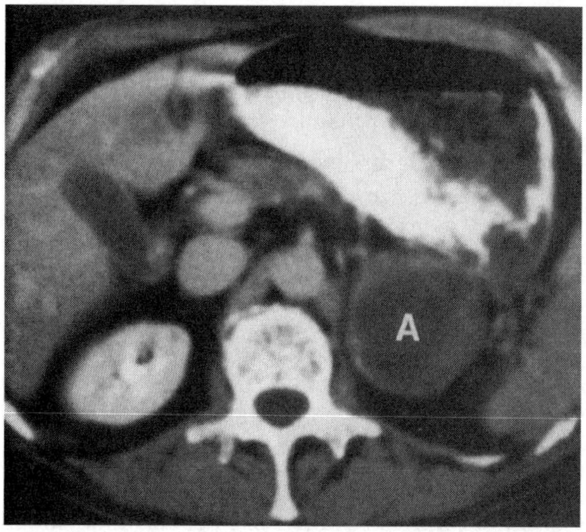

Figure 5b

Adrenal metastasis often is hyper-intense on T2 MRI

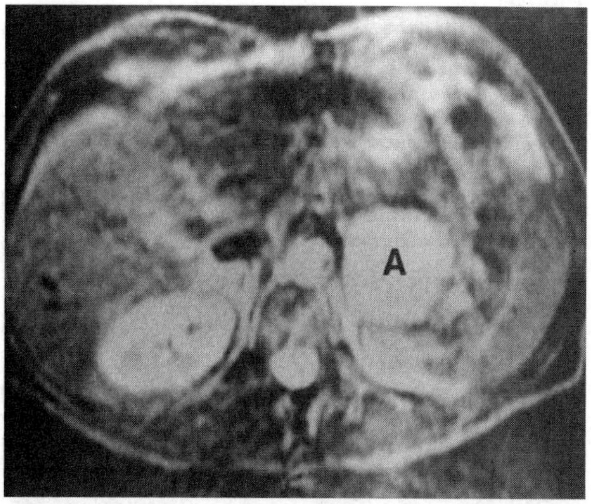

Figure 6

Classic findings of benign adenoma: Homogenous, smooth, distinct margins, lipid rich and nonenhancing on contrast CT

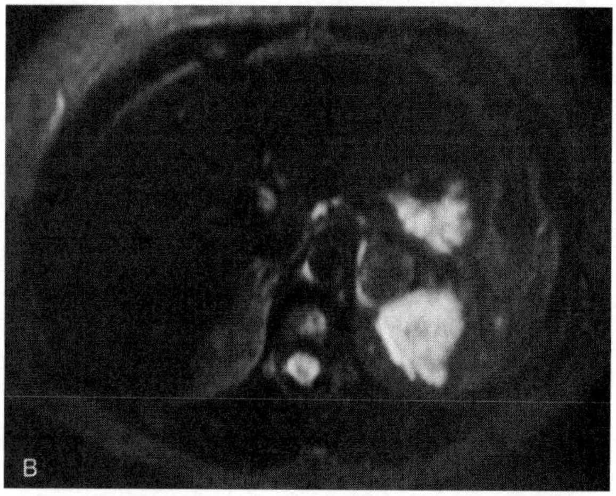

Diagnosis: Imaging Size Criteria

- 90% adrenal cortical carcinomas are usually >6 cm.
- It is rare for an adenoma to reach this size.
- However, CT underestimates actual size by as much as 20%.
- This is why many surgeons recommend surgical removal for tumors 5 cm or greater.
- As shown in the previous studies there is no cut-off with perfect accuracy.
- For test purposes it is recommended to remove adrenal glands ≥5 cm and treat them as adrenal cortical carcinomas.

Summary of Management Recommendations

- Hormonally active mass → surgical removal
- Hormonally inactive mass

  * If imaging suggests cancer → surgical removal

- If >5 cm at any age → surgical removal
- If <3 cm and nonfunctional → observe

Surveillance Recommendations for the Incidental Adrenal Mass

- Older consensus recommendation:
- CT at 6 months
- Annual endocrine evaluation for 4 years
- If the mass shows growth or develops detectable endocrine function then remove
- Newer emerging recommendations:
  * If mass stable on scans at 3 and 12 months and there is no function then routine follow-up is not required

9. Pheochromocytoma

Incidence and Presentation

- The clinical symptoms are directly caused by release of epinephrine and norepinephrine
- ***Hypertension is present in 90% of cases and may be paroxysmal, sustained or both.***
- ***Patients may also have orthostatic hypotension due to low plasma volume.***
- 30% of pheochromocytomas are found at autopsy and cause of death is often due to cardiovascular disease
- These tumors can arise anywhere in paraganglion system
- Can arise from the bladder and if in bladder is often associated with micturition syncope

Common Clinical Findings of Pheochromocytoma

- Classic triad:
  1. Episodic headache
  2. Tachycardia
  3. Diaphoresis
- Most commonly young to middle-age adults with unsustained HTN with superimposed paroxysms, but 10% are normotensive

Figure 7a

T1 weighted images of the bladder showing large mass

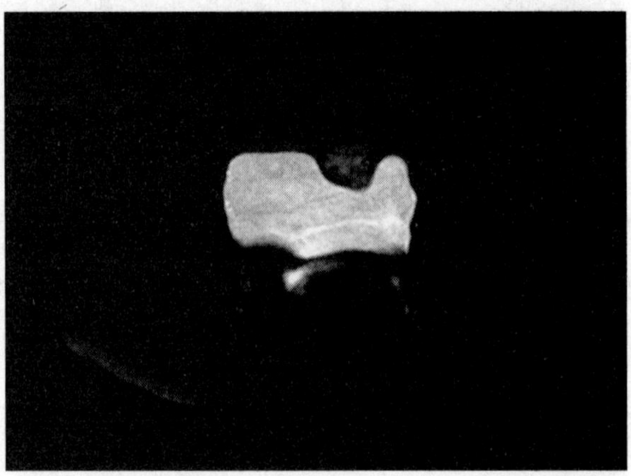

Figure 7b

T2 weighted image shows enhancement of the bladder pheochromocytoma

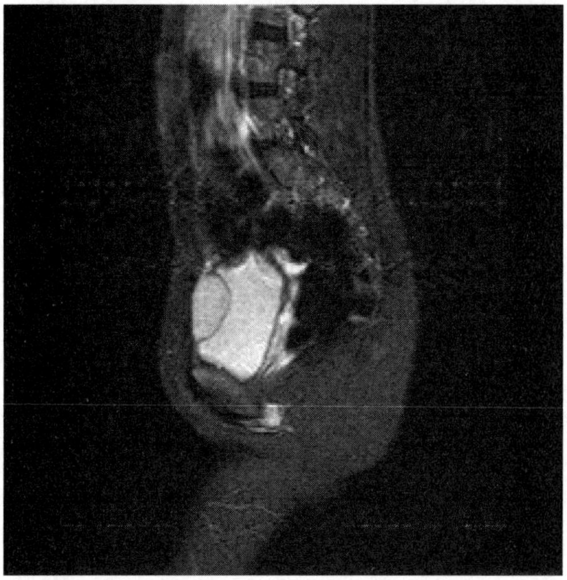

- Other commonly reported signs and symptoms
  * Sweating
  * Pallor
  * Flushing
  * Palpitations
  * Tachycardia
  * Abdominal pain
  * Chest pain
  * Weakness
  * Nausea
  * Emesis
  * Anorexia
  * Psychosis

- Diagnosis occasionally occurs during pregnancy and mimics pre-eclampsia and toxemia.

- The maternal and infant mortality is 40%.

- Small tumors may actually be more symptomatic than larger tumors, since large tumors are able to bind more of the catecholamines and metabolize them inside the tumor.

- Cardiomyopathy
  * Unexpected cardiovascular response during anesthesia is usually due to catecholamine-induced cardiomyopathy.
  * This entity is felt to be caused when catecholamine release results in small areas of myocardial necrosis, which leads to inflammation and fibrosis.
  * It is estimated that the mortality rate can be as high as 80% during surgery if cardiomyopathy is untreated.
  * It is recommended that all pheochromocytoma patients, regardless of age, have a complete cardiac work-up before surgery.

Pheochromocytoma and the Rule of 10s

- Bilateral in 10%
- Familial (nonsporadic) in 10%
- Pediatric in 10%
- Malignant in 10%
- Normotensive in 10%
- Extra-adrenal in 10%
- Multiple in 10%
- Childhood presentation breaks rules!
- 25% are bilateral, multiple, or extra-adrenal

Syndromes Associated With Pheochromocytoma

- Von Hippel-Lindau disease
- Von Recklinghausen's neurofibromatosis
- Multiple endocrine neoplasia
- Associated with MEN II but not MEN I

Pathophysiology of Pheochromocytoma

- Excessive secretion of catecholamines
- Norepinephrine
- Epinephrine
- Dopamine
- Levels that may be measured diagnostically
- Two different tests
- Breakdown products of the primary catecholamines
  * VMA
  * Metanephrines

Diagnosis: First Level

- Plasma free metanephrines—the most sensitive test!
- 99% of patients have elevated plasma metanephrines
- Next most sensitive test is 24° urinary catecholamines which if 2x normal is considered diagnostic.
- Most specific test:
  * 24° urinary metanephrines
  * Total metanephrines
  * Vanillyl mandellic acid (VMA)

Diagnosis: Second Level

- Clonidine suppression test (0.3 mg orally, test 3 hours later). Essential hypertensive patients will show a reduction in catecholamines by approximately 50% but in pheochromocytoma there will be no suppression.
- Glucagon stimulation test (2 mg IV and then 3 minutes later measure catecholamines). Pheochromocytoma patients increase catecholamines dramatically. Normal patients show no change.

Management

- Surgical excision is mainstay
- Evaluate for extra-adrenal, multiple, and bilateral sites
- Primarily search for extra-adrenal sites is radiographic
- Extent of disease staged preoperatively
- Unless metastatic disease apparent, cannot tell if will be malignant

Table 1

MEN Syndromes

MEN I ("Wermer's")	MEN IIA ("Sipple's")	MEN IIB
Parathyroid adenoma/carcinoma	Medullary thyroid carcinoma	Medullary thyroid carcinoma
Pituitary hyperplasia/adenoma	Pheochromocytoma	Pheochromocytoma
Pancreatic islet cell hyperplasia	Parathyroid hyperplasia/adenoma	Mucosal and GI neuroma
		Marfanoid features

Radiographic Localization

Imaging	Sensitivity	Specificity
CT	98%	70%
MRI *	100%	67%
MIBG †	86%-100%	85%-99%

* Hyper-intense on T2
† scintigraphy with 123 or 131I -meta-iodobenzylguanidine lights up even if not apparent on MRI

Preoperative Management

- There is some recent controversy over the early alpha blockade of patients before surgery. However, it is still widely recommended that patients be managed medically to control hypertension with a long-acting alpha blocker such as **phenoxybenzamine hydrochloride** before surgical resection.

- Initial alpha blockade may be followed by **beta blocker** if needed to control blood pressure and heart rate.

- ***It is accepted that beta blockers should not be used before alpha blockade treatment since beta blockade alone can cause increased vascular resistance and high blood pressure due to unopposed alpha adrenergic tone.***

Orthostatic Hypotension

- Liberalize water and salt intake

- IV hydration preoperative

- Invasive monitoring intra-operative

- Careful postoperative observation

Preoperative Preparation Required

- Mortality up to 80% in untreated patients with cardiomyopathy

- Consultation recommended: endocrinologist and anesthesiologist

- Preoperative goals:
  * Normalize blood pressure
  * Expand plasma volume
  * Prevent cardiac arrhythmias
  * Prevent intra-op hypertension
  * Minimize post-op hypotension

Preoperative Preparation

- Stepwise plan: pharmaceuticals

- Consider starting with long acting calcium-channel blocker

- Classic initial therapy is nonselective, long-acting **phenoxybenzamine**
  * Start 5 mg bid, ↑ 10 mg qod prn to 100 mg bid; beware postoperative hypotension

- If refractory arrhythmias (ie, sinus tachycardia), add a beta blocker

- Use only after alpha blockade (exacerbate HTN if unopposed)
  * Propranolol (20-40 mg tid)
  * Rarely will you need to add metyrosine (alpha-methyl paratyrosine) in severe cases to block the rate of catecholamine synthesis.

Intraoperative Management

- Pre-op anesthesia consultation

- Low threshold to postpone surgery if not prepared

- Certain popular agents are usually avoided:
  * Halothane, propofol, morpine sulfate, pancuronium

- To control intra-operative hypertension:
  * Phentolamine, nitroprusside, esmolol

Postoperative Management

- Hypotension is most common after surgery and is usually due to hypovolemia which resolves once the vasoconstrictive effects of catecholamines are no longer present and vascular tone is diminished.

- Hypotension may occur immediately after division of the adrenal vein.

Surgical Principles
- Ligate adrenal vein first!

- It prevents intra-operative catecholamine surge, by minimizing manipulation of the adrenal gland before the vein is ligated, thus the dogma: "Dissect the patient away from the tumor"

Surgical Outcomes
- Excision does not always lead to long-term cure; even in patients with a benign tumor

- Benign recurrence rate is 5%

- Malignant recurrence rate 10%

- Hypertension may persist due to vascular disease, age, or genetic predisposition

- 80% 20-year cause-specific survival

- Long-term follow-up required

10. Primary Hyperaldosteronism (Conn's Syndrome)

- Conn's syndrome was first described as a clinical syndrome in 1955

- Clinical presentation classically described in 1955:
  * Hypertension
  * Hypokalemia
  * Hypernatremia
  * Alkalosis
  * Periodic paralysis

Modern Clinical Presentation
- Hypokalemia

- Hypertension

- Depressed Renin

- High urine and plasma aldosterone

Typical Clinical Features
- Refractory hypertension

- Hypokalemia

- Profound hypokalemic response to diuretics

- Often asymptomatic

- May also manifest: muscle weakness, tetany, headache, polydipsia

- Patients often will have adapted a low-salt diet which helps to decrease potassium wasting, since less Na available for K exchange, and thus symptoms seem to improve.

Primary Hyperaldosteronism (Conn's Syndrome)
- A very rare cause of hypertension in ~ 0.5%

- Most commonly seen in Caucasians, 30-60 years of age

- Pathology:
  * 70% aldosteronoma
  * 30% bilateral adrenal hyperplasia
  * Bilateral adrenal hyperplasia mostly in men

Pathophysiology

- Primary hyperaldosteronism is the autonomous (without stimulation) secretion of aldosterone from the adrenal gland resulting in:
  * salt retention
  * hypertension
  * potassium wasting
  * may also be associated with the autonomous overproduction of cortisol

- Secondary hyperaldosteronism results from renovascular hypertension. The decreased renal blood flow causes increased aldosterone production secondary to over-production of renin.

Diagnosis: First Level

- Random Serum K <3.0 mEq/dL

- Plasma renin activity is suppressed (PRA) <2 ng/mL

- 25% of essential hypertensives have depressed PRA, but have normal serum potassium

- Plasma aldosterone >15 ng/dL

- Aldosterone: PRA >20:1

- Confirmation can be made by placing the patient on a high sodium diet for 3 days (>200 mEq/day) and measuring 24-hr urine aldosterone. This is diagnostic if:
  * Urine aldosterone >14 mcg/24°
  * Urine K >30 mEq/24°

Management

- *Bilateral adrenal hyperplasia*
  * Medical therapy indicated with spironolactone, which is an aldosterone antagonist
  * Side effects of spironolactone:
    - Normalizes serum K^+
    - Can result in painful gynecomastia
  * HCTZ normalizes blood pressure

- *Unilateral adrenal adenoma*
  * Adrenalectomy following control of HTN and hypokalemia (amiloride, triamterene, spironolactone)
  * Partial adrenalectomy has been reported and usually requires intraoperative ultrasound assessment of the adrenal gland

Result of Adrenalectomy

- 35% cured of hypertension

- 56% improved hypertension with need for fewer or milder medications

- All but 9% have cure or improvement

11. Cushing's Syndrome – Glucocorticoid Excess

Cushing's syndrome simply describes the symptoms from glucocorticoid excess, but does not distinguish one cause from another cause. This needs to be distinguished from Cushing's disease.

Cushing's syndrome is summarized in Table 2.

- Incidence: 1 per 100,000-500,000
- ACTH-dependent causes are the most common (82%)
- Also consider exogenous sources from therapeutic steroids

Table 2

Clinical Picture of Hypercorticolism or Cushing's Syndrome

Obesity	90%
Hypertension	80%
Diabetes	80%
Central obesity	80%
Weakness	80%
Muscle atrophy	70%
Hirsuitism	70%
Skin striae	70%
Moon facies	60%
Easy bruising	50%
Acne	50%
Psychological changes	50%

ACTH Dependent Causes of Cushing's Syndrome
- Cushing's disease = pituitary hypersecretion of ACTH – 70% of cases
- Ectopic ACTH – 12% of cases
- Most common sources of ectopic ACTH production:
  - * Carcinoma lung 52%
  - * Carcinoma pancreas 11%
  - * Thymoma 11%

ACTH-independent Causes (18%)
- Adrenal adenoma – 8%
- Adrenal carcinoma – 6%
- Bilateral adrenal hyperplasia – 4%

Pathophysiology
- ACTH-dependent = primary excessive ACTH secretion from the pituitary gland. Again this is Cushing's disease and is the most common ACTH-dependent cause.
- ACTH may also come from ectopic sources which also result in an increase in cortisol production from the adrenal gland
- ACTH-independent = Primary excessive cortisol secretion from an adrenal adenoma, adrenal carcinoma or bilateral adrenal hyperplasia inhibit production of ACTH

Diagnosis: Is this Pseudo-Cushing's?
- Rule out exogenous sources, glucocorticoids
- Topical creams, lotions
- Review of oral medications
- Nonendocrine causes of hypercorticolism
  - * Major depression
  - * Alcoholism

Diagnosis: A Three-Step Process

- Number One: Establish presence of excess glucocorticoids

- Number Two: Distinguish between ACTH-independent and ACTH-dependent causes

- Number Three: Determine specific etiology
  * ACTH-dependent
    - Cushing's disease
    - Ectopic ACTH secretion
  * ACTH-independent
    - Adrenal adenoma, carcinoma, or bilateral hyperplasia

Diagnosis Number One: Hypercorticolism?

- 24° urine free cortisol is the best initial diagnostic test: >100 mg/24 is diagnostic

- If equivocal: low-dose dexamethasone test
  * 1 mg at 11 PM, obtain plasma cortisol at 8 AM
  * Normal suppresses plasma cortisol to <5 ng/mL
  * If plasma cortisol is not suppressed = Cushing's syndrome

- Can also use salivary cortisol concentration.

Diagnosis Number Two: Relation to ACTH?

- Measure late afternoon ACTH >50 pg/mL = ACTH-dependent Cushing's because ACTH excess is causing overproduction glucocorticoids from the adrenal gland.

- <5 pg/mL =ACTH-independent Cushing's because excess glucocorticoids from the adrenal gland are causing suppression of ACTH.

Diagnosis Number Three: Specific Entity?

- ACTH-dependent Cushing's

- High-dose dexamethasone test
  * 8 mg at 11 PM
  * Obtain plasma cortisol at 8 AM

- < 50% reduction = ectopic ACTH

- 50% reduction = pituitary tumor and diagnostic of Cushing's disease because these patients have a relative resistance to negative feedback.

- (No reduction = ACTH-independent)

- ACTH-independent Cushing's imaging (CT) distinguishes:
  * Adenoma
  * Cancer
  * Bilateral hyperplasia

Management: Adenoma/Cancer

- Unilateral adrenalectomy

- May require preoperative reduction of cortisol secretion, if markedly elevated (see ectopic ACTH secretion)

- Excessive cortisol: Suppresses the other adrenal gland and will require intra-operative steroid support and a postoperative steroid taper may be needed while the contralateral gland recovers function.

Management: Bilateral Adrenal Hyperplasia

- Bilateral adrenalectomy

- After bilateral adrenalectomy, 10%-20% get Nelson's syndrome which is ACTH hyper-secretion by chromophobe adenoma resulting in:
  * Headache
  * Deep pigmentation
  * Visual disturbances

Management: Ectopic ACTH Secretion and Pituitary Tumor

- *Ectopic ACTH secretion*
  * Resection of tumor if possible
  * Medical therapy with metyrapone, ketoconozole, or aminoglutethimide

- *Pituitary Tumor*
  * Trans-sphenoidal hypophysectomy
  * For failure of pituitary surgery:
    - Bilateral adrenalectomy or radiation therapy

12. Adrenal Insufficiency (Addison's Disease)

• Rare but potentially fatal if not recognized and treated

• Incidence: 1 per 4,500-6,250 hospitalized pts

• Third-fifth decade of life is the most common age group

Primary Causes of Insufficiency
• Autoimmune adrenalitis

• Infection (TB, HIV most common)

• Adrenal hemorrhage

• *The most common cause in industrialized counties is autoimmune destruction of the adrenal gland. Diagnosis is made from finding 21-hydroxylase adrenal antibodies.*

• *The most common cause in nonindustrialized countries is TB*

Secondary Causes
• Metastatic disease

• Surgical removal of the adrenal gland

• Pituitary disease

• Sarcoidosis

• Exogenous steroid use

Pathophysiology and Clinical
• Deficiency of both glucocorticoid and mineralocorticoid

• Acute
  * Fever
  * Severe hypotension
  * Nausea/vomiting
  * Lethargy
  * Postoperative "crash" without apparent surgical complication

Pathophysiology and Clinical Presentation
• Deficiency of both glucocorticoid and mineralocorticoid

• Chronic presentation:
  * Fatigue
  * Weight loss
  * Anorexia
  * Nausea and vomiting
  * Abdominal pain

Diagnosis
• Clinical scenario, especially postoperative

• Labs: Hyponatremia, hyperkalemia, azotemia, hypoglycemia eosinophilia in 15%-20%

• The most common lab findings are:
  * ***Hyponatremia***
  * ***Hyperkalemia***

Screening Test
• ACTH stimulation 0.25 mg cosyntropin IV

• Measure plasma cortisol at 60 minutes

• Cortisol should be >18 ug/dL if normal

Management
• Adrenal crisis
  * IV access, blood for chemistry, ACTH and cortisol
  *Don't wait for result before treating
  * 2-3 liters D5 NS quickly
  * 4 mg dexamethasone IV
  * (IV cortisol will interfere with the diagnosis later during hospitalization)

• Subsequent

• Confirm diagnosis

• Determine and treat cause

• Maintenance therapy
  * Hydrocortisone 30 mg/day
  * Fluorohydrocortisone 0.05-0.1 mcg/day

13. Adrenal Cortical Carcinoma

- This a rare but very aggressive tumor
- Incidence: 1 per 1.7 million people
- It is the model cancers that invade into adjacent structures
- Suspicion of adrenal carcinoma should prompt consultation and team approach with other surgeons, vascular, or/and surgical oncology
- Accounts for 0.02% of cancers, and 0.2% of cancer deaths
- Can be difficult to diagnosis
- Weiss microscopic criteria for diagnosis
  * High mitotic rate and nuclear grade
  * Atypical mitosis
  * Eosinophilic cytoplasm
  * Diffuse architecture
  * Necrosis
  * Microscopic invasion

Clinical Findings
- Constitutional
- Weight loss, malaise, fever

Endocrine Evaluation Shows That 80% are Functional Tumors

Clinical Findings of Cushing's Most Common
- Sex steroid excess
- Oligomenorrhea
- Virilization/feminization
- Can present as incidentaloma

Diagnosis: Endocrine Evaluation
- 80% are functional
- Often secrete multiple hormones

* Glucocorticoids	72%
* Androgens	43%
* Precursors	22%
* Estradiol	8%
* Aldosterone	4%

- Endocrine function is useful in the diagnosis
- Finding of multiple hormones suggestive of carcinoma
- Carcinoma more often secretes sex steroids (Plasma DHEA, 24° urine 17-ketosteroids) than do adenomas
- Endocrine function is useful as a marker

Diagnosis: Radiography
- Cross-sectional imaging localization and staging
- CT or MRI can be helpful
- Over 90% are > 6 cm
- Irregular, inhomogeneous
- Can be distinguished from adrenal adenoma
- NP-59 adrenal scintigraphy
- CT ± washout curve
- MRI are bright or enhancing on T2 weighted images (Figure 8A and Figure 8B)

Adrenal Carcinoma Staging
- Common sites of metastases
  * Lung
  * Liver
  * Lymph nodes
- Staging studies
  * CXR
  * CBC, LFT, LDH, basic metabolic panel
  * CT and venogram versus MRI

Surgical Management
- Surgery is mainstay of treatment
- 5-year survival clinically localized disease 35%
- 5-year survival for pathologically confined disease 50%
- Frequently invading into adjacent structures!

Figure 8a

Adrenal mass is seen on MRI T1 weighted image with low signal intensity similar to liver

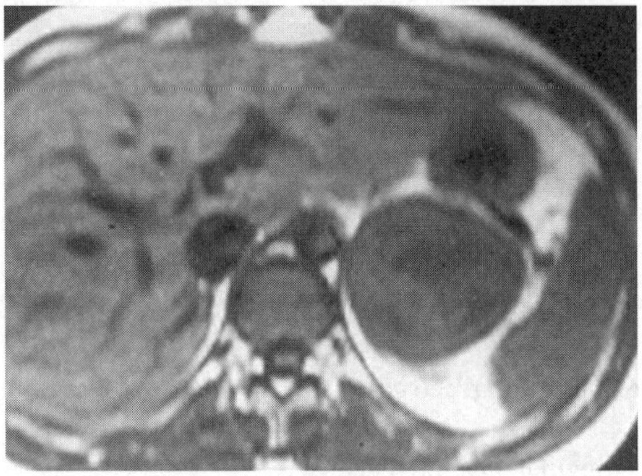

Figure 8b

T2 weighted images shows enhanced signal intensity of the adrenal mass consistent with adrenal cortical carcinoma

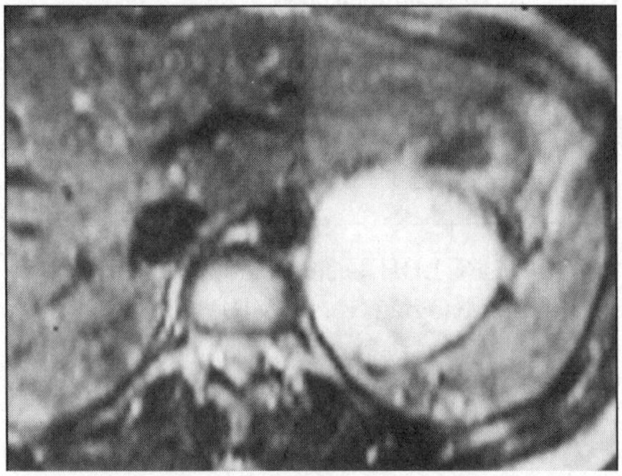

- Radical en-bloc adrenalectomy with regional lymphadenectomy and total or subtotal excision of adjacent organs (kidney, spleen, liver, colon, pancreas)

- May require cavotomy, bypass or other extensive reconstruction

Medical Management
- Metastatic or recurrent disease

- Mitotane (o,p'-DDD, a cogener of DDT)
  * Hormonal response in 75%
  * Response of tumor mass in 35%
  * No improvement in survival
  * All have significant toxicity
  * Trials of adjunctive use of mitotane

14. Metastatic Disease to the Adrenal Gland

- More common than adrenal cortical carcinoma 40%-50% of metastases from:
  * Melanoma
  * Breast
  * Lung
  * Kidney

- 8%-38% of patients with extra-adrenal malignancy will have adrenal metastases at autopsy

- *With known primary cancer*
  *Adrenal mass is metastasis in 32-73 (~50)%

Diagnosis
- In setting of widespread metastases (most common), diagnosis obvious

- If no other metastases, do work-up as for adrenal incidentaloma (see below), even with known primary cancer

- Findings suggestive of metastases

- No endocrine abnormalities

- Irregular/inhomogeneous on CT, bright on T2 images of MRI, cold spot on NP-59 scintigraphy

- Adrenal metastasis is the best indication for FNA of adrenal gland

- FNA cannot reliably distinguish adrenal adenoma vs. adrenal cortical carcinoma

- ***Must rule out pheochromocytoma biochemically before attempting FNA.***

- ***MRI appearance alone is not sufficient, since carcinoma, metastasis and pheo are all enhancing or bright on T2 weighted images.***

Management
- Solitary metastasis: May be benefit to adrenalectomy

- Decision in concert with oncologist

- Avoid direct gland manipulation
  * Hemorrhage
  * Tumor spillage

- Take generous peri-adrenal tissue, but resection into other organs not usually necessary

15. Principles of Adrenalectomy

- The laparoscopic approach is the standard of care for 90% of adrenal tumors.

- Large tumors >10 cm present unique challenges and can be carcinoma.

- These large tumors may be best approached through open incisions.

In testing situations, you must be prepared to discuss most of the different surgical options for organ removal. Since bleeding is the most common complication encountered during adrenalectomy, you must be prepared to discuss how you would covert from laparoscopic surgery to open surgery and control significant bleeding from the vena cava on the right side and the renal vein and aorta on the left side. Two sponge sticks and vascular clamps should be readily available for emergencies.

- Early division adrenal vein:
  Most important step = pheochromocytoma

- "Dissect patient away from gland"

- Traction on adjacent tissues

- For open surgery:
  * Divide superior and lateral attachments
  * Allow gland to be retracted into operative field

Open Surgical Adrenalectomy
- Approach determined by:
  * Adrenal pathology
  * Size
  * Associated conditions
  * Patient body habitus
  * Medical fitness
  * Surgeon experience

Anterior (Transperitoneal) Approach
- Chevron, hemi-chevron, or subcostal (not midline)

- Large masses, moderate-size cancers, or extra-adrenal involvement

Posterior Approach
- Rib-resecting or lumbotomy

- Small benign masses, bilateral adrenalectomy

- Lumbotomy causes less pain and seems easy, but can be difficult access without some prior experience!

Thoraco-abdominal Approach
- Through bed of 9th or 10th rib

- Diaphragmatic incision, with excellent extra- and intra-peritoneal exposure

- Large adrenal cancers

Laparoscopic Adrenalectomy
- Standard of care today

- Two different approaches
  * Transperitoneal
    - Most common
    - Most familiar anatomy
  * Retroperitoneal
    - Faster
    - Especially on left, once the surgeon has some experience

Options for Adrenalectomy

- Pheochromocytoma
  - * Variable in size
  - * Laparoscopy suitable according to the surgeon's experience
  - * Ligation of the adrenal vein can be easier with laparoscopy due to improved visualization compared to open surgery

- Aldosteronoma
  - * Usually small (<3 cm)
  - * Laparoscopy good choice

Figure 9

Chevron incision allows excellent exposure to both adrenal glands and can be useful when large tumors have the possibility of involving adjacent organs

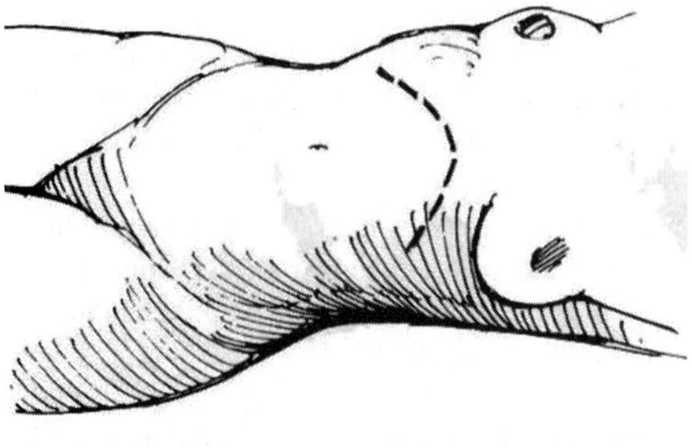

Figure 10

Surgical approach to the adrenal gland through the dorsal lumbotomy incisions

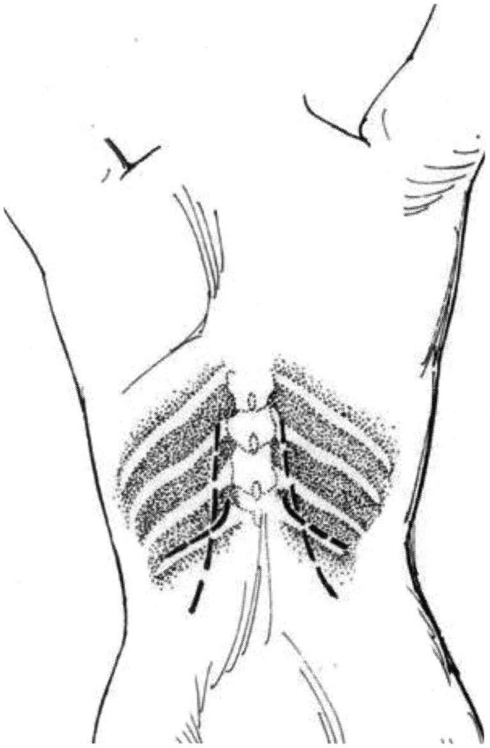

16. Complications of Adrenalectomy

- *Bleeding is the most common complication*

- Prevention—Find correct landmarks: left-sided dissection

  * Renal vein

  * Upper pole kidney

  * Adrenal vein is more medial

  * Adrenal is lateral to splenic artery

- Avoid hunting through fat!

- Harmonic Scalpel®/LigaSure Atlas™ best for hemostasis

Other Reported Complications During Adrenalectomy

- Bleeding: most common

- Endocrine imbalance

- Liver or spleen laceration

- Pneumothoax

- Trocar placement

- Diaphragm injury

18. References

Bauer SB. Anomalies of the kidney and ureteropelvic junction. In: Walsh PC, Retik AB, Vaughan ED Jr, Wein AJ, eds. *Campbell's Urology*. 7th ed. Philadelphia, Pa: WB Saunders; 1998:1708-1739.

Bravo EL. Primary aldosteronism: New approaches to diagnosis and management. *Cleve Clin J Med*. 1993;60:379-386.

Goeres R, Knappe G, Gerl H, et al. Diagnosis of Cushing's syndrome: Reevaluation of midnight plasma cortisol vs. urinary free cortisol and low dose dexamethasone suppression test in a large patient group. *J Endorcin Invest*. 1999:22:241-249.

Goldfarb DA. Contemporary evaluation and management of Cushing's syndrome. *World J Urol*. 1999;17:22-25.

Hilton S, Schwartz LH. Radiologic imaging of genitourinary neoplasms. In: Raghavan D, Scher HI, Leibel SA, Lange PH, eds. *Principles and Practice of Genitourinary Oncology*. Philadelphia, Pa: Lippincott-Raven; 1997:33-42.

Lenders JWM, Pacak K, Walther MM, et al. Biochemical diagnosis of pheochromocytoma: Which test is best? *JAMA*. 2002;287:1427-1434.

Vaughan ED Jr, Blumenfeld JD. The adrenals. In: Walsh PC, Retik AB, Vaughan ED Jr, Wein AJ, eds. *Campbell's Urology*. 7th ed. Vol 3. Philadelphia, Pa: WB Saunders Co; 1998:2915.

Vaughan ED Jr, Sosa RE. Renovascular hypertension and other renal diseases. In: Walsh PC, Retik AB, Vaughan ED Jr, Wein AD, eds. *Campbell's Urology*. 7th ed. Philadelphia, Pa: WB Saunders Co; 1998:423-459.

Vella A, Nippoldt TB, Morris JC. Adrenal hemorrhage: A 25-year experience at the Mayo Clinic. *Mayo Clin Proc*. 2001;76:161-168.

19. Questions

1. In a patient with Cushing's syndrome due to adrenal adenoma, the changes in hormone secretion following a high dose dexamethasone suppression test are best represented by:

A. ACTH: ↑ Urinary free cortisol: ↓

B. ACTH: ↑ Urinary free cortisol: ↑

C. ACTH: ↔ Urinary free cortisol: ↔

D. ACTH: ↓ Urinary free cortisol: ↓

E. ACTH: ↓ Urinary free cortisol: ↑

2. Which of the following is the most sensitive biochemical test for confirming the diagnosis of pheochromocytoma?

A. Plasma free metanephrines

B. Plasma catecholamines

C. Urinary metanephrines

D. Urinary vanillylmanelic acid

E. Urinary catecholamines

3. Adrenal hemorrhage is most frequently associated with:

A. Heparin-induced thrombocytopenia

B. Trauma

C. Warfarin therapy

D. Sepsis

E. Adrenal adenoma

4. A 45-year-old hypertensive man has an elevated 24-hour urinary aldosterone after a period of salt loading. CT scan of the adrenals is normal. The best study for localization of a surgically curable lesion is:

A. MRI scans

B. Adrenal venography

C. MIBG scan

D. Adrenal venous sampling

E. Iodocholesterol scan

5. A 55-year-old obese man with epigastric discomfort is noted to have a 5 cm right adrenal mass on CT scan. The mass measures -40 Hounsfield units. The next step is:

A. Observation

B. 24-hour urine for metanephrines

C. MRI scans

D. Right adrenalectomy

E. Dexamethasone suppression test

6. In the diagnostic evaluation of excess cortisol secretion, the administration of 2 mg of dexamethasone q.i.d. (high dose) for two days results in:

A. No suppression of urinary corticosteroid secretion in normal patients.

B. Suppression to less than half the baseline in patients with adrenal hyperplasia.

C. Suppression to less than the baseline in patients with benign cortical adenoma.

D. Suppression to less than half the baseline in patients with adrenal carcinoma.

E. Increased urinary secretion in patients with adrenal carcinoma.

7. In a patient with an absent right kidney and a left pelvic kidney, the right adrenal is:

A. Absent and the left is adjacent to the upper pole of the kidney.

B. Absent and the left is in the normal anatomic position.

C. In the normal anatomic position and the left is adjacent to the upper pole of the kidney.

D. In the normal anatomic position and the left is in the normal anatomic position.

E. In the normal anatomic position and the left is absent.

8. A 40-year-old woman undergoes bilateral adrenalectomy for Cushing's disease with complete resolution of her symptoms. Replacement therapy with cortisone and fludrocortisone is instituted. Three years later, she complains of visual disturbances and is noted to have skin hyperpigmentation. The most likely explanation is:

A. Addison's disease

B. Pituitary adenoma

C. Excessive cortisone replacement

D. Excessive ACTH production

E. Ectopic melanocyte-stimulating hormone secretion

9. Angiotensin II causes blood pressure elevation by its effect on:

A. Peripheral vascular tone and cardiac rate

B. Peripheral vascular tone and blood volume

C. Blood volume and cardiac output

D. Blood volume and renin substrate

E. The juxtaglomerular apparatus

10. Hypertension in Cushing's syndrome is primarily related to:

A. Elevated plasma catecholamines

B. Elevated plasma aldosterone

C. Retention of water and salt

D. ACTH-stimulated renin

E. Elevated angiotensin II

Answers

1. C.

Patients with adrenal Cushing's syndrome have autonomous adrenal production of cortisol which suppresses ACTH. Exogenous administration of either low-dose or high-dose dexamethasone is unable to alter the autonomous adrenal production. Therefore, it results in no change in either ACTH or urinary-free cortisol production.

2. A.

A number of biochemical tests are available to exclude or confirm the diagnosis of pheochromocytoma. Plasma-free metanephrines testing is the most sensitive test (99%). Other acceptable clinical tests with lower sensitivities include urinary fractionated metanephrines (97%), plasma catecholamines (84%), urinary catecholamines (86%), urinary total metanephrines (77%), and urinary vanillymandelic acid (64%).

3. A.

Adrenal hemorrhage is an uncommon condition that is infrequently diagnosed while patients are alive. It has classically been associated with meningococcal septicemia. Recent series, however, have demonstrated it is most often associated with heparin-induced thrombocytopenia. Sepsis, stress and warfarin therapy are rarer causes.

4. D.

Aldosterone secreting adenomas are unilateral and small in size (1-2 cm). They may be smaller than the resolution of CT scanning. In this setting, adrenal venous sampling for aldosterone levels is the most sensitive assessment to identify a unilateral adenoma. An MRI scan offers no advantage over CT scan in this setting. Adrenal venography can be complicated by adrenal infarction and is rarely used.

5. A.

A mass with Hounsfield units between -30/ -140 is characteristic of an adrenal myelolipoma. These tumors are benign and are composed of lipid and myeloid tissue. No additional therapy or evaluation is required. (Hilton S, Schwartz LH. Radiologic imaging of genitourinary neoplasms. In: Raghavan D, Scher HI, Leibel SA, Lange PH, eds. *Principles and Practice of Genitourinary Oncology*. Philadelphia, Pa: Lippincott-Raven; 1997:33-42.)

6. B.

The dexamethasone suppression test is known to have a false positive rate of 20%. However, false negative tests are rare. Dexamethasone administration should result in suppression of plasma cortisol values (50% of pretreatment value), urine 17-hydroxysteroids and urine-free cortisol in patients with Cushing's syndrome. Pituitary imaging with CT or MRI will disclose an adenoma in 50% of such cases. Cortisol levels fail to fall to these levels in patients with adrenal carcinoma or ectopic ACTH secretion.

7. D.

The adrenal glad is in the normal anatomic position, no matter whether the kidney is absent or ectopic. (Bauer SB: Anomalies of the kidney and ureteropelvic junction. In: Walsh PC, Retik AB, Vaughan ED Jr, Wein AJ, eds. *Campbell's Urology*. 7th ed. Philadelphia, Pa: WB Saunders Co; 1998: 1708-1739.)

8. B.

Ten percent to 20% of patients who have bilateral adrenalectomy for Cushing's syndrome later develop pituitary tumors which are almost always chromophobe adenomas (Nelson's syndrome). Progressive hyperpigmentation due to melanocyte stimulating hormone release by corticotropic releasing hormone, headaches, and visual disturbances, are due to the expanding adenoma that is shown by skull x-rays or CT scans of the sella turcica. Pituitary basophilic adenoma that was initially postulated by Cushing as causing the syndrome named for him has, in fact, rarely been a factor.

9. B.

Renin is a proteolytic enzyme secreted in the juxtaglomerular apparatus of the kidney and is physiologically inert. Antiotensinogen is a plasma globulin substrate of hepatic origin, upon which renin acts to produce angiotensin I. Angiotensin I is a decapeptide which is also physiologically inert. Angiotensin I is acted upon by converting enzyme to produce the octapeptide angiotensin II. Angiotensin II is the first effector hormone of the renin system, and is the only substance directly responsible for elevation in blood pressure in patients with renovascular hypertension. It acts upon the smooth muscle of the peripheral vasculature to cause vasoconstriction, and also stimulates the zona glomerulosa to produce aldosterone which causes sodium retention in the distal tubule and thus produces volume expansion.

10. C.

Cushing's syndrome is due to glucocorticoid excess while Cushing's disease is a pituitary adenoma. Approximately 80% of patients with Cushing's syndrome have hypertension at the time of presentation. Glucocorticoids have weak mineralocorticoid effects resulting in retention of salt and water.

Chapter 23: Interstitial Cystitis/ Sexually Transmitted Diseases/ Urinary Tract Infections

Deborah R. Erickson, MD
Daniel A. Shoskes, MD

Contents

Chapter 23A: Interstitial Cystitis

Deborah R. Erickson, MD

Contents

1. Introductory Definitions: Painful Bladder Syndrome (PBS)

A. There is still no well-established clinical definition of IC[1-3]

B. National Institute of Diabetes, Digestive and Kidney Diseases (NIDDK) research criteria for IC

1. Purpose: to form a group of patients who almost certainly have IC so they can be enrolled in research studies

2. The criteria are too strict for use as a clinical diagnosis of IC[4]

3. The criteria are found in many references.[2,5] Briefly, they are:
   a. Must have bladder pain or urgency
   b. Must have diffuse glomerulations (at least 10 per quadrant in at least 3 quadrants) on cystoscopy after bladder distention, or Hunner's ulcer
   c. Must void at least 8x/day and 1x/night
   d. On urodynamics, must have intense urge at <150 mL volume and capacity must be <350 mL, and involuntary bladder contraction excludes IC
   e. Known cause for symptoms (eg, UTI, vaginitis, herpes, radiation, stone, urethral diverticulum, etc.) excludes IC.
   f. IC is excluded if symptoms are relieved by antimicrobials, antispasmodics, anticholinergics, or urinary antiseptics

C. PBS definition from the international continence society: the complaint of suprapubic pain related to bladder filling, accompanied by other symptoms, such as increased daytime and nighttime frequency, in the absence of proven urinary infection or other obvious pathology[1]

D. Many IC patients do not meet the PBS definition because the pain location is not suprapubic and/or the pain is not uniquely related to bladder filling[6]

E. Bladder pain syndrome is the term recommended by the European Society for Study of IC (ESSIC) and they have a detailed diagnostic algorithm[3]

F. This presentation will use the term IC because most treatment trials used that term, and used some form of the NIDDK criteria

2. Patient Presentation

A. Symptoms

1. Classic: pelvic pain when holding urine, which results in urinary frequency and nocturia

2. Some patients have constant pain, made worse by holding urine

3. Some patients describe symptoms as "urgency," with or without pain

B. 90% of patients diagnosed with IC are female, but some men with "prostatodynia" may truly have IC[2,7]

C. The average age at onset is in the early 40s, but any age can be affected

D. Late deterioration of symptoms is unusual[2]

E. Many IC patients can identify certain factors that influence symptoms

1. Certain foods, especially citrus, tomatoes, ethanol, chocolate and spicy foods, exacerbate symptoms in some patients.[8] Some patients can avoid the food-induced irritative symptoms by using calcium glycerophosphate (Prelief®), an over-the-counter preparation (unpublished data). However, a controlled trial of intravesical solutions at pH 5.0 vs. 7.5 showed no difference in pain scores between the 2 solutions[9]

2. Many IC patients note worse symptoms before the menses. Certain objective measurements (eg, number of voids per day, cystometry) were found to vary during the menstrual cycle in controls and/or IC patients, suggesting that gonadal hormones affect bladder sensation[10]

3. Stress commonly makes IC symptoms worse[2,11]

3. Evaluation of Patients With IC Symptoms

A. Experts debate about the extent of evaluation needed

1. Agreed to be important: history, exam, UA, culture, voiding diary

2. Tests that some experts think are essential, while others use selectively, based on patient presentation and clinical judgment:
   a. Urodynamics
   b. Cystoscopy in office or under anesthesia with distention
   c. Bladder biopsy
   d. Urine cytology

3. Most experts agree that the potassium sensitivity test is not helpful for diagnosis and should not be used except in research settings.

4. Urine markers would be very useful, but currently they are still in the investigational stage

B. History: Key Features

1. Urinary frequency (day and night)

2. Relationship of pain to voiding: typically, IC involves pain withholding urine, improved after voiding. Pain while voiding may occur but is not the usual presentation for IC

3. Incontinence is not a typical feature of IC

4. Ask about prescription and recreational drug ingestion, as certain NSAIDs and ketamine can cause these cystitis symptoms[12-14]

C. Voiding Diary

1. Simple chart with time and amount of each void

2. 24-hour diary is equally valid to longer ones; doing it on a weekday or weekend is equally valid[15]

D. Physical Exam

1. Important to exclude other potential causes for symptoms (such as vaginitis, urethral diverticulum, etc.)

2. In typical IC, the pelvic exam is normal except the bladder is tender to palpate through the anterior vaginal wall

3. Check for pelvic floor dysfunction (levator muscles tight and/or tender), which often accompanies IC, contributes to pain and needs to be treated separately[16]

E. Urinalysis

1. Usually normal in IC, or may have pyuria.[17,18]

2. Benign hematuria is present in 24%-41% of IC patients.[19,20] However, a careful evaluation is needed. 2 recent papers found that 6 of 600[21] and 1 of 61[22] patients referred to tertiary centers with "IC" actually had transitional cell carcinoma

F. Urine Culture

G. Urine cytology was previously described as low-yield in women with irritative symptoms and no hematuria.[23] However, in the recent paper by Tissot et al, 2 of their 6 patients with transitional cell carcinoma had positive or suspicious cytology, but no hematuria.[21] Therefore, the yield of cytology is low but not zero

H. Urodynamics

1. Typical findings in IC
   a. Urge to void at <150 cc volume
   b. Capacity <350 cc volume
   c. No involuntary bladder contractions

2. Compliance is usually normal, but may be low[24]

I. Cystoscopy with bladder distention under anesthesia for diagnosis

1. Procedure
   a. General anesthesia or spinal at least T9 level (bladder pain can be carried by sympathetic fibers)[25]
   b. Distend at 80 cm water pressure 1-2 minutes[5]
   c. Drain the bladder, then refill and inspect cystoscopically
   d. A rare complication: total bladder necrosis[26]

2. Glomerulations (pinpoint petechial hemorrhages seen after bladder distention) were originally described as a classic feature of IC, but their diagnostic value is now being debated because:
   a. Glomerulations are not specific to IC. They can be seen in other conditions including radiation or chemical cystitis,[2] after urinary diversion,[2] severe stress incontinence,[27] or some people with no bladder complaints, including 20% of men having TURP.[28,29] The underlying mechanism is thought to be that glomerulations are the response of the bladder to distention after a chronic period of underfilling for any reason[2]
   b. Glomerulations are not "sensitive" for IC. If patients with symptoms of IC are divided into those with vs. without glomerulations, the two groups are very similar in terms of symptoms, physical exam findings, urodynamic findings, urine marker levels and bladder biopsy findings.[30] Only few exceptions to this statement have been published:
      1. Patients with glomerulations were more likely to have positive staining on bladder biopsies for platelet-derived endothelial growth factor/thymidine phosphorylase.[31]
      2. Patients with glomerulations were more likely to have levator ani muscle tenderness on exam[32] and had worse frequency (day and night),[30,32] higher PUF scores,[32] and smaller capacity under anesthesia[30,32]

c. Some patients who lack glomerulations on initial cystoscopy will have them on a later cystoscopy[33]

d. Some authors have described associations between severity of glomerulations and other clinical or endoscopic features.[34] However, these associations were within groups of IC patients and do not imply that lack of glomerulations means lack of IC.

3. Hunner's ulcer

   a. Unlike glomerulations, ulcers are often seen on cystoscopy without doing a bladder distention first[35]

   b. More common in Europe than in the USA. For example, in a paper from Sweden, 56% of the IC patients had ulcers[36]

   c. There are several clinical and pathologic differences between ulcer and nonulcer patients.[35-41] Therefore, these 2 patient groups are thought to represent different pathophysiologic subtypes of IC. Some of these differences are:

      1. Older age in ulcer patients. The ulcer patients are older at symptom onset, not just at diagnosis, so they probably have a different condition, not just a later stage of the nonulcer IC
      2. More severe bladder inflammation in ulcer patients
      3. Compared to nonulcer patients, ulcer patients are more likely to respond to TENS & DMSO, but less likely to respond to PPS[35]
      4. In general, urine marker levels are similar for ulcer vs. nonulcer patients[39,40]
      5. Ulcer patients secreted nitric oxide into the bladder, while nonulcer patients did not.[41]

   d. Descriptions vary as to what exactly is a Hunner's ulcer

      1. Photograph on page 353 in 2007 edition of *Campbell's Urology*[2]
      2. "...a reddened mucosal lesion with small vessels radiating toward a central pale scar, fibrin deposit or coagulum. This site ruptures with increasing bladder distention with petechial oozing of blood from the ulcer and mucosal margins"[36]
      3. "A velvet red patch that looks, for all practical purposes, like carcinoma *in situ*"[42]

J. Bladder Biopsy

   1. No bladder biopsy findings are specific to IC, nor required for the diagnosis of IC

   2. At this time, the main value of bladder biopsy is to exclude other pathologies, such as carcinoma *in situ*

   3. In the future, bladder biopsy findings may be used predict treatment response. No studies to date have divided patients into groups based on bladder biopsies and compared treatment responses. However, some studies selected patients with specific biopsy features for entry into treatment trials. For example, the cimetidine trial required significant inflammation on bladder biopsy[43] and the montelukast trial required detrusor mastocoytosis (at least 28 cells/mm^2)[44]

K. Cystoscopy awake is normal in most IC patients. However, cystoscopy (either awake or with anesthesia) is recommended in patients who are at higher risk for bladder cancer

L. Potassium Sensitivity Testing

   1. Not a standard diagnostic test for IC

   2. Not sensitive for IC. In several reports, the incidences of positive KCl test among IC patients ranged from 54%-83%.[45-51] (Note: only 1 of these studies used the complete NIDDK criteria including urodynamics and cystoscopy.[45] In this study 74% of IC patients had an increase in bladder pain or urgency after KCl instillation.)

3. Not specific for IC. Increase in bladder pain or urgency after KCl instillation can also be seen in patients with urodynamic detrusor overactivity (25%),[45] radiation cystitis (100%),[45] acute bacterial cystitis (100%),[45] men with lower urinary tract symptoms (16%),[48] men with prostatitis (84%),[52] men with CP/CPPS (50%)[53] and men with BPH (3%-4%).[45] Interestingly, a recent paper showed different rates of KCl test results for women with urodynamic detrusor overactivity, depending on whether or not their symptoms responded to anticholinergics.[54]
   a. 6 responded; 1 (17%) had a positive KCl test
   b. 25 did not respond; 24 (96%) had a positive KCl test

4. Rates in healthy controls: 3%-4% for women,[45] 36% for men[53]

5. Not likely to aid in diagnosis for patients who present with typical symptoms of IC[46]

6. Not correlated with urodynamic or cystoscopic findings for patients who presented with typical symptoms of IC (except, interestingly, 24 of 24 ulcer patients had positive KCl tests)[49,55]

7. Ability to predict treatment response in IC:
   a. Not predictive of having at least 50% improvement with oral heparinoid treatment[47,50]
   b. Did not predict response in a randomized trial of PPS vs. cyclosporine A[55]
   c. Did predict response to intravesical hyaluronic acid. This study used a lower dose of KCL; 0.3 M instead of 0.4 M[56]

8. For IC patients and patients seeing a gynecologist for pelvic pain, rates of positive KCl test were positively associated with PUF scores[51]

9. Currently not recommended except in a research context[57,58]

M. Variation on KCl test: comparative cystometry. The basic idea is to perform cystometry twice, once with physiologic saline and once with KCl, and compare the results.

1. One version: compare saline with 0.2 M KCl (less painful than the 0.4 M KCl used in the original KCl test). The test is positive if the capacity with KCl is >30% less than the capacity with saline.[59] This test predicted response to intravesical hyaluronic acid.[59,60]

2. Another version: compare saline with 0.3 M KCl. Using this test, patients with OAB are sensitive to KCl,[61] and patients with urodynamic detrusor overactivity were more sensitive to KCl than the IC patients.[62]

N. Intravesical anesthetic test[63-65]

1. A kinder alternative to KCl test: instead of provoking pain for a diagnosis, try to relieve it.

2. Instill local anesthetic into bladder; if pain resolves, this pinpoints bladder as pain source and also can be a treatment. Different combinations have been described, and to date there is no evidence to establish which is superior:

a. 8 ml 1% or 2% lidocaine, 8 ml 8.4% sodium bicarbonate, 40,000 units heparin.[63]
b. 20 ml 2% lidocaine jelly, 20 ml 0.5% bupivacaine.[64]
c. 5 ml 4% lidocaine followed directly by 5 ml 8.4% sodium bicarbonate, and catheter clamped for 10-15 minutes.[65]

3. Possible reasons why pain might persist:
   a. Insufficient dose, contact time and/or epithelial penetration.
   b. Bladder nerves may be unresponsive to lidocaine.
   c. Pain source may be outside the bladder, such as pelvic floor muscles or central sensitization.

O. Urine markers are still in the investigational stage

P. Bottom line: use the above tools as needed to achieve the following goals:

1. Establish (or rule out) the bladder as the source of pain

2. Look for other conditions that might be causing the symptoms, to be sure IC is really the correct diagnosis

3. Look for comorbid conditions that may accompany IC and also contribute to symptoms. These need to be treated separately along with IC[16,65]

4. Etiologies of IC

A. Many etiologies are proposed, and it is likely that some are interrelated. At this time, no specific primary cause of IC has been definitively proven

B. Most commonly stated etiologies (a detailed evaluation of the evidence for and against each one is beyond the scope of a review course:[2]

1. Abnormal bladder epithelium[66,67]

2. Bladder mast cell activation[68,69]

3. Allergic or autoimmune process[70,71]

4. Neurogenic inflammation[69,72]

5. Altered innvervation, either to the bladder[73] or generalized[74]

6. Toxic substance in urine: the best characterized is anti-proliferative factor, a 9-amino-acid glycosylated peptide that inhibits the growth of cultured bladder epithelial cells[75]

7. Increased urothelial release of ATP, which is a sensory neurotransmitter, in response to stretch[76,77]

C. Etiologies least likely to be true:

1. Infection
   a. Infection may, in theory, initiate a bladder epithelial injury or autoimmune process that leads to IC[78]
   b. After many studies, there is still no convincing evidence that ongoing infection is the cause of IC[79,80]
   c. Anecdotal reports describe patients who respond to antibiotics (for example, reference 81) but a randomized trial of long-term antibiotics for IC showed no significant advantages over placebo.[82]
   d. Keep in mind that IC patients can have episodes of bacterial infection, in addition to their chronic IC[65]

2. The many objective abnormalities found in IC research studies make it clear that IC is a physical disorder, not a psychologic problem

5. IC Treatments: General Principles

A. No single treatment is universally effective for all IC patients. If one treatment does not alleviate symptoms, try others

B. Many patients require combined treatments

C. In general, start with the most innocuous treatment, and progress to others (with more risk) if initial treatments fail. For example, a recent survey showed that invasive and intravesical treatments were more likely to make symptoms worse, and recommended starting with oral medications[83]

D. Many treatments are used, but few have been proven effective in randomized, double-blind controlled studies

E. The IC Association provides excellent resources for self-help measures including diet, exercise, and urinary alkalinization. Their web site address is www.ichelp.org

F. In some cases pain may persist due to other conditions outside the bladder, such as central sensitization[65]

6. Oral Medications for IC

For this review course, the only treatments included here are either superior to placebo in at least 1 controlled study, or commonly used by practitioners as "standard" IC treatments.

A. Pentosan polysulfate[84]

1. Second agent (and the only oral agent) to be FDA-approved for IC.
2. Superior to placebo in 3 trials conducted in the US between 1987 and 1993, before the drug was FDA-approved[85-87]
3. Not better than placebo in a European trial[71]
4. Not better than placebo in a recent USA trial, conducted when the drug was already FDA-approved and available[88]
5. Less effective than cyclosporine A in a randomized trial[90]
6. Usual dose: 100 mg PO TID. Larger doses up to 300 mg TID are not more effective.[91] This is not surprising because the oral bioavailability of PPS is extremely low[92,93]
7. At least 3-6 months are needed to achieve maximum benefit
8. Proposed mechanisms (none are proven to occur in human IC patients, but b. – d. below were demonstrated *in vitro* or in animal studies):
   a. Replace deficient glycoconjugates on bladder epithelium.
   b. Bind to and inactivate proinflammatory components in urine[94]
   c. Inhibit mast cell histamine secretion[95]
   d. PPS has several direct anti-inflammatory effects, including inhibition of complement activation[96-98]
   e. Inhibition of angiogenesis inhibition and VEGF production[99]
9. More effective in patients who start < 6 months after diagnosis, compared to those with longstanding diagnosis[100]

B. Amitriptyline (off-label use to treat IC)

1. Effective in open-label trials and a placebo-controlled study[101]

2. Usual dose: 25-75 mg PO QHS

3. Possible mechanisms include blocking histamine H1 receptors, anticholinergic effects, sedation (improves sleep), and modulating nociception in the central nervous system

4. Not all antidepressants are the same for IC. For example:
   a. Duloxetine was not effective[102]
   b. Imipramine helped only 9% of patients[103]
   c. SSRIs have not been specifically studied in IC, but in other chronic pain states, such as irritable bowel syndrome and fibromyalgia, SSRIs are clearly less effective than tricyclic antidepressants.[104] Therefore, there is no convincing rationale for using SSRIs to treat IC

C. Hydroxyzine (off-label use to treat IC)

1. Hydroxyzine was effective in an open-label study[105]

2. Not more effective than placebo in a recent trial.[89] However, the drug is already available, so the study had low enrollment, low statistical power, and possible selection bias

3. Proposed mechanisms: antihistamine, sedation (improves sleep)

4. Usual dose: 10-75 mg PO QHS. Start with low dose and increase gradually to avoid excessive sedation

D. Cimetidine (off-label use to treat IC)

1. Mechanism unknown, but cimetidine has direct immune modulating effects because T-cells have H_2 receptors

2. Originally described in open-label trials[43]

3. Cimetidine 400 mg BID was found to be more effective than placebo in a controlled trial.[43] However, that trial included only patients with significant inflammation on bladder biopsies, so the same good effects may not occur for patients with minimal or no inflammation

E. Immunosuppression (off-label use to treat IC).

1. Corticosteroids were originally deemed ineffective, but 2 recent trials showed improvement in about 50% of the patients.[41,106] Both of these trials enrolled only ulcer-type patients, so the value of corticosteroids in nonulcer patients is still undetermined

2. Cyclosporine A was effective in an open-label trial and a comparative trial with PPS.[90] Unlike the corticosteroid trials, these studies were not restricted to ulcer patients. In the randomized trial of cyclosporine A vs. PPS, 15 of 64 patients had ulcers

3. Bottom line: OK to try for refractory patients who understand the risks and will be compliant with follow-up

7. Intravesical Medications for IC

A. Dimethyl sulfoxide (DMSO)[107]

1. First agent to be FDA-approved for IC treatment.

2. Superior to saline placebo.[108]

3. Reported to be superior to intravesical BCG, but with a crossover study design, some of the benefits attributed to DMSO may have been delayed effects of BCG.[38]

4. Usual course: weekly for 6 weeks, then maintenance individualized.

5. Effective for both ulcer and nonulcer patients,[109] but ulcer patients respond even better to TUR of the ulcers[109] or laser fulguration

6. Many possible mechanisms, including anti-inflammatory, analgesic, free radical scavenger, and collagen dissolution, and alteration of bladder afferent innervation[108-110]

7. Some practitioners add other agents to DMSO. No studies have tested whether DMSO cocktails are more effective than DMSO alone, or which cocktail is best. Examples are DMSO plus:
   a. 40 mg methylprednisolone and 5000 units heparin[111]
   b. 100 mg hydrocortisone, 5000 units heparin and 1 ampule sodium bicarbonate[112]
   c. 10,000 units heparin, 10 mg triamcinolone and 44 mEq sodium bicarbonate[113]
   d. 40,000 units heparin, 10 mg triamcinolone and 44 mEq sodium bicarbonate[2]

B. Heparin (off-label use to treat IC)

1. No placebo-controlled studies, but heparin was effective in open-label trials[2,63]

2. Now usually used as part of an intravesical cocktail with local anesthetics. This makes sense because local anesthetics have anti-inflammatory as well as anesthetic properties.[114] Several different combinations are published, and there is no evidence on whether any of these is superior to the others. Examples include:
   a. 40,000 units heparin, 8 mL 1% or 2% lidocaine, 3 mL 8.4% Na bicarbonate.[63]
   b. 10,000 units heparin, 80 mg gentamicin, 50 mL 0.5% bupivacaine, 50 mL 8.4% Na bicarbonate, 100 mg hydrocortisone.[115]

C. Alkalinized lidocaine alone (off-label use to treat IC)

1. No studies have compared lidocaine with vs. without heparin

2. Alkalinized lidocaine was better than placebo[117]
   a. 5 ml 4% lidocaine followed by 5 ml 8.4% bicarbonate
   b. Active drug or saline given daily for 5 days
   c. At 8 days, rates of moderate or marked improvement were 30% with active drug group and 9.6 % with placebo

D. Intravesical PPS (off-label use to treat IC)

1. 300 mg twice a week for 10-12 weeks was beneficial in an open-label trial[118] and in a small placebo-controlled trial (good relief in 4 of 10 with PPS and 2 of 10 with placebo)[119]

2. Recent randomized trial[120]
   a. All patients got oral PPS and intravesical alkalinized lidocaine
   b. Comparison was for either 200 mg PPS or placebo given after the lidocaine solution.
   c. At 12 weeks, PPS group had significantly greater reduction in IC Symptom Index and total O'Leary-Sant score, but not IC Problem Index or any other symptom measurements

E. BCG (off-label use to treat IC)

1. Original impetus was a patient whose IC biopsy was misread as carcinoma in situ, received BCG and IC symptoms resolved. This prompted a small open-label trial, in which BCG was effective[121]

2. No statistically significant benefit over placebo in 2 trials[121,122]
The latter trial also found:
   a. In long-term follow-up, BCG responders and placebo responders did equally well.[123]
   b. If BCG or placebo nonresponders went on to open-label BCG, the response rate was 18% and was identical for the BCG and placebo treated groups[124]

3. Less effective than DMSO in one trial.[38]

4. Currently, little or no role in IC treatment.

F. Hyaluronic acid (off-label use to treat IC).

1. Effective in several open-label trials[125]
No placebo-controlled trials are published

2. Usual dose: 40 mg weekly for 4-6 weeks, then monthly maintenance

3. If pre-select with modified (lower-dose) potassium sensitivity test, excellent improvement in 17%-55% of patients[56,60]

G. Resiniferatoxin (under investigation:[126] Single dose not better than placebo, but multiple or prolonged dose regimens are under investigation in two trials

8. Non-medical, Non-surgical Treatments for IC

A. Physical Therapy

1. Rationale: some IC patients also have symptoms related to tension and spasm of the pelvic floor muscles

2. Effective in three open trials.[127-129] All 3 trials selected patients who had high pelvic muscle tone or pelvic muscle trigger points on physical examination

3. A multicenter controlled trial sponsored by the NIH is ongoing

4. The best plan for a urologist is to refer the patient to a physical therapists who has specific expertise in pelvic floor muscle spasms

B. Hyperbaric oxygen was effective in 3 of 14 patients, vs. 0 with sham Tx[130]

9. Surgery for IC

A. Bladder distention under anesthesia

1. After initial diagnostic distention, do a therapeutic bladder distention at 80 cm water pressure for 8 minutes.[2] Biopsy follows the second distention, to decrease the risk of bladder rupture

2. Published response rates:
   a. Any degree of improvement: 50%-61%[31,131,132]
   b. "Excellent" improvement: 12%-16%[132,133]
   c. One cannot predict which patients will improve[31,131,133]

3. Relief is usually transient (6 months or less)[2,31,131,132]

4. Mechanism of relief is unknown, but may be changes in bladder afferent nerve ending[2] or urine growth factors.[133,134]

B. Laser fulguration of Hunner's ulcer[135,136]

1. Applies to a minority of IC patients in US (most are nonulcer)

2. Risks include laser penetration through bladder with bowel injury

3. In Moldwin's study, all patients had a good response initially. 11 of 24 patients had relapse, but did well with re-treatment[136]

4. Similar results reported for transurethral resection of ulcers[137]

C. Intravesical Botox injections: experimental, off-label, efficacy is transient[138]

D. Sacral nerve stimulation

1. The Medtronic InterStim® is FDA-approved for "urinary urge incontinence, urinary retention, and significant symptoms of urgency-frequency in patients who have failed or could not tolerate more conservative treatments"

2. Some IC patients have urgency and frequency

3. The published literature to date includes four reports of successful short-term trials (3-14 days) in IC patients.[139-142] One of these also included improvement in urinary IC markers[140]

4. In 2 studies of long-term implants for IC patients, almost all patients who had a good result with the trial stimulation continued to have good results with mean 14-15 months follow-up.[143,144] However, another study of long-term stimulation for various indications found 2 of 2 IC patients failed[145]

5. Authors disagree as to whether IC patients need more reprogramming than other sacral nerve stimulator patients[146,147]

6. In a randomized trial of pudendal lead vs. sacral lead for IC, the pudendal lead was more effective[148]

E. Augmentation cystoplasty: not effective for IC, not recommended[149]

F. Cystectomy and orthotopic bladder substitution[150-156]

1. Opinions vary whether the trigone should be preserved. Linn et al found worse results when the trigone was resected, primarily because so many patients required intermittent catheterization.[151] In contrast, Christmas et al found worse results when the trigone was preserved, and they attributed this to persisting pain from the remnant trigone[152]

2. Results are better for patients who have the ulcer type of IC[150] and smaller bladder capacity under anesthesia[150,151,153,154]

3. Pain and recurrent ulcers can occur in the trigone or urethra[155]

4. Patients who describe the urethra as the main site of pain are more likely to fail[156]

5. Bottom line: patients who fail this can be miserable, the techniques are still being debated, and urologists who are not special experts should avoid these operations

G. Urinary diversion (with or without cystectomy): a last resort

1. Since a toxic urine factor may cause or promote IC, in theory a conduit would be better than a continent pouch. However, this has not been formally tested

2. Patients must understand that the pain may persist or recur; pain relief is NOT guaranteed even with cystectomy

3. Various authors have discussed ways to predict outcomes[2] but the only consistent finding is that patients with a small bladder capacity under anesthesia have better results[132,133]
   a. Patients with a large bladder capacity under anesthesia[157,158]
   b. Pain often persists in nonulcer IC, even after cystectomy[150]

10. References

1. Abrams P, Cardozo L, Fall M, et al. The standardisation of terminology in lower urinary tract function: report from the standardisation sub-committee of the International Continence Society. *Neurourol Urodynamics*. 2002; 21:16.

2. Hanno PM. Painful bladder syndrome/interstitial cystitis and related disorders. In: Wein AJ, Kavoussi LR, Novick AC, Partin AW, Peters CA, eds. *Campbell-Walsh Urology*. 9th ed. Philadelphia, PA: Saunders Elsevier; 2007: 330-370.

3. van de Merwe JP, Nordling J, Bouchelouche P, et al: Diagnostic criteria, classification, and nomenclature for painful bladder syndrome/interstitial cystitis: an ESSIC proposal. *Eur Urol. 2008;* 53: 60

4. Hanno PM, et al. The diagnosis of interstitial cystitis revisited: lessons learned from the National Institutes of Health Intersitial Cystitis Database Study. *J Urol*. 1999;161:553.

5. Stryker GE. KUH notes. *J Urol*. 1989;142:139.

6. Warren JW, Meyer WA, Greenberg P, et al. Using the International Continence Society's definition of painful bladder syndrome. *Urology*. 2006;67:1138.

7. Berger RE, Miller JE, Rothman I, et al. Bladder petechiae after cystoscopy and hydrodistention in men diagnosed with prostate pain. *J Urol*. 1998;159:83.

8. Shorter B, Lesser M, Moldwin RM et al.: Effect of comestibles on symptoms of interstitial cystitis. *J Urol*. 2007;178: 145

9. Nguan C, Franciosi LG, Butterfield NN, et al. A prospective, double-blind, randomized cross-over study evaluating changes in urinary pH for relieving the symptoms of interstitial cystitis. *BJU International*. 2005;95:91.

10. Powell-Boone T, Ness TJ, Cannon R, et al. Menstrual cycle affects bladder pain sensation in subjects with interstitial cystitis. *J Urol*. 2005;174:1832.

11. Lutgendorf SK, et al. Stress and symptomatology of patients with interstitial cystitis: a laboratory stress model. *J Urol*. 2000;l164:1205.
12. Cetinel S, Cetinel B, Ercan, F et al: Indomethacin-induced morphologic changes in the rat urinary bladder epithelium. *Urology*. 2003; 61: 236

13. Chu PS, Ma WK, Wong SC et al: The destruction of the lower urinary tract by ketamine abuse: a new syndrome? *BJU Int*. 2008; 102: 1616

14. Chen KT, Foo NP, Lin. HJ: Frequent visits with urinary symptoms: subtle signs of ketamine abuse. *Am J Emerg Med*.2008; 26: 1061

15. Mazurick CA, Landis JR: Evaluation of repeat daily voiding measures in the National Interstitial Cystitis Data Base Study. *J Urol*. 2000;163: 1208

16. Peters KM, Carrico DJ, Kalinowski SE, et al.: Prevalence of pelvic floor dysfunction in patients with interstitial cystitis. *Urology*. 2007;70: 16

17. Lynes WL, Flynn SD, Shortliffe LD, et al. Mast cell involvement in interstitial cystitis. *J Urol*. 1987;138:746.

18. Smith SD, Wheeler MA, Foster HE, et al. Improvement in interstitial cystitis symptom scores during treatment with oral L-arginine. *J Urol*. 1997;158:703.

19. Gomes CM, Sanchez-Ortiz RF, Harris C, et al. Significance of hematuria in patients with interstitial cystitis: review of radiographic and endoscopic findings. *Urology*. 2001;57:262.

20. Stanford EJ, Mattox TF, Parsons JK, et al. Prevalence of benign microscopic hematuria among women with interstitial cystitis: Implications for evaluation of genitourinary malignancy. *Urology*. 2006;67:946.

21. Tissot WD, et al: A referral center's experience with transitional cell carcinoma misdiagnosed as interstitial cystitis. *J Urol*. 2004 ;172:478.

22. Irwin P, Samsudin A. Reinvestigation of patients with a diagnosis of interstitial cystitis: common things are sometimes common. *J Urol*. 2005;174:584.

23. Duldulao KE, et al.: Value of urinary cytology in women presenting with urge incontinence and/or irritative voiding symptoms. *J Urol*. 1997;157:113.

24. Gillenwater JY, Wein AJ. Summary of the NIADDK workshop on interstitial cystitis, National Institutes of Health, Bethesda, Maryland, August 28-29, 1987. *J Urol*. 1988;140:203.

25. Lin WS, Wong KC. Anesthesia for genitourinary surgery. In: Barash PG, Cullen BF, Stoelting RK, eds. *Clinical Anesthesia*. 2nd ed. Philadelphia, PA: JB Lippincott; 1992: 1157-1168.

26. Zabihi N, Allee T, Maher MG, et al. Bladder necrosis following hydrodistention in patients with interstitial cystitis. *J Urol*. 2007;177: 149

27. Erickson DR. Glomerulations in women with urethral sphincter deficiency: report of 2 cases. *J Urol*. 1995;153:728.

28. Waxman JA, Sulak PJ, Kuehl TJ. Cystoscopic findings consistent with interstitial cystitis in normal women undergoing tubal ligation. *J Urol*. 1998;160:1663.

29. Furuya R, Masumori N, Furuya S, et al.: Glomerulation observed during transurethral resection of the prostate for patients with lower urinary tract symptoms suggestive of benign prostatic hyperplasia is a common finding but no predictor of clinical outcome. *Urology*.2007;70: 922.

30. Erickson DR, Tomaszewski JE, Kunselman AR, et al. Do the National Institute of Diabetes and Digestive and Kidney Diseases cystoscopic criteria associate with other clinical and objective features of interstitial cystitis? *J Urol*. 2005;173:93.

31. Tamaki M, Saito R, Ogawa O, et al. Possible mechanisms inducing glomerulations in interstitial cystitis: relationship between endoscopic findings and expression of angiogenic growth factors. *J Urol*. 2004 ;172:945.

32. Ottem DP, Teichman JMH. What is the value of cystoscopy with hydrodistension for interstitial cystitis? *Urology*. 2005;66:494.

33. Shear S, Mayer R. Development of glomerulations in younger women with interstitial cystitis. *Urology*. 2006;68:253.

34. Lamale LM, Lutgendorf SK, Hoffman AN, et al. Symptoms and cystoscopic findings in patients with untreated interstitial cystitis. *Urology*. 2006;67:242.

35. Braunstein R, Shapiro E, Kaye J, et al: The role of cystoscopy in the diagnosis of Hunner's ulcer disease. *J Urol*.2008180: 1383.

36. Peeker R, Fall M. Toward a precise definition of interstitial cystitis: further evidence of differences in classic and nonulcer disease. *J Urol*. 2002;167:2470.

37. Peeker R, Fall M. Interstitial cystitis – a time for revision of name and diagnostic criteria in the new millennium? (comment) *BJU. International*. 2002;89:635.

38. Peeker R, et al. Intravesical bacillus Calmette-Guerin and dimethyl sulfoxide for treatment of classic and nonulcer interstitial cystitis: a prospective, randomized double-blind study. *J Urol*.2000;164: 1912.

39. Erickson DR, Tomaszewski JE, Kunselman AR et al.: Urine markers do not predict biopsy findings or presence of bladder ulcers in interstitial cystitis/painful bladder syndrome. *J Urol*.2008;179: 1850.

40. Zhang CO, Li ZL, et al: APF, HBEGF, and EGF biomarkers in patients with ulcerative vs.non-ulcerative interstitial cystitis. *BMC Urology*.2005;5: 7

41. Hosseini A et al.: Nitric oxide as an objective marker for evaluation of treatment response in patients with classic interstitial cystitis. *J Urol*. 2004;172: 2261

42. Parsons CL. Interstitial cystitis: clinical manifestations and diagnostic criteria in over 200 cases. *Neurourology and Urodynamics*. 1990; 9:241.

43. Thilagarajah R, Witherow R O'N, Walker MM. Oral cimetidine gives effective symptom relief in painful bladder disease: a prospective, randomized, double-blind placebo-controlled trial. *BJU Int*. 2001;87:207.

44. Bouchelouche K, et al. The cysteinyl leukotriene D4 receptor antagonist montelukast for the treatment of interstitial cystitis. *J Urol*. 2001;166:1734.

45. Parsons CL, et al. The role of urinary potassium in the pathogenesis and diagnosis of interstitial cystitis. *J Urol*. 1998;159:1862.

46. Chambers GK, et al. An assessment of the use of intravesical potassium in the diagnosis of interstitial cystitis. *J Urol*. 1999 ;62:699.

47. Teichman JMH, Nielsen-Omeis BJ. Potassium leak test predicts outcome in interstitial cystitis. *J Urol*. 1999;161:1791.

48. Bernie JE. The intravesical potassium sensitivity test and urodynamics: implications in a large cohort of patients with lower urinary tract symptoms. *J Urol*. 2001;166:158.

49. Gregorie M, et al. Does the potassium stimulation test predict cystometric, cystoscopic outcome in interstitial cystitis? *J Urol.* 2002;168: 556.

50. Parsons CL, et al. Effect of pentosan polysulfate therapy on intravesical potassium sensitivity. *Urology.* 2002;59:329.

51. Parsons CL, et al. Increased prevalence of interstitial cystitis: previously unrecognized urologic and gynecologic cases identified using a new symptom questionnaire and intravesical potassium sensitivity. *Urology.* 2002;60:573.

52. Parsons CL, Albo M. Intravesical potassium sensitivity in patients with prostatitis. *J Urol.* 2002;168:1054.

53. Yilmaz U, Liu YW, Rothman I, et al. Intravesical potassium chloride sensitivity test in men with chronic pelvic pain syndrome. *J Urol.* 2004;172:548.

54. Minaglia S, Ozel B, Bizhang R, et al. Increased prevalence of interstitial cystitis in women with detrusor overactivity refractory to anticholinergic therapy. *Urology.* 2005;66:702.

55. Sairanen J, Tammela TL, Leppilahti M et al. Potassium sensitivity test (PST) as a measurement of treatment efficacy of painful bladder syndrome/interstitial cystitis: a prospective study with cyclosporine A and pentosan polysulfate sodium. *Neurourol Urodyn.*2007;26: 267.

56. Gupta SK, Pidcock L, Parr NJ. The potassium sensitivity test: a predictor of treatment response in interstitial cystitis. *BJU Int.* 2005;96:1063.

57. Hanno P. Is the potassium sensitivity test a valid and useful test for the diagnosis of interstitial cystitis? *Int Urogynecol J.* 2005;16: 428.

58. Hanno P. International Consultation on IC-Rome, September 2004/Forging an International Consensus: Progress in Painful Bladder Syndrome/Interstitial Cystitis. *Int Urogynecol J.* 2005;16:S2.

59. Daha LK, et al. Do cystometric findings predict the results of intravesical hyaluronic acid in women with interstitial cystitis? *Eur Urol.* 2005;47:393.

60. Riedl CR, Engelhardt PF, Daha KL et al.: Hyaluronan treatment of interstitial cystitis/painful bladder syndrome. *Int Urogynecol J.*2008.19: 717.

61. Philip J, Willmott S, Owen D, et al. A double-blind, randomized controlled trial of cystometry using saline versus 0.3 M potassium chloride infusion in women with overactive bladder syndrome. *Neurourol Urodyn.* 2007;26:110.

62. Philip J, Willmott S, Irwin P. Interstitial cystitis versus detrusor overactivity: a comparative, randomized, controlled study of cystometry using saline and 0.3 M potassium chloride. *J Urol.* 2006;175:566.

63. Parsons CL. Successful downregulation of bladder sensory nerves with combination of heparin and alkalinized lidocaine in patients with interstitial cystitis. *Urology.* 2005;65:45.

64. Forrest JB, Moldwin R: Diagnostic options for early identification and management of interstitial cystitis/painful bladder syndrome. *Int J Clin Pract.* 2008;62: 1926.

65. Nickel JC, Shoskes D, Irvine-Bird K: Clinical phenotyping of women with interstitial cystitis/painful bladder syndrome (IC/PBS): a key to classification and potentially improved management. *J Urol.* 2009;in press.

66. Hauser PJ, Dozmorov MG, Bane BL. et al.Abnormal expression of differentiation related proteins and proteoglycan core proteins in the urothelium of patients with interstitial cystitis. *J Urol.*2008;179: 764.

67. Zhang CO, Wang JY, Koch KR, et al. Regulation of tight junction proteins and bladder epithelial paracellular permeability by an antiproliferative factor from patients with interstitial cystitis. *J Urol*. 2005;174:2382.

68. Sant GR, Kempuraj D, Marchand JE. et al. The mast cell in interstitial cystitis: role in pathophysiology and pathogenesis. *Urology*. 2007;69(4 suppl): 34.

69. Elbadawi A: IC: a critique of current concepts with a new proposal for pathologic diagnosis and pathogenesis. *Urology*.1997; 49 (suppl 5A):14.

70. Peeker R, Atanasiu L, Logadottir Y. Intercurrent autoimmune conditions in classic and nonulcer interstitial cystitis. *Scand J Urol Nephrol*.2003;37: 60.

71. van de Merwe JP. Interstitial cystitis and systemic autoimmune diseases. *Nat Clin Pract Urol*.2007;4: 484.

72. Wesselmann U. Neurogenic inflammation and chronic pelvic pain. *World J Urol*. 2001;19: 180.

73. Hohenfeller M, et al. Interstitial cystitis: increased sympathetic innervation and related neuropeptide synthesis. *J Urol*. 1992;147:587.

74. Ness TJ, Powell-Boone T, Cannon R, et al. Psychophysical evidence of hypersensitivity in subjects with interstitial cystitis. *J Urol*. 2005;173:1983.

75. Keay SK, et al. An antiproliferative factor from interstitial cystitis patients is a frizzled 8 protein-related sailoglycopeptide. *Proc Nat Acad Sci*. 2004;101:11803.

76. Sun Y, Chai TC. Augmented extracellular ATP signaling in bladder urothelial cells from patients with IC. *Am J Physiol Cell Physiol*. 2006;290: C27.

77. Kumar V, Chapple CR, Surprenant AM. et al. Enhanced adenosine triphosphate release from the urothelium of patients with painful bladder syndrome: a possible pathophysiological explanation. *J Urol*.2007;178: 1533,.

78. Warren JW. Interstitial cystitis as an infectious disease. *Urol Clin North Am*. 1994;21(1):31.

79. Al-Hadithi HN, Williams H, Hart CA, et al. Absence of bacterial and viral DNA in bladder biopsies from patients with interstitial cystitis/chronic pelvic pain syndrome. *J Urol*. 2005;174:151.

80. Atug F, Turkeri L, Atug O, et al. Detection of Helicobacter pylori in bladder biopsy specimens of patients with interstitial cystitis by polymerase chain reaction. *Urol Res*. 2004;32:346.

81. Haarala M, et al. Urinary bacterial flora of women with urethral syndrome and interstitial cystitis. *Gynecol Obstet Invest*. 1999;47:42.

82. Warren JW, et al. Pilot study of sequential oral antibiotics for the treatment of intersitial cystitis. *J Urol*. 2000;163:1685.

83. Hill JR, Isom-Batz G, Panagopoulos G et al.: Patient perceived outcomes of treatments used for interstitial cystitis. *Urology.2008;*71: 62.

84. Anderson VR, Perry CM. Pentosan polysulfate: a review of its use in the relief of bladder pain or discomfort in interstitial cystitis. *Drugs*. 2006;66:821.

85. Parsons CL, Mulholland SG. Successful therapy of interstitial cystitis with pentosan polysulfate. *J Urol*. 1987;138:513.

86. Mulholland SG, et al. Pentosan polysulfate sodium for therapy of interstitial cystitis. *Urology*. 1990;35:552.

87. Parsons CL, et al. A quantitatively controlled method to study prospectively interstitial cystitis and demonstrate the efficacy of pentosan polysulfate. *J Urol*. 1993;150:845.

88. Holm-Bentzen M, et al. A prospective double blind clinically controlled multicenter trial of sodium pentosan polysulfate in the treatment of interstitial cystitis and related painful bladder disease. *J Urol.* 1987;138:503.

89. Sant GR, et al. A pilot clinical trial of oral pentosan polysulfate and oral hydroxyzine in patients with interstitial cystitis. *J Urol.* 2003; 170:810.

90. Sairanen J, Tammela TL, Leppilahti M, et al. Cyclosporine A and pentosan polysulfate sodium for the treatment of interstitial cystitis: a randomized comparative study. *J Urol.* 2005;174:2235.

91. Nickel JC, Barkin J, et al. Randomized, double-blind, dose-ranging study of pentosan polysulfate sodium for interstitial cystitis. *Urology.* 2005;65:654.

92. Erickson DR, Sheykhnazari M, Bhavanandan VP. Molecular size affects urine excretion of pentosan polysulfate. *J Urol.* 2006;175:1143.

93. Simon M, McClanahan RH, et al. Metabolism of [3H]pentosan polysulfate sodium (PPS) in healthy human volunteers. *Xenobiotica.* 2005;35:775.

94. Sadhukhan PC, et al. Sodium pentosan polysulfate reduces urothelial responses to inflammatory stimuli via an indirectmechanism. *J Urol.* 2002;168:289.

95. Chiang G, et al. Pentosan polysulfate inhibits mast cell histamine secretion and intracellular calciumion levels: an alternative explanation of its beneficial effect in interstitial cystitis. *J Urol.* 2000;164:2119.

96. Ghosh P. The pathobiology of osteoarthritis and the rationale for the use of pentosan polysulfate in its treatment. *Seminars Arthritis Rheum.* 1999;28:211.

97. Kilgore KS, et al. The semisynthetic polysaccharide pentosan polysulfate prevents complement-mediated myocardial injury in the rabbit perfused heart. *J Pharm Exp Ther.* 1998;285:987.

98. Bobadilla BA, et al. Pentosan polysulfate prevents glomerular hypertension and structural injury despite persisting hypertensin in 5/6 nephrectomy rats. *J Am Soc Nephrol.* 2001;12:2080.

99. Zaslau S, Sparks S, Riggs D, et al. Pentosan polysulfate (Elmiron): in vitro effects on prostate cancer cells regarding cell growth and vascular endothelial growth factor production. *Am J Surg.* 2006;192:640.

100. Nickel JC, Kaufman DM, Zhang HF et al.: Time to initiation of pentosan polysulfate sodium treatment after interstitial cystitis diagnosis: effect on symptom improvement. *Urology.* 2008;71: 57.

101. van Ophoven A, Pokupic S, Heinecke A, et al. A prospective, randomized, placebo-controlled, double-blind study of amitriptyline for the treatment of interstitial cystitis. *J Urol.* 2004;172: 533.

102. van Ophoven A, Hertle L. The dual serotonin and noradrenaline reuptake inhibitor duloxetine for the treatment of interstitial cystitis: results of an observational study. *J Urol.* 2007;177:552.

103. Nishijima S, Sugaya K, Yamada T, et al. Efficacy of tricyclic antidepressant is associated with beta2-adrenoceptor genotype in patients with interstitial cystitis. *Biomed Res.* 2006;27:163.

104. Jackson JL, O'Malley PG, Kroenke K. Antidepressants and cognitive-behavioral therapy for symptom syndromes. *CNS Spectr.* 2006;11:212.

105. Theoharides TC. Hydroxyzine in the treatment of interstitial cystitis. *Urol Clin North Am.* 1994;21(1):73.

106. Soucy F, Gregoire M. Efficacy of prednisone for severe refractory ulcerative interstitial cystitis. *J Urol.* 2005;173:841.

107. Dawson TE, Jamison J: Intravesical treatments for painful bladder syndrome/ interstitial cystitis. *Cochrane Database Syst Rev.* 2007 Oct 17;(4):CD006113.

108. Perez-Marrero R, Emerson LE, Feltis JT. A controlled study of dimethyl sulfoxide in interstitial cystitis. *J Urol.* 1988;140:36.

109. Rossberger J, Fall M, Peeker R. Critical appraisal of dimethyl sulfoxide treatment for interstitial cystitis: discomfort, side effects and treatment outcome. *Scand J Urol Nephrol.* 2005;39:73.

110. Melchior D, Packer CS, Johnson TC, et al. Dimethyl sulfoxide: does it change the functional properties of the bladder wall? *J Urol.* 2003;170:253.

111. Ghoneim GM, et al. Clinical experience with multi-agent intravesical therapy in interstitial cystitis patients unresponsive to single-agent therapy. *World J Urol.* 1993;11:178.

112. Parkin J, et al. Intravesical dimethyl sulfoxide (DMSO) for interstitial cystitis—a practical approach. *Urology.* 1997;49(suppl.5A):105.

113. Pontari MA, et al. Logical and systematic approach to the evaluation and management of patients suspected of having interstitial cystitis. *Urology.* 1997;49(suppl.5A):114.

114. Cassuto J, Sinclair R, et al. Anti-inflammatory properties of local anesthetics and their present and potential clinical implications. *Acta Anes Scand.* 2006;50:265.

115. Lukban JC, Whitmore KE, Sant GR. Current management of interstitial cystitis. *Urol Clin North Am.* 2002;29(3):649.

116. Welk BK, Teichman JM: Dyspareunia response in patients with IC treated with intravesical lidocaine, bicarbonate, and heparin. *Urology.* 2008;71: 67.

117. Nickel JC, Moldwin R, Lee S, et al. Intravesical alkalinized lidocaine (PSD597) offers sustained relief from symptoms of interstitial cystitis and painful bladder syndrome. *BJU Int*, 2009;in press.

118. Daha LK, Lazar D, Simak R, et al. The effects of intravesical pentosanpolysulfate treatment on the symptoms of patients with bladder pain syndrome/interstitial cystitis: preliminary results. *Int Urogynecol J. 2008;*19: 987.

119. Bade JJ, et al. A placebo-controlled study of intravesical pentosanpolysulphate for the treatment of interstitial cystitis. *Br J Urol.* 1997;79: 168.

120. Davis EL, El Khoudary SR, Talbott EO, et al.: Safety and efficacy of the use of intravesical and oral pentosan polysulfate sodium for interstitial cystitis: a randomized double-blind clinical trial. *J Urol.* 2008;179: 177

121. Peters K, et al. The efficacy of intravesical Tice strain bacillus Calmette-Guérin in the treatment of interstitial cystitis: a double-blind, prospective, placebo controlled trial. *J Urol.* 1997;157:2090.

122. Mayer R, et al. A randomized controlled trial of intravesical bacillus Calmette-Guérin for treatment refractory interstitial cystitis. *J Urol.* 2005;173:1186.

123. Propert KJ, Mayer R, Nickel JC, et al.: Followup of patients with interstitial cystitis responsive to treatment with intravesical bacillus Calmette-Guerin or placebo. *J Urol.* 2008;179: 552.

124. Propert KJ, Mayer R, et al. Did patients with IC who failed to respond to initial treatment with bacillus Calmette-Guerin or placebo in a randomized clinical trial benefit from a second course of open label BCG? *J Urol*. 2007;178: 886.

125. Iavazzo C, Athanasiou S, Pitsouni E, et al. Hyaluronic acid: an effective alternative treatment of interstitial cystitis, recurrent urinary tract infections, and hemorrhagic cystitis? *Eur Urol*. 2007;51: 1534.

126. Mourtzoukou EG, Iavazzo C, Falagas ME: Resiniferatoxin in the treatment of interstitial cystitis: a systematic review. *Int Urogynecol J*. 2008;19: 1571.

127. Weiss JM. Pelvic floor myofascial trigger points: manual therapy for interstitial cystitis and the urgency-frequency syndrome. *J Urol*. 2001;166:2226.

128. Doggweiler-Wiygul R, Wiygul JP. Interstitial cystitis, pelvic pain, and the relationship to myofascial pain and dysfunction: a report on four patients. *World J Urol*. 2002;20:310.

129. Oyama IA, Rejba A, Lukban JC, et al. Modified Thiele massage as therapeutic intervention for female patients with interstitial cystitis and high-tone pelvic floor dysfunction. *Urology*. 2004;64:862.

130. van Ophoven A, Rossbach G, Pajonk F, et al. Safety and efficacy of hyperbaric oxygen therapy for the treatment of interstitial cystitis: a randomized, sham controlled, double-blind trial. *J Urol*. 2006;176:1442.

131. Cole EE, et al. Are patient symptoms predictive of the diagnostic and/or therapeutic value of hydrodistention? *Neurourol Urodyn*. 2005;24:638.

132. Hanno PM, Wein AJ. Conservative therapy of interstitial cystitis. *Semin Urol*. 1991;9:143.

133. Erickson DR, Kunselman AR, Bentley CM, et al. Changes in urine markers and symptoms after bladder distention for interstitial cystitis. *J Urol*. 2007;177:556.

134. Chai TC, et al. Bladder stretch alters urinary heparin-binding epidermal growth factor and antiproliferative factor in patients with interstitial cystitis. *J Urol*. 2000;163:1440.

135. Malloy JR, Shanberg AM. Laser therapy for interstitial cystitis. *Urol Clin North Am*. 1994;21(1):141.

136. Rofeim O, et al. Use of the neodymium:YAG laser for interstitial cystitis: a prospective study. *J Urol*. 2001;166:134.

137. Peeker R, et al. Complete transurethral resection of ulcers in classic interstitial cystitis. *Int Urogynecol J*. 2000;11:290.

138. Giannantoni A, Porena M, et al. Botulinum A toxin intravesical injection in patients with painful bladder syndrome: 1-year followup. *J Urol*. 179: 2008;1031.

139. Maher CF, et al. Percutaneous sacral nerve root neuromodulation for intractable interstitial cystitis. *J Urol*. 2001;165:884.

140. Chai TC, et al. Percutaneous sacral third nerve root neurostimulation improves symptoms and normalizes urinary HB-EGF levels and antiproliferative activity in patients with interstitial cystitis. *Urology*. 2000;55:643.

141. Whitmore KE, Payne CK, et al. Sacral neuromodulation in patients with interstitial cystitis: a multicenter clinical trial. *Int Urogynecol J*. 2003;14: 305.

142. Peters KM, et al. Sacral neuromodulation for the treatment of refractory interstitial cystitis: outcomes based on technique. *Int Urogyn J Pelvic Floor Dysfunct*. 2003;14:223.

143. Comiter CV. Sacral neuromodulation for the symptomatic treatment of refractory interstitial cystitis: a prospective study. *J Urol.* 2003;169:1369.

144. Peters KM, Konstandt D. Sacral neuromodulation decreases narcotic requirements in refractory interstitial cystitis. *BJU Int.* 2004;93: 777.

145. Elhilali MM, Khaled SM, Kashiwabara T, et al. Sacral neuromodulation: long-term experience of one center. *Urology.* 2005;65:1114.

146. Maxwell KM, et al. Reprogramming requirements after sacral nerve stimulator implantation: correlation with preoperative indication. *J Urol.* 2008;179: 549.

147. Burks FN, Diokno AC, Lajiness MJ et al.: Sacral neuromodulation reprogramming: is it an office burden? *Int Urogynecol J.* 2008;19: 1137

148. Peters KM, et al. A prospective, single-blind, randomized crossover trial of sacral vs pudendal nerve stimulation for interstitial cystitis. *BJU Int.* 2007;100: 835.

149. Blaivas JG, et al. Long-term followup of augmentation enterocystoplasty and continent diversion in patients with benign disease. *J Urol.* 2005;173:1631.

150. Rössberger J, et al. Long-term results of reconstructive surgery in patients with bladder pain syndrome/IC: subtyping is imperative. *Urology.* 2007;70: 638.

151. Linn JF, et al. Treatment of interstitial cystitis: comparison of subtrigonal and supratrigonal cystectomy combined with orthotopic bladder substitution. *J Urol.* 1998;159:774.

152. Christmas TJ, et al. Bladder replacement by ileocystoplasty: the final treatment for intersitial cystitis. *Brit J Urol.* 1996;78:69.

153. Webster GD, Maggio MI. The management of chronic interstitial cystitis by substitution cystoplasty. *J Urol.* 1989;141:287.

154. Hughes OD, Kynaston HG, Jenkins BJ, et al. Substitution cystoplasty for intractable interstitial cystitis. *Br J Urol.* 1995;76:172.

155. Chakravarti A, Ganta S, Somani B, et al. Caecocystoplasty for intractable interstitial cystitis: long-term results. *Eur Urol.* 2004;46:114.

156. van Ophoven A, et al. Long-term results of trigone-preserving orthotopic substitution enterocystoplasty for interstitial cystitis. *J Urol.* 2002;167:603.

157. Lotenfoe RR, et al. Absence of neuropathic pelvic pain and favorable psychological profile in the surgical selection of patients with disabling interstitial cystitis. *J Urol.* 1995;154:2039.

158. Hohenfeller M, et al. Surgical treatment of interstitial cystitis. In: Sant GR, ed. *Interstitial Cystitis.* Philadelphia, PA: Lippincott-Raven; 1997:223-233.

11. Questions

1. The diagnosis of interstitial cystitis should not be made in patients with:

A. Male gender

B. Previous pelvic radiation

C. Age less than 18

D. No glomerulations or ulcers on cystoscopy

E. A large bladder capacity under anesthesia

2. Which statement about pentosan polysulfate is true?

A. It is the only FDA-approved oral treatment for IC

B. Alopecia is a common side effect

C. It was more effective than placebo in all trials published to date

D. Symptoms usually improve within one month

E. A potassium sensitivity test should be done before starting treatment

3. Which of the following is most consistent with interstitial cystitis?

A. Pain while voiding

B. Tender erythema of vaginal introitus

C. Urge incontinence

D. Urodynamic bladder capacity 500 mL

E. Normal office cystoscopy

4. Which of these is the worst treatment option for interstitial cystitis?

A. Cyclosporine

B. Sacral nerve stimulation

C. Bladder distention under anesthesia

D. Augmentation enterocystoplasty

E. Cystectomy and ileal conduit

5. Which statement about the NIDDK criteria for interstitial cystitis is false?

A. They were designed for research studies

B. They are not evidence-based

C. If a patient does not meet the criteria, he or she does not have interstitial cystitis

D. The criteria require both urodynamics and cystoscopy under anesthesia with distention

E. Presence of a ureteral stone is an exclusion criterion

Answers

1. B.

2. A.

3. E.

4. D.

5. C.

Chapter 23B: Sexually Transmitted Diseases

Deborah R. Erickson, MD

Contents

1. HIV/AIDS: General Information

A. Cause: human immunodeficiency virus (HIV)[1,2]

1. HIV-1 is the most common cause of AIDS

2. HIV-2: a related virus, causes some AIDS cases but these are rare in the developed world

B. Stages of HIV infection

1. Initial or primary infection may involve an acute illness "acute retroviral syndrome" 2-4 weeks after exposure. Patients are unlikely to see a urologist for this
   a. Symptoms resemble mononucleosis: fever, malaise, adenopathy, sore throat, and skin rash[1,3,4]
   b. Anti-HIV antibodies are usually not present this early. Therefore, standard laboratory tests for HIV are usually negative. Diagnosis is made by the following:[1]
      1) High plasma viremia, often >1 million RNA copies/mL
      2) Decreased blood CD4+ T-cell count
      3) Large increase in blood CD8+ T-cell count

2. Asymptomatic carriage of virus, with variable duration[1]
   a. Typical progressors (60%-70% of patients): 10-11 years
   b. Rapid progressors (10%-20% of patients): <5 years
   c. Slow progressors (5%-15% of patients): >15 years. Subsets include:
      1) Long-term nonprogressors (<2% of patients overall) remain asymptomatic and have low viral load
      2) Elite controllers have undetectable viral load

3. Eventual loss of cell-mediated immunity; AIDS is the end stage

4. AIDS case definition: an HIV+ person with no other known cause of cell-mediated immune deficiency, who has a total CD-4 T-cell count below 200 cells/microliter, and/or any one of 25 different "AIDS-defining"diseases.[2] Some well-known diseases on the list include:
   a. Candidiasis (bronchi, trachea, lungs or esophagus)
   b. Chronic herpes simplex ulcers (>1 month)
   c. Disseminated or extrapulmonary *Histoplasmosis, Coccidioidomycosis* or *Mycobacterium* infection
   d. Kaposi's sarcoma
   e. *Pneumocystis carinii* pneumonia
   f. Toxoplasmosis of the brain
   g. Invasive cervical cancer (HPV progresses rapidly in HIV-infected women)
   h. Non-Hodgkin's lymphoma

C. Diagnostic tests[1,6]

1. Most patients develop anti-HIV antibodies 3-6 weeks after infection. Standard lab tests, which are directed towards these antibodies, may be negative if done too early

2. Third-generation ELISA tests for anti-HIV antibodies have sensitivities and specificities approaching 100%.[1] However, even this accuracy leads to too many false-positive tests if widespread, indiscriminate screening is performed[7]

3. Positive ELISA should be confirmed with a more highly specific test (Western blot or immunofluorescence). ***Caveat***: it takes more time for a patient to become to seropositive by Western blot than by ELISA.[1] Therefore, if ELISA is positive and Western blot is negative, there are 2 possibilities:
   a. No HIV infection
   b. Recent onset of HIV infection

4. There are now 6 FDA-approved rapid point-of-service tests, using either blood or saliva[8] Sensitivity is high but false negative results can occur, for example:
   a. Like standard tests, these tests measure anti-HIV antibodies, so are negative if done too early
   b. Some, including the saliva test, are directed towards a single viral protein so are negative if the infecting virus has a mutated form[9]

D. Basic pathophysiology (targets of current anti-HIV drugs are in italics)[10]

1. HIV virus is a retrovirus, which means its genetic material is RNA

2. Certain inflammatory cells (especially T lymphocytes, monocytes and macrophages) have the CD4 receptor, which is essential for processing most types of foreign antigens

3. *HIV virus binds to the CD4 receptor and invades the cell*
   a. To invade the cell, the virus must bind not only the CD4 receptor, but also a chemokine receptor (most viral types use the receptor CCR5)[5,10]
   b. A naturally occurring deletion of 32 base pairs in the gene for CCR5 is present in up to 10%-20% of people of Northern European descent. The mutant CCR5 never reaches the cell membrane, therefore:
      1) Homozygotes (1%-2% of Caucasians) are almost completely resistant to HIV infection
      2) Heretozygotes may become infected but they have slower disease progression
   c. Other genetic differences also affect host response to HIV[5]

4. *Viral RNA is transcribed to DNA by the enzyme reverse transcriptase*

5. *Viral DNA is integrated into host cell genome*

6. Host DNA replicates, making new viral RNA

7. RNA is translated to protein precursors

8. *Viral protease cleaves precursors, leaving new viral proteins*

9. New virus particles are assembled and shed from host cells

10. Loss of CD4+ carrying cells leads to immune deficiency

11. Indices of disease severity:
    a. Low CD4+ cell count
    b. High amount of HIV RNA in bloodstream: "viral load," which also is useful for monitoring treatment response

2. HIV/AIDS Treatment

A. At present HIV cannot be completely eradicated, for 2 main reasons:[1]

1. Viral sanctuaries, where HIV virus can remain latent and sheltered, or where drugs do not penetrate, such as lymphoid tissue and the central nervous system

2. High genetic variability in virus, allowing escape from the immune response and development of drug resistance

B. Highly active antiretroviral therapy (HAART) drug regimens.

1. Improve immune function and decrease the rates of opportunistic infections and some AIDS-related malignancies. With HAART, average life expectancy is > 20 years.[3,11]

2. Currently, the goal of treatment is to keep the amount of HIV RNA in the blood (viral load) undetectable (<50 copies/mL). If HAART is

Table 1

Doses of Nucleoside Analog Reverse Transcriptase Inhibitors

Generic Name	Brand Name	Usual Oral Dose
Zidovudine[a]	Retrovir®	300 mg po bid
Didanosine	Videx®	200 mg po bid
Stavudine	Zerit®	40 mg po bid
Lamivudine	Epivir®	300 mg po bid
Abacavir[b]	Ziagen®	300 mg po bid
Emtricitabine	Emtriva®	200 mg po q day
Tenofovir[c]	Viread®	300 mg po q day
Emtricitabine/tenofovir	Truvada®	200 mg/300 mg q day
Zidovudine/ lamivudine	Combivir	300/150 mg bid
Lamivudine/abacavir	Epzicom	300/600 mg q day
Zidovudine/ lamivudine/abacavir	Trizivir	300/150/300 mg bid
Emtricitabine/tenofovir/efavirenz	Atripla[d]	200/300/600 a day

[a] Patent expired in 2005; generic forms are now available.

*[b] Severe hypersensitivity reactions can be fatal. Fortunately, a genetic test can identify who is susceptible (HLA-B*5701) and this screening is recommended before starting the drug (http://us.gsk.com/products/assets/us_ziagen.pdf).*

[c] Technically a nucleotide analog, not a nucleoside analog.

[d] This can be given alone because it is one of the recommended combinations: 2 nucleoside analog RT inhibitors (NRTI) and 1 non-nucleoside analog RT inhibitor (NNRTI).

Table 2

Non-nucleoside Analog Reverse Transcriptase Inhibitors

Generic Name	Brand Name	Usual Dose
Nevirapine	Viramune®	200 mg PO BID
Delavirdine[a]	Rescriptor®	400 mg PO TID
Efavirenz	Sustiva®	600 mg PO QHS
Etravirine[b]	Intelence	200 mg PO BID

[a]*Now rarely used because the other drugs in this table are superior.*
[b]*A second-generation drug, it can be effective for HIV strains resistant to efavirenz or nevirapine.*

stopped, viral load and CD4 cell counts return to pre-treatment levels, so treatment must be lifelong[12]

C. Classes of anti-HIV drugs[13,14]

1. Reverse transcriptase inhibitors stop conversion of viral RNA to DNA. There are 2 types:
   a. Nucleoside analogs or NRTIs (eg, zidovudine) (Tenofovir is technically a nucleotide analog, not a nucleoside analog.) (Table 1)
      1) Most are renally cleared and do not affect cytochrome P450 enzymes, so have fewer drug interactions than protease inhibitors or non-nucleoside reverse transcriptase inhibitors NNRTIs[15]

Table 3

Doses of Commonly Used Protease Inhibitors

Generic Name	Brand Name	Usual Oral Dose[a]
Ritonavir	Norvir®	n/a[b]
Indinavir	Crixivan®	800 mg PO TID
Nelfinavir	Viracept®	750 mg PO TID
Lopinavir/ritonavir	Kaletra®	400mg/100 mg BID
Saquinavir	Fortovase®	1200 mg PO TID
Saquinavir	Invirase®	1000 mg PO BID
Atazanavir	Reyataz®	400 mg po q day
Tipranavir	Aptivus®	500 BID†
Fosamprenavir	Levixa®	1400 mg PO BID
Darunavir	Prezista®	600 mg BID

[a]*Doses vary, depending on whether or not ritonavir is added. Since ritonavir is now recommended with all protease inhibitors, the doses here are the ones that apply to ritonavir coadministration. This is not always specified in the prescribing information, so consultation with a pharmacist is recommended*

[b]*Now rarely used as an anti-HIV drug per se, but is combined with other drugs to decrease their metabolism by inhibiting cytochrome P450 enzymes.*

2) Main toxicity: inhibit host mitochondrial DNA polymerase, leading to lactic acidosis, pancreatitis, subcutaneous lipoatrophy and peripheral neuropathy (the former 2 may be life-threatening).[11,12]

b. (Table 2). Main toxicities are skin reactions and liver toxicity.[11,12]

2. Protease inhibitors stop precursors from being cleaved into viral proteins (examples: indinavir, nelfinavir) (Table 3)
   a. Main toxicities: visceral fat accumulation, metabolic problems, such as insulin resistance and hyperlipidemia[12]
   b. Most are potent inhibitors of cytochrome P-450 enzymes, so they prolong the serum half-life of other drugs that use the same metabolism. However, the effects vary and are not generalizable (for example, paradoxically, tipranavir induces the enzymes).[16] Usually, a urologist's best option is to consult with a pharmacist
   c. Ritonavir is now recommended in all PI regimens as a "booster" to inhibit the metabolism (and thus increase the serum concentrations of) other anti-AIDS drugs.[14]
   d. PDE-5 inhibitors are metabolized by the same enzyme system, so dose reductions are recommended. Also, it is better to use a drug with a short half-life (eg, sildenafil) to decrease the risk of toxicity. Specific dose recommendations are as follows:[17]
      1) Sildenafil: maximum 25 mg Q 48 hours.
      2) Vardenafil: maximum 2.5 mg Q 72 hours.
      3) Tadalafil: maximum 10 mg Q 72 hours.
   e. Many other drugs are metabolized by the same enzymes, and require lower doses for patients on protease inhibitors. Some of the ones commonly used by urologists are ketoconazole, itraconazole and erythromycin

3. New drug: enfuvirtide (Fuzeon) inhibits fusion of the HIV virus with CD4 cells.[18]
   a. It must be given subcutaneously; 90 mg (1 mL) BID
   b. Indication: patients failing conventional anti-HIV therapy

4. New drug: maraivroc (Selzentry) CCR5 receptor blocker[13,14,19]
   a. Oral drug: dose depends on whether the drugs given along with it are CYP3A inhibitors or inducers
   b. Indication: in combination with other anti-HIV drugs, for treatment-experienced adult patients infected with only CCR5-tropic HIV-1, who have viral replication and HIV-1 strains resistant to multiple antiretroviral agents
   c. Black box warning: liver toxicity, may be preceded by systemic allergic reaction.

5. New drug: raltegravir (Isentress) integrase inhibitor; keeps viral DNA from being integrated into host cell genome[13,14,20]
   a. Oral drug: 400 mg BID (more if also on rifampin)
   b. Indication: in combination with other anti-HIV drugs, for treatment-experienced adult patients with viral replication and HIV-1 strains resistant to multiple antiretroviral agents

D. 2008 recommendation for initial treatment[13] is 2 NRTIs plus one of these:

1. Efavirenz (NNRTI)

2. One ritonavir-boosted protease inhibitor

E. After initial treatment, patients can get immune reconstitution syndrome, in which the restored immune response is excessive.[21] Two main types:

1. Response to pathogens that were present before treatment (symptomatic or asymptomatic): viruses, Mycobacteria, fungi, etc

2. Appearance of autoimmune disease (eg, Graves disease, sarcoid)

3. Urologic/Renal Manifestations of AIDS[1,2,20]

A. Almost any opportunistic infection can affect the urogenital tract or genital skin.[1,2,20] The most common ones include:

1. Tuberculosis

2. *Aspergillus*, *Candida* and other fungi

3. *Toxoplasma gondii*

4. Cytomegalovirus

5. Genital herpes

6. Genital warts

7. *Molluscum contagiosum* is usually self-limiting in healthy patients, but in AIDS patients the lesions can be larger, more numerous, and persistent. Treatments are the same as for genital warts[2]

B. AIDS patients are more likely to get bacterial UTIs and they require longer course of antibiotic treatment

C. With any infection, AIDS patients have a more severe presentation, so are more likely to develop renal or prostatic abscesses or Fournier's gangrene

D. Hemorrhagic cystitis may occur with viral infections, including BK virus, JC virus, adenovirus and cytomegalomirus[21,22]

E. AIDS patients have increased incidences of several types of malignancies. The ones most relevant to urologists are:

1. Kaposi's sarcoma (KS) (most common AIDS malignancy)
   a. Arises from lymphatic endothelium.[3]
   b. Caused by human herpes virus[8,3]
   c. Usually presents as a painless, pigmented (pink, red or blue) subcutaneous nodule
   d. Most common location is the lower extremities, but may occur on the genitalia. Penile KS can progress to gangrene by causing arterial occlusion.[2] Up to 2% of AIDS patients initially present with penile KS
   e. Penile KS treatment is palliative; options include HAART, local excision of small lesions, radiotherapy for large local lesions or systemic chemotherapy if metastatic[1-3]

2. Non-Hodgkin's lymphoma is the second most common AIDS malignancy. The testes are commonly involved, but kidneys or ureters also may be involved[2,3]

3. Invasive cervical cancer is one of the AIDS-defining conditions listed in "definitions" above

4. HIV+ patients have a higher incidence of testis cancer (seminomas and nonseminomas). The usual recommendation is to use the standard treatment for the tumor type and stage, if the patient can tolerate it[1-3]

5. Renal cell carcinoma is about 8 times more common in the HIV-infected population.[3]

6. Bowen's disease (carcinoma *in situ*) of the genitalia is more common in HIV+ patients. Squamous carcinomas have a more aggressive course in HIV+ patients[2,3]

7. It is still debated whether HIV patients have an increased incidence of prostate cancer[3,11]

F. Renal dysfunction is common in AIDS

1. Renal dysfunction has multiple causes including dehydration, sepsis, obstruction, thrombotic microangiopathy, immune complex-mediated glomerulonephritis and nephrotoxic drugs[2,24]

2. HIV-associated nephropathy (HIVAN).[1-3,24,25]
   a. Direct infection of glomerular podocytes and renal tubular cells with HIV
   b. Usual findings on histopathology:
      1) Focal segmental glomerular clerosis
      2) Tubulointerstitial disease is always present and often appears out of proportion to the degree of glomerular injury[25]

c. 12x more common in AfricanAmericans than Caucasians, 3rd leading cause of ESRD in AfricanAmericans ages 20-64 (after diabetes and hypertension)
d. Usual presentation: severe proteinuria, renal insufficiency, kidneys have increased echogenicity and may be enlarged or normal size[3,25]

G. Both the central and peripheral nervous systems can be affected, either by the HIV virus itself or by opportunistic infections such as toxoplasmosis and CMV. Thus, any type of neurogenic voiding dysfunction can occur

1. The most common problem is urinary retention

2. Neurogenic voiding dysfunction portends a poor prognosis, with mortality about 40% within 8 months after symptom onset[2]

H. Hypogonadism[2,26]

1. AIDS patients have testicular atrophy for many reasons, including the HIV virus itself, chronic illness/cachexia, drug side effects and, in the HAART era, the aging process

2. Hypogonadism causes not only decreased libido but also depression, low energy and muscle wasting

3. The Endocrine Society Clinical Practice Guidelines recommend short-term (3-6 months) testosterone replacement for HIV-infected men with low testosterone levels and weight loss[26]

4. Patients on testosterone therapy should be followed with PSA, DRE and blood counts (testosterone may cause polycythemia)

I. Electrolyte abnormalities[2]

1. Hyponatremia is the most common electrolyte abnormality (about 30% of hospitalized patients)
   a. Associated with poor prognosis
      50% survival rates:
      1) With hyponatremia, 11.5 month.
      2) Without hyponatremia, 39 months
   b. Many causes including volume depletion, salt-wasting renal tubular disease, SIADH, medications and adrenal insufficiency

2. Others: hypernatremia (much less common; about 5% of hospitalized patients), hypokalemia, hypomagnesemia, hypo- or hypercalcemia, hypo- or hyperphosphatemaia, hypo- or hyperuricemia, lactic acidosis

J. Adrenal insufficiency can be due to either CNS infection or adrenal infection/necrosis. HIV patients having stressful procedures should be monitored for this[2]

4. Aspects of AIDS Relevant to Urologic Practice

A. Indinavir can form stones that are not consistently seen on unenhanced CT scan[1-3,27]

1. These usually resolve with conservative treatment (stop drug temporarily, hydration)

2. There is no formal literature on alpha blockers, but they may help in this situation the same as for other types of stones

3. The bottom line on manipulating urine pH:
   a. Indinavir is most soluble at pH less than [5.3,28] Therefore, alkalinizing the urine is definitely the wrong plan
   b. In theory, acidifying the urine would help dissolve the crystals. In practice, it is difficult to get the urine pH below 5.5, and a low urine pH predisposes to uric acid stones. Therefore, the usual treatment is hydration and stopping the drug, without specific attempts to acidify the urine[2]

4. Reasons for intervention include persistent fever, intractable pain or solitary kidney

5. Often the "stones" are actually masses of crystals that disperse easily, so temporary stenting (plus hydration and stopping the drug) is usually sufficient[2,20]

6. Indinavir crystals may precipitate in the renal tubules and cause acute renal failure, without any definite stones.[28] Treatment is the same as for indinavir stones

7. Other drugs besides indinavir can also forms stones, including other protease inhibitors[29,30] and efavirenz (an NNRTI).[31]

B. AIDS patients also form the usual types of stones

1. In one series of 14 patients taking indinavir who had stones, only 4 patients' stones contained indinavir[32]

2. There are several reasons for stone formation in AIDS patients. For example, malnutrition and diarrhea lead to dehydration, urine acidification and hypocitraturia. A complete metabolic evaluation is indicated, including blood tests and 24-urine studies[3]

C. As described above in the section on treatment, some protease inhibitors increase the levels of other drugs by inhibiting cytochrome P-450 enzymes. Especially relevant to urology are:

1. PDE-5 inhibitors (sildenafil, vardenafil, tadalafil)

2. Some antibiotics (eg, ketoconazole, itraconazole, erythromycin)

D. Trimethoprim-sulfamethoxazole can cause rhabdomyolysis in AIDS patients, any time within two weeks of starting the drug[33]

E. HIV and prostate cancer

1. Life expectancy after starting HAART is usually >20 years. Therefore, prostate cancer screening should be done according to the AUA recommendations.[3]

2. With localized cancer, treatment outcomes appear similar for men with vs. without HIV.[11] If surgery is chosen, a laparoscopic approach involves less exposure to the operating team[3,34]

3. Effects of HIV drugs on cultured prostate cancer cells (the clinical relevance of these *in vitro* effects are still undetermined).

   a. Nelfinavir: growth arrest, apoptosis[35]

   b. Saquinavir: apoptosis, radiosensitization, inhibits proteosome function[36]

F. HIV-positive individuals are candidates for kidney transplantation if they meet certain criteria[37]

G. HIV and circumcision[38]

1. In 3 randomized trials in sub-Saharan Africa,

male circumcision protected men against HIV infection during vaginal sex with women. Infection rates for circumcised men were about 60% lower than for the uncircumcised control group

2. Possible reasons:
   a. Inner foreskin is rich in Langerhans cells and other HIV target cells near the epithelial surface, where there is no or minimal keratin protection
   b. Inner foreskin is susceptible to tears and abrasions
   c. In circumcised men, the penis is thought to have a greater keratin barrier

H. Being HIV+ does not require that a surgeon stop operating;[39,40] the American College of Surgeons web site at www.facs.org/fellows_info/statements/st13.html

I. Screening recommendations

1. Widespread community screening, regardless of risk group, is not recommended (too many false-positive tests)[7]

2. Recommendations from the US Preventive Services Task Force[41,42] are on their web site www.preventiveservices.ahrq.gov/, In summary, pregnant women and people in high-risk groups for HIV should be screened. High-risk groups include:
   a. Patients with other sexually transmitted diseases
   b. Past or present IV drug use
   c. Men who have had sex with men after 1975
   d. Unprotected sex with multiple partners
   e. People whose past or present partners are/were HIV-infected, IV drug users or men who had sex with men
   f. People who exchange sex for money or drugs (or their partners)
   g. Recipients of blood transfusions between 1978 and 1985
   h. Patients who request HIV testing
   i. People in high-risk settings, such as STD clinics, homeless shelters, correctional facilities, TB clinics and adolescent health clinics, that have a high prevalence of STDs.

3. New guidelines from the CDC[43] are found on their web site. http://www.cdc.gov/mmwr/preview/mmwrhtml/rr5514a1.htm. These are different from #2 above because they also recommend:
   a. In healthcare settings, routinely screen all patients aged 13-64 years (note: this applies to patients in health care settings, not the entire community population)
   b. Screen all patients initiating treatment for TB
   c. Screen after notifying the patient that an HIV test will be performed unless he/she declines (opt-out screening). Specific signed consent for HIV testing should not be required. General informed consent for medical care should be sufficient to encompass informed consent for HIV tests
   d. HIV test results should be provided in the same manner as results of other diagnostic or screening tests
   e. Prevention counseling should not be a required part of HIV screening programs in healthcare settings. Such counseling is strongly encouraged for high-risk persons in settings in which risk behaviors are assessed routinely (eg, STD clinics) but should not have to be linked to HIV testing

4. Rationale and advantages of the CDC guidelines, which are supported by the American College of Physicians and HIV Medicine Association[44]
   a. Many HIV-infected people do not think of themselves as at risk, so do not seek testing
   b. Many patients are infected for years before diagnosis, and they may unknowingly transmit the disease to others
   c. Early identification prolongs the patient's life, decreases risk of transmission to others, and is cost-effective at prevalence rates as low as 0.05%-0.2%

5. Disadvantages of CDC guidelines: legal and ethical concerns, also against the law in some states.[45-47] For example:
   a. An ethical principle is that the test must benefit the patient. A positive HIV test must lead to accessible HIV care[45]
   b. A positive HIV test may result in harm, such as domestic violence, loss of housing, employment or insurance, etc. Therefore, even if state law does not require informed consent, an uninformed patient who experiences these outcomes may claim that medical malpractice occurred[45]
   c. As of 2008, a separate written consent for HIV testing of nonpregnant adults is needed in Connecticut, Hawaii, Massachusetts, Michigan, Nebraska, New York, Pennsylvania, Rhode Island and Wisconsin[46]
   d. Many states require pre-test counseling and documentation of oral consent, even if written consent is not required[47]

5. Protection of Health Care Workers from HIV/AIDS

A. Though not part of HIV/AIDS, this is a good spot to emphasize that all health care workers should be immunized for hepatitis B

B. Universal precautions

1. All patients are considered potentially infected

2. Avoid direct contact with blood, semen, urine, mucous membranes or nonintact skin. (However, as of 2008 there were no documented cases of seroconversion from urine exposure)[3]

3. Care with passing sharps (use a Mayo stand as a way-station)

4. Do not recap needles (even clean ones cause injury)

5. Benefits of double gloving
   a. Decreases skin injury from large monofilament suture[39]
   b. If the surgeon's skin is penetrated, the simple action of the blade going through 2 layers of glove removes most or all of the patient's blood

C. Postexposure prophylaxis (PEP) for health care workers[1-3]

1. The risk of becoming HIV+ after a single sharps injury is low, even from a known HIV-positive source
   a. Overall risk from a single percutaneous injury involving a known HIV-positive source: 0.3%
   b. Risk is much greater for injection (hollow) needles than for knives or solid needles. As of 2004 there were no cases of seroconversion after injury with a solid needle
   c. As of 2008, the CDC had reports of 57 documented cases of seroconversion from occupational HIV exposure among US health care personnel; none were surgeons. There are an additional 140 seroconversions considered as possible occupational transmissions; 6 were surgeons[48]

2. PEP reduces the risk even further (but does not decrease it to zero)

3. A health care worker who has a sharps injury should be evaluated IMMEDIATELY at an employee health service or emergency department. If PEP is going to be used, it should begin within 2-4 hours of exposure

4. Most seroconversions occur within 3 months. If still negative 6 months after exposure, little residual risk[2]

5. The usual prophylaxis is 2 or 3 different antiviral medications (depending on the level of risk) taken for 4 weeks

6. Current CDC guidelines (basic summary; see reference 49 or websites www.cdc.gov/mmwr/PDF/rr/rr5409.pdf or http://www.cdc.gov/mmwr/preview/mmwrhtml/rr5409a1.htm
   a. If source is known to be HIV-negative, no PEP needed for any type of exposure
   b. If source is known to be HIV+, PEP recommended for percutaneous injuries, or exposure of source blood to health care worker's mucous membranes or nonintact skin
   c. If source status unknown, generally, no PEP recommended, but consider PEP if the source has HIV risk factors

6. Other STDs

For the other STDs, practical information for clinicians is well described in the Campbell's Urology chapter[50] and the CDC report.[4] The portions of the CDC report most relevant to urology are included in the handout. The entire report can be found online http://www.cdc.gov/mmwr/preview/mmwrhtml/rr5511a1.htm A few additional details are:

A. The CDC recommends that diagnosing a genital ulcer includes a culture or antigen test for HSV, but only a culture gives a definitive diagnosis, and culture is thought to be the gold standard[50]

B. Point of care (POC) tests for STDS[8]

   1. HIV tests were discussed earlier

   2. Syphilis tests: they all test for antibodies in the blood, but vary as to whether the antigen is specific to treponema or not
      a. Standard nontreponemal tests (eg, RPR, VDRL) correlate with disease activity.
      b. Standard treponemal tests (eg, FTA-ABS or TP-PA) are positive for live
      c. Current POC tests are treponemal, so are positive for life and cannot distinguish current from past infection

   3. POC tests for herpes simplex measure antibodies in the blood. They are sensitive and specific with two caveats:
      a. May be negative early in the disease, before antibodies have formed
      b. Usually positive for life, so cannot distinguish current from past infection

   4. POC tests for gonorrhea and chlamydia are not as sensitive as standard tests

C. Expedited partner therapy[51]

   1. Treating sex partners of patients diagnosed with chlamydia or gonorrhea by giving prescriptions or medications to the patient to take to his/her partner without the health care provider first examining the partner

   2. For CDC report, see http://www.cdc.gov/std/ept

3. Expedited partner therapy is allowed in some states, but not all. CDC has a great interactive web site with the rules in each state. http://www.cdc.gov/std/ept/legal/default.htm

D. Other good and recent reviews are for syphilis[52,53] and chlamydia[54]

7. Human Papilloma Virus (HPV)

A. Cause of cervical and anogenital cancers (also some head and neck cancers) and genital warts[55,56]

1. Types 16 and 18 cause about 70% of HPV-related cancers

2. Types 6 and 11 cause about 90% of cases of genital warts

B. Quadrivalent vaccine against these 4 types was 96%-100% effective in preventing HPV 6/11/16/18-related cervical and anogenital pre-cancers and genital warts.[55] The CDC recommends routine vaccination for females age 11-12 and catch-up vaccination for unvaccinated females
age 13-26.[7]
http://www.cdc.gov/mmwr/preview/mmwrhtml/rr5602a1.htm

C. Mechanisms of treatments for genital warts[58-60]

1. Podofilox (podophyllotoxin) (patient-applied) and podophyllin resin (physician-applied): antimitotic, cytotoxic

2. Imiquimod:
   a. No direct antiviral activity
   b. Works by increasing cytokines such as TNF-α and interferon, and stimulating cell-mediated immunity

3. Trichloracetic acid: coagulates proteins in wart tissue

4. New treatment Veregen (sinecatechins 15% ointment)[58]
   a. Mixture of 8 catechins derived from green tea
   b. Reduce expression HPV gene products E6 and E7, which lead to HPV-induced cell growth and neoplasia. May also inhibit proinflammatory enzymes and proteases
   c. FDA approved for external genital and perianal warts in women and men 18 years or older

5. Cryosurgery, laser, excision: mechanical destruction or removal

D. Which treatment for warts is best?

1. A nice algorithm for decision-making among the myriad treatments is too long to reproduce here but found in reference 59

2. Imiquimod alone equal to or better than ablation alone.[61,62] Imiquimod + ablation better than ablation alone[61]

3. Five-armed trial of provider-applied treatments.[63]
   a. Treatment arms were:
      1) Trichloroacetic acid
      2) Podophyllin 25%
      3) Cryotherapy
      4) Cryotherapy + podophyllin 25%
      5) Trichloroacetic acid + podophyllin 25%
   b. Arms 1 and 2 had worse results than 3,4 or 5
   c. Arms 3, 4 and 5 had similar results; 4 was slightly better

8. References

1. Krieger JN. Urologic implications of AIDS and HIV infection. In: Wein AJ, Kavoussi LR, Novick AC, Partin AW, Peters CA, eds. *Campbell-Walsh Urology*. 9th ed. Philadelphia, PA: Saunders Elsevier; 2007:386-404.

2. Heyns CF, Fisher M. The urological management of the patients with acquired immunodeficiency syndrome. *BJU International*. 2005;95:709.

3. Lebovitch S, Mydlo JH: HIV-AIDS: urologic considerations. *Urol Clin North Am*. 2008;35(1): 59.

4. Centers for Disease Control and Prevention. Sexually Transmitted Diseases Treatment Guidelines, 2006. *MMWR*. 2006;55 (No. RR-11).

5. Piacentini L, Biasin M, Fenizia C et al.: Genetic correlates of protection against HIV infection: the ally within. *J Intern Med*. 2009;265: 110.

6. Iweala O. HIV diagnostic tests: an overview. *Contraception*. 2004;70:141.

7. Meyer KB, Pauker SG. Screening for HIV: can we afford the false positive rate? *N Engl J Med*. 1987;317:238.

8. Greer L, Wendel GD Jr. Rapid diagnostic methods in sexually transmitted infections. *Infect Dis Clin North Am*. 2008;22(4): 601.

9. Brown P, Merline JR et al.: Repeatedly false-negative rapid HIV test results in a patient with undiagnosed advanced AIDS. *Ann Intern Med*. 149: 71, 2008.

10. Greene WC, Peterlin BM. Charting HIV's remarkable voyage through the cell: Basic science as a passport to future therapy. *Nature Medicine*. 2002;8:673.

11. Silberstein J, Downs T, Lakin C, et al. HIV and prostate cancer: a systematic review of the literature. *Prostate Cancer Prostatic Dis*. 12: 6.

12. Yeni P. Update on HAART in HIV. *J Hepatol*. 2006;44(1 suppl):S100.

13. Hammer SM, Eron JJ Jr, Reiss P, et al. Antiretroviral treatment of adult HIV infection: 2008 recommendations of the International AIDS Society-USA panel. *JAMA*. 2008;Aug 6; 300: 555.

14. Wilson LE, Gallant JE: HIV/AIDS: the management of treatment-experienced HIV-infected patients: new drugs and drug combinations. *Clin Infect Dis*. 2009;48: 214.

15. Back DJ, et al. The pharmacology of antiretroviral nucleoside and nucleotide reverse transcriptase inhibitors. *J Acquir Immune Defic Syndr.* 2005;39:S1.

16. Croom KF, Keam SJ. Tipranavir. *Drugs*. 2005;65:1669.

17. Crum NF, et al. A review of hypogonadism and erectile dysfunction among HIV-infected men during the pre- and post-HAART eras: Diagnosis, pathogenesis, and management. *AIDS Patient Care and STDS*. 2005;19:655.

18. Oldfield V, Keating GM, Plosker G. Enfuvirtide: a review of its use in the management of HIV infection. *Drugs*. 2005;65:1139.

19. https://www.pfizerpro.com/brands/selzentry.jsp

20. http://www.isentress.com/raltegravir/isentress/hcp/index.jsp

21. French MA: HIV/AIDS: immune reconstitution inflammatory syndrome: a reappraisal. *Clin Infect Dis*. 2009;48: 101.

22. Studmeister A. Cytomegalovirus-induced hemorrhagic cystitis in AIDS patient treated successfully with valganciclovir. *AIDS*. 2002; 16:1437.

23. Ghez D, Oksenhendler E, Scieux C, Lassoued K. Haemorrhagic cystitis associated with adenovirus in a patient with AIDS treated for a non-Hodgkin's lymphoma. *Am J Hematol*. 2000;63:32.

24. Roling J, Schmid H, et al. HIV-associated renal diseases and highly active antiretroviral therapy-induced nephropathy. *Clin Infect Dis*. 2006;42:1488.

25. Wyatt CM, Klotman PE, D'Agati VD. HIV-associated nephropathy: clinical presentation, pathology, and epidemiology in the era of antiretroviral therapy. *Semin Nephrol*. 2008;28: 513.

26. Bhasin S, Cunningham GR, Hayes FJ, et al. Testosterone therapy in adult men with androgen deficiency syndromes: an endocrine society clinical practice guideline. *J Clin Endocrinol Metab*. 2006;91:1995.

27. Schwartz BF, Schenkman N, Armenakas NA, Stoller ML: Imaging characteristics of indinavir calculi. *J Urol*. 1999;161: 1085.

28. Kalaitzis C, Passadakis P et al.: Urological management of indinavir-associated acute renal failure in HIV-positive patients. *Int Urol Nephrol*. 2007;39: 743.

29. Engeler DS, John H, Rentsch KM, Ruef C, Oertle D, Suter S: Nelfinavir urinary stones. *J Urol*. 2002;167: 1384.

30. Feicke A, Rentsch KM, Oertle D, et al. Same patient, new stone composition: amprenavir urinary stone. *Antivir Ther.* 2008;13: 733.

31. Wirth GJ, Teuscher J, Graf JD et al. Efavirenz-induced urolithiasis. *Urol Res*. 2006;34: 288

32. Nadler RB, Rubenstein JN, Eggener SE, et al. The etiology of urolithiasis in HIV infected patients. *J Urol*. 2003;169:475.

33. Walker S, Norwood J, Thornton C, et al. Trimethoprim-sulfamethoxazole associated rhabdomyolysis in a patient with AIDS: case report and review of the literature. *Am J Med Sci*. 2006;331:339.

34. Levinson A, et al. Approach to management of clinically localized prostate cancer in patients with human immunodeficiency virus. *Urology*. 2005;65:91.

35. Yang Y, et al. HIV-1 protease inhibitor induces growth arrest and apoptosis of human prostate cancer LNCaP cells *in vitro* and *in vivo* in conjunction with blockade of androgen receptor STAT3 and AKT signal. *Cancer Sci*. 2005;96:425.

36. Pajonk F, Himmelsbach J, Riess K et al.: The human immunodeficiency virus (HIV)-1 protease inhibitor saquinavir inhibits proteasome function and causes apoptosis and radiosensitization in non-HIV-associated human cancer cells. *Cancer Res*. 2002;62: 5230.

37. Bhagani S, Sweny P, Brook G, et al. Guidelines for kidney transplantation in patients with HIV disease. *HIV Med*. 2006;7:133.

38. Brooks RA, Etzel M, Klosinski LE et al.: Male circumcision and HIV prevention: looking to the future. *AIDS Behav*. 2009; in press.

39. Fry DE. Occupational blood-borne diseases in surgery. *Am J Surg*. 2005;190:249.

40. Centers for Disease Control and Prevention. Investigation of patients treated by an HIV-infected cardiothoracic surgeon--Israel, 2007. *MMWR*. 2009;Jan 9;57(53): 1413. http://www.cdc.gov/mmwr/preview/mmwrhtml/mm5753a3.htm

41. U.S. Preventive Services Task Force: Screening for HIV. Recommendation statement. *Ann Intern Med*. 2005;143:32.

42. Campos-Outcalt D. Clarifying the US Preventive Services Task Force's 2005 recommendations. *J Fam Pract*. 2006;55:425.

43. Branson BM, Handsfield HH, Lampe MA, et al. Revised recommendations for HIV testing of adults, adolescents, and pregnant women in health care settings. *MMWR Recomm Rep*. 2006;55(RR-14):1-17.

44. Qaseem A, Snow V, Shekelle P et al. Screening for HIV in health care settings: a guidance statement from the American College of Physicians and HIV Medicine Association. *Ann Intern Med*. 2009;150: 125.

45. Hanssens C. Legal and ethical implications of opt-out HIV testing. *Clin Infect Dis*. 2007;45 suppl 4):S232.

46. Bartlett JG, Branson BM et al.: Opt-out testing for human immunodeficiency virus in the United States: progress and challenges. *JAMA*. 2008;300: 945.

47. Wolf LE, Donoghoe A, Lane T. Implementing routine HIV testing: the role of state law. PLoS ONE 2(10):e1005, 2007.

48. Davison SP, Reisman NR, Pellegrino ED, et al.: Perioperative guidelines for elective surgery in the human immunodeficiency virus-positive patient. *Plast Reconstr Surg*. 121: 1831, 2008.

49. Panlilio AL, Cardo DM, et al. Updated U.S. Public Health Service guidelines for the management of occupational exposures to HIV and recommendations for postexposure prophylaxis. *MMWR Recomm Rep*. 2005;54(RR-9):1-17.

50. Frenkel T, Potts J. Sexually transmitted diseases. In: Wein AJ, Kavoussi LR, Novick AC, Partin AW, Peters CA, eds. *Campbell-Walsh Urology*. 9th ed. Philadelphia, PA: Saunders Elsevier; 2007:371-385.

51. Frenkl TL, Potts J: Sexually transmitted infections. *Urol Clin North Am.* 2008; 35(1): 33.

52. Eccleston K, Collins L, et al. Primary syphilis. *Int J STD.* AIDS. 2008;19: 145.

53. Domantay-Apostol GP, Handog EB, Gabriel MT. Syphilis: the international challenge of the great imitator. *Dermatol Clin.* 2008;26: 191.

54. Wagenlehner FM, Weidner W, Naber KG. Chlamydial infections in urology. *World J Urol.* 2006;24:4.

55. Barr E, Tamms G: Quadrivalent human papillomavirus vaccine. *Clin Infect Dis.* 2007;45: 609.

56. Giuliano AR, Tortolero-Luna G, Ferrer E, et al.: Epidemiology of human papillomavirus infection in men, cancers other than cervical and benign conditions. *Vaccine.* 2008;26 (suppl 10): K17, 2008.

57. Markowitz LE, Dunne EF, Saraiya M, et al. Quadrivalent Human Papillomavirus Vaccine: Recommendations of the Advisory Committee on Immunization Practices (ACIP). *MMWR Recomm Rep. 2007* 56(RR-2): 1.

58. Mayeaux EJ Jr, Dunton C. Modern management of external genital warts. *J Low Genit Tract Dis.* 2008;12: 185.

59. Kodner CM, Nasraty S. Management of genital warts. *Am Fam Phys.* 2004;70: 2335.

60. Scheinfeld N, Lehman DS. An evidence-based review of medical and surgical treatments of genital warts. *Dermatol Online J.* 2006;12: 5.

61. Schöfer H, Van Ophoven A, Henke U, et al.: Randomized, comparative trial on the sustained efficacy of topical imiquimod 5% cream versus conventional ablative methods in external anogenital warts. *Eur J Dermatol.* 2006;16: 642.

62. Stefanaki C, Katzouranis , et al. Comparison of cryotherapy to imiquimod 5% in the treatment of anogenital warts. *Int J STD AIDS.* 2008;19: 441.

63. Sherrard J, Riddell L. Comparison of the effectiveness of commonly used clinic-based treatments for external genital warts. *Int J STD AIDS.* 2007;18: 365.

9. Questions

1. Which statement about protease inhibitors is false?

A. Side effects include visceral fat accumulation and hyperlipidemia.

B. Protease inhibitors prolong the half-life of PDE-5 inhibitors and increase the risk of toxicity.

C. Indinavir stones are lucent enough to be missed on unenhanced CT scan.

D. Initial treatment for indinavir stones includes stopping the drug, hydration and urine alkalinization.

E. Recommended initial treatment for HIV/AIDS is two nucleoside analog reverse transcriptase inhibitors plus either a ritonavir-boosted protease inhibitor or efavirenz.

2. Which situation is not an indication for penicillin treatment?

A. Primary syphilis

B. Secondary syphilis

C. Tertiary syphilis

D. Tertiary syphilis in a patient with a penicillin allergy

E. Positive RPR found on prenatal screening

3. Which of the following STDs is least common among men in the United States?

A. Gonorrhea

B. Chancroid

C. Granuloma inguinale

D. Herpes simplex

E. Human papilloma virus

4. Which statement about HIV transmission is false?

A. Circumcision significantly decreases a man's risk of acquiring HIV from vaginal intercourse with women.

B. Patients undergoing surgery should be screened for HIV, and special precautions taken with infected patients to protect health care workers.

C. The risk of becoming HIV positive after a single sharps injury is low, even from a known HIV-positive source.

D. As of 2008, there were no documented cases of HIV seroconversion due to urine exposure.

E. Post-exposure prophylaxis is effective if it starts within 2-4 hours after exposure.

5. All of the following STDs have readily available, reliable diagnostic tests, except:

A. Syphilis

B. Gonorrhea

C. Chlamydia urethritis

D. Chancroid

E. Herpes simplex

Answers

1. D.

2. E.

3. C.

4. B.

5. D.

2006 MMWR STD Guidelines:

The following is excerpted from Morbidity and Mortality Weekly Report. *Recommendations and Reports. August 4, 2006; Volume 55: Number RR-11*

A. Genital Ulcers

Management of Patients Who Have Genital Ulcers

In the United States, the majority of young, sexually active patients who have genital ulcers have either genital herpes, syphilis, or chancroid. The frequency of each condition differs by geographic area and patient population; however, genital herpes is the most prevalent of these diseases. More than one of these diseases can be present in a patient who has genital ulcers. All three of these diseases has been associated with an increased risk for HIV infection. Not all genital ulcers are caused by sexually transmitted infections.

A diagnosis based only on the patient's medical history and physical examination frequently is inaccurate. Therefore, all patients who have genital ulcers should be evaluated with a serologic test for syphilis and a diagnostic evaluation for genital herpes; in settings where chancroid is prevalent, a test for *Haemophilus ducreyi* should also be performed. Specific tests for evaluation of genital ulcers include: 1) syphilis serology and either darkfield examination or direct immunofluorescence test for *T pallidum*; 2) culture or antigen test for HSV; and 3) culture for *H ducreyi*.

No FDA-cleared PCR test for these organisms is available in the United States; however, such testing can be performed by clinical laboratories that have developed their own tests and conducted a Clinical Laboratory Improvement Amendment (CLIA) verification study. Type-specific serology for HSV-2 might be helpful in identifying persons with genital herpes (see Genital Herpes, Type-Specific Serologic Tests). Biopsy of genital ulcers might be helpful in identifying the cause of ulcers that are unusual or that do not respond to initial therapy. HIV testing should be performed on all patients who have genital ulcers caused by *T pallidum* or *H ducreyi*, and should be strongly considered for those who have genital ulcers caused by HSV (see Diagnostic Considerations, sections: Syphilis, Chancroid, and Genital Herpes Simplex Virus).

Health care providers frequently must treat patients beforetest results are available because early treatment decreases the possibility of ongoing transmission and because successful treatment of genital herpes depends on prompt initiation of therapy. The clinician should treat for the diagnosis considered most likely, on the basis of clinical presentation and epidemiologic circumstances. In some instances, treatment must be initiated for additional conditions because of diagnostic uncertainty. Even after complete diagnostic evaluation, at least 25% of patients who have genital ulcers have no laboratory confirmed diagnosis.

Chancroid

In the United States, chancroid usually occurs in discrete outbreaks, although the disease is endemic in some areas. Chancroid is a cofactor for HIV transmission, as are genital herpes and syphilis; high rates of HIV infection among patients who have chancroid occur in the United States and other countries. Approximately 10% of persons who have chancroid that was acquired in the United States are coinfected with *T pallidum* or HSV; this percentage is higher in persons who have acquired chancroid outside the United States.

A definitive diagnosis of chancroid requires the identification of *H ducreyi* on special culture media that is not widely available from commercial sources; even when these media are used, sensitivity is <80%. No FDA-cleared PCR test for *H ducreyi* is available in the United States, but such testing can be performed by clinical laboratories that have developed their own PCR test and conducted a CLIA verification study.

The combination of a painful genital ulcer and tender suppurative inguinal adenopathy suggests the diagnosis of chancroid. A probable diagnosis of chancroid, for both clinical and surveillance purposes, can be made if all of the following criteria are met: 1) the patient has one or more painful genital ulcers; 2) the patient has no evidence of *T pallidum* infection by darkfield examination of ulcer exudate or by a serologic test for syphilis performed at least 7 days after onset of ulcers; 3) the clinical presentation, appearance of genital ulcers and, if present, regional lymphadenopathy are typical for chancroid; and 4) a test for HSV performed on the ulcer exudate is negative.

Treatment

Successful treatment for chancroid cures the infection, resolves the clinical symptoms, and prevents transmission to others. In advanced cases, scarring can result, despite successful therapy.

Recommended Regimens*

Azithromycin 1 g orally in a single dose

Or

Ceftriaxone 250 mg intramuscularly (IM) in a single dose

Or

Ciprofloxacin 500 mg orally twice a day for 3 days

Or

Erythromycin base 500 mg orally three times a day for 7 days

* Ciprofloxacin is contraindicated for pregnant and lactating women. Azithromycin and ceftriaxone offer the advantage of single-dose therapy. Worldwide, several isolates with intermediate resistance to either ciprofloxacin or erythromycin have been reported.

Other Management Considerations

Male patients who are uncircumcised and patients with HIV infection do not respond as well to treatment as those who are circumcised or HIV negative. Patients should be tested for HIV infection at the time chancroid is diagnosed. Patients should be retested for syphilis and HIV 3 months after the diagnosis of chancroid, if the initial test results were negative.

Follow-Up

Patients should be reexamined 3-7 days after initiation of therapy. If treatment is successful, ulcers usually improve symptomatically within 3 days and objectively within 7 days after therapy. If no clinical improvement is evident, the clinician must consider whether: 1) the diagnosis is correct; 2) the patient is coinfected with another STD; 3) the patient is infected with HIV; 4) the treatment was not used as instructed; or 5) the *H ducreyi* strain causing the infection is resistant to the prescribed antimicrobial. The time required for complete healing depends on the size of the ulcer; large ulcers might require >2 weeks. In addition, healing is slower for some uncircumcised men who have ulcers under the foreskin. Clinical resolution of fluctuant lymphadenopathy is slower than resolution for ulcers and might require needle aspiration or incision and drainage. Although needle aspiration of chancroid buboes is a simple procedure, incision and drainage might be preferred because of a reduced need for repeat drainage procedures.

Management of Sex Partners

Sex partners of patients who have chancroid should be examined and treated, regardless of whether symptoms of the disease are present if they had sexual contact with the patient during the 10 days preceding the patient's onset of symptoms.

Special Considerations

Pregnancy

The safety and efficacy of azithromycin for pregnant and lactating women have not been established. Ciprofloxacin is contraindicated during pregnancy and lactation. No adverse effects of chancroid on pregnancy outcome have been reported.

HIV Infection

HIV-infected patients who have chancroid should be monitored closely because, as a group, these patients are more likely to experience treatment failure and to have ulcers that heal more slowly. HIV-infected patients might require longer courses of therapy than those recommended for HIV negative patients, and treatment failures can occur with any regimen. Because evidence is limited concerning the therapeutic efficacy of the recommended ceftriaxone and azithromycin regimens in HIV-infected patients, these regimens should be used for such patients only if follow-up can be ensured. Some specialists prefer the erythromycin 7-day regimen for treating HIV-infected persons.

Genital HSV Infections

Genital herpes is a chronic, life-long viral infection. Two types of HSV have been identified, HSV-1 and HSV-2. The majority of cases of recurrent genital herpes are caused by HSV-2 although HSV-1 might become more common as a cause of first episode genital herpes. At least 50 million persons in the United States have genital HSV infection.

The majority of persons infected with HSV-2 have not been diagnosed with genital herpes. Many such persons have mild or unrecognized infections but shed virus intermittently in the genital tract. The majority of genital herpes infections are transmitted by persons unaware that they have the infection or who are asymptomatic when transmission occurs.

Diagnosis of HSV Infection

The clinical diagnosis of genital herpes is both insensitive and nonspecific. The classical painful multiple vesicular or ulcerative lesions are absent in many infected persons. Up to 50% of first-episode cases of genital herpes are caused by HSV-1 (63), but recurrences and subclinical shedding are much less frequent for genital HSV-1 infection than genital HSV-2 infection (64,65). Therefore, whether genital herpes is caused by HSV-1 or HSV-2 influences prognosis and counseling. Therefore, the clinical diagnosis of genital herpes should be confirmed by laboratory testing (66). Both virologic and type-specific serologic tests for HSV should be available in clinical settings that provide care for patients with STDs or those at risk for STDs.

Virologic Tests

Isolation of HSV in cell culture is the preferred virologic test for patients who seek medical treatment for genital ulcers or other mucocutaneous lesions. However, the sensitivity of culture is low, especially for recurrent lesions, and declines rapidly as lesions begin to heal. PCR assays for HSV DNA are more sensitive and have been used instead of viral culture (67,68); however, PCR tests are not FDA-cleared for testing of genital specimens. PCR is the test of choice for detecting HSV in spinal fluid for diagnosis of HSV infection of the central nervous system (CNS). Viral culture isolates should be typed to determine if HSV-1 or HSV-2 is the cause of the infection. Lack of HSV detection (ie, culture or PCR) does not indicate a lack of HSV infection, as viral shedding is intermittent. The use of cytologic detection of cellular changes of HSV infection is an insensitive and nonspecific method of diagnosis, both for genital lesions (ie, Tzanck preparation) and for cervical Pap smears and should not be relied upon.

Type-Specific Serologic Tests

Both type-specific and nontype-specific antibodies to HSV develop during the first several weeks after infection and persist indefinitely. Accurate type-specific HSV serologic assays are based on the HSV-specific glycoprotein G2 (HSV-2) and glycoprotein G1 (HSV-1). Such assays first became commercially available in 1999, but older assays that do not accurately distinguish HSV-1 from HSV-2 antibody (despite claims to the contrary) remain on the market. Therefore, the serologic type-specific glycoprotein G (gG)-based assays should be specifically requested when serology is performed (69–71).

The FDA-cleared glycoprotein G-based type-specific assays include the laboratory-based assays HerpeSelect™ -1 enzymelinked immunosorbent assay (ELISA) immunoglobulin G (IgG) or HerpeSelect-2 ELISA IgG and HerpeSelect 1 and 2 Immunoblot IgG (Focus Technology, Inc., Herndon, Virginia), and HSV-2 ELISA (Trinity Biotech USA, Berkeley Heights, New Jersey). Two other assays, Biokit HSV-2 and SureVue® HSV-2 (Biokit USA, Lexington, Massachusetts, and Fisher Scientific, Pittsburgh, Pennsylvania, respectively), are point-of-care tests that provide results for HSV-2 antibodies from capillary blood or serum during a clinic visit. The sensitivities of these glycoprotein G type-specific tests for the detection of HSV-2 antibody vary from 80%-98%, and false-negative results might be more frequent at early stages of infection. The specificities of these assays are ≥96%. False-positive results can occur, especially in patients with a low likelihood of HSV infection. Repeat or confirmatory testing might be indicated in some settings, especially if recent acquisition of genital herpes is suspected.

Because nearly all HSV-2 infections are sexually acquired, the presence of type-specific HSV-2 antibody implies anogenital infection and education and counseling appropriate for persons with genital herpes should be provided. The presence of HSV-1 antibody alone is more difficult to interpret. The majority of persons with HSV-1 antibody have oral HSV infection acquired during childhood, which might be asymptomatic. However, acquisition of genital HSV-1 appears to be increasing, and genital HSV-1 also might be asymptomatic. Lack of symptoms in an HSV-1 seropositive person does not distinguish anogenital from orolabial or cutaneous infection. Persons with HSV-1 infection, regardless of site of infection, remain at risk for HSV-2 acquisition.

Type-specific HSV serologic assays might be useful in the following scenarios: 1) recurrent genital symptoms or atypical symptoms with negative HSV cultures; 2) a clinical diagnosis of genital herpes without laboratory confirmation; and 3) a partner with genital herpes. Some specialists believe that HSV serologic testing should be included in a comprehensive evaluation for STDs among persons with multiple sex partners, HIV infection, and among MSM at increased risk for HIV acquisition. Screening for HSV-1 or HSV-2 in the general population is not indicated.

Principles of Management of Genital Herpes

Antiviral chemotherapy offers clinical benefits to the majority of symptomatic patients and is the mainstay of management. Counseling regarding the natural history of genital herpes, sexual and perinatal transmission, and methods to reduce transmission is integral to clinical management.

Systemic antiviral drugs can partially control the signs and symptoms of herpes episodes when used to treat first clinical and recurrent episodes, or when used as daily suppressive therapy. However, these drugs neither eradicate latent virus nor affect the risk, frequency, or severity of recurrences after the drug is discontinued. Randomized trials have indicated that three antiviral medications provide clinical benefit for genital herpes: acyclovir, valacyclovir, and famciclovir (72–80). Valacyclovir is the valine ester of acyclovir and has enhanced absorption after oral administration. Famciclovir also has high oral bioavailability. Topical therapy with antiviral drugs offers minimal clinical benefit, and its use is discouraged.

First Clinical Episode of Genital Herpes

Many persons with first-episode herpes have mild clinical manifestations but later develop severe or prolonged symptoms. Therefore, patients with initial genital herpes should receive antiviral therapy.

Recommended Regimens*

Acyclovir 400 mg orally three times a day for 7-10 days

OR

Acyclovir 200 mg orally five times a day for 7-10 days

OR

Famciclovir 250 mg orally three times a day for 7-10 days

OR

Valacyclovir 1 g orally twice a day for 7-10 days

* Treatment might be extended if healing is incomplete after 10 days of therapy.

Established HSV-2 Infection

The majority of patients with symptomatic, first-episode genital HSV-2 infection subsequently experience recurrent episodes of genital lesions; recurrences are less frequent after initial genital HSV-1 infection. Intermittent asymptomatic shedding occurs in persons with genital HSV-2 infection, even in those with longstanding or clinically silent infection. Antiviral therapy for recurrent genital herpes can be administered either episodically to ameliorate or shorten the duration of lesions or continuously as suppressive therapy to reduce the frequency of recurrences. Many persons, including those with mild or infrequent recurrent outbreaks, benefit from antiviral therapy; therefore, options for treatment should be discussed. Some persons might prefer suppressive therapy, which has the additional advantage of decreasing the risk of genital HSV-2 transmission to susceptible partners (81).

Suppressive Therapy for Recurrent Genital Herpes

Suppressive therapy reduces the frequency of genital herpes recurrences by 70%-80% in patients who have frequent recurrences (ie, ≥6 recurrences per year), and many patients report no symptomatic outbreaks. Treatment also is effective in patients with less frequent recurrences. Safety and efficacy have been documented among patients receiving daily therapy with acyclovir for as long as 6 years and with valacyclovir or famciclovir for 1 year. Quality of life frequently is improved in patients with frequent recurrences who receive suppressive therapy, compared with episodic treatment.

The frequency of recurrent genital herpes outbreaks diminishes over time in many patients, and the patient's psychological adjustment to the disease might change. Therefore, periodically during suppressive treatment (eg, once a year), providers should discuss the need to continue therapy with the patient.

Daily treatment with valacyclovir 500 mg daily decreases the rate of HSV-2 transmission in discordant, heterosexual couples in which the source partner has a history of genital HSV-2 infection (82). Such couples should be encouraged to consider suppressive antiviral therapy as part of a strategy to prevent transmission, in addition to consistent condom use and avoidance of sexual activity during recurrences. Suppressive antiviral therapy probably reduces transmission when used by persons who have multiple partners (including MSM) and by those who are HSV-2 seropositive without a history of genital herpes.

Recommended Regimens

Acyclovir 400 mg orally twice a day

OR

Famiciclovir 250 mg orally twice a day

OR

Valacyclovir 500 mg orally once a day

OR

Valacyclovir 1.0 g orally once a day

Valacyclovir 500 mg once a day might be less effective than other valacyclovir or acyclovir dosing regimens in patients who have very frequent recurrences (ie, ≥10 episodes per year). Several studies have compared valacyclovir or famciclovir with acyclovir. The results of these studies suggest that valacyclovir and famciclovir are comparable to acyclovir in clinical outcome (74,78,79,83). Ease of administration and cost also are important considerations for prolonged treatment.

Episodic Therapy for Recurrent Genital Herpes
Effective episodic treatment of recurrent herpes requires initiation of therapy within 1 day of lesion onset or during the prodrome that precedes some outbreaks. The patient should be provided with a supply of drug or a prescription for the medication with instructions to initiate treatment immediately when symptoms begin.

Recommended Regimens
Acyclovir 400 mg orally three times a day for 5 days

OR

Acyclovir 800 mg orally twice a day for 5 days

OR

Acyclovir 800 mg orally three times a day for 2 days

OR

Famciclovir 125 mg orally twice daily for 5 days

OR

Famciclovir 1000 mg orally twice daily for 1 day

OR

Valacyclovir 500 mg orally twice a day for 3 days

OR

Valacyclovir 1.0 g orally once a day for 5 days

Severe Disease
Intravenous (IV) acyclovir therapy should be provided for patients who have severe HSV disease or complications that necessitate hospitalization (eg, disseminated infection, pneumonitis, or hepatitis) or CNS complications (eg, meningitis or encephalitis). The recommended regimen is acyclovir 5-10 mg/kg body weight IV every 8 hours for 2-7 days or until clinical improvement is observed, followed by oral antiviral therapy to complete at least 10 days of total therapy.

Counseling
Counseling of infected persons and their sex partners is critical to the management of genital herpes. The goal of counseling is to: 1) help patients cope with the infection, and 2) prevent sexual and perinatal transmission (8). Although initial counseling can be provided at the first visit, many patients benefit from learning about the chronic aspects of the disease after the acute illness subsides.
Multiple resources, including web sites (http://www.ashastd.org and http://www.ihmf.org) and printed materials are available to assist patients, their partners, and clinicians in counseling.

HSV-infected persons might express anxiety concerning genital herpes that does not reflect the actual clinical severity of their disease; the psychological effect of HSV infection frequently is substantial. Common concerns regarding genital herpes include the severity of initial clinical manifestations, recurrent episodes, sexual relationships and transmission to sex partners, and ability to bear healthy children. The misconception that HSV causes cancer should be dispelled. The psychological effect of a serologic diagnosis of HSV-2 infection in a person with asymptomatic or unrecognized genital herpes appears small and transient (84).

The following recommendations apply to counseling of persons with HSV infection:

- Persons who have genital herpes should be educated concerning the natural history of the disease, with emphasis on the potential for recurrent episodes, asymptomatic viral shedding, and the attendant risks of sexual transmission.

- Persons experiencing a first episode of genital herpes should be advised that suppressive therapy is available and is effective in preventing symptomatic recurrent episodes and that episodic therapy sometimes is useful in shortening the duration of recurrent episodes.

- All persons with genital HSV infection should be

encouraged to inform their current sex partners that they have genital herpes and to inform future partners before initiating a sexual relationship.

- Sexual transmission of HSV can occur during asymptomatic periods. Asymptomatic viral shedding is more frequent in genital HSV-2 infection than genital HSV-1 infection and is most frequent during the first 12 months after acquiring HSV-2.

- All persons with genital herpes should remain abstinent from sexual activity with uninfected partners when lesions or prodromal symptoms are present.

- The risk of HSV-2 sexual transmission can be decreased by the daily use of valacyclovir by the infected person.

- Recent studies indicate that latex condoms, when used consistently and correctly, might reduce the risk for genital herpes transmission (15,16).

- Sex partners of infected persons should be advised that they might be infected even if they have no symptoms. Type-specific serologic testing of asymptomatic partners of persons with genital herpes is recommended to determine whether risk for HSV acquisition exists.

- The risk for neonatal HSV infection should be explained to all persons, including men. Pregnant women and women of childbearing age who have genital herpes should inform their providers who care for them during pregnancy and those who will care for their newborn infant. Pregnant women who are not infected with HSV-2 should be advised to avoid intercourse during the third trimester with men who have genital herpes. Similarly, pregnant women who are not infected with HSV-1 should be counseled to avoid genital exposure to HSV-1 during the third trimester (eg, oral sex with a partner with oral herpes and vaginal intercourse with a partner with genital HSV-1 infection).

- Asymptomatic persons diagnosed with HSV-2 infection by type-specific serologic testing should receive the same counseling messages as persons with symptomatic infection. In addition, such persons should be taught about the clinical manifestations of genital herpes.

Management of Sex Partners

The sex partners of patients who have genital herpes can benefit from evaluation and counseling. Symptomatic sex partners should be evaluated and treated in the same manner as patients who have genital lesions. Asymptomatic sex partners of patients who have genital herpes should be questioned concerning histories of genital lesions and offered type-specific serologic testing for HSV infection.

Special Considerations

Allergy, Intolerance, and Adverse Reactions

Allergic and other adverse reactions to acyclovir, valacyclovir, and famciclovir are rare. Desensitization to acyclovir has been described (85).

HIV Infection

Immunocompromised patients might have prolonged or severe episodes of genital, perianal, or oral herpes. Lesions caused by HSV are common among HIV-infected patients and might be severe, painful, and atypical. HSV shedding is increased in HIV-infected persons. Whereas antiretroviral therapy reduces the severity and frequency of symptomatic genital herpes, frequent subclinical shedding still occurs (86). Suppressive or episodic therapy with oral antiviral agents is effective in decreasing the clinical manifestations of HSV among HIV-positive persons (87-89). HIV-infected persons are likely to be more contagious for HSV; the extent to which suppressive antiviral therapy will decrease HSV transmission from this population is unknown. Some specialists suggest that HSV type-specific serologies be offered to HIV-positive persons during their initial evaluation, and that suppressive antiviral therapy be considered in those who have HSV-2 infection.

Recommended Regimens for Daily Suppressive Therapy in Persons Infected with HIV

Acyclovir 400-800 mg orally twice to three times a day

OR

Famciclovir 500 mg orally twice a day

OR

Valacyclovir 500 mg orally twice a day

Recommended Regimens for Episodic Infection in Persons Infected with HIV
Acyclovir 400 mg orally three times a day for 5-10 days

OR

Famiciclovir 500 mg orally twice a day for 5-10 days

OR

Valacyclovir 1.0 grams orally twice a day for 5-10 days

Acyclovir, valacyclovir, and famciclovir are safe for use in immunocompromised patients in the doses recommended for treatment of genital herpes. For severe HSV disease, initiating therapy with acyclovir 5-10 mg/kg body weight IV every 8 hours might be necessary.

If lesions persist or recur in a patient receiving antiviral treatment, HSV resistance should be suspected and a viral isolate should be obtained for sensitivity testing (90). Such patients should be managed in consultation with an HIV specialist, and alternate therapy should be administered. All acyclovir-resistant strains are resistant to valacyclovir, and the majority are resistant to famciclovir. Foscarnet, 40 mg/kg body weight IV every 8 hours until clinical resolution is attained, is frequently effective for treatment of acyclovir-resistant genital herpes. Topical cidofovir gel 1% applied to the lesions once daily for 5 consecutive days also might be effective. This preparation is not commercially available and must be compounded at a pharmacy.

Genital Herpes in Pregnancy
The majority of mothers of infants who acquire neonatal herpes lack histories of clinically evident genital herpes. The risk for transmission to the neonate from an infected mother is high (30%-50%) among women who acquire genital herpes near the time of delivery and is low (<1%) among women with histories of recurrent herpes at term or who acquire genital HSV during the first half of pregnancy. However, because recurrent genital herpes is much more common than initial HSV infection during pregnancy, the proportion of neonatal HSV infections acquired from mothers with recurrent herpes is substantial. Prevention of neonatal herpes depends both on preventing acquisition of genital HSV infection during late pregnancy and avoiding exposure of the infant to herpetic lesions during delivery.

Women without known genital herpes should be counseled to avoid intercourse during the third trimester with partners known or suspected of having genital herpes. In addition, pregnant women without known orolabial herpes should be advised to avoid receptive oral sex during the third trimester with partners known or suspected to have orolabial herpes. Some specialists believe that type-specific serologic tests are useful to identify pregnant women at risk for HSV infection and to guide counseling regarding the risk for acquiring genital herpes during pregnancy. Such testing should be offered to women without genital herpes whose sex partner has HSV infection. The effectiveness of antiviral therapy to decrease the risk for HSV transmission to pregnant women has not been studied.

All pregnant women should be asked whether they have a history of genital herpes. At the onset of labor, all women should be questioned carefully about symptoms of genital herpes, including prodromal symptoms, and all women should be examined carefully for herpetic lesions. Women without symptoms or signs of genital herpes or its prodrome can deliver vaginally. The majority of specialists recommend that women with recurrent genital herpetic lesions at the onset of labor deliver by cesarean section to prevent neonatal herpes. However, cesarean section does not completely eliminate the risk for HSV transmission to the infant.

The safety of systemic acyclovir, valacyclovir, and famciclovir therapy in pregnant women has not been definitively established. Available data do not indicate an increased risk for major birth defects compared with the general population in women treated with acyclovir during the first trimester (91).

These findings provide some assurance to women who have had prenatal exposure to acyclovir. The experience with prenatal exposure to valacyclovir and famciclovir is too limited to provide useful information on pregnancy outcomes. Acyclovir may be administered orally to pregnant women with first episode genital herpes or severe recurrent herpes and should be administered IV to pregnant women with severe HSV infection. Acyclovir treatment late in pregnancy reduces the frequency of cesarean sections among women who have recurrent genital herpes by diminishing the frequency of recurrences at term, and many specialists recommend such treatment (92-94). No data support the use of antiviral therapy among HSV seropositive women without a history of genital herpes. The risk for herpes is high in infants of women who acquire genital HSV during late pregnancy; such women should be managed in consultation with an infectious diseases specialist. Some specialists recommend acyclovir therapy in this circumstance, some recommend routine cesarean section to reduce the risk for neonatal herpes, and others recommend both.

Neonatal Herpes

Infants exposed to HSV during birth, as documented by maternal virologic testing or presumed by observation of maternal lesions, should be followed carefully in consultation with a specialist. Some specialists recommend that such infants undergo surveillance cultures of mucosal surfaces to detect HSV infection before development of clinical signs of neonatal herpes. In addition, some specialists recommend the use of acyclovir for infants born to women who acquired HSV near term because the risk for neonatal herpes is high for these infants. All infants who have neonatal herpes should be promptly evaluated and treated with systemic acyclovir. The recommended regimen for infants treated for known or suspected neonatal herpes is acyclovir 20 mg/kg body weight IV every 8 hours for 21 days for disseminated and CNS disease or for 14 days for disease limited to the skin and mucous membranes.

Granuloma Inguinale (Donovanosis)

Granuloma inguinale is a genital ulcerative disease caused by the intracellular gram-negative bacterium *Klebsiella granulomatis* (formerly known as *Calymmatobacterium granulomatis*). The disease occurs rarely in the United States, although it is endemic in some tropical and developing areas, including India; Papua, New Guinea; central Australia; and southern Africa. Clinically, the disease is commonly characterized as painless, progressive ulcerative lesions without regional lymphadenopathy. The lesions are highly vascular (ie, beefy red appearance) and bleed easily on contact. However, the clinical presentation also can include hypertrophic, necrotic, or sclerotic variants. The causative organism is difficult to culture, and diagnosis requires visualization of dark-staining Donovan bodies on tissue crush preparation or biopsy. No FDA-cleared PCR tests for the detection of *K granulomatis* DNA exist, but such an assay might be useful if a CLIA verification study has been conducted. The lesions might develop secondary bacterial infection or can coexist with other sexually transmitted pathogens.

Treatment

A limited number of studies on Donovanosis treatment have been published. Treatment halts progression of lesions, although prolonged therapy is usually required to permit granulation and reepithelialization of the ulcers. Healing typically proceeds inward from the ulcer margins. Relapse can occur 6-18 months after apparently effective therapy. Several antimicrobial regimens have been effective, but a limited number of controlled trials have been published (95).

Recommended Regimen

Doxycycline 100 mg orally twice a day for at least 3 weeks and until all lesions have completely healed

Alternative Regimens

Azithromycin 1 g orally once per week for at least 3 weeks and until all lesions have completely healed

OR

Ciprofloxacin 750 mg orally twice a day for at least 3 weeks and until all lesions have completely healed

OR

Erythromycin base 500 mg orally four times a day for at least 3 weeks and until all lesions have completely healed

OR

Trimethoprim-sulfamethoxazole one double-strength (160 mg/800 mg) tablet orally twice a day for at least 3 weeks and until all lesions have completely healed

Therapy should be continued at least 3 weeks and until all lesions have completely healed. Some specialists recommend the addition of an aminoglycoside (eg, gentamicin 1 mg/kg IV every 8 hours) to these regimens if improvement is not evident within the first few days of therapy.

Follow-Up
Patients should be followed clinically until signs and symptoms have resolved.

Management of Sex Partners
Persons who have had sexual contact with a patient who has granuloma inguinale within the 60 days before onset of the patient's symptoms should be examined and offered therapy. However, the value of empiric therapy in the absence of clinical signs and symptoms has not been established.

Special Considerations
Pregnancy
Pregnancy is a relative contraindication to the use of sulfonamides. Pregnant and lactating women should be treated with the erythromycin regimen, and consideration should be given to the addition of a parenteral aminoglycoside (eg, gentamicin). Azithromycin might prove useful for treating granuloma inguinale during pregnancy, but published data are lacking. Doxycycline and ciprofloxacin are contraindicated in pregnant women.

HIV Infection
Persons with both granuloma inguinale and HIV infection should receive the same regimens as those who are HIV negative. Consideration should be given to the addition of a parenteral aminoglycoside (eg, gentamicin).

Lymphogranuloma Venereum

Lymphogranuloma venereum (LGV) is caused by *C trachomatis* serovars L1, L2, or L3 (96). The most common clinical manifestation of LGV among heterosexuals is tender inguinal and/or femoral lymphadenopathy that is typically unilateral. A self-limited genital ulcer or papule sometimes occurs at the site of inoculation. However, by the time patients seek care, the lesions might have disappeared. Rectal exposure in women or MSM might result in proctocolitis (including mucoid and/or hemorrhagic rectal discharge, anal pain, constipation, fever, and/or tenesmus). LGV is an invasive, systemic infection, and if it is not treated early, LGV proctocolitis might lead to chronic, colorectal fistulas and strictures. Genital and colorectal LGV lesions might also develop secondary bacterial infection or might be coinfected with other sexually and nonsexually transmitted pathogens.

Diagnosis is based on clinical suspicion, epidemiologic information, and the exclusion of other etiologies (of proctocolitis, inguinal lymphadenopathy, or genital or rectal ulcers), along with *C trachomatis* testing, if available.

Genital and lymph node specimens (ie, lesion swab or bubo aspirate) may be tested for *C trachomatis* by culture, direct immunofluorescence, or nucleic acid detection. Nucleic acid amplification tests (NAAT) for *C trachomatis* are not FDA cleared for testing rectal specimens. Additional procedures (eg, genotyping) are required for differentiating LGV from non-LGV *C trachomatis* but are not widely available.

Chlamydia serology (complement fixation titers >1:64) can support the diagnosis in the appropriate clinical context. Comparative data between types of serologic tests are lacking, and the diagnostic utility of serologic methods other than complement fixation and some microimmunofluorescence procedures has not been established. Serologic test interpretation for LGV is not standardized, tests have not been validated for clinical proctitis presentations, and *C trachomatis* serovar-specific serologic tests are not widely available.

In the absence of specific LGV diagnostic testing, patients with a clinical syndrome consistent with LGV, including proctocolitis or genital ulcer disease with lymphadenopathy, should be treated for LGV as described in this report.

Treatment

Treatment cures infection and prevents ongoing tissue damage, although tissue reaction to the injection can result in scarring. Buboes might require aspiration through intact skin or incision and drainage to prevent the formation of inguinal/femoral ulcerations. Doxycycline is the preferred treatment.

Recommended Regimen

Doxycycline 100 mg orally twice a day for 21 days

Alternative Regimen

Erythromycin base 500 mg orally four times a day for 21 days

Some STD specialists believe that azithromycin 1.0 g orally once weekly for 3 weeks is probably effective, although clinical data are lacking.

Follow-Up

Patients should be followed clinically until signs and symptoms have resolved.

Management of Sex Partners

Persons who have had sexual contact with a patient who has LGV within the 60 days before onset of the patient's symptoms should be examined, tested for urethral or cervical chlamydial infection, and treated with a standard chlamydia regimen (azithromycin 1 gm orally x 1 or doxycycline 100 mg orally twice a day for 7 days). The optimum contact interval is unknown; some specialists use longer contact intervals.

Special Considerations

Pregnancy

Pregnant and lactating women should be treated with erythromycin. Azithromycin might prove useful for treatment of LGV in pregnancy, but no published data are available regarding its safety and efficacy. Doxycycline is contraindicated in pregnant women.

HIV Infection

Persons with both LGV and HIV infection should receive the same regimens as those who are HIV negative. Prolonged therapy might be required, and delay in resolution of symptoms might occur.

Syphilis

General Principles

Background. Syphilis is a systemic disease caused by *T pallidum*. Patients who have syphilis might seek treatment for signs or symptoms of primary infection (ie, ulcer or chancre at the infection site), secondary infection (ie, manifestations that include, but are not limited to, skin rash, mucocutaneous lesions, and lymphadenopathy), or tertiary infection (eg, cardiac or ophthalmic manifestations, auditory abnormalities, or gummatous lesions). Latent infections (ie, those lacking clinical manifestations) are detected by serologic testing. Latent syphilis acquired within the preceding year is referred to as early latent syphilis; all other cases of latent syphilis are either late latent syphilis or latent syphilis of unknown duration. Treatment for both late latent syphilis and tertiary syphilis theoretically might require a longer duration of therapy because organisms are dividing more slowly; however, the validity of this concept has not been assessed.

Diagnostic Considerations and Use of Serologic Tests

Darkfield examinations and direct fluorescent antibody (DFA) tests of lesion exudate or tissue are the definitive methods for diagnosing early syphilis. A presumptive diagnosis is possible with the use of two types of serologic tests: 1) nontreponemal tests (eg, Venereal Disease Research Laboratory [VDRL] and RPR), and 2) treponemal tests (eg, fluorescent treponemal antibody absorbed [FTA-ABS] and *T pallidum* particle agglutination [TP-PA]). The use of only one type of serologic test is insufficient for diagnosis because false-positive nontreponemal test results are sometimes associated with various medical conditions unrelated to syphilis.

Nontreponemal test antibody titers usually correlate with disease activity, and results should be reported quantitatively. A fourfold change in titer, equivalent to a change of two dilutions (eg, from 1:16-1:4 or from 1:8-1:32), is considered necessary to demonstrate a clinically significant difference between two nontreponemal test results that were obtained using the same serologic test. Sequential serologic tests in individual patients should be performed by using the same testing method (eg, VDRL or RPR), preferably by the same laboratory. The VDRL and RPR are equally valid assays, but quantitative results from the two tests cannot be compared directly because RPR titers frequently are slightly higher than VDRL titers. Nontreponemal tests usually become nonreactive with time after treatment; however, in some patients, nontreponemal antibodies can persist at a low titer for a long period of time, sometimes for the life of the patient. This response is referred to as the serofast reaction.

The majority of patients who have reactive treponemal tests will have reactive tests for the remainder of their lives, regardless of treatment or disease activity. However, 15%-25% of patients treated during the primary stage revert to being serologically nonreactive after 2-3 years (97). Treponemal test antibody titers do not correlate with disease activity and should not be used to assess treatment response.

Some clinical laboratories and blood banks have begun to screen samples using treponemal EIA tests (98). This strategy will identify both persons with previous treatment and persons with untreated or incompletely treated syphilis. False-positive results can occur, particularly among populations with a low prevalence of syphilis.

Persons with a positive treponemal screening test should have a standard nontreponemal test with titer to guide patient management decisions. If the nontreponemal test is negative, then a different treponemal test should be performed to confirm the results of the initial test. If a second trepomenal test is positive, treatment decisions should be discussed in consultation with a specialist. Some HIV-infected patients can have atypical serologic test results (ie, unusually high, unusually low, or fluctuating titers). For such patients, when serologic tests do not correspond with clinical syndromes suggestive of early syphilis, use of other tests (eg, biopsy and direct microscopy) should be considered. However, for the majority of HIV-infected patients, serologic tests are accurate and reliable for the diagnosis of syphilis and for following the response to treatment.

No single test can be used to diagnose neurosyphilis. The VDRL-cerebrospinal fluid (CSF) is highly specific, but it is insensitive. The majority of other tests are both insensitive and nonspecific and must be interpreted in relation to other test results and the clinical assessment. Therefore, the diagnosis of neurosyphilis usually depends on various combinations of reactive serologic test results, CSF cell count or protein, or a reactive VDRL-CSF with or without clinical manifestations. The CSF leukocyte count usually is elevated (>5 white blood cell count [WBC]/mm^3) in patients with neurosyphilis; this count also is a sensitive measure of the effectiveness of therapy. The VDRL-CSF is the standard serologic test for CSF, and when reactive in the absence of substantial contamination of CSF with blood, it is considered diagnostic of neurosyphilis. However, the VDRL-CSF might be nonreactive even when neurosyphilis is present. Some specialists recommend performing an FTA-ABS test on CSF. The CSF FTA-ABS is less specific (ie, yields more false-positive results) for neurosyphilis than the VDRL-CSF, but the test is highly sensitive. Therefore, some specialists believe that a negative CSF FTA-ABS test excludes neurosyphilis.

Treatment

Penicillin G, administered parenterally, is the preferred drug for treatment of all stages of syphilis. The preparation(s) used (ie, benzathine, aqueous procaine, or aqueous crystalline), the dosage, and the length of treatment depend on the stage and clinical manifestations of the disease. However, neither combinations of benzathine penicillin and procaine penicillin nor oral penicillin preparations are considered appropriate for the treatment of syphilis. Reports have indicated that inappropriate use of combination benzathine-procaine penicillin (Bicillin C-R®) instead of the standard benzathine penicillin product widely used in the United States (Bicillin L-A®) has occurred. Practitioners, pharmacists, and purchasing agents should be aware of the similar names of these two products and avoid use of the inappropriate combination therapy agent for treating syphilis (99).

The efficacy of penicillin for the treatment of syphilis was well established through clinical experience even before the value of randomized controlled clinical trials was recognized. Therefore, nearly all the recommendations for the treatment of syphilis are based on the opinions of persons knowledgeable about STDs and are reinforced by case series, clinical trials, and 50 years of clinical experience.

Parenteral penicillin G is the only therapy with documented efficacy for syphilis during pregnancy. Pregnant women with syphilis in any stage who report penicillin allergy should be desensitized and treated with penicillin. Skin testing for penicillin allergy might be useful in pregnant women; such testing also is useful in other patients (see Management of Patients Who Have a History of Penicillin Allergy).

The Jarisch-Herxheimer reaction is an acute febrile reaction frequently accompanied by headache, myalgia, and other symptoms that usually occur within the first 24 hours after any therapy for syphilis. Patients should be informed about this possible adverse reaction. The Jarisch-Herxheimer reaction occurs most frequently among patients who have early syphilis. Antipyretics may be used, but they have not been proven to prevent this reaction. The Jarisch-Herxheimer reaction might induce early labor or cause fetal distress in pregnant women, but this should not prevent or delay therapy (see Syphilis During Pregnancy).

Management of Sex Partners

Sexual transmission of *T pallidum* occurs only when mucocutaneous syphilitic lesions are present; such manifestations are uncommon after the first year of infection. However, persons exposed sexually to a patient who has syphilis in any stage should be evaluated clinically and serologically and treated with a recommended regimen, according to the following recommendations:

- Persons who were exposed within the 90 days preceding the diagnosis of primary, secondary, or early latent syphilis in a sex partner might be infected even if seronegative; therefore, such persons should be treated presumptively.

- Persons who were exposed >90 days before the diagnosis of primary, secondary, or early latent syphilis in a sex partner should be treated presumptively if serologic test results are not available immediately and the opportunity for follow-up is uncertain.

- For purposes of partner notification and presumptive treatment of exposed sex partners, patients with syphilis of unknown duration who have high nontreponemal serologic test titers (ie, ≥1:32) can be assumed to have early syphilis. However, serologic titers should not be used to differentiate early from late latent syphilis for the purpose of determining treatment (see Latent Syphilis, Treatment).

- Long-term sex partners of patients who have latent syphilis should be evaluated clinically and serologically for syphilis and treated on the basis of the evaluation findings.

For identification of at-risk sexual partners, the periods before treatment are: 1) 3 months plus duration of symptoms for primary syphilis; 2) 6 months plus duration of symptoms for secondary syphilis; and 3) 1 year for early latent syphilis.

Primary and Secondary Syphilis

Treatment

Parenteral penicillin G has been used effectively for more than 50 years to achieve clinical resolution (ie, healing of lesions and prevention of sexual transmission) and to prevent late sequelae. However, no comparative trials have been adequately conducted to guide the selection of an optimal penicillin regimen (ie, the dose, duration, and preparation). Substantially fewer data are available for nonpenicillin regimens.

Recommended Regimen for Adults*

Benzathine penicillin G 2.4 million units IM in a single dose

* Recommendations for treating HIV-infected persons and pregnant women for syphilis have been discussed in this report (see Syphilis, Special Considerations and Syphilis in Pregnancy).

Recommended Regimen for Children

After the newborn period (aged ≥1 month), children with syphilis should have a CSF examination to detect asymptomatic neurosyphilis, and birth and maternal medical records should be reviewed to assess whether such children have congenital or acquired syphilis (see Congenital Syphilis). Children with acquired primary or secondary syphilis should be evaluated (eg, through consultation with child-protection services) (see Sexual Assault or Abuse of Children) and treated by using the following pediatric regimen.

Benzathine penicillin G 50,000 units/kg IM, up to the adult dose of 2.4 million units in a single dose

Other Management Considerations
All patients who have syphilis should be tested for HIV infection. In geographic areas in which the prevalence of HIV is high, patients who have primary syphilis should be retested for HIV after 3 months if the first HIV test result was negative.

Patients who have syphilis and symptoms or signs suggesting neurologic disease (eg, meningitis) or ophthalmic disease (eg, uveitis, iritis, neuroretinitis, or optic neuritis) should have an evaluation that includes CSF analysis and ocular slitlamp examination. Treatment should be guided by the results of this evaluation.

Invasion of CSF by *T pallidum* accompanied by CSF abnormalities is common among adults who have primary or secondary syphilis. However, neurosyphilis develops in only a limited number of patients after treatment with the penicillin regimens recommended for primary and secondary syphilis. Therefore, unless clinical signs or symptoms of neurologic or ophthalmic involvement are present, CSF analysis is not recommended for routine evaluation of patients who have primary or secondary syphilis.

Follow-Up
Treatment failure can occur with any regimen. However, assessing response to treatment frequently is difficult, and definitive criteria for cure or failure have not been established. Nontreponemal test titers might decline more slowly for persons who previously had syphilis. Patients should be reexamined clinically and serologically 6 months and 12 months after treatment; more frequent evaluation might be prudent if follow-up is uncertain.

Patients who have signs or symptoms that persist or recur or who have a sustained fourfold increase in nontreponemal test titer (ie, compared with the maximum or baseline titer at the time of treatment) probably failed treatment or were reinfected. These patients should be retreated and reevaluated for HIV infection. Because treatment failure usually cannot be reliably distinguished from reinfection with *T pallidum*, a CSF analysis also should be performed. Clinical trial data have demonstrated that 15% of patients with early syphilis treated with the recommended therapy will not achieve a two dilution decline in nontreponemal titer used to define response at 1 year after treatment (100).

Failure of nontreponemal test titers to decline fourfold within 6 months after therapy for primary or secondary syphilis might be indicative of probable treatment failure. Persons for whom titers remain serofast should be reevaluated for HIV infection. Optimal management of such patients is unclear. At a minimum, these patients should receive additional clinical and serologic follow-up. HIV-infected patients should be evaluated more frequently (ie, at 3-month intervals instead of 6-month intervals). If additional follow-up cannot be ensured, retreatment is recommended. Because treatment failure might be the result of unrecognized CNS infection, many specialists recommend CSF examination in such situations.

For retreatment, the majority of STD specialists recommend administering weekly injections of benzathine penicillin G 2.4 million units IM for 3 weeks, unless CSF examination indicates that neurosyphilis is present. In rare instances, serologic titers do not decline despite a negative CSF examination and a repeated course of therapy. Additional therapy or repeated CSF examinations are not warranted in these circumstances.

Management of Sex Partners
See General Principles, Management of Sex Partners.

Special Considerations
Penicillin Allergy
Data to support the use of alternatives to penicillin in the treatment of early syphilis are limited. However, several therapies might be effective in non-

pregnant, penicillin-allergic patients who have primary or secondary syphilis. Doxycycline (100 mg orally twice daily for 14 days) and tetracycline (500 mg four times daily for 14 days) are regimens that have been used for many years. Compliance is likely to be better with doxycycline than tetracycline because tetracycline can cause gastrointestinal side effects. Although limited clinical studies, along with biologic and pharmacologic evidence, suggest that ceftriaxone is effective for treating early syphilis, the optimal dose and duration of ceftriaxone therapy have not been defined. Some specialists recommend 1 g daily either IM or IV for 8-10 days. Some patients who are allergic to penicillin also might be allergic to ceftriaxone; in these circumstances, use of an alternative agent might be required. Preliminary data suggest that azithromycin might be effective as a single oral dose of 2 g (101,102). However, several cases of azithromycin treatment failure have been reported, and resistance to azithromycin has been documented in several geographic areas (103). Close follow-up of persons receiving alternative therapies is essential. The use of any of these therapies in HIV-infected persons has not been well studied; therefore, the use of doxycycline, ceftriaxone, and azithromycin among such persons must be undertaken with caution.

Patients with penicillin allergy whose compliance with therapy or follow-up cannot be ensured should be desensitized and treated with benzathine penicillin. Skin testing for penicillin allergy might be useful in some circumstances in which the reagents and expertise are available to perform the test adequately (see Management of Patients Who Have a History of Penicillin Allergy).

Pregnancy

Pregnant patients who are allergic to penicillin should be desensitized and treated with penicillin (see Management of Patients Who Have a History of Penicillin Allergy and Syphilis During Pregnancy).

HIV Infection

See Syphilis Among HIV-Infected Persons.

Latent Syphilis

Latent syphilis is defined as syphilis characterized by seroreactivity without other evidence of disease. Patients who have latent syphilis and who acquired syphilis within the preceding year are classified as having early latent syphilis. Patients' conditions can be diagnosed as early latent syphilis if, within the year preceding the evaluation, they had: 1) a documented seroconversion or fourfold or greater increase in titer of a nontreponemal test; 2) unequivocal symptoms of primary or secondary syphilis; 3) a sex partner documented to have primary, secondary, or early latent syphilis; or 4) reactive nontreponemal and treponemal tests from a person whose only possible exposure occurred within the previous 12 months. Nontreponemal serologic titers usually are higher during early latent syphilis than late latent syphilis. However, early latent syphilis cannot be reliably distinguished from late latent syphilis solely on the basis of nontreponemal titers. All patients with latent syphilis should have careful examination of all accessible mucosal surfaces (ie, the oral cavity, the perineum in women, and perianal area, underneath the foreskin in uncircumcised men) to evaluate for internal mucosal lesions. All patients who have syphilis should be tested for HIV infection.

Treatment

Treatment of latent syphilis usually does not affect transmission and is intended to prevent late complications. Although clinical experience supports the effectiveness of penicillin in achieving this goal, limited evidence is available for guidance in choosing specific regimens.

The following regimens are recommended for penicillin nonallergic patients who have normal CSF examinations (if performed).

Recommended Regimens for Adults
Early Latent Syphilis
Benzathine penicillin G 2.4 million units IM in a single dose

Late Latent Syphilis or Latent Syphilis of Unknown Duration
Benzathine penicillin G 7.2 million units total, administered as 3 doses of 2.4 million units IM each

at 1-week intervals

After the newborn period, children with syphilis should have a CSF examination to exclude neurosyphilis. In addition, birth and maternal medical records should be reviewed to assess whether children have congenital or acquired syphilis (see Congenital Syphilis). Older children with acquired latent syphilis should be evaluated as described for adults and treated using the following pediatric regimens (see Sexual Assault or Abuse of Children). These regimens are for penicillin nonallergic children who have acquired syphilis and who have normal CSF examination results.

Recommended Regimens for Children
Early Latent Syphilis
Benzathine penicillin G 50,000 units/kg IM, up to the adult dose of 2.4 million units in a single dose

Late Latent Syphilis or Latent Syphilis of Unknown Duration
Benzathine penicillin G 50,000 units/kg IM, up to the adult dose of 2.4 million units, administered as 3 doses at 1-week intervals (total 150,000 units/kg up to the adult total dose of 7.2 million units)

Other Management Considerations
All persons who have latent syphilis should be evaluated clinically for evidence of tertiary disease (eg, aortitis and gumma) and syphilitic ocular disease (eg, iritis and uveitis). Patients who have syphilis and who demonstrate any of the following criteria should have a prompt CSF examination:

- neurologic or ophthalmic signs or symptoms,
- evidence of active tertiary syphilis (eg, aortitis and gumma),
- treatment failure, or
- HIV infection with late latent syphilis or syphilis of unknown duration.

If dictated by circumstances and patient preferences, a CSF examination may be performed for patients who do not meet these criteria. Some specialists recommend performing a CSF examination on all patients who have latent syphilis and a nontreponemal serologic test of ≥1:32 or if the patient is HIV infected with a serum CD4 count <350 (104). However, the likelihood of neurosyphilis in this circumstance is unknown. If a CSF examination is performed and the results indicate abnormalities consistent with neurosyphilis, the patient should be treated for neurosyphilis (see Neurosyphilis).

If a patient misses a dose of penicillin in a course of weekly therapy for late syphilis, the appropriate course of action is unclear. Pharmacologic considerations suggest that an interval of 10-14 days between doses of benzathine penicillin for late syphilis or latent syphilis of unknown duration might be acceptable before restarting the sequence of injections. Missed doses are not acceptable for pregnant patients receiving therapy for late latent syphilis; pregnant women who miss any dose of therapy must repeat the full course of therapy.

Follow-Up
Quantitative nontreponemal serologic tests should be repeated at 6, 12, and 24 months. Patients with a normal CSF examination should be retreated for latent syphilis if: 1) titers increase fourfold, 2) an initially high titer (≥1:32) fails to decline at least fourfold (ie, two dilutions) within 12-24 months of therapy, or 3) signs or symptoms attributable to syphilis develop. In rare instances, despite a negative CSF examination and a repeated course of therapy, serologic titers might still not decline. In these circumstances, the need for additional therapy or repeated CSF examinations is unclear.

Management of Sex Partners
See General Principles, Management of Sex Partners.

Special Considerations
Penicillin Allergy
The effectiveness of alternatives to penicillin in the treatment of latent syphilis has not been well documented. Nonpregnant patients allergic to penicillin who have clearly defined early latent syphilis should respond to therapies recommended as alternatives to penicillin for the treatment of primary and secondary syphilis (see Primary and Secondary Syphilis, Treatment). The only acceptable alternatives for the treatment of late latent syphilis or latent syphilis of unknown duration are doxycycline (100 mg orally twice daily) or tetracycline (500 mg orally four times daily), both for 28 days. These therapies

should be used only in conjunction with close serologic and clinical follow-up. Limited clinical studies, along with biologic and pharmacologic evidence, suggest that ceftriaxone might be effective for treating late latent syphilis or syphilis of unknown duration (105). However, the optimal dose and duration of ceftriaxone therapy have not been defined, and treatment decisions should be discussed in consultation with a specialist. Some patients who are allergic to penicillin also might be allergic to ceftriaxone; in these circumstances, use of an alternative agent might be required. The efficacy of these alternative regimens in HIV infected persons has not been well studied and, therefore, must be considered with caution.

Pregnancy
Pregnant patients who are allergic to penicillin should be desensitized and treated with penicillin (see Management of Patients Who Have a History of Penicillin Allergy and Syphilis During Pregnancy).

HIV Infection
See Syphilis Among HIV-Infected Persons.

Tertiary Syphilis

Tertiary syphilis refers to gumma and cardiovascular syphilis but not to all neurosyphilis. Patients who are not allergic to penicillin and have no evidence of neurosyphilis should be treated with the following regimen.

Recommended Regimen
Benzathine penicillin G 7.2 million units total, administered as 3 doses of 2.4 million units IM each at 1-week intervals

Other Management Considerations
Patients who have symptomatic late syphilis should be given a CSF examination before therapy is initiated. Some providers treat all patients who have cardiovascular syphilis with a neurosyphilis regimen. The complete management of patients who have cardiovascular or gummatous syphilis is beyond the scope of these guidelines. These patients should be managed in consultation with an infectious diseases specialist.

Follow-Up
Limited information is available concerning clinical response and follow-up of patients who have tertiary syphilis.

Management of Sex Partners
See General Principles, Management of Sex Partners.

Special Considerations
Penicillin Allergy
Patients allergic to penicillin should be treated according to treatment regimens recommended for late latent syphilis.

Pregnancy
Pregnant patients who are allergic to penicillin should be desensitized, if necessary, and treated with penicillin (see Management of Patients Who Have a History of Penicillin Allergy and Syphilis During Pregnancy).

HIV Infection
See Syphilis Among HIV-Infected Persons.

Neurosyphilis

Treatment
CNS involvement can occur during any stage of syphilis. A patient who has clinical evidence of neurologic involvement with syphilis (eg, cognitive dysfunction, motor or sensory deficits, ophthalmic or auditory symptoms, cranial nerve palsies, and symptoms or signs of meningitis) should have a CSF examination.

Syphilitic uveitis or other ocular manifestations frequently are associated with neurosyphilis; patients with these symptoms should be treated according to the recommendations for patients with neurosyphilis. A CSF examination should be performed for all such patients to identify those with abnormalities that require follow-up CSF examinations to assess treatment response.

Patients who have neurosyphilis or syphilitic eye disease (eg, uveitis, neuroretinitis, and optic neuritis) should be treated with the following regimen.

Recommended Regimen
Aqueous crystalline penicillin G 18-24 million units per day, administered as 3-4 million units IV every 4 hours or continuous infusion, for 10-14 days

If compliance with therapy can be ensured, patients may be treated with the following alternative regimen.

Alternative Regimen
Procaine penicillin 2.4 million units IM once daily

PLUS

Probenecid 500 mg orally four times a day, both for 10-14 days

The durations of the recommended and alternative regimens for neurosyphilis are shorter than that of the regimen used for late syphilis in the absence of neurosyphilis. Therefore, some specialists administer benzathine penicillin, 2.4 million units IM once per week for up to 3 weeks after completion of these neurosyphilis treatment regimens to provide a comparable total duration of therapy.

Other Management Considerations
Other considerations in the management of patients who have neurosyphilis are as follows:

- All patients who have syphilis should be tested for HIV.

- Many specialists recommend treating patients who have evidence of auditory disease caused by syphilis in the same manner as patients who have neurosyphilis, regardless of CSF examination results. Although systemic steroids are used frequently as adjunctive therapy for otologic syphilis, such drugs have not been proven beneficial.

Follow-Up
If CSF pleocytosis was present initially, a CSF examination should be repeated every 6 months until the cell count is normal. Follow-up CSF examinations also can be used to evaluate changes in the VDRL-CSF or CSF protein after therapy; however, changes in these two parameters occur more slowly than cell counts, and persistent abnormalities might be less important. If the cell count has not decreased after 6 months or if the CSF is not normal after 2 years, retreatment should be considered. Recent data on HIV-infected persons with neurosyphilis suggest that CSF abnormalities might persist for extended periods in these persons, and close clinical follow-up is warranted (105,106).

Management of Sex Partners
See General Principles, Management of Sex Partners.

Special Considerations
Penicillin Allergy
Ceftriaxone can be used as an alternative treatment for patients with neurosyphilis, although the possibility of cross-reactivity between this agent and penicillin exists. Some specialists recommend ceftriaxone 2 g daily either IM or IV for 10–14 days. Other regimens have not been adequately evaluated for treatment of neurosyphilis. Therefore, if concern exists regarding the safety of ceftriaxone for a patient with neurosyphilis, the patient should obtain skin testing to confirm penicillin allergy and, if necessary, be desensitized and managed in consultation with a specialist.

Pregnancy
Pregnant patients who are allergic to penicillin should be desensitized, if necessary, and treated with penicillin (see Syphilis During Pregnancy).

HIV Infection
See Syphilis Among HIV-Infected Patients.

Syphilis Among HIV-Infected Persons

Diagnostic Considerations
Unusual serologic responses have been observed among HIV-infected persons who have syphilis. The majority of reports have involved serologic titers that were higher than expected, but false-negative serologic test results and delayed appearance of seroreactivity also have been reported. However, unusual serologic responses are uncommon, and the majority of specialists believe that both treponemal and nontreponemal serologic tests for syphilis can be inter-

preted in the usual manner for the majority of patients who are coinfected with *T pallidum* and HIV.

When clinical findings are suggestive of syphilis but serologic tests are nonreactive or their interpretation is unclear, alternative tests (eg, biopsy of a lesion, dark-field examination, or DFA staining of lesion material) might be useful for diagnosis. Neurosyphilis should be considered in the differential diagnosis of neurologic disease in HIV-infected persons.

Treatment

Compared with HIV-negative patients, HIV-positive patients who have early syphilis might be at increased risk for neurologic complications and might have higher rates of treatment failure with currently recommended regimens. The magnitude of these risks is not defined precisely but is likely minimal. No treatment regimens for syphilis have been demonstrated to be more effective in preventing neurosyphilis in HIV-infected patients than the syphilis regimens recommended for HIV-negative patients (100). Careful follow-up after therapy is essential.

Primary and Secondary Syphilis Among HIV-Infected Persons

Treatment

Treatment with benzathine penicillin G, 2.4 million units IM in a single dose is recommended. Some specialists recommend additional treatments (eg, benzathine penicillin G administered at 1-week intervals for 3 weeks, as recommended for late syphilis) in addition to benzathine penicillin G 2.4 million units IM.

Other Management Considerations

Because CSF abnormalities (eg, mononuclear pleocytosis and elevated protein levels) are common in patients with early syphilis and in persons with HIV infection, the clinical and prognostic significance of such CSF abnormalities in HIV-infected persons with primary or secondary syphilis is unknown. Although the majority of HIV-infected persons respond appropriately to standard benzathine penicillin therapy, some specialists recommend intensified therapy when CNS syphilis is suspected in these persons. Therefore, some specialists recommend CSF examination before treatment of HIV-infected persons with early syphilis, with follow-up CSF examination conducted after treatment in persons with initial abnormalities.

Follow-Up

HIV-infected persons should be evaluated clinically and serologically for treatment failure at 3, 6, 9, 12, and 24 months after therapy. Although of unproven benefit, some specialists recommend a CSF examination 6 months after therapy.

HIV-infected persons who meet the criteria for treatment failure (ie, signs or symptoms that persist or recur, or persons that have fourfold increase in nontreponemal test titer) should be managed in the same manner as HIV-negative patients (ie, a CSF examination and retreatment). CSF examination and re-treatment also should be strongly considered for persons whose nontreponemal test titers do not decrease fourfold within 6-12 months of therapy. The majority of specialists would retreat patients with benzathine penicillin G administered as 3 doses of 2.4 million units IM each at weekly intervals, if CSF examinations are normal.

Special Considerations

Penicillin Allergy

Penicillin-allergic patients who have primary or secondary syphilis and HIV infection should be managed according to the recommendations for penicillin-allergic, HIV-negative patients. The use of alternatives to penicillin has not been well studied in HIV-infected patients.

Latent Syphilis Among HIV-Infected Persons

Diagnostic Considerations

HIV-infected patients who have early latent syphilis should be managed and treated according to the recommendations for HIV-negative patients who have primary and secondary syphilis. HIV-infected patients who have either late latent syphilis or syphilis of unknown duration should have a CSF examination before treatment.

Treatment

Patients with late latent syphilis or syphilis of unknown duration and a normal CSF examination can be treated with benzathine penicillin G, at weekly doses of 2.4 million units for 3 weeks. Patients who have CSF consistent with neurosyphilis should be treated and managed as patients who have neurosyphilis (see Neurosyphilis).

Follow-Up

Patients should be evaluated clinically and serologically at 6, 12, 18, and 24 months after therapy. If, at any time, clinical symptoms develop or nontreponemal titers rise fourfold, a repeat CSF examination should be performed and treatment administered accordingly. If during 12-24 months the nontreponemal titer does not decline fourfold, the CSF examination should be repeated and treatment administered accordingly.

Special Considerations

Penicillin Allergy

The efficacy of alternative nonpenicillin regimens in HIV-infected persons has not been well studied. Patients with penicillin allergy whose compliance with therapy or follow-up cannot be ensured should be desensitized and treated with penicillin (see Management of Patients Who Have a History of Penicillin Allergy). These therapies should be used only in conjunction with close serologic and clinical follow-up. Limited clinical studies, along with biologic and pharmacologic evidence, suggest that ceftriaxone might be effective (105). However, optimal dose and duration of ceftriaxone therapy have not been defined.

Syphilis During Pregnancy

All women should be screened serologically for syphilis during the early stages of pregnancy. The majority of states mandate screening at the first prenatal visit for all women. Antepartum screening by nontreponemal antibody testing is typical, but in some settings, treponemal antibody testing is being used. Pregnant women with reactive treponemal screening tests should have confirmatory testing with nontreponemal tests with titers. In populations in which use of prenatal care is not optimal, RPR-card test screening and treatment (ie, if the RPR-card test is reactive) should be performed at the time a pregnancy is diagnosed. For communities and populations in which the prevalence of syphilis is high or for patients at high risk, serologic testing should be performed twice during the third trimester, at 28 to 32 weeks' gestation and at delivery. Any woman who delivers a stillborn infant after 20 weeks gestation should be tested for syphilis. No infant should leave the hospital without the maternal serologic status having been determined at least once during pregnancy.

Diagnostic Considerations

Seropositive pregnant women should be considered infected unless an adequate treatment history is documented clearly in the medical records and sequential serologic antibody titers have declined. Serofast low antibody titers might not require treatment; however, persistent higher titer antibody tests might indicate reinfection and require treatment.

Treatment

Penicillin is effective for preventing maternal transmission to the fetus and for treating fetal infection. Evidence is insufficient to determine specific, recommended penicillin regimens that are optimal (107).

Recommended Regimen

Treatment during pregnancy should be the penicillin regimen appropriate for the stage of syphilis.

Other Management Considerations

Some specialists recommend additional therapy for pregnant women in some settings (eg, a second dose of benzathine penicillin 2.4 million units IM administered 1 week after the initial dose for women who have primary, secondary, or early latent syphilis). During the second half of pregnancy, syphilis management may be facilitated by a sonographic fetal evaluation for congenital syphilis, but this evaluation should not delay therapy. Sonographic signs of fetal or placental syphilis (ie, hepatomegaly, ascites, hydrops, or a thickened placenta) indicate a greater risk for fetal treatment failure (108); such cases should be managed in consultation with obstetricialists. Evidence is insufficient to recommend specific regimens for these situations.

Women treated for syphilis during the second half of pregnancy are at risk for premature labor and/or fetal distress, if the treatment precipitates the Jarisch-Herxheimer reaction. These women should be advised to seek obstetric attention after treatment, if they notice any contractions or decrease in fetal movements. Stillbirth is a rare complication of treatment, but concern for this complication should not delay necessary treatment. All patients who have syphilis should be offered testing for HIV infection.

Follow-Up

Coordinated prenatal care and treatment follow-up are vital. Serologic titers should be repeated at 28-32 weeks' gestation, at delivery, and following the recommendations for the stage of disease. Serologic titers can be checked monthly in women at high risk for reinfection or in geographic areas in which the prevalence of syphilis is high. The clinical and antibody response should be appropriate for the stage of disease. The majority of women will deliver before their serologic response to treatment can be assessed definitively. Inadequate maternal treatment is likely if delivery occurs within 30 days of therapy, if clinical signs of infection are present at delivery, or if the maternal antibody titer is fourfold higher than the pretreatment titer.

Management of Sex Partners.

See General Principles, Management of Sex Partners.

Special Considerations

Penicillin Allergy

For treatment of syphilis during pregnancy, no proven alternatives to penicillin exist. Pregnant women who have a history of penicillin allergy should be desensitized and treated with penicillin. Skin testing might be helpful (see Management of Patients Who Have a History of Penicillin Allergy).

Tetracycline and doxycycline usually are not used during pregnancy. Erythromycin should not be used because it does not reliably cure an infected fetus. Data are insufficient to recommend azithromycin or ceftriaxone for treatment of maternal infection and prevention of congenital syphilis.

HIV Infection

Placental inflammation from congenital infection might increase the risk for perinatal transmission of HIV. All HIV-infected women should be evaluated for infectious syphilis and treated. Data are insufficient to recommend a specific regimen (see Syphilis Among HIV-Infected Patients).

B. Management of Patients Who Have a History of Penicillin Allergy

No proven alternatives to penicillin are available for treating neurosyphilis, congenital syphilis, or syphilis in pregnant women. Penicillin also is recommended for use, whenever possible, in HIV-infected patients. Of the adult U.S. population, 3%–10% have experienced an immunoglobulin E (IgE) mediated allergic response to penicillin such as urticaria, angioedema, or anaphylaxis (i.e., upper airway obstruction, bronchospasm, or hypotension). Re-administration of penicillin to these patients can cause severe, immediate reactions. Because anaphylactic reactions to penicillin can be fatal, every effort should be made to avoid administering penicillin to penicillin-allergic patients, unless they undergo acute desensitization to eliminate anaphylactic sensitivity.

An estimated 10% of persons who report a history of severe allergic reactions to penicillin remain allergic. With the passage of time, the majority of persons who have had a severe reaction to penicillin stop expressing penicillin-specific IgE. These persons can be treated safely with penicillin. The results of many investigations indicate that skin testing with the major and minor determinants of penicillin can reliably identify persons at high risk for penicillin reactions. Although these reagents are easily generated and have been available for >30 years, only benzylpenicilloyl poly-L-lysine (Pre-Pen® [i.e., the major determinant]) and penicillin G have been available commercially. Testing with only the major determinant and penicillin G identifies an estimated 90%–97% of the currently allergic patients. However, because skin testing without the minor determinants would still miss 3%–10% of allergic patients and because serious or fatal reactions can occur among these minor-determinant–positive patients, specialists suggest exercising caution when the full battery of skin-test reagents is not available (Box 1). An additional challenge has occurred with the recent unavailability of Pre-Pen®; however, plans for future availability of this product have been made, as well as a companion minor determinant mixture.

Recommendations

If the full battery of skin-test reagents is available, including the major and minor determinants (see Penicillin Allergy Skin Testing), patients who report a history of penicillin reaction and who are skin-test negative can receive conventional penicillin therapy. Skin-test–positive patients should be desensitized.

If the full battery of skin-test reagents, including the minor determinants, is not available, the patient should be skin tested using benzylpenicilloyl poly-L-lysine (i.e., the major determinant) and penicillin G. Patients who have positive test results should be desensitized. Some specialists suggest that persons who have negative test results should be regarded as probably allergic and should be desensitized. Others suggest that those with negative skin-test results can be test-dosed gradually with oral penicillin in a monitored setting in which treatment for anaphylactic reaction can be provided.

If the major determinant (Pre-Pen®) is not available for skin testing, all patients with a history suggesting IgE mediated reactions (anaphylaxis, angioedema, bronchospasm, or urticaria) to penicillin should be desensitized in a hospital setting. In patients with reactions not likely to be IgE mediated, outpatient oral desensitization or monitored test doses may be considered.

BOX 1. Skin-test for identifying persons at risk for adverse reactions to penicillin*

Major Determinant
- Benzylpenicilloyl poly-L-lysine (Pre-Pen® [Taylor Pharmacal Company, Decatur, Illinois]) (6 x 10^{-5}M).

Minor Determinant Precusors†
- Benzylpenicillin G (10^{-2}M, 3.3 mg/mL, 6,000 units/mL),
- Benzylpenicilloate (10^{-2}M, 3.3 mg/mL), and
- Benzylpenicilloate (or penicilloyl propylamine) (10^{-2}M, 3.3 mg/mL).

Positive Control
- Commercial histamine for epicutaneous skin testing (1 mg/mL).

Negative Control
- Diluent used to dissolve other reagents, usually phenol saline.

* **Adapted from:** Saxon A, Beall GN, Rohr AS, Adelman DC. Immediate hypersensitivity reactions to beta-lactam antibiotics. Ann Intern Med 1987;107:204–15. Reprinted with permission from G.N. Beall and *Annals of Internal Medicine*.

† Aged penicillin is not an adequate source of minor determinants. Penicillin G should be freshly prepared or should come from a fresh-frozen source.

Penicillin Allergy Skin Testing

Patients at high risk for anaphylaxis, including those who 1) have a history of penicillin-related anaphylaxis, asthma, or other diseases that would make anaphylaxis more dangerous or 2) are being treated with beta-adrenergic blocking agents should be tested with 100-fold dilutions of the full-strength skin-test reagents before being tested with full-strength reagents. In these situations, patients should be tested in a monitored setting in which treatment for an anaphylactic reaction is available. If possible, the patient should not have taken antihistamines recently (e.g., chlorpheniramine maleate or terfenadine during the preceding 24 hours, diphenhydramine HCl or hydroxyzine during the preceding 4 days, or astemizole during the preceding 3 weeks).

Procedures

Dilute the antigens either 1) 100-fold for preliminary testing if the patient has had a life-threatening reaction to penicillin or 2) 10-fold if the patient has had another type of immediate, generalized reaction to penicillin within the preceding year.

Epicutaneous (Prick) Tests

Duplicate drops of skin-test reagent are placed on the volar surface of the forearm. The underlying epidermis is pierced with a 26-gauge needle without drawing blood. An epicutaneous test is positive if the average wheal diameter after 15 minutes is 4 mm larger than that of negative controls; otherwise, the test is negative. The histamine controls should be positive to ensure that results are not falsely negative because of the effect of antihistaminic drugs.

Intradermal Test

If epicutaneous tests are negative, duplicate 0.02-mL intradermal injections of negative control and antigen solutions are made into the volar surface of the forearm by using a 26- or 27-gauge needle on a syringe. The diameters of the wheals induced by the injections should be recorded.

An intradermal test is positive if the average wheal diameter 15 minutes after injection is >2 mm larger than the initial wheal size and also is >2 mm larger than the negative controls. Otherwise, the tests are negative.

Desensitization

Patients who have a positive skin test to one of the penicillin determinants can be desensitized (Table 1). This is a straightforward, relatively safe procedure that can be performed orally or IV. Although the two approaches have not been compared, oral desensitization is regarded as safer and easier to perform. Patients should be desensitized in a hospital setting because serious IgE-mediated allergic reactions can occur. Desensitization usually can be completed in approximately 4 hours, after which the first dose of penicillin is administered. After desensitization, patients must be maintained on penicillin continuouslyfor the duration of the course of therapy.

TABLE 1. Oral desensitization protocol for patients with a positive skin test*

Penicillin V suspension dose†	Amount§ (units/mL)	mL	Units	Cumulative dose (units)
1	1,000	0.1	100	100
2	1,000	0.2	200	300
3	1,000	0.4	400	700
4	1,000	0.8	800	1,500
5	1,000	1.6	1,600	3,100
6	1,000	3.2	3,200	6,300
7	1,000	6.4	6,400	12,700
8	10,000	1.2	12,000	24,700
9	10,000	2.4	24,000	48,700
10	10,000	4.8	48,000	96,700
11	80,000	1.0	80,000	176,700
12	80,000	2.0	160,000	336,700
13	80,000	4.0	320,000	656,700
14	80,000	8.0	640,000	1,296,700

Observation period: 30 minutes before parenteral administration of penicillin.

* Reprinted with permission from the *New England Journal of Medicine.* **SOURCE:** Wendel GO Jr, Stark BJ, Jamison RB, Melina RD, Sullivan TJ. Penicillin allergy and desensitization in serious infections during pregnancy. N Engl J Med 1985;312:1229–32.

† Interval between doses: 15 minutes; elapsed time: 3 hours and 45 minutes; and cumulative dose: 1.3 million units.

§ The specific amount of drug was diluted in approximately 30 mL of water and then administered orally.

C. Urethritis

Management of Male Patients Who Have Urethritis

Urethritis, as characterized by urethral inflammation, can result from infectious and noninfectious conditions. Symptoms, if present, include discharge of mucopurulent or purulent material, dysuria, or urethral pruritus. Asymptomatic infections are common. N. gonorrhoeae and C. trachomatis are clinically important infectious causes of urethritis. If clinicbased diagnostic tools (Gram stain microscopy) are not available, patients should be treated for both gonorrhea and chlamydia. Further testing to determine the specific etiology is recommended because both chlamydia and gonorrhea are reportable to state health departments, and a specific diagnosis might enhance partner notification and improve compliance with treatment, especially in exposed partners. Culture, nucleic acid hybridization tests, and nucleic acid amplification tests are available for the detection of both N. gonorrhoeae and C. trachomatis. Culture and hybridization tests require urethral swab specimens, whereas amplification tests can be performed on urine specimens. Because of their higher sensitivity, amplification tests are preferred for the detection of *C. trachomatis*.

Etiology

Several organisms can cause infectious urethritis. The presence of Gram-negative intracellular diplococci (GNID) on urethral smear is indicative of gonorrhea infection, which is frequently accompanied by chlamydial infection. Nongonoccocal urethritis (NGU) is diagnosed when microscopyindicates inflammation without GNID. *C. trachomatis* is a frequent cause of NGU (i.e., 15%–55% of cases); however, the prevalence varies by age group, with lower prevalence among older men. The proportion of NGU cases caused by chlamydia has been declining gradually. Complications of NGU among men infected with C. trachomatis include epididymitis, prostatitis, and Reiter's syndrome. Documentation of chlamydia infection is essential because of the need for partner referral for evaluation and treatment.

The etiology of the majority of cases of nonchlamydial NGU is unknown. Ureaplasma urealyticum and

Mycoplasma genitalium have been implicated as etiologic agents of NGU in some studies; however, detection of these organisms is frequently difficult (109–111). T. vaginalis, HSV, and adenovirus might also cause NGU (112–114). Diagnostic and treatment procedures for these organisms are reserved for situations in which these infections are suspected (e.g., contact with trichomoniasis and genital lesions or severe dysuria and meatitis, which might suggest genital herpes) or when NGU is not responsive to therapy. Enteric bacteria have been identified as an uncommon cause of NGU and might be associated with insertive anal sex.

Confirmed Urethritis

Clinicians should document that urethritis is present. Urethritis can be documented on the basis of any of the following signs or laboratory tests:

- Mucopurulent or purulent discharge.

- Gram stain of urethral secretions demonstrating >5 WBC per oil immersion field. The Gram stain is the preferred rapid diagnostic test for evaluating urethritis. It is highly sensitive and specific for documenting both urethritis and the presence or absence of gonococcal infection. Gonococcal infection is established by documenting the presence of WBC containing GNID, or

- Positive leukocyte esterase test on first-void urine or microscopic examination of first-void urine sediment demonstrating >10 WBC per high power field.

If none of these criteria are present, treatment should be deferred, and the patient should be tested for N. gonorrhoeae and C. trachomatis and followed closely if test results are negative. If the results demonstrate infection with either N. gonorrhoeae or C. trachomatis, the appropriate treatment should be given and sex partners referred for evaluation and treatment.

Empiric treatment of symptoms without documentation of urethritis is recommended only for patients at high risk for infection who are unlikely to return for a follow-up evaluation. Such patients should be treated for gonorrhea and chlamydia. Partners of patients treated empirically should be evaluated and treated.

Management of Patients Who Have Nongonococcal Urethritis

Diagnosis

All patients who have confirmed or suspected urethritis should be tested for gonorrhea and chlamydia. Testing for chlamydia is strongly recommended because of the increase utility and availability of highly sensitive and specific testing methods and because a specific diagnosis might enhance partne notification and improve compliance with treatment, especially in the exposed partner.

Treatment

Treatment should be initiated as soon as possible after diagnosis. Azithromycin and doxycycline are highly effective for chlamydial urethritis; however, infections with M. genitalium may respond better to azithromycin (115). Single-dose regimens have the advantage of improved compliance and directly observed treatment. To improve compliance, ideally the medication should be provided in the clinic or health-care provider's office.

Recommended Regimens

Azithromycin 1 g orally in a single dose

OR

Doxycycline 100 mg orally twice a day for 7 days

Alternative Regimens

Erythromycin base 500 mg orally four times a day for 7

days

OR

Erythromycin ethylsuccinate 800 mg orally four times a day for 7 days

OR

Ofloxacin 300 mg orally twice a day for 7 days

OR

Levofloxacin 500 mg orally once daily for 7 days

Follow-Up for Patients Who Have Urethritis

Patients should be instructed to return for evaluation if symptoms persist or recur after completion of therapy. Symptoms alone, without documentation of signs or laboratory evidence of urethral inflammation, are not a sufficient basis for retreatment. Patients should be instructed to abstain from sexual intercourse until 7 days after therapy is initiated, provided their symptoms have resolved and their sex partners have been adequately treated. Persistence of pain, discomfort, and irritative voiding symptoms beyond 3 months should alert the clinician

to the possibility of chronic prostatitis/chronic pelvic pain syndrome in men. Persons whose conditions have been diagnosed as a new STD should receive testing for other STDs, including syphilis and HIV.

Partner Referral

Persons with NGU should refer for evaluation and treatment all sex partners within the preceding 60 days. Because a specific diagnosis might facilitate partner referral, testing for gonorrhea and chlamydia is encouraged.

Recurrent and Persistent Urethritis

Objective signs of urethritis should be present before initiation of antimicrobial therapy. In persons who have persistent symptoms after treatment without objective signs of urethritis, the value of extending the duration of antimicrobials has not been demonstrated. Persons who have persistent or recurrent urethritis can be re-treated with the initial regimen if they did not comply with the treatment regimen or if they were reexposed to an untreated sex partner. Otherwise, a *T. vaginalis* culture should be performed using an intraurethral swab or a first-void urine specimen (112). Some cases of recurrent urethritis after doxycycline treatment might be caused by tetracycline-resistant U. urealyticum. Urologic examinations usually do not reveal a specific etiology. Approximately 50% of men with chronic nonbacterial prostatitis/chronic pelvic pain syndrome have evidence of urethral inflammation without any identifiable microbial pathogens. If the patient was compliant with the initial regimen and reexposure can be excluded, the following regimen is recommended.

Recommended Regimens

Metronidazole 2 g orally in a single dose

OR

Tinidazole 2 g orally in a single dose

PLUS
Azithromycin 1 g orally in a single dose (if not used for initial episode)

Special Considerations HIV Infection

Gonococcal urethritis, chlamydial urethritis, and nongonococcal, nonchlamydial urethritis might facilitate HIV transmission. Patients who have NGU and also are infected with HIV should receive the same treatment regimen as those who are HIV negative.

D. Gonococcal Infections

Gonococcal Infections in Adolescents and Adults

In the United States, an estimated 600,000 new *N gonorrhoeae* infections occur each year (123). Gonorrhea is the second most commonly reported bacterial STD. The majority of urethral infections caused by *N gonorrhoeae* among men produce symptoms that cause them to seek curative treatment soon enough to prevent serious sequelae, but treatment might not be soon enough to prevent transmission to others. Among women, several infections do not produce recognizable symptoms until complications (eg, PID) have occurred. Both symptomatic and asymptomatic cases of PID can result in tubal scarring that can lead to infertility or ectopic pregnancy.

Because gonococcal infections among women frequently are asymptomatic, an essential component of gonorrhea control in the United States continues to be the screening of women at high risk for STDs. The U.S. Preventive Services Task Force (USPSTF) recommends that clinicians screen all sexually active women, including those who are pregnant, for gonorrhea infection if they are at increased risk. Women aged <25 years are at highest risk for gonorrhea infection. Other risk factors for gonorrhea include a previous gonorrhea infection, other sexually transmitted infections, new or multiple sex partners, inconsistent condom use, commercial sex work, and drug use. The prevalence of gonorrhea infection varies widely among communities and patient populations. The USPSTF does not recommend screening for gonorrhea in men and women who are at low risk for infection (134).

Diagnostic Considerations

Because of high specificity (>99%) and sensitivity (>95%), a Gram stain of a male urethral specimen that demonstrates polymorphonuclear leukocytes with intracellular Gram negative diplococci can be considered diagnostic for infection with *N gonorrhoeae* in symptomatic men. However, because of lower sensitivity, a negative Gram stain should not be considered sufficient for ruling out infection in asymptomatic men. In addition, Gram stain of endocervical specimens, pharyngeal, or rectal specimens also are not sufficient to detect infection and, therefore, are not recommended. Specific testing for *N gonorrhoeae* is recommended because of the increased utility and availability of highly sensitive and specific testing methods and because a specific diagnosis might enhance partner notification.

Specific diagnosis of infection with *N gonorrhoeae* may be performed by testing endocervical, vaginal, male urethral, or urine specimens. Culture and nucleic acid hybridization tests are available for the detection of genitourinary infection with *N gonorrhoeae* (127). Culture and nucleic acid hybridization tests require female endocervical or male urethral swab specimens. NAAT offer the widest range of testing specimen types because they are FDA-cleared for use with endocervical swabs, vaginal swabs, male urethral swabs, and female and male urine. However, product inserts for each NAAT vendor must be carefully examined to assess current indications because FDA-cleared specimen types might vary. In general, culture is the most widely available option for the diagnosis of infection with *N gonorrhoeae* in nongenital sites (eg, rectum and pharynx). Nonculture tests are not FDA cleared for use in the rectum and pharynx. Some NAATs have the potential to cross-react with nongonococcal *Neisseria* and related organisms that are commonly found in the throat. Some noncommercial laboratories have initiated NAAT of rectal and pharyngeal swab specimens after establishing the performance of the test to meet CLIA requirements.

Because nonculture tests cannot provide antimicrobial susceptibility results, in cases of persistent gonococcal infection after treatment, clinicians should perform both culture and antimicrobial susceptibility testing.

All patients tested for gonorrhea should be tested for other STDs, including chlamydia, syphilis, and HIV.

Dual Therapy for Gonococcal and Chlamydial Infections

Patients infected with *N gonorrhoeae* frequently are coinfected with *C trachomatis*; this finding has led to the recommendation that patients treated for gonococcal infection also be treated routinely with a regimen that is effective against uncomplicated genital *C trachomatis* infection (135). Because the majority of gonococci in the United States are susceptible to doxycycline and azithromycin, routine cotreatment might also hinder the development of antimicrobial-resistant *N gonorrhoeae*.

Because of the high sensitivity of NAATs for chlamydial infection, patients with a negative chlamydial NAAT result at the time of treatment for gonorrhea do not need to be treated for chlamydia as well. However, if chlamydial test results are not available or if a non-NAAT was negative for chlamydia, patients should be treated for both gonorrhea and chlamydia.

Quinolone-resistant *N gonorrhoeae* (QRNG)
QRNG continues to spread, making the treatment of gonorrhea with quinolones such as ciprofloxacin inadvisable in many areas and populations (136). Resistance to ciprofloxacin usually indicates resistance to other quinolones as well. QRNG is common in parts of Europe, the Middle East, Asia, and the Pacific. In the United States, QRNG is becoming increasingly common. Previously, CDC had advised that quinolones not be used in California and Hawaii because of the high prevalence of QRNG in these areas (137). The prevalence of QRNG has increased in other areas of the United States, which has resulted in changes in recommended treatment regimens by other states and local areas. QRNG prevalence will continue to increase, and quinolones will eventually not be advisable for the treatment of gonorrhea. The CDC web site (http://www.cdc.gov/std/gisp) or state health departments can provide the most current information. In 2004, of 6,322 isolates collected by CDC's Gonococcal Isolate Surveillance Project (GISP), 6.8% were resistant to ciprofloxacin (minimum inhibitory concentrations [MICs] >1.0 mcg/mL). Excluding isolates from California and Hawaii, 3.6% of isolates were QRNG. QRNG was more common among MSM than among heterosexual men (23.9% versus 2.9%). In 2004, QRNG among heterosexual men outside of California and Hawaii was 1.4% (138).

Quinolones should not be used for the treatment of gonorrhea among MSM (139) or in areas with increased QRNG prevalence in the United States (eg, California and Hawaii) or for infections acquired while traveling abroad. Because oral alternatives to quinolones are limited, quinolones may continue to be used for heterosexual men and women in areas and populations not known to have elevated levels of resistance. Clinicians should obtain information on the sexual behavior and recent travel history (including histories from sex partners) of persons to be treated for gonorrhea to ensure appropriate antibiotic therapy.

Resistance of *N gonorrhoeae* to fluoroquinolones and other antimicrobials is expected to continue to spread; therefore, state and local surveillance for antimicrobial resistance is crucial for guiding local therapy recommendations. GISP, which samples approximately 3% of all U.S. men who have gonococcal infections, is a mainstay of surveillance. However, surveillance by clinicians also is critical. Clinicians who have diagnosed *N gonorrhoeae* infection in a person who was previously treated with a recommended regimen and who probably has not been reexposed should perform culture and susceptibility testing of relevant clinical specimens and report the case to the local health department.

Uncomplicated Gonococcal Infections of the Cervix, Urethra, and Rectum

Recommended Regimens*
Ceftriaxone 125 mg IM in a single dose

OR

Cefixime 400 mg orally in a single dose

OR

Ciprofloxacin 500 mg orally in a single dose*

OR

Ofloxacin 400 mg orally in a single dose*

OR

Levofloxacin 250 mg orally in a single dose*

PLUS

Treatment for Chlamydia if Chlamydia infection is not ruled out.

* Quinolones should not be used for infections in

MSM or in those with a history of recent foreign travel or partners' travel, infections acquired in California or Hawaii, or infections acquired in other areas with increased QRNG prevalence.

Recommended Regimens for MSM or Heterosexuals with a History of Recent Travel*
Ceftriaxone 125 mg IM in a single dose

OR

Cefixime 400 mg orally in a single dose

PLUS

Treatment for Chlamydia if Chlamydia infection is not ruled out.

* Quinolones should not be used for infections in MSM or in those with a history of recent foreign travel or partners' travel, infections acquired in California or Hawaii, or infections acquired in other areas with increased QRNG prevalence.

To maximize compliance with recommended therapies, medications for gonococcal infections should be dispensed on site.

Ceftriaxone in a single injecion of 125 mg provides sustained, high bactericidal levels in the blood. Extensive clinical experience indicates that ceftriaxone is safe and effective for the treatment of uncomplicated gonorrhea at all anatomic sites, curing 98.9% of uncomplicated urogenital and anorectal infections in published clinical trials (140).

Cefixime has an antimicrobial spectrum similar to that of ceftriaxone, but the 400 mg oral dose does not provide as high, nor as sustained, a bactericidal level as that provided by the 125 mg dose of ceftriaxone. In published clinical trials, the 400 mg dose cured 97.4% of uncomplicated urogenital and anorectal gonococcal infections (140). The advantage of cefixime is that it can be administered orally. Updates on the availability of cefixime are available from CDC or state health departments.

Ciprofloxacin is no longer universally effective against *N gonorrhoeae* in the United States (138). However, ciprofloxacin is safe, inexpensive, and can be administered orally. In published clinical trials of uncomplicated urogenital and anorectal infections in the absence of QRNG, a dose of 500 mg of ciprofloxacin provides sustained bactericidal levels with cure rates of 99.8% (140). If QRNG is suspected, ceftriaxone IM or cefixime PO (by mouth) should be used. If neither of these regimens are feasible options, then one of the alternative nonquinolone regimens in this report should be considered.

Similar to ciprofloxacin, ofloxacin is no longer universally effective against *N gonorrhoeae* in the United States. The 400 mg oral dose of ofloxacin has been effective for treatment of uncomplicated urogenital and anorectal infections; in clinical trials, 98.6% of infections were cured (140). Levofloxacin, the active l-isomer of ofloxacin, can be used in place of ofloxacin as a single dose of 250 mg.

Alternative Regimens
Spectinomycin 2 g in a single IM dose

OR

Single-dose cephalosporin regimens

OR

Single-dose quinolone regimens

Several other antimicrobials are active against *N gonorrhoeae*, but none have substantial advantages over the recommended regimens. Spectinomycin is expensive and must be injected; however, it has been effective in published clinical trials, curing 98.2% of uncomplicated urogenital and anorectal gonococcal infections (140). Spectinomycin is useful for the treatment of patients who cannot tolerate cephalosporins and quinolones.

Single-dose cephalosporin regimens (other than ceftriaxone 125 mg IM and cefixime 400 mg orally) that are safe and highly effective against uncomplicated urogenital and anorectal gonococcal infections include ceftizoxime (500 mg, administered IM), cefoxitin (2 g, administered IM with probenecid 1 g orally), and cefotaxime (500 mg, administered IM). None of the injectable cephalosporins offer any advantage over ceftriaxone.

Single-dose quinolone regimens include gatifloxacin 400 mg orally, norfloxacin 800 mg orally, and lomefloxacin 400 mg orally. These regimens appear to be safe and effective for the treatment of uncomplicated gonorrhea, but data regarding their use are limited. None of the regimens appear to offer any advantage over ciprofloxacin, ofloxacin, or levofloxacin, and they are not effective against QRNG.

Some evidence suggests that cefpodoxime and cefuroxime axetil 1 g orally might be additional oral alternatives in the treatment of uncomplicated urogenital gonorrhea; additional information on alternative oral regimens are available at http://www.cdc.gov/std. Cefpodoxime proxetil 200 mg PO is less active against N gonorrhoeae than cefixime and also does not quite meet the minimum efficacy criteria (demonstrated efficacy with lower 95% confidence interval [CI] of ≥95% in summed clinical trials) with cure rates, 96.5% (CI = 94.8%-98.9%) for urogenital and rectal infection; efficacy in treating pharyngeal infection is unsatisfactory, 78.9% (CI = 54.5%-94%). Clinical studies are being conducted to assess whether cefpodoxime 400 mg PO is an acceptable oral alternative. Treatment with cefuroxime axetil 1 g PO does not quite meet the minimum efficacy criteria for urogenital and rectal infection (95.9%; CI = 94.5%-97.3%) and its efficacy in treating pharyngeal infection is unacceptable (56.9%; CI = 42.2%-70.7%).

Azithromycin 2 g orally is effective against uncomplicated gonococcal infection but is expensive and causes gastrointestinal distress and is not recommended for treatment of gonorrhea. Although azithromycin 1 g theoretically meets alternative regimen criteria, it is not recommended because of concerns regarding the possible rapid emergence of antimicrobial resistance. *N gonorrhoeae* in the United States is not adequately susceptible to penicillins, tetracyclines, and macrolides (eg, erythromycin) for these antimicrobials to be recommended.

Uncomplicated Gonococcal Infections of the Pharynx

Gonococcal infections of the pharynx are more difficult to eradicate than infections at urogenital and anorectal sites. Few antimicrobial regimens can reliably cure >90% of gonococcal pharyngeal infections. Although chlamydial coinfection of the pharynx is unusual, coinfection at genital sites sometimes occurs. Therefore, treatment for both gonorrhea and chlamydia is recommended.

Recommended Regimens*
Ceftriaxone 125 mg IM in a single dose

OR

Ciprofloxacin 500 mg orally in a single dose

PLUS

Treatment for Chlamydia if Chlamydia infection is not ruled out.

* Quinolones should not be used for infections in MSM or in those with a history of recent foreign travel or partners' travel, infections acquired in California or Hawaii, or infections acquired in other areas with increased QRNG prevalence.

Recommended Regimens for MSM or Heterosexuals with a History of Recent Travel
Ceftriaxone 125 mg IM in a single dose

PLUS

Treatment for Chlamydia if Chlamydia infection is not ruled out.

Follow-Up
Patients who have uncomplicated gonorrhea and who are treated with any of the recommended or alternative regimens do not need a test of cure. Patients who have symptoms that persist after treatment should be evaluated by culture for *N gonorrhoeae,* and any gonococci isolated should be tested for antimicrobial susceptibility. Persistent urethritis, cervicitis, or proctitis also might be caused by *C trachomatis* or other organisms.

A high prevalence of *N gonorrhoeae* infection is observed in patients who have had gonorrhea in the preceding several months (141,142). The majority of infections identified after treatment with one of the recommended regimens result from reinfection rather than treatment failure, indicating a need for improved patient education and referral of sex partners. Clinicians should consider advising all patients with gonorrhea to be retested 3 months after treatment. If patients do not seek medical care for retesting in 3 months, providers are encouraged to test these patients whenever they next seek medical care within the following 12 months, regardless of whether the patient believes that their sex partners were treated. Retesting is distinct from test of cure to detect therapeutic failure, which is not recommended.

Management of Sex Partners

Effective clinical management of patients with treatable STDs requires treatment of the patients' recent sex partners to prevent reinfection and curtail further transmission. Patients should be instructed to refer their sex partners for evaluation and treatment. Sex partners of patients with *N gonorrhoeae* infection whose last sexual contact with the patient was within 60 days before onset of symptom or diagnosis of infection in the patient should be evaluated and treated for *N gonorrhoeae* and *C trachomatis* infections. If a patient's last sexual intercourse was >60 days before onset of symptoms or diagnosis, the patient's most recent sex partner should be treated. Patients should be instructed to avoid sexual intercourse until therapy is completed and until they and their sex partners no longer have symptoms.

For patients with gonorrhea whose partners' treatment cannot be ensured or is unlikely, delivery of antibiotic therapy (ie, either a prescription or medication) by heterosexual male or female patients to their partners is an option (see Partner Management). Use of this approach (25,27) should always be accompanied by efforts to educate partners about symptoms and to encourage partners to seek clinical evaluation. Male patients must inform female partners of their infection and be given accompanying materials about the importance of seeking medical evaluation for PID (especially if symptomatic). Possible undertreatment of PID in female partners and possible missed opportunities to diagnose other STDs are of concern and have not been evaluated in comparisons with patient-delivered therapy and partner referral. Patient-delivered therapy for patients with gonorrhea should routinely include treatment for chlamydia. This approach should not be considered a routine partner management strategy in MSM because of the high risk of coexisting undiagnosed STDs or HIV infection.

Special Considerations

Allergy, Intolerance, and Adverse Reactions Persons who cannot tolerate cephalosporins or quinolones should be treated with spectinomycin. Because spectinomycin is unreliable (52% effective) against pharyngeal infections, patients who have suspected or known pharyngeal infection should have a pharyngeal culture 3–5 days after treatment to verify eradication of infection.

Pregnancy

Pregnant women should not be treated with quinolones or tetracyclines. Those infected with N. gonorrhoeae should betreated with a recommended or alternate cephalosporin. Women who cannot tolerate a cephalosporin should be administered a single 2-g dose of spectinomycin IM. Either-azithromycin or amoxicillin is recommended for treatment of presumptive or diagnosed C. trachomatis infection during pregnancy (see Chlamydial Infections).

Administration of Quinolones to Adolescents

Fluoroquinolones have not been recommended for persons aged <18 years because studies have indicated that they can damage articular cartilage in some young animals. However, no joint damage attributable to quinolone therapy has been observed in children treated with prolonged ciprofloxacin regimens (143). Therefore, children who weigh >45 kg can be treated with any regimen recommended for adults (See Gonococcal Infections).

HIV Infection

Patients who have gonococcal infection and also are infected with HIV should receive the same treatment regimen as those who are HIV negative.

Gonococcal Conjunctivitis

In the only published study of the treatment of gonococcal conjunctivitis among U.S. adults, all 12 study participants responded to a single 1-g IM injection of ceftriaxone (144). The following recommendation reflects the opinions of consultants knowledgeable in the field of STDs.

Recommended Regimen

Ceftriaxone 1 g IM in a single dose

Consider lavage of the infected eye with saline solution once.

Management of Sex Partners

Patients should be instructed to refer their sex partners for evaluation and treatment (see Gonococcal Infections, Management of Sex Partners).

Disseminated Gonococcal Infection (DGI)

DGI results from gonococcal bacteremia. DGI frequently results in petechial or pustular acral skin lesions, asymmetrical arthralgia, tenosynovitis, or septic arthritis. The infection is complicated occasionally by perihepatitis and rarely by endocarditis or meningitis. Some strains of N. gonorrhoeae thatcause DGI may cause minimal genital inflammation. No studies on the treatment of DGI among adults have been published since publication of the last CDC STD treatment guidelines publication. DGI treatment recommendations reflect the opinions of consultants. No treatment failures have been reported with the recommended regimens.

Treatment

Hospitalization is recommended for initial therapy, especially for patients who might not comply with treatment, for those in whom diagnosis is uncertain, and for those who have purulent synovial effusions or other complications. Patients should be examined for clinical evidence of endocarditis and meningitis. Patients treated for DGI should be treated presumptively for concurrent C. trachomatis infection, unless appropriate testing excludes this infection.

Recommended Regimen

Ceftriaxone 1 g IM or IV every 24 hours

Alternative Regimens

Cefotaxime 1 g IV every 8 hours

OR

Ceftizoxime 1 g IV every 8 hours

OR

Ciprofloxacin 400 mg IV every 12 hours*

OR

Ofloxacin 400 mg IV every 12 hours*

OR

Levofloxacin 250 mg IV daily*

OR

Spectinomycin 2 g IM every 12 hours

*Quinolones should not be used for infections in MSM or in those with a history of recent foreign travel or partners' travel, infections acquired in California or Hawaii, or infections acquired in other areas with increased QRNG prevalence.

All of the preceding regimens should be continued for 24–48 hours after improvement begins, at which time therapy may be switched to one of the following regimens to complete at least 1 week of antimicrobial therapy.

E. Epididymitis

Acute epididymitis is a clinical syndrome consisting of pain, swelling, and inflammation of the epididymis of <6 weeks. Chronic epididymitis is characterized by a 3-month or longer history of symptoms of discomfort and/or pain in the scrotum, testicle, or epididymis that is localized on clinical examination. Chronic epididymitis has been subcategorized into inflammatory chronic epididymitis, obstructive chronic epididymitis, and chronic epididymalgia (192).

Among sexually active men aged <35 years, acute epididymitis is most frequently caused by *C trachomatis* or *N gonorrhoeae*. Acute epididymitis caused by sexually transmitted enteric organisms (eg, *Escherichia coli*) also occurs among men who are the insertive partner during anal intercourse. Sexually transmitted acute epididymitis usually is accompanied by urethritis, which frequently is asymptomatic and is usually never accompanied by bacteriuria. In men aged >35 years, sexually transmitted epididymitis is uncommon. However, bacteriuria secondary to obstructive urinary disease is relatively common. In this group, nonsexually transmitted epididymitis is associated with urinary-tract instrumentation or surgery, systemic disease, or immunosuppression.

Although the majority of patients can be treated on an outpatient basis, hospitalization should be considered when severe pain suggests other diagnoses (eg, torsion, testicular infarction, or abscess) or when patients are febrile or might be noncompliant with an antimicrobial regimen.

Diagnostic Considerations

Men who have acute epididymitis typically have unilateral testicular pain and tenderness; hydrocele and palpable swelling of the epididymis usually are present. Although the inflammation and swelling usually begin in the tail of the epididymis, they can spread to involve the rest of the epididymis and testicle. The spermatic cord is usually tender and swollen. Testicular torsion, a surgical emergency, should be considered in all cases, but it occurs more frequently among adolescents and in men without evidence of inflammation or infection. Emergency testing for torsion might be indicated when the onset of pain is sudden, pain is severe, or the test results available during the initial examination do not support a diagnosis of urethritis or urinary-tract infection. If the diagnosis is questionable, a specialist should be consulted immediately because testicular viability might be compromised. Radionuclide scanning of the scrotum is the most accurate radiologic method of diagnosis, although it is not routinely available. Color duplex doppler ultrasonography has a sensitivity of 70% and a specificity of 88% in diagnosing acute epididymitis.

The evaluation of men for epididymitis should include one of the following:

- Gram stain of urethral secretions demonstrating >5 WBC per oil immersion field. The Gram stain is the preferred rapid diagnostic test for evaluating urethritis. It is highly sensitive and specific for documenting both urethritis and the presence or absence of gonococcal infection. Gonococcal infection is established by documenting the presence of WBC containing intracellular Gram-negative diplococci on urethral Gram stain.

- Positive leukocyte esterase test on first-void urine or microscopic examination of first-void urine sediment demonstrating ≥10 WBC per high power field.

Culture, nucleic acid hybridization tests, and nucleic acid amplification tests are available for the detection of both *N gonorrhoeae* and *C trachomatis*. Culture and nucleic acid hybridization tests require urethral swab specimens, whereas amplification tests can be performed on urine specimens. Because of their higher sensitivity, amplification tests are preferred for the detection of *C trachomatis*. Depending on the risk, patients whose conditions have been diagnosed as a new STD should receive testing for other STDs.

Treatment

Empiric therapy is indicated before laboratory test results are available. The goals of treatment of acute epididymitis caused by *C trachomatis* or *N gonorrhoeae* are: 1) microbiologic cure of infection, 2) improvement of signs and symptoms, 3) prevention of transmission to others, and 4) a decrease in potential complications (eg, infertility or chronic pain). As an adjunct to therapy, bed rest, scrotal elevation, and analgesics are recommended until fever and local inflammation have subsided.

Recommended Regimens
For acute epididymitis most likely caused by gonococcal or chlamydial infection:

Ceftriaxone 250 mg IM in a single dose

PLUS

Doxycycline 100 mg orally twice a day for 10 days

For acute epididymitis most likely caused by enteric organisms or for patients allergic to cephalosporins and/or tetracyclines:

Ofloxacin 300 mg orally twice a day for 10 days

OR

Levofloxacin 500 mg orally once daily for 10 days

Follow-Up
Failure to improve within 3 days of the initiation of treatment requires reevaluation of both the diagnosis and therapy. Swelling and tenderness that persist after completion of antimicrobial therapy should be evaluated comprehensively. The differential diagnosis includes tumor, abscess, infarction, testicular-cancer, TB, and fungal epididymitis.

Management of Sex Partners
Patients who have acute epididymitis, confirmed or suspected to be caused by *N gonorrhoeae* or *C trachomatis,* should be instructed to refer sex partners for evaluation and treatment if their contact with the index patient was within the 60 days preceding onset of the patient's symptoms.

Patients should be instructed to avoid sexual intercourse until they and their sex partners are cured (ie, until therapy is completed and patient and partners no longer have symptoms).

Special Considerations
HIV Infection
Patients who have uncomplicated acute epididymitis and also are infected with HIV should receive the same treatment regimen as those who are HIV negative. Fungi and mycobacteria, however, are more likely to cause acute epididymitis in immunosuppressed patients than in immunocompetent patients.

F. Genital Warts

HPV types 6 or 11 are commonly found before, or at the time of, detection of genital warts; however, the use of HPV testing for genital wart diagnosis is not recommended.

Genital warts are usually flat, papular, or pedunculated growths on the genital mucosa. Diagnosis of genital warts is made by visual inspection and may be confirmed by biopsy, although biopsy is needed only under certain circumstances (eg, if the diagnosis is uncertain; the lesions do not respond to standard therapy; the disease worsens during therapy; the patient is immunocompromised; or warts are pigmented, indurated, fixed, bleeding, or ulcerated). No data support the use of HPV nucleic acid tests in the routine diagnosis or management of visible genital warts.

The application of 3%-5% acetic acid usually turns HPV-infected genital mucosal tissue to a whitish color. However, acetic acid application is not a specific test for HPV infection, and the specificity and sensitivity of this procedure for screening have not been defined. Therefore, the routine use of this procedure for screening to detect HPV infection is not recommended. However, some clinicians, who are experienced in the management of genital warts, have determined that this test is useful for identifying flat genital warts.

In addition to the external genitalia (ie, penis, vulva, scrotum, perineum, and perianal skin), genital warts can occur on the uterine cervix and in the vagina, urethra, anus, and mouth. Intra-anal warts are observed predominantly in patients who have had receptive anal intercourse; these warts are distinct from perianal warts, which can occur in men and women who do not have a history of anal sex. In addition to the genital area, HPV types 6 and 11 have been associated with conjunctival, nasal, oral, and laryngeal warts. Genital warts are usually asymptomatic, but depending on the size and anatomic location, genital warts can be painful, friable, or pruritic.

HPV types 16, 18, 31, 33, and 35 are found occasionally in visible genital warts and have been associated with external genital (ie, vulvar, penile, and anal) squamous intraepithelial neoplasia (ie, squamous cell carcinoma in situ, bowenoid papulosis, Erythroplasia of Queyrat, or Bowen's disease of the genitalia). These HPV types also have been associated with vaginal, anal, and CIN and anogenital and some head and neck squamous cell carcinomas. Patients who have visible genital warts are frequently infected simultaneously with multiple HPV types.

Treatment

The primary goal of treating visible genital warts is the removal of the warts. In the majority of patients, treatment can induce wart-free periods. If left untreated, visible genital warts might resolve on their own, remain unchanged, or increase in size or number. Treatment possibly reduces, but does not eliminate, HPV infection. Existing data indicate that currently available therapies for genital warts might reduce, but probably do not eradicate, HPV infectivity. Whether the reduction in HPV viral DNA, resulting from treatment, impacts future transmission remains unclear. No evidence indicates that the presence of genital warts or their treatment is associated with the development of cervical cancer.

Regimens

Treatment of genital warts should be guided by the preference of the patient, the available resources, and the experience of the health care provider. No definitive evidence suggests that any of the available treatments are superior to any other and no single treatment is ideal for all patients or all warts. The use of locally developed and monitored treatment algorithms has been associated with improved clinical outcomes and should be encouraged. Because of uncertainty regarding the effect of treatment on future transmission of HPV and the possibility of spontaneous resolution, an acceptable alternative for some persons is to forego treatment and wait for spontaneous resolution.

The majority of patients have <10 genital warts, with a total wart area of 0.5-1.0 cm2. These warts respond to various treatment modalities. Factors that might influence selection of treatment include wart size, wart number, anatomic site of wart, wart morphology, patient preference, cost of treatment, convenience, adverse effects, and provider experience. Factors that might affect response to therapy include the presence of immunosuppression and compliance with therapy. The majority of patients require a course of therapy rather than a single treatment. In general, warts located on moist surfaces or in intertriginous areas respond better to topical treatment than do warts on drier surfaces.

The treatment modality should be changed if a patient has not improved substantially. The majority of genital warts respond within 3 months of therapy. The response to treatment and its side effects should be evaluated throughout the course of therapy.

Complications occur rarely if treatments for warts are employed properly. Patients should be warned that persistent hypopigmentation or hyperpigmentation occurs commonly with ablative modalities. Depressed or hypertrophic scars are uncommon but can occur, especially if the patient has had insufficient time to heal between treatments. Rarely, treatment can result in disabling chronic pain syndromes (eg,vulvodynia or analdynia, and hyperesthesia of the treatment site) or, in the case of rectal warts, painful defecation or fistulas. A limited number of case reports of severe systemic effects from podophyllin resin and interferon have been documented.

Treatment regimens are classified into patient-applied and provider-applied modalities. Patient-applied modalities are preferred by some patients because they can be administered in the privacy of the patient's home. To use patient-applied modalities effectively, compliance with the treatment regimen is important along with the ability to identify and reach all genital warts.

Recommended Regimens for External Genital Warts

Patient-Applied:

Podofilox 0.5% solution or gel. Patients should apply podofilox solution with a cotton swab, or podofilox gel with a finger, to visible genital warts twice a day for 3 days, followed by 4 days of no therapy. This cycle may be repeated, as necessary, for up to four cycles. The total wart area treated should not exceed 10 cm^2, and the total volume of podofilox should be limited to 0.5 mL per day. If possible, the health care provider should apply the initial treatment to demonstrate the proper application technique and identify which warts should be treated. The safety of podofilox during pregnancy has not been established.

OR

Imiquimod 5% cream. Patients should apply imiquimod cream once daily at bedtime, three times a week for up to 16 weeks. The treatment area should be washed with soap and water 6-10 hours after the application. The safety of imiquimod during pregnancy has not been established.

Provider-Administered:
Cryotherapy with liquid nitrogen or cryoprobe. Repeat applications every 1-2 weeks.

OR

Podophyllin resin 10%-25% in a compound tincture of benzoin. A small amount should be applied to each wart and allowed to air dry. The treatment can be repeated weekly, if necessary. To avoid the possibility of complications associated with systemic absorption and toxicity, two important guidelines should be followed: 1) application should be limited to <0.5 mL of podophyllinor an area of <10 cm^2 of warts per session; and 2) no open lesions or wounds should exist in the area to which treatment is administered. Some specialists suggest that the preparation should be thoroughly washed off 1-4 hours after application to reduce local irritation. The safety of podophyllin during pregnancy has not been established.

OR

***Trichloroacetic acid* (TCA) or *Bichloroacetic acid* (BCA) 80%-90%.** A small amount should be applied only to the warts and allowed to dry, at which time a white "frosting" develops. If an excess amount of acid is applied, the treated area should be powdered with talc, sodium bicarbonate (ie, baking soda), or liquid soap preparations to remove unreacted acid. This treatment can be repeated weekly, if necessary.

OR

Surgical removal either by tangential scissor excision, tangential shave excision, curettage, or electrosurgery

Alternative Regimens
Intralesional interferon

OR

Laser surgery

Podofilox 0.5% solution or gel, an antimitotic drug that destroys warts, is relatively inexpensive, easy to use, safe, and self-applied by patients. The majority of patients experience mild-to-moderate pain or local irritation after treatment. Imiquimod is a topically active immune enhancer that stimulates production of interferon and other cytokines. Local inflammatory reactions are common with the use of imiquimod; these reactions include redness and irritation and are usually mild to moderate. Traditionally, follow-up visits are not required for patients using self-administered therapy. However, follow-up might be useful several weeks into therapy to determine the appropriateness of medication use and the response to treatment.

Cryotherapy destroys warts by thermal-induced cytolysis. Health care providers must be trained on the proper use of this therapy because over- and undertreatment might result in complications or low efficacy. Pain after application of the liquid nitrogen, followed by necrosis and sometimes blistering, is common. Local anesthesia (topical or injected) might facilitate therapy if warts are present in many areas or if the area of warts is large.

Podophyllin resin, which contains several compounds, including antimitotic podophyllin lignans, is another treatment option. The resin is most frequently compounded at 10%-25% in a tincture of benzoin. However, podophyllin resin preparations differ in the concentration of active components and contaminants. The shelf life and stability of podophyllin preparations are unknown. A thin layer of ophyllin resin must be applied to the warts and allowed to air dry before the treated area comes into contact with clothing; overapplication or failure to air dry can result in local irritation caused by spread of the compound to adjacent areas.

Both TCA and BCA are caustic agents that destroy warts by chemical coagulation of proteins. Although these preparations are widely used, they have not been investigated thoroughly. TCA solutions have a low viscosity comparable with that of water and can spread rapidly if applied excessively; therefore, they can damage adjacent tissues. Both TCA and BCA should be applied sparingly and allowed to dry before the patient sits or stands. If pain is intense, the acid can be neutralized with soap or sodium bicarbonate.

Surgical therapy has the advantage of usually eliminating warts at a single visit. However, such therapy requires substantial clinical training, additional equipment, and a longer office visit. After local anesthesia is applied, the visible genital warts can be physically destroyed by electrocautery, in which case no additional hemostasis is required. Care must be taken to control the depth of electrocautery to prevent scarring. Alternatively, the warts can be removed either by tangential excision with a pair of fine scissors or a scalpel or by curettage. Because the majority of warts are exophytic, this procedure can be accomplished with a resulting wound that only extends into the upper dermis. Hemostasis can be achieved with an electrocautery unit or a chemical styptic (eg, an aluminum chloride solution). Suturing is neither required nor indicated in the majority of cases if surgical removal is performed properly. Surgical therapy is most beneficial for patients who have a large number or area of genital warts. Carbon dioxide laser and surgery might be useful in the management of extensive warts or intraurethral warts, particularly for those patients who have not responded to other treatments.

Interferons, both natural or recombinant, have been used for the treatment of genital warts. They have been administered systemically (ie, subcutaneously at a distant site or IM) and intralesionally (ie, injected into the warts). Systemic interferon is not effective. The efficacy and recurrence rates of intralesional interferon are comparable to other treatment modalities. Administration of intralesional interferon is associated with stinging, burning, and pain at the injection site. Interferon is probably effective because of its antiviral and/or immunostimulating effects. Interferon therapy is not recommended as a primary modality because of inconvenient routes of administration, frequent office visits, and the association between its use and a high frequency of systemic adverse effects.

Because of the shortcomings associated with all available treatments, some clinics employ combination therapy (ie, the simultaneous use of two or more modalities on the same wart at the same time). No data support the use of more than one therapy at a time to improve efficacy of treatment, and some specialists believe that combining modalities might increase complications.

Recommended Regimens for Cervical Warts

For women who have exophytic cervical warts, high-grade SIL must be excluded before treatment is initiated. Management of exophytic cervical warts should include consultation with a specialist.

Recommended Regimens for Vaginal Warts

Cryotherapy with liquid nitrogen. The use of a cryoprobe in the vagina is not recommended because of the risk for vaginal perforation and fistula formation.

OR

TCA or BCA 80%-90% applied to warts. A small amount should be applied only to warts and allowed to dry, at which time a white "frosting" develops. If an excess amount of acid is applied, the treated area should be powdered with talc, sodium bicarbonate, or liquid soap preparations to remove unreacted acid. This treatment can be repeated weekly, if necessary.

Recommended Regimens for Urethral Meatus Warts

Cryotherapy with liquid nitrogen

OR

Podophyllin 10%-25% in compound tincture of benzoin. The treatment area must be dry before contact with normal mucosa. This treatment can be repeated weekly, if necessary. The safety of podophyllin during pregnancy has not been established.

Although data evaluating the use of podofilox and imiquimod for the treatment of distal meatal warts are limited, some specialists recommend their use in some patients.

Recommended Regimens for Anal Warts

Cryotherapy with liquid nitrogen

OR

TCA or BCA 80%-90% applied to warts. A small amount should be applied only to warts and allowed to dry, at which time a white "frosting" develops. If an excess amount of acid is applied, the treated area should be powdered with talc, sodium bicarbonate, or liquid soap preparations to remove unreacted acid.

This treatment can be repeated weekly, if necessary.

OR

Surgical removal

Warts on the rectal mucosa should be managed in consultation with a specialist. Many persons with warts on the anal mucosa also have warts on the rectal mucosa, so persons with anal warts can benefit from an inspection of the rectal mucosa by digital examination or anoscopy.

Counseling

Genital HPV Infection Education and counseling are vital aspects of managing patients with genital warts. Patients can be educated through patient education materials, including pamphlets, hotlines, and web sites (http://www.ashastd.org or http://www.cdc.gov/std/hpv).

Attempts should be made to convey the following key messages:

- Genital HPV infection is common among sexually active adults. The majority of sexually active adults will have it at some point in their lives, although the majority of them will never know because the infection usually has no symptoms and clears on its own.

- Genital HPV infection is usually sexually transmitted. The incubation period (ie, the interval between initial exposure and established infection or disease) is variable, and determining the timing and source of infection is frequently difficult. Within ongoing sexual relationships, sex partners usually are infected by the time of the patient's diagnosis, although they might have no symptoms or signs of infection.

- No recommended uses of the HPV test to diagnose HPV infection in sex partners have been established. HPV infection is commonly transmitted to partners but usually goes away on its own.

Genital Warts

- Genital warts are caused by specific types of HPV infection. The types that cause genital warts are different from the types that cause cervical and other anogenital cancers.

- Persons can possibly have infection with the types of HPV that cause genital warts but never develop symptoms. Why some persons with genital HPV infection develop warts and others do not is unclear. Immunity probably plays a key role.

- The natural history of genital warts is usually benign, but recurrence of genital warts within the first several months after treatment is common. Treatment for genital warts can reduce HPV infection, but whether the treatment results in a reduction in risk for transmission of HPV to sex partners is unclear. The duration of infectivity after wart treatment is unknown.

- Condoms might reduce the risk for HPV-associated diseases (eg, genital warts and cervical cancer). Consistent condom use also may reduce the risk for genital HPV (18). HPV infection can occur in areas that are not covered or protected by a condom (eg, scrotum, vulva, or perianus).

- The presence of genital warts is not an indication for HPV testing, a change in the frequency of Pap tests, or cervical colposcopy.

- HPV testing is not indicated for partners of persons with genital warts.

Follow-Up

After visible genital warts have cleared, a follow-up evaluation might be helpful. Patients should be cautioned to watch for recurrences, which occur most frequently during the first 3 months. External genital warts can be difficult to identify, so it might be useful for patients to have a follow-up evaluation 3 months after treatment. Earlier follow-up visits also might be useful for some patients to document the absence of warts, to monitor for or treat complications of therapy, and to provide an additional opportunity for patient education and counseling. Women should be counseled to undergo regular Pap screening as recommended for women without genital warts.

Management of Sex Partners

Examination of sex partners is not necessary for the management of genital warts because no data indicate that reinfection plays a role in recurrences. In addition, providing treatment for genital warts solely for the purpose of preventing future transmission cannot be recommended because the value of treatment in reducing infectivity is unknown. However, sex partners of patients who have genital warts might benefit from counseling and examination to assess the presence of genital warts and other STDs. The counseling of sex partners provides an opportunity for these partners to: 1) learn that HPV infection is common and probably shared between partners, and 2) receive STD evaluation and screening and Pap screening if they are female. Female sex partners of patients who have genital warts should be reminded that cytologic screening for cervical cancer is recommended for all sexually active women.

Special Considerations

Pregnancy

Imiquimod, podophyllin, and podofilox should not be used during pregnancy. However, because genital warts can proliferate and become friable during pregnancy, many specialists advocate their removal during pregnancy. HPV types 6 and 11 can cause respiratory papillomatosis in infants and children. The route of transmission (ie, transplacental, perinatal, or postnatal) is not completely understood. Whether cesarean section prevents respiratory papillomatosis in infants and children is unclear; therefore, cesarean delivery should not be performed solely to prevent transmission of HPV infection to the newborn. Cesarean delivery might be indicated for women with genital warts if the pelvic outlet is obstructed or if vaginal delivery would result in excessive bleeding. Pregnant women with genital warts should be counseled concerning the low risk for warts on the larynx (recurrent respiratory papillomatosis) in their infants or children (193). No controlled studies have suggested that cesarean section prevents this condition.

HIV Infection

No data suggest that treatment modalities for external genital warts should be different in the setting of HIV-infection. However, persons who are immunosuppressed because of HIV or other reasons might have larger or more numerous warts, might not respond as well as immunocompetent persons to therapy for genital warts, and might have more frequent recurrences after treatment (194,195). Squamous cell carcinomas arising in or resembling genital warts might occur more frequently among immunosuppressed persons, therefore, requiring biopsy for confirmation of diagnosis. Because of the increased incidence of anal cancer in HIV-infected homosexual men, screening for anal SIL by cytology in this population is recommended by some specialists. However, evidence is limited concerning the natural history of anal intraepithelial neoplasias, the reliability of screening methods, the safety and response to treatments, and the programmatic considerations that would support this screening approach. Until additional data are generated on screening for anal SIL, this screening approach cannot be recommended.

Squamous Cell Carcinoma in Situ

Patients in whom squamous cell carcinoma in situ of the genitalia is diagnosed should be referred to a specialist for treatment. Ablative modalities usually are effective, but careful follow-up is essential. The risk for these lesions leading to invasive squamous cell carcinoma of the external genitalia in immunocompetent patients is unknown but is probably low. Female partners of male patients who have squamous cell carcinoma in situ are at high risk for cervical abnormalities.

Chapter 23C: Urinary Tract Infections

Daniel A. Shoskes MD

Contents

1. Review of Antibiotics

Allergy, hypersensitivity, rash, GI upset, yeast vaginitis and pseudomembranous colitis can occur with any antibiotic, so the adverse reactions will list other issues that are more specific to each antibiotic

A. Ampicillin or amoxicillin (amoxicillin is less likely to cause diarrhea)

1. Mechanism of action: inhibit bacterial cell wall synthesis. Bacteriocidal

2. Usual spectrum: Strep, *Enterococcus*, *Proteus mirabilis*, *E coli*

3. Adverse reactions and disadvantages:
   a. More likely to disturb the normal vaginal flora than most other antibiotics; increases the risks of cystitis[2] and yeast vaginitis
   b. May cause acute interstitial nephritis
   c. Many GU pathogens such as *E coli* now have high resistance rates (up to 50% in some areas)[3]

B. Ampicillin/clavulanate: clavulanate inhibits beta-lactamase, so it expands the spectrum, but not a first-line treatment due to expense and GI side effects

C. Extended-spectrum penicillins

1. Usually combined with beta-lactamase inhibitors (eg, piperacillin/tazobactam or ticarcillin/clavulanate). Bacteriocidal

2. Spectrum varies; each drug should be considered individually

3. Advantages: broader spectrum for use in nosocomial infections or empiric sepsis treatment while awaiting culture results

4. Adverse reactions and disadvantages:
   a. Same as for ampicillin/amoxicillin
   b. Ticarcillin is given as the sodium salt (100 mg Na per gram Timentin; usual dose 3 g q 4-6 hours = 1200 to 1800 mg Na per day), so avoid in patients who need Na restriction[4]

D. Cephalosporins

1. Mechanism of action: inhibit bacterial cell wall synthesis. Bacteriocidal

2. Spectrum depends on the cephalosporin generation. Even within a generation, not all are the same so look up individually. None cover *Enterococcus* or MRSA. In general:
   a. First generation covers *Streptococcus, Staphylococcus* except MRSA, *E coli, Proteus mirabilis, Klebsiella*
   b. Second generation covers *Streptococcus, E coli, Proteus mirabilis, Klebsiella,* influenzae, some anaerobes
   c. Third generation covers *Streptococcus*, most Gram-negative rods including *Pseudomonas*

3. Adverse reactions and disadvantages:
   a. Similar to penicillins (including yeast vaginitis)
   b. Penicillin-allergic patients have about a 10% cross-reactivity rate; do not use for patients with immediate hypersensitivity to penicillin

E. Trimethoprim/sulfamethoxazole (TMP/SMX)

1. Mechanism of action: inhibit bacterial folate metabolism. Bacteriocidal

2. Usual spectrum: *Streptococcus, Staphylococcus*, most Gram-negative rods except *Pseudomonas*

3. Advantages: inexpensive, minimal adverse effects on fecal flora (good for prophylaxis)

4. Adverse reactions and disadvantages:
   a. Rapidly increasing resistance in *E coli* (20% in some areas)[2,3,5]
   b. Can interact with warfarin and elevate PT.
   c. Folate antagonism affects fetal development and can cause hematologic problems, especially in patients with AIDS or G6PD deficiency

5. Most (but not all) allergies are due to the sulfa component, and TMP alone can be as effective as the combination

F. Nitrofurantoin

1. Mechanism of action: binds to several bacterial proteins and inhibits several bacterial enzyme systems. These multiple actions make it harder for bacteria to develop resistance. Bacteriostatic

2. Usual spectrum
   a. The 2 organisms most reliably susceptible are *E coli* and *Staphylococcus saprophyticus*. Some strains of *Streptococcus* and *Klebsiella* also may be susceptible. Interestingly, most strains of *Enterococcus* including VRE are susceptible[6]
   b. *Proteus* and *Pseudomonas* are always resistant[1]

3. Advantages:
   a. Low impact on fecal and vaginal flora
   b. Very low incidence of resistance
   c. Less likely than other antibiotics to increase the anticoagulant effect of warfarin

4. Adverse reactions and disadvantages:
   a. Neurotoxicity (avoid in neurologic diseases, vitamin B deficiency, debilitation, anemia, diabetes mellitus, electrolyte imbalance)
   b. Pulmonary fibrosis or interstitial pneumonitis
   c. High levels in urine but not tissues, so do not use for tissue infections (eg, pyelonephritis, prostatitis)
   d. Do not use in patients with low creatinine clearance; will not get into urine, and increased risk of neurotoxicity
   e. Can cause hemolysis in patients with G6PD deficiency
   f. Recommended for 7 days in uncomplicated female cystitis (unlike most other antibiotics, which are for only 3 days)[1,3]

G. Tetracyclines

1. Mechanism of action: inhibit protein synthesis at ribosomal level. Bacteriostatic

2. Usual spectrum:
   a. Wide spectrum, but high incidence of resistance for the usual organisms that cause UTIs. Therefore, not good for empiric treatment, but OK if sensitivity is demonstrated
   b. Use with VRE and MRSA[6]
      1) Doxycycline can be effective against VRE (paradoxically, it is not effective against vancomycin-sensitive *Enterococcus*)
      2) Doxycycline is effective against community-acquired MRSA but not nosocomial MRSA
      3) Minocycline is effective against both community-acquired MRSA and nosocomial MRSA
   c. Good for several types of STDs. First-line drug for granuloma inguinale and lymphogranuloma venereum. Also good for *Chlamydia, Mycoplasma, Ureaplasma,* some strains of *N gonorrhoeae*
   d. Can be an alternative (with close follow-up) for primary and secondary syphilis in patients allergic to penicillin

3. Advantage: good penetration into the prostate

4. Adverse reactions and disadvantages:
   a. Can cause tooth discoloration and inhibit bone growth if used in pregnant women or young children
   b. Photosensitivity
   c. Higher incidence of vaginal yeast infections
   d. Can cause a rise in BUN without a concomitant rise in creatinine, so avoid in patients with high BUN

5. Doxycycline is unique because it is excreted mostly in the feces so does not need dose adjustment in renal failure

6. New tetracycline: tigecycline (Tygacil®)[7]
   a. A glycylcycline, it is a variant of minocycline
   b. Evades 2 most common bacterial resistance mechanisms to tetracyclines: ribosomal protection and efflux
   c. Broad spectrum including MRSA and VRE
   d. Must be given IV

e. 2007 indications: complicated skin and skin-structure infections, or complicated intra-abdominal infections, caused by susceptible strains of bacteria

H. Fluoroquinolones

1. Mechanism of action: inhibit bacterial DNA gyrase. Bacteriocidal

2. Usual spectrum: Most Gram-negative rods including pseudomonas, some strains of *N gonorrhoeae*, coverage for *Streptococcus* is not always reliable

3. Advantages: good tissue penetration, good oral bioavailability, low incidence of resistance (so far)

4. Adverse reactions and disadvantages:
   a. Affects cartilage development; avoid in children and pregnant women
   b. Can cause tendonitis and tendon rupture
   c. Lower seizure threshold; avoid in patients with epilepsy[1]
   d. Drug interactions
   e. False-positive urine opiate test

5. Specific problems with gatifloxacin[8]
   a. Life-threatening hypo- or hyperglycemia
   b. Can prolong the Q-T interval and should not be used in patients on anti-arrhythmic drugs

I. Aminoglycosides

1. Mechanism of action: inhibit ribosomal protein synthesis. Bacteriocidal

2. Usual spectrum: Most Gram-negatives, including *Pseudomonas*, also can cover staph in urine, but not adequate tissue levels for staph

3. Advantage: drug of choice for febrile UTI if combined with TMP/SMX or ampicillin[1]

4. Adverse reactions and disadvantages:
   a. Oto- and renal- toxicity
   b. Neuromuscular blockade with high levels, so be careful with myasthenia gravis patients
   c. Avoid in pregnancy

5. Once-daily dosing[1,9]

   a. Nephrotoxicity is due to uptake of the drug into the proximal tubular epithelium
      1) This uptake is saturable, so once the luminal concentration exceeds the limit, higher concentrations do not lead to more toxicity
      2) A time with low drug levels may let some of the drug leach back out of the tubular cells
      3) Much evidence shows that single daily doses are less toxic than continuous dosing
      4) Bacterial killing is equivalent or better with once-daily dosing
   b. Ototoxicity is related to the total daily dose, and most studies showed no difference in toxicity for once-daily vs. multiple-daily dosing
   c. Usual procedure: 1st dose 7 mg/kg (adjust if very overweight, very underweight or pre-existing renal insufficiency). Draw blood levels 6-14 hours after 1st dose, use a nomogram to guide future dosing[1]

J. Aztreonam

1. Mechanism of action: inhibit bacterial cell wall synthesis (this is a beta-lactam; same class as penicillin and cephalosporins). Bacteriocidal

2. Usual spectrum: most gram-negatives, including *Pseudomonas*. (Unlike other beta-lactams, has no Gram-positive coverage.)

3. Advantage: similar spectrum to aminoglycosides but not nephrotoxic

4. Adverse reactions and disadvantages: less than 1% cross-reactivity in patients allergic to penicillins or cephalosporins

K. Vancomycin

1. Mechanism of action: inhibit bacterial cell wall synthesis, at a different point than the beta-lactam antibiotics. Bacteriocidal

2. Usual spectrum: all gram-positives, including MRSA, except new strains of *Enterococcus* that are resistant. Vancomycin has no Gram-negative coverage

3. Advantages: excellent Gram Positive coverage including MRSA

4. Adverse reactions and disadvantages:
   a. Red-man syndrome (histaminic effect)
   b. Can be nephrotoxic or ototoxic if combined with other nephrotoxic/ototoxic drugs

L. Linezolid[10]

1. Mechanism: bind to bacterial ribosomes, inhibit initiation of protein synthesis. Bacteriocidal

2. Spectrum: Gram-positive, including most MRSA and VRE

3. Advantage: Excellent oral bioavailability

4. Adverse reactions and disadvantages:
   a. Myelosuppression (must monitor blood counts)
   b. Inhibition of monoamine oxidase (was originally developed as an antidepressant)
   c. High cost (mandated by FDA to limit outpatient use)

M. New drug: daptomycin[11]

1. New class of drugs: cyclic lipopeptides

2. Mechanism: bind to bacterial membranes and quickly depolarize membrane potential, inhibits protein, RNA and DNA synthesis

3. Spectrum: most Gram Positive including VRE and MRSA

4. 2007 indications: complicated skin or blood-borne infections by susceptible organisms

5. Must be given IV

2. Relevant Definitions

A. ***Bacteriuria***. Presence of bacteria in the urine[1]

1. May be symptomatic or asymptomatic

2. May be true infection or colonization (bacteriuria without pyuria implies colonization)

B. ***Pyuria***. Presence of white blood cells in urine

1. Indicates inflammatory response

2. Sterile pyuria with acute female dysuria suggests *Chlamydia*[12]

3. Chronic sterile pyuria suggests TB, stones or cancer

C. ***Urinary tract infection.*** Inflammatory response of the urothelium to bacterial invasion (usually includes both bacteriuria and pyuria)

D. ***Uncomplicated infection.*** Recent onset, community acquired infection in a healthy patient with a structurally and functionally normal urinary tract

E. ***Complicated infection.*** Infection associated with factors that increase the chance of acquiring bacteria and decrease the efficacy of therapy.[1] The urinary tract is structurally or functionally abnormal, the patient is compromised and/or the bacteria have increased virulence or antimicrobial resistance

F. ***Unresolved infection.*** One that does not resolve with antibiotic therapy. The most common reasons for this are:[1]

1. Bacteria resistant to the antibiotic (either resistant in the first place, or developed resistance during treatment, or emergence of a resistant strain while the sensitive strain was being eradicated)

2. Inadequate urine concentration of antibiotic (for example, azotemia or papillary necrosis, or malabsorption of oral antibiotics)

3. Inadequate tissue concentration of antibiotic (eg, nitrofurantoin does not penetrate tissue, or malabsorption of oral antibiotics)

4. Giant staghorn stone; "critical mass" of bacteria is too great for antibiotics to be effective

5. Patient behavior (self-inoculation or noncompliance)

G. ***Recurrent infection.*** An infection that occurs after documented, successful resolution of an antecedent infection. There are 2 types:

1. Reinfection: Each infection is a new event with different bacteria; the bacteria come from outside the urinary tract

2. Bacterial persistence: Multiple infection episodes are caused by the same bacteria, from a focus within the urinary tract such as a stone, fistula or the prostate

3. Bacterial Virulence Factors[1, 13-17]

A. The virulence factors most relevant to UTIs are adhesins, which promote bacterial attachment by binding to specific receptors on the tissue surface[1, 13-17]

1. Type 1 pili (Type 1 fimbriae)
   a. Have a FimH adhesion protein
   b. Bind to mannose residues on host cell glycoproteins, including uroplakins on bladder epithelial cells
   c. Since mannose inhibits this binding, these are also called mannose-sensitive pili. (Mannose is also used as a complementary/alternative treatment for recurrent UTIs.)
   d. Tamm-Horsfall protein prevents this adhesion, so is protective against UTIs[1,12,13]

2. *P pili (P fimbriae)*
   a. Bind to P blood group antigens, which are also expressed on uroepithelial cells
   b. Allow bacteria to ascend ureters and cause pyelonephritis in absence of reflux (the gene for these pili is on the pap operon, which stands for pyelonephritis-associated-pili)
   c. Mannose does not inhibit this binding, so also called mannose-resistant pili

3. Dr fimbriae bind to a complement regulatory protein on epithelial cells called "decay accelerating factor" (DAF)[13]

4. Bacteria also have other types of adhesions, but the above are the main ones relevant to UTIs

B. Examples of other virulence factors besides adhesins:

1. Hemolysins

2. Capsules to evade the host response

3. Systems that allow bacteria to sequester iron

4. Toxic bacterial proteins (such as the toxic shock toxin made by certain strains of staph and strep)

4. Host Defenses Against UTIs

A. Preventing bacteria from colonizing the vagina[1,13,14,17]

1. Normal flora (Lactobacillus) competes with other bacteria, and also maintains an acid vaginal pH, which may inhibit the growth of *E coli* in the vagina

2. Vaginal fluid influences bacterial adhesion, especially by its content of secretory IGA

B. Eliminating bacteria that enter the bladder

1. Normal urine flow and voiding (mechanical clearance)

2. Urine pH (acid), osmolarity, salts, organic acids and urea inhibit bacterial growth

3. Urine lactoferrin scavenges iron, which bacteria need for growth

4. Urine IgA, low-molecular-weight sugars and Tamm-Horsfall protein inhibit bacterial attachment to the epithelium.[13,14] Tamm-Horsfall protein also has other immune-modulating effects. Knock-out mice for Tamm-Horsfall protein get UTIs very easily[14]

5. The urothelium has Toll-like receptors, which recognize LPS and other specific molecules on pathogens, and activate the innate immune response.[1] This response includes several types of cells (PMNs, macrophages, eosinophils, mast cells, etc.)

6. Since some bacteria can persist and multiply within urothelial cells, exfoliation of infected cells is a defense mechanism[1]

5. Cystitis

A. Pathogenesis

1. Bacteria colonize vagina

2. Bacteria ascend urethra to bladder

3. Host defenses do not eliminate bacteria effectively due to:
   a. Impaired host defenses
   b. Bacterial virulence factors
   c. Bacterial persistence and growth within the epithelial cells[1,18]

B. Most common bacteria causing uncomplicated cystitis:

1. *E coli* about 80%[1,3,5]

2. *S saprophyticus* about 10%[1,3,5]

C. Risk factors

1. Factors that increase vaginal colonization by pathogens
   a. Epithelial cell receptivity (genetically determined). For example, Lewis blood group nonsecretors are more likely to get recurrent UTIs than secretors
   b. Menopause (increased vaginal pH and increased colonization by *E coli*). Topical estrogen is better than placebo for decreasing recurrent UTIs in postmenopausal women.[19-20] In an uncontrolled study, topical estrogen decreased UTI frequency in young women taking oral contraceptives[21]
   c. Spermicides alter the normal vaginal flora and increase colonization by pathogens
   d. Coitus (even without spermicides)[5]
   e. Recent antibiotic use (especially beta-lactams, which disturb the normal vaginal flora)[2]

2. Instrumentation/catheters can introduce bacteria into the bladder

3. Impaired host defenses
   a. Voiding dysfunction (high-pressure voiding and/or impaired bladder emptying)
   b. Immunosuppression

c. Diabetes (many are immunosuppressed and have incomplete bladder emptying)

D. Uncomplicated cystitis in 2007 is usually treated by primary care providers rather than urologists. Some primary care practices have protocols for over-the-telephone treatment (the phone interview includes screening for possible complicated UTIs)[5,22,23]

Rationale:

1. Healthy, nonpregnant women presenting with the triad of frequency, dysuria, and no vaginal symptoms have about a 96% chance of having a UTI, so empiric treatment is appropriate even with a negative urinalysis[21,23]

2. In a randomized trial of trimethoprim vs. placebo in women with uncomplicated UTI symptoms and a negative dipstick, symptom resolution at 3 days was 76% in the treatment group and 26% in the placebo group.[24] These results suggest a high probability of infection with these symptoms, even if the dipstick is negative

E. Uncomplicated cystitis as source for possible test questions:

1. History: acute onset irritative voiding symptoms, no flank pain, no fever, patient not systemically ill

2. Pelvic exam not needed unless:
   a. Symptoms of vaginitis
   b. Other symptoms to suggest comorbid pelvic conditions

3. Dipstick urinalysis
   a. Test for glucose (UTI has more morbidity in diabetics)
   b. Leukocoyte esterase is an enzyme produced by neutrophils
   c. Nitrites: Many strains of Gram-negative bacteria can convert urine nitrates to nitrites. However, most strains of Streptococcus and Enterococcus cannot. Therefore, a negative urine nitrite test does not rule out bacteriuria
   d. The sensitivity of a positive dipstick (LE or nitrites) is only about 75%,[1,5,22,23] so do not use this to rule out UTI in symptomatic patients. ***Corollary:*** patients with a high risk of missing asymptomatic bacteriuria (such as pregnant women) should be screened with culture, not dipstick[1]

4. Microscopic urinalysis
   a. False negative results can occur, especially for visualizing bacteria, so if the clinical scenario strongly suggests UTI, send a culture[1,25]
   b. Stamm showed that pyuria correlated with either bacterial or Chlamydial infection in women with acute dysuria.[12] His definition of pyuria was >10 WBC/mm^3 in an unspun specimen, counted with a hemacytometer. This is comparable to seeing 1-2 WBC/HPF on microscopy of acentrifuged specimen[1]
   c. If a symptomatic patient has visible bacteriuria but the culture is negative, possibilities include:
      1) Patient already taking antibiotics
      2) Infection with anaerobic bacteria
      3) Antiseptic solution used to clean the perineum may have entered the urine

5. Urine culture
   a. Original dogma: >100,000 colony-forming units/mL indicates UTI. However, this study compared asymptomatic people with pyelonephritis patients. Women with acute cystitis were not included[26]
   b. Modern knowledge: with acute female dysuria, >100 cfu/mL indicates infection, especially if the organism is *E coli* or *S saphrophyticus*[1,12,27]

6. Antibiotic treatment (the Infectious Diseases Society of America instituted guidelines for treatment of uncomplicated UTIs in 1999 They are on the IDSA web site: www.idsociety.org.) More recent recommendations are similar[3]
   a. Ampicillin/amoxicillin are not usual first-line treatments
      1) High rates of resistance in many areas
      2) Disrupts normal vaginal flora, increasing the risks of yeast vaginitis and future cystitis episodes

b. Good choices: TMP/SMX, TMP alone, or nitrofurantoin

c. Some areas have a high incidence of resistance to TMP/SMX (easy to call your local lab and ask)
   1) Quinolones are a good choice in these areas[1]
   2) Nitrofurantion is a good alternative (reliable coverage of the 2 most common organisms in uncomplicated UTIs, low incidence of developing resistance, and spares quinolone use)

d. In a randomized trial of 3-day therapy, ciprofloxacin was better than amoxicillin-clavulanate[28]

7. Treatment duration: 3 days for most uncomplicated cystitis
   a. In a recent Cochrane review, 3 days was similar to 5-10 days for symptomatic cure. 5-10 days had a higher bacteriologic cure rate, but also more adverse effects. Therefore, they recommended 3 days except in situations where eradication of bacteria is essential[29]
   b. A 7-day course is recommended if using nitrofurantoin, if symptoms have been present for >7 days, if the patient is a man or has complicating factors[1]

F. Evaluation of recurrent uncomplicated cystitis

1. For all: history, pelvic exam, urinalysis, urine culture

2. Further evaluation (eg, upper tract imaging, cystoscopy, urodynamics) is indicated only if the clinical scenario is suspicious for an underlying structural or functional abnormality, such as:
   a. Frequent infections with same bacterial species at short intervals (bacterial persistence)
   b. Abnormal urinalysis between infection episodes
   c. Voiding symptoms between infection episodes
   d. History of calculi (or infection with urea-splitting bacteria)
   e. Febrile UTIs or flank pain with UTIs
   f. Underlying illnesses such as diabetes, neurologic disorders, suspicion for fistula (history of diverticulitis, inflammatory bowel disease, etc.)

G. Treatment options for recurrent uncomplicated cystitis[1]

1. Change from spermicide to a different form of contraception

2. Topical estrogen in postmenopausal women[1,19,20]

3. Chronic low-dose antibiotic prophylaxis[1]
   a. Some of these drugs work because they have high urine concentrations at doses that do not affect the vaginal or bowel reservoirs, so there is little selection for resistant bacteria. Examples include:
      1) Nitrofurantion 50 or 100 mg q HS
      2) Cephalexin 250 mg or less, q HS
   b. Some of these drugs work by eradicating pathogens from the vagina. Examples include:
      1) TMP/SMX, 200/40 mg q HS (DS is 800/160)
      2) TMP alone (50 or 100 mg qHS) may be a better choice because:
         a) It avoids the problem of sulfa allergy
         b) It is likely to be equally effective. TMP is secreted into the vaginal fluid in high concentrations, while SMX is not secreted into the vaginal fluid at all[1]
      3) Quinolones (eg, norfloxacin 200 mg qHS) also eradicate vaginal pathogens but should be reserved for patients who fail the other regimens, due to expense, pregnancy concerns and risk of resistance

4. Postcoital prophylaxis for women with UTI episodes clearly related to intercourse; use same antibiotics as above

5. Chronic prophylaxis with methenamine hippurate

6. Intermittent self-start therapy
   a. Rationale: if a woman with previous cystitis has symptoms suggesting a recurrence, the chance of UTI is about 90%[1,5]
   b. Procedure from 2007 Campbell-Walsh: patients gets a dip slide and a 3-day course of full-dose antibiotics to keep at home. When UTI symptoms begin, start the dip slide culture at home before taking antibiotics, then bring the slide to the office as soon as possible.[1] Main advantages of this approach:
      1) If symptoms do not resolve, can do culture and sensitivity from the original dip slide
      2) If culture is negative, evaluate for other causes of irritative symptoms, such as carcinoma

7. Cranberry juice or cranberry extract pills
   a. Rationale: cranberries contain proanthocyanidins, which decrease adherence of P fimbriated *E coli*[1,30]
   b. Cochrane review in 2004 concluded there is evidence to support use of cranberry juice in nonelderly women (little or no data in that review for children or elderly)[31]
   c. Main problem: different pills and juices vary in their actual cranberry content[1]
   d. ONLY useful for cystitis caused by *E. Coli*

8. Mannose is used as a complementary prophylaxis for UTIs, with the rationale that it inhibits the binding of Type 1 pili to mannose residues on the urothelium, but there is no published literature about this

9. Campbell-Walsh p. 265: "Other factors, such as hygiene, frequency and timing of voiding, wiping patterns, use of hot tubs, and type of undergarments, have not been shown to predispose women to recurrent infection and there is no rationale for giving women specific instructions regarding them."

H. How is complicated cystitis different from what was just described?

1. Definition: patient is compromised and/or has a structural or functional urinary tract abnormality and/or bacteria with increased virulence, such as nosocomial infection. Also, men with UTIs should be suspected of having complicated UTIs[1,32]

2. Acute evaluation includes office visit, exam, urinalysis, urine culture. Start empiric antibiotics while waiting for culture results

3. Quinolones are good initial therapy while awaiting culture results

4. Antibiotics for at least 7 days

5. Besides just treating the cystitis, also do urologic evaluation based on the underlying abnormality (upper tract imaging, cystoscopy, urodynamics as appropriate to the clinical scenario)

6. Pyelonephritis

A. Pathogenesis

1. The most common route is ascending from the bladder. Therefore, the risk factors described above for cystitis also apply to pyelonephritis. For example, a recent case-control study found the following risk factors for acute pyelonephritis in healthy women[33]
   a. Frequency of coitus over past 30 days
   b. Recent UTI
   c. Diabetes
   d. Recent incontinence
   e. New sexual partner in previous year
   f. Recent spermicide use
   g. History of UTI in the participant's mother

2. Additional risk factors, which increase the chance that bladder infection will ascend to the kidneys:
   a. P pili on bacteria
   b. Vesicoureteral reflux
   c. Ureteral stasis or abnormal peristalsis

3. Less likely route: bloodborne (often leads to renal abscess)

B. Evaluation

1. For all patients: history, exam, urinalysis, urine culture

2. Upper tract imaging when indicated, such as:
   a. Known or suspected upper tract abnormalities
   b. History of stones or other conditions that predispose to upper tract abnormalities
   c. Severely ill or septic patient
   d. Symptoms present more than 5 days before treatment[1]
   e. Persistent fever after 72 hours of antibiotic treatment
   f. Infection with urea-splitting organisms[1]
   g. If planning outpatient treatment and the patient does not have reliable access to imaging if he/she fails to improve[1]

3. Blood cultures are indicated for men, pregnant women, patients with upper tract abnormalities, and severely ill or septic patients[1]

C. Outpatient treatment of acute uncomplicated pyelonephritis

1. Criteria: otherwise healthy woman, not pregnant, not septic, able to take oral fluids and antibiotics, compliant, reliable for follow-up

2. Treatment recommendations from IDSA guidelines:
   a. 14 days of quinolone has the best supportive evidence
   b. Moderate evidence supports treating 7 days for patients with milder cases
   c. Moderate evidence supports using TMP/SMX if the organism is known to be susceptible

D. In-patient treatment for uncomplicated pyelonephritis

1. Choices: parenteral quinolone, aminoglycoside ± ampicillin, or extended-spectrum cephalosporin ± aminoglycoside

2. Convert to oral regimen when patient is stable, treat 10-14 days

E. Inpatient treatment of complicated pyelonephritis[1,32]

1. Start with broad-spectrum IV antibiotics. Continue IV antibiotics at least 7 days if blood cultures are positive, otherwise 2-3 days, then change to oral based on culture results

2. Treat 14-21 days total

3. Low threshold for upper tract imaging

F. After treating pyelonephritis, get follow-up urine cultures at 5-7 days, 10-14 days and 4-6 weeks. 10%-30% of patients will relapse early after treatment. Treat for another 2 weeks; if relapse occurs, treat for 6 weeks[1]

G. Emphysematous pyelonephritis[1,32,34]

1. Definition: an acute necrotizing parenchymal and perirenal infection caused by gas-forming organisms

2. Most patients are diabetic and all are adults

3. Where does the gas come from? ***Theories:***
   a. With high tissue glucose levels, bacteria ferment sugar and produce carbon dioxide.
   b. Since most patients also have renal impairment, obstruction and/or papillary necrosis, another theory is that bacteria ferment necrotic tissue and produce gas

4. Overall mortality 20%-40%

5. *E coli* is the most common bacteria, then *Klebsiella* and *Proteus*

6. Radiologic evaluation
   a. Plain film may show gas in renal parenchyma
   b. Excretory urogram not a good choice; has risk of contrast toxicity in ill diabetic patient, and the poorly functioning kidney may not be seen
   c. Ultrasound shows echoes related to gas
   d. CT scan is best choice: clearly shows gas, also evaluates for hydronephrosis or abscess

7. Treatment: fluid resuscitation, antibiotics and prompt intervention. Intervention can be either nephrectomy or percutaneous drainage (which may progress to nephrectomy if fails). Different opinions about how to choose between nephrectomy vs. percutaneous drain:
   a. From Campbell-Walsh[1]
      1) If kidney is obstructed, can do either procedure
      2) If kidney is nonfunctioning and is not obstructed, the best choice is immediate nephrectomy
   b. From Huang (used by several centers worldwide)[34]
      1) If gas is limited to collecting system (class 1) or renal parenchyma (class2), do percutaneous drain
      2) If gas extends through Gerota's fascia, do percutaneous drain if has <2 other risk factors and ephrectomy if has 2 or more other risk factors. The other risk factors are thrombocytopenia, acute renal failure, altered mental status and shock
      3) If bilateral (class 4), start with bilateral drains, do nephrectomy if patient does not improve

H. Xanthogranulomatous pyelonephritis[1,35,36]

1. A rare, severe chronic renal infection with accumulation of lipid-laden foamy macrophages (xanthoma cells)

2. Usually begins in pelvis and calyces, then extends to destroy renal parenchyma and surrounding tissues

3. Classic radiographic triad:
   a. Unilateral renal enlargement (diffuse or mass effect)
   b. Stone in renal pelvis (may lack hydronephrosis because inflammatory fibrosis prevents collecting system dilation).
   c. Nonfunctioning or poorly functioning kidney

4. On CT scan may also see multiple cystic areas of necrosis and abscess ("bear paw sign")[35]

5. Most common bacteria: *Proteus*, and *E coli* is also common

6. Treatment: antibiotics to stabilize the patient, then surgery
   a. Localized lesions may be amenable to partial nephrectomy
   b. Nephrectomy in most cases. Surgery can be difficult when inflammatory mass extends into surrounding tissues. It is important to remove the entire inflammatory mass. Laparoscopic nephrectomy has good outcomes with experienced surgeons[36]
   c. Lipid-laden macrophages may resemble clear cell carcinoma on frozen section

7. Asymptomatic Bacteriuria

For recent ISDA guidelines,[37] see web site: www.idsociety.org

A. Incidence[1,37-40]

1. About 5% in healthy young sexually active women (incidence does not change with pregnancy, but clinical significance does)

2. 20%-50% of elderly women, 15%-30% of elderly men

3. High incidence in patients with catheters, stones, obstruction

B. Asymptomatic bacteriuria usually does not progress to clinically significant infection. One possible explanation is that the bacteria involved are nonpathogenic, and may actually prevent colonization by pathogenic strains[41]

C. Populations for whom no benefit to treatment has been demonstrated (assuming normal urinary tract with no stones or obstruction):

1. Nonpregnant young women

2. Diabetics (asymptomatic bacteriuria increases the risks of developing symptomatic UTIs, pyelonephritis and hospitalization, but treating asymptomatic bacteriuria doesn't reduce these risks)[39]

3. Elderly people, either in the community or institutionalized (***Caveat***: be sure they are truly asymptomatic! Symptoms of bacteriuria in the elderly can include incontinence, lethargy, anorexia, confusion)[40]

4. Patients with indwelling or intermittent catheterization (Same caveat, assuming they are truly asymptomatic)

5. Patients with spinal cord injuries[38]

D. Patients who do need treatment

2. Pregnant women (for details see next section)

3. Patients with stones, obstruction or other GU tract abnormalities

4. Patients who need the urine to be sterile for a procedure

8. UTIs in Pregnancy

A. Asymptomatic bacteriuria[1,38,42-44]

1. Incidence of asymptomatic bacteriuria in pregnancy is about 5% (the same as for nonpregnant women in the same age group)

2. Unlike nonpregnant women, pregnant women with asymptomatic bacteriuria need to be identified and treated
   a. Definitely known: if untreated, 20%-40% will develop pyelonephritis, which can lead to sepsis in the mother (1%-8% of pregnant women with pyelonephritis get ARDS)[42]
   b. Bacteriuria and pyelonephritis are associated with problems such as low birth weight and prematurity. Debated: does bacteriuria actually cause these problems, or is it simply associated with other poor prognosticators such as diabetes and low socioeconomic status?[37,42-44] Either way, treatment is recommended
   c. Women with Group B Strep bacteriuria may transmit it to the baby, which can cause sepsis, pneumonia, meningitis or death.[42,45] They need to be treated when diagnosed and also at time of delivery.[46] CDC guidelines are on the web at: www.cdc.gov/mmwr/PDF/RR/RR5111.pdf

3. Procedure to screen pregnant women for bacteriuria
   a. First prenatal visit: urine culture, not just urinalysis[1,38,42-44]
   b. Do midstream clean-catch voided urine (with catheter, risk of introducing bacteria outweighs benefits)
   c. If first culture is negative, repeat culture not recommended unless the patient has urologic abnormality or a history of recurrent UTIs[42]

4. Treatment: antibiotics 3-10 days, recheck culture 10 days later and periodically throughout pregnancy, consider daily suppression[38,44]

B. Treatment of symptomatic UTIs in pregnancy

1. Cystitis
   a. Duration of treatment still controversial: 3-7 days
   b. Not controversial: need to re-culture urine after treatment and be sure bacteriuria has resolved

2. Pyelonephritis
   a. Start with inpatient parenteral antibiotics (usual choices: ampicillin plus aminoglycoside, ampicillin-sulbactam, or broad-spectrum cephalosporin)
   b. After patient improves, continue culture-specific oral treatment for 10-14 days or longer.[1,43] Re-check culture to be sure bacteria are eradicated
   c. High risk of recurrent pyelonephritis, so continue suppressive therapy and check cultures monthly

C. Use of antibiotics in pregnancy

1. Agents considered safe throughout pregnancy (category B):
   a. Ampicillin, amoxicillin, penicillin V
   b. Cephalexin, cefaclor, ceftriaxone
   c. Clindamycin

2. Agents to avoid at certain times during pregnancy:
   a. If given in third trimester, sulfonamides can cause neonatal jaundice, and in G6PD patients can cause hemolytic anemia in the newborn
   b. If given in third trimester, nitrofurantion can cause hemolytic anemia due to immature fetal erythrocyte enzymes. Especially avoid in patients with G6PD

4. Agents to avoid throughout pregnancy:
   a. Quinolones cause abnormal cartilage development in animals. With rare exceptions,[47] most authors recommend avoiding quinolones during pregnancy
   b. Chloramphenicol ("gray baby syndrome")
   c. Trimethoprim (megaloblastic anemia and congenital malformations from folate antagonism)
   d. Erythromycin (maternal cholestatic jaundice).
   e. Tetracyclines (inhibit fetal bone growth, fetal tooth discoloration, may cause acute liver failure in mother)

9. Malakoplakia

A. An unusual inflammatory disease that was originally described in the bladder but can also affect the upper tracts, GI system, skin, lung, etc.[1,48]

B. Cause unknown, but the main theory is:

1 Starts with bacterial infection, most commonly *E coli*

2. Bacteria engulfed by macrophages, but phagocytosis is defective so bacteria are incompletely digested
   a. Bacterial fragments within macrophages form Michaelis-Gutman bodies. Pathognomonic when present, but may be absent in early disease so not required for diagnosis[1]
   b. The large macrophages containing the fragments are von Hansemann cells
   c. Macrophage staining for alpha-1-antitrypsin is generally specific to malakoplakia, and helps to distinguish it from other inflammatory conditions

C. Clinical features

1. Age usually >50, more common in females

2. Patients often debilitated and/or immunosuppressed

3. Symptoms: irritative bladder symptoms, hematuria

D. Cystoscopy: multiple plaques, may progress to large masses

E. Upper tract involvement: mass effect on IVP, ultrasound or CT scan

F. Treatment

1. Long-term antibiotics that kill intracellular bacteria, such as sulfonamides, TMP, doxycycline, rifampin and quinolones

2. Vitamin C and bethanechol may improve phagocytosis. A high ratio of cGMP to cAMP promotes phagocytosis. Bethancehol increases cGMP and vitamin C decreases cAMP[48]

3. Surgery if lesions do not respond to antibiotics

10. Prostatitis and Chronic Pelvic Pain Syndrome

A. Acute bacterial prostatitis (NIH category I)[49-51]

1. Pathogenesis
   a. 65%-80% are *E coli*; other organisms include enterococcus (5%-10%), *Pseudomonas, Serratia, Klebsiella, Enterobacter*
   b. The most likely route of infection is ascending, with reflux of urine and bacteria into the prostatic ducts
   c. Risk factors include UTI, indwelling or condom catheters, and transurethral surgery

2. Evaluation
   a. History: acute onset of perineal pain, obstructive or irritative voiding symptoms, and systemic symptoms (fever, chills, malaise, nausea, etc.)
   b. Exam: Prostate is hot, boggy, very tender, do not massage!
   c. Urinalysis, urine culture

3. Antibiotic treatment
   a. In acute prostatitis, most antibiotics achieve reasonable prostate concentration (unlike chronic prostatitis to be discussed below)
   b. Usual choices for acute treatment: ampicillin + gentamicin, 2nd or 3rd generation cephalosporin or quinolone
   c. After acute phase, treat with TMP or quinolone 2-4 weeks
   d. If acute symptoms do not improve within 36 hours of antibiotics, do a transrectal ultrasound or CT scan to look for prostate abscess. If abscess is present, transurethral drainage is usually the best route

4. Adjunct treatments
   a. If the patient cannot void, use a small urethral catheter (in/out or short term indwelling) or suprapubic
   b. Stool softeners

B. Unlike acute prostatitis, the chronic syndromes include prostatic massage as a recommended part of the evaluation[49]

1. 4-glass test from Meares and Stamey (1968)
   a. Voided bladder-1 (VB1) is the first 10 mL of urine voided and represents the urethral specimen

b. VB2 is a midstream voided urine (bladder urine)
c. Massage prostate, collect expressed prostatic secretions (EPS) into a sterile container
d. VB3 is the first 10 mL after massage, includes any EPS trapped in the prostatic urethra
e. All 4 specimens get microscopic exam and culture

2. In 2007, most urologists do only a 2-glass test
a. Midstream urine pre-massage
b. First 10 mL urine post-massage

3. Interpretation of 2-glass test
a. Both specimens have positive culture: cystitis. In this case, give a short course of an antibiotic that does not penetrate the prostate (eg, nitrofurantoin) and repeat the test
b. Pre-massage culture negative but post-massage culture positive: category II chronic bacterial prostatitis
c. Negative pre-massage for WBC and culture. Post-massage urine has negative culture but positive WBC in post-massage: inflammatory chronic pelvic pain syndrome (NIH category IIIa). d. Both specimens negative for WBC and culture: noninflammatory chronic pelvic pain syndrome (NIH category IIIb)

C. Chronic bacterial prostatitis (NIH category II)

1. ***Definition:*** documented recurrent UTIs, positive culture of EPS or post-massage urine in between episodes of acute UTI

2. Evaluation
a. History: it is important to document whether prior UTI's based on symptoms only or on culture
b. Exam: the prostate may be normal or boggy, normal size or enlarged, tender or not. Also palpate other potential areas of pain including groin, perineum, coccyx, external anal sphincter, internal pelvic side walls
c. Urinalysis and culture
d. Recommended: 2- or 4-glass test as described above
e. Flow rate, residual urine test, urine cytology recommended if hematuria
f. Optional tests depending on the clinical scenario: semen culture, urethral swab, urodynamics, cystoscopy, transrectal ultrasound, pelvic CT scan or MRI, serum PSA

3. Treatment
a. Antibiotics 4-12 weeks. Use one with good penetration into the prostate (quinolone is best, TMP an alternative)
b. For recurrent culture-positive episodes, consider transrectal ultrasound for abscess, cysts or obstructed seminal vesicles
c. Anecdotally, some patients may benefit from repeated prostate massage, but there is no evidence or consensus to support this[49]
d. No surgery unless specific indication!

D. Chronic pelvic pain syndrome (CPPS) NIH category III

1. ***Definition***: "Genitourinary pain in the absence of uropathogenic bacteria detected by standard microbiological methodology."

2. In a recent case-control study, CPPS patients more likely to have a history of nonspecific urethritis, cardiovascular disease, neurological disease, psychiatric conditions and hematopoetic, lymphatic or infectious diseases[51]

3. Evaluation is the same as described above for chronic prostatitis. NIH Chronic Prostatitis Symptom Index (CPSI) validated for symptom severity and treatment response but does not diagnose the condition. PSA and free PSA have small or no differences for men with CP/CPPS vs. normal men, so evaluation and treatment of elevated PSA is the same for men with or without CP/CPPS[52]

4. Two categories, based on results of 2- or 4-glass test
a. Inflammatory CPPS (IIIA) is defined as having a "significant number of white blood cells in EPS, post-prostatic massage urine, or semen."

b. Noninflammatory CPPS (IIIB) is defined as having an "insignificant number of white blood cells in EPS, post-prostatic massage urine, or semen." Some men in this category have primary bladder neck obstruction, so be sure to check uroflow and PVR, and have a low threshold for urodynamics with pressure-flow study[53]

c. Most treatment trials to date have enrolled patients with both types, and not separated them for data analyses. Those studies that did address the issue of IIIA or IIIB are identified in the descriptions below. Currently, there is no evidence that differentiation between IIIA and IIIB has any clinical relevance

5. Treatment options are listed below and were recently reviewed.[49,54] All of the drugs listed are off-label use for this condition
   a. A common treatment is to give antibiotics 4 weeks
      1) Some patients improve; may be a placebo effect, an eradication of fastidious organisms, or independent anti-inflammatory effects of some antibiotics[49]
      2) In two controlled trials, quinolones were no better than placebo.[55,56] These trials did not distinguish between inflammatory (IIIA) and noninflammatory (IIIB) CPPS. Also, these trials included chronic patients, who are likely to be the most refractory. Patients who had previously tried antibiotics were allowed into these trials, as long as they had no antibiotics in the previous 4 weeks
      3) Bottom line in 2007: may be OK to try a single course of empiric antibiotics for new patients in the absence of positive cultures, but definitely no benefit in chronic, previously treated patients.
   b. Alpha blockers: 4 placebo-controlled trials published
      1) Active drug was better than placebo in 3 trials.[57-59] Only 1 of these studies excluded men who had previously taken alpha blockers.[59] In the 4th trial, active drug not better than placebo, but that study included chronic, heavily pretreated patients.[55] These trials did not separate out inflammatory (IIIA) and noninflammatory (IIIB) CPPS
      2) Overall conclusion: alpha blockers are beneficial if used for more than 6 weeks in patients with recent symptom onset, and not heavily pre-treated[49]
      3) A recent meta-analysis also supported alpha blockers and recommended treatment >3 months[60]
   c. Finsateride was evaluated in 2 placebo-controlled trials for category IIIA CPPS. The first trial defined IIIA as 10 or more white blood cells in the post-massage urine, and found finasteride better than placebo for voiding symptoms but not for pain.[61] The second trial defined IIIA as any white blood cells in the EPS or post-massage urine. That study showed no significant benefit of finasteride over placebo, but was admittedly underpowered.[62] A third study compared finasteride with saw palmetto, and finasteride was more effective. That study separated their category IIIA and IIIB groups, and saw no differences in outcomes between these two groups.[63] Overall, the 2007 Campbell-Walsh recommends that finasteride not be used as monotherapy for CP/CPPS except perhaps in men with associated BPH[49]
   d. Anti-inflammatories: 2 studies, both enrolled IIIA and IIIB patients, neither study mention whether the two categories had different outcomes
      1) Rofecoxib was better than placebo for some, but not all, outcome measures in a recent study[64]
      2) Corticosteroids no better than placebo[65]
   e. Quercetin 500 mg twice a day was better than placebo in one study, with reduction in both CPSI and WBC count in the EPS[66]
   f. A complimentary/alternative terpene preparation was more effective than ibuprofen 600 mg TID[67]
   g. Physical therapy to pelvic floor has the rationale that pelvic floor muscle dysfunction is present in some CPPS patients.[68] It was effective in open-label trials[69-71]
   h. Pentosan polysulfate (PPS)
      1) Some overlap of symptoms between CPPS and IC men. Men with IC more likely to have pain improvement with voiding and suprapubic tenderness. If diagnosis is truly IC, then PPS would be an approved therapy

2) In a controlled trial of PPS in men with CPPS, 300 mg TID was better than placebo for some outcome measures, but not others.[72] This paper did not explain why the higher dose was chosen, especially since the higher dose is not more effective than the usual dose of 100 mg TID for interstitial cystitis

i. Extracorporeal magnetic therapy + terazosin was more effective than terazosin alone in a pilot study[73]

j. Topical capsaicin was effective for 16 of 22 patients in an open-label study[74]

k. Muscle relaxants

l. Neuroleptic pain medications (amitriptyline, gabapentin, pregabalin)

m. Reassurance and psychological support

n. Surgery or heat therapy only if specific indication!

E. Category IV: asymptomatic inflammatory prostatitis. No need to treat unless evaluating PSA, or if thought to be contributing to infertility[49]

11. Fungal UTI

About 80% of fungal UTIs are *Candida* so this outline will focus on *Candida*[1,75-77]

A. Risk factors

1. Indwelling catheters

2. Antibiotics

3. Diabetes mellitus

4. Impaired host (steroid therapy, malignancy, malnutrition, etc.)

5. GU tract anomaly (congenital, neurogenic, conduit diversion, etc.)

B. Review of antibiotics

1. Nystatin
   a. Mechanism of action: binds to sterols in cell membranes
   b. Some *Candida* species (not *albicans*) develop resistance to nystatin; if so they become resistant to amphotericin also

2. Amphotericin B
   a. Mechanism: binds to sterols in cell membranes. Has higher affinity for fungal cells (ergosterol component), but can also bind to cholesterol in mammalian cells (toxicity)
   b. Advantage: high efficacy, the gold standard for disseminated or invasive infections
   c. Many adverse effects including fever, rigors, hypokalemia, hypocalcemia, hyponatremia, hypomagnesemia, azotemia, liver toxicity, phlebitis
   d. Rigors/chills/fever may be due to stimulation of prostaglandin synthesis. Ibuprofen or corticosteroids may help symptoms. It isn't usually necessary to stop the drug
   e. Liposomal form has fewer side effects but can cause anaphylaxis

3. Imidazoles and triazoles are basically the same; imidazoles have two nitrogen atoms in the azole ring and triazoles have 3
   a. Mechanism: inhibit fungal cytochrome P-450 enzymes, so fungi cannot produce steroids for cell membranes
   b. Several are used topically, including butoconazole, clotrimazole, terconazole, tioconazole and miconazole. (In the past, miconazole could be used as a bladder irrigant, but in 2007 only the topical form is available in the United States.)
   c. Fluconazole
      1) Can be given orally or IV
      2) Fewer side effects than amphotericin, but higher rate of resistance
      3) Interacts with cytochrome P450 3A4,[78] so increases serum levels of drugs that share the same enzyme system such as oral hypoglycemics, warfarin, and other drugs as described below for ketoconazole
   d. Ketoconazole
      1) Good GI absorption but requires stomach acid, so absorption is poor in patients with achlorhydria, or taking H_2 blockers or proton pump inhibitors
      2) Inhibits mammalian cytochrome P-450 enzymes:
         a) Inhibits adrenal androgen synthesis
         b) Infrequent adrenal insufficiency
         c) Significant drug interactions: can increase to dangerous levels of terfenadine, astemizole, cisapride, cyclosporine, tacrolimus, methylprednisolone, phenytoin, etc.
      3) Poor renal excretion; may have insufficient urine levels to treat kidney or bladder infections (good use: blastomycosis or histoplasmosis in prostate)
      4) Hepatotoxicity is unusual but can be fatal
   e. Itraconazole: not used for *Candida*
   f. Voriconazole (a new triazole)
      1) Can be given orally or IV
      2) Indications relevant to urology include disseminated *Aspergillus*, Candidemia, and *Candida* infections of kidney, bladder wall and wounds

4. 5-fluorocytosine (flucytosine): converted to 5-fluorouracil by an enzyme (cytosine deaminase) that is present in some fungal species but minimal or absent in mammalian cells. Two different chapters in Campbell-Walsh have different opinions:

   a. A good choice for *Candida* cystitis without upper tract involvement[1]
   b. A poor choice for any *Candida* infection due to the rapid development of drug resistance in *Candida*, also risks of bone marrow toxicity and colitis[75]

5. Echinocandins (caspofungin, micafungin, anidulafungin)[78]
   a. Mechanism: inhibitors synthesis of beta-1,3-glucan, which is an essential component of the *Candida* cell wall
   b. Used for *Candida*; usually not effective for other fungal species (except caspofungin is effective for *Aspergillus*)[79]
   c. Must be given IV
   d. Few side effects; about 2% of patients have symptoms related to histamine release (these are basic polypeptides)
   e. Comparable efficacy to amphotericin B for invasive *Candida* infections

C. Skin infections (balanitis, vulvovaginitis):

1. Choice of several topical agents

2. For vulvovaginits or balanitis, 150 mg fluconazole as single oral dose is usually effective

D. Urine colonization

1. Asymptomatic Candiduria rarely leads to invasive disease

2. Most cases will resolve if the underlying risk factors are improved
   a. Remove or change catheter
   b. Stop antibiotics
   c. Improve nutritional status

3. Indications for treatment[77]
   a. Symptomatic patients
   b. Neutrop enic patients

c. Infants with low birth weight
d. Patients with renal allografts
e. Patients planned for urinary tract manipulation
f. Urine colonization in ICU patients is clearly associated with increased risk of invasive *Candida* infection, and with worse outcomes.[80] It is not definitively established whether treating *Candida* in these colonized patients improves outcomes

4. Treatment options
   a. Amphotericin B bladder irrigation (usually 50 mg in 1000 mL water at 42 mL/hour or 1000 mL/day). May work better in alkaline urine because *Candida* grows best at pH 5.1-6.4
   b. Oral or IV fluconazole (preferred because catheterization is not required)

E. Cystitis without upper tract involvement can be treated with oral or IV fluconazole, or amphotericin irrigation. If Candiduria persists, do upper tract imaging (if not done already) to rule out upper tract source[77]

F. Upper tract infection

1. IV amphotericin B is the best treatment

2. Upper tract imaging to look for fungus balls. If present, place a ureteral catheter or percutaneous nephrostomy tube. Irrigate the upper tract with amphotericin B and/or remove the obstructing fungus ball endoscopically or surgically

G. Systemic

1. Kidney infection may be a result or a cause of systemic *Candida*

2. IV amphotericin B is the gold standard

3. Caspofungin is a good choice also

H. *Candida* prostatic abscess may require TUR drainage as well as antimycotic therapy[81]

12. GU Tuberculosis

A. Epidemiology[75,82]

1. Prevalence in the United States decreased steadily from 1992 to 2002

2. Most cases in the United States are in AIDS patients or foreign-born people

3. Globally, TB is the most common opportunistic infection in AIDS patients

B. Microbiology

1. Almost all cases of GU tuberculosis are due to *Mycobacterium* tuberculosis. (Other species of *Mycobacterium* can cause disease, but they rarely infect the GU tract.)

2. The human is the only reservoir of *M tuberculosis*

C. Pathogenesis

1. Almost all TB infections are acquired by inhalation

2. Initial infection lasts about 4 weeks
   a. Bacteria multiply in the lungs
   b. Bacteria disseminate through lymphatics and blood

3. After about 4 weeks, host response (mostly T lymphocytes and macrophages) contains the infection. At this point, positive reaction to PPD test occurs

4. In 90%-95% of competent hosts, bacteria remain dormant in the lungs, and no clinical disease ever develops

5. Active disease develops with immunocompromising disorders such as debilitation, trauma, steroids or other immunosuppressive therapy, diabetes or AIDS

6. For most cases of GU TB:
   a. Kidneys become colonized during the initial dissemination
   b. Renal foci are activated when local immune response fails

c. Ureteral or bladder TB is "always" secondary to renal TB[75,82] (one case report of bladder TB alone[83])

7. Epididymal TB is generally thought to be from hematogenous spread, and usually starting in the globus minor (the part of the epididymis with the greatest blood supply). However, more recently this is debated, and some cases are now thought to be extensions of renal involvement.[84] Either way, all men with epididymal TB should have upper tract evaluation to check for upper tract involvement

8. Testis TB is usually local spread from epididymal TB

9. Rare kinds of GU TB:
   a. Prostate TB is rare and due to hematogenous spread
   b. TB of penis is very rare and is acquired by coitus with infected partner or by infected clothing
   c. Urethral TB is very rare; pathogenesis uncertain

10. GU TB is rare in immunocompetent children because the symptoms of renal TB usually do not appear for 3 to 10 years (or longer, 20 years or more) after the primary infection

D. Progression of renal TB

1. Bloodborne bacteria settle in capillaries near glomeruli

2. Cellular response is PMNs at first, then macrophages

3. Caseating granulomas develop with Langhans giant cells, lymphocytes, fibroblasts. These may progress to either fibrous tissue (leading to calyceal strictures) or necrotic areas (destroying the calyces)

4. Fibrous tissue may become calcified, and renal calcification is a common sign of TB

5. Reduced renal blood flow may lead to hypertension

6. Ureteral involvement is most commonly at the ureterovesical junction. This indicates extensive renal TB, and complete destruction ensues rapidly[82]

7. Bladder involvement usually begins around the ureteral orifice. Fibrosis may lead to stricture or reflux

E. Diagnosis of GU TB

1. Symptoms are often minimal and vague
   a. Frequent painless micturition
   b. Malaise, weight loss, lethargy, low-grade fevers
   c. Flank pain, suprapubic pain and colic are rare
   d. Painful epididymal or scrotal swelling
   e. With epididymal TB, hematospermia may be the only sign. Men with repeated episodes should be evaluated for TB[75]

2. Urine studies
   a. Sterile pyuria classic, but up to 20% of patients lack pyuria
   b. Up to 50% have microhematuria (this isn't specific to TB)
   c. 3 to 5 early am urine specimens for culture and AFB stain
   d. PCR techniques to identify GU TB are being evaluated[75,82]

3. PPD skin testing
   a. The exact definition of a positive reaction depends on the clinical scenario (eg, >15 mm is positive for a person with no risk factors, but with risk factors, 5 mm or 10 mm may be considered positive)[75]
   b. People born outside the United States may have been vaccinated with BCG, if so they may have a severe positive reaction

4. Plain abdominal films often show calcifications

5. Typical findings on excretory urogram[75,85,86]
   a. Irregular "moth-eaten" calyces
   b. Hydronephrosis, hydrocalyx and/or hydroureter

c. Scarring with superior displacement of UPJ ("hiked-up pelvis" resembles high-insertion UPJ obstruction)[85]

d. Nonvisualization of calyx from infundibular stricture

e. Scarring of ureters

1) Most common site: distal ureter

2) The finding of multiple ureteral scars is "almost pathognomonic" for GU TB[86]

f. Nonvisualization of kidney from extensive scarring ("autonephrectomy")

g. Small, contracted bladder

6. CT scan will usually show the same findings, especially with modern 3D reconstruction, and also has the advantage of evaluating other areas outside the GU tract[75]

7. Cystoscopy is rarely indicated in the diagnosis of GU TB, except in rare situations such as passing ureteral catheters to determine which kidney is involved[75]

8. Bladder biopsy is contraindicated with active TB, unless you think a bladder lesion is really cancer. Since bladder TB almost always starts at the ureteral orifices, suspect cancer if lesions are far away from the orifices and the orifices are normal[82]

F. Drug treatment

1. Recommendations are continually changing and depend on the patient's compliance, HIV status and extent of disease. It is best to consult with an infectious disease specialist

2. The most recent published CDC guidelines[87] are from 2003 and are on their web site at www.cdc.gov/mmwr/PDF/rr/rr5211.pdf

3. Basic idea from 2003 guidelines:

a. 6 months treatment for GU TB (9 months if slow to respond). Take all drugs together as single dose at night[75]

b. First 2 months should include 4 drugs: INH, rifampin, pyrazinamine and ethambutol. (If sensitivity results confirm susceptibility to both INH and rifampin; OK to stop ethambutol)

c. Next 4 months: INH and rifampin (if TB sensitive to both)

4. Isoniazid (INH)

a. First-line drug unless organism is resistant

b. Bactericidal to rapidly dividing bacteria Inhibits synthesis of mycolic acids, components of the cell wall

c. High urine concentrations, passes freely into renal cavities and prostate[75]

d. Adverse reactions

1) Liver toxicity (risk increased if also drink alcohol)

2) Neurotoxicity is due to enhanced excretion of pyridoxine (vitamin B6) and is prevented by pyridoxine supplements[75]

e. Drug interactions: may increase levels of phenytoin and carbamazepine

5. Rifampin

a. First-line drug unless organism is resistant. Effective against both rapidly dividing and semidormant bacteria

b. Mechanism of action: inhibits bacterial RNA polymerase

c. High urine concentrations, passes freely into renal cavities, high prostate concentrations, also enters macrophages[75]

d. Adverse reactions

1) Major risk is liver toxicity[75]

2) All get orange discoloration of body fluids (urine, sweat, tears, sputum)

e. Drug interactions: induces cytochrome P450 enzymes, so can reduce levels of many other drugs to subtherapeutic. Relevant drugs include several anti-AIDS drugs, also steroids, cyclosporine and tacrolimus[82]

6. Pyrazinamine

a. First-line drug unless resistant; especially active against dormant and semidormant bacteria. Exact mechanism unknown; may inhibit fatty acid synthase[75]

b. High concentrations in urine and prostate

c. Adverse reactions

1) Serious reactions uncommon

2) Up to 40% get arthralgia; most respond to NSAIDs

3) It is expected to increase serum uric acid levels

a) Known gout is a contraindication to use

b) Serum uric acid levels demonstrate compliance

c) European guidelines recommend giving a xanthine oxidase inhibitor[82]

7. Ethambutol

a. First-line drug unless resistant. Active against actively dividing bacteria. Exact mechanism unknown, may inhibit mycobacterial cell wall synthesis[75]

b. About 80% excreted unchanged in urine, also enters macrophages

c. The only major adverse reaction is retrobulbar neuritis. Follow visual acuity and red/green color discrimination

8. Second-line drugs are used if the organism is resistant to the first-line drugs or if the patient cannot tolerate the first-line drugs. Examples: cycloserine, ethionamide, streptomycin, amikacin, kanamycin, capreomoycin, para-amino salicylic acid, levofloxacin

G. Surgery

In all situations except stent or percutaneous drainage to relieve renal obstruction, patients should have at least 4 weeks of extensive drug therapy before surgery.[75,82,88,89]

1. Indications for nephrectomy

a. Persistent symptoms

b. Coexisting renal carcinoma

c. Extensive disease with hypertension and UPJ obstruction

d. Nonfunctioning kidney used to be an indication for nephrectomy, but recent thought is that an asymptomatic nonfunctioning kidney can be left in place[75]

2. Role of partial nephrectomy is controversial

a. Usually used only for calcified lesions

b. The clearest indications are a localized calcified lesion that does not respond to drug therapy,[75,82] or is growing and threatening to destroy the entire kidney[75]

3. Epididymectomy is indicated if the lesion fails drug therapy or if the exam is suspicious for testis cancer. Procedure:[75]

a. Remove epididymis through scrotal incision, starting with the globus minor

b. Bring the vas end out through a separate stab incision in the groin, to prevent abscess formation

4. Ureteral stricture:

a. Stent is the best initial treatment (or percutaneous tube if stent cannot be passed)

b. Oral drug therapy ± percutaneous irrigation with drugs

c. If distal stricture does not improve after 3 weeks drug therapy, some authors add corticosteroids[75]

d. For persistent distal strictures, reimplant (psoas hitch or Boari flap if needed)

5. Augmentation cystoplasty or conduit diversion may be considered for persistent contracted bladder after intensive drug therapy[75,89,90]

6. Open surgery for abscesses should not be attempted. Abscess should be drained percutaneously[75,82]

13. References

1. Schaeffer AJ and Schaeffer EM. Infections of the urinary tract. In: Wein AJ, Kavoussi LR, Novick AC, Partin AW, Peters CA, eds. *Campbell-Walsh Urology*. 9th ed. Philadelphia, PA: Saunders Elsevier: 2007:223-303.
2. McLaughlin SP, Carson CC. Urinary tract infections in women. *Med Clin North Am*. 2004;88(2):417.
3. Nicolle L, Anderson PA, Conly J, et al. Uncomplicated urinary tract infection in women. Current practice and the effect of antibiotic resistance on empiric treatment. *Can Fam Physician*. 2006;52:612.
4. *Physicians' Desk Reference*. 61st ed. 2007; 1578.
5. Fihn SD. Acute uncomplicated urinary tract infection in women. *N Engl J Med*. 2003;349:259.
6. Cunha BA. New uses for older antibiotics: nitrofurantoin, amikacin, colistin, polymyxin B, doxycycline, and minocycline revisited. *Med Clin North Am*. Nov 2006;90(6):1089.
7. *Physicians' Desk Reference*. 61st ed. 2007; 3488.
8. Schaeffer AJ. The expanding role of fluoroquinolones. *Am J Med*. 2002;113(suppl 1A):45S.
9. Turnidge J. Pharmacodynamics and dosing of aminoglycosides. *Inf Dis Clin North Am*. 2003; 17:503.
10. Moellering RC. Linezolid: the first ozaxolidinone antimicrobial. *Annals Int Med*. 2003;138:135.
11. *Physicians' Desk Reference*. 61st ed. 2007; 1026.
12. Stamm WE, et al. Causes of the acute urethral syndrome in women. *N Engl J Med*. 1980;303:409.
13. Kucheria R, Dasgupta P, Sacks SH, et al. Urinary tract infections: new insights into a common problem. *Postgrad Med J*. 2005;81:83.
14. Saemann MD, Weichhart T, et al. Tamm-Horsfall protein: a multilayered defence molecule against urinary tract infection. *Eur J Clin Invest*. 2005;35:227.
15. Kaper JB, Nataro JP, Mobley HLT. Pathogenic *Escherichia coli*. *Nature Reviews/Microbiology*. 2004;2:123.
16. Johnson JR. Microbial virulence determinants and the pathogenesis of urinary tract infection. *Inf Dis Clin North Am*. 2003;17:261.
17. Stapleton A. Novel approaches to prevention of urinary tract infections. *Inf Dis Clin North Am*. 2003;17:457.
18. Anderson GG, et al. Host subversion by formation of intracellular bacterial communities lin the urinary tract. *Microbes and Infection*. 2004;6:1094.
19. Cardozo L, Lose G, McClish D, et al. A systematic review of estrogens for recurrent urinary tract infections: third report of the hormones and urogenital therapy (HUT) committee. *Int Urogynecology J*. 2001;12:15.
20. Ballagh SA. Vaginal hormone therapy for urogenital and menopausal symptoms. *Sem Reprod Med*. 2005;23:126.
21. Pinggera GM, et al. Effects of local estrogen therapy on recurrent urinary tract infections in young females under oral contraceptives. *Eur Urol*. 2005;47:243.
22. De Alleaume L, et al. Clinical inquiries: When are empiric antibiotics appropriate for urinary tract infection symptoms? *J Fam Pract*. 2006;55:338.
23. Wright OR, Safranek S. Urine dipstick for diagnosing urinary tract infection. *Am Fam Physician*. 2006;73:129.

24. Richards D, Toop L, Chambers S, Fletcher L. Response to antibiotics of women with symptoms of urinary tract infection but negative dipstick urine test results: double-blind randomized controlled trial. *BMJ*. 2005;331:143.

25. Ravel R. *Clinical Laboratory Medicine*. St. Louis, MO: Mosby Year-Book; 1995:54.

26. Kass EH. Asymptomatic infections of the urinary tract. *Trans Assoc Am Physicians*. 1956;69:56.

27. Stamm WE, et al. Diagnosis of coliform infection in acutely dysuric women. *N Engl J Med*. 1982;307:463.

28. Hooton TM, et al. Amoxicillin-clavulanate vs ciprofloxacin for the treatment of uncomplicated cystitis in women: a randomized trial. *JAMA*. 2005;293:949.

29. Milo G, Katchman EA, Paul M, et al. Duration of antibacterial treatment for uncomplicated urinary tract infection in women. *Cochrane Database Syst Rev*. 2005 Apr 18;(2)CD 004682.

30. Di Martino P, Agniel R, David K, et al. Reduction of *Escherichia coli* adherence to uroepithelial bladder cells after consumption of cranberry juice: a double-blind randomized placebo-controlled cross-over trial. *World J Urol*. 2006;24:21.

31. Jepson RG, Mihaljevic L, Craig J. Cranberries for preventing urinary tract infections. *Cochrane Database Syst Rev*. 2004;(2):CD001321.

32. Rubenstein JN, Schaeffer AJ. Managing complicated urinary tract infections: the urologic view. *Inf Dis Clin North Am*. 2003;17:333.

33. Scholes D, Hooton TM, Roberts PL, et al. Risk factors associated with acute pyelonephritis in healthy women. *Ann Intern Med*. 2005;142:20.

34. Huang JJ, et al. Emphysematous pyelonephritis: clinicoradiological classification, management, prognosis, and pathogenesis. *Arch Intern Med*. 2000;160:797.

35. Dwivedi US, Goyal NK, Saxena V, et al. Xanthogranulomatous pyelonephritis: our experience with review of published reports. *ANZ J Surg*. 2006;76:1007.

36. Vanderbrink BA, Ost MC, Rastinehad A, et al. Laparoscopic versus open radical nephrectomy for xanthogranulomatous pyelonephritis. *J Endourol*. 2007;21:65.

37. Nicolle LE, et al. Infectious Diseases Society of America guidelines for diagnosis and treatment of asymptomatic bacteriuria in adults. *Clin Inf Dis*. 2005;40:643.

38. Colgan R, Nicolle LE, McGlone A, Hooton TM. Asymptomatic bacteriuria in adults. *Am Fam Physician*. 2006;74:985.

39. Ooi ST, Frazee LA. Gardner WG. Management of asymptomatic bacteriuria in patients with diabetes mellitus. *Ann Pharmacother.* 2004;38:490.

40. Stalam M, Kaye D. Antibiotic agents in the elderly. *Inf Dis Clin North Am*. 2004;18(3):533.

41. Roos V, Ulett GC, Schembri MA, Klemm P. The asymptomatic bacteriuria *Escherichia coli* strain 83972 outcompetes uropathogenic *E coli* strains in human urine. *Infect Immun*. 2006;74:615.

42. Le J, Briggs GG, McKeown A, Bustillo G. Urinary tract infections during pregnancy. *Ann Pharmacother.* 2004;38:1692.

43. Mittal P, et al. Urinary tract infections in pregnancy. *Clin Perinat*. 2005;32(3):749.

44. Macejko A, Schaeffer AJ. Asymptomatic bacteriuria and symptomatic urinary tract infections during pregnancy. *Urol Clin North Am*. 2007 Feb;34:35.

45. Muller AE, Oostvogel PM, Steegers EA, Dorr PJ. Morbidity related to maternal group B streptococcal infections. *Acta Obstet Gynecol Scand*. 2006;85:1027.

46. Centers for Disease Control and Prevention. Prevention of Perinatal Group B Streptococcal Disease. *MMWR*. 2002;51(no. RR-11):1-28.

47. Shrim A, Garcia-Bournissen F, Koren G. Pharmaceutical agents and pregnancy in urology practice. *Urol Clin North Am*. 2007;34:27.

48. No authors listed: Case records of the Massachusetts General Hospital. Weekly clinicopathological exercises. Case 31-2000. A 32-year-old man with a lesion of the urinary bladder. *N Engl J Med*. 2000;343:1105.

49. Nickel JC. Inflammatory conditions of the male genitourinary tract: prostatitis and related conditions, orchitis and epididymitis. In Wein AJ, Kavoussi LR, Novick AC, Partin AW, Peters CA, eds. *Campbell-Walsh Urology*. 9th ed. Philadelphia, PA: Saunders Elsevier; 2007: 304-29.

50. Nickel JC. Recommendations for the evaluation of patients with prostatitis. *World J Urol*. 2003;21:75.

51. Pontari MA, McNaughton Collins M, O'Leary MP, et al. A case control study of risk factors in men with chronic pelvic pain syndrome. *BJU Int*. 2005;96:559.

52. Nadler RB, McNaughton Collins M, Propert KJ, et al. Prostate-specific antigen test in diagnostic evaluation of chronic prostatitis/chronic pelvic pain syndrome. *Urology*. 2006;67:337.

53. Hruz P, Danuser H, Studer UE, Hochreiter WW. Non-inflammatory chronic pelvic pain syndrome can be caused by bladder neck hypertrophy. *Eur Urol*. 2003;44:106.

54. Dimitrakov JD, Kaplan SA, et al. Management of chronic prostatitis/chronic pelvic pain syndrome: an evidence-based approach. *Urology*. 2006;67:881.

55. Alexander RB, Propert KJ, Schaeffer AJ, et al. Ciprofloxacin or tamsulosin in men with chronic prostatitis/chronic pelvic pain syndrome: a randomized, double-blind trial. *Ann Intern Med*. 2004;141:581.

56. Nickel JC, et al. Levofloxacin for chronic prostatitis/chronic pelvic pain syndrome in men: a randomized placebo-controlled multicenter trial. *Urology*. 2003;62:614.

57. Nickel JC, et al. Treatment of chronic prostatitis/chronic pelvic pain syndrome with tamsulosin: a randomized double-blind trial. *J Urol*. 2004;171:1594.

58. Mehik A, Alas P, Nickel JC, et al. Alfuzosin treatment for chronic prostatitis/chronic pelvic pain syndrome: a prospective, randomized, double-blind, placebo-controlled pilot study. *Urology*. 2003;62:425.

59. Cheah PY, et al. Terazosin therapy for chronic prostatitis/chronic pelvic pain syndrome: a randomized placebo-controlled trial. *J Urol*. 2003; 169:592.

60. Yang G, Wei Q, Li H, et al. The effect of alpha-adrenergic antagonists in chronic prostatitis/chronic pelvic pain syndrome: a meta-analysis of randomized controlled trials. *J Androl*. 2006;27:847

61. Leskinen M, Lukkarinen O, Marttila T. Effects of finasteride in patients with inflammatory chronic pelvic pain syndrome: a double-blind, placebo-controlled pilot study. *Urology*. 1999;53:502.

62. Nickel JC. et al. A randomized placebo-controlled multicenter study to evaluate the safety and efficacy of finasteride for male chronic pain syndrome (category IIIA chronic nonbacterial prostatitis). *BJU International* .2004;93:991.

63. Kaplan SA, Volpe M, Te AE. A prospective, 1-year trial using saw palmetto versus finasteride in the treatment of category III prostatitis/chronic pelvic pain syndrome. *J Urol*. 2004;171:284.

64. Nickel JC, Pontari M, Moon T, et al. A randomized, placebo-controlled multicenter study to evaluate the safety and efficacy of rofecoxib in the treatment of chronic nonbacterial prostatitis. *J Urol*. 2003;169:1401.

65. Bates SM, et al. A prospective, randomized, double-blind trial to evaluate the role of a short reducing course of oral corticosteroid therapy in the treatment of chronic prostatitis/chronic pelvic pain syndrome. *BJU Int*. 2007;99:355.

66. Shoskes DA, Zeitlin SI, Shahed A, Rajfer J. Quercitin in men with category III chronic prostatitis: a preliminary prospective, double-blind, placebo-controlled trial. *Urology*. 1999;54:960.

67. Lee CB, Ha US, Lee SJ, et al. Preliminary experience with a terpene mixture versus ibuprofen for treatment of category III chronic prostatitis/chronic pelvic pain syndrome. *World J Urol*. 2006;24:55.

68. Hetrick DC, Glazer H, et al. Pelvic floor electromyography in men with chronic pelvic pain syndrome: a case-control study. *Neurourol Urodyn*. 2006;25:46.

69. Anderson RU, Wise D, Sawyer T, Chan C. Sexual dysfunction in men with chronic prostatitis/chronic pelvic pain syndrome: improvement after trigger point release and paradoxical relaxation training. *J Urol*. 2006;176:1534.

70. Clemens JQ, Nadler RB, et al. Biofeedback, pelvic floor re-education, and bladder training for male chronic pelvic pain syndrome. *Urology*. 2000;56:951.

71. Cornel EB, van Haarst EP, et al. The effect of biofeedback physical therapy in men with chronic pelvic pain syndrome type III. *Eur Urol*. 2005;47:607.

72. Nickel JC, Forrest JB, Tomera K, et al. Pentosan polysulfate sodium therapy for men with chronic pelvic pain syndrome: a multicenter, randomized, placebo controlled study. *J Urol*. 2005;173:1252.

73. Paick JS, Lee SC, Ku JH. More effects of extracorporeal magnetic innervation and terazosin therapy than terazosin therapy alone for non-inflammatory chronic pelvic pain syndrome: a pilot study. *Prostate Cancer Prostatic Dis*. 2006;9:261.

74. Turini D, et al. Heat/burning sensation induced by topical application of capsaicin on perineal cutaneous area: new approach in diagnosis and treatment of chronic prostatitis/chronic pelvic pain syndrome? *Urology*. 2006;67:910.

75. McAleer SJ, Johnson CW, Johnson WD. Tuberculosis and parasitic and fungal infections of the genitourinary system. In: Wein AJ, Kavoussi LR, Novick AC, Partin AW, Peters CA, eds. *Campbell-Walsh Urology*. 9th ed. Philadelphia, PA: Saunders Elsevier; 2007: 436-70.

76. Kauffman CA. Candiduria. *Clin Infect Dis*. 2005;41: S371.

77. Pappas PG, Rex JH, Sobel JD, et al. Guidelines for treatment of candidiasis. *Clin Infect Dis*. 2004;38: 161.

78. Bennett JE. Echinocandins for candidemia in adults without neutropenia. *N Engl J Med*. 2006;355:1154.

79. Boucher H, Groll AH, Chiou CC, Walsh TJ. Newer systemic antifungal agents: pharmacokinetics, safety and efficacy. *Drugs*. 2004;64:1997.

80. Magill SS, Swoboda SM, Johnson EA, et al. The association between anatomic site of Candida colonization, invasive candidiasis, and mortality in critically ill surgical patients. *Diagn Microbiol Infect Dis*. 2006;55:293.

81. Bastide C, Carcenac A, Arrova F, Rossi D. Prostatic abscess due to *Candida tropicalis*. *Prostate Cancer Prostatic Dis*. 2005;8:296.

82. Cek M, Lenk S, Naber KG, et al. EAU guidelines for the management of genitourinary tuberculosis. *Eur Urol*. 2005;48:353.

83. Pommerville PJ, Zakus P, van der Westhuizen N, et al. Tuberculosis of the bladder without previous renal infection. *Can J Urol.* 2006;13:3044.

84. Madeb R, Marshall J, Nativ O, Erturk E. Epididymal tubersulosis: case report and review of the literature. *Urology.* 2005;65:798.

85. Kim SH: Urogenital tuberculosis. In: Pollack HM, McClennan BL, eds. *Clinical Urography.* 2nd ed. Philadelphia, PA: W.B. Saunders Co; 2000,:1192-1228.

86. Wang LJ, Wu CF, Wong YC, et al. Imaging findings of urinary tuberculosis on excretory urography and computerized tomography. *J Urol.* 2003;169:524.

87. Centers for Disease Control and Prevention. Treatment of Tuberculosis, American Thoracic Society, CDC, and Infectious Diseases Society of America. *MMWR.* 2003;52(no.RR-11);1-88.

88. Porter MP, Eubank WB, Krieger JN. Genitourinary tuberculosis: a focused review. *Contemp Urol.* 2001;13:34.

89. Gupta NP, Kumar R, Mundada OP, et al. Reconstructive surgery for the management of genitourinary tuberculosis: a single center experience. *J Urol.* 2006;175:2150.

90. de Figueiredo AA, Lucon AM, Srougi M. Bladder augmentation for the treatment of chronic tuberculous cystitis. Clinical and urodynamic evaluation of 25 patients after long term follow-up. *Neurourol Urodyn.* 2006;25:433.

14. Questions

1. Which operation for GU tubercuclosis does not require extensive drug therapy first?

A. Complete nephrectomy

B. Partial nephrectomy

C. Stent for ureteral stricture

D. Reimplant ureter for stricture

E. Epididymectomy

2. Which antituberculous agent decreases blood levels of anti-HIV protease inhibitors?

A. Isoniazid (INH)

B. Rifampin

C. Pyrazinamine

D. Ethambutol

E. Cycloserine

3. Which antibiotic may cause severe peripheral neuropathy?

A. Nitrofurantoin

B. TMP/SMX

C. Amoxicillin/clavulanate

D. Levofloxacin

E. Cephalexin

4. All of the following are good choices for acute uncomplicated cystitis, except:

A. 3 days fluoroquinolone

B. 3 days TMP/SMX

C. 3 days trimethoprim

D. 3 days ampicillin

E. 7 days nitrofurantoin

5. Asymptomatic bacteriuria needs to be treated in which population?

A. Patients with indwelling catheters

B. Diabetics

C. Elderly people

D. Mentally retarded people

E. Pregnant women

6. A patient with invasive *Candida* pyelonephritis started treatment with amphotericin B and is miserable with rigors, chills and fever. All of the following are good options for this patient, except:

A. Continue amphotericin B and pre-treat with ibuprofen

B. Change to the liposomal form of amphotericin B

C. Change to 5-fluorocytosine

D. Change to caspofungin

E. Change to voriconazole

Answers

1. C.

2. B.

3. A.

4. D.

5. E.

6. C.

Chapter 24: Renal and Ureteral Trauma

Allen F. Morey, MD, FACS

Contents

1. Renal Trauma

Mechanism of Injury

Blunt Trauma

Cause of more than 90% of renal injuries (usually motor vehicle collisions, vehicle pedestrian accidents, sports injuries); usually contusions or minor lacerations amenable to nonoperative management. Major blunt renal injuries usually associated with other major injuries of the head, chest and/or abdomen (avg 3+).

Penetrating Renal Injuries

Penetrating renal injuries (stab wounds, gunshot wounds) associated with a much higher degree of renal damage than blunt injuries.

Diagnosis of Renal Injury

Clinical Indicators of Major Renal Injury

- Rib or vertebral body fractures
- Direct blow to flank
- Abdominal mass or tenderness
- Flank pain or ecchymosis

Hematuria is an Imperfect Indicator of Renal Injury

- Amount of hematuria does not correlate to severity of renal injury
- Minor, completely benign renal injuries (contusion) often present with gross hematuria
- While deep renal lacerations are often found to produce gross hematuria, major renal injury (or renovascular injury may occur in the absence of hematuria as well

Children

- More susceptible to renal trauma than adults: less cushioning by perirenal fat, underdeveloped rib cage, less protection by muscles of flank and abdomen. Abnormal kidneys, such as those with congenital hydronephrosis due to UPJ obstruction, are more prone to major injury in the context of seemingly trivial trauma
- Hypotension not reliable in children: outpouring of catecholamines can maintain BPin spite of significant blood loss
- Consider UPJ disruption (more common in children because of their increased flexibility and renal mobility; Table 1)

Contrasted Renal CT: Imaging Study of Choice

- 2 phase study with initial vascular/cortical phase roughly 30 seconds after IV contrast infusion, second (delayed) phase scan at 10 minutes to document the finding of perirenal or ureteral contrast extravasation
- Advantages: excellent anatomic detail, depth and location of renal laceration, magnitude of perirenal hematoma or urinoma, associated abdominal injuries; presence and location of contralateral kidney, appropriate for blunt or penetrating trauma in stable patients (Figure 1)
- Beware that rapid sequence helical CT scans may miss urinary extravasation without delayed cuts. Repeat CT imaging for Grade 4 injuries is warranted after 48 hours due to the potential for perirenal fluid accumulation

Figure 1

Left renal stab wound with Grade 3 injury successfully managed nonoperatively

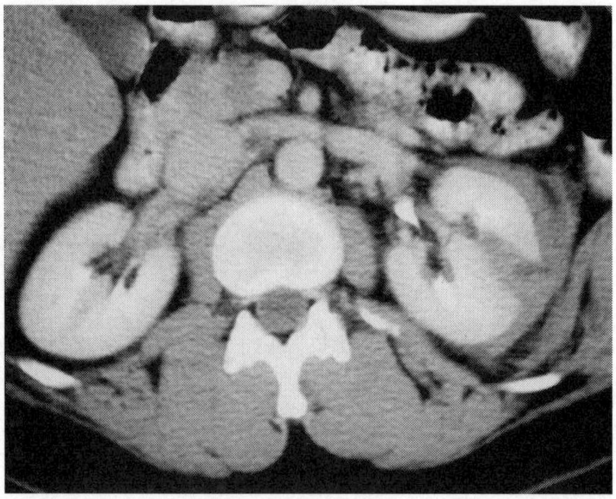

Table 1

Suspected Renal Injury?

Indications for Imaging

Blunt Trauma: Adults	
Gross hematuria	
Microhematuria (5+ RBC/HPF) plus hypotension (systolic BP <90 mm Hg)	
Rapid deceleration	
Blunt Trauma: Children	
Gross hematuria or significant microhematuria (50+ RBC/HPF)	
Multisystem trauma	
Penetrating Trauma	
All with any degree of hematuria after penetrating abdominal, flank or thoracic injury.	
Clinical suspicion based on entrance or exit wound (regardless of hematuria)	
When is Immediate Imaging Not Required (Significant Renal Injury <2%)?	
Adults with isolated microhematuria (no evidence of shock)	
Children with isolated insignificant microhematuria (<50 RBC/HPF) without signs of multisystem trauma	

- IVP has an extremely low yield and rarely alters patient management in blunt trauma

- Ultrasound not reliable for imaging renal trauma

Major Renal Injury, Such as UPJ Disruption or Arterial Thrombosis, May Occur Without Hematuria

However, these injuries are almost always due to rapid deceleration injury or multisystem trauma which warrant abdominal imaging.

- UPJ disruption: look for nonvisualization of distal ureter on 10 minute delayed scan

- Traumatic thrombosis of the renal artery (Figure 2) or its branches occurs because the media and adventitia of the renal artery are more elastic than the intima. Intimal tear produces thrombosis and occlusion with complete or segmental renal ischemia

Unstable Patients

Penetrating abdominal trauma is associated with a higher incidence of associated intraabdominal injury, many of which require immediate laparotomy.

Figure 2

Traumatic thrombosis of left renal artery results in renal ischemia

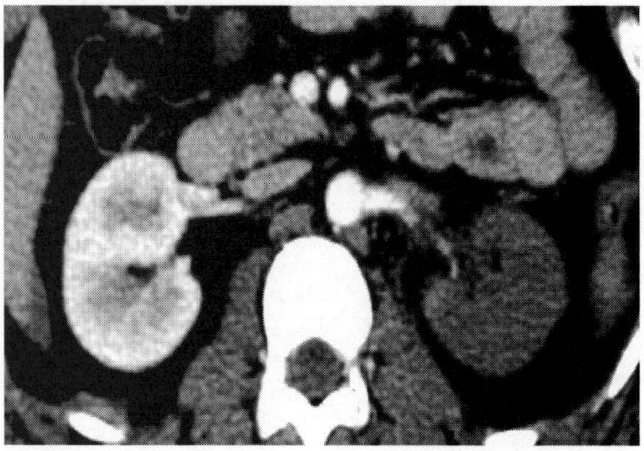

Patient remained stable without intervention

(Grade 4 injury) due to peripheral perfusion from capsular collateral vessels; found at least 8 hours after the time of injury. A conservative approach is warranted since renal salvage is unlikely after prolonged ischemia of this duration.

Forniceal Rupture

Forniceal rupture is a benign finding after blunt trauma which may masquerade as a major renal injury because it produces medial urinary extravasation on CT scan (Figure 3). In forniceal rupture, renal laceration is absent, perirenal hematoma is absent and the ureter is well visualized. No therapy is warranted.

Therapeutic Angioembolization

Therapeutic angioembolization has become recognized as a safe and effective means of controlling significant bleeding after renal trauma. This strat-

- *Single shot IVP.* Best performed intraoperatively, when no preliminary CT obtained—bolus IV injection of 2 cc/kg contrast followed by single 10 minute film; helpful in staging patients with multiple penetrating abdominal wounds, or in presence of unexpected retroperitoneal hematoma discovered during trauma laparotomy. Obscured renal outline suggests injury. Single shot IVP is best used to guide exploration of penetrating injuries (ie, solitary or ectopic kidney) or confirm nonoperative management of blunt injuries

Injury Classification and Interventions

The American Association forthe Surgery of Trauma Renal Injury Scaling System

The American Association for the Surgery of Trauma renal injury scaling system is used widely with well established prognostic value. Injury classification is accomplished by either abdominal CT or direct renal exploration (Table 2). The odds of renal surgery are increased by 15-fold for every increase in grade; the odds of nephrectomy increase by 7-fold with each increase in grade.

Cortical Rim Sign

The "cortical rim sign" is a radiographic finding associated with acute renal arterial thrombosis

Table 2

AAST Renal Injury Grading Scale

Grade	
Grade 1	Contusion or subcapsular hematoma (no laceration)
Grade 2	Cortical laceration <1 cm deep, no extravasation
Grade 3	Cortical laceration >1 cm, no extravasation
Grade 4	Laceration: >1cm deep, into collecting system, or Vascular: Thrombosed renal artery or segmental vein injury
Grade 5	Laceration: Shattered kidney, or Vascular: Renal pedicle avulsion

egy is generally employed in stable patients who demonstrate persistant bleeding from a segmemntal arterial injury. More significant injuries require operative intervention to prevent life-threatening hemorrhage.

Indications For Exploration

The only absolute indication for renal exploration is hemodynamic instability from renal injury with associated findings such as large, expanding or pulsatile retroperitoneal hematoma.

Renal Exploration After Trauma is Undertaken Selectively

Goals of renal exploration are either: a) treatment of major renal injuries, or b) evaluation of suspected renal injury when detailed imaging is unavailable. Unnecessary or prolonged renal exploration must be avoided in the critically ill patient.

GU Management of Renal Injury

GU management of renal injury is influenced, but not dictated by the decision of trauma surgeons to explore or observe associated abdominal injuries. It is perfectly acceptable to decline exploration of an injured kidney even when the abdomen is open if radiographic features are indicative of an injury that may be safely observed. Unnecessary renal exploration may result in unnecessary nephrectomy.

- If immediate laparotomy is otherwise unnecessary, a conservative urological approach is selected ini tially. Observation alone is appropriate for all minor renal injuries (Grade 1-3), which will resolve spontaneously nearly always

- The presence of an expanding or pulsatile hematoma in an unstable patient should warrant immediate renal exploration. If laparotomy is undertaken, relative indications for renal exploration include major renal injuries (Grade 4+) or renal imaging. which is absent or inconclusive.

Associated/Predictive Features of Failed Non-operative Management

- Increasing AAST Organ Injury Scale grade

- Nephrectomy is performed in 4% of blunt and 21% of penetrating injuries

Figure 3

Forniceal rupture and renal contusion in solitary right kidney after blunt trauma

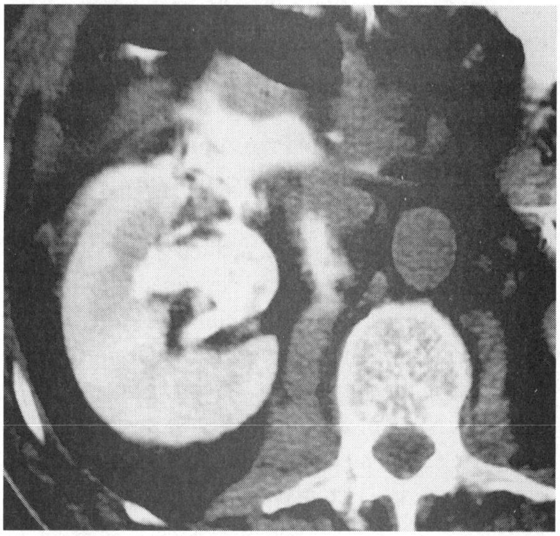

- Gunshot wounds are 6 times more likely to result in nephrectomy than stab wound.

- Transfusion requirement.

- Presence of shock at admission.

- Nonrenal abdominal operation or major abdominal vascular injury.

- Increased perirenal hematoma size (>3 cm) and presence of intravascular contrast extravasation into hematoma are radiographic signs on CT which appear to be associated with need for therapeutic angioembolization to control ongoing renal bleeding.

- Gunshot wounds often produce extensive tissue destruction via blast effect; clinical course often unpredictable and usually warrants exploration unless imaging suggests renal injury is minor.

- Stab wounds of the abdomen and flank increasingly being successfully managed nonoperatively (roughly 50%), particularly if the entrance wound is posterior to the anterior axillary line.

Renal Exploration and Reconstruction

Midline Transabdominal Incision

Repair of major visceral and vascular injuries other than those involving the kidney should usually be performed first. If renal hemorrhage is massive and life threatening, the kidney must be explored initially and other injuries secondarily.

Early Vascular Control Proximal to Injury

Early vascular control proximal to injury has been associated with increased rates of renal salvage. Access to the renal vascular pedicle is best obtained through the posterior parietal peritoneum, which is incised over the aorta, just medial to the inferior mesenteric vein. The aorta is traced superiorly until the left renal vein is identified crossing anteriorly. The left renal vein is then elevated exposing both underlying renal arteries. Vessel loops are placed around the vessels supplying the injured kidney to facilitate occlusion, should the need arise.

Once control of the vessels is obtained, the colon is reflected medially to expose the kidney. Should a great deal of blood loss be encountered, immediate vascular control may be obtained by occlusion of the ipsilateral renal artery. Warm ischemia time should be limited to 30 minutes. Once the kidney is exposed, the hematoma is swept away and the entire surface and collecting system of the kidney are inspected systematically.

Renal lacerations are debrided and oversewn with 30 absorbable capsular sutures. Large segmental vessels are suture ligated, and exposed collecting system is closed primarily with fine absorbable suture. Hemostasis is facilitated by application of absorbable collagen or gelatin sponge bolsters. Once the bleeding has been controlled, the open margins of the kidney are reapproximated and the renal capsule closed. If polar lacerations produce large areas of devitalized tissue, heminephrectomy is the best course of action. The area of reconstruction is covered by perirenal fat or a pedicle flap of omentum in order to insure against urinary leakage. A Penrose (nonsuction type) drain is placed in the dependant portion of the wound. Suction drains may promote or exacerbate urinary leakage.

Renal vascular injuries require prompt and efficient treatment. In the event of traumatic renal artery occlusion, arterial reconstruction is performed via end to end anastomosis, autotransplantation, or various graft techniques. These maneuvers must be performed within 3 hours of the time of injury to be successful, and even in the best of hands often yield poor outcomes. Renal vein injuries may be managed be simple ligation or direct repair. Cooling of the kidney during vascular reconstruction is not appro priate during the trauma setting. In the event of penetrating injury to the renal pedicle, immediate nephrectomy is often the best solution in the presence of a normal contralateral kidney.

Nephrectomy is performed as a life-saving maneuver undertaken in the event of irreparable renal laceration or pedicle injury in the setting of hemodynamic instability. As an alternative to immediate nephrectomy, if the patient is hypothermic, acidotic, and coagulopathic, a "damage control" approach may be employed with initial packing of the renal fossa and subsequent pack removal, irrigation, and repair after correction of metabolic disturbances in selected cases.

Complications of Renal Trauma

Urinary Extravasation After Blunt Trauma

Urinary extravasation after blunt trauma usually resolves spontaneously and warrants no specific immediate therapy; if persistent after 3+ days, ureteral stent placement with foley catheter is indicated. Percutaneous drainage is usually not justified.

- Presence of >25% devitalized renal tissue with extravasation has higher risk of complications and has been noted as a relative indication for exploration although perirenal abscess or urinoma are now usually well managed by percutaneous drainage.

Delayed Retroperitoneal Bleeding

Delayed retroperitoneal bleeding may occur within several weeks of an injury and be life threatening. Arteriovenous fistulas present with delayed onset of significant gross hematuria; audible bruit may be noted on abdominal auscultation. Penetrating injuries account for most cases of renal AV fistula.

- Arteriography: use indicated in stable patients with delayed or persistent bleeding from a renal laceration or stab wound (and no other indication for laparatomy), in conjunction with selective embolization (devitalized tissue <20%) Percutaneous angiographic embolization is the initial treatment of choice for symptomatic AV fistulas (80% effective); surgical correction may be required for larger fistulas.

Hypertension After Renal Injury

Although cortical scars often develop after high grade renal injuries, hypertension after renal injury is rare, but may occur either acutely as a result of external compression (Page kidney) or may be renin mediated as a late complication. Medical management is preferable and usually successful. If medical control proves difficult, surgical correction or nephrectomy are indicated. Nuclear renal scans are useful as a means of documenting recovery of function after trauma.

2. Ureteral Trauma

Injury Detection (Table 3)

Diagnosis of Ureteral Injury

Ureteral injury may be difficult to diagnose since hematuria and retroperitoneal hematoma may be absent in about one third of cases). Most occur in the context of penetrating abdominal injury or in conjunction with major abdominal or pelvic surgery

- Although no single test reliably excludes a ureteral laceration, a CT with 10 minute delayed films is likely to demonstrate extravasation (Figure 4). If IVP is obtained, delayed films are usually necessary to establish the diagnosis. Retrograde pyelography is excellent but often impractical in the setting of acute trauma.

- Missed or delayed diagnosis carries with it substantial morbidity and mortality. High index of suspicion is required to detect contusion, especially if bullet path near ureter. Penetrating injury to common iliac vessels or bladder should arouse suspicion of ureteral injury.

- Direct inspection during laparotomy is ideal when ureteral injury is suspected. Antegrade (intrapelvic) or retrograde (intraureteral) injection of methylene blue or indigo carmine with gentle ureteral occlusion may be used to distend the ureter and identify leak. If normal efflux seen from ureteral orifice during cystotomy, ureteral injury is unlikely.

Table 3

Ureteral Injuries at a Glance

1. High index of suspicion warranted—often not associated with hematuria
2. Rarely isolated injury, nearly always iatrogenic or due to penetrating trauma
3. Often missed by IVP or rapid sequence CT—remember delayed films!
4. Direct inspection during laparotomy is best when ureteral injury is suspected

UPJ Disruption
Radiographic hallmarks of diagnosis on CT are a medial and periureteral pattern of contrast extravasation with nonvisualization of ipsilateral distal ureter.

Management

Immediate diagnosis and immediate repair is best, whenever possible, whether in the setting of iatrogenic ligation or laceration.or in the setting of external trauma. Delayed diagnosis often occurs, however, and thus requires individualized treatment based on patient condition and length of delay.

- <5 days, consider immediate repair

- >5+ days since injury, sepsis, debilitated patient? Best to drain urinoma percutaneously and place nephrostomy tube or ureteral stent in conjunction with delayed elective repair as needed

Ureteral Contusion
Because endoscopic stent placement is often unwieldly during trauma laparotomy, empiric ureteral stent placement through a small cystotomy is prudent when ureteral contusion is noted after trauma. If ischemia of ureteral wall appears more pronounced, consider focal defect resection with stented primary ureteroureterostomy.

Ureteral Exploration
Midline incision most versatile. Allows all types of repair from ureteroureterostomy to autotransplantation to nephrectomy. Minimize ureteral mobilization to preserve blood supply. Easily located crossing common iliac artery.

Types of Repair
Ureteroureterostomy. Judicious debridement, direct repair over ureteral stent is preferred approach for cases with short defect in abdominal ureter. Goal of primary repair is tension-free, spatulated, stented, watertight, end-to-end anastomosis. Fine absorbable sutures (such as 5-0 PDS) are best. Generally avoided below iliac vessels in lieu of ureteral reimplantation due to less robust ureteral blood supply distally. Usually performed in the setting of penetrating traumatic injury.

Psoas hitch and reimplant. Recommended procedure for extensive distal injuries, with or without a Boari bladder flap. Requires normal bladder capacity and elasticity; should easily reach to level of L-5. May be combined with downward nephropexy to engage bladder flap onto higher levels of the ureter. Direct ureteral reimplant may be performed without psoas hitch when distal ureter is injured near bladder. A large caliber, tension-free, stented, refluxing ureteral reimplant anastomosis is preferred.

Transureteroureterostomy. Best used only for long ureteral defects in the mid or lower ureter complicated by severe scar, abscess, extravasation, or delayed diagnosis. Should not be used in patient with history of stone disease or advanced pelvic malignancy.

Autotransplant. Rarely needed, but is alternative to nephrectomy in the event of extensive ureteral injuries, such as ureteral avulsion consequent to ureteroscopic extraction of impacted upper tract stone.

Ileal or appendiceal interposition. May be useful for delayed reconstruction of extensive middle or upper ureteral defects. As a general rule, it is best to use other urinary tract structures for ureteral preferentially over bowel segments due to potential risks of mucous production, infection, malignancy and bowel complications.

Damage control. In unstable patients, delayed reconstruction often advised after initial stabilization by ureteral ligation over feeding tube or long (90 cm) single J stent brought out to skin. Delayed ureteral reconstruction may then be perfomred when the patient is stable.

Ureterocalycostomy. Recommended after failed UPJ repair where proximal renal pelvis cannot be engaged. Ureter is sewn to lower pole calyx after resection of overlying parenchyma.

3. References

1. McAninch JW, Carroll PR, Klosterman PW. Renal reconstruction after injury. *J Urol.* 1991;145:932-937.

2. Miller KS, McAninch JW. Radiographic assessment of renal trauma: Our 15 year experience. *J Urol.* 1995;154:352.

3. Morey AF, Bruce JE, McAninch JW. Efficacy of radiographic imaging in pediatric blunt renal trauma. *J Urol.* 1996;156:2014-2018.

4. Boone TB, Gilling PJ, Husmann DA. Uretero-pelvic junction disruption following blunt abdominal trauma. *J Urol.* 1993;150:33-36.

5. Perez Brayfield MR, Keane TE, Krishnan A, Lafontaine P, Feliciano DV, Clarke HS. Gunshot wounds to the ureter: a 40 year experience at Grady Memorial Hospital. *J Urol.* 2001;166;119-121.

6. Brown SL, Hoffman DM, Spirnak JP. Limitations of routine spiral computerized tomography in the evaluation of blunt renal trauma. *J Urol.* 1998;160:1979-1981.

7. Armenakas NA, Duckett CP, McAninch JW. Indications for nonoperative management of renal stab wounds. *Journal of Urology.* 1999;161:768-771.

8. Morey AF, McAninch JW, Tiller BK, Duckett CP, Carroll PR. Single shot intraoperative excretory urography for the immmediate evaluation of renal trauma. *J Urol.* 1999;161:1088-1092.

9. Santucci RA, McAninch JW, Safir M, Mario LA, Service S, Segal MR. Validation of the American Association for the Surgery of Trauma Organ Injury Severity Scale for the Kidney. *J Trauma.* 2001;50:195-200.

10. Ali ali M, Haddad LF. The late treatment of 63 overlooked or complicated ureteral missile injuries: the promise of nephrostomy and role of autotransplantation. *J Urol.* 1996;156:1918-1921.

11. Brandes S, Coburn M, Armenakas N, McAninch JW. Diagnosis and management of ureteric injury: an evidence based analysis. *BJU Intl.* 2004;94:277-283.

12. Elliott SP, McAninch JW. Ureteral injuries from external violence: The 25 year experience at San Francisco General Hospital. *J Urol.* 2003;170:1213.

13. Wright JL, Nathens AB, Rivara FP, Wessels H. Renal and extrarenal predictors of nehprectomy from the National Trauma Data Bank. *J Urol.* 2006;175:970-975.

14. Buckley JC, McAninch JW. Selective management of Isolated and nonisolated Grade IV renal injuries. *J Urol.* 2006;176:2498-2502.

4. Questions

1. A 1 cm segment of left middle third ureter is lacerated completely during an elective left colectomy. The injury is recognized intraoperatively, the tissues appear viable, and the patient is stable. The best choice for management is:

   A. Transureteroureterostomy over a stent

   B. Ureteroneocystostomy

   C. Ileal ureter interposition

   D. Ureteroureterostomy over a stent

   E. Ureteral ligation with percutaneous nephrostomy

2. What is the best technique to evaluate microhematuria in a stable patient with a transthoracic gunshot wound?

   A. Abdominal sonography

   B. Intravenous pyelography

   C. Intraoperative one shot IVP

   D. Immediate abdominal CT without IV contrast

   E. Immediate CT with intravenous contrast

3. A stab wound victim is found to have a Grade 2 laceration of the lateral left kidney on abdominal CT with a small perirenal hematoma. Laparotomy is required due to bleeding from a concomitant splenic injury. The patient has received 2 units of blood and is now stable. What is the best course of action for the urologist?

   A. Immediate nephrectomy

   B. Intraoperative one shot IVP

   C. Renal exploration with repair of the laceration

   D. Observation with repeat imaging

   E. Renal angiography with superselective embolization

4. A victim of a posterior stab wound is found to have a lateral Grade 4 right renal laceration on abdominal CT. No other abdominal injuries were identified and no contrast extravasation was identified. The patient has received 3 units of blood and now appears stable. What is the best course of action?

   A. Immediate nephrectomy

   B. Intraoperative one shot IVP

   C. Cystoscopy and retrograde pyelogram

   D. Observation with repeat imaging

   E. Renal angiography with superselective embolization

Answers

1. D.

2. E.

3. D.

4. E.

Chapter 25: Bladder, Urethra and Genital Trauma

Richard A. Santucci, MD

Contents

Introduction

It is the goal of the urologist in a trauma situation to successfully diagnose and treat genitourinary injuries. However, it must be remembered (in practice as well as on the written exams) that the patient's level of hemodynamic stability, the need to search for associated injuries such as spinal cord injury, and the need to mesh urologic studies/treatments together with other required treatments (such as emergency laparotomy) demand a coordinated effort between all the members of the trauma team.

1. Bladder Trauma

Injury Grade

As with all other organs, the American Association for the Surgery of Trauma (AAST) has developed a 5-point injury severity scale. Table 1 lists the AAST organ injury severity scale for the bladder.

Blunt Bladder Injuries

- Rare: <2% of abdominal injuries requiring surgery.[1] Rarity is owed to the protected position of the bladder deep in the bony pelvis[1]
- Severe associated injuries are seen.[2] Mortality occurs frequently (12%-22%)[1,3,4]
- Most commonly after such high-energy situations as automobile versus pedestrian accidents[5]
- Occurs in association with urethral rupture in 10%-29% of patients[6]
- Overwhelmingly associated with pelvic fracture, occurring in 6%-10%[4,5] of pelvic fracture cases, specifically with fracture of the pubic arch[5]

Table 1

American Association for the Surgery of Trauma (AAST) Five-point Injury Severity Scale

Grade[a]		
I	Hematoma Laceration	Contusion, intramural hematoma Partial thickness
II	Laceration	Extraperitoneal bladder wall laceration <2 cm
III	Laceration	Extraperitoneal (≥2 cm) or intraperitoneal (<2cm) bladder wall laceration
IV	Laceration	Intraperitoneal bladder wall laceration ≥2 cm
V	Laceration	Intraperitoneal or extraperitoneal bladder wall laceration extending into the bladder neck or ureteral orifice (trigone)

[a]Advance one grade for multiple lesions up to grade III.
From Moore, et al.[70]

Figure 1

Algorithm for the management of major pelvic trauma

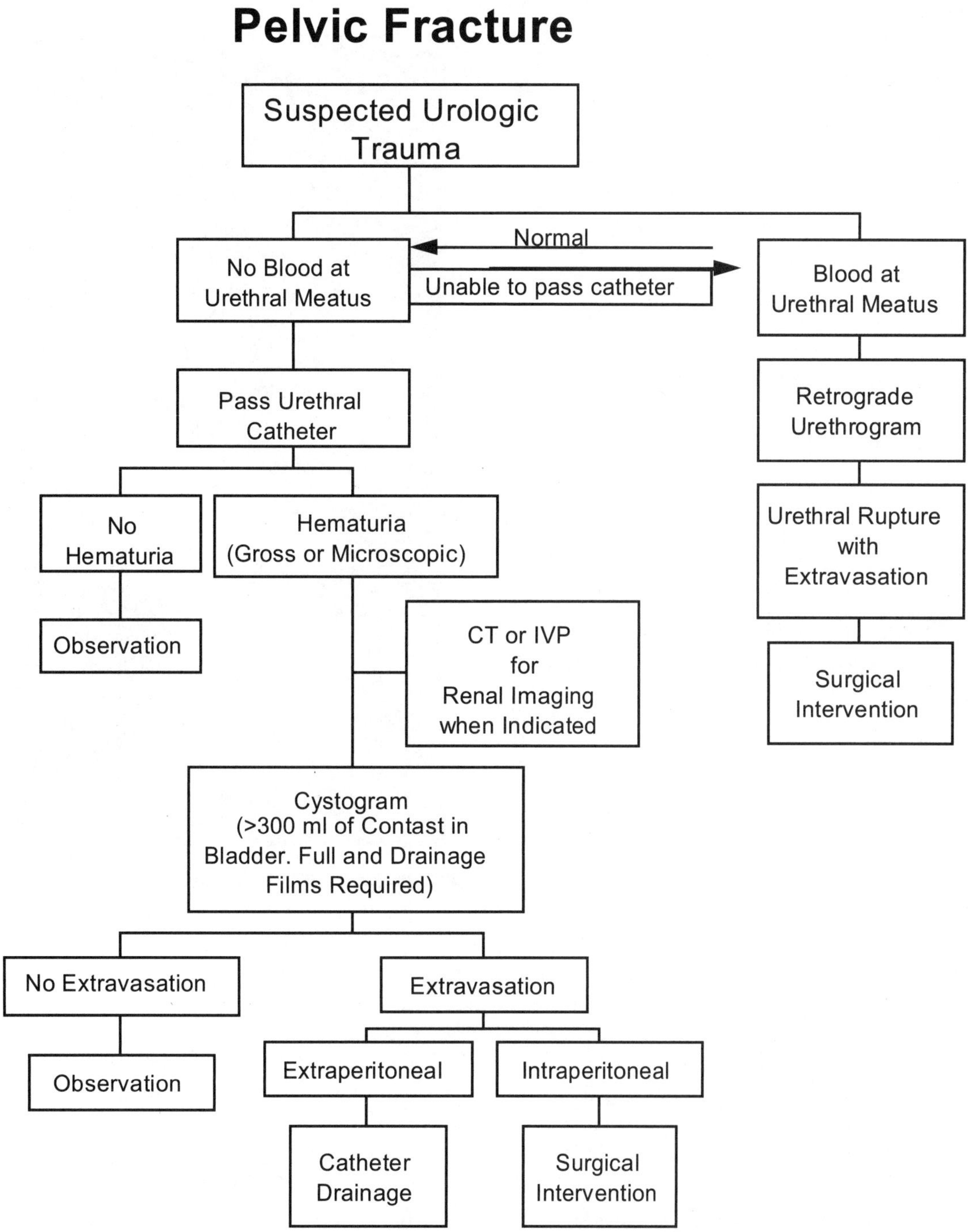

Our algorithm for the management of major pelvic trauma is found in Figure 1

It underscores the major diagnostic goals in these patients:

1. Determine if urethral injury is present.

2. Determine if bladder rupture is present, and classify it as intraperitoneal (requires exploration and repair) or extraperitoneal (can usually be managed by bladder drainage alone) injury.

3. Determine if associated renal injuries are present, and if these injuries require surgical exploration.

Penetrating Bladder Injury

- Wartime incidence 15%-20%.[7] Civilian closer to 2%

- Commonly have associated major abdominal injuries (35%) and often are in shock (22%)[8]

- Mortality in this population is high (12%), usually from acute exsanguination secondary to major pelvic blood vessel transection[8]

Diagnosis

1. Suspicion
   - Usually bladder injury will be implied by the trajectory of the knife or missile wound, and all patients with hematuria at risk for bladder involvement must have formal cystography or intraoperative exploration to rule out bladder involvement

2. Physical signs
   - After blunt trauma, lower abdominal pain, tenderness, and bruising can be present. Often difficult to differentiate from the sequellae of pelvic fracture
   - Some intraperitoneal ruptures are discovered because a urethral catheter does not return urine
   - Delayed diagnosis heralded by fever, absence of voiding, peritoneal irritation, and elevated blood urea nitrogen (BUN)

Figure 2

Plain film cystogram showing intraperitoneal bladder rupture

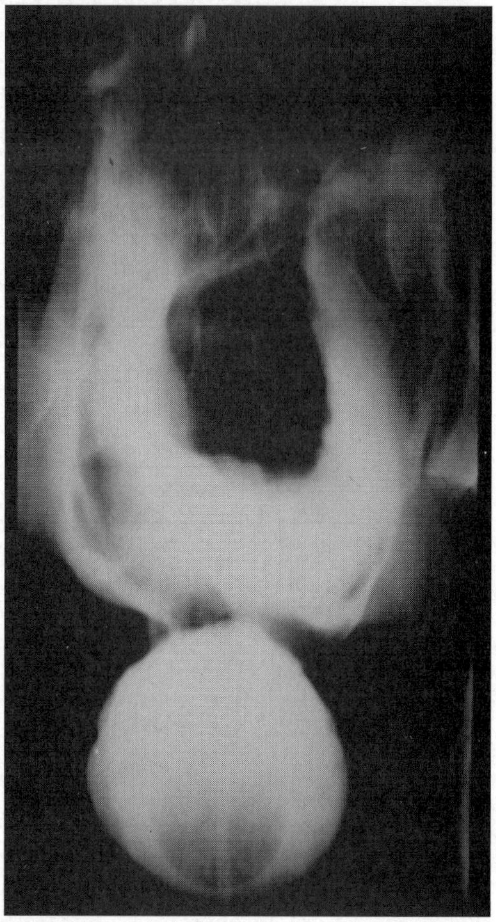

3. Hematuria
   - Most (>95%) will have gross hematuria.[1,2] Usually associated with more severe injury (rupture)
   - VERY rare to have no hematuria. Minority (5%) microscopic hematuria. Associated with less severe injury (contusion)[2]

4. Plain cystography
   - Near 100% accurate when drainage films obtained[1]

- Complete filling a must (at least 350 cc 30% contrast, or stop for pain)

- Using only 250 cc has been associated with false negatives.[4] ***Test Question***

- Figure 2 shows intraperitoneal bladder rupture as seen on plain cystography

5. CT cystography
   - Preferred (patient is often already in the CT room)

   - Use retrograde filling just like plain film cystogram (clamping the Foley and letting IV contrast filter into the bladder anterograde via the kidneys is associated with missed injuries and is NOT okay)[9,10]

   - Must dilute contrast to 2%-4% (dilute 6:1 with saline)[11]

   - 1 in 10 will be positive (blunt injury)[11]

   - Figures 3 and 4 show bladder ruptures as seen on CT cystography

Figure 3

CT image of extraperitoneal bladder rupture

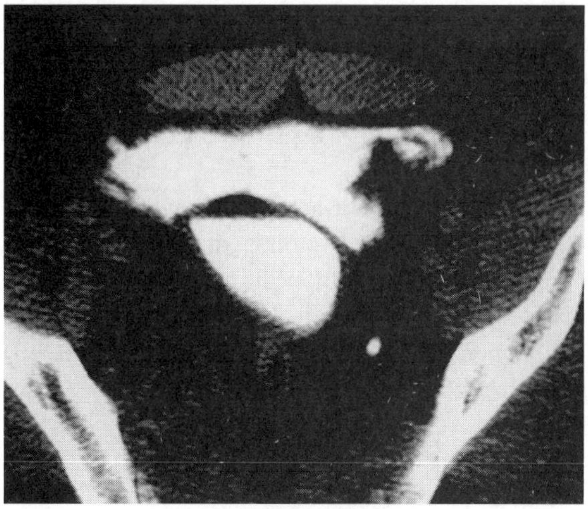

Figure 4

CT image of intraperitoneal bladder rupture

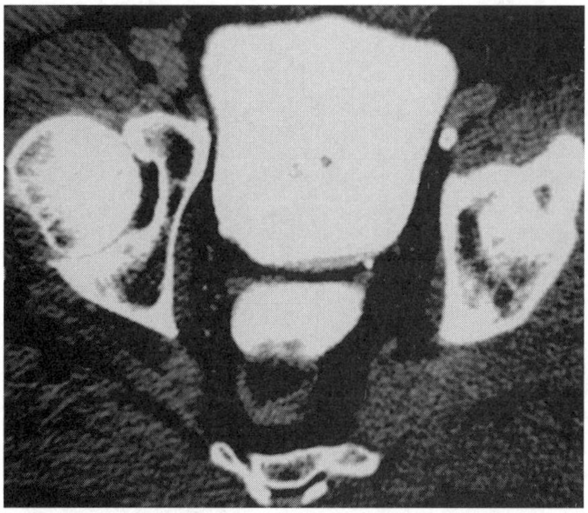

Management

1. Extraperitoneal
   - Found alone in 62% of cases, in combination with intraperitoneal rupture in 12%[1]

   - Mechanism thought to be direct laceration with pelvic bone[4] although this has been seen in only 35% of patients in some series[1]

   - Basically, can treat "nonoperatively," with catheter drainage only.[4,12] CAUTION: complications can be high (up to 26%).[13] ***Test Question***

   - There are several cases where open repair is suggested:

     * bone fragment projecting into the bladder (which is unlikely to heal, rare)[14]

     * open pelvic fracture (high risk of infection, vesicocutaneous fistula)[15]

     * rectal perforation (high risk of infection)[15]

* poor drainage of bladder secondary to blood clots in the first 48 hours (theoretically increases infectious/nonhealing complications)[13,16]

* patient undergoing laparotomy for other reasons (such as open exploration by General Surgery for intraabdominal injuries). Increases risk of vesico-cutaneous fistula[13]

* planned anterior-approach open reduction of pelvic fracture by orthopedic team. Keeps urine leak off orthopedic hardware

* open repair is associated with significantly less complications[15]

  • early 5% vs. 12%

  • late 5% vs. 21%

Figure 5

Open injured bladders, inspect and repair extraperitoneal ruptures in one layer *from the inside*

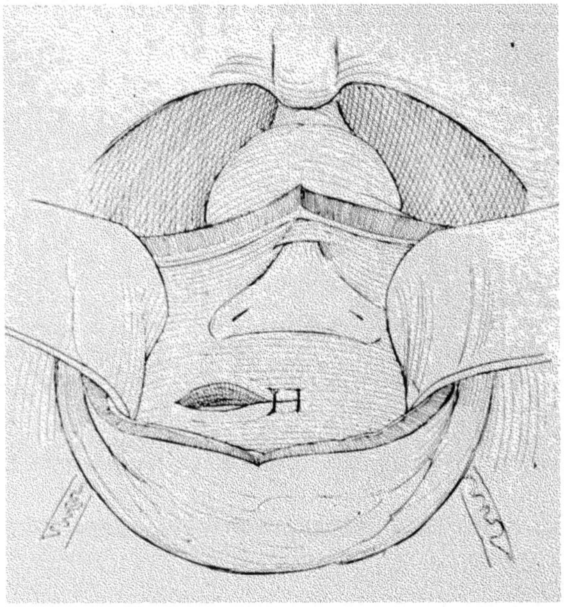

Figure 6

Close extraperitoneal bladder ruptures with 2 layers

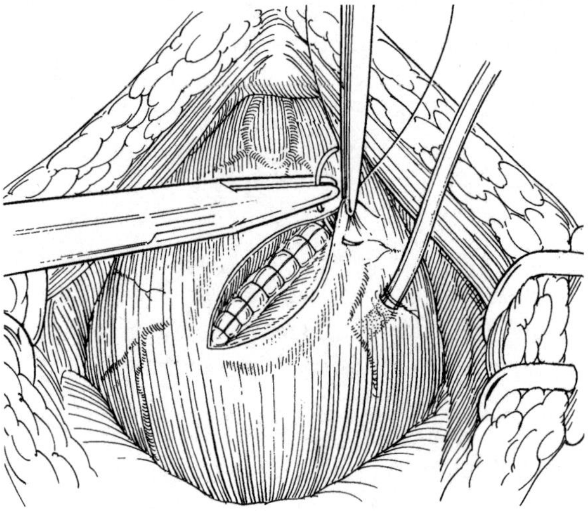

• Technique

* Open bladder and inspect from the inside out, as shown in Figure 5. ***Test Question***

* Be mindful of associated urethral, bladder neck, prostate, associated rectal injuries

* Extraperitoneal: close from the inside in 1 layer

* Cystotomy and intraperitoneal, 2 layer closure, as seen in Figure 6

* Drain

* ± suprapubic tube

2. Intraperitoneal

- 25% of all bladder injuries; seen together with extraperitoneal ruptures in another 12%[1]

- It is generally accepted that intraperitoneal ruptures occur after blunt trauma because rapidly rising intraperitoneal pressure causes the bladder to burst[3,5,17]

- Must be repaired:

  * Often larger than suggested on cystogram (mean 6 cm): unlikely to heal spontaneously

  * Continued urine leak causes chemical peritonitis in 2-3 days

Post-Op

- ***Catheter.*** Traditional to leave a large-bore suprapubic catheter in addition to a urethral Foley catheter after repair. However, no clinical advantage to adding a suprapubic tube[18]

- Complications rare

- Acute, self-limited urinary frequency is commonly seen but usually improves by 2 months. Persistent frequency rare (2%)[1]

2. Posterior Urethral Trauma

Etiology

- 4%-14% of pelvic fracture cases[19]

- Associated with bilateral pubic rami fractures ("straddle" fractures) especially with diastasis of the sacroiliac joint (odds ratio = 24)[20,21]

- Mostly males, <2% are females[22-24]

- Girls younger than 17 have a significantly increased risk when compared to older females (greater compressibility of the pelvic bones?)[25]

- Associated bladder rupture in 10%-17%.[4,6] May make the diagnosis of associated bladder injuries difficult: a catheter often cannot be placed acutely for cystogram, and extravasated contrast from the urethral injury can mask further extravasation from an extraperitoneal bladder rupture[6]

Figure 7

Urethral injury can cause a (late) perineal hematoma

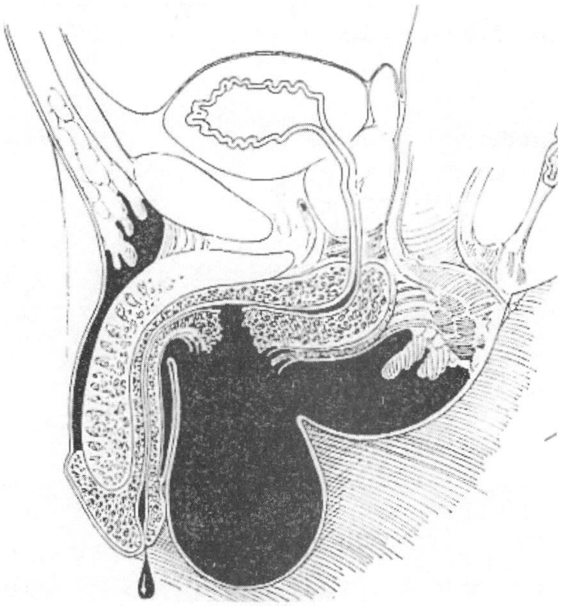

- Urethral-rectal fistula can occur in up to 8%[26]

- Can rarely occur without pelvic fracture,[27,28] usually as a result of direct perineal blunt trauma

Clinical Diagnosis

- Exam: blood at meatus (50%).[6,21,28] The amount of meatal bleeding does not correlate to the severity of injury[19]

- "High riding prostate" (34%).[28] False positives are common: pelvic hematoma can obscure the prostate.[20] Often the exam is not done, or not recorded[29]

- Clinically: triad of blood at the urethral meatus, inability to urinate, and the presence of a palpably full bladder

- Often discovered only when a urethral catheter cannot be placed, or when it is misplaced into pelvic hematoma

- Perineal hematoma may be seen if sufficient time has passed from the time of injury, as depicted in Figure 7[20]

Urethrography

- Use 16F Foley catheter, place it 1-2 cm into the fossa navicularis, inflate the balloon with a small amount (1-2 cc) of water until a snug fit[30]

- Alternatively, use Brodney or Knudson clamp

- Use 30% diatrizoate meglumine (Hypaque-M) or similar, injected gently in small 10cc increments using a 60 cc catheter-tip syringe. Lateral decubitus view static films are acceptable, but simpler to perform under fluoroscopy

Classification of Injury

- Colopinto scheme (old, but still referred to)[19]

  * Type I: Urethral stretch injury

Table 2

Urethra Injury Scale

Grade[a]	Injury Type	Description of Injury
I	Contusion	Blood at urethral meatus; urethrography normal
II	Stretch injury	Elongation of urethra without extravasation on urethrography
III	Partial disruption	Extravasation of urethrography contrast at injury site with visualization in the bladder
IV	Complete disruption	Extravasation of urethrography contrast at injury site without visualization in the bladder; <2 cm of urethra separation
V	Complete disruption	Complete transaction with ≥2 cm urethral separation, or extension into the prostate or vagina

[a]Advance 1 grade for bilateral injuries up to grade III
From Moore, et al.[70]

* Type II: Urethral disruption proximal to the genitourinary diaphragm

* Type III: Urethral disruption both proximal to and distal to the genitourinary diaphragm

- AAST organ injury severity scale is in Table 2

Complete vs. Partial Rupture

- Accurate diagnosis of exact nature of urethral injury is difficult

- There may be no radiologic differences on urethrogram between partial and complete transections[31]

- Some with "complete disruption" heal without stricture—likely these patients actually had partial urethral disruption

- Don't worry too much about whether it's partial or complete!

Management

Primary *open* realignment

- Never do it

- Increased impotence, incontinence[32], stricture formation[33] and operative blood loss

Primary *endoscopic* realignment

- Allows healing without stricture in 50%-65%.[22,3-36] Most strictures that do occur are mild (dilation or DVIU may cure it)[22,28,37,38]

- Patients not aligned (s/p tube only) nearly always (96%) develop a urethral stricture requiring posterior urethroplasty,[37] (while in series of patients treated with early urethral stenting, as few as 7% ultimately required open urethroplasty[28,34])

- Even in those who need urethroplasty, catheter placement may align the two ends of the urethra, making surgery easier, or even shorten the ultimate stricture[39]

- Immediate (as is practical), certainly within 72 hours suggested.[40] Some successful 11-19 days after injury[41-45]

- Does not worsen rates of impotence, anejaculation or incontinence[28,34,36,46]

- No traction! (increases the risk of bladder neck injury and subsequent incontinence)[31,36]

- Methods to pass catheter:

  * First try a single, gentle Foley attempt by the urologist

  * Second, consider bedside cystoscopy. Pass wire retrograde under direct cystoscopic vision, the pass Council catheter over wire[28]

  * Third. Go to OR. Attempt anterograde flexible cystoscopy. Often this is possible when retrograde cystoscopy fails. Place guidewire through the distraction injury

  * Fourth, give up and place a suprapubic tube

- Catheterize for 6 weeks, then cystourethrogram[22,28] or pericatheter RUG[48] to prove it's healed

- Some have catheterized for only 21 days with good results (probably too short!)[49]

- Suprapubic tube is left in after the urethral catheter is removed, as many patients will develop symptomatic urethral stricture after catheter removal. If the patient voids satisfactorily via the urethra, the suprapubic tube is removed 7-14 days later

Placement of Foley by Urologist

- Make 1 gentle attempt to place a urethral Foley catheter in cases of suspected partial urethral disruption

- No evidence that you "can turn an incomplete transection into a complete one"[29,34]

- Works even with radiographic evidence for "complete tear"[34,37,38]

- Confirm placement by CT or cystogram

Suprapubic Tube

- Can do open cystotomy if unable to get a bedside urethral catheter in

- Also consider open cystotomy to facilitate bladder inspection, urethral catheterization (if possible) and suprapubic tube placement

- No evidence that suprapubic tube causes pelvic fracture hardware infection, although orthopedic authors worry over it[22,50]

- Absolute indication: Associated rectal injuries = open exploration, repair, irrigation, and placement of drains. Area of urethral dislocation need not be explored or even exposed[51]

Figure 8

Combined cystogram and retrograde urethrogram showing stricture after posterior urethral distraction injury

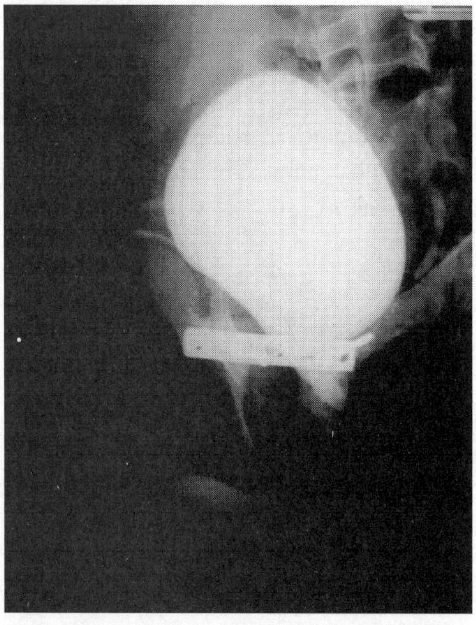

- Some have also advocated open exploration in cases of a high-riding or "pie in the sky" bladder, and in cases of associated bladder neck tear,[32] however these are not absolute indications for surgery and will heal in a majority of cases

Delayed Open Reconstruction

- Wait 3 months (some do wait more, but no evidence it's better)

- Difficult. Consider transfer to a center with experience in the operation[35,52]

- Combined retrograde urethrogram and simultaneous cystogram ("up and down-o-gram" as seen in Figure 8) is mandatory

- Pubectomy required historically 10%-30% of the time, but increased familiarity with the perineal approach makes it rare now. Only use in:

  * Really long strictures

  * Some recurrent strictures

  * Very complex strictures (urethro-rectal fistulae, etc.)

Delayed Endoscopic Treatment ("Cut to the Light")
- Requires an average of 1.5-3.4[28,36] procedures in those reports that actually found it helped

- May be associated with unacceptable complication rates, including accidentally coring a false passage that inadvertently bypasses the bladder neck[26]

- Avoid in cases of long strictures or significant dislocation of the prostate from the anatomic position

- Failure rate is significant[54-56]

- May be most useful mostly in patients who cannot tolerate open urethroplasty second to comorbidity[57]

- Probably you should refer these patients to a center of excellence for urethral reconstruction for definitive (open) reconstruction

Complications

Impotence

- Impotence rates of at least 13%-30%, likely due to original pelvic trauma[22,28,34,36]
- Patients with severe distraction runs higher (48%-72%)[52,58]
- Another 32% report poorer quality erections after injury, although not fully impotent[58]
- Some will recover erectile function as long as a year or 2 after injury[26,31]
- *Etiology.* Reported as injury to the penile parasympathetic nerves,[26] but studies have found evidence for arterial insufficiency[59,60]

Incontinence

- Many posterior urethral distraction injury patients have damage or denervation of external (striated) sphincter
- In these cases, continence is provided by the bladder neck[61]
- Patients with open bladder neck have a significantly higher rate (53%) of incontinence when compared to patients with a closed bladder neck[62]
- Yet, total incontinence overall is rare (2%-4%)[28,58]
- Mild incontinence in 6%[58]
- Up to 10% have areflexic bladder from the original injury[58]

3. Anterior Urethral Trauma

Etiology

- Rare
- 10% of all urethral injuries[63]
- 5%-25% of all GU injuries in wartime series[7]
- Often isolated injuries[64]
- The majority of disruptions occur after straddle injury[65]
- Remainder from gunshot wounds[66]

Diagnosis

- High index of suspicion required
- Urethrography should be performed in suspected cases[67,68]
- May be associated with swelling/eccymosis under Buck's fascia, causing classic "eggplant deformity" of penile shaft only, as seen in Figure 9
- If Buck's fascia is also ruptured, then hematoma gets contained by Colles' fascia. In this case swelling of the entire scrotum and a small perirectal "butterfly hematoma" may be evident. ***Test Question***

Initial Management

- Anterior urethral injuries are rare, and the literature is not clear on the best way to treat them
- Literature avors open anastomotic repair over simple catheter alignment, or (alternatively) suprapubic tube without any attempt at repair. [67,69] 12% failure rate overall. ***Test Question***

Principles of repair: Tensionless
Minimal debridement
Spatulated
Watertight
"Stented" (Foley)

- Debride only minimally[64,67]

4. Penile Trauma

The AAST organ injury severity scale for the penis is found in Table 3

Penile Amputation

- Self-mutilation most common etiology[71]
- Most (87%) are actively psychotic
- Reimplant if possible. Formalize the amputation if not. ***Test Question***
- Preserve amputated penis. Keep in wet sterile gauze, in a sterile baggy. Put baggy on ice
- <24 cold ischemia time to be viable
- Many do well: 18%-25% strictures, fistula rate[71,72]

Penile Gunshot

- Rare[73]
- Urethrography is suggested. 50% have urethral involvement[73-75]

Figure 9

"Eggplant deformity" after penile fracture

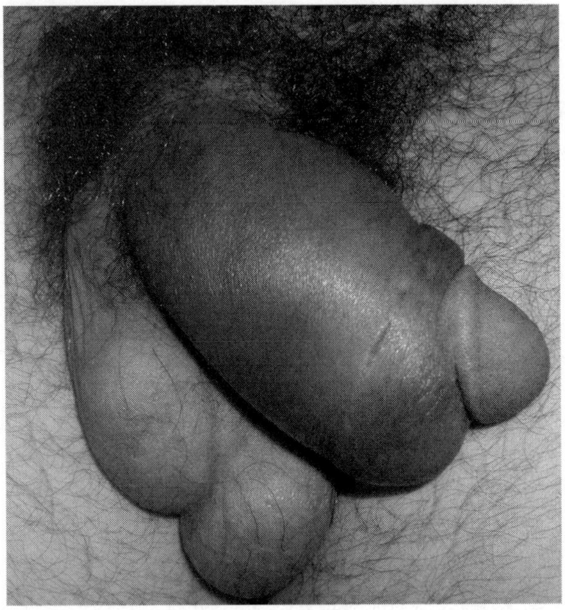

Classic "eggplant deformity" after penile fracture where blood (and possibly urine) is contained by Buck's fascia.

Table 3

Penis Injury Scale

Grade[a]	Description of Injury
I	Cutaneous laceration/contusion
II	Buck's fascia (cavernosum) laceration without tissue loss
III	Cutaneous avulsion Laceration through glans/meatus Cavemosal or urethral defect <2 cm
IV	Partial penectomy Cavarnosal or urethral defect ≥2 cm
V	Total penectomy

[a]Advance 1 grade for multiple injuries up to grade V From Moore, et al.[70]

- Look for associated injuries: present 80% of the time. 75% will be hemodynamically unstable[76]

- Repair most primarily,[77] but massive injury such as from close range shotgun wound are treated with wet dressing in a staged fashion[73,78]

- Superficial penetration or trivial wound? Nonoperative Rx[74,78,79]

- Repair corporal injures with buried nonabsorbable[74] or absorbable (preferred)[79] sutures

- Associated anterior urethral injuries should be closed primarily with a watertight, spatulated, catheter-stented technique using absorbable suture[74]

- Posterior urethral injuries should be managed in a staged fashion, with suprapubic catheterization[74] and placement of a urethral catheter (if possible)

- ***Complications.*** True incidence unknown (poor follow-up) but most get erection back 1-6 weeks after repair[73,75] and do not develop stricture[75]

Penile Fracture

- As infrequent as 1/175,000 hospital admissions in the United States,[80] but significantly more common in some centers abroad[81-83]

- Usually from some blow to the erect penis: falling on the penis,[84] rough masturbation,[85,86] being struck in the penis,[83] and even rolling over in bed[82,85]

- Size of cavernosal rupture varies between 0.5-5 cm.[83,85] Bilateral injuries can also occur[87]

Diagnosis

- History is often constant: a blow to the erect penis, accompanied by a snapping or popping sound, penile pain, and immediate detumescence[88], although these classic findings are not universally seen[89]

- Because of embarrassment, delay in presentation to the hospital is common[85,90]

- ***Physical exam.*** Penile swelling and eccymosis are nearly always present. A palpable corporal defect may be appreciable,[87] but this can be obscured by swelling and hematoma

  * The "rolling clot sign" where clot lying near the fracture site is palpable as a firm, immobile, discrete swelling over which the penile skin can be rolled. This sign appears to be reliably associated with the location of cavernosal rupture[83,91]

  * Extruded blood combined with tissue swelling can create a hugely deformed eccymotic penis, which is referred to as an "eggplant" deformity.[87] This sign is highly diagnostic[83]

  * If Buck's fascia is ruptured, blood and urine will extravasate around Colle's fascia, giving a characteristic scrotal swelling and a "butterfly sign" in the perineum[92]

Associated Injury

- Associated with urethral injury 0%-38% of the time. (The wide range in associated urethral injury is likely because penile fractures in some Middle Eastern areas are often due to low-energy injuries such as manual bending of the penis with the hand, while those in the West are most often due to high energy injuries such as those that occur during vigorous intercourse or falls)[83]

- Urethrography must be performed in cases of suspected urethral injury (blood at meatus, inability to void, gross hematuria),[83,93] although urethral bleeding without associated urethral injury has been reported after penile fracture[94]

- Difficulty voiding or gross hematuria is present in 20% of cases[87]

- Rare cases of false-negative urethrography in patients with penile fracture and urethral injury have been reported,[95] so direct inspection of the urethra during exploration is a good practice

- Ultrasound has been used to aid in the diagnosis of penile fracture,[87] although the clinical picture is usually so clear that such imaging techniques are not necessary

- MRI has been used to image the injured corpora cavernosa.[89] Necessary?

- Cavernosography is a sensitive tool,[85] but seldom adds anything to the usually unambiguous presentation.[83] Most only use cavernosography if the diagnosis is somehow in doubt,[88,96] which it seldom appears to be[93]

- 1% of cases actually have rupture of the dorsal vein only, and no corporal rupture is present

Management

- Surgical repair recommended.[82,86,87,89,90,93,94,97-99]

- Circumcising incision[82,83,93]

- Absorbable sutures[82,86,93]

- Place a Foley to aid in identification of the urethra, and prevent urethral injury during repair.[83,94] The urethral catheter may be removed when penile swelling decreases enough to allow micturition

- Avoid compression dressing after repair

- No need for medications, such as diazepam, amyl nitrate, or diethylstilbesterol, to eliminate erections after surgery[81,100]

Outcomes/Complications

- A certain number of patients become impotent, due to traumatic corporeal veno-occlusive dysfunction, persistent venous leak, or arterial insufficiency[101]

- Unrepaired penile fractures can result in functional inability to have intercourse, often because of angulation at the site of injury[80]

- Patients who undergo early repair of penile fracture have a low complication rate.[81,86] Mild curvature was present in less than 5% of cases, and most often this complication occurred in patients who did not present to the hospital immediately after injury[94]

Penis Caught in Zipper Injury

- First step: cut the zipper slider with an orthopedic pin cutter or similar metal snips. ***Test Question***

- Alternatively: local anesthetic, lubrication of the zipper with mineral oil, and a single manual attempt at opening the zipper[102,103]

- Second step: zipper teeth should be individually pulled apart from each other using hemostats[104]

5. Testes Trauma

- Rare, as the tough tunica albuginea usually protects[105]

- The AAST organ injury severity scale for the testes is found in Table 4

Table 4

Testis Injury Scale

Grade[a]	Description of Injury
I	Contusion/hematoma
II	Subclinical laceration of tunica albuginea
III	Laceration of tunica albuginea with <50% parenchymal loss
IV	Major laceration of tunica albuginea with ≥50% parenchymal loss
V	Total testicular destruction or avulsion

[a]Advance one grade for multiple injuries up to grade V
From Moore, et al.[70]

Blunt

- Testicular rupture after a direct blow to the testicle is as high as 50%[106]

- Most unilateral, both testes in 1.5% of cases[107]

- Most common etiology is assault[108] and sports injuries,[109,110] but motor vehicle accidents account for a significant minority (10%)

- Exact mechanism of testicular injury is unknown, but hypothesized that the testicle is driven against and trapped against the thigh or bony pelvis. Once trapped, the force can transmit to the testicle and cause rupture[109,111]

- Rarely, testicular injury is self-inflicted (50% of reported cases of genital mutilation involve the testicles)[112]

- Examination may be limited by pain. Use 1% lidocaine spermatic cord block

- There are no specific symptoms,[108] however history of trauma in association with scrotal pain, eccymosis, and (at times) hematocele are often found. Associated epididymal ruptures can occur, but are extremely rare[108]

- Testes injuries which do not require operative exploration should be managed with analgesics, scrotal elevation to promote veno-lymphatic drainage, and ice to control pain and swelling[113]

- Ruptured? Operate. Think it may be ruptured? Operate. ***Test Question***

Penetrating

- Civilian male victims of gunshot wounds will suffer injury to the scrotum approximately 2% of the time[76]

- Assault is the most common, but self-inflicted gunshot incurred by patients placing a loaded handgun in pants pocket do occur

- Penetrating trauma caused bilateral injury with an incidence nearly 15 times that of blunt injury[106]

- Use physical examination primarily and ultrasound secondarily to rule out testicular injury. Equivocal cases should be explored

- Most cases ultimately require exploration: 92%-97%[75,114]

- Testicular salvage is only possible in 35%-65%[73,75,115] of testicular (or cord) gunshot wounds, but every attempt to save those cases with ≥ 40% of spared parenchyma should be made (as seen in Figures 10a and 10b)

Clinical Findings

- Associated injuries are common (83%),[73] mostly surrounding structures: thigh (75%), penis (37%), perineum (25%), urethra (18%)[115]

- A significant minority have an associated injury to the femoral vessels with attendant significant bleeding—vigilance for this injury is warranted[73]

- Bilateral injury is present in as many as 31% (penetrating)[107]

- Transection of the vas is not uncommon after blunt trauma to the testes, occurring in 10% of patients in 1 series[73]

Imaging

Sonography

- A useful adjunct, but in no case should a "normal" sonogram dissuade exploration of a grossly abnormal testicle on physical exam

- Perform immediate exploration without obtaining a sonogram in those cases where the physical examination clearly shows significant testicular trauma: large hematocele, gross testicular rupture, or testicular dislocation

- Abnormal sonographic findings: heterogeneity of the parenchyma which may indicate intratesticular hematoma,[116] loss of continuity of the tunica albuginea which may indicate tunica rupture,[116-118] or hematocele[118,119]

- Testicular rupture can be difficult to diagnose with ultrasound, and in one series sonography incorrectly diagnosed this entity more commonly than it correctly diagnosed it[120]

- Added benefit of ultrasound in some testis trauma cases: diagnose unexpected associated conditions, such as testicular torsion, or testicular tumors associated with a history of trauma

Radionucleotide Scans

- Useful to evaluate the painful testicle not associated with previous trauma,[121] but usually not indicated for trauma[122]

Figure 10a

Close range, low-velocity testicular gunshot wound

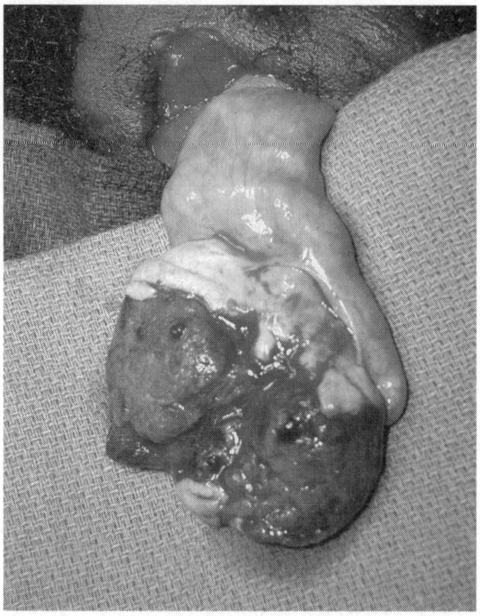

Figure 10b

Same testicle is preserved after minimal parenchymal debridement and suture closure of the capsule

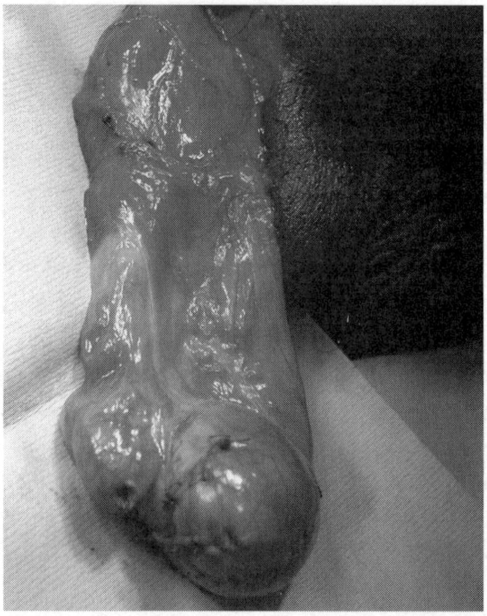

Surgical Management

- Explore and repair all cases of significant hematocele,[123] intratesticular hematoma, or frank rupture of the tunica albuginea

- Lack of evidence for tunica rupture on ultrasound is not sufficient reason to delay exploration as tunica fracture lines are rarely detected[124]

- Do not delay—increases orchidectomy rate between 3- to 8-fold[106,108]

- Even small tears can ultimately result in testicular loss if ignored: intratesticular swelling results in extrusion of seminiferous tubules, forcing the friable tissue out of the breached capsule like toothpaste out of a tube[109]

- Midline raphe incision

- At exploration, necrotic testicular tissue should be debrided and the capsule closed with running absorbable suture. In some cases, loss of capsule will require removal of intratesticular tissue to allow closure. ***Test Question***

- In blunt injury, significant intratesticular hematoma should be drained, as increased intratesticular pressure from these collections can result in testicular atrophy later[106]

- Leave drains when the operative field cannot be made absolutely hemostatic

- Antibiotics, such as cefazolin, are continued until drains are removed, although there are no randomized trials supporting this approach

- Bilateral injury? Debride conservatively and preserve as much functioning testicular tissue as possible[107]

- Injuries to the vas should be tied off with nonabsorbable suture for reconstruction, if necessary, at a later time[73]

- Postoperatively, gentle pressure dressings can be applied, usually by fluffed gauze held in place by an athletic supporter

Nonoperative Management

- Nonoperative therapy of significant testicular injuries was used historically,[106,111] but now is out of favor

- Results in higher orchidectomy rates. Often patient deterioration forces delayed scrotal exploration

- Results in longer hospital stays and period of debility than prompt surgical therapy[111]

- Only appropriate for insignificant scrotal injuries not resulting in testicular hematoma or rupture

- Specifically, patients with intratesticular hematoma do poorly without operation. 40% develop testicular infection and/or testicular necrosis, often requiring orchidectomy[125]

Outcome

- After repair of even bilateral rupture, preservation of adequate sperm production has been documented[76,126]

- A small percentage of patients with testicular injury will have complications such as wound infection,[78] the majority do well[76]

6. Genital Skin Loss

Etiology

Penetrating

- Not common
- Can often be closed primarily even with >50% skin loss, owing to scrotal skin distensibility

Burns

- Burns involve the perineum 1% of cases
- Often full thickness, as penile skin is thin[127]
- Treat like other burns, with early resection of burn eschar and coverage with split thickness skin grafts, when possible

Constricting Bands

- Can result from prescription venous return constriction devices used to prolong erection,[128] or sadomasochistic sex play
- Rarely result in significant skin loss, although the more common injury involves direct pressure necrosis under the band (which usually heals well)

Avulsion

- Resultant from traction by mechanical devices such as farm machinery, industrial machinery, or by suction devices (vacuum cleaners)
- Subdermal penile tissue is loose areolar tissue, so it is often torn free without damage to the underlying structures

The AAST Organ Injury Severity Scale for the scrotum is found in Table 5

Initial Management

- Wet gauze dressings, which are changed frequently (every nursing shift, or 8 hours), and urinary drainage. Silvadene dressings preferred for burns. ***Test Question***
- Daily inspection by the surgical team is mandatory
- Coexisting infection? Plan intervals of operative debridement, up to daily, until active infection is controlled

Surgical Management of Penile Skin Wounds

- The algorithm for penile skin wounds is found in Figure 11
- Foreskin flaps can be used to cover distal penile skin loss such as would occur with burns to the shaft of the penis[127]

Table 5

Scrotum Injury Scale

Grade[a]	Description of Injury
I	Contusion
II	Laceration <25% of scrotal diameter
III	Laceration ≥25% of scrotal diameter
IV	Avulsion <50%
V	Avulsion ≥50%

[a] *From Moore et al.*[70]

Figure 11

Algorithm for the treatment of penile skin wounds

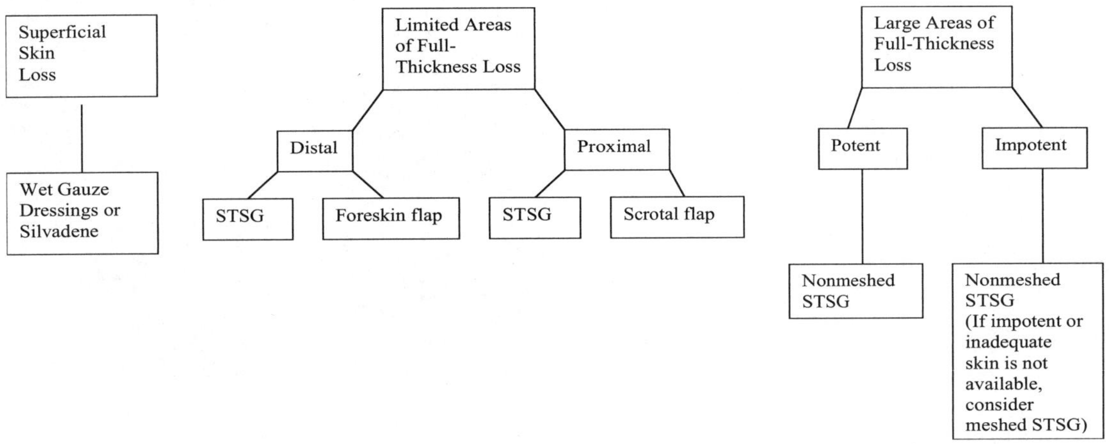

- Scrotal rotation flaps for more proximal defects. Risk of unacceptable cosmetic result because the scrotum is hair-bearing skin

- Local flaps such as from the abdomen and thigh can also be used, but they have a less acceptable cosmetic result than STSG[129]

- Skin coverage using the avulsed skin which can sometimes be retrieved from the scene of the accident should be avoided, as some authors have stated that it "inevitably" becomes necrotic and infected[113]

- Treatment of choice for penile skin coverage is thick (0.15 inch), unmeshed, split-thickness skin grafts from a thigh donor site

  * Remove subcoronal skin, even to the point of excising unaffected subcoronal skin. Lymphatic obstruction of this skin, if not excised, will result in circumferential lymphedema[127]

  * Grafts will never regain normal sensation,[130] although sexual function is often preserved because of intact sensation in the skin of the glans

  * Meshed skin grafts should not be used on the penis in potent patients except in extreme cases where there is a paucity of donor skin in cases of large-area burns. Meshed grafts have a tendency towards contracture,[129] and are cosmetically less acceptable than unmeshed skin grafts

- Treat donor site with large semi-occlusive dressing such as Op-Site® or Tegaderm™. Speeds healing (mean 9 days to re-epithelialization), lowers rates of infection (3-5%), decreases subjective pain scores, and costs least,[131] as in Figure 12

- Wound exudates under the dressing are removed with a tiny (7F) silicone wound drain (TLS Evacuated Tube Drainage System; Porex; Newnan, GA)

  * The dressing is removed if infection is suspected[132]

Figure 12

OpSite dressing

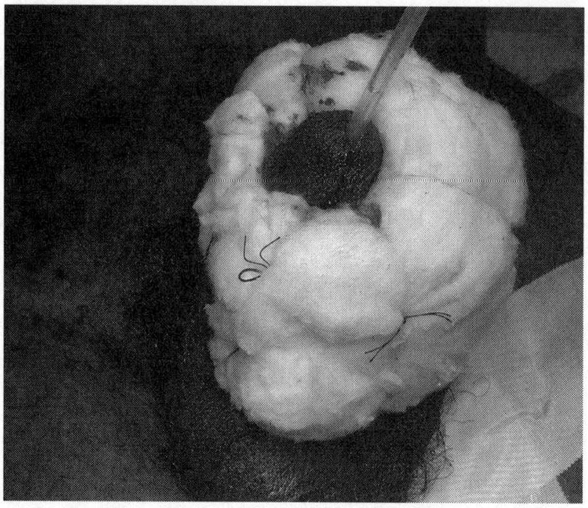

Large OpSite dressing to cover skin graft donor site, and small drain to remove exudate while occlusive dressing is in place.

  * If healing is not complete after dressing removal, the residual wounds can be treated with petroleum-impregnated gauze until completely healed[133]

Postoperative Penile Skin Graft Wound Management

- Use dilute, sprayed, fibrin glue to glue down the skin graft (much more reliable skin take)

- The wound is inspected, "deblebbed" and redressed at 24 hours. Bed rest X for 72 hours. Allow patient activity and self-dressing of wound on POD #4. Soft, dry gauze dressings are continued for another 3 weeks

- Intercourse is avoided for at least another 6 weeks until the graft is completely healed

Surgical Management: Scrotum

- The algorithm for management of scrotal skin loss is found in Figure 14

- Scrotal skin loss involving less than 60% of the skin can often be closed acutely/primarily

- In more significant loss, the testes may either be placed in thigh pouches, or treated with wet dressings until the time for reconstruction. (Thigh pouches have been classically used to protect the testes until definitive reconstruction can be completed,[134] some have used saline dressings for up to 3 weeks in small numbers of patients with good results)[78]

- Consider **primary** closure. After 2-3 weeks of dressing changes, some even with significant scrotal skin loss can have primary closure and avoid the need for scrotal reconstruction[78]

- Split thickness skin grafts, meshed 2:1, give excellent cosmetic result when necesary. The meshing allows exudates to escape from the interstices thus improving graft take, and decreases the size of the donor site wound. The method of graft is to create a pouch and place the testicles inside. If the skin graft is merely placed over the testes, than a pouch-like scrotum that allows free testicular movement is not created

- Third option: thigh flaps. Particularly useful if the testes have already been buried in the thighs after traumatic or surgical scrotal removal. The thigh flaps can be left as a permanent solution, or rotated into a neo-scrotum if desired

Figure 13

Algorithm for management of scrotal skin loss

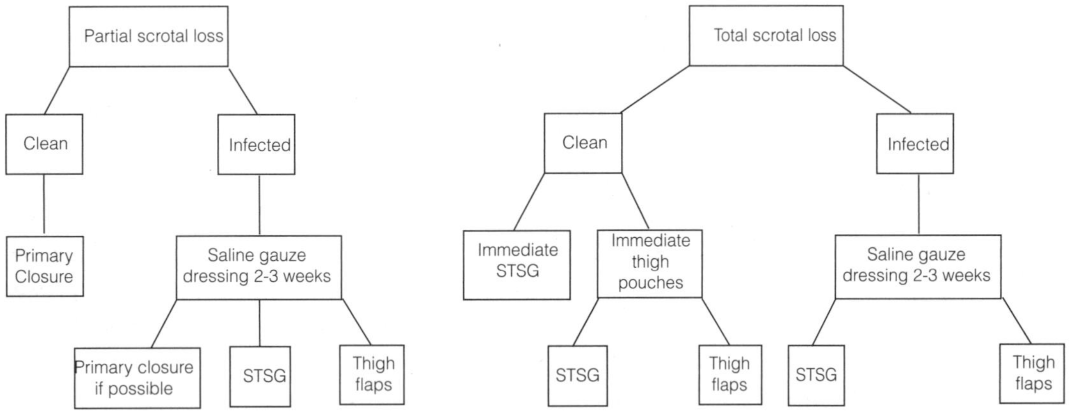

7. References

1. Carroll PR, McAninch JW. Major bladder trauma: mechanisms of injury and a unified method of diagnosis and repair. *J Urol.* 1984;132: 254-257.

2. Cass AS. The multiple injured patient with bladder trauma. *J Trauma.* 1984;24:731-734.

3. Corriere JN, Jr, Sandler CM. Management of the ruptured bladder: seven years of experience with 111 cases. *J Trauma.* 1986;26: 830-833.

4. Cass AS, Luxenberg M. Features of 164 bladder ruptures [see comments]. *J Urol.* 1987;138:743-745.

5. Hochberg E, Stone NN. Bladder rupture associated with pelvic fracture due to blunt trauma. *Urology.* 1993;41:531-533.

6. Cass AS, Gleich P, Smith C. Simultaneous bladder and prostatomembranous urethral rupture from external trauma. *J Urol.* 1984;132:907-908.

7. Selikowitz SM. Penetrating high-velocity genitourinary injuries. Part I. Statistics mechanisms, and renal wounds. *Urology.* 1977;9:371-376.

8. Duncan AO, Phillips TF, Scalea TM, Maltz SB, Atweh NA, Sclafani SJ. Management of transpelvic gunshot wounds. *J Trauma.* 1989;29:1335-1340.

9. Mee SL, McAninch JW, Federle MP. Computerized tomography in bladder rupture: diagnostic limitations. *J Urol.* 1987;137:207-209.

10. Haas CA, Brown SL, Spirnak JP. Limitations of routine spiral computerized tomography in the evaluation of bladder trauma. *J Urol.* 1999; 162:51-52.

11. Peng MY, Parisky YR, Cornwell EE 3rd, Radin R, Bragin S. CT cystography versus conventional cystography in evaluation of bladder injury. *AJR.* 1999;173:1269-1272.

12. Hayes EE, Sandler CM, Corriere JN Jr. Management of the ruptured bladder secondary to blunt abdominal trauma. *J Urol.* 1983; 129:946-948.

13. Kotkin L, Koch MO. Morbidity associated with nonoperative management of extraperitoneal bladder injuries. *J Trauma.* 1995;38:895-898.

14. Corriere JN Jr, Sandler CM. Mechanisms of injury, patterns of extravasation and management of extraperitoneal bladder rupture due to blunt trauma. *J Urol.* 1988;139:43-44.

15. Cass AS, Luxenberg M. Management of extraperitoneal ruptures of bladder caused by external trauma. *Urology.* 1989;33:179-183.

16. Skinner EC, Parisky YR, Skinner DG. Management of complex urologic injuries. *Surg Clin North Am.* 1996;76:861-878.

17. Peters PC. Intraperitoneal rupture of the bladder. *Urol Clin North Am.* 1989;16:279-282.

18. Volpe MA, Pachter EM, Scalea TM, Macchia RJ, Mydlo JH. Is there a difference in outcome when treating traumatic intraperitoneal bladder rupture with or without a suprapubic tube? *J Urol.* 1999;161:1103-1105.

19. Colapinto V, McCallum RW. Injury to the male posterior urethra in fractured pelvis: a new classification. *J Urol.* 1977;118:575-580.

20. Koraitim MM, Marzouk ME, Atta MA, Orabi SS. Risk factors and mechanism of urethral injury in pelvic fractures. Br J Urol. 1996;77:876-880.

21. Lowe MA, Mason JT, Luna GK. Maier RV, Copass MK, Berger RE. Risk factors for urethral injuries in men with traumatic pelvic fractures. *J Urol.* 1988;140:506-507.

22. Routt ML, Simonian PT, Defalco AJ, Miller J, Clarke T. Internal fixation in pelvic fractures and primary repairs of associated genitourinary disruptions: a team approach [published erratum appears in *J Trauma*. 1997 May;42(5):981] [see comments]. *J Trauma*. 1996;40:784-790.

23. Hemal AK, Dorairajan LN, Gupta NP. Post-traumatic complete and partial loss of urethra with pelvic fracture in girls: an appraisal of management. *J Urol*. 2000;163:282-287.

24. Persky L. Childhood urethral trauma. *Urology*. 1978;11:603-606.

25. Hemal AK, Singh I, Chahal R, Gupta NP. Core through internal urethrotomy in the management of post-traumatic isolated bladder neck and prostatic urethral strictures in adults. A report of 4 cases. *Int Urol Nephrol*. 1999;31:703-708.

26. Turner-Warwick R. Prevention of complications resulting from pelvic fracture urethral injuries—and from their surgical management. *Urol Clin North Am*. 1989;16:335-358.

27. Cass AS. Urethral injury in the multiple-injured patient. *J Trauma*. 1984;24:901-906.

28. Elliott DS, Barrett DM. Long-term follow-up and evaluation of primary realignment of posterior urethral disruptions [see comments]. *J Urol*. 1997;157:814-816.

29. Jackson DH, Williams JL. Urethral injury: a retrospective study. *Br J Urol*. 1974;46: 665-676.

30. Sandler CM, Corriere JN Jr. Urethrography in the diagnosis of acute urethral injuries. *Urol Clin North Am*. 1989;16:283-289.

31. Morehouse DD, Belitsky P, Mackinnon K. Rupture of the posterior urethra. *J Urol*. 1972;107:255-258.

32. Webster GD, Mathes GL, Selli C. Prostatomembranous urethral injuries: a review of the literature and a rational approach to their management. *J Urol*. 1983;130: 898-902.

33. Coffield KS, Weems WL. Experience with management of posterior urethral injury associated with pelvic fracture. *J Urol*. 1977;117:722-724.

34. Kotkin L, Koch MO. Impotence and incontinence after immediate realignment of posterior urethral trauma: result of injury or management? *J Urol*. 1996;155:1600-1603.

35. Morehouse DD, Mackinnon KJ. Management of prostatomembranous urethral disruption: 13-year experience. *J Urol*. 1980;123: 173-174.

36. Asci R, Sarikaya S, Buyukalpelli R, Saylik A, Yilmaz AF, Yildiz S. Voiding and sexual dysfunctions after pelvic fracture urethral injuries treated with either initial cystostomy and delayed urethroplasty or immediate primary urethral realignment. *Scand J Urol Nephrol*. 1999;33:228-233.

37. Herschorn S, Thijssen A, Radomski SB. The value of immediate or early catheterization of the traumatized posterior urethra [see comments]. *J Urol*. 1992;148:1428-1431.

38. Al-Ali IH, Husain I. Disrupting injuries of the membranous urethra—the case for early surgery and catheter splinting. *Br J Urol*. 1983;55:716-720.

39. Devine CJ Jr, Jordan GH, Devine PC. Primary realignment of the disrupted prostatomembranous urethra. *Urol Clin North Am*. 1989; 16:291-295.

40. Rehman J, Samadi D, Ricciardi R Jr, Kreutzer E. Early endoscopic realignment as primary therapy for complete posterior urethral disruptions. *J Endourol*. 1998;12:283-289.

41. Porter JR, Takayama TK, Defalco AJ. Traumatic posterior urethral injury and early realignment using magnetic urethral catheters. *J Urol*. 1997;158:425-430.

42. Towler JM, Eisen SM. A new technique for the management of urethral injuries. *Br J Urol*. 1987;60:162-166.

43. Londergan TA, Gundersen LH, Van Every MJ. Early fluoroscopic realignment for traumatic urethral injuries. *Urology*. 1997;49:101-103.

44. Cohen JK, Berg G, Carl GH, Diamond DD. Primary endoscopic realignment following posterior urethral disruption. *J Urol*. 1991;146:1548-1550.

45. Turner-Warwick R. A personal view of the immediate management of pelvic fracture urethral injuries. *Urol Clin North Am*. 1977;4: 81-93.

46. Follis HW, Koch MO, McDougal WS. Immediate management of prostatomembranous urethral disruptions. *J Urol*. 1992;147: 1259-1262.

47. Gheiler EL, Frontera JR. Immediate primary realignment of prostatomembranous urethral disruptions using endourologic techniques. *Urology*. 1997;49:596-599.

48. Jepson BR, Boullier JA, Moore RG, Parra RO. Traumatic posterior urethral injury and early primary endoscopic realignment: evaluation of long-term follow-up. *Urology*. 1999;53: 1205-1210.

49. Patterson DE, Barrett DM, Myers RP, DeWeerd JH, Hall BB, Benson RC Jr. Primary realignment of posterior urethral injuries. *J Urol*. 1983;129:513-516.

50. BM P. Pelvic ring injury and associated urologic trauma: An orthopaedic perspective. *Sem Urol*. 1995;13:25-33.

51. Koraitim MM. Pelvic fracture urethral injuries: the unresolved controversy. *J Urol*. 1999;161:1433-1441.

52. Dhabuwala CB, Hamid S, Katsikas DM, Pierce JM Jr. Impotence following delayed repair of prostatomembranous urethral disruption. *J Urol*. 1990;144:677-678.

53. Dixon CM, Hricak H, McAninch JW. Magnetic resonance imaging of traumatic posterior urethral defects and pelvic crush injuries. *J Urol*. 1992;148:1162-1165.

54. Levine LA, Eckrich PC. Endoscopic repair of the completely disrupted urethra. *J Endourol*. 1993;7:225-227.

55. Gupta NP, Gill IS. Core-through optical internal urethrotomy in management of impassable traumatic posterior urethral strictures. *J Urol*. 1986;136:1018-1021.

56. el-Abd SA. Endoscopic treatment of posttraumatic urethral obliteration: experience in 396 patients. *J Urol*. 1995;153:67-71.

57. Chiou RK, Gonzalez R, Ortlip S, Fraley EE. Endoscopic treatment of posterior urethral obliteration: long-term follow-up and comparison with transpubic urethroplasty. *J Urol*. 1988;140:508-511.

58. Corriere JN Jr, Rudy DC, Benson GS. Voiding and erectile function after delayed one-stage repair of posterior urethral disruptions in 50 men with a fractured pelvis. *J Trauma*. 1994;37:587-589; discussion 589-590.

59. Armenakas NA, McAninch JW, Lue TF, Dixon CM, Hricak H. Posttraumatic impotence: magnetic resonance imaging and duplex ultrasound in diagnosis and management. *J Urol*. 1993;149:1272-1275.

60. La M, Te H, Ad S. Impotence associated with blunt pelvic and perineal trauma: Penile revascularization as a treatment option. *Semin Urol*. 1995;13:66-72.

61. Morey AF, McAninch JW. Reconstruction of traumatic posterior urethral strictures. *Tech Urol.* 1997;3:103-107.

62. Iselin CE, Webster GD. The significance of the open bladder neck associated with pelvic fracture urethral distraction defects. *J Urol.* 1999;162:347-351.

63. Mitchell JP. Injuries to the urethra. *Br J Urol.* 1968;40:649-670.

64. Kiracofe HL, Pfister RR, Peterson NE. Management of non-penetrating distal urethral trauma. *J Urol.* 1975;114:57-62.

65. Pierce JM Jr. Disruptions of the anterior urethra. *Urol Clin North Am.* 1989;16:329-334.

66. Pontes JE, Pierce JM Jr. Anterior urethral injuries: four years of experience at the Detroit General Hospital. *J Urol.* 1978;120:563-564.

67. Husmann DA, Boone TB, Wilson WT. Management of low velocity gunshot wounds to the anterior urethra: the role of primary repair versus urinary diversion alone. *J Urol.* 1993;150:70-72.

68. Devine CJ Jr, Devine PC, Horton CE. Anterior urethral injury: etiology, diagnosis, and initial management. *Urol Clin North Am.* 1977;4:125-131.

69. Lucey DT, Smith MJ, Koontz WW Jr. Modern trends in the management of urologic trauma. *J Urol.* 1972;107:641-646.

70. Moore EE, Malangoni MA, Cogbill TH, Peterson NE, Champion HR, Jurkovich GJ, Shackford SR. Organ injury scaling VII: cervical vascular, peripheral vascular, adrenal, penis, testis, and scrotum. *J Trauma.* 1996;41: 523-524.

71. Aboseif S, Gomez R, McAninch JW. Genital self-mutilation. *J Urol.* 1993;150:1143-1146.

72. Lowe MA, Chapman W, Berger RE. Repair of a traumatically amputated penis with return of erectile function [see comments]. *J Urol.* 1991;145:1267-1270.

73. Gomez RG, Castanheira AC, McAninch JW. Gunshot wounds to the male external genitalia. *J Urol.* 1993;150:1147-1149.

74. Miles BJ, Poffenberger RJ, Farah RN, Moore S. Management of penile gunshot wounds. *Urology.* 1990;36:318-321.

75. Cline KJ, Mata JA, Venable DD, Eastham JA. Penetrating trauma to the male external genitalia. *J Trauma.* 1998;44:492-494.

76. Brandes SB, Buckman RF, Chelsky MJ, Hanno PM. External genitalia gunshot wounds: a ten-year experience with fifty-six cases. *J Trauma.* 1995;39:266-271; discussion 271-262.

77. Selikowitz SM. Penetrating high-velocity genitourinary injuries. Part II: Ureteral, lower tract, and genital wounds. *Urology.* 1977;9:493-499.

78. Bertini JE Jr, Corriere JN Jr. The etiology and management of genital injuries. *J Trauma.* 1988;28:1278-1281.

79. Monga M, Moreno T, Hellstrom W. A strategy for success: Managing gunshot wounds to the male genitalia. *Contemp Urology.* 1995; January:58-63.

80. Farah RN, Stiles R, Cerny JC. Surgical treatment of deforminty and coital difficulty in healed traumatic rupture of the corpora cavernosa. *J Urol.* 1978;120:118-120.

81. el-Sherif AE, Dauleh M, Allowneh N, Vijayan P. Management of fracture of the penis in Qatar. *Br J Urol.* 1991;68:622-625.

82. Al-Saleh BM, Ansari ER, Al Ali IH, Tell JY, Saheb A. Fractures of the penis seen in Abu Dhabi. *J Urol.* 1985;134:274-275.

83. Zargooshi J. Penile fracture in Kermanshah, Iran: Report of 172 cases. *J Urol.* 2000;164:364-366.

84. Al Saleh BM.S, Ansari ER, Al Ali IH, Tell JY, Saheb A. Fractures of the penis seen in Abu Dhabi. *J Urol.* 1985;134:274-275.

85. Karadeniz T, Topsakal M, Ariman A, Erton H, Basak D. Penile fracture: differential diagnosis, management and outcome. *Br J Urol.* 1996;77:279-281.

86. Nicolaisen GS, Melamud A, Williams RD, and McAninch JW. Rupture of the corpus cavernosum: surgical management. *J Urol.* 1983;130:917-919.

87. Cendron M, Whitmore KE, Carpiniello V, Kurzweil SJ, Hanno PM, Snyder HM, Duckett JW. Traumatic rupture of the corpus cavernosum: evaluation and management. *J Urol.* 1990;144:987-991.

88. Orvis BR, McAninch JW. Penile rupture. *Urol Clin North Am.* 1989;16:369-375.

89. Fedel M, Venz S, Andreessen R, Sudhoff F, Loening SA. The value of magnetic resonance imaging in the diagnosis of suspected penile fracture with atypical clinical findings. *J Urol.* 1996;155:1924-1927.

90. Agrawal SK, Morgan BE, Shafique M, Shazely M. Experience with penile fractures in Saudi Arabia. *Br J Urol.* 1991;67:644-646.

91. VN, GCR. Fracture of the penis. *Br J Surg.* 1985;72:305-306.

92. Gottenger EE, Wagner JR. Penile fracture with complete urethral disruption. *J Trauma.* 2000;49:339-341.

93. Fergany AF, Angermeier KW, Montague DK. Review of Cleveland Clinic experience with penile fracture. *Urology.* 1999;54:352-355.

94. Asgari MA, Hosseini SY, Safarinejad MR, Samadzadeh B, Bardideh AH. Penile fractures: Evaluation, therapeutic approaches and long-term results. *J Urol.* 1996;155:148-149.

95. Mydlo JH, Hayyeri M, Macchia RJ. Urethrography and cavernosography imaging in a small series of penile fractures: a comparison with surgical findings. *Urology.* 1998;51:616-619.

96. Dever DP, Saraf PG, Catanese RP, Feinstein MJ, Davis RS. Penile fracture: operative management and cavernosography. *Urology.* 1983;22:394-396.

97. Meares EM. Traumatic rupture of the corpus cavernosum. *J Urol.* 1971;105:407-408.

98. Kalash, SS and Young, JD., Jr.: Fracture of penis: controversy of surgical versus conservative treatment. *Urology.* 24: 21-24, 1984.

99. Tan LB, Chiang CP, Huang CH, Chou YH, Wang CJ. Traumatic rupture of the corpus cavernosum. *Br J Urol.* 1991;68:626-628.

100. Tan LB, Chiang CP, Huang CH, Chou YH, Wang CJ. Surgical treatment of the ruptured bladder: 22 years reviewed. *J Formos Med Assoc.* 1990;89:986-991.

101. Penson DF, Seftel AD, Krane RJ, Frohrib D, Goldstein I. The hemodynamic pathophysiology of impotence following blunt trauma to the erect penis. *J Urol.* 1992;148:1171-1180.

102. Cass AS, Gleich P, Smith C: Male genital injuries from external trauma. *British Journal of Urology.* 1985;57:467-470.

103. Kanagaye JT. Penile zipper entrapment: A simple and less threatening approach using mineral oil. *Ped Emerg Care.*1993; 90-91.

104. Nolan JF, Stillwell TJ, Sands JP. Acute management of the zipper-entrapped penis. *J Emerg Med.* 1990;305-307.

105. Wesson MB. Traumatism of the testicle: Report of a case of a rupture of a solitary testicle. *Urol Cutaneous Rev*. 1946;50:16-19.

106. Cass AS, Luxenberg M. Testicular injuries. *Urology*. 1991;37:528-530.

107. Cass AS, Ferrara L, Wolpert J, Lee J. Bilateral testicular injury from external trauma. *J Urol*. 1988;140:1435-1436.

108. Schuster G. Traumatic rupture of the testicle and a review of the literature. *J Urol*. 1982;127:1194-1196.

109. MacDermott JP, Gray BK, Stewart PA. Traumatic rupture of the testis. *Br J Urol*. 1988;62:179-181.

110. Vacarro JA, Davis R, Belville WD. Traumatic hematocele: Association with rupture of the testicle. *J Urol*. 1986;136:1217-1218.

111. Cass AS. Testicular trauma. *J Urol*. 1983;129:299-300.

112. Romilly CS, Isaac MT. Male genital self-mutilation. *British Journal of Hospital Medicine*. 1996;55:427-431.

113. Culp DA. Genital injuries: Etiology and initial management. *Urologic Clinics of North America*. 1977;4:143-156.

114. Monga M, Moreno T, Hellstrom WJ. Gunshot wounds to the male genitalia. *J Trauma*. 1995;38:855-858.

115. Bickel A, Mata J, Hochstein LM, Landreneau MD, Aultman DF, Culkin DJ. Bowel injury as a result of penetrating scrotal trauma: review of associated injuries. *J Urol*. 1990;143: 1017-1018.

116. Fournier GR Jr, Laing FC, Jeffrey RB, McAninch JW. High resolution scrotal ultrasonography: a highly sensitive but nonspecific diagnostic technique. *J Urol*. 1985;134:490-493.

117. Wessells H, McAninch JW. Testicular trauma. *Urology*. 1996;47:750.

118. Herbener TE. Ultrasound in the assessment of the acute scrotum. *J Clin Ultrasound*. 1996;24:405-421.

119. Cunningham JJ. Sonographic findings in clinically unsuspected acute and chronic scrotal hematoceles. *AJR*. 1983;140:749-752.

120. Corrales JG, Corbel L, Cipolla B, Staerman F, Darnault P, Guille F, Lobel B. Accuracy of ultrasound diagnosis after blunt testicular trauma [see comments]. *J Urol*. 1993;150:1834-1836.

121. Chen DC, Holder LE, Melloul M. Radionuclide scrotal imaging: further experience with 210 new patients. Part 2: Results and discussion. *J Nucl Med*. 1983;24:841-853.

122. Barloon TJ, Weissman AM, Kahn D. Diagnostic imaging of patients with acute scrotal pain. *Am Fam Physician*. 1996;53:1734-1750.

123. Altarac S. Management of 53 cases of testicular trauma. *Eur Urol*. 1994;25:119-123.

124. McAninch JW, Kahn RI, Jeffrey RB, Laing FC, Krieger MJ. Major traumatic and septic genital injuries. *J Trauma*. 1984;24:291-298.

125. Cass AS, Luxenberg M. Value of early operation in blunt testicular contusion with hematocele. *J Urol*. 1988;139:746-747.

126. Pohl DR, Johnson DE, Robison JR. Bilateral testicular rupture: report of a case. *J Urol*. 1968;99:772-773.

127. Horton CE, Dean JA. Reconstruction of traumatically acquired defects of the phallus. *World J Surg*. 1990;14:757-762.

128. Meinhardt W, Kropman RF, Lycklama à Nijeholt AAB, Zwartendijk J. Skin necrosis caused by the use of negative pressure device for erectile impotence. *J Urol*. 1990;983.

129. Wheeler JSJ, Steinberg J. Penile skin avulsion managed by scrotal flaps. *Surgical Rounds*. 1997;426-430.

130. Horton CE, McCraw JB, Devine CJJ, Devine PC. Secondary reconstruction in the genital area. *Urologic Clinics of North America*. 1997;4:133-141.

131. Revis DRJ, Seagle MB. Skin grafts, split thickness. *eMedicine*; 2000.

132. Barnett A, Berkowitz RL, Mills R, Vistnes L M. Comparison of synthetic adhesive moisture vapor permeable and fine mesh gauze dressing for split-thickness skin graft donor sites. *Am J Surg*. 1983;145:379-381.

133. Genecov DG, Schneider AM, Mrykwas MJ, Parker D, White WL, Argenta LC. A controlled subatmospheric pressure dressing increases the rate of skin graft donor site re-epithelialization. *Ann Plastic Surg*. 1998;40:219-225.

134. McDougal WS. Scrotal reconstruction using thigh pedicle flaps. *J Urol*. 1983;129:757-759.

8. Questions

All questions are taken verbatim from AUA practice exams before 2001.

A. Bladder Trauma

1. Following an automobile accident, a 30-year-old comatose man has a blood pressure of 110/70 mm hg, plus of 80/min, CVP of 12 cm H_2O and a urinary output of 40 ml/hour. There is gross blood in the urine. Nasotracheal intubation has been performed. The first x-ray obtained should be:

A. Skull

B. Cervical spine

C. Chest

D. IVP

E. Cystogram

2. A 26-year-old woman has a pelvic fracture, collapsed lung and a severe closed head injury following an automobile accident. A retrograde cystogram reveals an extraperitoneal bladder rupture. The next step in management is:

A. Catheter drainage

B. Immediate surgical repair

C. Diagnostic peritoneal lavage

D. Abdominal and pelvic CT scan

E. Suprapubic cystotomy

3. An intoxicated 45-year-old man with a history of chronic alcoholism is evaluated in the emergency room. Physical examination reveals no abnormalities other than ecchymoses over the lower abdomen. The blood pressure is 160/80 mm Hg, pulse 70, respirations 20, temperature 37.5° C and the CVP is 10 mm H_2O. A plain film of the abdomen shows a "ground glass" appearance. Initial blood studies reveal: HCT 32%, WBC 15,800/cu mm, Na 122 mEq/L, K 6.0 mEq/L, Cl 109 mEq/L, CO2 13 mEq/L, BUN 80 mg/dL and creatinine 4.3 mg/dL. A Foley catheter is placed but there is no urine output. The next step in management should be:

A. Kayexalate® and furosomide

B. Cystogram

C. Renogram

D. Noncontrast CT scan

E. Tap the abdomen

4. A 24-year-old man is struck by a car and sustains multiple injuries including a pelvic fracture. He has blood at the meatus and a retrograde urethrogram is normal. A catheter is passed and the bladder is filled with 200 cc of contrast. A full and post-drainage film are normal. The next step should be:

A. Evaluation of the upper tracts by CT scan

B. Repeat the cystogram

C. Leave catheter and irrigate as needed to clear clots

D. Flexible cystoscopy to exclude a urethral or bladder injury

E. Intravenous urogram with tomograms

5. A 43-year-old woman sustains a single gunshot wound to the abdomen. You are consulted at the time of emergency laparotomy for an obvious bullet hole in the dome of the bladder. You should:

A. Open the bladder anteriorly and inspect the inside of the bladder

B. Perform an intraoperative cystogram

C. Debride the bullet hole and close it in two layers

D. Perform an intraoperative IVP

E. Place a ureteral stent

B. Urethral Trauma

1. A 25-year-old pedestrian is struck by an automobile. On arrival in the emergency room, a plain film of the pelvis reveals a left superior and inferior pubic ramus fracture as well as a fracture of the sacroiliac joint. Examination of the patient reveals a suprapubic mass. No blood is noted at the meatus and the prostate is in the normal position on digital examination. The most appropriate initial diagnostic test is:

A. IVP

B. Retrograde urethrogram

C. Cystogram

D. Pelvic CT scan

E. Peritoneal lavage

2. A 26-year-old uncircumcised boy is shot in the penis with a low velocity bullet from a .22 caliber handgun. He has voided a small amount of grossly bloody urine and is now in urinary retention. A urethrogram shows disruption of 1 cm of the penile urethra with extravasation of contrast material. The best next step is debridement of the wound and:

A. Suprapubic tube

B. Patch graft urethroplasty

C. Urethral catheter

D. Island flap urethroplasty

E. End-to-end reanastomosis

3. A 14-year-old boy has a straddle injury to the perineum. Physical examination reveals ecchymosis limited to the penis and scrotum. The fascia that contains the extravasated blood is:

A. Buck's

B. Dartos

C. Colles'

D. External spermatic

E. Transversalis

C. Genital Trauma

1. A 22-year-old man sustains a severe burn of his genitalia. There is marked bullous edema and eschar formation of the entire penis and much of the scrotum. He has had a Foley catheter in his urethra to monitor urine output. The most appropriate initial management is:

A. Radical eschar debridement

B. Split thickness skin grafts as soon as possible

C. Antibiotic therapy and topical cleansing with water

D. Remove the Foley and insert a suprapubic tube

E. Observe until the wound begins to granulate

2. The preferred management of ruptured testis is:

A. Orchidectomy

B. Closure of the tunica albuginea

C. Orchidectomy and prosthesis infection

D. Bedrest, scrotal elevation, and ice packs

E. Incision and drainage of scrotum

3. A 23-year-old man suffers severe scrotal, penile and buttock burns. 4 days later the scrotal skin appears necrotic and malodorous with the testes visible. After giving antibiotics and performing local debridement, the next step in management is to:

A. Perform local wound care and delayed reconstruction

B. Perform split thickness skin grafts to cover testes

C. Place testes in subfascial thigh pouches

D. Create lateral subcutaneous flaps to cover the scrotum

E. Place testes under subpubic subcutaneous space

4. A 3-year-old boy is seen because his foreskin is caught in his zipper. The best treatment is:

A. Circumcision

B. Manipulation of the zipper under general anesthesia

C. Manipulation of the zipper under local anesthesia

D. Divide the median bar of the zipper with a bone cutter

E. Excision of the piece of penile skin caught

5. At the time of a newborn circumcision, the distal one-half of the glans penis is amputated, including the urethra. The prepuce and glans have been kept in iced saline for 4 hours. The best management is:

A. Primary anastomosis

B. Graft of preputial skin for coverage

C. Discard glans tip and allow secondary healing

D. Discard the glans tip and re-configure remaining glans

E. Primary anastomosis with microvascular reconstruction

6. A 16-year-old uncircumcised boy is shot in the penis with a low velocity bullet from a .22 caliber handgun. He has voided a small amount of grossly bloody urine and is now in urinary retention. A urethrogram shows disruption of 1 cm of the penile urethra and extravasation of contrast material. The best next step is debridement of the wound and:

A. Suprapubic tube

B. Patch graft urethroplasty

C. Urethral catheter

D. Island flap urethroplasty

E. End-to-end anastomosis

2005 SESAP 5/150 Questions

1. An intoxicated 45-year-old man is evaluated in the emergency room for abdominal pain. Physical examination reveals no abnormalities other than ecchymosis over the lower abdomen. The blood pressure is 160/80 mm Hg, puls 70, respirations 20, temperature 37.5 degrees Celsius. A plain film of the abdomen shows a "ground glass" appearance. Initial blood studies reveal: HCT 32, WBC 15,800, Na 122 MEq/L, K 6.0 mEq/L, Cl 109 meEq/L, CO2 13 mEq/L, BUN 80 mg/dL, and creatinine 4.3 mg/dL. A Foley catheter is placed but there is no urinary output. The next step is:

A. Kayexalate and furosemide

B. Cystogram

C. Renogram

D. Noncontract CT scan

E. Paracentesis

2. A 13-year-old boy falls from a tree and develops gross hematuria. CT scan shows a left renal laceration extending into the collecting system with significant urinary extravasation. Contrast is seen in the distal ureter. 3 weeks following the injury, he develops a low grade fever, an ileus and a tender distended abdomen. CT scan shows a large left urinoma. The next step is:

A. Placement of a urethral catheter

B. Percutaneous nephrostomy drainage

C. Open surgical drainage and renorrhaphy

D. Percutaneous drainage of the urinoma

E. Placement of a ureteral stent

3. A 4-year-old boy fell from a second-story window. On examination his vital signs are stable, but he has right flank and upper quadrant abdominal tenderness and fullness. He does not have peritoneal signs. Urinalysis is negative. The next step is:

   A. Observation

   B. Abdominal paracentesis

   C. Abdominal and renal ultrasound

   D. IVP

   E. Abdominal CT scan

4. The most definitive study to rule out traumatic bladder rupture is:

   A. Pelvic CT scan

   B. Cystoscopy

   C. Pelvic ultrasound

   D. CT cystogram

   E. IVP

2004 SESAP 3/150 Questions

1. A 20-year-old man sustains a circumferential avulsion of the skin of the midshaft of the penis. There is intact skin on both the proximal and distal aspects of the penile shaft, with a denuded area 4 cm in length. The most appropriate treatment is:

   A. Primary approximation of the skin

   B. Split-thickness skin graft to the denuded area

   C. Split thickness skin graft and removal of distal penile skin

   D. Full thickness skin graft to the denuded area

   E. Scrotal rotational flap covering the denuded area

2. A 23-year-old man notes a cracking noise and subsequent penile pain during intercourse, followed by progressive penile swelling and ecchymosis. He is initially embarrassed to seek medical attention despite persistent penile pain. 36 hours after the traumatic event, he is afebrile with stable vital signs. A retrograde urethrogram is normal. The next step is:

   A. Reassurance and cold compresses

   B. Cavernosal-spongiosal shunt

   C. Surgical exploration

   D. Foley catheter splinting

   E. Corporeal aspiration and Foley catheter drainage

3. A 10-year-old boy has a perineal "butterfly" hematoma following a straddle injury. This suggest rupture of the:

   A. Tunica albuginea

   B. Corpus spongiosum

   C. Corpus cavernosum

   D. Posterior urethra

   E. Colles' fascia

2003 SESAP 5/150 Questions

1. A 25-year-old male pedestrian is struck by an automobile. He has a left superior and inferior pubic ramus fracture as well as a fracture of the sacroiliac joint. He has a palpable bladder. No blood is noted at the meatus and the prostate is in the normal position on digital examination. The next stop is:

   A. IVP

   B. Retrograde urethrogram

   C. Cystogram

D. Pelvic CT scan

E. Peritoneal lavage

2. A 23-year-old man suffers severe scrotal, penile and buttock burns. 4 days later, the scrotal skin appears necrotic and malodorous and testes are visible. After administering antibiotics and performing local debridement, the next step is:

A. Local wound care and delayed reconstruction

B. Split-thickness skin grafts to cover testes

C. Place testes in subfascial thigh pouches

D. Create lateral subcutaneous flaps to cover scrotum

E. Place testes into infrapubic subcutaneous space

3. A 42-year-old man is undergoing laparotomy for intra abdominal injuries and bladder rupture. Bleeding is noted in the perivesical area. After repair of bladder rupture, pelvic pressure does not stop the persistent oozing. Multiple blood transfusions are given and his core temperature is 35.5 degrees Celsius. The next step is:

A. Intraoperative arteriography

B. Ligation of the hypogastric arteries

C. Intravenous aminocaproic acid

D. Close the abdomen and place patient in a MAST suit

E. Pack pelvis and close abdomen

2002 SESAP 5/150 Questions

1. The optimal tissue for early coverage of the perineum following an avulsion skin injury is a(n):

A. Island skin flap

B. Musculocutaneous flap

C. Full-thickness skin graft

D. Split-thickness skin graft

E. Dermal graft

2. A 23-year-old woman suffers a complex pelvic fracture in a motor vehicle accident. A cystogram reveals limited extraperitoneal extravasation of contrast at the bladder neck. The bladder is compressed by a pelvic hematoma and an anterior vaginal laceration is also present. No other injuries are noted and the patient is hemodynamically stable. Treatment should be:

A. Urethral catheter drainage

B. Percutaneous suprapubic cystostomy

C. Open bladder repair

D. Suprapubic cystostomy and perivesical drainage

E. Repair of vaginal and bladder laceration

2001 SESAP 5/150 Questions

1. A 12-year-old prepubertal boy has severe right scrotal pain 1 day after being kicked in the groin. There is a blue area over the superior portion of the testis, but the examination is difficult due to a hydrocele. Urinalysis is normal. The next step is:

A. Immediate exploration

B. Scrotal ultrasound with Doppler

C. Scrotal nuclear scan

D. Manual detorsion, exploration

E. Observation, anti-inflammatory medications

2. A 22-year-old man sustains a severe burn of his genitalia. There is marked bullous edema and eschar formation of the entire penis and much of the scrotum. He has had a catheter in his urethral for 3 days to monitor urine output. The next step is:

A. Radical eschar debridement

B. Split-thickness skin graft as soon as possible

C. Antibiotic therapy and topical cleansing with water

D. Remove the urethral catheter and insert a suprapubic tube

E. Observe until the wound begins to granulate

Answers

Bladder Trauma

1. B.

2. A.

3. B.

4. B.

5. A.

Urethral Trauma

1. B.

2. E.

3. A.

Genital Trauma

1. B.

2. B.

3. A.

4. D.

5. A.

6. E.

2005 SESAP 5/150

1. B.

2. D.

3. E.

4. D.

2003 SESAP 3/150

1. C.

2. C.

3. B.

2003 SESAP 5/150

1. B.

2. A.

3. E.

2002 SESAP 1/150

1. D.

2. E.

2001 SESAP 5/150

1. D.

2. E.

Chapter 26: Physiology and Complications of Laparoscopy

Jeffrey A. Cadeddu, MD

Contents

1. Physiologic Changes of Pneumoperitoneum

Initially, laparoscopy was utilized for minor and rapid gynecological interventions, but after 2 decades it is now used to treat many urological conditions. Laparoscopic and robotic-assisted laparoscopic interventions are now lengthy, complex and are often utilized to treat high-risk patients who present with multiple comorbid conditions. In addition to common surgical complications, such as bleeding and infection, laparoscopy may result in a unique set of physiological disturbances and complications. Many of these can cause significant morbidity if not recognized and treated promptly. This chapter will review the physiological changes associated with abdominal laparoscopy and will discuss common complications of laparoscopic urological surgery emphasizing their recognition and management.

Respiratory Changes

Hypercarbia

Carbon dioxide (CO_2), used for peritoneal insufflation, is noncombustible and is highly soluble in blood. However, it may be rapidly absorbed through the peritoneum and induce hypercarbia and acidosis. The absorption is increased with high intraabdominal pressures (IAP) and prolonged procedures. The compensatory renal excretion of H^+ is too slow to correct the low bicarbonate levels in the extracellular fluid, and acidosis results. The deep head-down position (Trendelenburg), often utilized in laparoscopic prostate and bladder surgery, causes a significant rise in the intracranial pressure and may worsen CO_2 accumulation and hypercarbia. The alternatives to CO_2 insufflation include nitrous oxide and inert gases such as helium, argon and xenon. Nitrous oxide, however, supports combustion and can cause distention of the bowel, while inert gases are not readily soluble in blood and risk an embolus.

Changes in Ventilatory Dynamics

High IAP decreases diaphragmatic motion, elevating intrathoracic pressure and limiting expansion of the lungs. The functional residual capacity and pulmonary dynamic compliance are decreased and peak inspiratory pressures are elevated. That in turn leads to increasing ventilation-perfusion mismatch and shunting, which may result in hypoxemia, especially in patients with compromised pulmonary reserves. High peak and plateau inspiratory pressures can also cause ventilator induced lung injury.

Pulmonary Complications

Hypoxemia

Adequate ventilation and oxygenation can limit hypoxemia, but in patients with COPD, conversion to open surgery may be required.

Atelectasis

Presents with low grade fever in the first 24-48 hours following the procedure and is treated with the intensive use of incentive spirometers, deep breathing and coughing.

Table 1

Respiratory Effects of Pneumoperitonium

Parameter	Change
Peak inspiratory pressure	↑
Chest wall mechanical resistance	↑
Pulmonary compliance	↓
Pulmonary dead space	↔
Functional residual capacity	↓
Vital capacity	↓
Shunting	↑
Ventilation-perfusion mismatch	↑

Pneumothorax/Pneumomediastinum/ Pneumopericardium

Results from the barotrauma sustained during elevated inspiratory pressures. The diagnosis is made with a chest x-ray, and a chest drain may be necessary for resolution. Capnothorax is a CO_2 accumulation in the intrapleural space. It is suspected when the mean airway pressure suddenly rises and oxygen saturation declines. Capnothorax often resolves spontaneously as CO_2 is rapidly reabsorbed once the pneumoperitoneum is released. Chest tubes are usually not necessary and treatment with oxygen is often sufficient.

Subcutaneous Emphysema

Subcutaneous emphysema results from CO_2 passing into subcutaneous tissues and retroperitoneum and presents with skin crepitus upon palpation. It is often self-limited, but massive subcutaneous emphysema involving the face and neck can cause pneumomediastinum and result in respiratory compromise requiring intubation.

Gas Embolism

This is the most serious pulmonary complication that can result in rapid cardiovascular collapse and death. It is extremely rare and is often caused by direct insufflation of a vessel with a Veress needle or rapid absorption of large amount of CO_2 through an injured vessel due to raised IAP. It presents with sudden hypotension, cyanosis, increasing concentration of end-tidal CO_2 and a "mill wheel" murmur over the right ventricle. If a gas embolism is suspected the following interventions must be initiated immediately to prevent the embolus from going into the right ventricle outflow tract and pulmonary vasculature:

- Release pneumoperitoneum
- Place the patient in the left lateral decubitous, head-down position
- Increase minute ventilation and administer 100% O_2
- Place a central venous line in an attempt to aspirate the gas
- Cardiopulmonary resuscitation may be necessary

Hemodynamic Changes

Decrease in Cardiac Preload

Compression of the inferior vena cava secondary to increased IAP decreases venous return and therefore reduces preload. Low volume status can exacerbate this effect.

Increase in Cardiac Afterload

Hypercarbia enhances sympathetic activity and may stimulate the renin-angiotensin cascade with resultant vasoconstriction and increase in systemic vascular resistance (SVR).

Decrease in Cardiac Output

Decrease in cardiac preload and rise in SVR may decrease cardiac output despite tachycardia and increased cardiac contractility arising from increased sympathetic tone.

Arrhythmias

Rapid insufflation and stretching of peritoneum can induce vagal-stimulated cardiovascular response with significant bradyarrhythmias such as bradycardia, bigeminy, unifocal and multifocal ventricular ectopy, nodal rhythm, AV dissociation and asystole. Most arrhythmias will respond to release of pneumoperitoneum and increase in minute ventilation.

Table 2

Physiologic Effects of Pneumoperitonium

Parameter	Change
Heart rate	↔ ↑
Mean arterial pressure	↑
Systemic vascular resistance	↑
Venous return	↓
Central venous pressure	↑
Cardiac output	↔ ↑
Glomerular filtration rate	↓
Urine output	↓
Intracranial pressure	↑

Renal Changes

Oliguria

Oliguria during laparoscopy results from several physiological derangements induced by intraperitoneal insufflation. Several distinct mechanisms, such as direct compression of renal parenchyma and vasculature, decreased cardiac output, increased activity of renin-angiotensin system and increase in antidiuretic hormone release, are postulated to cause decreased urine production during abdominal insufflation. Using warm CO_2 for insufflation may help with local renal vasodilation and limit the deleterious effects of pneumoperitoneum on urine production. However, the best prevention strategy is maintenance of adequate intravascular volume preoperatively and throughout the procedure.

2. Complications

Complications of Patient Positioning

Laparoscopic procedures require longer surgical time and often rely on gravity to facilitate intra-abdominal organ retraction. Patients frequently spend a significant time in a modified flank or Trendelenburg position and, therefore, proper positioning and padding is critical to avoid neuro-muscular injuries.

- The nerves most prone to injury are brachial plexus, femoral, sciatic and lateral popliteal

- To avoid injury to the brachial plexus the upper side arm should be supported by a pillow or a folded blanket and care must be taken to ensure that the arm is not overly abducted or externally rotated to prevent the humeral head from applying pressure on the brachial plexus

- The downside leg must be padded and gently flexed as the upside leg must be supported by pillows and elevated to minimize adduction at the hip and limit stretching of the sciatic nerve

- Patients must be secured to the table with either padded straps or padded tape at the level of the ankles, hips and shoulders to prevent falling and shifting during rotation of the table

- Neuro-muscular injuries usually present with paresthesias and weakness in the affected extremity. Mild injuries will respond to physical therapy and will frequently resolve over several weeks, however, severe stretch injuries may result in permanent neurological dysfunction

- Rhabdomyolysis is a serious complication of improper positioning and involves muscle ischemia following prolonged compression. Rhabdomyolysis may result in acute renal failure secondary to myoglobinuria and tubular obstruction by myoglobin casts. The risk factors for development of rhabdomyolysis include morbid obesity, exaggerated intraoperative position, hypovolemia with intraoperative hypotension, operative time more than 5 hours, diabetes, compromised renal function and hypertension. The condition should be suspected in patients presenting postoperatively with excessive muscular pain, oliguria, dark urine and rising creatinine. The mainstay of therapy is vigorous hydration. Urine alkalinization has been shown to be beneficial in animal studies, but clear evidence of clinical efficacy has not been established. The best prevention strategy is careful padding of all pressure points, minimizing the use of kidney rest and limiting operative times

Complications of Access

- Intraperitoneal access and establishment of pneumoperitoneum is most commonly achieved by 2 distinct techniques: the Veress closed technique and the Hasson open technique

- The closed technique consists of placing the Veress insufflation needle into the abdomen (most commonly through the umbilicus) blindly followed by insufflation and insertion of the first trocar either blindly or using an optical trocar system

- With the Hasson method an opening is created in the peritoneum under direct vision and a blunt tip trocar is introduced, and pneumoperitoneum is established

- Both approaches are relatively safe, with the closed technique having a slightly higher incidence of vascular injury

- Correct placement of Veress needle is confirmed with the following maneuvers:

    * Two "pops" should be felt as the needle traverses the fascia and the peritoneum

    * Aspiration of blood or bowel contents indicates improper position

    * Injection of 5-10 cc of saline and inability to aspirate back indicates that the needle is in the correct position

    * "Drop test": a bleb of saline left in the hub of the needle should fall freely down the needle

    * Initial low pressure reading (<10 mm Hg) upon insufflation confirms proper needle position

Vascular Injuries Due to Access

Common iliac artery can be injured by blind Veress needle insertion, as the bifurcation of the great vessels is located approximately at the level of the umbilicus. If blood is aspirated initially upon Veress needle placement, the needle must be withdrawn slightly and the new position retested prior to insufflation. Management of vascular injuries due to Veress needle depends on amount of bleeding. Many are small and at most will require a laparoscopic suture repair. Major vascular injuries, however, may require immediate open conversion and formal repair. Injuries to epigastric vessels occur during trocar placement through the lateral portion of the rectus muscle. This injury is diagnosed by observing bleeding from the trocar site on the inside of the anterior abdominal wall. Management involves placement of full thickness suture ligature through the fascia and the peritoneum under laparoscopic guidance using a fascial closure device.

Visceral Injuries Due to Access

An injury to colon, stomach or bladder is suspected when colored or malodorous fluid is aspirated through the Veress needle. These organs must be carefully examined once pneumoperitoneum is established to see whether a formal repair is necessary. Injuries to these organs secondary to Veress needle placement are usually self-limited and rarely require intervention. However, even a small perforation in the gall bladder may result in a bile leak and peritonitis and therefore a cholecystectomy is usually necessary. Veress needle injuries to the liver or spleen can usually be controlled by direct pressure or application of hemostatic agents such as FloSeal® or fibrin glue. Argon beam coagulation is usually adequate to control bleeding from these small punctures as well.

Intraoperative Complications

Vascular Injuries

Vascular injuries are the most commonly reported complication of urologic laparoscopy and can result in minor bleeding or severe life-threatening hemorrhage. Preventive measures include good exposure, careful dissection and precise ligation of blood vessels, clear visualization of the tip of dissecting struments, and care not to manipulate hemostatic clips.

- Bleeding resulting from injury to small vessels (<4 mm) can be controlled with the use of LigaSure™ or Harmonic® scalpel devices. Hem-o-lock® or metal clips can be used to ligate bleeding vessels unless the clips will interfere with application of a vascular stapler. Minor bleeding from the renal vein and even vena cava can be controlled by increasing the pneumoperitoneum to 20 mm Hg and applying direct pressure over the defect. Placement of additional trocars may sometimes be necessary to provide retraction or to place a suction/irrigator device. Once the injury is clearly visualized, the adjunctive maneuvers may include application of FloSeal and oxidized cellulose. Intracorporeal suturing can be utilized as well, and Lapra-Ty® clips can save valuable time by eliminating the need for knot tying. Major vascular injuries resulting in severe hemorrhage, expanding hematoma or hemodynamic instability require immediate open conversion and formal repair

Injuries to Abdominal Viscera

Injuries to liver and spleen often occur when the instrument is outside the field of view. To prevent these complications, it is important to follow the instruments with the camera during insertion, especially when a novice surgeon is operating. Minor tears can be FloSeal controlled with application of oxidized cellulose, fibrin glue and gelatin thrombin matrix (Baxter, Inc., Deerfield, IL). Argon beam coagulation is very useful as well. Major lacerations with significant bleeding may require conversion to open surgery and consultation with a general surgeon. Bleeding secondary to large splenic tears is very difficult to control and a splenectomy may be necessary.

- Distal pancreas can be injured during left-sided nephrectomy and adrenalectomy. Cautery must be avoided in close proximity to the tail of the pancreas, and if retraction of the pancreas is necessary, blunt wide surface retractors must be utilized. If pancreatic injury is recognized intraoperatively, a general surgery consultation must be obtained to establish whether distal pancreatectomy is necessary

Gastrointestinal Injuries

- Unrecognized bowel injuries during abdominal laparoscopy can cause significant morbidity and even result in a fatality. The bowel is often injured during applications of monopolar electrocautery and during blind passage of instruments. Breaks in insulation coating and poor visualization of cautery contact points can result in thermal injuries to bowel "off screen" which remain unrecognized. Thermal spread from monopolar cautery can extend several centimeters from the operative site resulting in sufficient temperature elevations to cause tissue destruction

- Patients with unrecognized bowel injuries often present 1-2 days postoperatively and lack the typical signs and symptoms of peritonitis. If the diagnosis is missed, patients can succumb to sepsis and cardio-pulmonary collapse within 96 hours of surgery. Clinicians must have a low threshold for ordering abdominal CT in patients presenting in the following fashion:

    * Low grade temperature

    * Abdominal distention and diarrhea with persistent bowel sounds and absence of peritoneal signs

    * Severe trocar site pain without purulence or erythema

    * Nausea and vomiting are uncommon

    * Leucopenia with a left shift

- CT of the abdomen and pelvis with oral contrast has very high sensitivity for diagnosis of a bowel injury. If CT is indicative of a bowel perforation, an immediate exploration with bowel repair and/or resection is necessary

- Rectal injury is a rare complication of laparoscopic radical prostatectomy. If recognized intraoperatively and gross fecal spillage is absent, the perforation can be closed primarily in 2 layers. Closed suction drain must be placed near the repair and the patient's antibiotic coverage must be broadened for several days. However, gross fecal contamination, or inability to complete a primary repair require open conversion and a diverting colostomy

- Occasionally, when developing a plane between the colonic mesentery and Gerota's fascia, inadvertent incision in the mesentery creates a sufficient opening for small bowel herniation. To prevent an internal hernia, which may lead to small bowel obstruction, all mesenteric windows must be closed with clips or intracorporeal suturing. If internal hernia is suspected, a CT is helpful in establishing the diagnosis

- Trocar site hernias causing small bowel obstruction are rare complications of abdominal laparoscopy. 5 millimeter and 12 mm radially dilating trocars in adults do not require formal fascial closure; however, the fascia of 12 mm bladed trocar sites, especially in the midline, should be closed using absorbable suture, a fascial closure device. Trocar site hernia is suspected when a patient presents with a bulge at the trocar site with or without signs of small bowel obstruction. CT is usually diagnostic. Management consists of open or laparoscopic exploration and reduction of the hernia. Bowel resection may be necessary if the incarcerated loop appears nonviable

Diaphragmatic Injuries

- Diaphragm is usually injured by electrocautery during laparoscopic renal and adrenal surgery. Diaphragmatic injuries can range from subtle, presenting with increasing airway pressures and hypercarbia to severe, causing a rapid cardiovascular collapse secondary to tension pneumothorax. Tension pneumothorax must be treated immediately by release of pneumoperitoneum and decompression of the chest with a needle or tube thoracostomy. If pleurotomy is identified intraoperatively, but the patient remains stable, the injury can be suture repaired at the end of the procedure once all the air is expelled from the pleural cavity

Ureteral Injuries

- Ureteral injuries usually result from electrocautery burns that frequently remain unrecognized intraoperatively. Patients present with increased output from the drains, pain secondary to urinoma formation, or urinary ascites. Diagnosis is made with retrograde pyelography or intravenous urography. Minor injuries with minimal extravasation can be managed with retrograde or antegrade stent insertion or percutaneous nephrostomy drainage. Large injuries with significant tissue loss may require open reconstruction. If ureteral burn is recognized intraoperatively, the affected segment must be widely excised and ureteral continuity reestablished. Location of the injury dictates the method of repair that should be utilized

3. Special Circumstances

Extraperitoneoscopy

- Hypercarbia secondary to CO_2 absorption is more pronounced, with extraperitoneal laparoscopy, as compared to the intraperitoneal approach, especially in the presence of subcutaneous emphysema

- Hemodynamic changes are similar to thosc of intraperitoneal approach; however, decrease in renal vein flow, oliguria and the rise in mean arterial pressure are less pronounced

Hand-Assisted Laparoscopy

- Analgesic requirements, corrected 2-week abdominal/flank pain scores, and duration of convalescence is not affected by the presence of the hand-port incision

- Physiologic derangements and complications of hand-assisted laparoscopy are similar to those of the standard laparoscopic approach. However, the incidence of postoperative ileus and delayed bowel function seems to be higher

- The unique complications of hand-assisted laparoscopy include herniation and dehiscence involving the hand port incision, although both are rare

Laparoscopy in Neonates and Infants

- Young patients absorb proportionally more CO_2 than older individuals and have a higher risk for developing hypercarbia, which in turn could stimulate the sympathetic nervous system and sensitize the myocardium to the arrhythmogenic effects of catecholamines

- Cardiovascular physiology of infants differs from that of adults. Their blood pressure and systemic vascular resistance are usually lower, where heart rate, O_2 consumption and cardiac output are higher. High IAP in neonates and young children may increase pulmonary vascular resistance resulting in increased right-to-left cardiac shunting and decreased cardiac index

- It is prudent to preheat CO_2 to maintain normothermia, especially during high flow insufflation and in small babies. Cases of hypothermia due to CO_2 insufflation have been reported in neonates

Laparoscopy During Pregnancy

- Insufflation of an abdomen containing a gravid uterus can result in physiological changes that exceed those normally seen during laparoscopy. Diaphragmatic expansion is significantly reduced resulting in exaggerated changes in peak airway pressure, functional residual capacity and ventilation-perfusion mismatching

- The primary concern regarding the safety of laparoscopic surgery during pregnancy is the physiologic consequences of the CO_2 insufflation to the fetus. Elevation of maternal partial pressure of arterial CO_2 could potentially impair fetal CO_2 excretion across the placenta and could exacerbate fetal acidosis. Perioperative monitoring of arterial blood gases as well as perioperative fetal and uterine monitoring is recommended even for healthy parturients

4. Complications of Kidney Tumor Ablation

- Both laparoscopic and percutaneous kidney tumor ablation is an increasingly popular and viable alternative to surgery for treatment of small renal tumors. Complications associated with cryoablation and radiofrequency ablation techniques are increasing and require familiarity by the urologist

- **Minor Complications include:**
  - Elevated serum creatinine
  - Hematuria
  - Minor hemorrhage (small perinephric hematoma)
  - Pain or paresthesia at the probe site

- **Major Complications include:**
  - Bowel injury — eg, nephrocolic fistula
  - Ileus
  - Open conversion
  - Significant hemorrhage (large or expanding hematoma – more common with cryoablation of tumors >3 cm)
  - Urinary extravasation – collecting system injury (reported with cryoablation and RFA)
  - UPJ obstruction (reported with cryoablation and RFA)

Conclusions

Practical knowledge of physiological changes and potential complications of laparoscopy, as well as their prevention, timely diagnosis and proper management, is essential to get patients safely through the complex and often prolonged urologic laparoscopic procedures. Thorough preoperative assessment, careful perioperative monitoring, meticulous technique and good communication between surgeons and anesthesiologists are critical to minimizing surgical complications and improving patient outcomes.

5. Further Reading

Book Chapters

1. Lee BR, Jarrett TW. Prevention and management of laparoscopic complications. In: Smith AD, Badllani G, Bagley D, et al, eds. *Smith's Textbook of Endourology.* London, England: BC Decker Inc; 2007:475-484.

2. Dunn MD, Monk TG. Anesthetic considerations. In: Smith AD, Badllani G, Bagley D, et al, eds. *Smith's Textbook of Endourology.* Hamilton, London, England: BC Decker Inc; 2007:385-394.

3. Pearle MS, Cadeddu JA. Physiologic effects of pneumoperitoneum. In: Smith AD, Badllani G, Bagley D, et al, eds. *Smith's Textbook of Endourology.* London, England: BC Decker Inc; 2007:395-405.

4. Eichel L, McDougall EM, Clayman RV. Basics of laparoscopic urologic surgery. In: Wein AJ, Kavoussi LR, Novick AC, Partin AW, Peters CA, eds. *Campbell-Walsh Urology.* Philadelphia, PA: Saunders Elsevier; 2007:171-220.

Review Articles

1. Conachar ID, Soomro NA, Rix D. Anaesthesia for laparoscopic urological surgery. *Brit J Anaes.* 2004;6:859-64.

2. Bird VG, Winfield HN. Laparoscopy in urology: Physiologic considerations. *Urol Board Rev Man.* 2002;10:1-21.

3. Gerges FJ, Kanazi GE, Jabbour-Khoury SI. Anesthesia for laparoscopy: a review. *J Clin Anest.* 2006;18: 67-78.

4. Hedican SP. Complications of hand-assisted laparoscopic urologic surgery. *J Endo.* 2004;18:387-396.

5. Henny CP, Hofland J. Laparoscopic surgery: Pitfalls due to anesthesia, positioning and pneumoperitoneum. *Surg Endo.* 2005;19: 1163-1171.

6. Matsumoto ED, Cadeddu JA. Laparoscopic access: one goal, many choices. *AUA Update Series.* 2006:25(Lesson 5).

7. O'Rourke N, Kodali B. Laparoscopic surgery during pregnancy. *Curr Opin Anest.* 2006;19: 254-259.

8. Truchon R. Anaesthetic considerations for laparoscopic surgery in neonates and infants: a practical review. *Best Pract Res Clin Anaesthe.* 2004;2:343-355.

9. Venkatesh R, Landman J, Sundaram C, Clayman RV. Prevention, recognition, and management of laparoscopic complications of urologic surgery. *AUA Update Series.* 2003;22 (Lesson 40).

Original Articles

1. Reisiger K, Landman J, Kibel A, Clayman RV. Laparoscopic renal surgery and the risk of rhabdomyolysis: diagnosis and treatment. *Urology.* 2005; 66(Suppl. 5A):29-35.

2. Bishoff JT, Allaf ME, Kirkels W, et al. Laparoscopic bowel injury: incidence and clinical presentation. *J Urol.* 1999;161: 887-890.

3. Vallancien G, Cathelineau X, Baumert H, et al. Complications of transperitoneal laparoscopic surgery in urology: review of 1,311 procedures in a single center. *J Urol.* 2002;168:23-26.

4. McDougal EM, Monk TJ, Wolf JS, et al. The effect of prolonged pneumoperitoneum on renal function in animal model. *J Amer Coll Surg.* 1996;182: 317-28.

5. Strup SE, Trabulsi EJ, McGinnis ED, et al. Complications of hand-assisted laparoscopic nephrectomy: a review of 118 consecutive cases. *J Urol.* 2002;167(suppl.):168.

6. Gill IS, Strzempkowski B, Kaouk J, et al. Prospective randomized comparison: transperitoneal versus retroperitoneal laparoscopic radical nephrectomy. *J Urol*. 2002; 167(suppl):19.

7. Guillonneau B, Rozet F, Cathelineau X, et al. Perioperative complications of laparoscopic radical prostatectomy: The Montsouris 3-year experience. *J Urol*. 2002;167:51-56.

8. Cadeddu JA, Regan F, Kavoussi LR, et al. The role of computerized tomography in the evaluation of complications after laparoscopic urological surgery. *J Urol*. 1997;158:1349-1352.

9. Chiu AW, Azadzoi KM, Hatzichristou DG, et al. Effects of intra-abdominal pressure on renal tissue perfusion during laparoscopy. *J Endo*. 1994:99-103.

10. Bergesio R, Habre W, Lanteri C, et al. Changes in respiratory mechanics during abdominal laparoscopic surgery in children. *Anaes Inten Care*. 1999;27:245-248.

11. Steinbrook RA, Bhavani-Shankar K. Hemodynamics during laparoscopic surgery in pregnancy. *Anesthe Anal*. 2001;93: 1570-1571.

12. Bhavani-Shankar K, Mushlin P. Arterial to end-tidal gradients in pregnant subjects. *Anesthesiology*. 1997;87:1596.

13. Johnson DB, Solomon SB, Shingleton WB, et al. Defining the complications of cryoablation and radiofrequency ablation of small renal tumors: a multi-institutional review. *J Urol*. 2004;172:874..

6. Questions

1. All of the following are properties of nitrous oxide insufflant, except:

A. It doesn't cause hypercarbia

B. It is readily soluble in blood

C. It may cause bowel distention

D. It doesn't support combustion

E. It does not irritate the diaphragm or peritoneum

2. Which of the following are signs of a gas embolism?

A. Sudden hypotension

B. Cyanosis

C. Increasing end-tidal CO_2

D. "Mill wheel" murmur

E. All of the above

3. All of the following maneuvers must be performed immediately if one suspects a gas embolism, except:

A. Release pneumoperitoneum

B. Increase minute ventilation and administer 100% oxygen

C. Place patient in a head-down, right lateral decubitous position

D. Place a central venous line and attempt to aspirate the gas

E. Initiate CPR as indicated

4. All of the following mechanisms account for oliguria during laparoscopy, except:

A. Direct compression of the renal parenchyma

B. Compression of renal vasculature

C. Decrease in cardiac output

D. Compression of the ureter

E. Increased activity of renin-angiotensin access and antidiuretic hormone release

5. Which of the following is not true about diagnosis and treatment of perioperative rhabdomyolysis?

A. It may present with muscular pain, oliguria, and dark urine

B. Morbid obesity is a risk factor for developing rhabdomyolysis

C. It may result in acute renal failure

D. Vigorous hydration is a mainstay of therapy

E. Urinary alkalinization has been shown to be beneficial in human studies

6. Laparoscopic bowel injury is associated with all of the following, except:

A. Peritoneal signs

B. High fever

C. Severe nausea and vomiting

D. High white blood cell count

E. All of the above

7. The nerves most prone to injury secondary to positioning for laparoscopy are all of the following, except:

A. Brachial plexus

B. Lateral popliteal

C. Sciatic

D. Femoral

E. None of the above

8. All of the following confirm correct placement of the Veress needle, except:

A. 2 "pops" are heard as the needle traverses the fascia and the peritoneum

B. Inability to aspirate back 5-10cc of saline injected through the needle

C. Low pressure reading at initiation of insufflation

D. A decrease in pressure with elevation of the abdominal wall

E. None of the above

9. Which of the following are true of the laparoscopic diaphragmatic injuries?

A. They are usually due to electrocautery

B. They always result in a tension pneumothorax and cardiovascular collapse

C. They cannot be repaired laparoscopically

D. When recognized, they must be repaired immediately

E. All of the above

10. Regarding trocar site hernias, all of the following are true, except:

A. To prevent hernias the fascia of 12 mm radially dilating trocar sites must always be closed

B. They can present as a tender or non-tender bulge at the trocar site

C. They can cause small bowel obstruction

D. They can be repaired laparoscopically

E. All of the above

Answers

1. D.
Nitrous oxide supports combustion.

2. E.
All choices are correct and are common presenting signs of gas embolus.

3. C.
Patient should be placed in a head-down, left lateral decubitous position.

4. D.
Ureteral compression has not been shown to be a mechanism of oliguria of pneumoperitoneum.

5. E.
Alkalinization was found to be beneficial only in animal studies.

6. E.
None of the choices are part of common presentation of laparoscopic bowel injury.

7. E.
All of the listed nerves are commonly affected.

8. E.
All of the choices indicate correct placement of the Veress needle.

9. A.
Diphragmatic injuries are usually secondary to electrocautery.

10. A.
Fascia of dilating trocar sites doesn't need to be closed. The actual diameter of the fascial opening is about one-half of the trocar size.

Chapter 27: Evaluation and Treatment of Male Factor Infertility

Paul J. Turek MD, FACS, FRSM

Contents

1. Introduction

The Problem

1.) Approximately 25% of couples will become pregnant after one month of trying to conceive. However, only **85% of couples will be pregnant after one year.**

2.) Approximately 15% of couples will therefore have difficulty conceiving.

3.) During the infertility evaluation, **a male factor alone may be found in approximately 30% of couples**, and both a male and female factor in an additional 20% such that a male factor may be involved in the infertility problem in approximately 50% cases.

2. Reproductive Anatomy and Physiology

Embryology

1.) Genital organs are observed during the **5th gestational week** and include an indifferent gonad, a **mesonephric duct** and the mullerian ducts.

2.) The indifferent gonad forms from a thickening in the **urogenital ridge** near the mesonephros; germ cells migrate from the yolk sac and populate the urogenital ridge. These cells are **primordial germ cells** and are very closely related to **embryonic stem cells.**

3.) Sexual differentiation of the embryo stems from the presence or absence of **sex determining region-Y (SRY)** on the **Y chromosome.** The **SRY** gene product is a protein that harbors a high mobility group box (HMG) sequence, a **DNA-binding motif** that kinks DNA. This DNA bending effect alters gene expression, leading to formation of a testis and subsequently to the male phenotype. Notably, XY individuals who lack the SRY gene on the Y chromosome are phenotypic females. Other genes are also involved in determining gonadal sex, including ***WT1, SOX-9, Wnt4 and DAX-1,*** and their expression patterns may account for phenotypic **sex reversal** cases (Figure 1).

4.) Induced to form a testis, the gonad develops clustered cords of germ cells that converge to form the **rete testis** at the hilum of the testis. These are testis stem cells and serve as the renewing source of germ cells for spermatogenesis throughout life. To further underscore their stem cell like character, adult human testicular stem cells can
be "coaxed" into embryonic-like stem cells.

5.) During the **8th week** of gestation, **testosterone** is made by differentiating **Leydig cells** and then declines in production after the 12th week during which external genital development occurs.

6.) In response to testosterone, the **mesonephric duct** forms the ureter in both sexes and regionally specializes to form the **vas deferens, epididymis, ejaculatory ducts** and **seminal vesicle** in the male, joining with the testis in the form of ductuli efferentes testis.

Figure 1

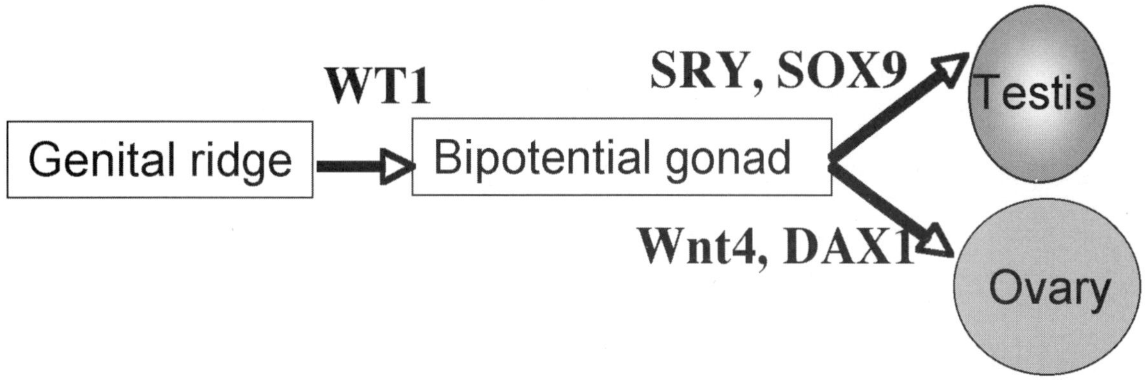

Genes involved in the early development cascade that determines gonadal sex. Abnormal expression of *Wnt-4* or *DAX-1* may account for cases of sex reversal in which *SRY* is not involved.

Abnormal development of mesonephric duct structures is relatively common, clinically presenting as infertility with **azoospermia** due to **congenital absence of the vas deferens (CAVD)**, a *form fruste* of **cystic fibrosis** that is associated with ***CFTR*** gene mutations but not necessarily with disease symptoms.

7.) The **Müllerian duct** develops into fallopian tubes, the uterus and the upper portion of the vagina in the female; in the male this development is inhibited by a **müllerian-inhibiting substance (MIS)** produced by the primitive testis (Figure 2). Except for the **appendix testis** and **prostatic utricle**, regression is otherwise complete. If MIS is not secreted, an intersex condition termed **Persistent Müllerian Duct Syndrome** can result. This familial X-linked or autosomal dominant disorder presents as a male patient with normal male external and internal genitalia, but also a fully developed uterus and fallopian tubes due to incomplete involution of mullerian derivatives. Clinically, there may be a hernia that contains a uterus and fallopian tubes **(hernia uteri inguinalis)** or cryptorchidism.

8.) Later in gestation, Leydig cells also synthesize **Insulin-Like-3** to promote transabdominal testis migration that begins **testis descent** into the scrotum. The testis descends as a result of differential growth of the gubernaculum testis. Descent into the scrotum is usually completed by birth, although descent can still occur during the 1st year of life. **Dihydrotestosterone (DHT),** a testosterone metabolite, masculinizes the genital anlage to form the external genitalia, including the penis, scrotum, and prostate.

Gross Anatomy

1.) The male reproductive system includes the following components: the testes and seminiferous tubules, efferent ductules and rete testis, epididymides, vasa deferentia, ejaculatory ducts, seminal vesicles, prostate, penis, and urethra.

2.) To understand infertility, any consideration of anatomy must also include the hypothalamic/pituitary/gonadal axis.

Reproductive Hormonal Axis (Figure 3)

1.) Components

a. Extrahypothalamic central nervous system

b. Hypothalamus

c. Pituitary

Figure 2

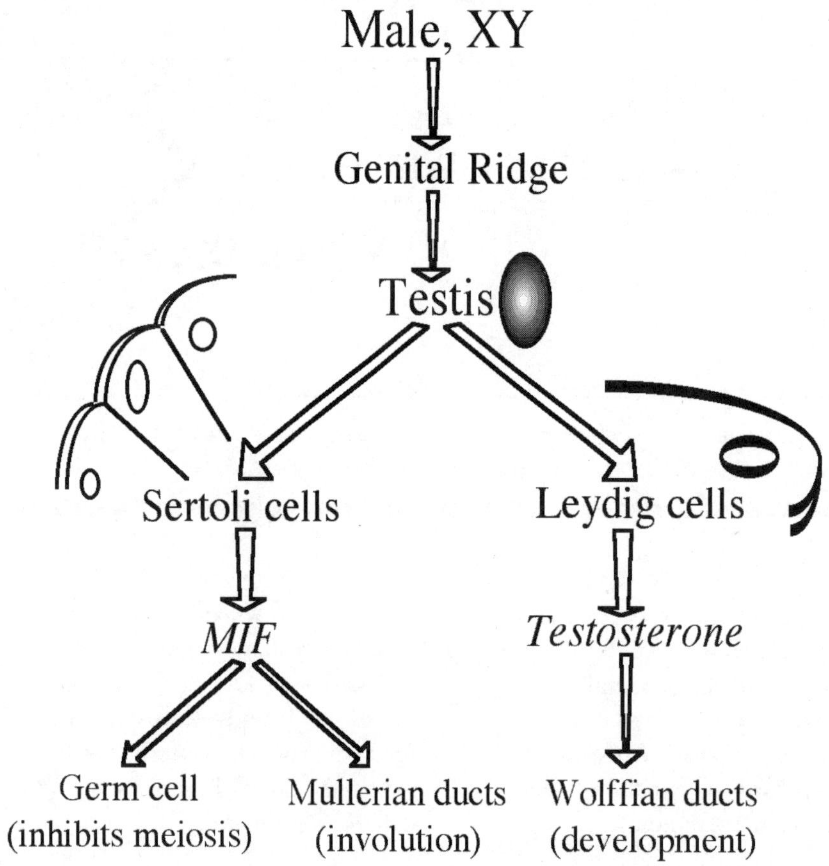

Pathway of male gonadal development. Secretion of MIS (Müllerian-inhibiting substance) from Sertoli cells within the early male gonad governs germ cell allocation and Müllerian duct inhibition. Testosterone leads to Wolffian duct development.

d. Testes

e. Steroid sensitive organs

2.) Functions

a. Normal male sexual development

b. Maintenance of secondary sexual characteristics

c. Male sexual behavior

d. Sperm production and maturation

Extrahypothalamic Central Nervous System

1.) The extrahypothalamic central nervous system is responsible for a variety of stimulatory and inhibitory influences on fertility including stress and catecholamines.

2.) In humans, the effects of **stress** of both a physical and/or emotional nature are mediated through this system, but the mechanisms are unknown. In studies of acute physical stress in military recruits, testosterone LH along with testosterone decreases.

Figure 3

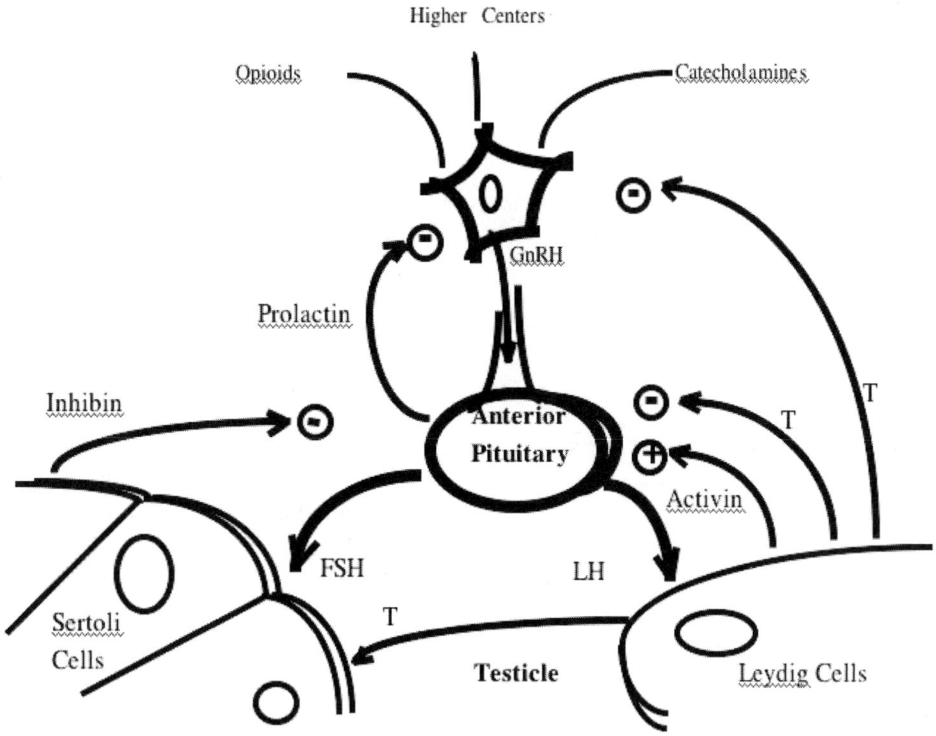

The hypothalamic-pituitary-gonadal hormone axis. Both inhibitory and stimulatory feedback loops within the axis. Testosterone balance occurs in a negative feedback loop. GnRH – gonadotropin-releasing hormone; PRL - prolactin; T – testosterone; LH – luteinizing hormone; FSH – follicle-stimulating hormone.

Hypothalamus—Gonadotropin-Releasing Hormone (GnRH)

1.) The hypothalamus is the center of integration for neuronal and humoral messages in the brain. The anterior and ventromedial nuclei are most important for male fertility.

2.) The hypothalamus is responsible for production of **GnRH**, the **primary releasing substance involved in male sexual function.**

Pituitary—Luteinizing Hormone (LH) and Follicle-Stimulating Hormone (FSH)

1.) The **effect of GnRH** is the **production and release of LH and FSH** from the anterior pituitary gland.

2.) Both LH and FSH are **glycopeptides** with 2 molecular chains. They share a common alpha chain; specificity is determined by a unique **beta chain.**

3.) **LH and FSH are secreted episodically.** LH is rapidly metabolized, causing wide swings in concentration in the bloodstream. When more accurate LH levels are needed, pooled blood samples are used. FSH is more slowly metabolized, resulting in a more constant serum levels.

4.) **The testes are the primary target for LH and FSH.** No other target organs for these hormones have been found.

The Testes

1.) Microscopic anatomy

a. **Seminiferous tubules comprise the bulk (80%) of the testis** and are responsible for sperm production. Thus, testis atrophy generally suggests a low sperm count.

b. The **interstitium** between the seminiferous tubules contains blood vessels, lymphatics and **Leydig cells.**

2.) Seminiferous tubule structural organization

a. The tubules are long ducts lined by **Sertoli cells** that engulf and nurture the developing germ cells.

b. Sertoli cells contain membrane receptors that bind FSH, resulting in increased intracellular cAMP and subsequent cytoskeletal reorganization for protein synthesis.

c. The primary secretion products from Sertoli cells include **Müllerian-inhibiting substance** in the fetus, **androgen-binding protein (ABP), transferrin** and **inhibin** (a nonsteroidal glycoprotein) in the adult.

d. Sertoli cells regulate of the tubule microenvironment. They govern fluid secretions, phagocytosis, steroid metabolism (in part), sperm production and sperm movement during development.

e. Sertoli cells are also responsible for the **"blood-testis barrier."** In addition, a selective physiologic barrier is created by active transport processes across Sertoli cells. Further compartmentalization is established as Sertoli cells divide developing germ cells into two areas, the **basal compartment** for immature germ cells and stem cells and the **adluminal compartment** for germ cells undergoing differentiation and maturation. This complex barrier provides an **immunologically privileged site for mature spermatozoa,** as these haploid cells harbor unique and specific antigens that are not otherwise recognized as **"self"** by the body's immune system.

3.) Seminiferous tubules—spermatogenesis

a. **LH, FSH and testosterone** are all **required** for **normal spermatogenesis.**

b. Sertoli cells, lining 250m of seminiferous tubules in the average testis, regulate the complex process of spermatogenesis.

c. A variety of germ cell types exist, including **spermatogonia, primary spermatocytes, secondary spermatocytes, spermatids and spermatozoa.** 14 germinal cell subtypes are recognized histologically and are associated with 6 distinct stages of spermatogenesis. Early stage spermatogonia are actually adult testis **stem cells** and are the source of the constantly self-renewal germ cell lineage. Spermatids and spermatozoa have a **haploid** complement of chromosomes.

d. The process of spermatogenesis takes about **60 days** to complete. The average **daily output is 125 million spermatozoa**, which declines with age. A normal man makes **1200 sperm** for every heartbeat.

e. **Spermiogenesis is the maturation process**

of a spermatid to a spermatozoan. This includes nuclear condensation and programmed repackaging of DNA from **histones** to **protamines**, acrosome formation, residual body separation from the sperm, and tail formation. It is one of the most complex morphological changes undertaken by any mammalian cell.

4.) Interstitium--Leydig cells

a. Leydig cells contain membrane receptors that bind LH, resulting again in cAMP production, protein kinase activation, and protein phosphorylation.

b. LH stimulation results in the conversion of cholesterol to testosterone in a steroidogenic pathway.

c. Testosterone diffuses into the plasma (**endocrine** function) or into the seminiferous tubule lumen (**paracrine** function). In the plasma, **testosterone is bound (98 percent) to sex hormone binding globulin (SHBG) or albumin.** Within the seminiferous tubules, testosterone is bound to Androgen binding protein (ABP).

d. Depending on the target tissue, testosterone may be active itself or may be reduced to **dihydrotestosterone (DHT)** by the enzyme **5-alpha reductase.**

e. Testosterone is responsible in part for sexual differentiation, spermatogenesis, gonadotropin regulation, sexual maturation and behavior.

Feedback Mechanisms

1.) GnRH, LH and FSH drive the production of testosterone and spermatozoa as noted above. There are also feedback mechanisms that regulate the production and release of these substances.

2.) LH regulation

a.) Testosterone and estradiol are the major **negative feedback** substances that control the formation and release of LH.

b. **Testosterone therefore regulates its own production** and release by acting on the pituitary and in hypothalamus. Thus, exogenous testosterone supplements will suppress both endogenous testosterone (through decreased LH) and sperm production (through decreased FSH).

c. **Estradiol is produced within the testicle and the liver upon conversion from testosterone (5-alpha reductase).** It is found in smaller amounts within the blood stream (testosterone:estrogen ratio is typically 10:1) but is potent in action. The site of regulation is also at the level of the pituitary and hypothalamus.

3.) FSH regulation

a. Testosterone and estradiol are the major modulators of pituitary FSH secretion. This is why exogenous testosterone supplements suppress spermatogenesis.

b. In man, Sertoli cells produce **inhibin**, a 2-subunit hormone in the transforming growth factor family, which has an inhibitory effect on pituitary FSH output. In contrast, activin, a glycoprotein formed as a homodimer of either inhibin chain, has a stimulatory effect on pituitary FSH. Neither inhibin nor activin affects pituitary LH release.

Testicular Transport

1.) Human sperm production, unlike most mammalian species, **occurs in a patchwork pattern** and not in a **wave-like manner** within the seminiferous tubules. This, in combination with constantly renewing cycles of spermatogenesis, **insures that sperm production is continuous in nature.**

2.) Movement of the spermatozoa from the testis to

the epididymis is controlled by: fluid pressure within the seminiferous tubule, myoepithelial contractions of the seminiferous tubules and tunica albuginea, and cilia within the efferent ductules.

Epididymal Functions

1.) Transport and storage

a. The spermatozoa traverse the length of the epididymis in approximately 12 days. This process is governed by regular slow contractions of the muscular wall in a fashion similar to intestinal peristalsis.

b. Approximately **700 million sperm are stored within the epididymides and vasa deferentia.** Approximately 60% of sperm are stored within the tail (cauda) of the epididymides. Sperm become progressively more motile as they traverse the epididymal tubules, an important fact in harvesting sperm from the epididymis for *in vitro* fertilization (IVF) with intracytoplasmic sperm injection (ICSI).

c. At **emission,** coordinated contractions of the tails of the epididymides and the vasa deferentia occur, mediated by the sympathetic nervous system, propelling sperm into the prostatic urethra. During **ejaculation,** the somatic nervous system stimulates rhythmic contractions of periurethral and pelvic floor muscles propel the sperm through the urethra.

2.) Sperm maturation

a. Motility and fertilizing capacity are gained during transport through the epididymis.

b. **Sperm capacitation** takes place after the sperm have been ejaculated and are in contact with the female reproductive tract. **Fertilizing capacity** lasts approximately **48 hours** within the female internal genitalia, important for counseling patients on the optimum frequency of sexual intercourse during ovulation.

Semen Composition

1.) The bulk of seminal fluid originates from the accessory ducts, with the spermatozoa adding a small (<10%) amount to the total volume.

2.) Prostatic fluid

a. The **prostatic fluid** is usually found in the first part of the ejaculate and contributes approximately **10%-20% of the total volume. This fluid is acidic (pH <6.5)**

b. Specific prostate products include liquefaction factors like prostate specific antigen (PSA), zinc, citric acid, acid, phosphatase, and spermine. The latter substance, when oxidized to aldehydes, produces the characteristic odor of semen.

c. **PSA, a 33 kd molecular weight serum protease in the family of glandular kallikreins, serves to liquefy the coagulum** of human semen after 5-20 minutes following ejaculation.

3.) Seminal vesicle fluid

a. The **seminal vesicle** fluid is usually found in the second part of the ejaculate and contributes approximately **two-thirds of the total volume. This fluid is basic (pH >7.0)**

b. Specific substances secreted by the seminal vesicles include coagulation factors, prostaglandins, and fructose. **Fructose** is measured on a semen analysis to investigate the diagnosis of seminal vesicle agenesis or ejaculatory duct obstruction.

3. Clinical Evaluation of the Subfertile Male

Fertility History (Figure 4)

1.) Present partner history:

a. Duration of infertility.

b. Contraceptive methods and time used.

c. Length of time trying to conceive.

d. Number of pregnancies, including miscarriages and abortions, which are indication of the potential to conceive.

2.) Previous partner history.

a. In past relationships, the number of pregnancies achieved should be determined.

b. If conceptions occurred in past relationships, but none in the current one, then the infertility is considered primary.

3.) Sexual history

a. Frequency of intercourse and masturbation. Overly frequent (daily) or infrequent (> 48 hours apart around the time of ovulation) can adversely conception.

Figure 4

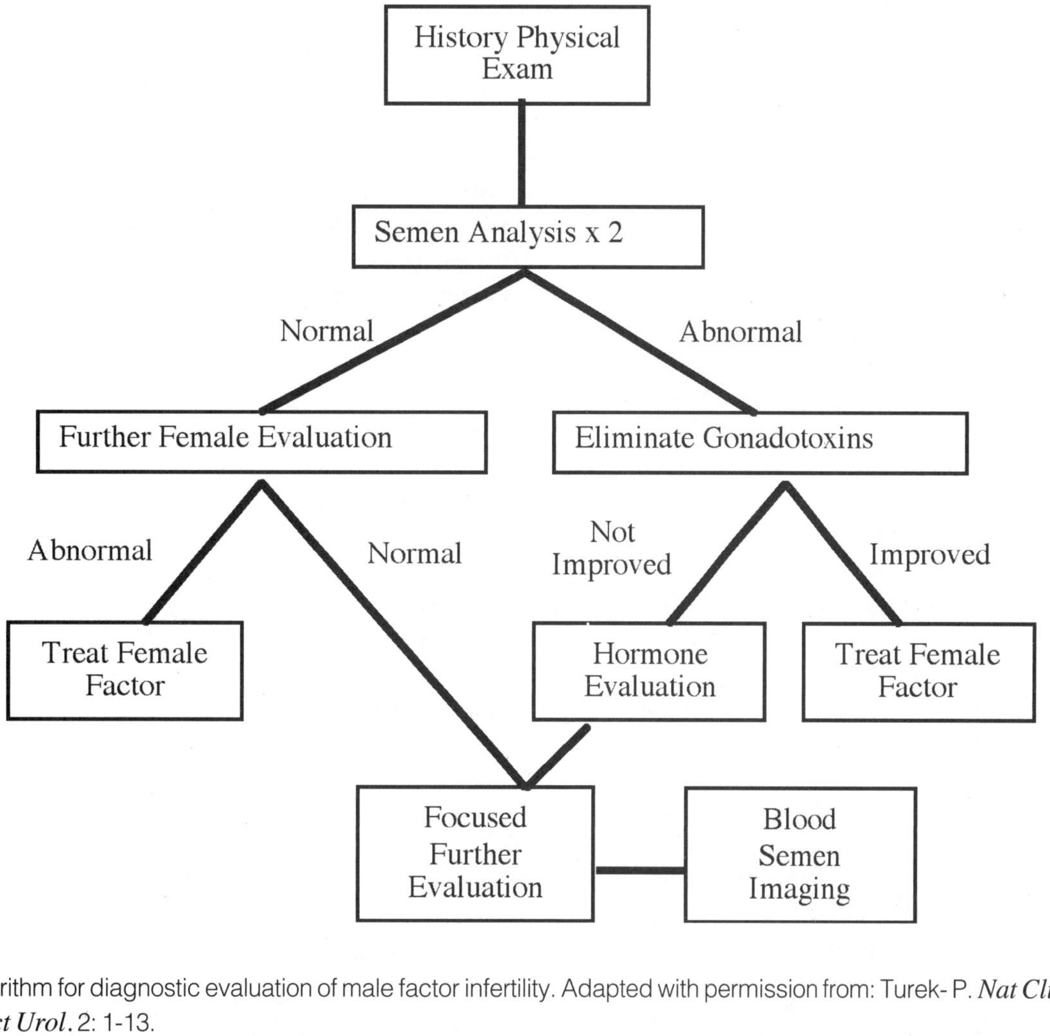

Algorithm for diagnostic evaluation of male factor infertility. Adapted with permission from: Turek- P. *Nat Clin Pract Urol*. 2: 1-13.

b. Libido, potency and sexual technique. Problems in these areas are often overlooked by clinicians. **Situational erectile dysfunction** due to stress is common among couples trying to conceive and is easily treated with **phosphodiesterase inhibitors.**

c. Ejaculation. Ejaculation needs to occur deep within the vagina. Severe problems with **premature ejaculation, chordee or severe hypospadias** may prevent proper deposition of sperm.

d. **Dyspareunia** and the use of lubrication. Inadequate natural vaginal lubrication can produce painful intercourse for either partner. Most lubricants are spermicidal. The use of vegetable oil based substances are safe for sperm viability.

e. The **ovulatory cycle**. It is important that the couple understand when ovulation occurs and have timed intercourse during this time. Evidence suggests that having more sex before rather than after ovulation-improves pregnancy rates.

4.) Genitourinary history

a. Testicular descent. Bilateral **cryptorchidism** is associated with impaired spermatogenesis and fertility. With unilateral maldescent, there is a slight decrease in fertility potential.

b. Sexual development and onset of puberty. **Delayed puberty** can indicate syndromes (eg, Kallmann) or chromosomal issues (eg, XXY)

c. Infections. Venereal, nonvenereal, mumps (at puberty or later), recent febrile illness or other infectious problems that directly involve the genitalia or urogenital duct system may be associated with a significant scarring and subsequent fertility problems. Viral infections and other febrile illnesses not specifically involving the genitalia may also decrease spermatogenesis and temporarily lower sperm counts.

d. **Trauma or torsion.** Either condition may injure the duct system or result in ischemic damage to the seminiferous tubules.

e. Exposure to chemicals (Table 1). A variety of drugs and industrial compounds may be associated with abnormal semen analyses. **Industrial solvents** are the most concerning. Chemotherapy agents are also gonadotoxic (Table 2).

f. Exposure to heat. Prolonged exposure to high temperatures may adversely affect spermatogenesis. **Hot tubs and hot baths on a regular basis may have significance in this regard.**

g. Exposure to **radiation**. Even small amounts of ionizing radiation, particularly that used for medical radiation therapy, may destroy sperm forming cells. **Spermatogonia are particularly radiosensitive.**

Table 1

Drugs and Chemicals with Potential Adverse Fertility Effects

Alcohol
Chemotherapy (see Table 2)
Arsenic
Aspirin (large doses)
Caffeine
Cimetidine
Colchicine
Dibromochloropropane (pesticide)
DES
Heavy metals: lead, cadmium, mercury
Monoamine oxidase inhibitors
Marijuana
Medroxyprogesterone
Nicotine
Nitrofurantoins
Phenytoin
Spironolactone
Sulfasalazine
Testosterone

Table 2

Chemotherapeutic Agents and Effects on Male Infertility

Condition	Testosterone	FSH	LH	Prolactin
Normal	Normal	Normal	Normal	Normal
Primary Testicular Failure	Low	High	High	Normal
Hypogonadotropic Hypogonadism	Low	Low	Low	Normal
Hyperprolactinemia	Low	Low	Low	High
Androgen Resistance	High	High	High	Normal

5.) Previous infertility evaluation

a. Patient. Previous semen analyses and medical or surgical treatment is important for prognosis and the diagnosis of infertility etiology.

b. Wife/partner. It is wise to understand the fertility potential of the female partner. Obviously, conception involves two partners and if an irreversible problem exists in the female partner, pregnancy is not likely. The evaluation of each partner should be carried out simultaneously; the male evaluation should be completed prior to any invasive procedures on the female partner. **At least 1 year of maternal reproductive potential should exist for the best outcomes after male infertility treatment.**

General Medical History

1.) While most conditions causing male infertility do not lead to long-term medical consequences, **1%-2% of men undergoing evaluation for infertility will have a significant underlying medical condition.**

a. Medical illnesses. Medical problems such as **diabetes** and **hypertension** or their pharmacologic treatments may adversely affect erectile and ejaculatory function and hence fertility.

b. Abnormal sex steroid metabolism may be associated with various liver and renal diseases and interfere with spermatogenesis. Rare medical illnesses like **Young syndrome** (Immotile cilia syndrome) and **Kartagener syndrome** (ciliary defect with situs inversus) can adversely affect fertility.

2.) Surgical history

a. **Inguinal herniorrhaphy**, particularly when performed on a young child and when performed bilaterally, may be associated with injury to the vas deferens in 1%-2% of patients.

b. Surgery on the ureter, bladder, bladder neck or urethra may result in problems with emission and/ or ejaculation.

c. **Retroperitoneal surgery** and major pelvic procedures may result in **failure of emission** and/or problems with retrograde ejaculation. Men with testis cancer are cured with great success. Those with nonseminomatous tumors treated with retroperitoneal lymphadenectomy may have fertility problems due to absent ejaculation from either failure of emission or from retrograde ejaculation. 2 or 3 adjuvant cycles of chemotherapy given in lieu of retroperitoneal lymphadenectomy does not have a significant impact on fertility.

3.) Current and past medications

a. A variety of drugs and chemotherapeutic agents may adversely affect sperm production and/or function. The adverse affects are usually reversible upon discontinuation of the medication (Table 1).

4.) Occupation and habits

a. Occupation and stress. The effects of daily stress on fertility are poorly quantified. **Severe, acute stress has been associated with decreases in testosterone, ejaculate volume and sperm count.** This difficult to treat. Encouraging regular exercise, yoga, or acupuncture may help.

b. The active ingredients in **cigarettes, marijuana, coffee, tea, alcohol** and some naturopathic herbs have all been demonstrated in laboratory studies to be gonadotoxic. The susceptibility of individuals to these substances varies widely and is difficult to quantify.

5.) Family history

a. Sibling fertility status may help to identify familial conditions like cystic fibrosis, genetic infertility due to Y chromosome deletions and congenital adrenal hyperplasia.

b. In utero exposure to **diethylstilbestrol (DES)** may result in testicular, epididymal, and penile anatomic abnormalities. Despite the finding of impaired semen quality in DES-exposed men, proof of decreased fertility is not obvious in extensive follow-up studies.

Physical Examination

1.) General examination. The general examination evaluates the patient's **body habitus** and secondary sex characteristics. In particular, the pattern of hair distribution and **gynecomastia** can be evidence of general endocrine disorders.

2.) Genitalia. The genitalia are the most important aspect of the examination. This should be performed in a systematic fashion, taking care to evaluate the areas listed below:

a. Penis. The size of the penis and location of the meatus are important in assuring the delivery of spermatozoa deep within the vagina at ejaculation.

b. Testes. The **location, size, and consistency** of the testes should be noted. The testes should be in a dependent part of the scrotum. Testicular size is particularly important, as the bulk of the testicle (80%) relates to sperm production. Note the length and width of the testicle or or quantify the volume by comparison to plastic models of known volumes. The normal testicle in the adult is greater than 4 cm in length and greater than **2.5 cm in width (20 mL).** Each testicle should have a firm consistency. Ethnic variations in testis size are well described.

c. Epididymides. The epididymides should be examined for size and consistency. The **obstructed epididymis feels enlarged and firm.** The epididymis that is scarred from either trauma or chronic infection may be hard and irregular. Part of the epididymis may be missing in association with congenital absence of the vas deferens.

d. Vasa deferentia. Each vas deferens should be palpable as a distinct, firm, cord-like structure in the scrotum. In **1-2% of infertile men, one or both vasa are not palpable in**

the scrotum, a condition termed congenital absence of the vas deferens (CAVD).

e. Spermatic cords. Each should be evaluated for size and consistency with the patient in upright and supine positions. The patient should perform a Valsalva maneuver while standing to accentuate differences in blood volume within the cord, characteristic of a varicocele. The internal spermatic veins fill while standing and this filling may be increased with this maneuver. In the supine position, these veins drain more easily and hence the **varicocele** is not as easily palpable. Persistent fullness in the spermatic cord upon reclining is suggestive of **cord lipoma** and not varicocele. Other abnormalities involving the spermatic cord include **hydrocele and spermatocele.**

f. Inguinal region. The inguinal canals are palpated for evidence of hernias. In addition, the inguinal regions should be inspected to assess if previous surgery in this area may have injured the vasa deferentia or testicular blood supply.

3.) Rectal examination. A general rectal examination can detect lower gastrointestinal pathology and palpate the prostate and seminal vesicles. The prostate should be small and benign in consistency without tenderness or inflammation. The seminal vesicles are generally not palpable under normal conditions but may be palpable with **ejaculatory duct obstruction.**

Semen Analyses

1.) Collection. Generally **2 semen analyses** are needed to establish a baseline. If significant discrepancy exists, a third or perhaps even a fourth specimen may be needed. Each semen analysis is collected after **2 to 3 days of sexual abstinence.** The specimen is generally collected by masturbation into a clean, dry container and examined within 1 hour. If the specimen is collected at home, it should be kept near body temperature during transportation to the laboratory (shirt pocket). Lubricants should be avoided during specimen collection. If needed, silicone condom devices are available.

2.) Minimal standards of adequacy. While there is no absolute measure of fertility on semen analysis, minimal standards of semen adequacy have been defined with expert consensus by the World Health Organization (Table 3).

3. Additional physical parameters. Other semen properties examined on a routine semen analysis include:

a. Coagulation. This occurs immediately after ejaculation.

b. Liquefaction. This occurs 5 to 30 min following ejaculation. **Prostatic specific antigen (PSA)** is the serine protease responsible for this process.

c. Viscosity. This parameter refers to the fluid consistency of the semen after coagulation and liquefaction have occurred. Viscosity is normal if it is possible to pour the semen in a drop by drop fashion.

d. **pH.** The pH of semen normally ranges from 7.2 to 8.0. A low pH implies absence or blockage of the seminal vesicles, as the ejaculate consists entirely of acidic prostatic fluid.

e. **Fructose.** As noted above, fructose is produced by the seminal vesicles. Fructose is checked in low volume (<1.5mL) azoospermia. Absence of fructose in semen suggests absence of the vasa deferentia and seminal vesicles, ejaculatory duct obstruction or dysfunction of the seminal vesicles.

Other Laboratory Tests

1.) Urinalysis. This is useful to rule out infection of the lower genitourinary tract and associated glandular structures.

Table 3

Semen Analysis: Minimal Standards of Adequacy

Seen on at least 2 occasions:

Ejaculate volume	1.5-5.0 ml
Sperm density	>20 million/ml
Motility	>60% motile
Forward progression	>2.0 (scale 0-4)
Morphology (WHO)	>30% normal morphology
(Strict)	>14% normal morphology

And:

No significant sperm agglutination
No significant pyospermia
No hyperviscosity

2.) Endocrine evaluation. **99% of endocrine conditions can be detected through the initial measurement of serum FSH and testosterone. Prolactin and LH** can be included if the initial evaluation is abnormal. Hormonal testing can differentiate between hypogonadism due to hypothalamic or pituitary disease and that due to primary testicular failure.

3.) Other tests regularly recommended in the past are now unnecessary on a routine basis. These include testing **thyroid** and **adrenal function** (<0.5% of cases). **Prolactin** should be determined if a low testosterone is found or if the patient has gynecomastia, severe headaches or visual disturbances. Prolactin secreting pituitary tumors produce high levels of circulating prolactin, and these lesions tend to reduce LH and FSH levels by altering regulation or by mass effect.

4.) Genetic testing. **Karyotype analysis is critical for all men with azoospermia and severe oligospermia (<5 million sperm/mL) who are planning IVF/ICSI.** In addition, specific deletions in the Y-chromosome are found in approximately 15% of men with azoospermia and 5%-8% of men with severe oligospermia. Several regions of the long arm of the Y chromosome have been classified as **Azoospermic Factor (AZF) regions. Most deletions are found in the AZFc region in a specific gene complex termed DAZ (Deleted in Azoospermia). Deletions in these regions appear specific for infertility.** Deletions of AZFa and AZFb have a much poorer prognosis for sperm retrieval from the testis than patients with AZFc deletions.

5.) Tests of sperm function

a. **Sperm morphology.** Sperm cytology is another measure of semen quality. By assessing the dimensions and shape characteristics of the sperm head, midpiece, and tail, sperm can be classified as "normal" or not. In the strictest classification system (Kruger morphology), only 14% of sperm are normal. In fact, this number correlates with the success of egg fertilization *in vitro* (IVF) and thus is ascribed clinical significance. In addition, **sperm morphology is an indicator of testicular health,** because shape characteristics are determined during spermatogenesis. Sperm morphology complements other information to estimate the chances of fertility.

b. **Sperm chromatin assay.** The structure of sperm chromatin (the DNA-associated proteins) is independent of semen quality and can be measured by **COMET** and **TUNNEL** assays and by flow cytometry after acid treatment and staining of sperm with acridine orange. These tests assess the degree of DNA fragmentation that occurs after chemically stressing the sperm DNA-chromatin complex, and can indirectly reflect the quality of sperm DNA integrity. **Abnormally fragmented sperm DNA rarely occurs in fertile men, but can be found in 5% of infertile men with normal semen analyses and 25% of infertile men with abnormal semen analyses.** This test can detect infertility that is missed on a conventional semen analysis. Often reversible, causes of DNA fragmentation include tobacco use, medical disease, hyperthermia, air pollution, infections, and varicocele.

6. **Antisperm antibodies.** A link between infertil-

ity and antisperm antibodies has been recognized for years. **The effect of antibodies is to disturb either sperm transport through the female reproductive tract or sperm-egg interaction.** Enzyme-linked immunosorbent assay (ELISA) and immunobead binding assays are two commonly used tests to detect the presence of antibodies on sperm.

7. **White blood cells.** Reproductive tract infections are a treatable cause of infertility and are often heralded by the presence of excessive white blood cells in the ejaculate. Special stains are needed to distinguish white cells from immature germ cells, the latter of which are not pathologic.

Radiologic procedures

1.) Transrectal Ultrasound (TRUS). TRUS is indicated in infertile men with low volume ejaculates (<1.5 mL) **Ejaculatory duct obstruction** (EDO) may be identified by seminal vesicle dilatation (>1.5 cm in diameter); seminal vesicle hypoplasia or absence is also easily diagnosed. Frequently, the causes of EDO, including stones, scar, cysts or a persistent utricle, can be diagnosed by TRUS. In addition, seminal vesicle fluid can be sampled to confirm the presence of sperm in patients with suspected obstruction and **seminal vesiculography** or **chromotubation** (antegrade injection of diluted indigo carmine monitored by flexible cystoscopy) can be performed to demonstrate obstruction.

2.) **Vasography.** Classically, intraoperative, transcrotal vasography is used to detect abdominal vas deferens, seminal vesicle and ejaculatory duct patency prior to definitive surgery for obstruction. It is usually performed at the same setting as reconstruction as there is a 5%-10% chance of vasal scarring after the procedure.

3. **Scrotal ultrasound.** A scrotal ultrasound is indicated when the testes are not easily palpable due to coexistent hydrocele, to confirm the origin and character (solid vs. cystic) of intrascrotal masses, and for confirming the presence of a clinically suspicious varicocele. There is level I evidence to suggest that finding and treating subclinical varicoceles does not improve fertility.

4. Classification of Abnormalities

General Information

1.) A variety of classification schemes exist to categorize fertility problems. One of the most useful is based on the findings on semen analyses with initial classification of problems into one of four categories: 1.) all parameters normal, 2.) azoospermia, 3.) a single abnormal parameter and 4.) multiple abnormal parameters. The decision to treat a semen abnormality to improve fertility depends in part on maternal reproductive potential and also on how correctable the problem is, as outlined in Figure 5.

2.) Distribution of semen abnormalities among infertile men:

Azoospermia	8%
Single abnormal parameter	37%
Multiple abnormal parameters	55%

Among the single abnormal parameters, isolated abnormalities in **motility** account for the majority of cases.

All Parameters Normal

1.) Further evaluation of the female partner is recommended. This may include assessment of **menstrual history, cycle day 3 FSH and estradiol** levels, an **antral follicle count** by ultrasound and a **hysterosalpingogram** to assess uterine anatomy.

2.) If the female partner is normal, sperm function tests may be useful. Most couples with unexplained infertility will go on to be treated with intrauterine **insemination (IUI) or *In Vitro* fertilization (IVF).**

Azoospermia

1.) When no sperm are found on semen analysis, the specimen should be **centrifuged** to confirm the absence of any sperm **(pellet analysis).** In addition, a **collection error** and/or retrograde ejaculation must be ruled out as causes of azoospermia.

Figure 5

Algorithm for treatment of male infertility

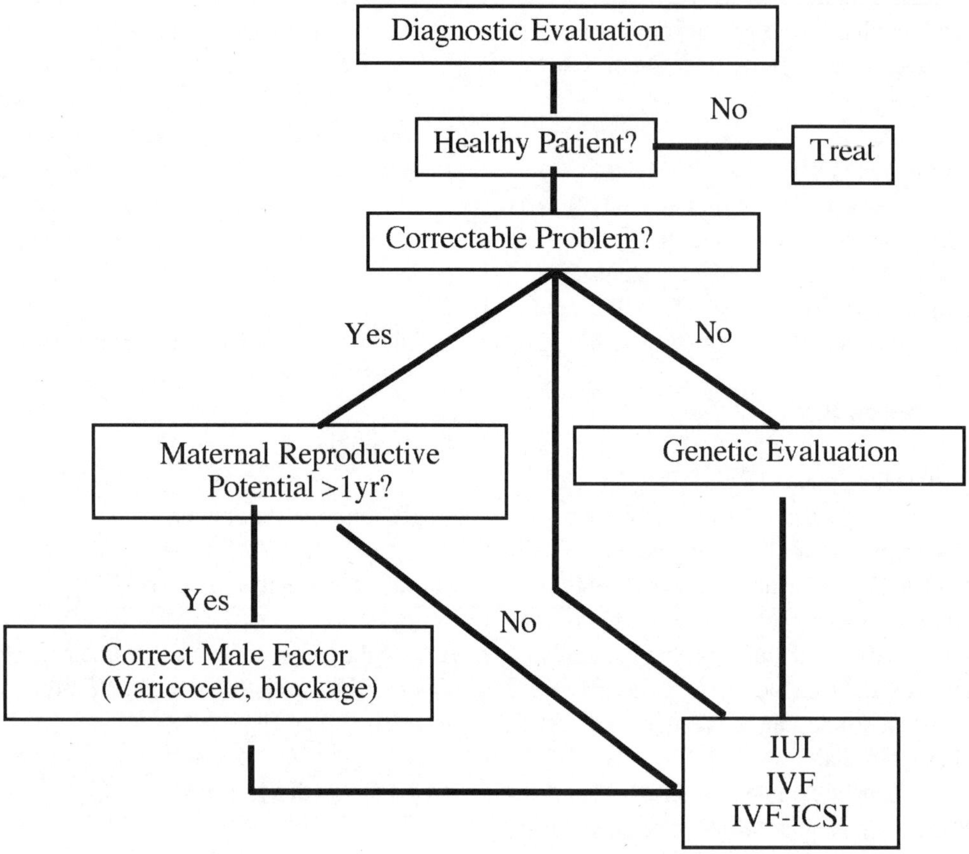

Algorithm for treatment of male infertility. Used with permission from P. Turek. Nat Clin Pract Urol. *2005;2:1-13.*

Table 4

Techniques for Testis Biopsy

Technique	Advantages	Disadvantages	Harvest
Fine needle aspiration	Office procedure/local	Minimal tissue – Yes/no sperm	Y
Needle core biopsy	Office/good tissue prep	Painful/decrease control	?
Open biopsy "window"	Office procedure/ adequate tissue	Painful/some testicular injury	Y

2.) The results of gonadotropin levels determine what additional evaluation and treatment is necessary.

a. LH, FSH, and testosterone levels differentiate **primary testicular failure** from **secondary testicular failure** caused by either pituitary or hypothalamic dysfunction.

b. A serum **FSH >3 times normal** along with atrophic testicles on physical examination is a **"medical biopsy"** and indicates severe testicular failure. **This does not mean that there is no sperm in the testis, as fully one half of men can have low numbers of sperm on more extensive evaluation.** However, this finding obviates the need for a surgical biopsy to rule out obstructive conditions. Sperm found in these men can be used with IVF/ICSI by testicular sperm extraction techniques (TESE).

3.) After ruling out a major endocrine abnormality, the major differential diagnosis is **ductal obstruction** or testicular failure.

a. Negative fructose test. 3 possibilities exist in the azoospermic patient with normal hormone studies and a negative fructose test. These are congenital bilateral absence of the vas deferens (CAVD), bilateral ejaculatory duct obstruction and, rarely, **seminal vesicle dysfunction** similar to bladder myopathy. The treatment of CAVD is direct sperm aspiration from the epididymis. The sperm are then processed and used in combination with *in vitro* fertilization (IVF) and intracytoplasmic injection (ICSI) techniques. Ejaculatory duct obstruction is managed by transurethral resection.

b. Positive fructose test. A positive fructose test rules out complete obstruction of the ejaculatory ducts and severe dysfunction of the seminal vesicles but does not give an indication of the patency of the ductal system. Thus, a positive fructose test in azoospermia does not differentiate between proximal ductal obstruction and testicular failure.

c. Testicular biopsy. A testicular biopsy is important in the azoospermic patient with normal hormones and normal sized testes with fructose in the ejaculate. The microscopic examination of the biopsy will indicate whether spermatogenesis is progressing normally. With the advent of IVF and ICSI, sperm found on testicular biopsy can be cryopreserved for future use (Table 4).

d. Alternatively, nonsurgical **fine needle aspiration (FNA) "mapping"** of the testis under local anesthesia can provide diagnostic information on 1) whether sperm are being produced in the testis, 2) the location of sperm and 3) the relative quantity of sperm. This can inform men with testicular failure, who often showing **"patchy"** or **"focal"** areas of sperm production, about the chances of successful subsequent sperm retrieval for IVF-ICSI.

e. If the testicular biopsy or FNA mapping indicates complete spermatogenesis, scrotal exploration and vasography are indicated. A **vasogram** is performed by injecting contrast material through one vas deferens to determine patency. If patency is demonstrated, then exploration of the epididymis is undertaken to localize the site of obstruction. Fluid within the vas deferens lumen at **vasotomy** should be examined microscopically to determine if sperm are present or absent. A microscopic **vasoepididymostomy** is necessary to correct epididymal obstruction. If no spermatozoa are detected in the tubules of the epididymis during this exploration, then intratesticular ductal obstruction may be the cause of azoospermia. Since these cases are difficult to correct, IVF and ICSI with testicular sperm is recommended.

4.) Vasectomy is one cause of azoospermia amenable to surgical repair with microsurgery. It is well established that 1.) surgeon experience and 2.) use of optical magnification, improve outcomes after vasectomy reversal. In experienced hands, **a return of sperm to the ejaculate should be possible in 90%-95% of cases of vasovasostomy, with pregnancy rates from**

35%-60% depending on partner fertility potential. In older vasectomies, it is often necessary to perform a **vasoepididymostomy** for secondary epididymal obstruction that is acquired due to prolonged obstruction after vasectomy.

Multiple Abnormal Parameters on the Semen Analysis

1.) Diffuse abnormalities of all or many of the seminal parameters are the most common pathologic pattern identified (55%). Determination of the LH, FSH, and testosterone levels can rule out endocrine causes.

2.) Stress, infections and other environmental factors, such as wet heat, drugs and toxin exposures may produce a transient abnormality of all seminal parameters. Therefore, when other specific factors cannot be identified, it may be beneficial to follow these patients for 3 months to assess for self-correction of the abnormality. If spontaneous correction has not occurred, nonspecific therapy can be instituted as discussed below or, more commonly, couples can be offered assisted reproductive technology (IUI, IVF).

3. Varicoceles

a. **A varicocele** is defined as **dilated, varicose internal spermatic veins** producing fullness, dilatation, and **poor drainage of the pampiniform plexus.** A varicocele is found in **15%** of males in the general population but is found in **35% to 40% of men presenting with primary infertility** and results in abnormal semen parameters.

b. Varicoceles are **classified according to size as either large (grade III), medium (grade II), or small (grade I).**
Large varicoceles can be seen as a "bag of worms" under the scrotal skin. Medium varicoceles are readily detected by **palpation,** especially on standing. Small varicoceles can only be identified by feeling an impulse in the scrotum with the Valsalva maneuver or a difference in the size and fullness of the spermatic cord when the patient moves from the standing to the supine position. The majority (90%) of varicoceles occur on the left side, but bilateral varicoceles are more common than previously believed. Repair of **subclinical varicoceles** (ie, those detected by ultrasound but not by palpation) is ineffective.

c. The exact mechanism through which the varicocele exerts a detrimental effect is unclear; the leading theory is that it causes **increased intrascrotal temperature** through retrograde venous blood flow. There is a characteristic decrease in normal sperm morphology, with an increase in immature and tapered sperm forms. There may also be decreased sperm motility and varying degrees of oligospermia.

d. Treatment of varicocele involves surgical ligation or transvenous angiographic identification and embolization of the involved internal spermatic veins. The usual surgical approach is **retroperitoneal, inguinal or subinguinal ligation** of the internal spermatic and collateral veins. Laparoscopy may be useful in cases of bilateral varicoceles. Newer interventional **angiographic techniques** and catheters allow for selective catheterization of the internal spermatic veins. For venous occlusion, a variety of techniques are used, including sclerosing solutions, balloons and stainless-steel coils.

e. Results of varicocele ligation from several case series indicate approximately a **70% improvement in semen quality** associated with a **40% pregnancy rate.** With initial sperm counts >10 million sperm per milliliter, the improvement in pregnancy rates is significantly better than if the initial counts are lower. Both surgical and angiographic techniques for occlusion of varicoceles have a small failure rate with persistence and/ or recurrence of the varicocele noted during follow-up. **Pregnancies, when they occur, are generally noted a mean of 7-8 months after varicocelectomy.**

Isolated Abnormal Parameter on Semen Analysis

1.) Abnormal semen volume

a. Large ejaculate volume. A volume greater than 5.5 mL may dilute the spermatozoa and cause poor cervical placement of seminal fluid during intercourse. Mechanical concentration of the spermatozoa and intrauterine insemination may be employed.

b. Absent or low ejaculate volume. Once a collection error has been ruled out, it is essential to consider **retrograde ejaculation, absence or blockage of the accessory sex glands, or endocrine dysfunction (low testosterone)** as causes of low ejaculate volume. Retrograde ejaculation is confirmed by the finding of large quantities of spermatozoa in the postejaculatory urine sample (>15 sperm/HPF). Sympathomimetic drugs with **alpha-adrenergic activity** can reverse this problem in one-third of patients, generally those without scar tissue at the bladder neck from prior surgery. In others, it may be necessary to obtain, wash, and inseminate (IUI) sperm collected from the postejaculate urine sample. Endocrine abnormalities and infections are treated with the appropriate hormones and antibiotics.

2. Hyperviscosity. Problems with hyperviscous semen are rare and may reflect enzymatic imbalance in the semen. Mechanical disruption of the sample in the laboratory to decrease viscosity, followed by IUI may be useful.

3. Decreased motility and forward progression (asthenospermia)

a. This is the most common isolated abnormality found on semen analysis and can be due to endocrine dysfunction, infection of accessory glands, varicocele, epididymal dysfunction, genetics, reactive oxygen species (oxidants), or environmental exposures. Specific therapy is available for the some of these problems. Empirical treatment with **antioxidants (vitamins A, C and E, zinc and folate)** may be tried.

b. Sperm motility and forward progression may also be adversely affected by the presence of **antisperm antibodies** that agglutinate or immobilize the spermatozoa. Special sperm tests are available to determine the levels of antisperm antibodies in semen. Several treatments are available for antibodies, including IUI, IVF and ICSI and treatment of the male with systemic steroids for 6-9 months. The latter treatment has been associated with decreased antibody levels but not necessarily increased natural pregnancy rates.

4.) Oligospermia

a. Decreased sperm numbers as an isolated problem may be secondary to endocrine dysfunction, genetic or idiopathic conditions. Occasionally the absolute number of sperm is relatively normal, but the number of sperm per milliliter may appear to be low due to a large ejaculate volume. **With sperm densities <5 X 10^6 /mL, a karyotype analysis and specific deletions in the Y chromosome should be evaluated.**

b. In general, there are 2 treatments for oligospermia. One attempts to stimulate the testes with a variety of drugs to increase the output of spermatozoa (see section on idiopathic infertility). Alternatively, with advances in assisted reproduction, spermatozoa can be concentrated for use with IUI. In addition, IVF and ICSI are available when simpler approaches fail.

5.) Abnormal morphology. An isolated problem with morphology is unusual. This may result from gonadotoxic exposures (eg, tobacco), systemic illness, fevers, varicocele or idiopathic causes.

Empirical Treatment of Idiopathic Infertility

1.) Second only to the large proportion of patients with varicoceles, **idiopathic infertility** is the second largest group of infertility patients. Essentially, idiopathic infertility refers to men who have an abnormal parameter or parameters on the semen analyses with a normal history, physical examination, and screening hormone analysis. The etiology of the abnormal semen quality is unclear and reflects our incomplete knowledge about the genetics of spermatogenesis. Many of these cases are likely to have genetic etiologies.

2.) Nonpharmacologic treatments. A variety of nonpharmacologic treatments have been suggested, but their efficacy has not been rigorously demonstrated. These include:

a. **Vitamins/diet.** Specific vitamins and changes in dietary habits have not been associated with improved semen quality and fertility. Antioxidant therapy has been shown to increase motility of *in vitro* isolated sperm, but treatment of men with unexplained severe asthenospermia with high dose vitamin E and C did not improve motility in a large, randomized study. However, this therapy is likely to specifically help tobacco smokers to reduce the oxidative effects on sperm.

b. Jockey shorts to **boxer shorts.** A recent study has refuted the idiom that a switch from jockey to boxer shorts improves spermatogenesis and semen parameters.

c. Antibiotics for "occult infection."

d. Varicocelectomy for the "occult" or **subclinical varicocele.** There are 3 randomized, controlled clinical trials suggesting no benefit to varicocelectomy in cases of nonpalpable, ultrasound-detected varicoceles.

3.) Drug therapy for idiopathic infertility

a. The use of **human menopausal gonadotropin (hMG)** or **recombinant FSH, human chorionic gonadotropin (hCG,** essentially LH), or the combination of FSH and hCG does not result in significant improvements in sperm counts or fertility with idiopathic infertility. GnRH therapy, when given in a pulsatile fashion, has the potential to raise LH and FSH levels, but its administration is complex and costly.

b. **Clomiphene citrate** is an antiestrogen that has been used nonspecifically for idiopathic infertility for 40 years. As a **selective estrogen receptor modulator (SERM),** this medication blocks the negative feedback of estradiol on the hypothalamic-pituitary axis, resulting in increased LH and FSH levels. Overall improvement in the semen analysis is noted in approximately 50% of patients and pregnancies occur in 25%-30% of patients in uncontrolled studies. Men with low-normal testosterone and FSH levels, indicative of mild central hypogonadism, may respond best to this therapy.

c. **Tamoxifen** is also an antiestrogen. This agent, however, lacks the estrogenic activities of clomiphene and may provide equal efficacy.

d. **Aromatase inhibitors** block the conversion of testosterone to estrogens in men. They may be useful in oligospermic or azoospermic men with a **testosterone:estrogen ratio of <10:1** to increase sperm yield from the ejaculate or from testis sperm extraction procedures.

e. **L-Carnitine** is found in high concentrations in the normal epididymis and is postulated to be important for sperm motility. Oral L-Carnitine is currently available from several popular fertility supplements and there is early evidence that some men with low motility will show improvement, especially those with varicoceles.

Assisted reproductive technology (ART)

1.) ART attempts to improve the conception by bypassing many or all of the barriers associated with normal fertilization. The simplest techniques involve sperm processing and insemination of the female; the more sophisticated ones involve manipulation of the sperm and ova extracorporeally. Fertilization with these procedures can occur *in vitro* or *in vivo*.

2.) Semen processing is used as an isolated procedure or in conjunction with oocyte processing.

Sperm washing, swim-ups, sedimentations, and gradient centrifugations are commonly employed to remove seminal plasma and leukocytes and to select for and concentrate highly motile sperm. Theoretically, with these procedures, fewer sperm than normal are needed since they are placed higher within the female reproductive tract than the ejaculate during intercourse.

3.) **Intrauterine insemination (IUI)** is used to treat male factor infertility. A small catheter is used to inject processed sperm through the cervix and into the uterine cavity. By bypassing the cervical mucus, more motile sperm can progress to the fallopian tubes where normal fertilization occurs. Indications for IUI include male factor infertility due to mechanical or anatomical problems (eg, erectile dysfunction, hypospadias) or low semen quality, and cervical mucus problems. **Usually, more than 5 million motile sperm are required for IUI. Pregnancy rates are variable with these techniques, but average 30%-35% in couples who try 3-4 times.**

4.) **IVF,** first introduced in 1978, was developed to manage fallopian tube obstruction. It is now used routinely for male factor infertility. Female partners undergo ovarian hyperstimulation to induce the maturation of multiple oocytes which are then harvested ultrasonographically, just prior to ovulation. Processed semen and recovered oocytes are mixed in vitro. If fertilization occurs, embryos are placed back into the uterus transcervically. Usually only 20%-30% percent of replaced embryos survive and become clinical pregnancies. Of those couples who fail the first IVF attempt, 10%-18% percent will fertilize on the second cycle. Depending on the cause of infertility, and the number of embryos replaced, pregnancy rates can approach 40%-50% per IVF attempt.

5.) Micromanipulation. Sperm and oocyte micromanipulation by **intracytoplasmic sperm injection (ICSI) has become the mainstay of addressing the poor fertilizing capacity of sperm often seen in male infertility.** By injecting a single sperm directly into an oocyte, multiple barriers of fertilization are bypassed and success rates (when compared to standard IVF) are greatly improved. Pregnancy rates of 40%-50% have been obtained using this technique even in the most severe cases of male infertility.

a. ICSI allows only ejaculated sperm but sperm retrieved from the male reproductive tract to produce pregnancies. **Vasal, epididymal and even testicular sperm, from both obstructed and nonobstructed men, are now routinely used with IVF and ICSI.**

Table 5

Techniques for Sperm Harvest in Assisted Reproduction

Technique	Advantages	Disadvantages
Percutaneous epididymal sperm aspiration (PESA)	Office/minimally invasive large numbers of sperm	Damage to epididymis
Testicular sperm extraction (TESE)	Office/easily repeatable	Lower numbers of sperm
Microsurgical epididymal Sperm aspiration (MESA)	Large numbers/controlled	Anesthetic required/invasive
Testicular microdissection	Search for active spermatogenesis In Klinefelter's/NOA	Anesthetic/lengthy/invasive

b. Consequently, **sperm retrieval techniques** (Table 5) have been developed to harvest sperm from male reproductive tract organs. In cases of ejaculatory failure, **vasal sperm aspiration (VASA)** is possible. For men with epididymal obstruction including those with vasectomy, epididymal sperm aspiration by microscope **(MESA)** or percutaneously **(PESA)** is possible. For obstructed men, testis sperm needle aspiration **(TESA)** or biopsy **(TESE)** is also indicated. For men with nonobstructive azoospermia or testis failure, TESE or **Microdissection TESE** are generally needed. There is a measurable risk of testis atrophy and hormone failure after microdissection TESE.

6.) **IVF with ICSI** should not be performed without **karyotype analysis on both partners.** Despite its great success, there remain concerns with ICSI.

a. **Multiple gestations occur in 35% of pregnancies compared to 1%-2% of naturally conceived pregnancies.** Multiple gestations are associated with lower birth weights, higher overall complication rates and increased learning disabilities relative to singletons. In addition, the **delivery costs** associated with managing multiple, often premature, gestations are at least **10-20 times higher** than that associated with the singleton deliveries. There is also strong evidence to suggest that the incidence of low birth weight singletons is also increased after ICSI. Among respectable ART programs, there is a trend to transfer as few embryos back as possible to reduce the multiple gestation rate.

b. **ICSI bypasses many mechanisms of natural selection such that many men who would not be able to conceive under normal circumstances are now able to father children.** Although overall rates of **major birth defects (3.3%)** associated with IVF and ICSI may be similar to intercourse, there is concern about elevated risks of specific malformations, including **hypospadias**, with this technology. In addition, there are concerns regarding possible **developmental issues.** There is a significant **increase in sex chromosomal abnormalities** among ICSI offspring **(0.8% vs 0.2% naturally)** that is likely attributable to the chromosomal status of the fathers rather than to the technique itself. As previously mentioned, from 5%-8% of men with severe oligospermia have deletions in the AZF region of the Y chromosome. It has been shown conclusively that these genetic deletions are passed to the male offspring produced by these fathers through IVF/ICSI.

c. More recently, concerns have arisen regarding whether **rare imprinting diseases such as Beckwith-Weideman Syndrome** and Anglemann Syndrome are increased along with autism in children conceived with ICSI. For these reasons, genetic counseling is recommended for all couples considering IVF-ICSI.

7.) Preimplantation genetic diagnosis **(PGD)** is now possible by sampling a single cell from an 8-cell developing embryo *in vitro* and performing either fluorescent in situ hybridization (FISH) or single-cell polymerase chain reaction (PCR) to **examine for aneuploidy, chromosomal translocations, or even specific diseases caused by point mutations.** Current indications for PGD include lethal disease prevention and aneuploidy screening in advanced maternal age couples.

5. References

Goldstein M, ed. *Surgery of Male Infertility.* Philadelphia, PA: WB Saunders Co.; 1995.

Jarow JP, Sharlip ID, Belker AM, et al for the Male Infertility Best Practice Policy Committee of the American Urological Association Inc. *J Urol.* 2002; 167:2138-2144.

Schlegel PN, Chang TSK. Physiology of Male Reproduction. In: Walsh PC, Retik A, Vaughan ED Jr, Wein A, eds. *Campbells Urology.* 7th ed. Philadelphia, PA: Saunders; 1998, chap: 42; 1254-1286.

Sigman M, Howards SS. Male infertility. In: Walsh PC. Retik A. Vaughan ED Jr, Wein A, eds. *Campbells Urology.* 7th ed. Philadelphia, PA: Saunders; 1998: chapter 1287-1330.

Sigman M, Jarow JP. Endocrine evaluation of infertile men. *Urology.* 1997; 50(5):659-664.

Turek PJ. Male Infertility. In: EA Tanagho and JC McAninch, eds. *Smith's Urology,* 15th ed. Stamford, CT: Appleton and Lange; 2003; chapter 46.

Turek PJ, Reijo Pera RA. Current and Future Genetic Screening for Male Infertility. *Urol Clin North Am.* 29:767-792.

Turek PJ. Practical approach to the diagnosis and management of male infertility. *Nature Clin Pract Urol.* 2005; 2: 1-13.

6. Questions

1. Embryologically, the vas deferens and body of the epididymis are derived from what developmental structure?

A. Müllerian ducts

B. Wolffian ducts

C. Urogenital ridge

D. Gubernaculum testis

E. Metenephros

2. The vast majority of the fluid in the male ejaculate is derived from the:

A. Epididymides

B. Ejaculatory ducts

C. Seminal Vesicles

D. Testicles

E. Vas deferens

3. The most common and correctable identifiable problem causing male infertility is:

A. Infection

B. Obstruction

C. Gonadotoxin exposure

D. Varicocele

E. Genetic

4. A 25-year old bodybuilder eschews the merits of "natural" bodybuilding and cycles and stacks injectable anabolic steroids regularly to maximize muscle bulk. His fertility potential would be expected to be:

A. Normal, because exogenous testosterone does not impair production of endogenous testosterone

B. Low, because exogenous testosterone stimulates pituitary production of FSH and LH

C. Low, because exogenous testosterone inhibits pituitary production of FSH and LH

D. Low, because exogenous testosterone is not as potent as endogenous testosterone at nurturing spermatogenesis

E. Normal, because intratesticular testosterone concentrations are 50x higher than serum levels, whether or not the blood contains exogenous testosterone

5. The role of PSA in the ejaculate is:

A. To coagulate the ejaculate

B. To serve as a marker for prostate cancer

C. To serve as a liquefaction factor

D. To give semen its characteristic odor

E. To agglutinate the ejaculate

6. What genetic mutation is involved with congenital absence of the vas deferens (CAVD)?

A. Klinefelter syndrome (47,XXY)

B. Reifenstein syndrome

C. 3p1

D. CFTR (delta f 508)

E. 45XO

7. Low serum testosterone, LH and FSH characterize what type of hypogonadism?

A. Hypergonadotropic hypogonadism

B. Young syndrome

C. Hypoprolactinism

D. Kallman syndrome

E. Klinefelter syndrome

8. How do elevated levels of prolactin influence testosterone production?

A. Inhibits GnRH and LH

B. Indirectly inhibits Sertoli cells

C. Directly inhibits Leydig cells

D. Upregulates inhibin

E. Downregulates activin

9. What testicular hormone is the major feedback inhibitor of LH secretion?

A. Testosterone

B. Inhibin

C. Activin

D. Prolactin

E. Sertolin

10. What is the initial evaluation for a man with one semen analysis that shows low volume ejaculate?

A. Semen pH

B. Postejaculate urinalysis

C. Semen fructose

D. TRUS

E. Repeat semen analysis

11. What is the normal size for adult human testes?

A. 5 mL

B. 10 mL

C. 20 mL

D. 30 mL

E. 40 mL

12. In the absence of genital tract infection, "round cells" in the semen analysis are most likely what kind of cell?

A. Squamous epithelial cells

B. Immature germ cells

C. Prostatic epithelial cells

D. Leydig cells

E. Sertoli cells

13. Hormonal screening of infertility patients below what sperm concentration will pick up most endocrinopathies?

A. <1 million/mL

B. <5 million/mL

C. <10 million/mL

D. <20 million/mL

E. <60 million/mL

14. Vasography is routinely performed by all of the following methods EXCEPT which one?

A. Scrotal

B. Transperineal

C. Transrectal

D. Transurethral

E. Transabdominal

15. Why is performing varicocelectomy at the same time as vasectomy reversal discouraged?

A. Venous congestion

B. Arterial compromise

C. Increased risk of sperm granuloma

D. All of the above

E. None of the above

16. A man has the following semen analysis profile after vasectomy reversal. This pattern is typical of what problem?

Timepoint after surgery	Volume	concentration	Motility
6 weeks	3.0	45 million/mL	45%
3 months	3.5	50 million/mL	15%
6 months	2.5	20 million/mL	0%

A. Antisperm antibodies

B. Testicular injury

C. Stricture formation at anastomosis

D. Primary hypogonadism

E. Ejaculatory duct obstruction

17. What percentage of oligospermic infertile males will have genetic microdeletions of the Y chromosome?

A. 1%

B. 5%

C. 25%

D. 50%

E. 75%

18. Which of the following has the highest impact on pregnancy rates with *in vitro* fertilization (IVF)?

A. Oligospermia-male factor infertility

B. Tubal obstruction-female factor infertility

C. Female age

D. Epididymal sperm

E. Testis sperm

19. What patency rates are achievable from contemporary series of microscopic vasovasostomies?

A. 90%-99%

B. 80%-90%

C. 50%-60%

D. 40%-50%

E. 25%-35%

20. Which fluid characteristic(s) from the testis vas deferens predict the best success for vasectomy reversal?

A. Clear with no sperm

B. Creamy with sperm fragments

C. Creamy with no sperm

D. Cloudy with motile sperm

E. Cloudy with fragmented sperm

Answers

1. B.
Müllerian ducts regress in the male. The indifferent gonad migrates to the urogenital ridge to become the testicle. The gubernaculum testis is responsible for pulling the testis into the scrotum during development.

2. C.
At least 65%-70% of ejaculate volume is derived from the seminal vesicles, with the remainder from the vas deferens (with sperm) and prostatic secretions. Periurethral glands may also contribute a small amount of fluid to the normal ejaculate.

3. D.
Infection and obstruction occur in 5%-10% of male infertility. The prevalence of gonadotoxin exposure is not well known. Varicocele occurs in 40% of infertile men.

4. C.
Because of negative feedback inhibition that maintains homeostatic balance in the pituitary-gonadal axis, excess testosterone of any type will cause anterior pituitary production of LH and FSH to fall. This results in azoospermia in most of men on anabolic steroids, but the effect will vary based on the dose, frequency and duration of the cycles and stacking regimen

5. E.
PSA is a serine protease that enzymatically breaks down the seminal coagulum after ejaculation.

6. D.
CFTR mutations, most commonly delta 508, are involved with CAVD

7. D.
Kallmann syndrome, a form of hypogonadotropic hypogonadism

8. A.
Hyperprolactinemia causes hypogonadotropic hypogonadism

9. A.
Testosterone.

10. E.
Low volume ejaculates are commonly due to collection error.

11. C.

12. B.

13. C.
99% of endocrinopathies will be detected if screening is done in men with <10 million sperm/mL

14. E.
Vasography is not routinely done transabdominally

15. A.
With varicocele repair, all venous drainage from the testis is ligated except for the vasal veins. With vasectomy reversal, injury to the vasal veins may occur.

16. C.
Anastomotic strictures after vasectomy reversal typically cause a decrease in sperm motility followed by a decrease in sperm concentration over time.

17. B.
5%. The range is from 3%-8%.

18. C.

19. A.

20. D.

Chapter 28: Erectile Dysfunction, Peyronie's Disease and Priapism

Dana A. Ohl, MD
Susanne A. Quallich, MD
Jens Sønksen, MD

Contents

I. Erectile Dysfunction

1. **Normal Sexual Function**
2. **Erectile Dysfunction (ED): General Considerations**
3. **Evaluation of a Man Presenting with ED**
4. **ED Treatments**

1. Normal Sexual Function

Neuroanatomic considerations

Sexual activity is initiated in the central nervous system. The brain is the most poorly understood component of the sexual response, but is of great importance. Some important areas that are known to contribute to sexual response include the medial preoptic nucleus and paraventricular nucleus, which reside near the hypothalamus. The exact function and interaction of these structures are not known. The effects of neurochemicals in the brain are generally understood as follows: serotonin and norepinephrine inhibit libido, erectile response, and ability to climax; dopamine, conversely, generally improves all of these functions. The effects of antidepressants that may increase CNS serotonin or norepinephrine levels thus commonly cause sexual dysfunction. ***The most common sexual adverse effect of the frequently prescribed selective serotonin reuptake inhibitors (SSRIs) is anorgasmia,*** although decreased libido and isolated erectile dysfunction may also occur.

Descending neural pathways controlling erection exit the brain and travel in the spinal cord to the level of S2-4, where they exit as peripheral parasympathetic nerves. These penile erection effector nerves are perilously close to the prostate and rectum as they travel through the pelvis, making them prone to injury from surgical extirpative procedures. The final cavernous nerves enter the corpora cavernosa just below the prostate at the divergence of the crura. ***Activation of these parasympathetic nerves causes vascular changes that lead to erection.***

Conversely, ***the detumescence mechanism is under control of the sympathetic nervous system.*** The nerves responsible for this function, as well as for the basic sympathetic tone resulting in baseline flaccidity, arise from T10-L3. After leaving the spinal cord and sympathetic chain, these nerves typically travel out of the superior hypogastric plexus in close proximity to the cavernous nerves and enter the penile tissue in the same location.

Interestingly, ***ejaculation is a completely different neurological event from penile erection.*** The nerves controlling seminal emission are also sympathetic and arise from T10-L3. They travel out of the sympathetic chain, through the superior hypogastric plexus and then through the pelvis to the ejaculatory organs, including the vas deferens, seminal vesicles, prostate and bladder neck. ***The locations of the sympathetic chain just lateral to the aorta and of the hypogastric plexus anterior to the aorta make these structures prone to surgical injury from aortic surgery or retroperitoneal lymphadenectomy for testis cancer.*** Indeed, prior to nerve sparing procedures for testis cancer, a radical lymph node dissection in this area nearly always caused absence of seminal emission or (less commonly) retrograde ejaculation. Aortic surgery still carries with it a significant risk of ejaculatory dysfunction.

Penile anatomy and vascular supply (Figure 1)

The penile deep structures consist of 3 erectile bodies, 2 corpora cavernosa and a single corpus spongiosum. Surrounding the entire package of erectile bodies is Buck's fascia. All 3 bodies contain erectile tissue. Practically speaking, in normal anatomic circumstances, there is free flow of blood between the corpora cavernosa and they function together as a unit. That is why injection of a drug into only 1 side can effect erection on both sides. The 2 units may not function together in cases of anatomic problems, such as repaired diphallus from exstrophy/epispadias syndrome. The corpora cavernosa are responsible for the primary structural integrity of the erection, due to their ability to become rigid when filled with blood. The rigidity is due to limitation of the swelling that can occur due to the tough nature of the containing tissue layer, the tunica albuginea.

The corpus spongiosum surrounds the urethra and distally enlarges to become the glans penis. Although the corpus spongiosum becomes engorged during sexual stimulation, it does not contain a tough fascial covering and thus cannot become rigid. The lack of a tough fascial covering prevents blood trapping due to lack of venoocclusive function (see below). The inability to trap blood in the tissue can be exploited in cases of priapism by intentionally shunting blood from the corpus cavernosum to the spongiosum so that it may escape into the systemic circulation.

Microscopically, it is difficult to differentiate the tissue within the different erectile bodies. In this tissue, blood flows thorough lacunar spaces, which are endothelial-lined and surrounded by the trabecular smooth muscle. It is on this smooth muscle that is activated or relaxed by the final neural pathways leading to erection and detumescence.

The arterial blood supply to the penis is from the common iliac → internal iliac (hypogastric) → internal pudendal → common penile artery. After giving off branches to the scrotum and urethral bulb, the common penile artery bifurcates into the dorsal penile artery (which supplies the glans and skin of the penis) and the deep penile artery (syn., cavernosal artery, profunda artery), supplying the corpus cavernosum. The deep arteries enter each corpus cavernosum and course down the center, giving off branches into the erectile tissue. Blood then flows radially toward the tunica albuginea toward the venules that give egress.

These arterial systems are present on both sides and are usually both functioning. Normal blood flow on one side is usually enough to keep things functioning properly. However, there can be individual variation in the anatomy. In some men, only one side provides the majority of blood, and in other, the

Figure 1

Penile anatomy and vascular supply

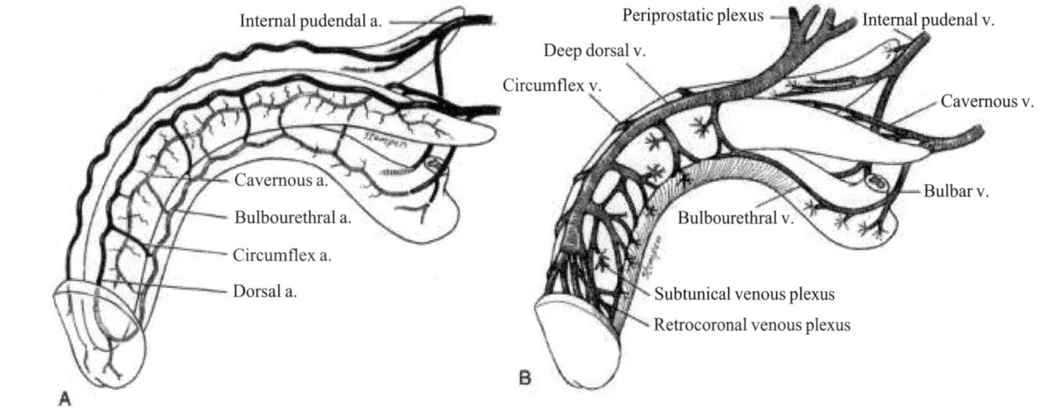

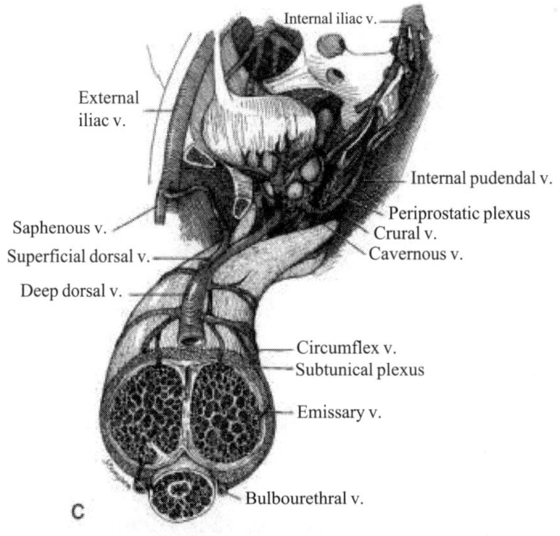

A. Penile arterial supply
B. Venous drainage
C. Cross section of penis showing corpora cavernosa, corpus spongiosum and their relationship to the vascular supply

From Lue TF. Physiology of penile erection and pathophysiology of erectile dysfunction and priapism. In: Walsh PC, ed. Campbell's Urology. *8th ed. Philadelphia, PA: Saunders; 2002.*

dorsal arteries may provide intracavernosal flow via perforating vessels more distally than normal. This anatomic variation may have importance in planning Peyronie's disease surgery, in which the neurovascular bundle is elevated.

The venous drainage of the penis is redundant and plentiful. The largest vein is the deep dorsal, originating at the glans and running deep to Buck's fascia. Circumflex veins coming up from the side and a few direct cavernosal perforators join the deep dorsal vein in its proximal course. After leaving the penis, the deep dorsal vein perforates the urogenital diaphragm and courses toward the apex of the prostate, where it can be problematic during radical prostatectomy. At the cavernosal crura, large cavernosal veins also drain the corpora cavernosa. It is a common misconception that veno-occlusive dysfunction is caused by vascular anomalies. Rather, this is a physiological problem in the tissue, rather than anatomic.

Neurovascular changes of erection

In the flaccid state, there is very little blood flow into the penis. The predominant basic neural tone is sympathetic. The smooth muscle surrounding the lacunar spaces are held in a state of contraction from this sympathetic tone, and therefore, as each unit of space holds less blood, the penis as a whole contains less blood volume and is smaller. The baseline sympathetic tone also keeps the blood supply in a relatively vasoconstricted state.

The actual process of erection involves filling and trapping of blood in the penile tissue. Blood flow increases 20-40 fold through the cavernosal arteries. Smooth muscle relaxation of the cavernosal smooth muscle surrounding the lacunar spaces also occurs, creating a permissive increase in blood volume stored in each space. Therefore, penile blood volume increases and the penis grows. The increase in penile size is checked by the limitation of stretch of the tunica albuginia surrounding the corpus cavernosum. As this limit is reached, an increase in blood volume pushed into the penis results in an increase in pressure, since size has reached its maximum.

This increase in intracavernosal pressure is also responsible for the veno-occlusive function of the penis. In the flaccid state, the low blood flow into the corpus caversosum courses radially from the center, eventually exiting by small venules that perforate the tunica albuginia. During the low flow flaccid state, this egress proceeds in an unimpeded fashion. When the intracavernosal pressure increases to more blood coming in at the limit of the tunica capacity, these venules are compressed against the underside for the tunica, resulting in blood trapping.

The smooth muscle relaxation is controlled by well-known neurochemical cascades. The major control system is the nitric oxide/cyclic GMP (NO/cGMP) system. NO is released by nitrergic end-neurons and endothelial cells in the cavernosal tissue in response to sexual stimulation. NO is produced by the cleavage of l-arginine by nitric oxide synthase (NOS). In the neurons, neuronal NOS (nNOS) is the active enzyme and endothelial NOS (eNOS) is the active form in the vascular lining. Production of NO causes the conversion of GTP into cGMP by the action of guanylate cyclase. Interaction of cGMP with protein kinase G causes calcium shifts and resultant smooth muscle relaxation.

Cyclic nucleotides of all types are broken down by phophodiesterases (PDEs) in the body. The most important PDE in the penile tissue is PDE5, which is present in high concentration, is specific for cGMP and plays a central role in inactivation of the NO/ cGMP pathway. As soon as cGMP is produced, PDE5 begins breaking it down. There is a catalytic domain of the PDE5 molecule that breaks the compound down, and a regulatory domain that makes the enzyme even more efficient in breaking down cGMP, when levels of substrate increase. Therefore, as soon as the chemical reaction takes place to produce cGMP, PDE5 begins turning it off. Preventing the breakdown of cGMP by PDE5 inhibitors form the basis for the drugs sildenafil, vardenafil and tadalafil.

Although PDE5 is clearly the predominant PDE in the penis, and its relative importance in the penis compared to the rest of the body is substantial, allowing an oral agent to be given to get an effect in the penis without exaggerated systemic adverse events. One must remember that PDE is present throughout the body. It is present in systemic and pulmonary vascular beds and the gastroesophageal sphincter, among other areas. PDE5 inhibitors may cause adverse effects from such systemic inhibition, as well cross-reactivity with other PDE families.

Although less important than the cGMP system, a parallel cAMP system is present in the penile tissue, as well. cAMP is degraded by several cAMP specific PDEs (not PDE5, which is cGMP-specific). When present, cAMP also causes smooth muscle relaxation via protein kinase A and calcium flux in much the same way as cGMP. Although not necessarily so important in normal physiological functioning, this system is exploited during intraurethral suppository or intracavernosal injection administration of prostaglandin E1, as this drug initiates the production of cAMP.

Both cyclic nucleotide systems can be manipulated by non-specific PDE inhibitors, such as papaverine. Injection of this drug into the penis causes prolonged smooth muscle relaxation by preventing the degradation of both cGMP and cAMP. However, oral administration cannot achieve a targeted response in the penis without insurmountable systemic adverse effects of PDE inhibition.

Following sexual activity, activation of the sympathetic supply to the penis results in arterial vasoconstriction, contraction of lacunar smooth muscle, defeat of the venoocclusive mechanism as intrapenile pressure decreases, and reversal of the changes mentioned above. This results in return to the baseline flaccid state.

Physiology of ejaculation

After a period of sexual stimulation, coordination of psychic and physical stimulation results in climax and ejaculation. The brain component of this stimulation is poorly understood. Sensory input into the reflex is mostly from the glans and is carried via the dorsal nerves of the penis, which enter the cord at levels S2-4. Sacral input into the reflex causes contraction of the periurethral muscles and proprioception from these muscles may give further to promote reaching climax. Following high pressure contraction of the pelvic/periurethral muscles, ascending pathways meet those descending from the brain at the thoracolumbar junction at levels T10-L3. From there, sympathetic nerves exit the cord and course via the route above, culminating in the ejaculatory organs. The vas deferens propels sperm distally, and the prostate and seminal vesicles contract, expelling the semen into the posterior urethra. At the same time, sympathetic nerves also cause extremely tight contraction of the bladder neck, preventing retrograde ejaculation. After a short delay, involuntary rhythmic skeletal muscle contraction of the bulbocavernosus and bulbospongiosus result in the projectile ejaculation phase.

Since ejaculation is a separate neurological event from penile erection, climax and ejaculation can occur in the absence of an erection.

2. Erectile Dysfunction (ED): General Considerations

Epidemiology of ED

Erectile dysfunction has been defined by several consensus conferences, with the most often quoted being the NIH Consensus Development Panel on Impotence, convened in 1993. This panel suggested ED should be defined as: ***"Inability of the male to attain and maintain erection of the penis to permit satisfactory sexual intercourse."*** This and the other panel definitions have some commonalities. First, the term "erectile dysfunction" should be used instead of "impotence," as the latter can be construed as derogatory and is not as descriptive of the actual condition. The dysfunction should be recurrent or persistent. The ability either to obtain and/ or maintain an erection may be affected. Finally, the definition weighs heavily on patient satisfaction. It is important to remember that sexual function and expectation is not homogeneous across a patient population, so the definition of dysfunction must add in an element of patient expectation/ satisfaction

The Massachusetts Male Aging Study of men ages 40-70, suggested that nearly 50% of men suffer some degree of erectile dysfunction. This study has been criticized of overstating the numbers due to inclusion of men with "mild" ED. Other studies have examined broader age ranges and have come up with a lower incidence. A paper published by Selvin et al, in 2007 suggested that 18.4% of men over age 20 had ED. This was from data obtained by the National Health and Nutrition Examination Survey.

The Selvin study also re-demonstrated the link between ED and cardiovascular disease. Sexual dysfunction was positively correlated with age, hypertension and presence of preexisting cardiovascular disease. Diabetics have a particularly high rate of problems with a crude incidence rate of greater than 50%. The recent study has corroborated a great deal of prior information suggesting this inextricable link. Previous reports have linked ED to hypertension, dyslipidemia, smoking, diabetes, obesity, depression and preexisting cardiovascular disease.

Men with ED are also at risk for developing manifestations of cardiovascular disease when followed over time, suggesting that ED represents the first manifestation of the generalized condition. A small amount of plaque in the 1mm penile arteries can lead to functional impairment that may pre-date any functional problem in larger arteries, such as coronaries and carotids. Thompson showed this to be true in the Prostate Cancer Prevention Trial, where men presenting with no cardiovascular disease at study entry were examined over the follow-up period. Those presenting with ED at study entry had a near-doubling of the rate of cardiovascular events.

General types of ED

As one can surmise from the functional requirements for sexual function, there are several general ED variants.

Arteriogenic: If one cannot increase blood flow the 20-40 fold that is necessary to fill the penis, inadequate blood supply will be the cause of ED. This can be due to atherosclerotic disease, diabetic small vessel disease, or trauma, which may either be a major pelvic injury or chronic compression, such as that seen in bicycle riders. Arteriogenic contribution is the most common type of ED.

Veno-occlusive dysfunction: Blood trapping is an essential part of the erectile process. Lack of smooth muscle relaxation in the cavernosal bodies, due to tissue degeneration from ischemia, trauma, inadequate neurotransmitter release (diabetic microneuropathy), or Peyronie's Disease can cause ED, even in the face of normal arterial inflow.

Neurogenic: Conditions such as diabetic or alcoholic neuropathy, multiple sclerosis, spinal cord injury, or radical prostatectomy can lead to a situation where the signal to cause vascular changes never gets to the penile tissues.

Hormonal: Testosterone deficiency has been shown in multiple animal models to result in decreased production of nitric oxide synthase, NO and cGMP production, and worsened erectile function. This has been corroborated in human case series. It is clear now that in addition to effects on libido, testosterone deficiency may result in an unfavorable change in penile tissue function. While hypogonadism may not be the primary cause of ED, it may compound the problem.

Anatomic: Peyronie's Disease can lead to sexual difficulty due to deformity, decreased flexibility of the penile tissue or from the development of veno-occlusive dysfunction (see more in the section on Peyronie's Disease).

Drug-induced: Many drugs can lead to erectile dysfunction, and the list is too long to print here. The most commonly implicated drugs are antihypertensives (which may cause ED simply by doing what they are intended to do—lower blood pressure) and antidepressants, due to the CNS effects.

Psychogenic: Although with our current understanding of ED we believe that 90% of cases have a predominantly organic cause, there remains a large subset of patients with a psychogenic source. Differentiation of these cases is usually by history, but other testing may be necessary. Since these patients should be treated with therapy, rather than organic treatments with potential adverse effects, it is important to identify them.

3. Evaluation of a Man Presenting with ED

The evaluation of a man with ED follows the typical model for most medical evaluations, history, physical examination, basic lab tests, specialized testing, and finally, treatment. How the ED evaluation differs, however, is that treatment is many times introduced prior to having a specific diagnosis. For instance, it may not be necessary to know if a patient has arterial inflow disease, if an arterial bypass procedure may not be indicated in such a man. An oral agent for treatment may be given to that man to achieve his goals of treatment, with no specialized testing done at all.

The goal-oriented approach to erectile dysfunction treatment is a widely accepted concept. There have been several consensus panels convened that have verified this idea. One must remember that consensus panels on the definition of ED have focused on putting the definition in terms of "satisfactory" sexual activity, and the goal-oriented treatment approach follows along that same line. Nevertheless, some basic evaluation should be done in all men and specialized tests are appropriate for some.

History

The extent and duration of the ED should be ascertained. The degree of current function may guide the physician in predicting what level of therapy might be needed to circumvent the problem. For instance, if the patient states he retains 70% of his natural function, an oral agent will likely be successful in treating the problem. Whether the dysfunction is intermittent or consistent is important. Prior treatments for the problem should be listed and the exact method of administration of such treatments should be elucidated, as incorrect administration may by the central reason for failure of the previous treatment. There have been two large studies that demonstrated re-education alone resulted in changing PDE5 inhibitor failures into successes.

The history is essential in determining whether the ED appears predominantly organic or psychogenic.

Components of the ED history that would support the diagnosis of organic ED include:

- Older age
- Presence of organic risk factors, such as diabetes or hypertension
- Gradual onset and progressive worsening
- Pelvic or retroperitoneal surgery, such as radical prostatectomy
- Consistent dysfunction—no difference between intercourse and masturbation
- Sleep erections and morning erections are absent or significantly diminished in quality
- Orgasm present, even without penile tumescence

Conversely, ***components of the history that should make the clinician suspect psychogenic source include:***

- Younger age
- Absence of risk factors
- Abrupt onset, especially in relation to a psychologically traumatic event
- Inconsistent and varying dysfunction, with differences between sexual situations
- Sleep and morning erections present
- Orgasm absent

Individuals with psychogenic ED should be identified in the history, so that they may receive proper psychological treatment. In those patients that have a confusing history that is not quite clear, further testing can be carried out.

A general medical history should be performed on all men presenting with ED. Drug interactions are possible with ED treatments, and it is important to have a complete list of patient medications.

Previous surgeries, such as prostatectomy, can lead to ED. Others, such as retroperitoneal lymph node dissection, can lead to disorders of ejaculation.

Evaluation of the person's cardiovascular risk and risk reduction program is important. Many men with ED may not have good general medical care, and with the Internet providing a convenient avenue for supporting self-diagnosis, they may present to the urologist without having seen a physician for many years. Assessment for obesity, hypertension, dyslipidemia and diabetes may be deficient. Presentation for ED may represent an opportunity for improving the general health of a patient. Many urologists will not wish to order blood tests assessing such cardiovascular risk, but should at least inform the patient of the relationship between ED and other conditions, and facilitate the referral to a general doctor for such care. Alternatively, basic blood tests, such as lipid profile and fasting blood sugar might be ordered in anticipation of a primary care office visit.

The other cardiac history that is necessary in the urologist's office is whether the patient can tolerate the physical rigors of sexual activity. There is a possibility that an ED patient has not had an erection for many years, and has not been subjected to any physical challenge close to that of sexual intercourse. If he is then given a method to have an erection, he may be at risk for a cardiac event during sex. Questions regarding ability to successfully perform activities of about 3-5 MET will predict success with sexual activity.

The Princeton Guidelines is a good reference that allows the stratification of men into certain cardiac risk classes. When a man presents with ED, a clinical assessment of risk factors allows him to be placed into low, intermediate and high risk groups. The low risk patients can be given an ED treatment and allowed to have sexual activity. The high risk patients should be counseled that sexual activity should not even be attempted until their clinical situation is changed, ie, with cardiac medications, or revascularization, etc. The intermediate risk group should be delayed in their treatment until further cardiac evaluation is done, re-stratifying them into low or high risk (Figure 2).

Figure 2

Princeton Guidelines algorithm for interaction between erectile dysfunction treatment and cardiac risk

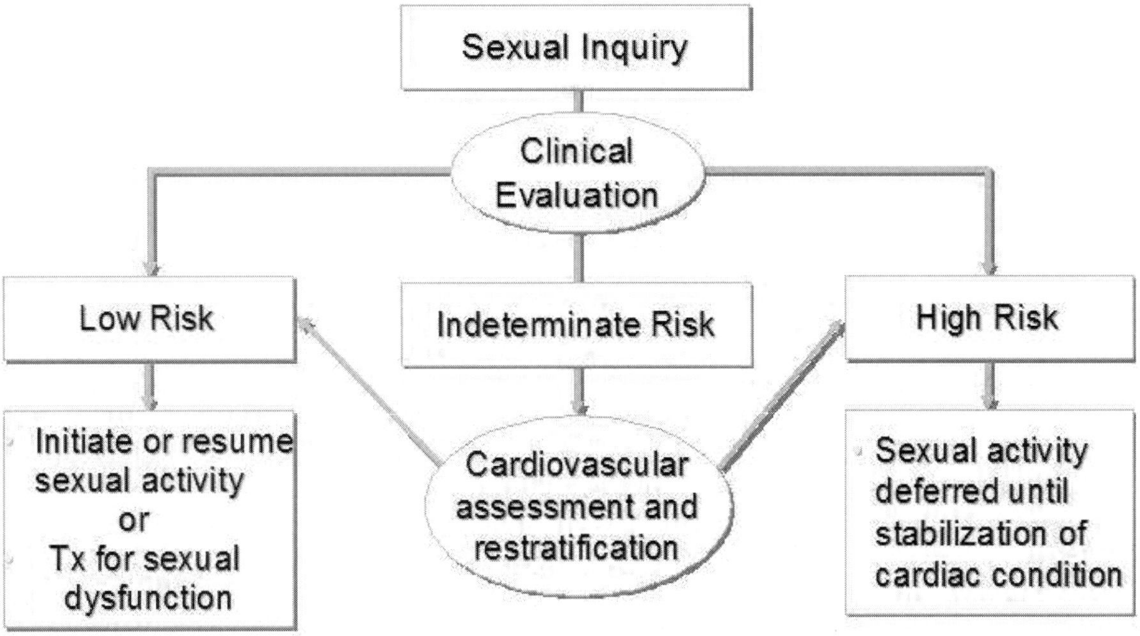

Adapted from DeBusk R, Drory Y, Goldstein I, Jackson G, et al. Management of sexual dysfunction in patients with cardiovascular disease: recommendations of the Princeton Consensus Panel. Am J Card. *2000;86:62F-68F.*

Finally, the history should include queries about what the patient's goals are in treatment of erectile dysfunction. This may change the choice of treatment plan.

Physical examination

The degree of virilization should be noted, and if abnormal, may make the clinician suspect hypogonadism. Peripheral pulses should be palpated. If abnormal, there may an increased likelihood of vasculogenic ED. Neurological examination can tip off CNS disease or peripheral neuropathies that may be the cause of the dysfunction. Detailed examination of the penis for hypospadias, disproportion of the corporal bodies, and plaque is performed. The diagnosis of Peyronie's Disease can be suspected by history, but corroborative findings on physical examination are essential. If a plaque is palpated, it is essential to determine if it is present deep within the cavernosal tissue, as this may be suspicious for an infiltrative process, such as a penile metastasis.

Basic laboratory testing

Because of the potential effects on libido and also penile tissue function, ***a testosterone level should be performed in all men presenting with ED.*** It is unlikely that testosterone deficiency will be the entire cause sexual dysfunction, but may be a contributing cause. Whether or not to obtain a total testosterone (low cost) or free testosterone (more accurate) is controversial. It is probably best to obtain the level in the morning, especially if the patient is a younger man, as there is a diurnal variation with peaks in the morning. In men with hypogonadism on initial testing, further evaluation should include a prolactin level, and LH. It is also possible to check another pituitary axis (eg, thyroid) to look for global pituitary dysfunction.

In men without good prior medical care, assessment for cardiovascular risk factors with blood testing is recommended. These include lipid profile and assessment for diabetes with either fasting blood glucose or hemoglobin A1C. These will uncommonly be ordered by the urologist, but patients should be encouraged to work with a primary care doctor to have these assessments done.

Specialized testing

As mentioned previously, specialized tests are not necessary in all patients. They should be used selectively, and in those patients for whom the results will alter clinical care decisions. Some of the potential tests that may be used in men with ED are as follows:

Nocturnal penile tumescence (NPT) monitoring: Men will normally have several erections during sleep. This is related to sleep pattern, and not to sexual stimulation. Because men with a psychogenic source of ED will continue to have such sleep pattern-related erections, this test represents an opportunity to differentiate men with organic from those with predominantly psychogenic problems. The men with organic ED will have poor responses noted during sleep, in concert with their organic dysfunction. Men with psychogenic problems will have a discrepancy between sleep and conscious erections. They are psychologically preventing the erectile response during conscious sexual encounters, but in the absence of their anxiety during sleep will function perfectly fine.

NPT testing can be done in a supervised sleep laboratory or in an ambulatory setting. The disadvantages of the laboratory setting are cost and difficulty sleeping in a strange surrounding The advantage of the lab is the ability to monitor for rapid eye movement (REM) sleep by lab personnel. Absence of such sleep may lead to false positive testing.

Many urologists utilize the RigiScan ambulatory NPT monitor. Advantages include low cost and the ability of patient to sleep in his own surroundings. Another advantage is the ability of the machine to measure penile rigidity. REM sleep is not measured in the ambulatory setting and false positive tests may be encountered. There are many standards for what constitutes a normal test, but most would consider 2-3 erectile events per night, duration of greater than 15 minutes per event and rigidity of 50%-60% a normal test (Figure 3).

Duplex doppler ultrasonography: This has uniformly replaced other gross screening tests for penile blood flow used in the past, such as determination of the penile brachial index. Advantages of duplex ultrasound over prior tests include ability to visualize the artery being measured, identification of Peyronie's plaques, and direct measurement of blood flow in response to pharmacologic injection.

Injection of a vasoactive drug into the penis is essential to glean useful information from the test. As noted previously, penile blood in the flaccid state is extremely low, and nearly non-measurable by ultrasound scanning. It is the ***increase*** in blood flow that needs to be measured to assess for arteriogenic erectile dysfunction. There are a wide number of protocols for type and dose of injected medicines, including 10-40 micrograms of prostaglandin E1, 30-60 mg of papaverine, and combinations of papaverine, phentolamine and prostaglandin E1.

Normal ranges vary from author to author, but peak systolic blood greater than 25-35 cm per second in the cavernosal artery following injection represents normal arterial inflow. End-diastolic flows should be less than 3 cm per second and resistive index >0.85. These suggest normal veno-occlusive function. The patient should achieve a normal erection.

If during such a test, the patient notes that the erection obtained is much poorer than his normal baseline erection, the test may be a false-positive. Epinephrine that is released in response to the penile injection activates the detumescence mechanism and may be the cause. A patient with sufficient anxiety can also create a false-positive.

Cavernosometry/ cavernosography: The test is invasive, with 2 needles in the penis, 1 for infusion of medications and saline, and the other for pressure measurements. A pharmacologic agent is injected to achieve full smooth muscle relaxation, and saline infusion is begun. Salient data obtained from the study are flow necessary to obtain erection and maintain erection and pressure degradation curves. What is considered a normal test varies with authors. Injection of contrast at the end of the study may identify the extremely rare patient with a focal large leak from the corpus cavernosum that may be amenable to surgical therapy.

In men whom veno-occlusive dysfunction is suspected, this test can give more specific information, but is rarely carried out, as specific treatment of

Figure 3

NPT monitoring

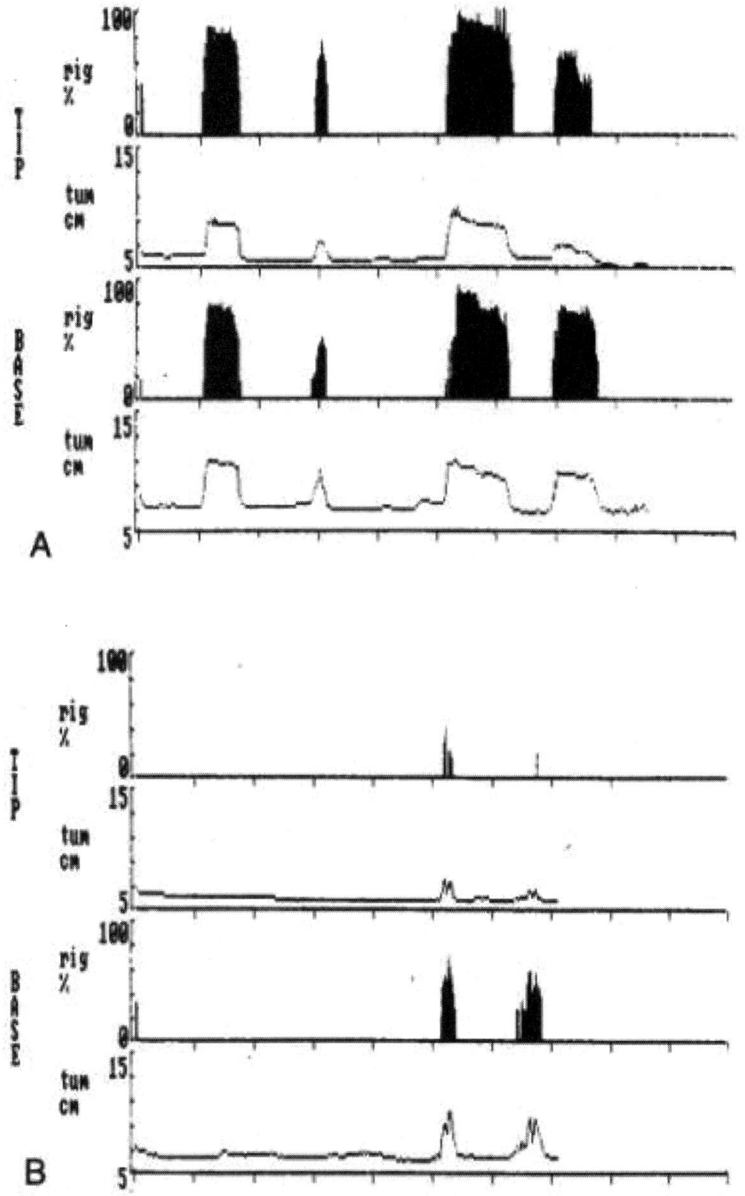

A. Normal Rigiscan study showing several episodes of prolonged tumescence during a night of sleep

B. Abnormal Rigiscan study with short-lived episodes of tumescence. The tip does not have adequate rigidity

From Broderick GA, Lue TF. Evaluation and nonsurgical management of erectile dysfunction and priapism. In: Walsh PC, ed. Campbell's Urology. *8th ed. Philadelphia, PA: Saunders; 2002: Chapter 46.*

such dysfunction is rarely performed. When venous ligation procedures were first introduced, this test was more common, but such surgery has fallen out of favor due to the poor durability of the results.

Penile arteriography: Specific arteriography of the internal pudendal system is reserved for those individuals in whom penile revascularization is being considered. Thc arteriogram is performed under pharmacologically stimulated erection. Penile arterial supply, as well as patency of potential donor arteries (usually inferior epigastrics) is carefully examined. Also, it is important to note the presence or absence of generalized atherosclerosis, the presence of which may lessen enthusiasm for a revascularization procedure. This very uncommon test should be performed by angiographers with expertise in this area, to maximize the chance that useful information will be gleaned.

4. ED Treatments

Sex Therapy

After identification of a psychogenic source for ED, referral to a therapist with expertise in treating sexual dysfunction is in order. Organic treatments may be used in conjunction with the therapist's recommendations, but they should have a good safety profile, so as to not put the patient at undue risk. It is wise to let the therapist guide introduction of organic treatments. Otherwise the patient may rely on the organic treatment and not have little incentive for working on the psychogenic side.

Yohimbine

Yohimbine is a supplement that has a historical place in the treatment of ED. Its proposed role in the treatment of ED is to increase parasympathetic and decrease sympathetic activity. Many OTC "male enhancement" supplements may contain some amount of yohimbine. In high enough doses it can lead to diaphoresis, palpitations and elevated heart rate. The AUA does not recommend yohimbine for the treatment of ED, and patients with a history suggestive of cardiovascular disease should be cautioned against these supplements.

PDE5 inhibitors

This class of drug is considered first line therapy for those men presenting with ED without a contraindication to their administration. Administration results in inhibition of PDE throughout the body, but due to the relative importance of the enzyme in the penile tissue, a favorable environment in the penile tissue of prolonged cGMP effect is seen without major change in systemic homeostasis. This is due to direct inhibition of the breakdown of cGMP produced by the NO/cGMP system described earlier.

Drugs available include sildenafil citrate (25, 50 and 100 mg), vardenafil hydrochloride (5, 10 and 20 mg), and tadalafil (5, 10 and 20 mg for demand dosing, and 2.5 or 5 mg for daily use). All are highly specific for PDE5, and all are efficacious in promoting penile erection capability in men with ED. Vardenafil is the most potent agent in laboratory testing, followed by sildenafil and then tadalafil, but laboratory potency does not necessarily translate into clinical effectiveness.

Success rates for improvement of erection is approximately 70%-80%, and improvement to the point where the drugs are suitability for monotherapy of ED is seen in approximately 60% of cases. The drugs are more effective in men with mild ED, and men with severe ED may not respond to these agents. They are permissive agents—they do not work autonomously, but require sexual stimulation to initiate the processes leading to nitric oxide production in the penis. Without such production, the drugs have no effect, as they do not turn on the process—they merely stop it from turning off. PDE5 inhibitors are taken prior to sexual activity to obtain tissue levels prior to sexual stimulation, and the effectiveness of each drug is dependent on pharmacokinetics.

Sildenafil and vardenafil each achieve peak plasma concentrations in about 1 hour, and tadalafil peaks in 2 hours. The half lives of sildenafil and vardenafil are 4-5 hours, and for tadalafil, the half-life is 18 hours in young men and longer in elderly men. Choice of agent must take into consideration the sexual pattern of the patient, without the physician making assumptions about such things. The advent of daily tadalafil presents the option for continuous treatment for ED, equivalent to that of other organic diseases, without suffering a decline in erectile improvement due to the lower dose.

There are class-related side effects due to systemic inhibition of PDE5. Most of these are vasodilatory effects, with systolic and diastolic blood pressures decreasing in range of low single digits. Other vasodilatory side effects commonly seen are skin flushing, rhinitis and headache. Inhibition of PDE5 at the gastroesophageal sphincter may lead to acid reflux and dyspepsia.

Although the drugs are highly specific for PDE5, there are 2 important cross-class PDE interactions. Sildenafil, at clinical doses inhibits PDE6 in the retina of the eye to a lesser degree than PDE5, and this results in 5%-10% of men reporting a bluish discoloration in their color perception. This stops as the drug level goes down, and no long term problems have been associated with this vision change. Tadalafil at clinical doses inhibits PDE11, but the effect of this inhibition is not known. The muscular pain associated specifically with tadalafil administration is of unknown etiology.

Because these agents inhibit the PDE5 systemically, it is essential they NOT be given in conjunction with organic nitrates. Nitrates active the NO/cGMP system in the systemic circulation and these agents stop it from turning off. Profound drops in blood pressure may be seen. To a lesser degree, alpha blockers may synergistically drop blood pressure with PDE5 inhibitors, and caution must be used in this drug interaction in conjunction with published prescribing information.

There have been recent reports of non-arteritic ischemic optic neuropathy (NAION) associated with PDE5 inhibitors. Caution needs to be exercised in men with acute vision loss on these agents, with discontinuation the safe option. However, men with vascular disease are exactly those people at risk for both NAION and ED. It is likely that the association, if any, is due to the underlying medical condition and not a drug effect.

Advantages of PDE5 inhibitors include oral administration, safety and effectiveness. Disadvantages include cost, systemic administration as opposed to local effect, potential for interaction with nitrates, and poor efficacy in men with severe ED. Cost is becoming an issue as well, as some insurance companies offer extremely limited coverage for any ED medications.

Penile injection therapy

It was noted quite by accident by the famous French surgeon, Virag, that injection of papaverine into the penis can result in erection. Early work by Brindley verified this finding, as his memorable presentation at the Las Vegas AUA meeting will attest to. Thoughout the intervening years from this early report to the present, many vasoactive agents have been used for ED therapy. Only alprostadil (PGE1) has been approved by the FDA for this indication. Alprostadil, when introduced into the corpus cavernosum, actives the cAMP system described earlier, leading to calcium flux and smooth muscle relaxation.

Alprostadil is available commercially in preparations up to 60 micrograms. It is stored as a powder and needs to be reconstituted prior to use. Direct injection of the drug results in a suitable erection for intercourse in 60%-80% of ED cases. In distinction to PDE5 inhibitors, alprostadil is an actual initiator of erection, and does not depend on sexual activity for erection to occur (although sexual activity may augment the response). The initial injection procedure should done under medical supervision.

Adverse events associated with PGE1 injection include priapism and penile pain. The pain is present in about 35%-40% of cases and may be a cause for discontinuation of the treatment. Priapism usually occurs at the time of the first injection, when sensitivity to the drug in the individual patient is not yet known. The priapism associated with penile injection therapy is easily treated with sympathomimetic agents, if addressed in a timely fashion. Fibrosis can occur in a small number of cases, but with PGE1, the fibrosis rate is much less than with off-label use of papaverine.

Advantages of PGE1 injection therapy include higher efficacy in difficult cases, its ability to initiate erection. Disadvantages include cost, invasiveness, penile pain, and the possibility of priapism and penile fibrosis.

Intraurethral alprostadil

In hopes of decreasing invasiveness of injectable PGE1, the urethral suppository form of the drug is available in doses from 125 to 1000 micrograms. The efficacy is approximately 30%-40%, but in responsive individuals, this system avoids the need for penile injection. Penile pain is also a problem with this method of administration, although priapism is extremely uncommon. The initial administration should be performed under medical supervision.

Advantages of intraurethral alprostadil include less invasive administration compared to injection and ability to initiate erection. Disadvantages include low efficacy, penile pain and cost.

Vacuum constriction devices

The concept of these devices is actually quite simple—instead of positive arterial pressure bringing blood into the penis, an external negative pressure device pulls the blood in. A constriction band is placed at the base of the penis prior to removal of the vacuum to keep the blood there. The band is allowed to remain in place for up to 30 minutes. These devices can cause discoloration of the penis, decrease in temperature, discomfort with ejaculation and loss of erection during intercourse. However, the adverse events are mild and limited, and FDA has taken away the requirement for a prescription that was in place several years ago, due to the track record of safety. There is a high drop-out rate in people that begin using these devices, usually due to the less-than-optimal sexual experience. However, there are some long-term users, and for the patient who is a non-interventionalist, a vacuum device may be a satisfactory choice.

Advantages of vacuum constriction devices include safety, non-invasiveness, rapid initiation of therapy with little training and no prescription is required. Disadvantages include poor sustenance of erection, change in color or temperature of the penis, ejaculatory pain and a high drop-out rate among users.

Penile prosthesis

Penile implants have been available since the 1970s. Initial devices had an extremely high failure rate, with the expectation that reoperation would be necessary in the majority of cases. The devices have improved substantially since then. ***Advantages of penile prosthesis are high efficacy in all patient severities, and high patient and partner satisfaction rates. Disadvantages include the need for surgery, and potential complication of infection, erosion and need for reoperation.***

There are 4 major types of penile prosthesis:

Malleable or semirigid devices (Figure 4) remain firm all the time, but can usually be molded into conformation with the clothing. They are very simple and have a low failure rate, but concealment is many times a problem. Furthermore, since there is

Figure 4

Malleable penile prosthesis

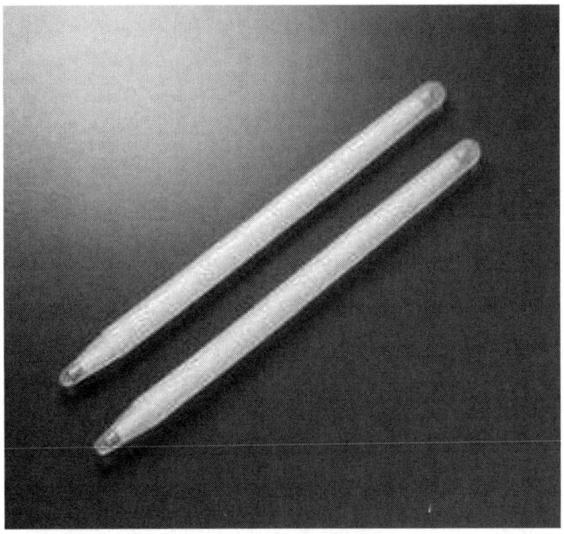

American Medical Systems, Minneapolis, MN

Figure 5

2-piece inflatable penile prosthesis

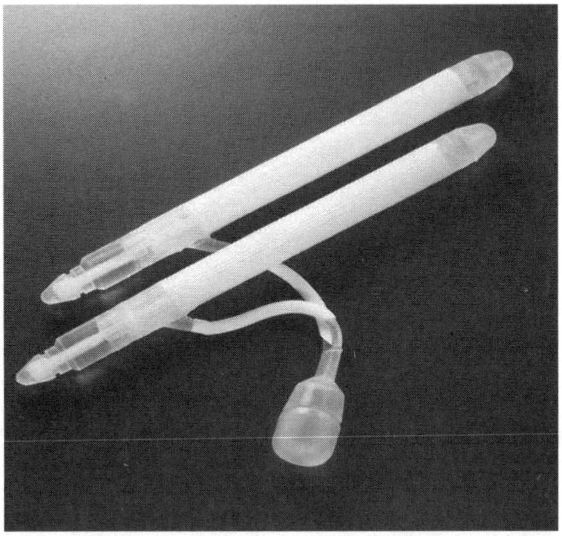

American Medical Systems, Minneapolis, MN

no excursion in girth, many patients are unhappy with the erection quality.

Mechanical devices are similar to semirigids in that they are in a fixed degree of penile girth, so erection quality is a complaint of these devices. However, since they are arranged with stacked disks that allow a total of more movement, they are much more malleable and easier to conceal. The flexibility sometimes allows the penis to assume some rather odd shapes and occasionally be overflexible during sexual activity.

2-piece inflatable devices (Figure 5) were designed to meet the advantages of inflatables, as far as girth expansion and rigidity, while allowing flaccidity and concealment, while also capitalizing on the advantages of semirigid—lack of the need for a reservoir implantation. There is only one 2-piece inflatable available on the market. It has 2 cylinders which are filled in the center, allowing for fluid insertion just under the surface of the cylinders. The fluid source is partly from a small reservoir at the base of each cylinder (deep in the corporal body) and partly from the scrotal pump used to activate the device.

Some investigators have reported very high satisfaction rates with the two-piece inflatable, while other are more pessimistic. While the manufacturers have successfully developed a product with simplicity and inflatability, some patients find the excursion limited, and erection not acceptable and/ or the deflatability limited and concealment difficult.

3-piece inflatable devices (Figure 6) are most commonly reported in series in the literature. They consist of 2 cylinders, a reservoir in the pelvis and a pump in the scrotum. They are the most complicated devices and require a larger surgical procedure to implant the device. However, they give the best flaccidity and the best rigidity of all the devices available.

Figure 6

3-piece inflatable penile prosthesis with paired cylinders, reservoir and scrotal pump

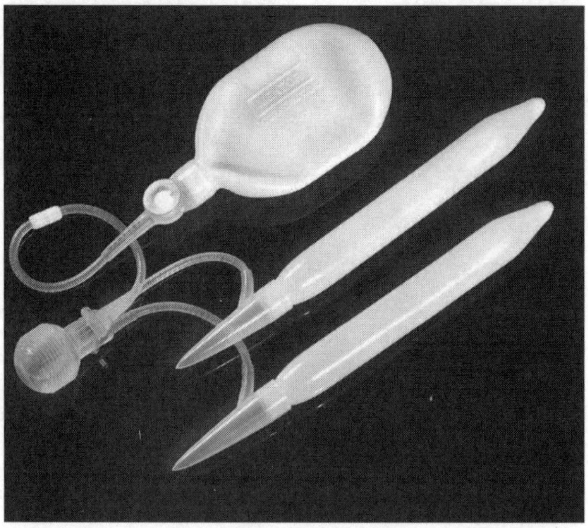

Coloplast, Copenhagen, Denmark

Surgical approaches for penile implants

There are a variety of ways to place a penile prosthesis, but most surgeons utilize the infrapubic or penoscrotal approaches.

In the infrapubic approach, an incision is made at the base of the penis. The corporal bodies are approached dorso-laterally, and the cylinders placed there, after dilation. The pump is placed lateral to the penis as low in the scrotum as possible. A fascial incision is made to place the reservoir and the connections are made to complete the implantation. ***Advantages of the infrapubic approach include avoidance of the urethra, and ability to directly open the abdominal fascia for reservoir placement. Disadvantages include longer operative time, abdominal fascial incision pain, and possibility of dorsal neurovascular bundle injury.***

In the penoscrotal approach, an incision is made at the penoscrotal angle over the urethra. The corporal bodies are approached lateral to the urethra and the cylinders placed there. The pump is placed in the inferior dependent portion of the scrotum. The reservoir is placed blindly through the internal ring into the retropubic space, and inflated after insertion. ***Advantages of the penoscrotal approach include decreased operative time, decreased postoperative pain due to no fascial incision, and better access to the corporal bodies for dilation. Disadvantages include the possibility of bladder or vascular injury during blind reservoir placement.***

Complications of penile prosthesis surgery include infection, erosion and mechanical failure, necessitating re-operation. Erosion is thought to be due to subclinical infection in nearly all cases.

Infection can be acute after placement of prosthesis, or indolent, presenting well after the initial surgery. Acute infection tends to be with virulent organisms, such as *S aureus* creating purulent infection. Late infection tends to be most commonly due to *S epidermidis*. ***With current improvement in coating of prosthetic devices, the infection rate should be less than 1%.***

One can never be faulted for removing a device to treat infection. However, the fibrosis and shrinkage seen following explantation dictates that one considers a salvage operation in such cases. This procedure, popularized by Mulcahy, involves removal of the infected device, followed by irrigation of a series of solutions of peroxide, betadine, and antibiotics. The operative field is re-prepped and draped with an entire new set of instruments, as if it were a new operation. The new device is then inserted. The rate of a successful outcome in a salvage prosthesis operation is approximately 80%.

Mechanical malfunctions may be due to cylinder or tubing leak, connector failure, autoinflation due to pressure on the reservoir, or cylinder aneurysm formation. ***If mechanical malfunction is seen in a prosthesis, the entire device should be replaced with a new one.*** Recent data from Henry and other suggest that some modification of a salvage operation be done in all re-do implants, as the rate of subclinical bacterial colonization is substantial. The two companies currently producing 3-piece inflatables have made significant improvements in recent years to lower the failure rate. These include: Dacron buttressing and parylene coating of silicone cylinders, improvement of connector system, lock-out systems in the reservoir and/or pump to prevent autoinflation, and coating of the devices with antibiotics or bacterial resistant materials to lower the risk of infection.

Penile Revascularization

Revascularization of the penis to correct erectile difficulty is uncommonly performed. This is due to the rather stringent criteria for patient selection, including a young age, a history of significant pelvic/perineal trauma, and no preexisting erectile complaints. Angiography is a prerequisite to the surgery. Because ED in older men coexists with other comorbidities and commonly involves some degree of venous leak, revascularization is not an option.

II. Peyronie's Disease

1. **Epidemiology and Etiology of PD**
2. **Clinical Course of PD**
3. **Office Evaluation and Medical Management**
4. **Surgical Therapy**

1. Epidemiology and Etiology of PD

Introduction

Peyronies's Disease (PD) was first described by Francois de la Peyronie in 1743, and the disease still carries his name. The disease is manifested by development of penile plaque, pain and deformity of erection due to disproportion of the tunica albuginea from the plaque. There are large voids in our understanding of this condition, and thus we are lacking specific treatments to reverse the condition. Many patients with this condition will tolerate it until it reaches stability, and then decide whether or not surgical intervention is indicated. It represents a frustrating condition for both the patient and treating physician.

Older studies have underestimated the rate of PD in the population. Many of the older reports were simply case series or simple calculations based on number of patients seen vs. number of cases of the condition. Incidences in these studies were ranging from 0.3% up to 1%. Dr. Charles Devine estimated that 1% of male physicians in his patient population suffered from the condition. Autopsy studies with evidence of penile plaque suggest a prevalence as high as 22% of men.

More recent studies have reported a higher incidence and may be more accurate due to their methodology. Sommer in 2002 reported results of a survey of 8000 men, with a self-reported rate of 3.2%. Mulhall looked for evidence of PD in men attending a mass prostate cancer screening event, and found that 8.9% of men had objective findings on evaluation. ***The true incidence of Peyronie's Disease is higher than previously thought and is most likely between 3 and 10%.***

Most investigators believe that Peyronie's Disease results from a combination of a scar-forming tendency coupled with penile trauma as the direct inciting event.

Evidence for the genetic predisposition is present. There is an association between Dupuytren's contracture and PD; men are prone to PD if their father had Dupuytren's contracture. There is an association seen between PD and plantar fasciitis. Gene expression studies in PD tissue and normal tunica albuginea show differences in genes that control scar modification.

In a man with a predisposition to PD, penile trauma during intercourse results in an injury to the tissue. Cytokines and fibrin in the tissue launch an initial attempt at healing. In men with a PD tendency, the normal migration of fibroblasts occurs, but these cells then differentiate into myofibroblasts, and contribute to abnormal healing and abnormal scar formation. Scar remodeling proceeds in an abnormal fashion in PD patients, resulting in a plaque.

2. Clinical Course of PD

In the early stages of the condition, there is development of a (sometimes) painful plaque. As the plaque remodels, pain may persist as penile deformity evolves. In nearly everyone, the pain eventually abates, and this is usually associated with plaque stabilization. This occurs in about 12-18 months. Once stabilization occurs, it is less likely that the situation will worsen or improve.

Early reports of PD suggested a very optimistic outlook for spontaneous improvement or even resolution of the condition. In 1970, Williams reported that 76% of people with PD either improved or resolved their condition within 4 years. Gelbard was less optimistic in 1990, reporting only 13% resolving the situation, and ½ of patients stabilizing, with the rest continuing to worsen. A large recent study by Mulhall agreed with these numbers with 12% improving, and a little less than ½ of patients stabilizing with at least 1 year of follow-up. Thus is appears that ***spontaneous improvement of Peyronie's Disease occurs at a relatively low rate, probably between 10%-15%.***

Erectile dysfunction is a common problem, and PD, based on recent reports is also common. Thus, it may be difficult to decipher whether there is an association between the 2 conditions. It appears that the rate of ED in PD patients is increased. Hellstrom suggested that 20%-40% of men with PD will suffer from erectile dysfunction. Investigators examining the etiology have found abnormal veno-occlusive function in a large number of patients, suggesting that the plaque creates abnormal tissue function and pliability underneath.

3. Office Evaluation and Medical Management

In men presenting with PD, one should try to elicit a history of penile trauma during intercourse, but commonly, no history can be found. Other scar forming manifestations in the past history, family history or on physical examination should be sought. The degree of erectile function should be documented, and objective testing is sometimes indicated to serve as a baseline prior to therapy. A history of prior surgeries, and treatment for ED, particularly intracavernosal injection therapy should be noted.

On physical examination, one should define the extent and location of the plaque. This is a challenge in itself, as the plaque can extend distally, proximally, laterally, through the septum or some combination of these. Ultrasound may be used to corroborate the physical exam findings. As patients tend to overestimate the degree or curvature, a photograph of the deformity in the erect state is an excellent tool to allow the clinician to appreciate the degree of physical impairment associated with the condition. In-office pharmacologic erection also can be used to document the deformity. Accurate measurements help aid in determining the response to therapy.

Duplex ultrasound following intracavernosal injection can detect the degree of arterial inflow disease, or, more importantly, the degree of veno-occlusive impairment. Documentation of baseline impairment may be helpful in addressing concerns after surgical therapy when patients complain of decline in function.

Most importantly, it is important to document the source of intracavernosal flow prior to planning surgical therapy. During Peyronie's plaque incision and grafting, the neurovascular bundle is commonly elevated from the tunica to allow access to the plaque. If an individual supplies his cavernosal bodies with blood from the dorsal arteries (Figure 7), such an operation may result in interruption of this important collateral supply, with resultant arteriogenic ED.

There have been a variety of medical managements put forth for the treatment of PD. Most reports on such therapies are simple case series, where all patients have received the treatment, and the "success rate" is published. Since there is no control group in most studies, the placebo effect cannot be quantified, nor can the background rate of spontaneous resolution. Treatments that have been suggested as effective in PD through the years have included: vitamin E, colchicines, Potaba, tamoxifen, as well as injectable corticosteroids, collagenases and verapamil.

Perhaps the best studied and most promising medical management is intralesional verapamil. Scar formation has calcium-dependent processes, and the theory is that a calcium channel blocker, such as verapamil may have benefit. The largest experience is in an uncontrolled series of Levine, which suggested that penile deformity improved in more than 60% of cases, with worsening in only 10%, very favorable to historical thinking. There are 2 small placebo-controlled studies showing some benefit from this therapy.

Figure 7

Duplex ultrasound of a man with aberrant penile blood supply

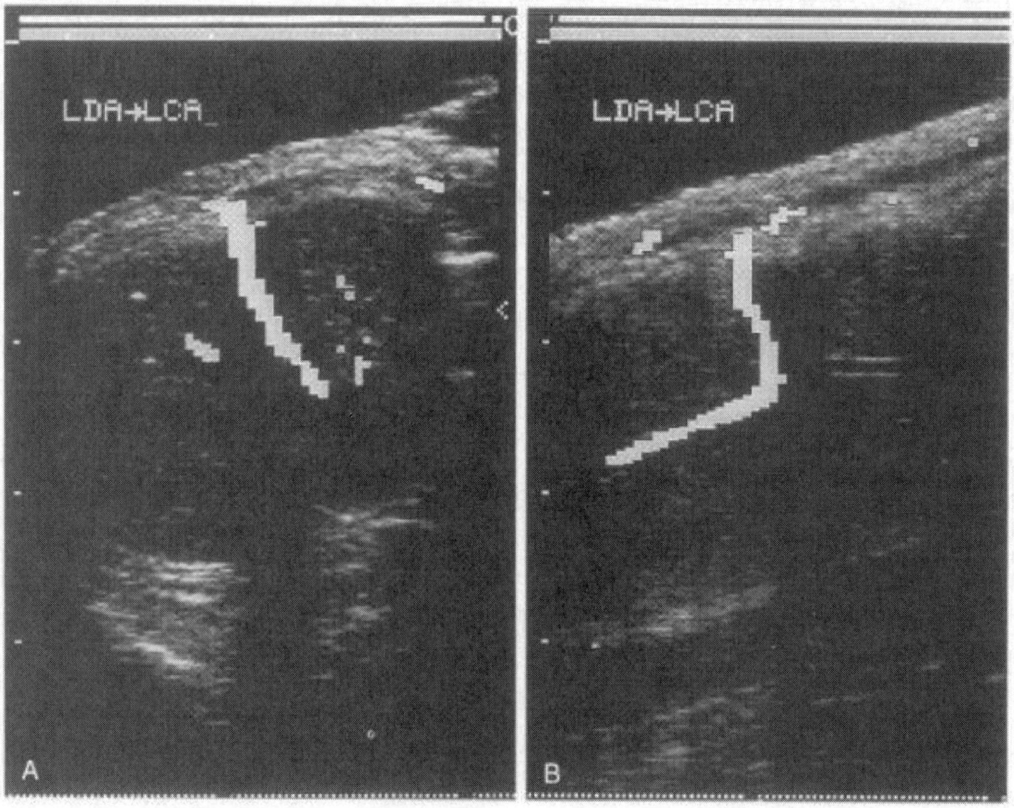

His cavernosal arteries are supplied by perforators from the dorsal arteries. This man would be at high risk for arteriogenic erectile dysfunction if the neurovascular bundle were elevated in a surgical procedure.

4. Surgical Therapy

Prior to performing surgery on PD, it must be stable for a minimum of 6 months time. One does not want to miss the opportunity for spontaneous resolution, but more importantly, if the deformity is changing, it may continue to change after surgery. Therefore, the penis may be straight at the end of the operation, only to have a recurrence of a deformity some weeks later. If the patient has excellent erections, and the deformity does not preclude sexual intercourse, the wisdom of such surgery is suspect, as the patient may end up worse after surgery than his presurgical condition.

Figure 8

Penile plication procedure

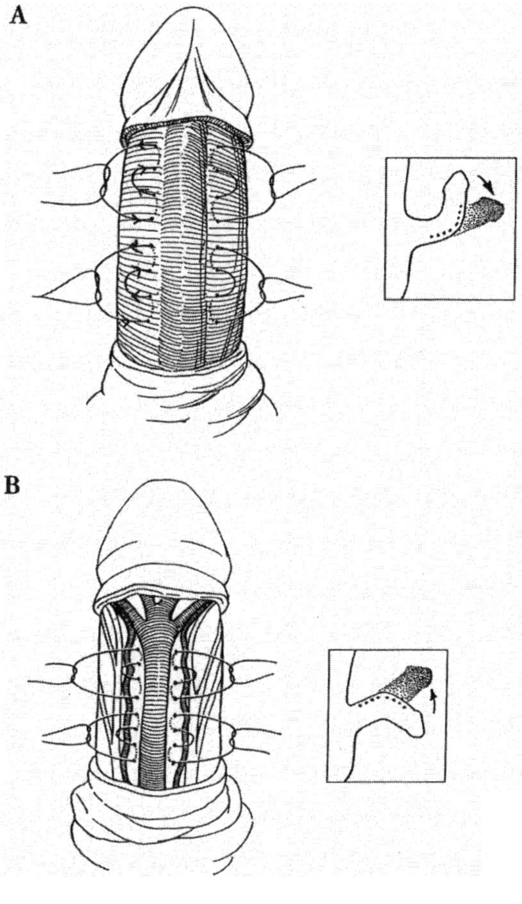

From Gholami SS, Lue TF. Correction of penile curvature using the 16-dot plication technique: a review of 132 patients. J Urol. *2002;167:2066-2069.*

The first group of surgical procedures for PD are the penile shortening procedures, commonly referred to a plication procedures, or Nesbit procedure (Figure 8). The idea is that the tunica albuginia opposite the plaque is shortened to match the shortening from the disease. The resultant erection will be straight, as both sides are restricting expansion of the penis equally. ***Advantages of penile shortening procedures are: lower incidence of post-op ED; and lower incidence of penile numbness, since the neurovascular bundle is usually not mobilized. The disadvantage is that an already shortened penis (shortened from the PD) is made even shorter by the surgery.***

Penile lengthening procedures involve plaque incision (and rarely excision) with grafting of the tunica defect (Figure 9). Since most plaques are located dorsally, access must be gained by elevation of the neurovascular bundle, opening up the possibility of post-operative glans numbness. The fact that the intracavernosal tissue is exposed opens up the possibility of destroying some degree of tissue function, resulting in post-operative erectile dysfunction. Graft materials used were originally dermis, followed by synthetics, such as Dacron and Gore-Tex. Currently many PD surgeons have gravitated to the cadaveric pericardium or porcine small intestinal submucosa grafts. ***The advantage of penile lengthening procedures is reversal of some degree of penile shortening. The disadvantages include a higher rate of penile numbness and post-operative erectile dysfunction.***

In men presenting with PD with deformity and concomitant decline in erectile function, the rate of post-operative ED is expected to be higher. Such men would be better served with implantation of a three-piece penile prosthesis to treat the ED and also to help correct the penile deviation. In the operating room, after placement of the prosthesis, a penile molding procedure consisting of forceful shaping of the penis with the device inflated can be performed. Rarely, prosthesis implantation needs to be combined with a formal straightening procedure described above.

Figure 9

Grafting of the tunica defect

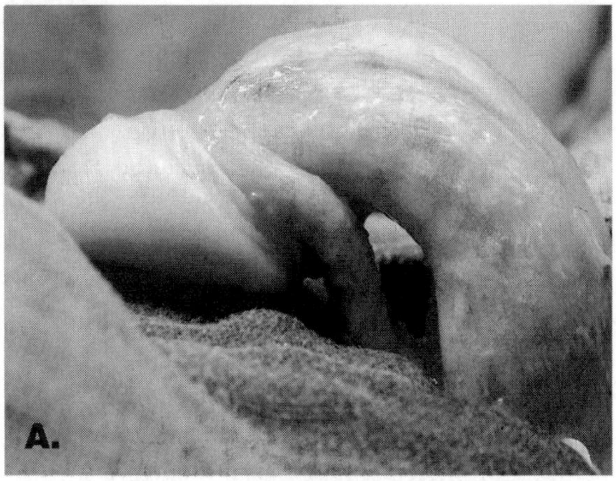

After elevation of the neurovascular bundle, an artificial erection test shows severe deformity

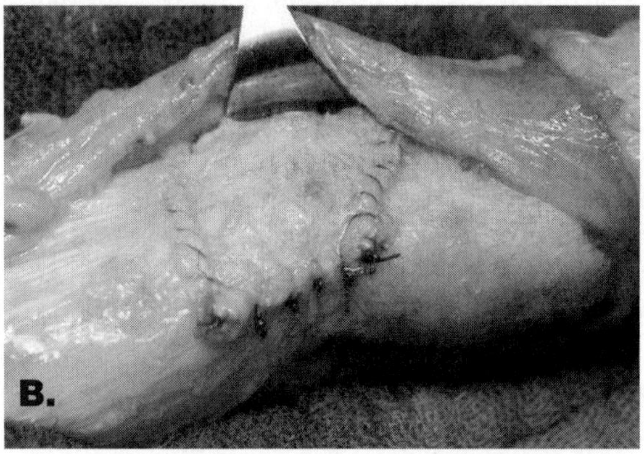

The graft (in this case dermis) has been sutured into place to fill the defect caused by plaque incision

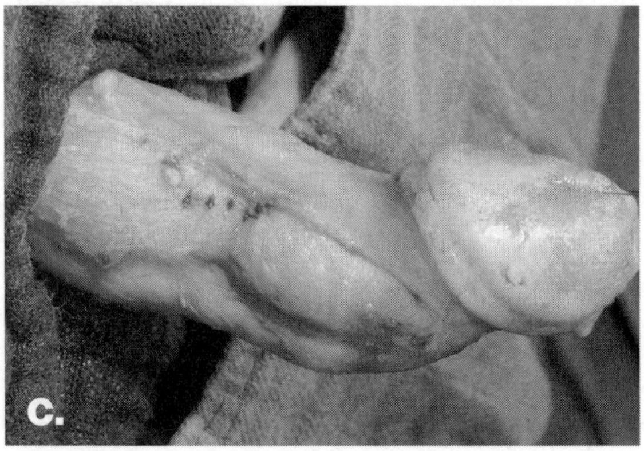

Final artificial erection test shows corretion of the deformity

From: Backhaus BO, Muller SC, Albers P: Corporoplasty for advanced Peyronie's disease using venous and/or dermis path grafting: new surgical technique and long-term patient satisfaction. J Urol. *2003;169:981-984.*

III. Priapism

Introduction

Priapism is a pathological prolonged erection, unassociated with sexual stimulation. It is one of the true urological emergencies. If this condition persists without treatment, permanent penile tissue damage may result with loss of erectile function.

1. Ischemic vs. Non-ischemic Priapism

One of the immediate challenges that faces the treating physician is determining if the priapism is ischemic.

Ischemic priapism is a hypoxic, low-flow state and is due to lack of drainage of blood from the corpus cavernosum. It is quite painful to the patient, and leads to cavernosal damage if not treated. The erection is usually very firm and non-compressible. There is very little, if any, flow on duplex ultrasonography. Blood gases obtained from corpus cavernosum show low PO_2 (<30 mm Hg), high PCO_2 (>60 mm Hg), and low pH (<7.25). Etiologies of low-flow priapism include penile injection therapy (usually low-flow after several hours), sickle cell anemia, psychotropic drugs, pelvic malignancies with obstruction of venous outflow, metastatic tumors of the penis, heparin and intravenous fat emulsion.

In contrast, ***non-ischemic priapism*** is a high-flow state, caused by unchecked blood flow into the corpus cavernosum, but with preserved outflow. There is continuous turnover of oxygenated blood, and lack of ischemia. Although the patient might be troubled by the fact that he has a continuous erection, it tends to not be painful. On examination it is usually compressible, but fills rapidly after the pressure is relieved. Cavernosal blood gases show a normal arterial pattern, and duplex Doppler ultrasound shows high continuous flows through the cavernosal arteries. Etiologies of non-ischemic priapism are penile trauma, with laceration of the cavernosal artery, intracavernosal pharmacotherapy (early after injection), and certain neurological condition, such as acute spinal cord injury.

Ischemic priapism IS an emergency, but non-ischemic priapism is not.

Initial assessment includes attempting to find the source of the problem on history. Has the patient used penile injection therapy or psychotropic drugs? Is there a history of sickle cell? Is the problem recurrent? Examination may give clues as to whether ischemia is present. Blood may be obtained for blood gas determination to make a final determination. One should determine on physical exam which compartments of the penis are erect. Usually the corpus spongiosum is not involved, and allows surgical shunting into the spongiosal space a possibility. If the entire penis is involved, one needs to consider the possibility of an infiltrative process, rather than simple priapism.

Laboratory assessment includes cavernosal blood gas determination. One should also order a complete blood count, to look for hematological malignancies and hemoglobin electrophoresis. A toxicology screen may give insight into drug-induced priapism. Color Doppler ultrasound may assist in determining state of ischemia.

Initial management of ischemic priapism is aimed at treating the underlying cause, if identified, and clearing the cavernosum of the ischemic blood and restoring oxygenated blood flow. Aspiration of blood, coupled with saline irrigation will uncommonly be curative. In cases of priapism due to penile injection therapy, this may work. However, after irrigation is attempted, injection of a sympathomimetic agent is the next step. ***The best agent is phenylephrine, 500 micrograms per mL, to inject 1-2 mL (500-1000 micrograms for adult patients).*** This can be repeated every 3-5 minutes for an hour. Blood pressure should be monitored during this administration. Phenylephrine is the drug of choice due to its pure alpha agonist effect, and lack of secondary neurotransmitter release.

If sympathomimetic drugs do not resolve the situation, surgical shunting should be performed. The idea is to shunt blood from the corpus cavernosum into either the corpus spongiosum or the systemic circulation. Distal shunts (Winter, Ebbehøj, as shown in Figure 10, or al-Ghorab) should be performed first, followed by proximal shunts (Quackles or Grayhack, as shown in Figure 11). Success rates for shunting procedures in rectifying the priapism situation are between 60%-70%.

Figure 10

Ebbehøj shunt

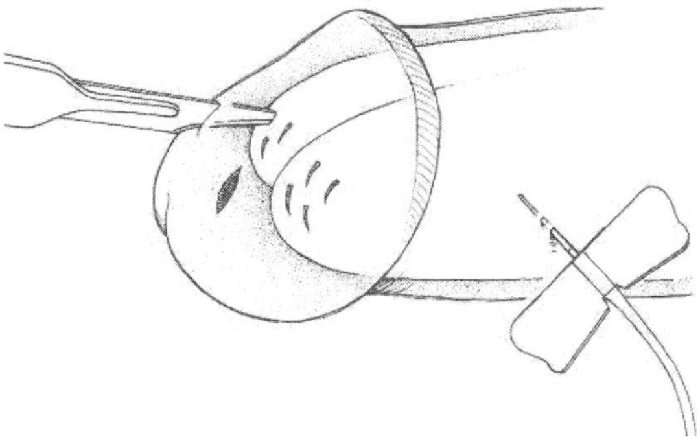

This is one variety of distal cavernosal-spongiosal shunt for priapism

From Bochinski DJ, Deng DY, Lue TF. The treatment of priapism—when and how? Int J Impotence Res. *2003;15 (suppl 5):S86-S90.*

Erectile dysfunction occurs after many cases of priapism, and the likelihood for permanent dysfunction increases as the time from the onset of the priapism increases. The rate is low in men who promptly respond to irrigation or injection of phenylephrine. Those who require surgical shunting have a higher rate of permanent dysfunction. Those responding to distal shunts have a 50% rate of ED and those requiring proximal shunts retain erectile function in only about 25% of cases. This is not to imply that distal shunts are less successful in rectifying the problem, but more a reflection of longer duration of refractory priapism, causing further damage while increasingly complex procedures are introduced over time to treat it.

Men with non-ischemic priapism can be followed over time for resolution of the problem. Angioembolization with autologous clot can give a temporary cessation of blood flow to break the cycle and fix the problem. Permanent ED following clot embolization is uncommon. Permanent angioembolization or ligation of the offending blood supply gives a higher rate of ED.

Figure 11

Quackles shunt (A.) and Grayhack shunt (B.)

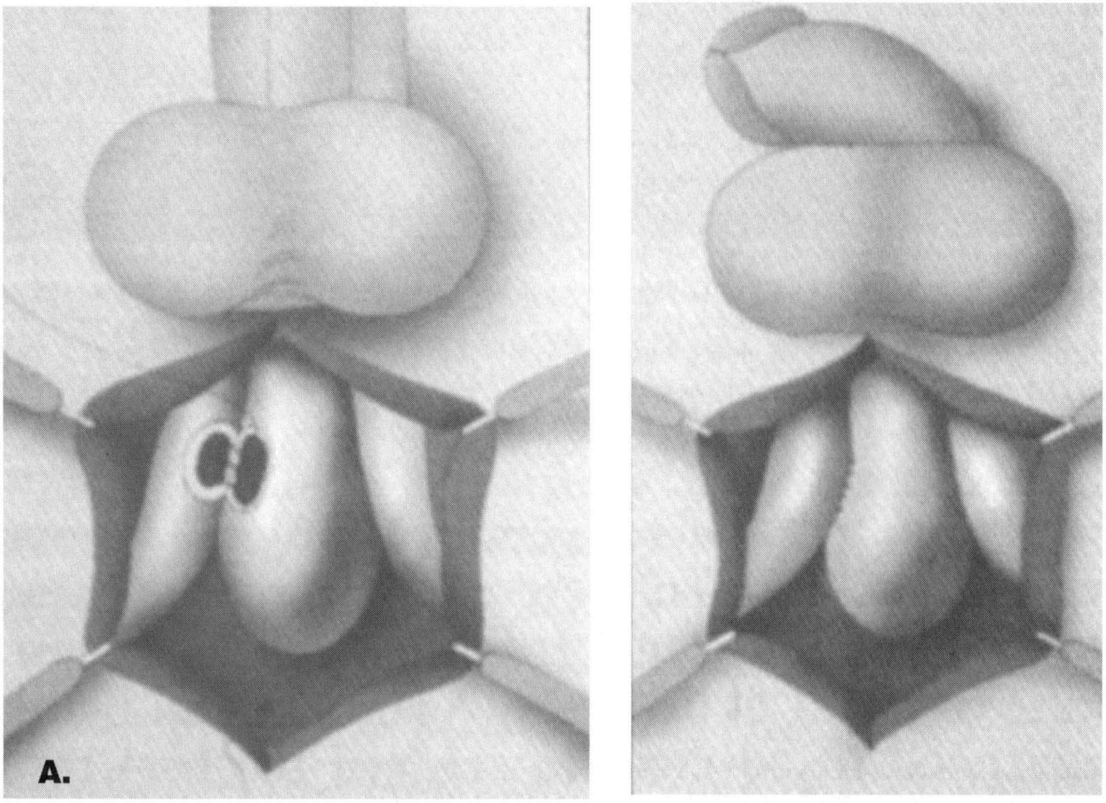

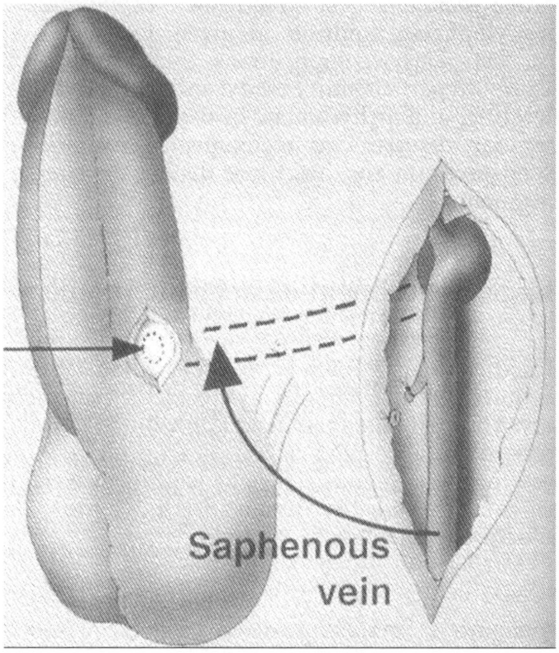

B.

Proximal cavernosal-spongiosal shunts, utilized if distal shunts fail to relieve the priapism

From Bochinski DJ, Deng DY, Lue TF. The treatment of priapism—when and how? Int J Impotence Res. *2003; 15 (suppl 5):S86-S90.*

Figure 12

Angioembolization of a case of high-flow priapism with autologous clot

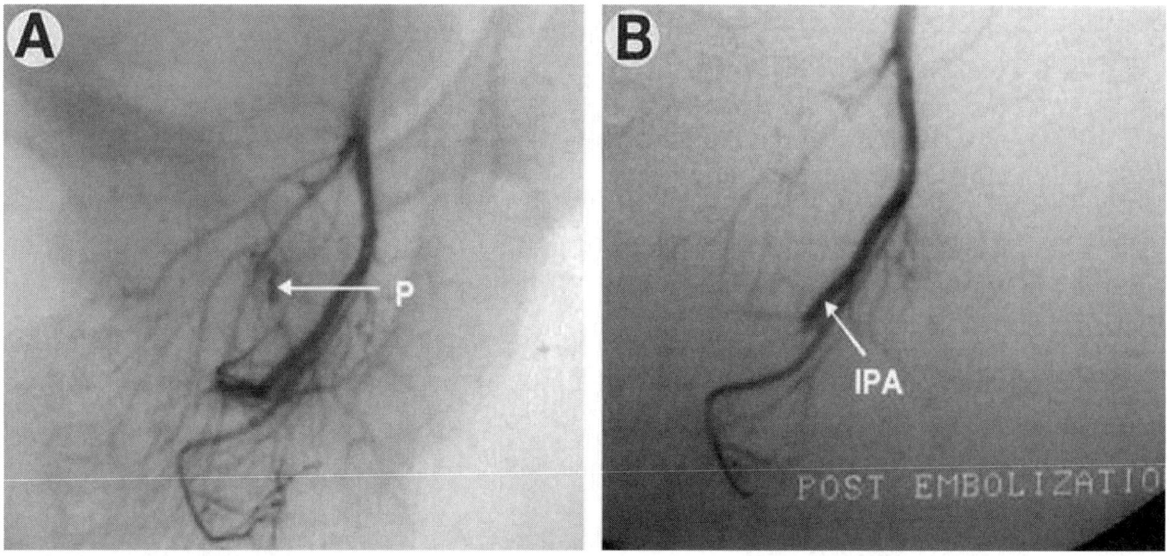

A. Initial contrast injection shows pseudoaneurysm of the carvernosal artery from trauma
B. After autologous clot is injected, there is no longer flow from the injured vessel. This patient regained his potency after his treatment

From Park JK, Jeong YB, Han YM. Recanalization of embolized caverenosal artery: restoring potency in the patient with high flow priapism. J Urol. *2001;165:2002-2003.*

The AUA Guidelines algorithm for the treatment of priapism is shown in Figure 13.

Limited studies from Burnett suggest a novel use for phosphodiesterase type 5 inhibitors in the prevention of recurrent, or "stuttering," priapism. The proposed action is via altered signaling in the nitric oxide pathway, which is corrected by the administration of the PDE5 medication, resulting in relaxation of the smooth muscle and subsequent correction of the priapism. Burnett's case reports demonstrated success with tadalafil 5 mg daily, and also sildenafil citrate at 50 mg daily.

Figure 13

AUA Guidelines Panel algorithm for the treatment of priapism

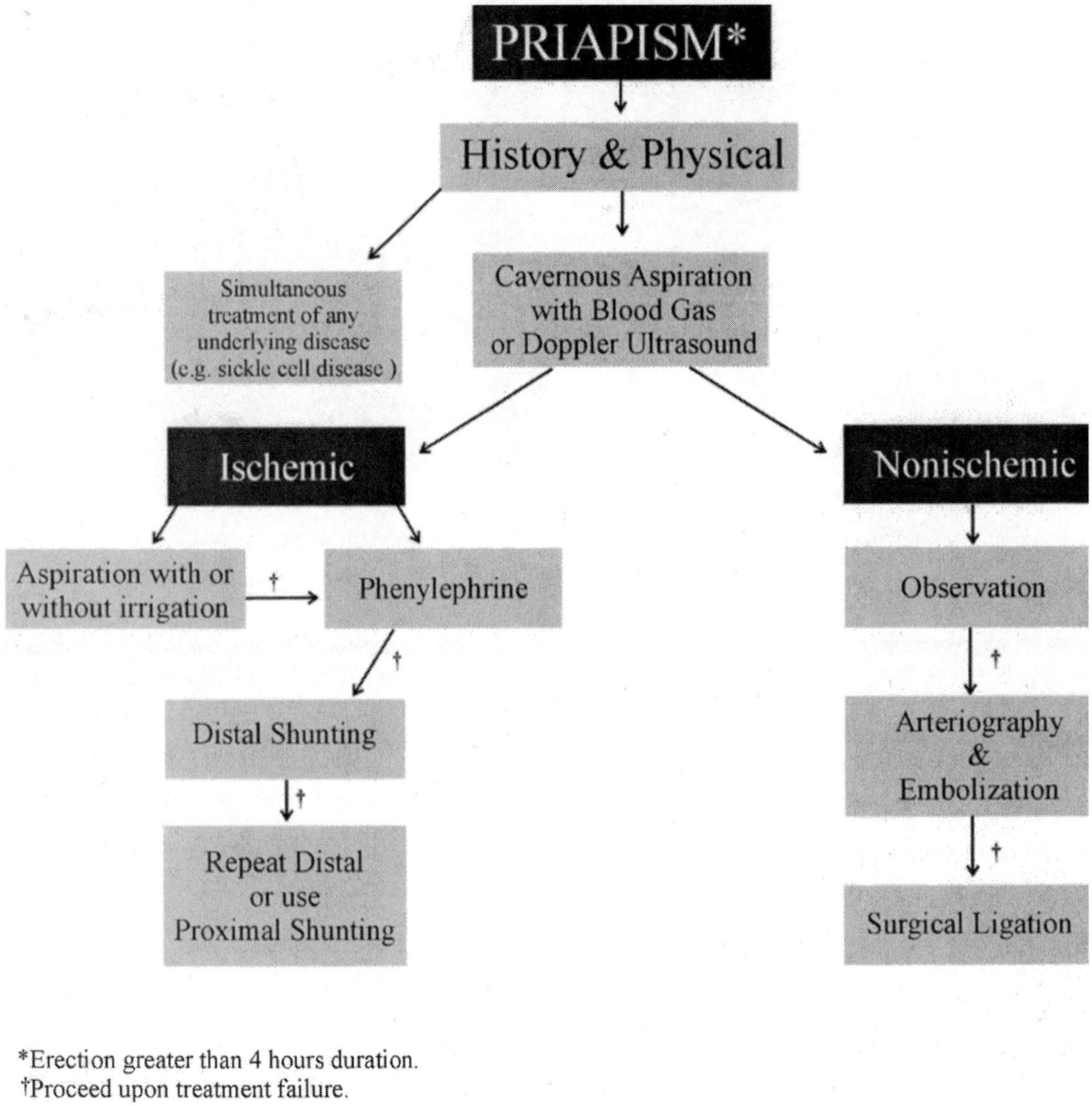

From: Montague DK, Jarow J, Broderick GA, et al. American Urological Association guideline on the management of priapism. J Urol. *2003;170:1318-1324.*

3. Questions

1. The nitric oxide/cyclic GMP (NO/cGMP) system in the penis is of the utmost importance in the generation of penile erection. cGMP produced by this cascade is inactivated by which of the following?
(*Note:* NOS = nitric oxide synthase; PDE = phosphodiesterase)

A. PDE 2, 3 and 4

B. PDE 5

C. Norepinephrine

D. Neuronal NOS

E. Endothelial NOS

2. Which of the following statements is the most accurate regarding the source of the blood that results in erection of the corpora cavernosa?

A. The blood supply comes from the cavernosal (deep) penile arteries

B. The blood supply comes from the deep dorsal arteries

C. The blood supply comes from both the cavernosal and deep dorsal arteries

D. The blood supply does not come from the cavernosal or deep dorsal arteries

3. Which of the following is the most common sexual adverse effect of selective serotonin reuptake inhibitors (SSRIs)?

A. Decreased libido

B. Premature ejaculation

C. Erectile dysfunction

D. Anorgasmia

E. Orchalgia

4. All of the following characteristics in an erectile dysfunction patient's history suggest a primary psychogenic problem, except:

A. Sudden onset

B. Young age

C. Sleep erections present

D. Varying degree of dysfunction

E. Orgasm is preserved

5. Which of the following agents cause partial inhibition of PDE6?

A. Sildenafil

B. Tadalafil

C. Vardenafil

D. Prostaglandin E1

E. Apomorphine

6. Which of the following erectile dysfunction treatments results in the highest satisfaction rates?

A. Sildenafil

B. Intraurethral prostaglandin E1

C. Penile injection therapy with prostaglandin E1

D. Vacuum constriction device

E. Inflatable penile prosthesis

7. The penoscrotal approach for inflatable penile prosthesis placement offers which of the following advantages over the infrapubic approach?

A. Safer reservoir placement

B. Preservation of glans tumescence

C. Less risk of penile contracture

D. Less risk of penile sensory loss

E. Larger girth implant is possible

8. A man presents with Peyronie's disease and very significant penile shortening. Intercourse is impossible due to a 90-degree dorsal deformity. He has firm erections, but is quite upset with how short the penis has become. Length preservation is the primary goal of the patient. Which of the following procedures should be avoided to try to help achieve his goals?

A. Penile placation procedure (eg, Nesbit)

B. Penile prosthesis placement

C. Penile prosthesis placement with a molding procedure

D. Plaque excision with dermal graft

E. Plaque incision with pericardial graft

9. A 48-year-old-man present with Peyronie's disease with a 90-degree dorsal deformity. Erections are perfectly firm by history. He undergoes a plaque incision and grafting, with elevation of the neurovascular bundle. Sensation returns to normal, but he is completely unable to achieve erection following the surgery. Which of the following pre-operative tests might have predicted this complication from surgery?

A. Serum testosterone level

B. Nocturnal penile tumescence study

C. Duplex Doppler ultrasound of the penile vessels

D. Biothesiometry

E. Penile-brachial index

10. Which of the following injectable agents is recommended by the AUA Guidelines on priapism, due to its pure alpha adrenergic effect and lack of secondary neurotransmitter release?

A. Epinephrine

B. Phenylyephrine

C. Metaraminol

D. Norepinephrine

E. Dopamine

Answers

1. B

2. A

3. D

4. E

5. A

6. E

7. D

8. A

9. C

10. B

4. Further Reading

AUA Guidelines available online:

Management of Erectile Dysfunction:
http://www.auanet.org/guidelines/edmgmt.cfm

Management of Priapism:
http://www.auanet.org/guidelines/priapism.cfm

Also:

Burnett AL, Bivalacqua TJ, Champion HC, Musicki B. Feasibility of the use of phosphodiesterase type 5 inhibitors in a pharmacologic prevention program for recurrent priapism. *J Sexual Med*. 2006;3(6):1077-1084.

Burnett AL, Bivalacqua TJ, Champion HC, Musicki B. Long-term oral phosphodiesterase 5 inhibitor therapy alleviates recurrent priapism. *Urology*. 2006;67(5):1043-1048.

Francis SH. Corbin JD. Phosphodiesterase-5 inhibition: the molecular biology of erectile function and dysfunction. *Urol Clin North Am*. 2005;32:419-429.

Gholami S, Gonzalez-Cadavid NF, Lin CS, Rajfer J, Lue TF. Peyronie's disease: a review. *J Urol*. 2003;169:1234-1241.

Greenfield JM, Levine LA. Peyronie's disease: etiology, epidemiology and medical treatment. *Urol Clin North Am*. 2005;32:469-478.

Lue TF: Erectile dysfunction. *N Engl J Med*. 2000;342:1802-1813.

Montague DK, Jarow J, Broderick GA, et al. American Urological Association guideline on the management of priapism. *J Urol*. 2003;170:1318-1324.

Mulhall JP, Schiff J, Guhring P. An analysis of the natural history of Peyronie's disease. *J Urol*. 2006;175:2115-2118.

Porst H, Rajfer J, Casabe A, et al. Long-term safety and efficacy of tadalafil 5 mg dosed once daily in men with erectile dysfunction. *J Sexual Med*. 2008;5(9):2160-2169.

Selvin E, Burnett AL, Platz EA. Prevalence and risk factors for erectile dysfunction in the US. *Am J Med*. 2007;120:151-157.